CRITICAL CARE
NURSING

Assessment & Intervention

Sharon L. Roberts, RN, PhD, FAAN
Professor of Nursing
California State University, Long Beach
Long Beach, California

Appleton & Lange
Stamford, Connecticut

Copyright © 1996 by Appleton & Lange
A Simon & Schuster Company

96 97 98 / 10 9 8 7 6 5 4 3 2 1

Prentice Hall International (UK) Limited, *London*
Prentice Hall of Australia Pty. Limited, *Sydney*
Prentice Hall Canada, Inc., *Toronto*
Prentice Hall Hispanoamericana, S.A., *Mexico*
Prentice Hall of India Private Limited, *New Delhi*
Prentice Hall of Japan, Inc., *Tokyo*
Simon & Schuster Asia Pte. Ltd., *Singapore*
Editora Prentice Hall do Brasil Ltda., *Rio de Janeiro*
Prentice Hall, *Englewood Cliffs, New Jersey*

Library of Congress Cataloging-in-Publication Data

Roberts, Sharon L., 1942–
    Critical care nursing : assessment and intervention / Sharon L. Roberts
        p.   cm.
    Includes bibliographical references
    ISBN 0-8385-3604-2 (pbk. : alk. paper)
    1. Intensive care nursing—Handbooks, manuals, etc.   I. Title.
    [DNLM: 1. Critical Care—handbooks.   2. Nursing Care—handbooks.
WY 49 R647c 1996]
RT120.I5R613 1996
616′.028—dc20
DNLM/DLC
for Library of Congress   95-31492
                                                         CIP

Acquisitions Editor: David Carroll
Production Editor: Todd Miller
Designer: Mary Skudlarek

PRINTED IN THE UNITED STATES OF AMERICA

ISBN 0-8385-3604-2

9 780838 536049

90000

TABLE OF CONTENTS

PREFACE

The portable handbook is divided into 10 chapters covering 141 topics and 51 tables. When appropriate, each chapter is divided into three parts. Part I concerns health problems and nursing management; Part II, surgical corrections and nursing management; and Part III, supportive procedures and nursing management. This three-part separation allows the critical care nurse to find the information directly from the table of contents or indirectly from within the chapter. Information on a particular surgical intervention or supportive procedure is covered separately, so the content can be developed in greater detail than in other handbooks. As a result, the critical care nurse can focus on a particular health problem, including medical and surgical and nursing management, by means of nursing diagnoses and collaborative problems. When appropriate, the nurse is referred within the nursing management section to Part II and part III for additional information. The nurse may also be referred to Part II or Part III in another chapter. For example, in the discussion of acute myocardial infarction (AMI) under the headings for diagnostic data, medical and surgical management, specific nursing diagnosis, or collaborative problem, the reader is directed to a diagnostic table, drug table, surgical intervention (coronary artery bypass surgery), or supportive procedure (percutaneous transluminal coronary angioplasty). Other critical care handbooks include a surgical or supportive procedure only under a specific health problem, requiring the critical care nurse or student to refer to a specific health problem or index to find the limited information.

■ HEALTH PROBLEMS AND NURSING MANAGEMENT

Health problems confronting critical care patients are discussed in Part I. Information is presented hierarchically so the critical care nurse can delineate nursing diagnoses and collaborative problems and formulate a range of appropriate nursing interventions. Each specific health problem discussed in Part I is organized according to the following framework: case management basis including diagnostic category and length of stay; definition; pathophysiology; nursing assessment; medical and surgical management; nursing management according to nursing diagnoses and collaborative problems; and when appropriate, discharge planning.

CASE MANAGEMENT BASIS

The restructuring of health care services and the reimbursement system has been the catalyst for the advancement of professional nursing practice. Primary nursing as a unit-based model implemented to achieve continuity of patient care was the best model for professional practice until the health care industry turned its attention to case-types in the form of diagnostic related groups (DRGs).[1] Therefore, when possible, each health problem, surgical intervention, or supportive procedure will begin with a DRG and length of stay (LOS) subsumed under the heading Case Management Basis. The LOS is the framework of time within which the management of a patient with a specific DRG must be accomplished. For example, with DRG:140 Angina pectoris, the LOS is 3.70 days.[2] The critical care nurse identifies common nursing diagnoses, collaborative problems, and expected patient outcomes and designs a management plan to be accomplished within 3.70 days. The LOS may vary regionally somewhat as the DRG categories are reevaluated.

DEFINITION AND PATHOPHYSIOLOGY

Once the case management basis has been delineated, the entry continues with a brief definition of the health problem. The pathophysiological basis of the health problem is then briefly described. Essential pathophysiological information is presented so that common nursing diagnoses and collaborative problems can be developed. It is beyond the scope of the handbook to provide an in-depth discussion of pathophysiological mechanisms surrounding each health problem. The reader can obtain a more detailed discussion of this information in core critical care or pathophysiology textbooks.

NURSING ASSESSMENT

The nursing assessment section consists of four subcategories. First, the primary causes of each health problem are given. Second, risk factors that pertain specifically to the individual's history with a particular health problem are covered, as appropriate. Third, cardinal signs and symptoms are presented in the physical assessment format of inspection, palpation, percussion, and auscultation. Fourth, the critical care nurse collects data from diagnostic test results. The diagnostic test results provide information that enables the physician and nurse to diagnose the patient's health problem. Critical care nurses also use diagnostic test results to identify the patient's progress or to recognize the development of a potential complication. Throughout each nursing diagnosis and collaborative problem and its interventions, hemodynamic parameters and a variety of other measurements are given. The critical care nurse is to relate these parameters, measurements, and values to the patient's specific problem and compare them to the normal parameter, measurement, or value. Should additional information be needed about a particular hemodynamic parameter, laboratory test, or diagnostic test, the critical care nurse will be referred to a specific table.

MEDICAL AND SURGICAL MANAGEMENT

Medical and surgical management focuses on treatments that are delegated interventions or physician-prescribed, such as intravenous therapy, oxygenation, ventilatory support, medications, diet, physical activity, invasive procedures, or surgical interventions. These interventions are presented separately before the nursing management section so they can be integrated into specific nursing diagnoses or collaborative problems.

NURSING MANAGEMENT: NURSING DIAGNOSIS AND COLLABORATIVE PROBLEMS

A major focus of the handbook is on nursing management through the use of nursing diagnoses and collaborative problems. North

American Nursing Diagnosis Association (NANDA)-approved nursing diagnoses are used, with the wording-related factors and secondary factors completing the statement. Critical care nurses manage a wide range of collaborative problems on a daily basis, but there has not always been a way to record this data. The purpose of including collaborative problems is to allow for inclusion of physiological data using Carpenito's Bifocal Clinical Practice Model. According to Carpenito, "Collaborative problems are certain physiological complications that nurses monitor to detect onset or changes in status. Nurses manage collaborative problems utilizing physician-prescribed and nursing-prescribed interventions to minimize the complications of the events."[3] Since the original creation of the nursing diagnosis taxonomy, times have changed and critical care nursing has become a highly technical, advanced area of practice in which many nursing diagnoses are physiological or collaborative.[4] Critical care nurses work closely with physiological phenomena and, in a research-based practice, may independently and successfully manipulate variables such as left ventricular afterload, right ventricular preload, impaired ejection fraction, unbalanced ventilation-perfusion, and increased intracranial pressure.[5]

Collaborative problems are written, as Carpenito suggests, with the diagnostic label "Potential Complication." The prescription for definitive treatment of collaborative problems depends on both nursing and medicine. In treating a critically ill patient with a cardiac problem, the physician initiates hemodynamic monitoring so that cardiac output, cardiac index, pulmonary artery pressure, and pulmonary capillary wedge pressure can be monitored. The critical care nurse draws upon her or his knowledge of hemodynamics to delineate potential complications related to changes in cardiac output or oxygen supply and demand. Examples of collaborative problems or potential complications that necessi-

tate physician–nurse collaboration consist of the following:

Potential Complication: Decreased cardiac output related to decreased myocardial oxygen supply secondary to

Potential Complication; Decreased oxygen supply related to reduced coronary artery perfusion secondary to

Potential Complication: Dysrhythmia related to increased sympathetic tone or myocardial ischemia secondary to

Potential Complication: Hypoxemia related to pulmonary congestion secondary to

The treatment of collaborative problems in the handbook differs from Carpenito's Bifocal Model in two respects. First, Carpenito does not believe the *related-to* statement is necessary.[3] However, it is this author's opinion that the *related-to* statement helps the critical care nurse specifically delineate what is wrong with the patient. The *related-to* statement helps the critical care nurse identify causes, expected patient outcomes, and ultimately independent and delegated interventions.

A second deviation from Carpenito's Bifocal Clinical Practice Model is in the area of desired outcome criteria for collaborative problems. According to Carpenito, "Client outcome criteria are inappropriate for collaborative problems. They represent criteria that cannot be used to evaluate the effectiveness or appropriateness of nursing interventions.[3] In the handbook, the terms *expected patient outcomes* (EPO) and *desired outcomes* are the same. With collaborative problems, the prescription for definitive treatment comes from both nursing and medicine. The author therefore believes it is relevant to include the expected patient outcome criteria for collaborative problems. The expected patient outcomes become the measurable evaluative finding that lets the critical care nurse know whether interventions have corrected the nursing diagnosis or collaborative problem. The handbook includes expected patient outcomes for each potential complication, subsumed under the heading Collaborative Problem. New collaborative problems are presented throughout each chapter. The resource used for collaborative problems and nursing diagnosis was *Nursing Diagnosis Application to Clinical Practice.*[6]

Under each nursing diagnosis and collaborative problem or potential complication, the nursing management entry contains a variety of interventions. While an array of interventions is covered, they should be adapted to the specific patient and his or her critical health problem. When possible, interventions are organized as: consulting with other professional disciplines, reviewing results of laboratory or diagnostic data, promoting or limiting physical activity, providing diet, obtaining and monitoring patient care data, implementing a wide range of patient care interventions, and teaching. Within some interventions, the critical care nurse may be referred to a specific table or other sections within the chapter for additional information. For example, if a particular drug, such as dopamine, is mentioned, the nurse is referred to Table 1–10. Positive Inotropes and Sympathomimetics, for more details about the drug. Likewise, a specific surgical intervention or supportive procedure may be mentioned within a nursing diagnosis or the intervention for a potential complication. The nurse is then directed to Part II or Part III. The references to specific tables and Part II or Part III within a chapter will greatly expand the information available to the critical care nurse.

DISCHARGE PLANNING

As nurses endeavor to safely expedite safe movement of a patient through the health care delivery system in a timely manner, discharge planning will become even more vital to the patient's and family's well-being. Critically ill patients are being hospitalized for a shorter length of stay; therefore critical care nurses will become increasingly involved in initiat-

ing early phases of discharge planning. Patient care and teaching will need to be consolidated into a shorter span of time to ensure that important information has been given to the patient and family.

SURGICAL INTERVENTIONS AND NURSING MANAGEMENT

The organizing framework for Part II; Surgical Interventions and Nursing Management, differs from the format of Part I. Pathophysiology, primary causes, risk factors, physical assessment, and diagnostic test results are not covered. Instead, the section is organized as follows: Case management basis, including diagnostic category and length of stay; definition; patient selection; procedure; complications; medical and surgical management; nursing management according to nursing diagnoses and collaborative problems; and discharge planning.

SUPPORTIVE PROCEDURES AND NURSING MANAGEMENT

Part III, Supportive Procedures and Nursing Management, is organized as follows: Case management basis including diagnostic category and length of stay when applicable; definition; patient selection including indications and contraindications; procedures; complications; nursing management according to nursing diagnoses and collaborative problems; and discharge planning. Content in Part III focuses on such topics as percutaneous transluminal coronary angioplasty, hemodynamic monitoring, ultrafiltration, et cetera.

When appropriate, tables consisting of standard laboratory tests, invasive diagnostic procedures, noninvasive diagnostic procedures, and medications applicable to that particular system are cross-referenced. Selected references used in the chapter are also cited.

In summary, the handbook is designed to be a portable reference for critical care nurses. The book provides the nurse with on-the-scene information regarding health problems, nursing diagnoses, collaborative problems, and nursing interventions until additional literature can be obtained.

■ REFERENCES

1. Zander K, Etheredge, ML, Bower K. *Nursing Case Management: Blueprints for Transformation.* Waban, Mass.: Winslow Printing Systems, 1987.

2. Neal MC, Paquette M, Mirch M. Nursing Diagnosis Care Plans for DRGs. Venice, Ca: General Medical Publishers, 1990.

3. Carpenito L. *Nursing Diagnosis Application to Clinical Practice.* 4th ed. Philadelphia, Pa: JB Lippincott Co., 1992:36–45.

4. Roberts SL. Physiological nursing diagnoses are necessary and appropriate for critical care. *Focus Crit Care* 1988; 5(15):42.

5. Thelan LA, Davie JK, Urden LD. *Textbook of critical Care Nursing Diagnosis and Management.* St. Louis, Mo: CV Mosby, 1990.

6. Carpenito L. *Nursing Diagnosis Application to Clinical Practice.* 5th ed. Philadelphia, Pa: JB Lippincott Co; 1993.

1

Cardiac Deviations

PART I: HEALTH PROBLEMS AND NURSING MANAGEMENT

■ ACUTE CHEST PAIN

(For related information see Part I: Acute myocardial infarction, p. 38; Congestive heart failure, p. 87; Acute cardiac tamponade, p. 117; Acute pericarditis, p. 123; Dysrhythmias, p. 184. Part II: Coronary artery bypass graft, p. 194. Part III: Hemodynamic monitoring, p. 219; Percutaneous transluminal coronary angioplasty, p. 226; Coronary laser angioplasty, p. 228; Coronary atherectomy, p. 234; Intracoronary stents, p. 237; Intra-aortic balloon pump, p. 254; ST segment monitoring, p. 264; Thrombolytic therapy, p. 265. See also Respiratory Deviations, Part III: Pulse oximetry, p. 426; Mechanical ventilators, p. 428.)

Diagnostic Category and Length of Stay
DRG: 140 Angina pectoris
LOS: 3.70 days

Definition
Acute chest pain is due to myocardial ischemia, which is the result of an imbalance between myocardial oxygen supply and demand. Anmbalance between myocardial oxygen supply and demand can occur from either a primary decrease in coronary blood flow or a disproportionate increase in myocardial oxygen demand. There are three types of acute chest pain: stable angina, unstable angina, and variant or Prinzmetal's angina. Angina occurs in coronary atherosclerosis and can occur in patients with normal coronary arteries. Stable angina is a syndrome of several weeks' duration that is provoked by activities that increase myocardial oxygen demand. The pain lasts 1 to 5 weeks and is relieved by rest. Unstable angina is also known as crescendo angina or preinfarction angina. The pain is effort-induced, intense, and lasts for more than 30 minutes. Unstable angina occurs as a result of an increased demand for oxygen by the myocardium and a transient reduction in coronary blood flow. Oxygen supply may have been compromised by fixed obstructive lesions in the coronary vessels. Finally, variant or Prinzmetal's angina is pain that occurs at rest and can be associated with ST segment elevations on the electrocardiogram (ECG). The pain is severe and is due to decreased coronary blood flow secondary to coronary artery spasm.

Pathophysiology

Acute chest pain results from hypoxia of cardiac muscle that occurs when there is an imbalance between myocardial oxygen supply and demand. As blood flow decreases, the myocardium avoids ischemia through autoregulation of coronary blood flow. This is thought to be the result of relaxation of the smooth muscle of the arterioles in response to release of adenosine. Adenosine, a powerful vasodilator of the coronary vasculature, decreases resistance in the coronary arteriolar bed. When the autoregulation mechanisms fail to meet the metabolic needs of the myocardium, pain occurs. Lactic acid accumulation can impair left ventricular function, resulting in decreased strength of cardiac contraction and impaired wall motion. The degree of impairment is dependent on the size of the ischemic area and the general contractility of the left ventricular myocardium. In stable angina, the thrombus that may form within the atherosclerotic plaque remains within the vessel wall and does not rupture. In unstable angina, the plaque ruptures, causing not only a partial thrombolic occlusion in the coronary artery but also increased platelet aggregation and further thrombogenesis.

Nursing Assessment

PRIMARY CAUSES

- Cardiovascular mechanisms include coronary artery disease, aortic valve disease, cardiomyopathy, pericarditis, aortic dissection and aneurysm, mitral valve prolapse, pulmonary embolism, and pulmonary hypertension.
- Gastrointestinal causes consist of esophageal disorders, peptic ulcer disease, gastritis, or cholecystitis.
- Neuromusculoskeletal changes leading to acute chest pain are costochondritis, chest wall pain, cervical or thoracic radiculopathy or shoulder arthropathies, pneumothorax, mediastinitis, pleuritis, or intrathoracic malignancy.

RISK FACTORS

- Family history of coronary artery disease
- Lifestyle factors such as cigarette smoking, obesity, stress, lack of physical activity, or aging
- Other conditions such as hyperlipidemia, hypertension, hypercholesterolemia, or diabetes
- Male sex, age 35 to 55
- Postmenopausal women.

PHYSICAL ASSESSMENT

- Inspection: Complaints of tightness or fullness in the middle or lower sternum, over the left precordium, or left shoulder or upper arm pain extending down the arm to the fourth and fifth finger; fatigue; weight gain; skin color pale dusky-ashen or cyanotic; or presence of peripheral edema.
- Palpation: Apical impulses show widening of apical impulse, which implies left ventricular enlargement; presystolic impulse implies a vigorous atrial contraction into a poorly compliant left ventricle; sustained impulse signifies large akinetic or dyskinetic left ventricular segment or left ventricular hypertrophy; triple impulse can represent hypertrophic obstructive cardiomyopathy; peripheral pulses diminished secondary to peripheral vascular occlusive disease; skin clammy and cool.
- Auscultation: Carotid or femoral bruits signifying arteriosclerosis; split S_2; S_3 to S_4; systolic nonejection click; or systolic and diastolic murmur.

DIAGNOSTIC TEST RESULTS

Standard Laboratory Tests. (See Table 1–1)

- Blood studies: hemoglobin $\leq$ 12 g/100 mL
- Serum chemistry: cholesterol $\geq$330 mg/dL, triglycerides $\geq$190 mg/dL (age-related), blood urea nitrogen (BUN) $\geq$20 mg/dL, and creatinine $\geq$1.2 mg/dL.
- Serum enzymes: increased

TABLE 1–1. STANDARD LABORATORY TESTS

TABLE 1-1

Test	Purpose	Normal Value	Abnormal Findings
Arterial Blood Gases pH	Measure of hydrogen ion concentration (pH) indicates the acid-base level of the blood	7.35–7.42	pH ≤7.35 can indicate acidosis pH ≥7.42 can indicate alkalosis
PaO_2	Measure of partial pressure exerted by the small amount of oxygen dissolved in the arterial blood indicates how much oxygen the lungs are delivering to the blood	80–100 mm Hg	PaO_2 ≤60 mm Hg can indicate hypoxemia
$PaCO_2$	Measure of partial pressure exerted by carbon dioxide dissolved in the arterial blood indicates how efficiently the lung eliminates carbon dioxide	35–45 mm Hg	$PaCO_2$ ≥45 mm Hg can indicate hypoventilation (hypercarbia) and respiratory acidosis $PaCO_2$ ≤35 mm Hg can indicate hyperventilation (hypocarbia), respiratory alkalosis, compensation
HCO_3	Measures the amount of bicarbonate or alkaline substance dissolved in blood Influenced by metabolic changes HCO_3 is under renal control	22–26 mEq/L	HCO_3 ≥26 mEq/L can indicate metabolic alkalosis HCO_3 ≤22 mEq/L can indicate metabolic acidosis
Blood Studies White blood cell (WBC) count	Used to determine infection or inflammation	4100–10,900/μL	≥10,900 /μL can indicate AMI, infection, inflammation, leukemia, burns ≤4100/μL can indicate bone marrow depression, influenza, measles, infectious hepatitis, mononucleosis
WBC differential	Used to determine the stage and severity of an infection Used to identify the various types of leukemia		
Neutrophil	Used to evaluate the body's reaction to inflammation	Relative value: 47.6%–76.8% Absolute value: 1950–8400/μL	≥8,400/μL can indicate AMI, infection, ischemic necrosis, metabolic disorders, stress response of inflammatory disease

TABLE 1-1

TABLE 1–1. CONTINUED

Test	Purpose	Normal Value	Abnormal Findings
			≤1950/μL can indicate bone marrow depression, hepatic disease, collagen vascular disease, deficiency of folic acid or vitamin B_{12}
Eosinophils	Used to diagnose allergic infections, severity of infestations with worms and other large parasites	Relative value: 0.3%–0.7% Absolute value 12–760/μL	≥760/μL can indicate allergic disorders, parasitic infections, skin diseases, neoplastic diseases, collagen vascular disease, ulcerative colitis, pernicious anemia, excessive exercise
			≤12/μL can indicate stress from trauma, shock, burns, surgery, Cushing's syndrome
Basophils	Used to study allergic reactions	Relative value: 0.5%–1.0% Absolute value: 12–200/μL	≥200/μL can indicate chronic myelocytic leukemia, polycythemia vera, hemolytic anemia, myxedema, ulcerative colitis, nephrosis
			≤12/μL can indicate hyperthyroidism or stress
Lymphocytes	Used to detect viral infections	Relative value: 20%–40% Absolute value: 1000–4000/μL	≥4000/μL can indicate AMI, infections, thyrotoxicosis, ulcerative colitis, immune diseases, hypoadrenalism, lymphocytic leukemia
			≤1000/μL can indicate debilitating diseases such as CHF or renal failure, high levels of corticosteroids, immunodeficiency
Monocytes	Used to detect severe infections	Relative value: 2%–6% Absolute value: 100–600/μL	≥600/μL can indicate AMI, infections, collagen vascular disease, carcinomas

TABLE 1–1. CONTINUED

TABLE 1-1

Test	Purpose	Normal Value	Abnormal Findings
Red blood cell (RBC) count erythrocytes	Used to determine the total number of red blood cells Used to support the diagnosis of anemia or polycythemia	Men: 4.2–5.4 million/mm^3 Women: 3.6–5.0 million/mm^3	M≥4 million/mm^3 and W≥5 million/mm^3 can indicate polycythemia vera, severe diarrhea, dehydration, pulmonary fibrosis, or immediately following hemorrhage M≤4.2 million/mm^3 and W≤3.6 million/mm^3 can indicate anemia, disease of bone marrow function, hemolytic and pernicious anemia, SLE, Addison's disease, subacute endocarditis
Red cell indices	Used to differentiate anemias Used to evaluate mean corpuscular volume (MCV), hemoglobin (MCH) and hemoglobin concentration (MCHC)		
Mean corpuscular volume (MCV)	An index that expresses the volume occupied by a single red cell	84–99µ^3/red cell	≥99µ^3/red cell can indicate macrocytic anemias, reticulocytosis, liver disease, alcoholism, vitamin B$_{12}$ deficiency ≤84µ^3/red cell can indicate iron deficiency anemia, pernicious anemia, macrocytic anemia
Mean corpuscular hemoglobin (MCH)	An index used in diagnosing severely anemic patients	27–32 picograms (pg)	≥32 pg can indicate macrocytic anemia
Mean corpuscular hemoglobin concentration (MCHC)	Used to evaluate therapy for anemia Measures the concentration of hemoglobin in the red blood cells	32%–36%	≥36% can indicate spherocytosis ≤32% can indicate microcytic anemias, iron deficiency, pyridoxine-responsive anemia, thalassemia

TABLE 1-1

TABLE 1–1. CONTINUED

Test	Purpose	Normal Value	Abnormal Findings
Erythrocyte sedimentation rate (ESR)	Used to determine the progress of an inflammatory disease such as AMI and to differentiate pain of pericarditis and Dressler's syndrome for anginal pain	0–20 mm/h	≥20 mm/h can indicate inflammatory disease, anemia, tissue destruction, nephritis, toxemia ≤0 mm/h can indicate polycythemia, CHF, low plasma protein
Hematocrit (HCT)	Measures percentage of volume of packed red blood cell in a whole blood sample Used to assist in the diagnosis of hydration, polycythemia, and anemia	Men: 42%–54% Women: 38%–46%	M≥54% and W≥46% can indicate polycythemia, dehydration, hemoconcentration, erythrocytosis M≤42% and W≤38% can indicate anemia or hemodilution, leukemia, hyperthyroidism, cirrhosis, massive blood loss
Hemoglobin (Hgb)	Measures blood's capacity to transport oxygen Used to measure the severity of anemia in polycythemia	Men: 14.0–16.5 g/100 mL Women: 12–15 g/100mL	≥15g/100 mL can indicate polycythemia, dehydration, COPD, CHF ≤12g/100 mL can indicate anemia, recent hemorrhage, cirrhosis, hyperthyroidism, hemolytic reaction
Coagulation Studies Platelet Count	To evaluate platelet production and functions, which consist of coagulation and clotting of blood Vascular integrity and vasoconstriction Adherence and aggregation activity in the formation of a platelet plug that occludes breaks in small vessels	150,000 to 350,000/mm^3	≥350,000/mm^3 can indicate cancer, polycythemia vera, splenectomy, trauma, RA, acute infection, heart disease, cirrhosis, chronic pancreatitis ≤150,000/mm^3 can occur after massive blood transfusion, pneumonia, aplastic or hypoplastic bone marrow, allergic reactions, infection, DIC

TABLE 1–1. CONTINUED

TABLE 1-1

Test	Purpose	Normal Value	Abnormal Findings
Prothrombin time (PT)	Used to measure the extrinsic coagulation system Monitor response to more anticoagulant therapy	Men: 9.6–11.8 s Women: 9.5–11.3 s	≥11.8 s can indicate deficiencies in fibrinogen; prothrombin; factors V, VII, or X; vitamin K deficiency; hepatic disease; ongoing oral anticoagulant therapy
Partial thromboplastin time (PTT) Activated partial thromboplastin time (APTT)	Used to test for coagulation disorders, detect deficiencies of stage II clotting mechanism, or detect deficiencies of the components of the intrinsic thromboplastin system	PTT 30–45 s APTT 16–25 s	≥25 s can indicate coagulation defect of stage I, von Willebrand's disease, hemophilia, vitamin K deficiency, liver disease, DIC ≤16 s can indicate extensive cancer, acute hemorrhage, very early stages of DIC
Fibrinogen	Used to diagnose suspected bleeding disorders	195–365 mg/dL	≥365 mg/dL can indicate cancer of the stomach or breast or inflammatory disorders ≤195 mg/dL can indicate hypofibrinogenemia; DIC; fibrinolysis; hepatic disease; cancer of the prostate, pancreas, or lung; bone marrow lesions; recent trauma
Activated clotting time (ACT)	Used to monitor heparin therapy	70–120 s	Desirable range for anticoagulation may be 150–109 s > 120 s can signify coagulation deficiencies
Fibrin split products (FSP)	Used to determine the amount of fibrinolysis during coagulation Used to detect FSP in the circulation	Serum contains ≤10 μg/mL of FSP (screening assay) Quantitative assay is ≤3 μg/mL	≥10 μg/mL may indicate primary or secondary fibrinolytic states, alcohol cirrhosis, congenital heart disease, deep vein thrombosis, AMI after 1–2 days

Immunodiagnostic Studies

Test	Purpose	Normal Value	Abnormal Findings
Rheumatoid factor (RF)	Used to confirm RA	Titer is ≤1:20	Titer ≥1:80 is positive for RA

TABLE 1-1

TABLE 1–1. CONTINUED

Test	Purpose	Normal Value	Abnormal Findings
Antistreptolysin-O-test (ASO)	Used to help diagnose rheumatic fever Used to confirm infection with beta-hemolytic streptococci	ASO titer ≤85 Todd units/mL	≥500–5000 Todd units/mL can indicate acute rheumatic fever
Blood cultures	Used to confirm bacteremia Used to determine the causative organism	Blood cultures are negative with no growth	Positive blood cultures are due to bacteremia or septicemia
Serum Chemistries			
Electrolytes Sodium	Used to detect changes in water and salt balance	135–145 mEq/L	≤135 mEq/L (hyponatremia) can be associated with severe burns, diarrhea, vomiting, nephritis, malabsorption syndrome, diabetic acidosis, edema, or excessive sweating ≥145 mEq/L (hypernatremia) can be associated with dehydration, Conn's syndrome (primary aldosteronism), coma, Cushing's syndrome, diabetes mellitus
Potassium	Used to evaluate the presence of hypokalemia or hyperkalemia Used to monitor renal function, acid-base balance, and glucose metabolism Used to evaluate neuromuscular and endocrine disorders	3.8–5.5 mEq/L	≥5.5 mEq/L (hyperkalemia) can indicate burns, crushing injuries, diabetic ketoacidosis, AMI, renal failure, Addison's disease ≤3.8 mEq/L (hypokalemia) can reflect diarrhea, starvation, malabsorption, vomiting, burns, primary aldosteronism, renal tubular acidosis, liver disease with ascites, chronic fever

TABLE 1–1. CONTINUED

TABLE 1-1

Test	Purpose	Normal Value	Abnormal Findings
Chloride	Influences the osmotic pressure of the blood, tissues, interstitial fluid and monitors electrical activity	100–108 mEq/L	Chloride >108 (Hyperchloremia) can indicate dehydration, Cushing's syndrome, hyperventilation, anemia, cardiac decompensation
			Chloride <100 (hypochloremia) can indicate severe vomiting, gastric suctioning, severe diarrhea, ulcerative colitis, Addison's disease, fever, acute infection, CHF
Carbon dioxide content (CO_2)	Used to evaluate acid-base balance	22–34 mEq/L	Increased CO_2 can indicate severe vomiting, continuous gastric drainage, emphysema, aldosteronism
			Decreased CO_2 can indicate severe diarrhea, starvation, acute renal failure, diabetic acidosis
Amylase	Used to differentiate diagnosis of acute pancreatitis from other acute abdominal problems	60–180 Somogyi units/dL	>180 Somogyi units/dL can indicate obstruction of the common bile duct, acute versus chronic pancreatitis, cirrhosis, hepatitis
Lipase	Used to aid in the diagnosis of acute pancreatitis	32–80 U/L	≥80 U/L may indicate acute pancreatitis, pancreatic duct obstruction, high intestinal obstruction, renal disease with impaired excretion

TABLE 1-1

TABLE 1–1. CONTINUED

Test	Purpose	Normal Value	Abnormal Findings
End products of metabolism, blood urea nitrogen (BUN)	Used as a gross index of glomerular function and production and excretion of urea Aid in the assessment of hydration	8–20 mg/dL	Increased BUN can indicate impaired renal function, shock, dehydration, gastrointestinal hemorrhage, infection, excessive protein uptake, urinary tract obstruction Decreased BUN can indicate liver failure, malnutrition, impaired absorption, overhydration
Creatinine	Used to diagnose impaired renal function or renal glomerular filtration	Men: 0.8–1.2 mg/dL Women: 0.6–0.9 mg/dL	Increased creatinine can indicate impaired renal function, chronic nephritis, muscle disease Decreased creatinine can indicate muscular dystrophy
Serum enzymes Creatine kinase (CK)	Used as an index of injury to myocardium and skeletal muscle such as muscular dystrophy CK is divided into three isoenzymes: CK-MM (skeletal muscle), CK-MB (cardiac muscle) and CK-BB (brain)	Men: 50–1801 U/L Women: 50–1601 U/L	Increased CK begins within 4–6 hours and reaches a peak several times the normal within 30 hours Extensive increase in CK can indicate severe myocardial infarction with a poor prognosis, acute cardiovascular disease, progressive muscular dystrophy, myxedema, cardiac surgery or defibrillation, hypokalemia, central nervous system trauma, pulmonary infarction
CK-MB(CK$_3$) isoenzyme	Released from myocardial tissue	<31 U/L or 0%	≥31U/L occurs in MI and chest pain increases 4–6 hours after an MI, not demonstrable after 24–36 hours

TABLE 1-1

TABLE 1–1. CONTINUED

Test	Purpose	Normal Value	Abnormal Findings
Lactate dehydrogenase (LDH)	Used to help confirm myocardium or pulmonary infarction	Men: 63 to 155 units Women: 62–131 units	≥ 155 u after an MI with high levels within 12–24 hours of infarction and 2–10 times the normal range
			Elevated LDH can continue for 6–10 days. LDH levels return to normal within 8–14 days
			Other clinical conditions causing increased LDH include acute leukemia, hemolytic anemia, hepatic disease, pulmonary infarction, acute renal infarction, shock, myxedema
			≤ 63 units can indicate a positive response to cancer therapy
LD-1	Found in the heart, red blood cells, kidneys, and is the fraction observed after AMI	LD-1 18%–29% of total	With AMI, one concentration of LDH_1 is greater than LDH_2 within 12 to 48 hours after onset of symptoms. The reversal of normal isoenzyme patterns is typical of myocardial damage and is referred to as "flipped LDH"
Serum glutamic-oxaloacetic transaminase (SGOT) (aspartate aminotransferase, aspartate transaminase)	Used to detect recent MI Used to aid detection of acute hepatic disease	8–20 U/L	≥ 20 U/L can indicate MI; may be increased 4–10 times the normal values
			SGOT reaches a peak in 24 hours and returns to normal by day 3–4
			Other reasons for increased SGOT include liver disease, acute pancreatitis, trauma, hemolytic anemia, severe trauma, recent brain trauma, crushing injuries

TABLE 1-1

TABLE 1–1. CONTINUED

Test	Purpose	Normal Value	Abnormal Findings
Lipoprotein Tests			
Cholesterol	Used to assess the risk of coronary artery disease Used to diagnose nephrotic syndrome, pancreatitis, hepatic disease, and hypo- and hyperthyroidism	120–200 mg/dL	≥200 mg/dL can indicate cardiovascular disease, hepatitis, type II familial hypercholesterolema, hypothyroidism, lipid disorders, bile duct blockage, nephrotic syndrome, pancreatitis ≤120mg/dL can indicate malnutrition, cellular necrosis of the liver, hyperthyroidism, anemia, sepsis, severe infection, terminal stage of cancer, hypoproteinemia
High-density lipoprotein (HDL)	Used to assess the risk of coronary artery disease	Men: 26–63 mg/dL Women: 55 mg/dL	M≥44 mg/dL and W≥55 mg/dL can indicate a chronic liver disorder, biliary cirrhosis, chronic hepatitis, or alcoholism
cholesterol	Used to monitor persons with known low levels of HDL		M≤44mg/dL and W≤55mg/dL can indicate high risk for coronary heart disease when HDL is <45mg/dL in mean and <55mg/dL in women, biliary cirrhosis, chronic hepatitis or alcoholism
Low-density lipoproteins (LDL)	Used to determine the risk of CHD and atherosclerosis	62–185 mg/100mL	0%–24% is associated with type II hyperlipidemia 25%–50% is consistent with type III hyperlipidemia 51%–100% is consistent with type IV hyperlipidemia

TABLE 1–1. CONTINUED

TABLE 1-1

Test	Purpose	Normal Value	Abnormal Findings
Triglycerides	Used to evaluate patients with suspected atherosclerosis Used as an indicator of the body's ability to mobilize fats and of hyperlipemia	40–150 mg/dL	≥150 mg/dL can indicate liver disease, risk of biliary obstruction, CAD, diabetes, nephrotic syndrome, pancreatitis, MI, types I, IIb, III, IV and V hyperlipoproteinemias, hypothyroidism ≤40 mg/dL can indicate malnutrition and abetalipoproteinemia
Protein Tests			
Total serum protein	Used to aid diagnosis of hepatic disease, protein deficiency, blood dyscrasias, renal disorders and gastrointestinal disease	6.6–7.9 g/dL	≥7.9 g/dL can indicate dehydration, vomiting, infection, multiple myeloma, chronic diarrhea, chronic or inflammatory disease ≤6.6 g/dL can indicate malnutrition, gastrointestinal disease, blood dyscrasias, essential hypertension, Hodgkin's disease, diabetes mellitus, hepatic dysfunction, malabsorption, severe burns, hemorrhage, CHF
Albumin	Used to aid diagnosis of hepatic disease protein deficiency, blood dyscrasias, renal disorders, and gastrointestinal disease	3.3–4.5 g/dL	≥4.5 g/dL can indicate multiple myeloma ≤3.3 g/dL can indicate malnutrition, nephritis, diarrhea, hepatic disease, Hodgkin's disease, peptic ulcer, cholecystitis, collagen disease, essential hypertension, hyperthyroidism, RA
Globulins	Used to aid diagnosis of hepatic disease, protein deficiency, blood dyscrasias, renal disorders, and gastrointestinal disease	0.1–0.4 g/dL	≥0.4 g/dL can indicate subacute bacterial endocarditis, multiple myeloma, RA, diabetes mellitus ≤0.1 g/dL can indicate neoplastic disease, renal or hepatic dysfunction, blood dyscrasias

TABLE 1-1

TABLE 1–1. CONTINUED

Test	Purpose	Normal Value	Abnormal Findings
Urinalysis			
Creatinine	Used to assess glomerular filtration	Men: 1.0–1.9 g/24 h Women: 0.8–1.7g/24 hours	M≤1.0 g/24 h and W≤0.8 g/24 h can indicate impaired renal perfusion, renal disease, bilateral pyelonephritis, acute or chronic glomerulonephritis, polycystic kidney disease
Creatinine clearance	Used to assess renal function and monitor progression of renal insufficiency	Men: 95–135 mL/min/1.73 m² of body surface Women: 85–125 mL/min/1.73 m²	M≤90 mL/min and W84 mL/min/1.73 m₂ can indicate clinical conditions causing reduced renal perfusion (shock, CHF, or severe dehydration), acute tubular necrosis, glomerulonephritis, pyelonephritis, bilateral renal lesions

AMI, acute myocardial infarction; CAD, coronary artery disease; CHF, congestive heart failure; COPD, chronic obstructive pulmonary disease; DIC, disseminated intravascular coagulation; MI, myocardial infarction; RA, rheumatoid arthritis; SLE, systemic lupus erythematosus.

From Bustin D, 1986; Ford RD, 1987; Dossey BM, Guzzetta CE, Kenner CV, 1992; Corbett JV, 1992; Stillwell SB, 1992; Loeb S, 1993.

Invasive Cardiac Diagnostic Procedures. (See Table 1–2)

- Cardiac catheterization: May show extensive coronary heart disease (three vessel or left main coronary artery disease) and marked left ventricular dysfunction.
- Coronary arteriography: Reveals the location of lesions causing angina; the degree of obstruction, with a 50% reduction in diameter equal to a 75% reduction in cross-sectional area, a 75% reduction in diameter equal to a 90% reduction in cross-sectional area, or a 100% reduction being total occlusion; the status of vessels distal to a point of obstruction and the presence of collateral circulation.
- Ventriculography: Marked regional left ventricular dysfunction or marked fall in ejection fraction.

Noninvasive Cardiac Diagnostic Procedures. (See Table 1–3)

- Cardiac scans: Thallium 201: Where coronary artery blood flow is decreased, thallium fails to localize in that segment of the myocardium. This is called a perfusion deficit or cold spot, which is a negative image, and occurs in unstable angina patients. Multigated nuclear ventriculogram (MUGA) provides information about the size, contraction pattern, and ejection fraction of the left ventricle.
- Chest roentgenogram: Chest roentgenograms may be normal in patients with coronary artery disease yet cardiomegaly may be found.
- Echocardiography: Can view the left ventricle and reveal segmental wall motion abnormalities, which may indicate ischemia

TABLE 1–2. INVASIVE CARDIAC DIAGNOSTIC PROCEDURES

TABLE 1-2

Test	Purpose	Abnormal Findings
Aortography	Used to visualize the aorta, valve leaflets, and major vessels of the aorta	Aortic valve insufficiency, aneurysms or dissections of ascending aorta, coarctation of the aorta, injuries to the aorta or major branches
Cardiac catheterization	Used to evaluate valvular insufficiency or stenosis, septal defects, congenital anomalies, myocardial function, myocardial blood supply, and cardiac wall motion	CAD, impaired wall motion, valvular heart disease, and septal defect
	Used to compare the size of the cardiovascular system in systole and diastole, assess segmental wall motion, assess chamber size, and evaluate ejection fraction	
Right heart catheterization	Performed to measure right heart pressures, evaluate the pulmonic and tricuspid valves, sample blood oxygen content of right heart chambers for detection of left-to-right shunt, determine cardiac output by the direct Fick method, and evaluate mitral valve stenosis or mitral valve insufficiency by transseptal approach	
Left heart catheterization	Performed to obtain pressure measurement, to evaluate mitral and aortic valve and left ventricular function, evaluate mitral and aortic valve disease, and conduct left ventriculography	
Coronary angiogram	Used to examine the endothelial surfaces of the coronary arteries	Noncomplex atheroma: smooth-surface atheroma without hemorrhage or ulceration causing chronic, unstable angina
Coronary arteriography	Used to visualize the coronary arterial circulation and evaluate the extent of CAD	Complex atheroma: plaque ulceration with a ragged surface and intimal hemorrhage causing accelerated angina
	Used to perform intracoronary thrombolysis and to perform percutaneous transluminal coronary angioplasty	Partially occluded thrombus causes unstable angina at rest
		Ischemic heart disease, atypical angina, coronary artery spasm
Endomyocardial biopsy	Used to identify cardiac transplant rejection, myocardial and adriamycin-induced cardiomyopathy, and to differentiate restrictive from constrictive cardiac disease	

TABLE 1-2

TABLE 1-3

TABLE 1-2. CONTINUED

Test	Purpose	Abnormal Findings
Ventriculogram	Used to delineate areas of poor ventricular contractility: hypokinesis (reduction in wall movement); akinesis (absence of wall movement}; dyskinesis (paradoxic expansion of the ventricular wall with contraction [aneurysm]) Used to determine the degree of valvular incompetence or regurgitation by observing the amount of reflex into the atrium and to determine if the valve is thickened, stenotic, or prolapsed	Ventricular hypertrophy, MI, bundle branch block, myocardial ischemia, or metabolic disturbance

CAD, coronary artery disease; MI, myocardial infarction.

TABLE 1–3. NONINVASIVE CARDIAC DIAGNOSTIC PROCEDURES

Test	Purpose	Abnormal Findings
Cardiac Scans		
Multigated Nuclear Ventriculogram (MUGA)	Used to evaluate left ventricular function such as ejection fraction, ejection velocity, and motion of left ventricle Used to detect intracardiac shunting	CAD, indicated by decreased wall motion (hypokinesis), systolic bulging (dyskinesis), no wall motion (akinesis) to areas supplied by the obstructed coronary artery; cardiomyopathies, CHF; and ejection fraction ≤50% reflecting ventricular dysfunction
Positron-Emission Tomography (PET) Scan	Used to measure regional myocardial blood flow, fatty acid metabolism, glucose metabolism, and blood volume Used to determine whether treatment such as thrombolytic therapy or coronary artery bypass graft is needed	Separates normal myocardium, ischemic but viable tissue, and dead tissue in AMI patients
Technetium Tc-99m stannous pyrophosphate	A MI indicator Used to demonstrate location, size, and extent of MI 24–48 h after suspected MI Used to differentiate between old and new infarcts	Hot spots, indicating acute MI, seen within 48–72 h after onset. Apparent 12 hours after onset and disappear after 1 wk

TABLE 1–3. CONTINUED

Test	Purpose	Abnormal Findings
Thallium myocardial imagery	Used for myocardial perfusion imaging in which normal myocardium will have greater thallium activity than abnormal myocardium	Decreased uptake in areas of decreased myocardial perfusion caused by obstructed coronary arteries
	Used in conjunction with treadmill stress ECG to diagnose ischemic heart disease	Ischemic areas show normal uptake at rest and decreased "cold spots" on exercise
	Used to reveal wall motion defects and heart pump performance during increased oxygen demands	Infarcted areas show no uptake in rest or exercise
	Used to demonstrate location and extent of acute or chronic MI	
	Used to evaluate patency of grafts after coronary artery bypass surgery	
Chest roentgenogram	Used to detect mediastinal abnormalities, such as tumors and cardiac disease	Shift, hypertrophy of right heart, cardiac borders obscured by stringy densities
	Used to detect pneumonia, atelectasis, pneumothorax, and tumors	Atelectasis, cor pulmonale, CHF, or cystic fibrosis
Echocardiography	Generally, used to study structural cardiac abnormalities and blood flow dynamics	Mitral stenosis, mitral valve prolapse, aortic insufficiency, aortic stenosis, subaortic stenosis, tricuspid valve disease, left atrial tumor, pericardial effusion, or enlarged heart chamber
	Specifically, used to identify abnormalities of valve, cardiac tumors, pericardial effusion, mural and atrial thrombi, abnormal aortic size from dilation or aneurysm, aortic dissection, congenital cardiac lesions, hemodynamic alteration such as pulmonary hypertension, and abnormal ventricular size and wall movement resulting from infarction, aneurysm, or cardiomyopathy	
M-mode echocardiography	Measures intracardiac structures using a single ultrasound beam, giving narrow segmental view of heart	
Two-dimensional echocardiography	Provides for real-time imagery of cardiac structure using a planar ultrasound beam, giving wider view of the heart and its structure	

TABLE 1-3

TABLE 1-3

TABLE 1–3. CONTINUED

Test	Purpose	Abnormal Findings
Graded Exercise Test (Stress Test)	Used to evaluate cardiovascular function of patients with or without known heart disease	1 mm depression of ST segment for 0.08 seconds after the junction of QRS complex and S-T segment
	Used to determine functional capacity of the heart after surgery or myocardial infarction, set limitations for exercise program, identify cardiac dysrhythmias that develop during physical exercise, or evaluate effectiveness of antiarrhythmial or antianginal therapy	Depressed J-point, with an upsloping but depressed ST segment of 1.5 mm below the baseline 0.08 second after the J-point
		Hypotension, ST segment depression of 3 mm, down-sloping ST segments and ischemic ST segments appearing within the first 3 minutes of exercise and lasting 8 minutes into the recovery period
		Dyskinetic left ventricular wall motion or severe transmural ischemia: ST segment elevation
Magnetic resonance imaging (MRI)	Used to view heart in multitude of planes and yields visualization of cardiac chambers, ventricular wall, aorta, pulmonary artery, and septum during systole and diastole	Cerebral edema, demyelinating disease, plaque formation, infarctions, tumors, blood clots, hemorrhage, or abscesses
	Detects changes in the chemistry of tissues before they become structural changes	
Phonocardiography (PCG)	Used to identify timing and configuration of heart sounds and their relation to each other	Valvular disorders, hypertrophic cardiomyopathies, or left ventricular failure
Vectorcardiography (VCG)	Used to detect ventricular hypertrophy, interventricular conduction disturbances, and MI	

AMI, acute myocardial infarction; CAD, coronary artery disease; CHF, congestive heart failure; MI, myocardial infarction.

From Ford RD 1987; Loeb, S 1991; Dossey BM, Guzzetta CE, Kenner CV, 1992; and Corbett JV, 1992.

or previous infarction. Also assesses left ventricular function.

- Graded exercise test (Stress ECG): Reveals onset of ST depression within the first 3 minutes of exercise, persistent ST segment depression 8 minutes after exercise, downward sloping or 2 mm ST depression for at least 0.8 seconds in hypotension, abnormalities after exercise, and exercise-induced S_3 gallop.

ECG

- Specific changes including 1 mm or more of horizontal or downsloping ST depression or T wave inversion during chest pain are suggestive of ischemia.
- Other changes reveal left bundle branch block, left anterior hemiblock, ventricular premature beats, and ST and T wave changes.

MEDICAL AND SURGICAL MANAGEMENT

PHARMACOLOGY

- Nitrates: Used for both angina and coronary spasm. Nitrates (intravenous, oral, sublingual, or topical nitroglycerin [NTG]) acts by dilating vascular and selected smooth muscle, causing venous dilatation and, to a lesser degree, arterial dilatation. The venous dilatation decreases venous return (preload), decreases afterload, decreases myocardial oxygen demand, and increases myocardial oxygen supply (Table 1–4).

- Beta-adrenergic blocking agents: Used solely or in combination with nitrates for managing stable and unstable angina. Beta blockers, such as propranolol, inhibit the binding of catecholamines at receptor sites, inhibiting both inotropic and chronotropic actions. The result is a reduction in the resting and exercise heart rate, reduction in myocardial contractility, and a reduction in myocardial oxygen demand (Table 1–5).
- Calcium channel blocker: Used to treat angina by inhibiting the movement of calcium ions across myocardial and vascular smooth muscle. This effect produces the following: vasodilation of the coronary arteries and collateral vessels, decrease myocardial contractility and subsequent decrease in myocardial oxygen demand, peripheral vasodilation, causing decreased systemic blood pressure and a decrease in cardiac conduction. Three calcium channel blockers are used: verapamil, nifedipine, or diltiazem (Table 1–6).
- Morphine Sulfate: Used, if necessary, in small increments to reduce pain (Table 1–7).

PHYSICAL ACTIVITY

- Activity is limited, based upon the patient's activity tolerance and effect upon myocardial oxygen supply and demand.

OXYGEN THERAPY

- Supplemental oxygen 2 to 4L (24% to 36% O_2) is given, depending upon the patient's arterial blood gases (ABG).

DIET

- The dietary plan involves lowering cholesterol levels by restricting total fat, saturated fat, and cholesterol. Some patients may also require weight reduction.

PERCUTANEOUS TRANSLUMINAL CORONARY ANGIOPLASTY (PTCA)

- May be used in patients with one- or two-vessel disease. The procedure reduces coronary obstruction, relieves symptoms, and improves myocardial perfusion and function (see PTCA, p. 226.)

CORONARY LASER ANGIOPLASTY

- Used to restore blood flow distal to the lesion (see Coronary Laser Angioplasty, p. 238.)

SURGICAL INTERVENTION

- Coronary Artery Bypass Surgery (CABG): The surgery is indicated in patients with left main coronary artery disease, three-vessel disease with left ventricular dysfunction and greater than mild angina (see CABG, p. 194).

NURSING MANAGEMENT: NURSING DIAGNOSES AND COLLABORATIVE PROBLEMS

Nursing Diagnoses

Common nursing goals in patients with acute chest pain are to reduce pain, provide knowledge, and foster effective coping behavior.

Pain related to imbalanced myocardial oxygen supply/demand secondary to decreased cardiac output.

Expected Patient Outcome. Patient experiences diminished or resolved chest pain.

- Review results of ECG and serum enzymes.
- Obtain baseline creatinine kinase (CK) isoenzymes when the patient first experiences chest pain.
- Reduce the patient's physical activity to the level of activity before chest pain occurrence.
- Provide small portions of easily digested food and avoid foods containing caffeine.
- Monitor quality of the patient's chest pain: sensation of pressure or heavy weight in the chest, burning sensation, tightness in chest, shortness of breath, visceral nature

TABLE 1-4

TABLE 1–4. VASODILATORS

Medications	Route/Dose	Uses and Effects
Arterial Dilators		
Hydralazine hydrochloride (Apresoline Hydrochloride)	IV/IM: 10–40 mg repeated q 4–6 h 5–100 mg bolus titrated to effect PO: Initial 10 mg four times daily up to 50 mg four times daily	Management of hypertension and CHF Decrease blood pressure by direct relaxation of vascular smooth muscle Decreases afterload Increases heart rate Increases cardiac output
Minoxidil (Loniten)	PO: (Hypertension) 5 mg/d, increased q 3–5 d up to 40 mg/d in single or divided doses as needed; maximum of 100 mg/d	Management of hypertension associated with damage to target organs
Dipyridamole (Persantine)	PO: 150–400 mg/d in divided doses IV: 0.142 mg/kg/min, infused over 4 min	Used to reduce the rate of reinfarction following an MI Non-nitrate coronary vasodilator Increases coronary blood flow by dilating coronary arteries, which can increase myocardial oxygen supply
Venodilators		
Isosorbide dinitrate (Isordil)	Sublingual/chew: 2.5–10 mg may be repeated q 5–10 min for 3 doses in 15–30 min PO: 5 to 30 mg qid	Management of angina pectoris and chronic CHF Decreases preload Decreases myocardial oxygen consumption Increases coronary blood flow by dilating coronary arteries and improving collateral flow to ischemic regions
Erythrityl tetranitrate (Cardilate)	PO: Prophylaxis for angina 5–10 mg	Management of long-term angina pectoris Relaxes vascular smooth muscle with resulting vasodilation Dilates peripheral blood vessels, which causes peripheral pooling of blood, decreased venous return to heart and decreased LVEDP
Pentaerythritol tetranitrate (Peritrate)	PO: 10–20 mg tid or qid up to 40 mg qid; or 80 mg sustained release q 12 h	Management of angina pectoris

TABLE 1-4

Preparation/Administration	Side Effects	Nursing Implications
	Headache, peripheral neuropathy, dizziness, tachycardia, angina, arrhythmias, nausea, vomiting, diarrhea, rashes, sodium retention arthritis, palpitation, orthostatic hypotension, tremors, constipation	Monitor BP, HR, and ECG to determine the drug's effectiveness
	Tachycardia, angina, rebound hypertension, edema, hypersensitivity rash, nausea, headache, fatigue	May be taken without regard to meals or food Take BP and apical pulse before medication and at regular intervals during therapy Monitor daily weight and I & O. Observe patient for edema
Before IV administration, dilute to at least 1:2 ratio with 0.5 N NaCl injection	Headache, dizziness, faintness, syncope, weakness, flushing, nausea, vomiting, diarrhea, skin rash	Take on an empty stomach 1 hour before or 2 hours after meals with a full glass of water
	Headache, apprehension, dizziness, hypotension, syncope, nausea, vomiting, abdominal pain, flushing, tachycardia, pallor	Monitor effectiveness of therapy by evaluating the severity and frequency of anginal pain Monitor patient's BP, HR and rhythm in response to the drug Minimize orthostatic hypotension by having patient slowly change to upright position
	Headache, dizziness, weakness, blurred vision, syncope, tachycardia, hypotension, flushing, pallor, rash, vomiting	Monitor BP and presence of chest pain
Administered 30 min before, 1 h after meals, and at bedtime Sustained release forms also taken on an empty stomach		Avoid sudden discontinuation of medication to reduce risk of coronary vasospasm

TABLE 1–4. CONTINUED

TABLE 1-4

Medications	Route/Dose	Uses and Effects
Nitroglycerin	IV low dose: 5–50 μg/min for preload reduction	Management of angina, hypertension, and CHF or AMI
	IV high dose: 50–100 μg/min has a balanced effect on preload and afterload	Increases coronary blood flow by dilating coronary arteries
	Maximum rate of 300 μg/min	Decreases preload
	Sublingual: 0.15–0.6 mg, repeat, if necessary, q 5 min for 15 min	Decreases myocardial oxygen consumption
	Lingual spray: 0.4 mg/spray 1–2 sprays; can repeat 3–5 min for total of 3 sprays	Decreases peripheral vascular resistance
	Ointment: 1 in=15 mg up to 5 in in 4 h	Decreases BP
	Transdermal patch: 2.5–15.0 mg/ 24 h	Increase cardiac output
	PO: 2.5–9.0 mg 3–4 times/d as extended release capsules	
Balanced Arterial/Venous Dilators		
Nitroprusside (Nipride)	IV: 0.25–6.0 μg/kg/min, not to exceed 8 μg/kg/min	Management of hypertension
	Adjust 0.5 μg increments can be made in 3–5 minutes	Acts directly on the vascular smooth muscle to decrease resistance and dilate vessels
		Decreases BP
		Increases HR slightly
		Reduces systemic vascular resistance moderately
		Decreases left ventricular filling pressure
		Increases cardiac output
Prazosin hydrochloride (Minipress)	PO: Initial dose 1 mg; maintenance dose 6–15 mg in divided doses; up to 40 mg/d	Dilates both arteries and veins by blocking postsynaptic alpha 1-adrenergic receptors
	Maximum daily dose is 20 mg	Decreases preload
		Decreases afterload
		Decreases BP

AMI, acute myocardial infarction; BP, blood pressure; CHF, congestive heart failure; D₅W, 5% dextrose in water; ECG, electrocardiogram; HR, heart rate; I&O, intake and output; IV, intravenous; LVEDP, left ventricular end-diastolic pressure; MI, myocardial infarction; NaCl, sodium chloride; NS, normal saline; PCWP, pulmonary capillary wedge pressure; PO, by mouth; PP, pulse pressure; SBP, systolic blood pressure.

From Deglin JH, Vallerand AH, Russin MM, 1988; Govoni LE, Hayes JE, Shannon MT, et al., 1992; Loeb S, 1993; Scherer JC, 1985; Vallerand AH, & Deglin JH, 1991; Kuhn M, 1992.

TABLE 1-4

Preparation/Administration	Side Effects	Nursing Implications
Preparation: 25–500 µg/mL diluted in D$_5$W or NS Administration: Use proper tubing as recommended by manufacturer	Headache, apprehension, weakness, dizziness, hypotension, light-headedness, restlessness, blurred vision, hypotension, tachycardia, syncope, nausea, vomiting, abdominal pain, flushing	Closely monitor HR, BP, PCWP, PP to evaluate the efficiency of therapy Patient with a low PCWP may be sensitive to the hypotensive effects of nitrate Stop infusion and lift patient's lower extremities if SBP ≤90 mm Hg should patient complain of dizziness
Administration: Via a controlled infusion pump and protected by an opaque covering such as aluminum foil to prevent degradation and loss patency	Abdominal pain, apprehension, coma, diaphoresis, dizziness, dyspnea, headache, muscle twitching, nausea, palpitations, restlessness, hypotension, retrosternal discomfort, irritation at the infusion site Cyanide toxicity: confusion, weakness, tinnitus, muscular twitching	Infusion for longer than 72 h at rate ≥ 6 µg/kg/min increases possibility of thiocyanate toxicity Thiocyanate levels are checked after 24 h and infusion is stopped should level exceed 12 mg/ 100 mL
	Dizziness, drowsiness, syncope, headache, weakness, blurred vision, angina, edema, nausea, vomiting, diarrhea, abdominal cramps, impotence, dyspnea, urinary frequency, diaphoresis	Monitor effectiveness by checking BP and HR At initial dose ≥1 mg, patient may develop severe syncope and loss of consciousness Slowly increase drug dose

TABLE 1-5

TABLE 1–5. BETA-ADRENERGIC BLOCKERS

Medications	Route/Dose	Uses and Effects
Cardioselective		
Acebutolol (Sectral)	PO: Initial 200–1200 mg single or divided doses for hypertension	Management of hypertension, angina pectoris, AMI, ventricular ectopy
	PO: Initial 200 mg bid	Blocks stimulation of beta$_1$ (myocardial) and beta$_2$ (pulmonary, vascular, uterine) receptor sites
	Maintenance 600–1200 mg single or divided doses	Decrease cardiac output
Metoprolol tartrate (Lopressor)	IV: Three boluses, 5 mg each at q 2 min intervals; after 15 min, 50 mg every 6 h for 48 hours orally for AMI	Management of hypertension, angina pectoris, AMI, ventricular dysrhythmias
	PO: Initial 100 mg daily, single or divided doses, then maintenance dose of 100 to 400 mg daily for hypertension	Blocks stimulation of beta$_1$ (myocardial) and beta$_2$ (pulmonary, vascular, uterine) receptor sites
Atenolol (Tenormin)	PO: 50–100 mg/d	Management of hypertension, angina pectoris, AMI supradysrhythmias
		Blocks stimulation of beta$_1$ (myocardial) and beta$_2$ (pulmonary, vascular, uterine) receptor sites
Nonselective		
Nadolol (Corgard)	PO: 40–320 mg/d	Management of hypertension, angina pectoris, AMI, ventricular dysrhythmias
Pindolol (Visken)	PO: Initial 5 mg bid; maintenance dose 10–15 mg/d in 2–3 divided doses up to 60 mg/d; usual dose 10–30 mg/d in 3 divided doses	Management of hypertension
		Blocks stimulation of beta$_1$ (myocardial) and beta$_2$ (pulmonary, vascular, uterine) receptor sites
Propranolol hydrochloride (Inderal)	Angina PO: 10–20 mg 3–4 times daily or 80 mg once daily of extended-release preparation. Maintenance dose is 160–240 mg, up to 320 mg	Blocks stimulation of beta$_1$ (myocardial) and beta$_2$ (pulmonary, vascular, uterine) receptor sites Decreases HR Decreases BP
	Hypertension PO: 40 mg bid or 80 mg extended-release preparation. Maintenance dose 160–480 mg/d in 2 divided doses or 120–160 mg/d of extended-release preparation up to 640 mg/d	Management of angina, hypertension, ventricular and supraventricular ectopy, AMI, hypertrophic subaortic stenosis
	Myocardial Infarction PO: 180–240 mg/d in 2–4 divided doses starting 5–21 days after AMI	

TABLE 1-5

Preparations/Administration	Side Effects	Nursing Implications
	Bradycardia, fatigue, bronchospasm, sleep disturbance, cold extremities, impotence, increased triglycerides, decreased HDL cholesterol	Meals will not interfere with the drug's effectiveness Monitor HR, rhythm, and pulse quality Monitor ECG
	Bradycardia, fatigue, bronchospasm, sleep disturbance, cold extremities, impotence, increased triglycerides, decreased HDL cholesterol, bronchial asthma, muscle aches, dizziness, headache, depression, palpitations, dry skin, pruritus, nausea, gastric pain, dry mouth	Monitor HR, rhythm, and pulse quality Monitor ECG
	Bradycardia, fatigue, bronchospasm, sleep disturbance, cold extremities, impotence, increased triglycerides, decreased HDL cholesterol, dizziness, vertigo, lethargy, drowsiness, hypotension, nausea, vomiting, visual disturbances	May need to administer 50 mg dose after dialysis Monitor HR, rhythm, and pulse quality Monitor ECG
	Bradycardia, fatigue, bronchospasm, sleep disturbance, cold extremities, impotence, increased triglycerides, decreased HDL cholesterol, rash, pruritus, fever, dizziness, headache, behavioral changes	Meals will not interfere with drug's effectiveness Monitor HR, rhythm, and pulse quality
	Bradycardia, fatigue, bronchospasm, sleep disturbance, cold extremities, impotence, hyperthyroidism, increased triglycerides, decreased HDL cholesterol	Meals will not interfere with drug's effectiveness Monitor HR, rhythm, and pulse quality
	Bradycardia, fatigue, bronchospasm, sleep disturbance, cold extremities, impotence, increased triglycerides, decreased HDL cholesterol, pruritus, vertigo, confusion, depression, syncope, weakness, drowsiness, visual disturbances	Teach patient to take drug with food to enhance absorption Monitor HR, rhythm, and pulse quality

TABLE 1-5

TABLE 1–5. CONTINUED

Medications	Route/Dose	Uses and Effects
Propranolol hydrochloride (continued)	Dysrhythmias PO: 10–30 mg 4 times daily up to 160–480 mg daily Intravenous: 1–3 mg not more than 1 mg/min	
Timolol maleate (Blocadren)	Hypertension PO: Initial 10–60 mg/d in 2–3 divided doses MI prophylaxis PO: 10 mg bid	Management of hypertension, AMI, ventricular dysrrhythmias Blocks stimulation of $beta_1$ (myocardial) and $beta_2$ (pulmonary, vascular, uterine) receptor sites
Labetalol hydrochloride (Normodyne, Trandate)	IV: 0.25 μg/kg then 40–80 mg at 10 min intervals; 20 mg slowly over 20 min PO: Initial 100 mg bid; maintenance dose 200–400 mg twice daily	Management of hypertension Blocks stimulation of $beta_1$ (myocardial) and $beta_2$ (pulmonary, vascular, uterine) receptor sites
Esmolol (Brevibloc)	IV: 500 μg/kg/min for 1 minute; give 50 μg/kg/min for 4 minutes Not to exceed 200 μg/kg/min	Management of supraventricular tachyarrhythmias Blocks stimulation of $beta_1$ (myocardium) with less effect on $beta_2$ (pulmonary and vascular) receptor sites

AMI, acute myocardial infarction; BP, blood pressure; ECG, electrocardiogram; HR, heart rate; IV, intravenous; PO, by mouth.

From Deglin JH, Vallerand AH, Russin MM, 1988; Govoni LE, Hayes JE, Shannon MT, et al, 1992; Loeb S, 1993; Scherer JC, 1985; Vallerand AH, Deglin JH, 1991; Clark BK, 1992.

such as deep, heavy, squeezing or aching, and gradual increases in intensity followed by gradual fading away.

- Monitor location of the patient's chest pain: over the sternum, between epigastrium and pharynx, radiating to left shoulder and left arm, lower cervical or upper thoracic spine, or left intercapsular or supracapsular area.
- Obtain a 12-lead ECG during episodes of chest pain.
- Monitor duration of the patient's chest pain: 0.5 to 30 minutes.
- Encourage patient to describe how the pain radiates: medial aspect of the left arm, left shoulder, jaw, and occasionally right arm.
- Administer prescribed intravenous (IV), oral, sublingual or topical NTG at a dose of 0.3 to 0.4 mg sublingual, to be repeated every 5 minutes for a total of 3 tablets given in 15 minutes, or NTG 50 μg IV bolus followed by an infusion rate of 10 to 20 μg/min. The rate may be increased by 5 to 10 μg/min every 5 to 10 minutes until the desired clinical response is achieved. The goal is to relieve or reduce chest pain, and achieve heart rate (HR) $\leq$100 bpm, respiratory rate (RR) 12 to 20 bpm, systolic blood pressure (SBP) $\geq$90 mm Hg, and have ST segment and T wave revert to preangina pattern. (see Table 1–4)

- Monitor patient for side effects of NTG: headache, hypotension, syncope, facial flushing, and nausea.
- Assess HR and rhythm, RR and rhythm, BP, and skin for presence of pallor or cyanosis and diaphoresis during the pain episode and treatment with NTG.

TABLE 1-5

Preparations/Administration	Side Effects	Nursing Implications
	Bradycardia, fatigue, bronchospasm, sleep disturbance, cold extremities, impotence, increased triglycerides, decreased HDL cholesterol, lethargy, weakness, anxiety, rash	Monitor HR, rhythm, and pulse quality
Administration: Do not infuse with sodium bicarbonate	Bronchoconstriction, heart block, orthostatic hypotension, palpitation, bradycardia, syncope, rashes, fatigue, headache, paresthesia, impotence, nasal stuffiness	Administer on an empty stomach Keep patient supine Monitor BP before and 5–10 minutes after infusion
Preparation: Dose of 5g/500 ml D5W yields 10 mg/ml Incompatible with sodium bicarbonate	Dizziness, headache, confusion, agitation, weakness, visual disturbance, bronchospasm, wheezing, hypotension, nausea, vomiting, constipation, abdominal pain, dyspepsia, rash or urinary retention	Monitor HR, rhythm, and pulse quality

- Assess heart rate and rhythm with continuous ECG monitoring. Document ECG rhythm strips every 2 to 4 hours in patients experiencing chest pain episode: ST depression and T wave inversion.
- Administer prescribed beta-adrenergic blockers (propranolol, metoprolol, atenolol, timolol, nadolol, or pindolol) to reduce the disparity between myocardial oxygen demand and supply (see Table 1–7).
- Administer prescribed calcium channel blockers as needed (verapamil, nifedipine, or diltiazem) to maintain coronary artery perfusion pressure (CAPP) at 60 to 80 mm Hg, BP $\geq$90 mm Hg, and urinary output (UO) $\geq$0.5 mL/kg/h (see Table 1–6).
- Monitor side effects of beta blockers and calcium channel blockers: HR $\leq$60 bpm and BP $\leq$90/60 mm Hg.

- Administer prescribed morphine sulfate 2 to 5 mg IV, repeated every 5 to 30 minutes until the desired clinical response is achieved.
- Administer prescribed heparin 500 U IV bolus followed by infusion rate of 1000 U/h, which is titrated according to partial prothrombin time (PTT) (Table 1–8).
- Should chest pain occur during eating, advise small feedings rather than larger meals.
- Provide a restful environment and encourage patient to rest between interventions. This can decrease myocardial oxygen demand.
- Administer prescribed FIO_2 at 50% or oxygen 2 to 4 L/min by means of nasal cannula or mask.
- Administer prescribed IV fluids to maintain adequate hydration.

TABLE 1-6

TABLE 1–6. CALCIUM CHANNEL BLOCKERS

Medication	Route/Dose	Uses and Effects
First Generation		
Phenylalkylamines Verapamil hydrochloride (Calan, Isoptin)	IV: 5–15 mg/kg bolus over 2 min; can repeat in 30 min followed by 5 mg/h infusion PO: 40–120 mg q 6–8 h	Management of supraventricular tachyarrhythmias, temporary control of rapid ventricular rate in atrial flutter, atrial fibrillation, angina, or hypertension Inhibits calcium transport into myocardial and vascular smooth muscle cells Decreases SA and AV conduction Prolongs AV node refractory periods in cardiac conduction tissue Dilates coronary arteries and arterioles Suppresses supraventricular tachyarrhythmias Decreases BP Decreases myocardial contractility Decreases HR
Dihydropyridines Nifedipine (Adalat, Procardia)	Sublingual: 10–20 mg prn PO: 30–60 mg tid; not to exceed 180 mg/d	Management of angina and hypertension Decreases myocardial oxygen utilization Decreases BP Acts on slow calcium channels in vascular smooth muscle and myocardium, leading to coronary vasodilation Relaxes arterial smooth muscle and dilates arterial resistance vessels
Benzothiazepines Diltiazem hydrochloride (Cardizem)	PO: 30–120 mg tid–qid or 60–120 mg bid as SR tablets; up to 240 mg/d IV: 0.25–0.35 mg/kg initially as bolus, followed by 10–15 mg/h infusion up to 24 h	Management of angina Inhibits transport of calcium into myocardial and vascular smooth muscle cells Decreases SA-AV node conduction Increases coronary vasodilation Decreases peripheral vascular resistance
Second Generation		
Isradipine	PO: 2.5–10.0 mg bid, maximum dose of 20 mg/d	Management of angina, coronary artery spasm, hypertension Increases systemic vasodilation Increases coronary vasodilation Increases HR
Nicardipine hydrochloride (Cardene)	PO: 20–40 mg tid	Increases coronary vasodilation Increases peripheral vasodilation Increases HR

AV, atrioventricular; BP, blood pressure; CO, cardiac output; ECG, electrocardiogram; HR, heart rate; IV, intravenous; PO, by mouth; SA, sinoatrial; SBP, systolic blood pressure.

From Deglin JH, Vallerand AH, Russin MM, 1988; Govoni LE, Hayes, JE, Shannon MT, et al, 1992; Loeb S, 1993; Scherer JC, 1985; Vallerand AH, Deglin JH, 1991; White P, 1992.

TABLE 1-6

Preparation/Administration	Side Effects	Nursing Implications
	Dizziness, headache, fatigue, bradycardia, hypotension, edema, asystole, constipation, nausea, abdominal discomfort, depression, bradycardia, flushing, diaphoresis	Monitor ECG continuously Measure serial PR interval and HR Monitor BP and HR before administration; if SBP ≤90 mm Hg or HR ≤50 bpm, notify physician Schedule drug 1 h before or 2 h after meals; meals can decrease drug metabolism Monitor hemodynamic parameters
	Dizziness, light-headedness, headache, nervousness, sore throat, dyspnea, cough, wheezing, hypotension, syncope, tachycardia, nausea, abdominal discomfort, diarrhea, flatulence, muscle cramps, flushing, rashes, diaphoresis	For patient experiencing vasodilatory side effects, make prescribed dosage adjustment Measure serial PR interval, CO, HR, BP. If SBP ≤90 mm Hg and HR ≤50, notify physician Monitor serum potassium levels Observe for peripheral edema, which can be dose-related
	Dizziness, headache, fatigue, arrhythmias, edema, hypotension, syncope, palpitations, second and third degree heart block, anorexia, constipation, nausea, abdominal discomfort, rash, petechiae, bradycardia, vomiting, nervousness, drowsiness, confusion	Regularly evaluate severity and frequency of patient's angina Monitor BP, HR, ECG Notify physician if SBP ≤90 mm Hg or HR ≤50 bpm Maintain safety precautions should dizziness occur
	Ankle edema, fatigue, facial flushing, headache	

TABLE 1-7

TABLE 1–7. NARCOTICS AND ANALGESICS

Medication	Route/Dose	Uses and Effects	Side Effects
Narcotics			
Morphine sulfate	IV: 2.5–15.0 mg q 4 h or infusion initiated with a loading dose of 15 mg, followed by 0.8–10.0 mg/h PO: 10–30 mg q 4 h or 30 mg q 8–12 h as extended-release preparation Subcutaneous/ intramuscular: 5–20 mg every 4h	Management of severe pain, pulmonary edema Relief of pain	Sedation, confusion, headache hallucination, dizziness, diplopia, blurred vision, hypotension, bradycardia, nausea, vomiting, constipation, diaphoresis, flushing, marked miosis
Analgesics			
Ibuprofen (Motrin)	PO: 200–400 mg q 4–6 h, not to exceed 2400 mg/d	Management of inflammatory disorders Inhibits prostaglandin synthesis	Headache, drowsiness, blurred vision, tinnitus, edema, nausea, dyspepsia, vomiting, constipation, gastrointestinal bleeding, renal failure, rashes, light-headedness, fatigue, malaise, anorexia, diarrhea, bloating, abdominal pain
Indomethacin (Indocin)	PO: 25–50 mg bid/tid or 75 mg extended-release capsule once or bid, not to exceed 200 mg or 150 mg of SR/d	Management of inflammatory disorders Inhibits prostaglandin synthesis	Headache, drowsiness, dizziness, edema, rashes, blurred vision, nausea, vomiting, dyspepsia, constipation, blood dyscrasias, prolonged bleeding time, increased blood pressure, palpitation, tachycardia, light-headedness

IV, intravenous; PO, by mouth.

From Deglin JH, Vallerand AH, Russin MM, 1988; Govoni LE, Hayes JE, Shannon MT, et al, 1992; Loeb S, 1993; Scherer JC, 1985; and Vallerand AH, Deglin JH, 1991.

- Administer prescribed analgesic and narcotic to reduce chest discomfort.
- Teach patient to report any chest pain.
- Teach patient to report side effects of NTG: headache, hypotension, syncope, facial flushing, or nausea.
- Teach patient the significance of limiting activity during pain experience to minimize oxygen required and chest pain.

Knowledge deficit related to risk factors associated with angina, diagnostic procedures or treatment alternatives.

Expected Patient Outcome. Patient verbalizes an understanding of risk factors associated with angina and an understanding of diagnostic or treatment procedures.

- Consult with cardiologist about the type and amount of information to be presented to the patient.
- Develop an individualized teaching plan that includes the pathophysiological process causing angina, risk factors associated with angina, and purposes behind diagnostic or treatment procedures.

- Discuss with patient a pain reduction protocol: note quality, location, and duration of chest pain; take one NTG, wait 5 minutes and take up to three NTGs if pain is not relieved; lie down because of possible orthostatic hypotension; and, if pain is not relieved with 3 NTG over 15 minutes, call for emergency service.
- Include patient's family in the teaching program.
- Encourage patient to gradually increase physical activity and cease if chest pain occurs.
- Teach patient the relationship between coronary artery disease and modification of specific risk factors: low cholesterol, low saturated-fat diet, cessation of smoking, progressive exercise, and stress reduction through guided imagery, progressive relaxation and meditation.
- Teach patient that physical activity progresses from complete bed rest, to being up in chair for 20 to 30 minutes, to standing at bedside, to being up and about in room, to ambulation in hallway 150 feet; the amount of metabolic equivalent (MET) or oxygen consumed varies from approximately 1 MET, or 3.5 mL/kg/min, to 5 MET, or 17.0 mL/kg/min.
- Teach patient to report any episodes of chest pain.
- Teach patient stress reduction techniques: guided imagery, meditation, or muscle relaxation.
- Teach patient self-management during acute chest pain: stop activity and rest, take nitrates as ordered, and report if pain lasts ≥ 20 min, diaphoresis, or shortness of breath occur.
- Teach patient about the common side effect of nitroglycerin: headache.

Denial, ineffective related to fear of the diagnosis and need for possible surgery.

Expected Patient Outcome. Patient acknowledges pain and seeks appropriate treatment while experiencing chest pain.

- Assist the patient in identifying why he or she is denying the pain.
- Explore with patient reasons for delaying treatment.
- Encourage patient to discuss his or her concerns about chest pain and its immediate and future implications. Sharing concerns can reduce tension and encourage support for others.
- Confront patient's behavior, when appropriate, and assist to accept the chest pain so the patient will be motivated to seek earlier care. This allows for feelings of acceptance and establishment of more adaptive behaviors.
- Instruct patient about the importance of follow-up care in order to provide ongoing assessment of disease's progress and benefits of treatments.
- Teach the patient to acknowledge the chest pain, take NTG, and call for emergency service should the pain continue, and to seek help rather than delay treatment.
- Teach patient's family about the need for early evaluation and treatment when chest pain occurs.
- Instruct patient about the benefits of CABG should emergency surgery be required.

(For additional nursing diagnosis, see Acute myocardial infarction, p. 38: **Activity intolerance** related to chest pain, hypotension, or tachycardia secondary to coronary artery occlusion.)

Collaborative Problems

Common collaborative goals in patients with acute chest pain are to increase myocardial oxygen supply and decrease myocardial oxygen demand.

Potential Complication: Decreased Myocardial Oxygen Supply. Decreased myocardial oxygen supply related to reduced coronary artery perfusion or decreased diastolic filling time secondary to coronary artery disease or tachycardia.

TABLE 1-8

TABLE 1–8. ANTICOAGULANTS AND ANTIPLATELETS

Medications	Route/Dose	Uses and Effects
Thrombolytic Agents		
Urokinase (Abbokinase) Non–clot-specific	IV: 6000 IU/min into occluded artery for up to 2 min	Lysis of coronary artery thrombosis and pulmonary embolism
Streptokinase (Streptase) Non–clot-specific	Myocardial infarction IV: 250,000 IU bolus over 20–30 min Intracoronary: 20,000 IU bolus followed by 2000 IU/min infusion Deep vein thrombosis, pulmonary emboli, arterial embolism or thrombosis IV: 250,000 IU loading dose, followed by 100,000 IU/h for 24 h for pulmonary embolism, 72 h for recurrent pulmonary emboli or deep vein thrombosis	Activates plasminogen, which dissolves fibrin deposits Increases lysis of thrombi or emboli with systemic effect Decreases blood and plasma viscosity and erythrocyte aggregation Increases perfusion of collateral blood vessels Acute management of deep vein thrombosis, acute arterial thrombosis or embolism, acute pulmonary embolus, coronary artery thrombus
Tissue plasminogen activator (t-PA) (Activase) Clot-specific	IV: >65kg: 60 mg 1st hour (6–10 mg given as bolus over first 1–2 min), 20 mg 2nd and 3rd hour; total of 100 mg <65 kg: 1.25 mg/kg with total dose over 5 h given as 0.75 mg/kg over 1st hour and 0.25 mg/kg over 2nd and 3rd hours	Stimulates conversion of plasminogen in thrombi to plasmin by binding to fibrin; clot-specific
APSAC (Eminase) Clot-specific	IV: 30 units over 3–5 min	Lysis of coronary artery thrombi following AMI
Anticoagulants		
Heparin sodium (Lipo-Hepin)	IV bolus: 10,000 U, followed by 5000–10,000 U q 4–6 h IV: 5000 U (35–70 U/kg) followed by 20,000–40,000 U infused over 24 h SC: 5000 U IV, followed by 8000–10,000 U q 8 h or 15,000–20,000 U q 12 h	Management of various thromboembolic disorders Potentiates effect of antithrombin III Can neutralize thrombin, preventing conversion of fibrinogen to fibrin

TABLE 1-8

Preparation/Administration	Side Effects	Nursing Implications
Preparation: Reconstitute with 5.2 mL of sterile water for a solution of 50,000 IU/mL Dilute solution further with 0.9% NaCl or dextrose 5% or water using 2 mL of 0.9% NaCl injection or dextrose 5% injection for each 250,000 IU of streptokinase	Reperfusion arrhythmias, periorbital edema, urticaria, flushing, bleeding, fever, bronchospasm, headache, itching, nausea	Monitor for bleeding every 15 min for the first h, every 30 min for next 7 h, then once each shift Monitor effectiveness by regularly checking vital signs, Hgb, Hct, PT and PTT
Administration: Use an infusion pump to slowly deliver 250,000 IU of reconstituted drug into each occluded cannula over 25–30 min. Clamp off cannula for 2 h, aspirate contents of cannula, and flush with 0.9% NaCl. For continuous infusion, deliver 30 mL/h (750,000 IU vial) or 90 mL/h (250,000 IU vial)	Bleeding, transient lowering or elevation of BP, periorbital edema, urticaria, phlebitis, hypersensitivity to drug	Monitor drug's effectiveness through BP and clotting status Monitor percutaneous puncture site for oozing
Preparation: Reconstitute to 1 mg/mL by adding 20 or 50 mL of preservative-free sterile water for injection Administration: Can be continuous infusion, direct injection, or intermittent infusion	Intracranial bleeding, headache, arrhythmias, epistaxis, nausea, vomiting, ecchymosis, urticaria, itching, flushing, bleeding, musculoskeletal pain, fever	Monitor drug's effectiveness by regularly checking ECG, BP, pulse, respirations Obtain coagulation studies before therapy Avoid IM injections, venipuncture, and arterial puncture during therapy because of risk of bleeding
Preparation: Do not mix with other drugs Administration: Discard drug if not administered within 30 min after reconstitution Administer 6 h after onset of symptoms	Dysrhythmias, hypotension, hemoptysis, bleeding, hematuria, urticaria, itching, flushing	Monitor for reperfusion dysrhythmias such as sinus bradycardia, accelerated idioventricular rhythm, VT, PVC Monitor ECG to determine effectiveness of the drug
Administration: Administer diluted or undiluted intermittent or continuous infusion Preparation: In 50–100 mL of 0.9% NaCl solution for intermittent infusion	Hepatitis, bleeding, rashes, urticaria, fever, spontaneous bleeding, chills, numbness, hypertension, headache, chest pain, diarrhea	Monitor drug's effectiveness by regularly checking PTT or APTT Monitor platelet count regularly Check patient for bleeding gums, bruises on arms, or petechiae

TABLE 1-8

TABLE 1–8. CONTINUED

Medications	Route/Dose	Uses and Effects
Dihydroergotamine mesylate (Embolex) and heparin sodium	IM: DHE 0.5 mg/2500 USP units heparin IM: DHE 0.5 mg/5000 USP units heparin	DHE is an alpha-adrenergic blocking agent with a direct stimulating effect in the smooth muscle of peripheral blood vessels Thromboprophylactic effect Heparin inhibits reactions leading to clotting of blood and formation of fibrin clots
Warfarin (Coumadin)	IV/IM: 10–15 mg/d for 2–5 d, then adjust daily dose by PT PO: 5–15 mg/d for 2–5 days, then adjust daily dose by result of PT	Management of thromboembolic disorders Adjunct to management of coronary occlusion Interferes with hepatic synthesis of vitamin K-dependent clotting factors (II, VII, IX, X)
Antiplatelet Agent		
Dipyridamole (Persantine)	PO: 100–400 mg/d in 2–4 divided doses	Management of angina Used in combination with anticoagulants to prevent thromboembolism in patients with prosthetic heart valves

AMI, acute myocardial infarction; APTT, activated partial thromboplastin time; BP, blood pressure; ECG, electrocardiogram; Hct, hematocrit; Hgb, hemoglobin; IM, intramuscular; IV, intravenous; NaCl, sodium chloride; PO, oral; PT, prothrombin time; PTT, partial thromboplastin time; PVC, premature ventricular contraction(s); SC, subcutaneously; VT, ventricular tachycardia.

From Deglin JH, Vallerand AH, Russin MM, 1988; Govoni LE, Hayes JH, Shannon MT, et al, 1992; Loeb S, 1993; Scherer JC, 1985; and, Vallerand AH, Deglin JH, 1991.

Expected Patient Outcomes. Patient maintains adequate myocardial oxygen supply, as evidenced by arterial oxygen content (CaO_2) 18 to 20 mL/100mL, arterial oxygen delivery (DO_2) 900 to 1200 mL/min, arterial oxygen delivery index (DO_2I) 500 to 600 mL/min/m², coronary artery perfusion pressure (CAPP) 60 to 80 mm Hg, cardiac output (CO) 4 to 8 L/min, cardiac index (CI) 2.7 to 4.0 L/min/m², systemic vascular resistance (SVR) 900 to 1200 dynes/s/cm⁻⁵, systemic vascular resistance index (SVRI) 1970 to 2390 dyness/cm⁻⁵ ≠ m², continuous mixed venous oxygen saturation (SvO_2) 60% to 80%, BP ≥90/60 mm Hg or within the patient's normal range, hemoglobin within normal range, HR ≤90 bpm, capillary refill ≤3 seconds, arterial oxygen saturation (SaO_2) ≥95%, PaO_2 ≥80 mm Hg, absence of dysrhythmias, and absence of chest pain.

- Consult with cardiologist to validate the expected outcomes used to determine whether or not patient's myocardial oxygen supply is sufficient.
- Consult with physician about underlying factors that decrease myocardial oxygen supply.
- Consult with cardiac rehabilitation as to the appropriate activity program for the patient.
- Review results from coronary angiogram, echocardiogram, ECG, graded exercise test, thallium 201 scan, MUGA scan, serum enzymes, BUN and creatinine.
- Limit patient's physical activity when chest discomfort occurs in response to decreased myocardial oxygen supply.
- Provide small portions of low-saturated-fat and low-cholesterol diet as ordered.
- Maintain CI at 4.5 L/min/m² or greater and oxygen delivery of ≥1200 mL/min (or 600

TABLE 1-8

Preparation/Administration	Side Effects	Nursing Implications
	Hemorrhage, numbness, tingling of toes and fingers, muscle pain in extremities, weakness in legs, localized edema, hypersensitivity	
	Nausea, cramps, bleeding, fever, anorexia, diarrhea, dermatitis, ulcer	Monitor for evidence of bleeding or bruising
Administration: Administer 1 h before meals	Headache, dizziness, weakness, syncope, flushing, hypotension, nausea, vomiting, diarrhea, gastric distress, faintness, skin rash	Monitor BP, heart rate and rhythm Monitor for prolonged bleeding

mL/min/m^2 indexed for body size) in order to maximize oxygen supply.

• Calculate arterial oxygen delivery (Do_2), which is determined by the amount of oxygen in the blood (Cao_2) and the amount of blood delivered to the tissue (CO/CI). Report value ≤900 mL/min.

• Monitor myocardial oxygen consumption (MVo_2) by multiplying systolic blood pressure (SBP) with HR. Coronary artery perfusion occurs during diastole, and increased HR will decrease diastolic filling time and subsequent coronary artery perfusion and increase MVo_2.

• Monitor and report hemodynamic findings reflective of decreased myocardial tissue oxygen supply resulting from decreased cardiac output: BP ≤ 90/60 mm Hg, CAPP ≤60 mm Hg, CO ≤4 L/min, CI ≤2.7 L/min/m^2, Do_2 ≤900 mL/min and Do_2I ≤500 mL/min/m^2.

• Obtain, document, and report other findings suggestive of decreased myocardial oxygen supply: HR ≥100 bpm, which decreases diastolic filling time; SBP ≤90/60 mm Hg; capillary refill ≥3 seconds, peripheral pulses ≤2+, presence of dysrhythmia and chest pain.

• Monitor BP, capillary refill, and HR; a slow HR increases diastolic filling time, which extends the time during which oxygenated blood is available to the coronary vasculature.

• Monitor continuous ECG monitoring to assess HR, rhythm, ST or T wave changes that may indicate ischemia or injury. Document ECG rhythm strips every 2 to 4 hours in patients with dysrhythmias.

- Administer prescribed oxygen 2 to 4 L/min (24% to 36% O_2) by means of nasal cannula or mask to maintain $Pao_2 \geq 80$ mm Hg, $Sao_2 \geq 95\%$, or $S\bar{v}o_2 \geq 60\%$.
- Administer prescribed IV fluids to maintain adequate circulating volume.
- Administer prescribed IV nitroglycerin 5 $\mu g/min$ titrated to maintain SBP ≥ 90 mm Hg, CAPP ≥ 60 mm Hg, $Do_2 \geq 900$ mL/min and $Do_2I \geq 500$ mL/min/m^2. Contraindicated in unstable angina patients with hypotension (see Table 1–4)
- Administer prescribed calcium channel blockers (diltiazem or nifedipine) to decrease myocardial oxygen demand, increase myocardial oxygen supply, and decrease coronary artery vasospasm. Contraindicated in unstable angina patients with hypotension, congestive heart failure (CHF), or high-grade heart block (see Table 1–6)
- Administer prescribed beta-blockers with calcium channel blockers in unstable angina patients. Be careful in patients with left ventricular dysfunction or conduction disturbance because of the potential increase in the incidence and severity of CHF. Contraindicated in unstable angina patients with hypotension, CHF, high-grade heart block, or bradycardia (see Table 1–5)
- Administer prescribed thrombolytic therapy (streptokinase or tissue plasminogen activator) to maintain CAPP ≥ 60 mm Hg, CO ≥ 4 L/min, and CI ≥ 2.7 L/min/m^2 (see Table 1–8)
- Administer prescribed analgesic or narcotic to maintain HR ≤ 100 bpm and reduce chest pain.
- Should pharmacological therapy be ineffective in increasing myocardial tissue oxygen supply, prepare patient for PTCA insertion and coronary laser angioplasty. (See PTCA, p. 226 and Coronary laser angioplasty, p. 228.)
- Should PTCA and thrombolytic therapy be ineffective, prepare patient for emergency CABG. (See CABG, p. 194.)
- Teach patient the importance of reporting chest pain. Mild to severe aching, sharp, tingling, or burning sensation or pressure described as heavy, squeezing, heartburn, or tight chest lasting 5 to 10 minutes.
- Teach patient to pace activities so as not to decrease HR and subsequently decrease myocardial tissue oxygen supply.

Potential Complication: Increased Myocardial Oxygen Demand. Increased myocardial oxygen demand related to increased systolic left ventricular wall tension, tachycardia, increased myocardial contractility secondary to atherosclerotic lesions or inotropic drug therapy.

Expected Patient Outcomes. Patient maintains reduced myocardial oxygen demand, as measured by oxygen extraction ratio (O_2ER) of 22% to 30%, mean arterial pressure (MAP) 70 to 90 mm Hg, pulmonary capillary wedge pressure (PCWP) 6 to 12 mm Hg, pulse pressure (PP) 30 to 40 mm Hg, continuous mixed venous oxygen saturation ($S\bar{v}o_2$) 60% to 80%, rate pressure product (RPP) $\leq 12,000$, SVR 900 to 1200 dynes/s/cm^{-5}, SVRI 1970 to 2300 dynes/s/cm$^{-5} \cdot m^2$, stroke volume (SV) 60 to 130 mL/beat, stroke volume index (SVI) 45 to 85 mL/m^2/beat, oxygen consumption (Vo_2) ≥ 200 or ≤ 250 mL/min, oxygen consumption index (Vo_2I) ≥ 115 or ≤ 165 mL/min/m^2, BP within patient's normal range, HR ≤ 100 bpm, and temperature $\leq 100°F$.

- Confer with cardiologist to validate expected patient outcomes that reflect decreased myocardial oxygen demand.
- Consult with dietitian about the patient's diet: small, frequent, easily digested meals and no caffeine.
- Review results from coronary angiogram, echocardiogram, ECG, graded exercise test, thallium 201 scan, MUGA scan, serum enzymes, BUN and creatinine.
- Review results of 12-lead ECG.
- Limit physical activity to bed rest during acute chest pain so as not to increase HR and increase myocardial oxygen demand or consumption.
- Patient feeds self while sitting with head of bed (HOB) 45 degrees. Patient requires 1 to

1.5 metabolic equivalents or oxygen consumption of approximately 3.5 mL/kg/min.

- Provide prescribed diet consisting of low-sodium and low-saturated-fat foods.
- Calculate arterial oxygen demand, which is the product of CO and the difference between arterial oxygen content and venous oxygen content $C(a - v)o_2$.
- Calculate oxygen utilization coefficient or oxygen extraction ratio (o_2ER) by dividing the arteriovenous oxygen content difference ($C[a - v]o_2$) by arterial oxygen content (Cao_2).
- Calculate the RPP by multiplying HR with SBP. This value correlates well with myocardial oxygen consumption or demand (MVo_2). Report RPP $\geq$ 12,000.
- Obtain Vo_2 and Vo_2I in relationship to Do_2 and Do_2I. When Vo_2 (oxygen consumption) is limited by Do_2 (oxygen delivery), the Vo_2 is thought of as being supply-dependent. The rate of oxygen consumed is limited by the rate of oxygen delivered to the tissues.
- Continuously monitor $S\bar{v}o_2$ to evaluate oxygen supply and demand. An $S\bar{v}o_2$ of $\leq$60 % can indicate decreased oxygen supply and increased oxygen demand.
- Obtain and report hemodynamic parameters reflecting increased myocardial oxygen demand resulting from decreased CO: $o_2ER \geq 25\%$, PP $\leq$30 mm Hg, RPP $\geq$12,000, $S\bar{v}o_2 \leq$60%, SVR $\geq$1200 dynes/s/cm^{-5}, SVRI $\geq$ 2390 dynes/s/cm$^{-5} \cdot$ m^2, SV $\leq$60 mL/beat, SVI $\leq$45 mL/m^2/beat, $Vo_2 \geq$250 mL/min and $Vo_2I \geq$165 mL/min/m^2.
- Initiate continuous ECG monitoring to assess HR and rhythm. Document ECG rhythm strips every 2 to 4 hours in patients with tachydysrhythmias or premature ventricular contractions.
- Provide passive range of motion (ROM) exercises without increasing myocardial oxygen demand to maintain muscle tone.
- Administer prescribed Fio_2 at 50% or oxygen 2 to 4 L/min by means of nasal cannula or mask to maintain $Pao_2 \geq$80 mm Hg, $Sao_2 \geq$95%, and $S\bar{v}o_2 \geq$60%.

- Administer IV fluids to maintain adequate hydration and UO $\geq$30 mL/h.
- Administer prescribed peripheral nitrates (IV nitroglycerin) to maintain SVR $\leq$1200 dynes/s/cm^{-5}, SVRI $\leq$2390 dynes/s/cm$^{-5} \cdot$m^2, and RPP $\leq$12,000 (see Table 1–6).
- Administer prescribed beta-adrenergic blockers to reduce the disparity between myocardial oxygen demand and supply (propranolol, metoprolol, atenolol, timolol, nadolol, or pindolol) to maintain o_2ER 25%, PP 30 to 40 mm Hg, RR $\leq$12,000, SVo_2 60% to 80%, SV 60 to 130 mL/beat, SVI 45 to 85 mL/m^2/beat, Vo_2 200 to 250 mL/min, Vo_2I 115 to 165 mL/min/m^2 or HR $\leq$100 bpm (see Table 1–5).
- Inform patient that increased physical activity, increased heart rate, straining while having a stool, suctioning, or moods such as irritability, anxiety, or nervousness can increase myocardial oxygen demand.
- Teach patient techniques to reduce myocardial oxygen consumption: guided imagery, meditation, or progressive relaxation.
- Teach patient the common side effects of beta-adrenergic blockers and vasodilators.

(For additional collaborative problems, see Acute myocardial infarction, p. 38: **Potential Complication: Dysrhythmias** related to increased sympathetic tone or myocardial ischemia secondary to coronary artery disease, p. 184.)

DISCHARGE PLANNING

The critical care nurse provides the patient and significant other(s) with verbal or written discharge notes regarding the following subjects.

1. Allowances and limitations: Avoiding isometric-type activity such as heavy lifting or pushing. Use of home exercise program. Teach patient and significant other(s) activity schedule. A postdischarge exercise program to keep HR $\leq$100 bpm as follows. (1) first week, walk 0.25 miles within 8 to 10 minutes; (2) second week, walk 0.25 miles within 5 minutes; (3) third week, walk

0.50 miles within 15 minutes; and (4) fourth week, walk 1.0 miles within 30 minutes.

2. Sexual activity guidelines: Avoid sexual activity when fatigued, or if acute chest pain occurs during sexual activity, stop and take nitrate if ordered. Should acute chest pain persist, report symptoms to physician.

3. Names of medications, purpose, dosage, schedule, and side effects.

4. Following prescribed low-sodium, low-cholesterol, and low-saturated-fat diet.

5. Names of community agencies that can help patient stop smoking and maintain controlled exercise program.

■ ACUTE MYOCARDIAL INFARCTION

(For related information see Part I: Cardiogenic shock, p. 72; Congestive heart failure, p. 87; Acute chest pain, p. 1; Dysrhythmias, p. 184. Part II: Coronary artery bypass graft, p. 194. Part III: Hemodynamic monitoring, p. 219; Percutaneous transluminal coronary angioplasty, p. 226; Coronary laser angioplasty, p. 228; Coronary atherectomy, p. 234; Intracoronary stents, p. 237; Intra-aortic balloon pump, p. 254; ST segment monitoring, p. 264; Thrombolytic therapy, p. 265. See also Behavioral Deviations, p. 725.)

Diagnostic Category and Length of Stay

DRG: 121 circulatory disorders with AMI and CV complications, discharged alive
LOS: 8.2 days
DRG: 122 circulatory disorders with AMI and no CV complications, discharged alive
LOS: 6.20 days
DRG: 123 circulatory disorders with AMI, expired
LOS: 3.0 days

Definition

Acute myocardial infarction (AMI) is the rapid ischemic necrosis of myocardial tissue resulting from oxygen deprivation. AMI is caused by complete obstruction of a coronary artery or is subsequent to an increase in myocardial tissue oxygen demand that a partially obstructed coronary artery cannot meet. An AMI can be classified according to the degree of tissue destruction: transmural injury or nontransmural injury. Transmural injury is a lesion involving the full myocardial thickness. Nontransmural injury is tissue damage involving partial thickness of the myocardium and can be categorized into three types. Subendocardial MI damages the inner ventricular lining, subepicardial MI damages the outer ventricular lining, and intramural MI does not involve the full thickness of the heart muscle.

Pathophysiology

Physiological events cause disruption of the intima covering the plaque. Thrombosis forms, spasm may occur, and blood flow to the involved areas of the myocardium ceases. Infarction results from the mechanical obstruction caused by thrombus, plaque rupture, dissection, and spasm. An AMI is characterized by three zones of myocardial damage: ischemia, injury, and infarction. The zone of ischemia borders the area of injury. Ischemia is defined as oxygen deprivation accompanied by inadequate removal of metabolites because of inadequate perfusion. There can be an actual decrease in blood flow (oxygen supply) or an increase in oxygen demand when supply is fixed. In this zone there is a temporary interruption of blood flow that usually does not involve tissue death. The cells in this area are weakened by decreased oxygen supply; however, function can return within 2 to 3 weeks after the onset of the occlusion. The zone of injury surrounds the area of infarction and results in tissue damage from prolonged interruption of blood supply. This area may extend the area of infarction or, with adequate collateral circulation, regain its function within 2 to 3 weeks. The zone of infarction involves cell destruction (necrosis). Infarction results from the mechanical obstruction caused by thrombosis, plaque rupture, dissection, or spasm. Necrosis in this area occurs within 5 to 6 hours after the occlusion. The larger the infarcted area, the greater the loss of contractility, which causes the following: reduced contractility with abnormal wall motion, altered left ventricular compliance, reduced stroke volume, reduced stroke work, reduced ejection fraction, elevated left ventricular end-diastolic pressure (LVEDP) or preload, elevated afterload, reduced myocardial tissue perfusion, decreased myocardial oxygen supply, increased myocardial oxygen demand, pulmonary congestion with hypoxemia, and reduced renal arterial perfusion with reduced glomerular filtration rate.

Nursing Assessment

PRIMARY CAUSES

- Gradual occlusion of a coronary artery resulting from atherosclerotic processes, cardiovascular thrombus formation, or coronary artery vasospasm.

RISK FACTORS

- History of earlier AMI or family history of coronary artery disease (CAD); other conditions such as hyperlipidemia, hypertension, or diabetes mellitus; life-style factors such as obesity, smoking, lack of physical activity or stress; men or postmenopausal women.

PHYSICAL ASSESSMENT

- Inspection: Patient complains of substernal chest pain lasting more than 30 minutes. Typically the pain may be described as radiating to the lower jaw and teeth, neck, left shoulder, upper back, or down the left arm to the two fingers innervated by the ulnar nerve. The patient may also experience apprehension, restlessness, confusion, anxiety, or agitation; orthopnea or dyspnea; pallor, ashen skin, or cyanosis; lightheadedness or syncope; diaphoresis; nausea or vomiting; and decreased urinary output.
- Palpation: Skin cool and moist; peripheral pulses normal to decreased; abnormally located ventricular impulse; capillary refill decreased; systolic outward impulse or bulge

seen in patients with an anterior myocardial infarction and may indicate the development of left ventricular aneurysm; presystolic impulse and occasionally palpable S_3.
- Auscultation: Hypotension; bradycardia to tachycardia; tachypnea, basilar rales, or diffuse wheezing; systolic murmur; presystolic gallop (S_4); paradoxic splitting S_1, S_2, and S_3 heart sounds; transient pericardial friction rub.

DIAGNOSTIC TEST RESULTS

Hemodynamic Parameters. (See Table 1–9)

- Cardiac output (CO) ≤ 4 or ≥ 8 L/min; cardiac index (CI) ≤ 2.7 or ≥ 4.3 L/min/m^2; mixed venous oxygen saturation (S$\bar{v}$o$_2$) $\leq 60\%$, pulmonary artery pressure (PAP) systolic ≥ 25 mm Hg and diastolic ≥ 15 mm Hg; pulmonary capillary wedge pressure (PCWP) ≥ 12 mm Hg; systemic vascular resistance (SVR) ≥ 1200 dynes/s/cm^{-5}; right ventricular stroke work (RVSW) ≤ 10 or ≥ 15 g-m/beat; or left ventricular stroke work (LVSW) ≤ 60 or ≥ 80 g-m/beat.

Standard Laboratory Tests. (See Table 1–1)

- Blood studies: Elevated erythrocyte sedimentation rate (ESR) within a few hours of infarction, peaks in the fourth or fifth day after AMI and remains elevated for several weeks. Elevated white blood cell count (WBC) within a few hours after the onset of chest pain or AMI, peaks 2 to 4 days later, and returns to normal within a week. The peak is usually 12,000 to 15,000 cells/mm^3 and can become as high as 20,000 cells/mm^3.
- Serum chemistries: Elevated blood urea nitrogen (BUN), cholesterol, low-density lipoprotein (LDL), and triglycerides readings. High-density lipoprotein (HDL) may be decreased.
- Serum enzymes: Elevated creatinine kinase (CK) appears in 4 to 8 hours, peaks within 24 hours, and lasts for 3 to 4 days. Elevated total lactic dehydrogenase (LDH) appears within 24 to 48 hours, peaks in 3 to 6 days,

TABLE 1-9

TABLE 1–9. HEMODYNAMIC PARAMETERS

Test	Purpose	Normal Value	Formulas	Abnormal Findings
Arterial-alveolar oxygen tension ratio (P[a/A]O$_2$)	Measurement of the efficiency of gas exchange in the lung	0.75–0.90	Pao$_2$/Pao$_2$	≤0.75 can indicate ventilation-perfusion (V/Q) inequalities, shunt abnormalities, or diffusion problems
Arterial oxygen content (CaO$_2$)	Measurement of oxygen content in arterial blood including oxygen bound to hemoglobin and oxygen dissolved in blood	18–20 mL/100mL	Cao$_2$ = (Sao$_2$ × Hgb × 1.34) + Pao$_2$ × 0.003	A decreased value may indicate a low Pao$_2$, Sao$_2$, or hemoglobin (Hgb)
Arterial oxygen saturation (Sao$_2$)	The percentage of oxyhemoglobin saturation of arterial blood	95.0%–97.5%		≤95% can indicate impaired respiratory function or insufficient oxygen from inspired air
Arteriovenous oxygen content difference C(a − v)o$_2$	Reflects tissue extraction of oxygen Used to measure oxygen uptake at the tissue level	4–6 mL/100mL	Arterial O$_2$ content in arterial blood (Cao$_2$) − O$_2$ content in venous blood (Cvo$_2$)	≥6 mL/100 mL can indicate decreased cardiac output or impaired ventricular performance
Cardiac output (CO)	Measurement of blood pumped out of ventricles each minute The product of stroke volume and heart rate	4–8 L/min	(SV)(HR)	≤4L/min can indicate impaired myocardial contractility resulting from myocardial infarction; drugs such as procainamide, quinidine, or propranolol; acidosis, hypoxia; increased left ventricular filling produced by fluid depletion; or increased SVR from arteriosclerosis, hypertension, valvular heart disease leading to decreased blood flow from the ventricle
Cardiac index (CI)	Cardiac output adjusted for body size	2.7–4.3 L/min/m^2	CI = CO/BSA	≤2.2 L/min/m^2 indicates hypoperfusion ≤1.8 L/min/m^2 indicates cardiogenic shock

TABLE 1-9

TABLE 1–9. CONTINUED

Test	Purpose	Normal Value	Formulas	Abnormal Findings
Central venous pressure (CVP)	Measurement created by volume in the right side of the heart, reflects filling pressure of right ventricle Indicator of right atrial preload	2–6 mm Hg 5–12 cm H_2O	(CVP diastolic $\times$ 2) + (CVP systolic) = 3	$\leq$2 mm Hg can indicate hypovolemia, vasodilation, myocardial contractility $\geq$6 mm Hg can indicate increased circulatory volume, vasoconstriction, decreased contractility of myocardium, right ventricular failure, tricuspid insufficiency, positive-pressure breathing, pericardial tamponade, pulmonary embolus, obstructive pulmonary disease
Coronary artery perfusion pressure (CAPP)	Measurement of the perfusion of the coronary arteries during diastole	60–80 mm Hg	MAP $-$ PCWP or DBP $-$ PAWP	$\geq$80 mm Hg can indicate increased resistance to flow through the coronary arteries from reflex coronary artery vasoconstriction $\leq$60 mm Hg can indicate hypoperfusion
Continuous mixed venous oxygen saturation ($S\bar{v}_{O_2}$)	Measurement of overall tissue utilization of oxygen and patient's ability to balance oxygen supply and demand at the tissue level The net result of overall cardiopulmonary function and tissue perfusion, measured by PAP	60%–80%	$(CO \times Ca_{O_2} \times 10)$ $- \ddot{V}_{O_2}$	$\leq$60% can indicate lactic acidosis or poor cardiac output > 80% can indicate hyperdynamic state

TABLE 1-9

TABLE 1–9. CONTINUED

Test	Purpose	Normal Value	Formulas	Abnormal Findings
Ejection fraction (EF)	Measurement of the ratio of the amount of blood ejected from the left ventricle to the amount of blood remaining in the ventricle at end-diastole An indirect measure of contractility	60%–75%	SV/end-diastolic volume (EDV) × 100	≤50% can indicate impaired myocardial contractility or cardiogenic shock
Left atrial pressure (LAP)	A direct measure-ment of left ventricular end-diastolic pressure (LVEDP) Used after cardiac surgery to determine how well the left ventricle is ejecting its volume	8–12 mm Hg		≥12 mm Hg can indicate a lower ejection fraction for the left ventricle
Left ventricular stroke work (LVSW)	Measurement of the pressure generated by left ventricular contraction is systolic arterial pressure minus pulmonary capillary wedge pressure Indicator of left ventricular contractility	60–80 g-m/beat	(SBP − PCWP) SV × 0.0136	≤80 g-m/beat can indicate left ventricular failure and increased contraction <60 g-m/beat can indicate decreased contractility
Left ventricular stroke work index (LVSWI)	Measurement of amount of work performed by the left ventricle per cardiac contraction adjusted for body size Indicator of left ventricular contractility	35–85 g-m/beat/m²	SVI(MAP − PCWP) × 0.0136/CI	≤45 g-m/beat/m² occurs with decreased contractility
Mean arterial pressure (MAP)	Measurement of the average arterial pressure that determines blood flow to the tissues	70–100 mm Hg	SBP + (2 × DBP) = 3	≥70 mm Hg can signify increased cardiac output ≥70 mm Hg can signify decreased systemic vascular resistance and cardiac output

TABLE 1–9. CONTINUED

TABLE 1-9

Test	Purpose	Normal Value	Formulas	Abnormal Findings
Oxygen utilization coefficient (O_2ER)	Measurement that indicates the balance between oxygen supply and oxygen demand	25%	$C(a - v)o_2/Cao_2$	$\geq$25% indicates that an increased O_2 supply is needed
Oxygen consumption (Vo_2)	Measurement of the volume of oxygen used each minute at the tissue level	200–250 mL/min	$CO \times 10 \times C(a - v)o_2$	$\leq$200 mL/min can indicate the metabolic needs of tissues not met, inadequate O_2 transportation $\geq$250 mL/min can indicate hypermetabolic states such as hyperthermia, fever, seizures, trauma
Oxygen consumption index (Vo_2I)	Measurement of Vo_2 adjusted for body size	115–165 mL/min/m²	$CI \times 10 \times C(a - v)o_2$	
Oxygen (arterial) delivery (Do_2)	Measurement of the volume of oxygen delivered each minute at the tissue level	900–1200 mL/min	$CO \times 10 \times Cao_2$	$\leq$900 mL/min can indicate decreased cardiac output as in cardiogenic shock or decreased O_2 content $\geq$1100 mL/min can indicate increased oxygen content and increased blood flow
Oxygen (arterial) index (Do_2I)	Measurement of DO_2 adjusted for body size	500–600 mL/min/m²	$CI \times 10 \times Cao_2$	
Pulmonary artery pressure (PAP)	Measurement of venous pressure in the lungs and mean filling pressure in the left atrium and left ventricle In the absence of pulmonary stenosis, systolic PAP usually equals right ventricular systolic pressure	Systolic 15–25 mm Hg Diastolic 8–15 mm Hg Mean 10–20 mm Hg		$\geq$25/15 mm Hg can indicate increased left ventricular failure, increased pulmonary blood flow, pulmonary hypertension, mitral stenosis, chronic obstructive pulmonary disease, pulmonary edema, left ventricular failure, pulmonary embolus

TABLE 1-9

TABLE 1–9. CONTINUED

Test	Purpose	Normal Value	Formulas	Abnormal Findings
Pulmonary capillary/ artery wedge pressure (PCWP/PAWP)	Measurement of pressure created by volume in the left side of the heart Reflects filling pressure of left ventricle if no obstruction exists between catheter balloon tip and left ventricle Indicator of left atrial preload	6–12 mm Hg		≥12 mm Hg can increase left ventricular failure, mitral stenosis and regurgitation, cardiac tamponade, cardiac insufficiency ≤6 mm Hg can indicate hypovolemia
Pulmonary vascular resistance (PVR)	Measurement of the resistance against which the right ventricle must pump to eject the volume Indicator of right ventricular resistance or afterload	155–255 dynes/s/ cm^{-5}	PAM − PCWP × 80 CO	≥250 dynes/s/cm^{-5} may indicate pulmonary hypertension, hypoxia, lung disease, pulmonary embolism, shock ≤100 dynes/s/cm^{-5} can indicate arterial dilation produced by drugs (nitroprusside, nitroglycerin, amrinone, or calcium channel blockers)
Pulmonary vascular resistance index (PVRI)	Measure of PVR adjusted for body size Indicator of right ventricular resistance or afterload	200–450 dynes/s/ $cm^{-5} \cdot m^2$	PAM − PCWP × 80 CI	≤450 dynes/s/ $cm^{-5} \cdot m^2$ may indicate pulmonary hypertension, hypoxia, lung disease, pulmonary embolism, shock ≤200 dynes/s/ $cm^{-5} \cdot m^2$ can indicate arterial dilation produced by drugs (nitroprusside, nitroglycerin, amrinone, or calcium channel blockers)
Pulse pressure (PP)	Measurement of stroke volume and arterial compliance	30–40 mm Hg	SBP − DBP	≤40 mm Hg can occur in decreased peripheral resistance or increased SV ≥30 mm Hg occurs in increased peripheral resistance or decreased SV

TABLE 1-9

TABLE 1–9. CONTINUED

Test	Purpose	Normal Value	Formulas	Abnormal Findings
Rate pressure product (RPP)	Indirect measure of myocardial oxygen demand.	≤12,000	HR × SBP	Activities performed with lower heart rate and SBP are better tolerated by patient with coronary heart disease
Right atrial pressure (RAP)	Measurement of right atrial pressure	4–6 mm Hg		Increased RAP can indicate pulmonary disease, right ventricular failure, fluid overload, cardiac tamponade, tricuspid stenosis and regurgitation, pulmonary hypertension
Right ventricular pressure (RVP)	Measurement of right ventricular pressure with right ventricular systolic pressure equals pulmonary artery systolic pressure Right ventricular end-diastolic pressure reflects right ventricular function and equals right atrial pressure	Systolic 15–25 mm Hg Diastolic 0–8 mm Hg		Increased RVP ≥25/8 mm Hg can indicate mitral stenosis or insufficiency, pulmonary disease, hypoxemia, constrictive pericarditis, chronic congestive heart failure, atrial and ventricular septal defects, patent ductus arteriosus
Right ventricular stroke work (RVSW)	Measurement of the pressure generated by right ventricular contraction is pulmonary artery systolic pressure minus the right atrial mean pressure	10–15 g-m/beat	(PA sys − RA) × SV × 0.0136	Decreased RVSW can indicate right ventricular failure
Right ventricular stroke work index (RVSWI)	Measurement of amount of work right ventricle does per cardiac contraction, adjusted for body size Indicator of right ventricular contractility	7–12 g-m/beat/m²	(PAD − CVP) × SI × 0.0136	Decreased RVSWI can indicate right ventricular failure

TABLE 1-9

TABLE 1–9. CONTINUED

Test	Purpose	Normal Value	Formulas	Abnormal Findings
Stroke volume (SV)	The volume of blood ejected from the ventricle per beat Indicator of contractility	60–130 mL/beat	CO/HR	Factors that alter preload, afterload, or contractility
Stroke volume index (SVI)	Stroke volume adjusted for body size Indicator of contractility	45–85 mL/m^2/beat	SV/CI	Factors that alter preload, afterload, or contractility
Systemic vascular resistance (SVR)	Measure of the resistance against which the left ventricle must pump to eject volume Resistance to flow is also referred to as afterload	900–1200 dynes/s/cm^{-5}	MAP − CVP × 80 CO	Increased SVR can indicate peripheral vasoconstriction that might occur with hypovolemia Decreased SVR can indicate peripheral vasodilation, such as in septic shock
Systemic vascular resistance index (SVRI)	The SVR adjusted for body size Indicator of left ventricular afterload	1970–2390 dynes/s/cm^{-5} · m^2		Increased SVRI can indicate arterial constriction produced by drugs (epinephrine, norepinephrine, dopamine, phenylephrine), hypovolemia, cardiogenic shock Decreased SVRI can indicate arterial dilatation produced by drugs (nitroprusside, nitroglycerine, amrionone, or calcium channel blockers); septic, anaphylactic, or neurogenic shock
Venous oxygen content (Cvo$_2$)	Measurement of oxygen content in the venous blood	15.5 mL/100mL	Cvo$_2$ = (Svo$_2$ × Hgb × 1.34) + (Pvo$_2$ × 0.003)	A decreased value may indicate decreased Svo$_2$, Pvo$_2$, and hemoglobin

BSA, body surface area; g − m; SBP, systolic blood pressure.

From Bustin D, 1986; Ford RD, 1987; Dossey BM, Guzzette CE, Kenner CV, 1992, Flynn JB, Bruce NP, 1993; Stillwell SB, 1992.

and lasts for 18 to 36 days. Elevated serum glutamic-oxalacetic transaminase (SGOT) is present within 8 to 12 hours, peaks in 18 to 36 hours, and lasts for 3 to 4 days. Elevated isoenzyme creatine kinase-myocardial muscle (CK-MB) appears 4 to 8 hours, peaks within 16 to 24 hours, and lasts for less than 2 to 3 days.

- Urinalysis: Elevated creatinine clearance.

Invasive Cardiac Diagnostic Procedures. (See Table 1–2)

- Cardiac catheterization and coronary angiography: The procedure is used to visualize the coronary arteries, evaluate valvular function, and evaluate ventricular function. Coronary artery occlusion is graded according to the following system: (1) Normal shows no decrease in lumen diameter; (2) A 25% occlusion is a decrease in lumen diameter of 25%; (3) A 50% occlusion is a decrease in lumen diameter of 26% to 50%; (4) A 75% occlusion is a decrease in lumen diameter of 51% to 75%; (5) A 90% occlusion is a decrease in lumen diameter of 76% to 90%; (6) A 99% occlusion is a hairwidth lumen with greater than 90% narrowing; and (7) A 100% occlusion is a total occlusion. Left ventriculography is used to assess regional endocardial wall motion and systolic thickening and global left ventricular function by means of ejection fraction. Wall motion analysis involves the dividing of an outline of the left ventricular cavity into five segments. Inward systolic endocardial motion of each segment toward the center of the ventriculographic image normally occurs in a smooth, concentric manner. Regional wall motion abnormalities occur when there is a reduction in systolic wall thickening in conjunction with various degrees of hypokinesis, akinesis, or dyskinesis. The analysis of left ventricular function allows correlation of prior ischemic myocardial damage with angiographic assessment of the vessels supplying these segments. The left ventricular ejection fraction is an objective measure of left ventricular function. An ejection fraction less than 55% is suggestive of myocardial incompetency and an ejection fraction of less than 35% can indicate poor surgical prognosis.

Noninvasive Cardiac Diagnostic Procedures. (See Table 1–3)

- Chest roentgenogram: May reveal cardiomegaly and signs of left ventricular failure signifying AMI with 25% left ventricular muscle loss. Chest roentgenogram is useful in differentiating AMI from other conditions, such as pericarditis, pulmonary embolus, dissecting thoracic aortic aneurysm, pleurisy, pneumonia, Pancoast's tumor, or cervical arthritis.
- Echocardiography: M-mode echocardiography is used to assess the function of the posterior left ventricular wall and the interventricular septum. In addition, small segments of the anterior wall can also be involved. Two-dimensional echocardiography can be used to visualize a larger portion of the left ventricle and to diagnose abnormal regional wall motion. It is also used to diagnose mechanical complications of AMI such as left ventricular aneurysm, ventricular septal defect, myocardial rupture, papillary muscle or chordae tendineae rupture, pericardial effusion, or left ventricular thrombus.
- Magnetic Resonance Imaging (MRI): The technique can detect, localize, and determine the size of an infarct. It can also quantify chamber size and identify damaged myocardium, evaluate segmental wall motion, and detect abnormalities such as edema, fibrosis, or wall thinning.
- Multigated nuclear ventriculogram (MUGA) scanning: IV isotope technetium 99m pertechnetate is used to evaluate left ventricular function and ejection fraction. The procedure is also used to detect intracardiac shunting or to detect aneurysms of the left ventricle and other myocardial wall motion

abnormalities, such as areas of akinesia or dyskinesia.

- Positron emission tomography (PET): The technique is used to assess regional perfusion and myocardial metabolism noninvasively through direct measurement of fuel uptake and use. The scan can localize and facilitate the understanding of ischemia in areas of myocardium resulting from an imbalance of oxygen and demand.

- Radionuclide angiography: IV technetium Tc 99m pyrophosphate tracer combines with calcium in the necrotic myocardium to form a "hot spot," or increased level of radioactivity on the scan, signifying an infarcted area. The tracer is concentrated in and around the area of infarction, showing a distinct area of isotope activity on the cardiac image. Thallium 201 is used for perfusion imaging. The radioactive substance is distributed to the myocardium in proportion to blood flow. Normally the perfused myocardium shows an accumulation of isotope on a scintigram. Infarcted areas show "cold spots" or decreased uptake in exercise, signifying areas of decreased myocardial perfusion resulting from blocked coronary arteries. Infarcted myocardium will show no uptake in either rest or exercise.

ECG

- General changes: Acute myocardial infarction can be either transmural or subendocardial. The evolving AMI will progress through ischemia and injury to necrosis. The pathological changes in ECG are reflected as inverted T wave, elevated ST segment, and Q waves in the ECG leads over the infarct. The leads in the wall opposite the infarct may show reciprocal changes: depressed ST segment, tall R waves, and tall T waves. A *myocardial ischemia* shows ST segment depression and T wave inversion in all leads. A *myocardial injury* in subendocardial injury reveals ST segment depression ≥ 1 mm which usually returns to normal when the chest pain ceases. Subepi-

cardial injury shows ST segmental T wave elevation. A *myocardial infarction* reveals Q waves ≥ 0.04 seconds (1 mm) wide in leads facing the infarction, ST segment elevation in leads over or facing the infarcted area, and reciprocal ST depression in leads 180 degrees from the area of infarction. Non-Q wave infarction is revealed by ST depression and inverted T waves in leads facing the epicardial surface overlying the infarction, ST elevation and upright T waves in opposite leads.

- Specific changes: An *anterior infarction* is revealed by Q wave ≥ 0.04 seconds duration in leads V_1 and V_2, Q waves in V_3 and V_4, loss of R waves in V_2 through V_6, ST segment elevation in leads V_1 to V_4 and T wave inversion in leads V_1 to V_4. Reciprocal changes are seen in leads II, III and aVF. An *anterolateral infarction* shows Q wave and inverted T wave in leads I, aVL and V_4 to V_6. An *anteroseptal infarction* reveals Q wave, ST segment elevation, and T wave inversion in one or more of leads V_1 to V_4. An *inferior infarction* reveals Q wave ≥ 0.04, ST segment elevation, and T wave inversion in leads II, III and aVF. Pericordial ST segment depression can indicate a larger infarction with possible posterolateral involvement. Reciprocal changes are found in leads V_1 to V_3 and precordial leads of the anterior chest. A *lateral infarction* shows Q wave, ST segment elevation, and T wave inversion in leads I, aVL and V_5 to V_6. Reciprocal changes are seen in leads V_1 and V_3. A *posterior infarction* shows ST segment depression in leads V_1 to V_3, tall R waves in V_1 and V_2, and tall T waves in leads V_1 to V_3. Inferred diagnosis is made from reciprocal changes in anterior chest leads V_1 to V_3.

MEDICAL AND SURGICAL MANAGEMENT

PHARMACOLOGY

- Morphine sulfate: Used to relieve pain, anxiety, restlessness, reduce myocardial oxygen demand or consumption, dilate the arteries and veins, reduce the work of breathing, and slow the heart rate (see Table 1–7).

- Nitrates: Vasodilators, such as nitroglycerin and nitroprusside, are used to decrease arteriolar resistance by reducing the impedance to ejection (afterload) and decrease filling pressure (preload) by redistributing intravascular volume from the central to the peripheral vasculature (see Table 1–4).
- Calcium channel blockers: Used to inhibit the entry of calcium into cardiac and vascular smooth muscle cells through voltage sensitive channel. Calcium channel blockers include nifedipine, verapamil, and diltiazem (see Table 1–6).
- Positive inotropes: Used to increase contractility, decrease afterload, and decrease preload (dopamine or dobutamine) (see Table 1–10).
- Beta-adrenergic blocking agents: Used to decrease myocardial oxygen demand, decrease heart rate, decrease blood pressure, decrease stroke volume, and treat dysrhythmias (propranolol, metoprolal, atenolol, timolol, nadolol, or pindolol) (see Table 1–5).
- Thrombolytic therapy: Used to improve collateral blood flow to decrease hypoperfusion, increase myocardial oxygen supply, decrease myocardial oxygen demand, and reestablish blood flow by recannulizing the occluded coronary artery, thereby limiting the infarct size. Thrombolytic agents used are streptokinase, tissue plasminogen, or anisoylated plasminogen streptokinase activator complex (APSAC) (see Table 1–8 and Thrombolytic therapy, p. 265).
- Anticoagulant therapy: Used to prevent venous thrombolism, reduce arterial embolization from mural thrombi in the left ventricle, reduce the potential for extension of AMI, and reduce death from AMI. Anticoagulants act by inhibiting the clotting of blood by interfering with the conversion of prothrombin to thrombin and of fibrinogen to fibrin (heparin) (see Table 1–8).
- Antidysrhythmia agents: To prevent primary ventricular dysrhythmias (see Table 1–11 and Dysrhythmias, p. 184).

OXYGEN THERAPY
- Oxygen therapy 2 to 4 L/min of 100% oxygen by mask or nasal cannula for 2 to 4 days to reduce hypoxemia. Hypoxemia is varied and is influenced by pulmonary congestion resulting from left ventricular failure or other existing health problems, such as chronic obstructive pulmonary disease (COPD), pneumonia, or atelectasis.

PHYSICAL ACTIVITY
- Bed rest for the first 24 to 36 hours in uncomplicated AMI patient to decrease myocardial work load and oxygen demand.
- Progress of physical activity in uncomplicated AMI is (day #1) bed rest with complete bed bath and bedside commode; (day #2) sit in chair for 30 minutes twice a day and be assisted with meals; (day #3) sit in chair for 1 hour twice a day and be assisted with bed bath; (days 4 and 5) walk in room for 5 minutes and be assisted with bath; and (day #6) activity according to patient's tolerance, including showering while sitting in a chair.

DIET
- A full liquid diet given in small multiple feedings for first 24 hours after AMI, followed by a 1200-to-1500-calorie, 2-g-sodium, low-saturated-fat, soft diet, which is divided into small meals.

PERCUTANEOUS TRANSLUMINAL CORONARY ANGIOPLASTY (PTCA)
- Angioplasty decreases or eliminates resistance at the site of coronary artery stenosis and increases blood flow to ischemic myocardial tissue. The increased coronary perfusion, rather than decreased myocardial oxygen consumption (MVo_2), is the beneficial factor in angioplasty. PTCA increases the luminal diameter of the decreased vessel (see PTCA, p. 226.)

CORONARY LASER ANGIOPLASTY
- May be used as an adjunct to PTCA and coronary bypass surgery in the revascular-

TABLE 1-10

TABLE 1–10. POSITIVE INOTROPES AND SYMPATHOMIMETICS

Medications	Route/Dose	Uses and Effects
Positive Inotropes		
Cardiac glycosides Digoxin (Lanoxin)	IV: Initial dose 0.5 mg given over 10–20 min; 0.25 mg or 0.125 mg administered after 3 h; total dose of 1.00–1.25 mg PO: 1.00–1.25 mg in divided doses over initial 24 h; 0.5 mg is added during the second 24 h; maintenance is 0.125–0.500 mg/d	Management of CHF, atrial fibrillation, atrial flutter, or paroxysmal atrial tachycardia Increases contractility of myocardium Decreases CVP Decreases PCWP Increases cardiac output Improves renal blood flow Increases oxygen delivery to myocardium Decreases myocardial oxygen demand Increases force of myocardial contraction Depresses SA node and prolongs conduction to AV node by vagal stimulation
Sympathomimetric amines		
Dobutamine (Dobutrex)	IV: 5–15 µg/kg/min up to 40 µg/kg/min 2–3 µg/kg/min with 2–3 µg/kg/min increments every 10–30 min High is ≥20 µg/kg/min	Management of heart failure Facilitation of AV conduction in atrial fibrillation Increases contractility without increasing BP or HR Increases cardiac output Less increase in myocardial oxygen consumption Decreases preload or PCWP Dilates vascular and bronchial smooth muscle Increases ejection fraction
Dopamine (Intropin)	IV: 1–5 µg/kg/min initially. Increase by 1 to 4 µg/kg/min at 10–30 min increments up to 50 µg/kg/min Low dose: 3–5 µg/kg/min Moderate dose: 5–10 µg/kg/min High dose: 1–20 µg/kg/min	Management of shock resulting from cardiogenic shock, trauma, sepsis or CHF Vasodilation and increases blood flow through renal and mesenteric blood vessels Increases cardiac output Increases HR Increases strength of myocardial contraction Increases cardiac output
Norepinephrine (Levophed)	IV: 0.01–0.02 µg/min; titrate to maintenance dose of 2–4 µg/min	Causes peripheral vasoconstriction and increased BP Restores BP in hypotensive states associated with shock Increases CO

TABLE 1-10

Preparation/Administration	Side Effects	Nursing Implications
	Fatigue, weakness, headache, fibrillation, blurred vision, bradycardia, constrictive pericarditis, nausea, vomiting, anorexia, diarrhea, paresthesia, confusion, drowsiness, hypotension, diaphoresis, malaise	Obtain baseline HR, rhythm, BP, and electrolyte level before giving first dose Monitor effectiveness by taking an apical-radical pulse for 1 min before each dose Monitor serum digoxin levels, not to exceed 0.5–2.0 mg/mL
Preparation: Dilute 250-mg vial with 250 mL for concentration of 1000 μg/ml Vial reconstituted with 10–20 mL sterile water or D_5W Administration: Incompatible with alkaline solution; use large veins for administration and infusion pump to regulate flow rate	Headache, shortness of breath, stenosis, atrial tachycardia, hypertension, preexisting PVCs, nausea, vomiting, palpitations, nervousness, mild leg cramps	Monitor BP and HR every 2–5 min during initial administration and titration of the drug Monitor CP, PCWP, and UO to determine drug's effectiveness
Preparation: Dilute 200 mg (5 mL) in 250 mL for concentration of 800 μg/mL or 400 mg (10 mL) in 250 mL for concentration of 1600 μg/mL Administration: Crystallizes when administered with alkaline solutions; use large vein	Headaches, mydriasis, dyspnea, arrhythmias, hypotension, angina, vomiting, widening QRS, piloerection, tachycardia, aberrant conduction, bradycardia	Observe vein for blanching or pallor indicating extravasation and report. Treat with phentolamine (5–10 mg in 10–15 mL NS) by local infiltration Do not use proximal port of PA catheter to administer drug if cardiac output readings are being obtained Monitor BP, HR, pulse pressure, and UO to determine effectiveness
Preparation: Dilute 4 mg (4 mL) ampule of norepinephrine bitartrate in 250 mL for concentration of 16 μg/mL Administration: Oxidizes on exposure to light or air Slowly taper infusion when stopping the drug	Headache, palpitation, dizziness, hypertension, reflex bradycardia, fatal dysrhythmias, fatigue, nausea, respiratory difficulty, restlessness, anxiety, tremor, diarrhea, vomiting	Monitor BP every 3 to 5 min and evaluate CO Observe skin for symptoms of excessive vasoconstriction

TABLE 1-10

TABLE 1–10. CONTINUED

Medications	Route/Dose	Uses and Effects
Epinephrine (Adrenalin)	IV: 0.5–1.0 mg q 5 min as needed or followed by infusion at 0.001 mg/min (1 μg/min); may be increased to a maximum of 0.004 mg/min (4 μg/min) Intracardiac: 0.1–1.0 mg, repeat q 5 min as needed IM: 0.5 mg may be followed by IV administration	Treatment of anaphylaxis or cardiac arrest Strengthens myocardial contraction Increases systolic BP but may decrease diastolic BP Increases HR and CO
Phosphodiesterase inhibitor (PDI), Inodilator		
Amrinone lactate (Incocar lactate)	IV: 0.75 mg/kg over 2–3 min loading dose; repeated, if necessary, in 30 min; not to exceed 10 mg/kg/24 h Continuous maintenance infusion: 5–10 μg/kg/min PO: 1 to 3 mg/kg at 8 h intervals	Management of CHF Increases myocardial contractility Decreases preload Decreases afterload Increases CO Increases stroke volume
Other PDI Medications Milrinone lactate (Primacor) Enoximone (Investigational)		

AV, atrioventricular; BP, blood pressure; CHF, congestive heart failure; CO, cardiac output; CP; CVP, central venous pressure; D_5W, 5% dextrose in water; HR, heart rate; IM, intramuscular; IV, intravenous; MAP, mean arterial pressure; NS, normal saline; PA, pulmonary artery; PCWP, pulmonary capillary wedge pressure; PO, by mouth; PVC, premature ventricular contraction; PVR, pulmonary vascular resistance; SA, sinoatrial; SVR, systemic vascular resistance; UO, urinary output.

From Deglin JH, Vallerand AH, Russin MM, 1995; Govoni LE, Hayes JE, Shannon MT, et al, 1992; Loeb S, 1993; Scherer JC, 1992; Vallerand AH, Deglin JH, 1991; Clements JV, 1992.

ization of occluded vessels. The laser can be transmitted through an optical fiber to direct it precisely and to use it for tissue photocoagulation (see Coronary laser angioplasty, p. 228.)

INTRA-AORTIC BALLOON PUMP (IABP)

• Counterpulsation's outcome is achieved by reducing myocardial oxygen consumption (demand) and enhancing coronary artery tissue perfusion. Myocardial oxygen demand is reduced when left ventricular (LV) afterload is reduced. When LV afterload increases, there is a corresponding increase in intramyocardial wall tension, causing in-creased LV work and increased subendocardial ischemia. Subendocardial tissue is sensitive to changes in myocardial oxygen supply and demand. Counterpulsation, which enhances coronary artery blood flow during diastolic augmentation, can minimize the extent of myocardial necrosis. The overall effect is to augment oxygen supply and decrease oxygen demand by minimizing afterload (see IABP, p. 254.)

CARDIAC ASSIST DEVICE

• The cardiac assist device facilitates the limitation of infarct size by salvaging myocardial tissue that is severely ischemic but

TABLE 1-10

Preparation/Administration	Side Effects	Nursing Implications
Preparation: 1 mg ampule 1:1000 solution in 250 mL for concentration of 4 μg/mL	Nervousness, restlessness, tremor, headache, nausea, vomiting, urinary retention	Monitor BP and HR every 2–5 min during the initial infusion
Administration: Solution should be clear, not brown, which indicates oxidation		Do not use proximal port of a PA catheter for infusion if CO readings are being obtained
		Monitor CO to evaluate drug's effectiveness
Administration: Incompatible with solutions containing furosemide and will form a precipitate	Arrhythmias, hypotension, dyspnea, vomiting, diarrhea, hepatotoxicity, hypokalemia, fever function, hypersensitivity to amrione or bisultites, thrombocytopenia, abdominal cramps, ascites, chest pain	Monitor BP, PCWP, MAP, SVR, PVR, HR, and CO during infusion as the level of the drug may rise during continuous infusion and its effect can increase
		Observe patient for 4 h after adjusting the dose

viable. The cardiac assist device allows the severely ischemic myocardium to reduce activity to basal rates, resulting in acute realignment of myocardial oxygen consumption with available supply (see Cardiac assist device, p. 248.)

SURGICAL INTERVENTION

- Coronary artery bypass graft surgery (CABG): Surgical revascularization or aortocoronary bypass grafting is used to restore adequate blood flow or blood supply and to provide nutritional support to the myocardial tissue. The harvested vessel or conduit is anastomosed between the aortic root and a point distal to the obstructing coronary lesion or stenosis (see CABG, p. 194.)

NURSING MANAGEMENT: NURSING DIAGNOSES AND COLLABORATIVE PROBLEMS

Nursing Diagnoses

Common nursing goals for patients with AMI are to restore myocardial tissue perfusion, reduce chest pain, prevent complication such as activity intolerance, provide adequate nutritional intake, encourage appropriate individual coping, and provide information about the illness or treatment.

TABLE 1-11

TABLE 1–11. ANTIARRHYTHMIA AGENTS

Medication	Route/Dose	Uses and Effects
Class IA **Sodium Channel** **Blockers:** **Delayed** **Repolarization** **Increasing Action** **Potential Duration**		
Quinidine sulfate (Apo-Quinidine)	IV: 5–8 mg/kg at 0.3 mg/kg/min PO: 200 mg q 2–3 h for 5–8 doses; may increase dose daily as needed, then 200–300 mg q 6–8 h, not to exceed 4 g/d	Management of atrial and ventricular arrhythmias including premature atrial contraction, premature ventricular contractions, and ventricular tachycardia Decreases systemic vascular resistance Decreases BP Decreases myocardial excitability Slows conduction Decreases atrial and ventricular arrhythmias
Procainamide hydrochloride (Pronestyl hydrochloride)	IV: Continuous infusion 2–6 mg/min; slowly 100 mg q 5 min, slow push at 20–50 mg/min PO: 250–500 mg q 3–4 h; 250–1000 mg q 6 h	Management of ventricular and supraventricular arrhythmias Decreases atrial and ventricular arrhythmias Decreases myocardial excitability Slows conduction velocity Depresses myocardial contractility Decreases systemic vascular resistance
Disopyramide phosphate (Norpace)	PO: 100–200 mg q 6–8 h; 300 mg loading dose followed by 150 mg q 6 h	Decreases conduction velocity Increases action potential duration in myocardial tissue Prolongs P wave, QRS complex, or PR interval Reduces automaticity Suppresses ventricular, atrial, and supraventricular arrhythmias
Moricizine hydrochloride (Ethmozine)	PO: 600–900 mg tid	Management of ventricular dysrhythmias
Class IB **Accelerated** **Repolarization,** **Thereby Shortening** **Action Potential** **Duration**		
Lidocaine (Xylocaine)	IV: 50–100 mg bolus followed by 0.5 mg/kg in 10–15 min Continuous infusion 1–4 mg/min	Depresses myocardial cells Reduces action potential amplitude Abolishes automatic and reentrant arrhythmias Suppresses ventricular arrhythmias

TABLE 1-11

Preparation/Administration	Side Effects	Nursing Implications
Administration: Avoid IM administration; concomitant use with digoxin increases digoxin level	Vertigo, headache, dizziness, blurred vision, photophobia, diplopia, hypotension, tachycardia, diarrhea, nausea, cramping, anorexia, rashes, fever, tinnitus, confusion, syncope, gastric distress, dyspnea	Monitor patient for urinary retention Monitor ECG for prolonged QRS and QT intervals; PR interval remains normal
Administration: When converting from IV to PO, administer oral dose 3–4 h after last IV dose	Confusion, seizures, dizziness, hypotension, ventricular arrhythmias, asystole, heart block, nausea, vomiting, rashes, fever, chills, depression, tachycardia, bitter taste, diarrhea	Monitor BP and cardiac rhythm continuously Monitor ECG for QRS and QT intervals prolonged by 50% Report severe hypotension
	Blurred vision, dizziness, headache, fatigue, dyspnea, hypotension, dry mouth, constipation, nausea, abdominal pain, flatulence, urinary hesitancy, retention, dry mouth, muscle weakness, bradycardia, tachycardia, pruritus, paresthesia	Monitor for urinary retention Monitor ECG for minor prolongation of QRS and moderate increase QT interval
	Fatigue, dyspnea, dizziness, nausea, headache, palpitations, AV block, intraventricular conduction defect, possible dysrhythmias	Monitor ECG for slight increase in PR and QRS interval, QT increase as a result of widened QRS
Use infusion pump for continuous administration	Drowsiness, dizziness, lethargy, confusion, hypotension, nausea, vomiting, bradycardia, restlessness, irritability, blurred vision, muscular twitching	Monitor ECG, which usually reveals no changes in PR, QRS, and QT intervals

TABLE 1-11

TABLE 1–11. CONTINUED

Medication	Route/Dose	Uses and Effects
Mexiletine hydrochloride (Mexitil)	PO: 200–400 mg every 8 h; then maintenance of 200–400 mg q 8 h; not to exceed 1200 mg/d IV: Loading dose 150–250 mg over 5–10 min, followed by 0.5–1.5 mg/min	Decreases duration of the action potential and refractory period in the Purkinje fibers Suppresses ventricular dysrhythmias, PVC, and nonsustained VT
Tocainide hydrochloride (Tonocard)	PO: 400 mg q 6–8 h; maintenance dose 1.2–1.8 g/d in divided doses q 8 h up to 2–4 g/d	Used to manage ventricular dysrhythmias Decreases action potential duration Increases shortening of the effective refractory period Suppresses automaticity of conduction tissue Suppresses spontaneous depolarization of the ventricles during diastole
Class IC **Inhibition of His-Purkinje System, thus QRS Prolongation**		
Encainide hydrochloride (Enkaid)	PO: 25 mg q 8 h initially and may increase to 35 mg q 8 h after 3–6 days, not to exceed 75 mg/dose	Malignant ventricular arrhythmias Slow depolarization in atrial, ventricular, and Purkinje's fibers Prolonged refractory periods in accessory pathways Prolongs QRS complex
Flecainide monoacetate (Tambocor)	PO: 100 mg q 12 h initially, not to exceed a total daily dose of 400 mg	Suppresses ventricular arrhythmias Slows conduction in the His-Purkinje system
Propafenone hydrochloride (Rythmol)	PO: 300 mg q 12 h, then 300 mg q 8 h to a maximum of 900 mg daily	Ventricular and supraventricular dysrhythmias including AV nodal entry
Class III		
Amiodarone hydrochloride (Cordarone)	PO: 800–1600 mg/d in 1–2 doses for 1–3 wk; then 600–800 mg/d in 1–2 doses for 1 mo; maintenance dose 400 mg/d IV: 5–10 mg/kg/d	Control supraventricular arrhythmias Prolongs the action potential and refractory period in myocardial tissue Slows sinus rate Increases PR and QT intervals Decreases peripheral vascular resistance

TABLE 1-11

Preparation/Administration	Side Effects	Nursing Implications
Administration: Administered with meals to decrease GI irritation	Dizziness, light-headedness, blurred vision, arrhythmias, palpitations, headache, fatigue, confusion, edema, nausea, vomiting, rashes, tremor, dyspnea, convulsive seizures, abnormal taste sensation, pruritus	
Administration: Administer before meals, since food delays the drug's absorption	Light-headedness, vertigo, tremor, headache, restlessness, sedation, depression, blurred vision, hypotension, tachycardia, palpitations, arrhythmias, nausea, vomiting, anorexia, diarrhea, constipation, abdominal discomfort, urinary retention, rashes, flushing, numbness, complete heart block, chest pain, hearing loss, ataxia, agitation, confusion	Monitor ECG for increases in QRS and QT intervals; minor decrease in sinus node conduction
Administration: Administer with meals to decrease GI irritation Available for compassionate use only	Headache, dizziness, blurred vision, dyspnea, palpitations, arrhythmias, anorexia, vomiting, rash, hypokalemia, hyperglycemia	Monitor ECG for prolonged PR and QRS intervals May worsen PVC or cause new dysrhythmias
	Dizziness, nervousness, headache, fatigue, tremor, blurred vision, diplopia, dyspnea, arrhythmias, nausea, vomiting, dyspepsia, impotence, rashes, urinary retention, malaise, fever, tinnitus, nasal congestion, dry mouth	Monitor ECG for prolongation of PR and QRS intervals
	Dizziness, headache, altered taste, nausea, constipation, CHF	Monitor ECG for slight increase in PR and QRS intervals Increased QT resulting from widened QRS
Administration: Take with food to reduce GI reaction	Malaise, fatigue, dizziness, headache, bradycardia, photosensitivity, hypothyroidism, nausea, vomiting, constipation, anorexia, tremor, poor coordination, paresthesia, abnormal gait, ataxia, muscle weakness, numbness, hypotension, abdominal pain, sinoatrial block	Monitor ECG for sinus bradycardia, slight increase in PR interval, marked prolongation of QT and prominent U wave

TABLE 1-11

TABLE 1–11. CONTINUED

Medication	Route/Dose	Uses and Effects
Bretylium tosylate (Bretylate)	IV: 5–10 mg/kg over 1 min repeated every 15–30 min until 30 mg/kg has been given IV drip: 5–10 mg/kg over 10–30 min IM: 5–10 mg/kg; repeat q 1–2 h if arrhythmia persists; then q 6–8 h	Refractory ventricular fibrillation Suppresses ventricular tachycardia and fibrillation
Sotalol hydrochloride (Beta-Cardone)	PO: 160–480 mg bid IV: 0.2–1.5 mg/kg	Supraventricular dysrhythmias including atrial flutter and fibrillation Wolff-Parkinson-White dysrhythmias Ventricular dysrhythmias
Class IV Atropine	IV (bradycardia): 0.5–1.0 mg q 1–2 h prn to a maximum of 2 mg	Treatment of sinus bradycardia or asystole during CPR Sinus node dysfunction and in evaluation of coronary artery disease during atrial pacing

AV, atrioventricular; BP, blood pressure; CHF, congestive heart failure; CPR, cardiopulmonary resuscitation; D_5W, 5% dextrose in water; ECG, electrocardiogram; GI, gastrointestinal; IM, intramuscular; IV, intravenous; NS, normal saline; PO, by mouth; PVC, premature ventricular contraction(s); VT, ventricular tachycardia.

From Deglin JH, Vallerand AH, Russin MM, 1988; Govoni LE, Hayes JE, Shannon MT, et al, 1992; Loeb S, 1993; Scherer JC, 1985; Vallerand AH, Deglin JH, 1991; Stier F, 1992.

Altered myocardial tissue perfusion related to coronary artery occlusion, increased heart rate, or reduced aortic pressure secondary to coronary artery disease.

Expected Patient Outcomes. Patient maintains adequate myocardial tissue perfusion, as evidenced by coronary arterial perfusion pressure (CAPP) 60 to 80 mm Hg, CO 4 to 8 L/min, CI 2.7 to 4.3 L/min/m², heart rate (HR) ≤ 90 bpm, blood pressure (BP) ≥ 90/60 mm Hg, absence of dysrhythmias, and absence of chest pain.

- Collaborate with cardiologist on expected results of clinical indicators used to evaluate reperfusion after thrombolytic therapy. The indicators include resolution of chest pain, resolution of ST segment elevation, and appearance of reperfusion dysrhythmias.
- Review results of prothrombin time, partial thromboplastin time, platelet count, and cardiac enzymes in relation to thrombolytic therapy.
- Limit physical activity to bed rest to reduce myocardial work load and HR, to avoid decrease of the diastolic filling time and subsequent myocardial tissue perfusion.
- Use active or passive leg exercises to enhance venous return.
- Obtain, document, and report hemodynamic parameters that indicate decreased myocardial tissue perfusion: CAPP ≤60 mm Hg, CO ≤4 L/min, and CI ≤2.7 L/min/m². In AMI, the CAPP is especially important, since a value ≤40 mm Hg can result in collapse of the coronary arteries.
- Obtain, document, and report other clinical findings suggestive of decreased myocardial tissue perfusion: HR ≥100 bpm, which decreases diastolic filling time, dysrhythmias, or chest pain.
- Monitor, document, and report the presence of three clinical indicators of reperfusion:

TABLE 1-11

Preparation/Administration	Side Effects	Nursing Implications
Preparation: IV drip 500 mg diluted in 50 mL D$_5$W or NS and infused at 5–10 mg/kg over 10–30 min	Syncope, faintness, vertigo, dizziness, nasal stuffiness, postural hypotension, bradycardia, nausea, vomiting, rash, abdominal pain, lethargy, anxiety	Keep patient supine when administering IV bolus and observe for hypotension
		Monitor ECG for transient increase in sinus rate, AV conduction, ventricular automaticity
		Reduce drug gradually
	Bradycardia, hypotension, atrioventricular block, CHF	Monitor ECG for prolonged PR, QRS, and QT interval
		Monitor potassium levels in presence of hypokalemia
	Hypertension, ventricular tachycardia, palpitation, paradoxical bradycardia, AV dissociation, atrial or ventricular fibrillation, headache, weakness, ataxia, excitement, fatigue, weakness, disorientation	

resolution of chest pain, resolution of ST segment elevation, and appearance of reperfusion dysrhythmias.

- Initiate continuous ECG for indication that coronary artery occlusion has resolved: resolution of ST segment elevation ≤1 mm, diminished chest pain and dysrhythmias, such as ventricular tachycardia, sinus bradycardia, and accelerated idioventricular rhythm (see ST segment monitoring, p. 264).
- Administer prescribed IV fluids to maintain adequate circulating volume.
- Administer prescribed oxygen 2 to 4 L/min by means of nasal cannula or mask to maintain Pao$_2$ ≥80 mm Hg, Sao$_2$ ≥95%, or Svo$_2$ ≥60%.
- Administer prescribed thrombolytic therapy (streptokinase, tissue plasminogen activator [t-PA] or anisoylated plasminogen streptokinase activator complex [APSAC, Eminase]) to lyse clots within coronary artery, which increases blood flow to ischemic myocardial tissue, and to improve and maintain CAPP ≥60 mm Hg, CO ≥4 L/min, and CI ≥2.7 L/min/m^2 (see Table 1–5 and Thrombolytic therapy, p. 265).

- Obtain vital signs every 15 minutes during thrombolytic therapy or for 2 hours after initiation of treatment and then every 4 hours for 24 hours.
- Obtain, document, and report clinical findings indicating allergic reactions: hives, chilling, fever, or flushing.
- For patients receiving thrombolytic therapy, observe for oral, nasal, gastrointestinal, or genitourinary bleeding as well as oozing from puncture sites.
- Administer prescribed heparin immediately after streptokinase and 1 hour after t-PA infusion to prevent occlusion of the coronary artery and recurring thrombus formation.
- Administer prescribed vasodilators (nitroprusside, nitroglycerin, (NTG) or calcium channel blockers such as verapamil, nifedi-

TABLE 1-12

TABLE 1–12. ANGIOTENSIN CONVERTING ENZYMES (ACE) INHIBITORS

Medication	Route/Dose	Uses and Effects
Captopril (Capoten)	PO: Initial 6.25–12.5 mg tid; for CHF, with a maintenance dose of 50–100 mg tid 25 mg bid-tid to a maximum of 450 mg/d for hypertension	Management of hypertension and CHF Vasodilation of peripheral vessels Prevents production of angiotensin II or vasoconstriction Decreases BP Decreases preload Decreases afterload Increases glomerular filtration rate Increases renal blood flow Increases cardiac output
Enalapril maleate (Vasotec)	IV: 0.625 over 5 min with maintenance dose of 0.625 q 6 h PO: Initial 5 mg/d; range of 5–20 mg in 1–2 doses. Maintenance dose of 10–40 mg/d	Indicated for management of hypertension Prevents production of angiotensin II Decreases systemic vascular resistance Decreases BP Decreases preload Decreases afterload
Ramipril (Altace)	PO: 2.5 mg/d with a maintenance dose of 2.5–20.0 mg daily; may require a diuretic	Treatment of hypertension
Lisinopril (Prinivil, Zestril)	PO: 10 mg/d; maintenance dose 20–40 mg/d Reduce dose in patients with renal dysfunction	Treatment of hypertension and CHF

From Kuhn M, 1992.

BP, blood pressure; CBC, complete blood count; CHF, congestive heart failure; HR, heart rate; IV, intravenous; PO, by mouth.

pine, or diltiazem) to maintain CAPP ≥60 mm Hg, CO ≥4 L/min, and CI ≥2.7 L/min/m^2 (see Table 1–4 and Table 1–6).
- In patients receiving diltiazem or verapamil, initiate monitoring of PR interval to determine the presence of atrioventricular (AV) nodal conduction disturbance and the HR for effects on the sinus node.
- Administer prescribed beta-blocker (propranolol) to maintain BP within patient's normal range and HR ≤90 bpm (see Table 1–5).
- Administer prescribed narcotic (morphine) to maintain HR ≤100 bpm and reduce chest pain (see Table 1–12)
- Should pharmacological therapy be ineffective in increasing myocardial tissue perfusion, assist with PTCA insertion or laser angioplasty (see PTCA, p. 226, and Laser angioplasty, p. 228.)
- Should PTCA and thrombolytic therapy be ineffective, prepare patient for coronary atherectomy, intracoronary stent, or CABG (see Transluminal coronary atherectomy, p.

TABLE 1-12

Preparation/Administration	Side Effects	Nursing Implications
Administration: Do not use with antacids Administer 1 h before meals, since food may reduce absorption	Dizziness, cough, hypotension, tachycardia, angina, anorexia, loss of taste perception, proteinuria, rashes, fever, gastric irritation, abdominal pain, nausea, vomiting, diarrhea, fatigue, dry mouth, dyspnea	Monitor drug's effectiveness by evaluating BP and HR before administration Evaluate potassium level for hyperkalemia or hypokalemia Change patient's position slowly Evaluate CBC every 2 wk for 3 mo
	Headache, dizziness, fatigue, cough, hypotension, tachycardia, angina, anorexia, diarrhea, nausea, impotence, rashes, hyperkalemia	Monitor effectiveness of drug by evaluating BP; hypotension can occur after the initial dose Observe BP for 2 h, then 1 h after BP is stable Monitor potassium level for hyperkalemia or hypokalemia Can be given with or without food
	Dizziness, cough, hypotension, tachycardia, angina, anorexia, loss of taste perception, proteinuria, rashes, fever, gastric irritation, abdominal pain, nausea, vomiting, diarrhea, fatigue, dry mouth, dyspnea	Monitor drug's effectiveness by evaluating BP and HR before administration Evaluate potassium level for hyperkalemia or hypokalemia Change patient's position slowly
Can be given with or without food	Dizziness, cough, hypotension, tachycardia, angina, anorexia, loss of taste perception, proteinuria, rashes, fever, gastric irritation, abdominal pain, nausea, vomiting, diarrhea, fatigue, dry mouth, dyspnea	Monitor drug's effectiveness by evaluating BP and HR before administration Evaluate potassium level for hyperkalemia or hypokalemia Change patient's position slowly

234, Intracoronary stent, p. 237, or CABG, p. 194.)

- Teach patient the importance of reporting chest pain.
- Teach patient the common side effects of calcium channel blockers: hypotension, dizziness, headache, ankle edema, flushing, nausea, palpitations, and fatigue.
- Instruct patient to alleviate hypotension and its resulting dizziness or faintness by sitting or lying down when the medication is taken and for 15 to 20 minutes afterword.

Pain related to impaired myocardial oxygen supply secondary to myocardial ischemia or coronary artery occlusion.

Expected Patient Outcomes. Patient experiences relief of chest pain, as evidenced by absence of facial grimacing, verbalization of pain relief, and HR within normal range for patient.

- Obtain, document, and report patient's description of chest pain including location, radiation, duration, intensity, quality, and precipitating factors. This helps to quantify pain by comparing the episode with previous experiences of pain.

- Obtain baseline LDH and CK isoenzymes when the patient first experiences chest pain in order to determine whether extension of the myocardial infarction is occurring.

- Obtain and review a 12-lead ECG daily for 3 days to note myocardial changes. Should chest pain occur, obtain a 12-lead ECG during the episode to determine whether the pain is caused by ischemia or extension of the existing infarction.

- Provide prescribed diet of small, easily digested portions of food to decrease myocardial oxygen demand.

- Limit the patient's physical activity to bed rest or level of activity before the episode of chest pain. This will reduce myocardial oxygen demand.

- Obtain and report hemodynamic changes during the pain episode: CO $\leq$4 L/min, BP $\leq$90/60 mm Hg, and HR $\geq$120 bpm.

- During the pain episode, assess the HR and rhythm, respiration rate (RR) and rhythm, BP, and the skin for the presence of pallor, cyanosis, and diaphoresis. Pain may increase RR, while stress-induced catecholamines can increase HR and BP.

- Administer prescribed morphine, 2 to 4 mg IV initially in 2 μg increments to relieve decreased myocardial work load, chest pain, and maintain BP within patient's normal range, PAP systolic $\leq$30 mm Hg or diastolic $\leq$15 mm Hg, PCWP 6 to 12 mm Hg, pulmonary vascular resistance (PVR) 155 to 255 dynes/s/cm^{-5}, and SVR 900 to 1200 dynes/s/cm^{-5} (see Table 1–7).

- Observe patient for the presence of complaints of chest pain lasting more than 20 to 30 minutes unrelieved by NTG, shortness of breath, pallor or cyanosis, diaphoresis, weakness, anxiety, nausea, vomiting, palpitations, or restlessness.

- Observe, document, and report clinical findings suggesting extension of AMI: chest pain, shortness of breath, perspiration, weakness not relieved by medication or rest, and pain not always associated with physical exercise.

- Monitor and report clinical findings suggesting acute chest pain or angina. Chest pain or pressure resulting from ischemia usually is relieved by rest or vasodilators and pain is associated with physical or emotional stress.

- Administer prescribed IV NTG infusion of 10 μg/min at 10 minute intervals to achieve a 10% reduction in systolic blood pressure (SBP) or attainment of a SBP of 95 mm Hg, up to a maximum dosage determined by agency protocol to control pain by causing coronary vasodilation. Coronary artery vasodilation increases coronary blood flow and myocardial perfusion. Other effects are rate pressure product (RPP) $\leq$12,000, arterial oxygen delivery (Do$_2$) $\geq$900 mL/min, arterial oxygen delivery index (Do$_2$I) $\geq$600 mL/min/m^2, and relief of chest pain. The peripheral vasodilation effects decrease preload and subsequently decrease myocardial work and oxygen demand (see Table 1–4).

- During each titration of NTG, monitor patient's BP and resolution of chest pain. Should SBP $\leq$90 mm Hg occur, decrease the flow rate to a predetermined rate. If patient's SBP $\leq$80 mm Hg or sweating, tachydysrhythmias, bradydysrhythmias occur, stop the infusion and consult with the physician for further directions.

- Administer other prescribed coronary vasodilators as needed (isosorbide dinitrate, verapamil, nifedipine, or diltiazem) to reduce pain by dilating coronary arteries, increase coronary perfusion, and decrease oxygen demand. This is accomplished by inhibition of the influx of calcium through the muscle cells. Other goals of these drugs are to maintain CAPP at 60 to 80 mm Hg, BP $\geq$90 mm Hg, urinary output (UO) $\geq$0.5 mL/kg/h, and relieve chest pain (see Table 1–4).

- Administer prescribed thrombolytic medications to enhance myocardial perfusion and subsequent myocardial tissue oxygen supply (see Table 1–8 and Thrombolytic therapy, p. 265).

- Administer prescribed beta blockers (propranolol) to reduce HR, lower SBP, and reduce myocardial oxygen demand. Beta blockers may be contraindicated in AMI patients with severely compromised myocardial contractility because of their negative inotropic effects, which compromise contractility (see Table 1–4).
- Administer prescribed oxygen at 2 to 4 L/min by means of nasal cannula or mask to enhance oxygen delivery to ischemic tissue and reduce myocardial oxygen demand.
- Administer prescribed IV fluids to maintain adequate circulating volume.
- Administer prescribed stool softeners.
- Assist patient to assume a position of comfort.
- Assist patient with activities of daily living (ADL).
- Teach patient to describe pain using a scale of 1 to 10, with 10 being severe pain.
- Instruct the patient to report increased or decreased chest pain immediately.
- Instruct the patient in the use of alternative pain relief measures: relaxation, repositioning, guided imagery, and distraction.
- Teach patient to exhale with physical movement to avoid increasing intrathoracic pressure and compromising myocardial tissue perfusion.

Activity intolerance related to chest pain, hypotension, or tachycardia secondary to coronary artery occlusion.

Expected Patient Outcome. Patient gradually increases tolerance of physical activity without experiencing chest pain or intolerance.

- Consult with cardiologist about clinical parameters used to evaluate the patient's tolerance of gradual increases in physical activity.
- Confer with the cardiac rehabilitation specialist to individualize the patient's exercise and daily activity program.
- Consult with cardiologist about applying antiembolic hose to reduce venous stasis,

improve venous return, and reduce risk of thromboembolism.

- Provide appropriate progressive physical activity for patients with uncomplicated AMI: (day #1) Use a bedside commode, feed self, and be assisted with bathing; (day #2) includes sitting in a chair and self-bathing from a basin; (day #3) includes sitting in a chair for various lengths of time; (day #4) patient is walking in the hall or taking a bath or shower.
- Monitor patient's cardiac tolerance of gradual but progressive increases in physical activity: RR ≤24 BPM; normal sinus rhythm on ECG; HR ≤120 bpm, which is within 20 bpm of resting HR; BP within 20 mm Hg of patient's normal range; absence of chest pain; and serum enzymes peaked and returning toward normal.
- Document and report clinical indicators that suggest activity intolerance: angina, fatigue, tachypnea, shortness of breath, dizziness, unsteady gait, HR ≥120 bpm, ST depression of ≥1.5 mm, decreased systolic blood pressure, and dysrhythmias such as PVCs ≥10/min.
- Provide passive range of motion (ROM) exercises to maintain muscle tone and enhance circulation.
- Teach patient how to conserve energy while performing ADL to avoid increasing myocardial oxygen demand.
- Teach patient to pace physical activities and to avoid isometric work.
- Instruct patient as to the importance of scheduling rest periods before and after periods of activities.
- Instruct patient to stop activity if fatigue or chest pain develop, signifying decreased myocardial oxygen supply or increase myocardial oxygen demand.
- Teach patient to consult with physician before changing physical activity schedule after discharge.

Nutrition, altered: less than body requirements related to fatigue, chest pain, increased myocardial oxygen demand, or loss of appetite.

Expected Patient Outcomes. Patient maintains adequate nutrition as evidenced by stable weight, BUN 8 to 20 mg/dL, hematocrit M: 42% to 54% or F: 38% to 46%, hemoglobin M: 14.0 to 16.5 g/100 mL or W: 12 to 15 g/100 mL, lymphocytes 20% to 40%, serum albumin 3.3 to 4.5 g/dL, total serum protein 6.6 to 7.9 g/dL, electrolytes within normal range, and caloric intake ranging from 35 to 45 calories/kg of normal body weight.

- Consult with dietitian to individualize the patient's specific low-cholesterol, low-fat diet.
- Consult with the patient about his or her food preferences.
- Review the patient's BUN, total serum protein, and electrolytes.
- Encourage patient to eat the prescribed low-sodium, low-cholesterol, low-saturated-fat and low-calorie diet that reflects the patient's weight and needs.
- Monitor the patient's daily weight to evaluate whether weight maintenance is being achieved within a prescribed range.
- Administer prescribed IV fluids and oral fluids to maintain hydration.
- Instruct the patient regarding the relationship between diet and cardiac disease.
- Teach the patient to avoid using or use in modification caffeine products such as coffee, certain teas, and cola drinks.
- Explain the importance of dietary limitations if no specific diet is recommended: limit intake of eggs, cream, butter, and foods high in animal fat.

Denial, ineffective related to patient's unwillingness to accept consequences of his or her behaviors as evidenced by failure to acknowledge symptoms, risk factors, and lifestyle changes associated with AMI.

Expected Patient Outcome. Patient acknowledges his/her denial, by recognizing and changing factors contributing to AMI.

- Assess patient for behaviors reflective of denial: (1) The patient does not follow the nursing or medical plan of care; (2) the patient does not talk about the episode of AMI; and (3) The patient makes statements that are unrealistic for someone who has survived an AMI. For example the patient plans to return to work upon discharge from the hospital or plans to continue a pre-MI high-saturated-fat diet.
- Discuss with the patient positive health behaviors: following prescribed diet, taking medications, increasing physical activity, and seeking early treatment for reoccurrence of chest pain.
- Encourage the patient to discuss fears regarding MI and heart disease.
- Encourage patient to use relaxation techniques such as guided imagery and relaxation breathing to enhance sense of control and sense of a positive coping response.
- Monitor physiological parameters such as BP and HR during conversations that involve stressful topics. The topics can increase BP and HR, which may reflect the patient's coping ability.
- Instruct the patient about the signs and symptoms of myocardial infarction so when these occur, the patient can recognize the problem and seek health care: crushing chest pain, facial grimacing, cool, clammy skin, increased heart rate, lightheadedness, nausea, or diaphoresis.

Knowledge deficit related to the causes, course of treatment, and life-style changes associated with AMI.

Expected Patient Outcomes. Patient and family will be able to discuss the causes of MI and life-style changes to be made after discharge.

- Consult with the dietitian to develop a low-cholesterol and low-saturated-fat diet tailored to the age, sex, physical condition, life-style, and likes and dislikes of the patient.
- Refer the patient to the dietitian when the diet has been developed.
- Arrange consultation between the dietitian, patient, and family regarding the prescribed hospital and discharge diet.

- Develop a teaching plan that includes standardized information about anatomy and physiology or the heart muscle, coronary arteries, atherosclerotic process contributing to AMI, and the normal myocardial healing process.
- Provide the patient with information about risk factors, medications, progressive ADL, diet, sexual activity, work, and stress reduction.
- Help the patient identify alternative approaches to reducing the risk factors.
- Teach the patient to avoid isometric activity, Valsalva's maneuver, and activities necessitating arms positioned above head. These activities increase cardiac work, increase myocardial oxygen demand, and decrease CO.
- Explain purpose of planned rest periods.
- Teach the patient stress reduction techniques: meditation and guided imagery.
- Instruct patient about prescribed medications including purposes, dosage, schedule, and common side effects.
- Explain the importance of controlling any coexisting disease that may aggravate recovery: hyperlipidemia, hypertension, or diabetes.

Collaborative Problems

Common collaborative goals in patients with AMI are to restore myocardial oxygen supply, reduce myocardial oxygen demand, increase CO, correct dysrhythmias, and improve oxygenation.

Potential Complication: Decreased Myocardial Oxygen Supply. Decreased myocardial oxygen supply related to reduced coronary artery perfusion secondary to hypotension, coronary ischemia, coronary vasospasm, or coronary artery disease.

Expected Patient Outcomes. Patient maintains adequate myocardial oxygen supply, as evidenced by arterial oxygen content (CaO_2) 18 to 20 mL/100 mL, arterial oxygen delivery (DO_2) 900 to 1200 mL/min, arterial oxygen delivery index (DO_2I) 500 to 600 mL/min/m², CAPP 60 to 80 mm Hg, CO 4 to 8 L/min, CI 2.7 to 4.L/min/m², SVR 900 to 1200 dynes/s/cm⁻⁵, systemic vascular resistance index (SVRI) 1970 to 2390 dynes/s/cm⁻⁵ · m², continuous mixed venous oxygen saturation ($S\bar{v}O_2$) 60% to 80%, SBP ≥90 mm Hg or within the patient's normal range, hemoglobin within normal range, HR ≤100 bpm, capillary refill ≤3 seconds, arterial oxygen saturation (SaO_2) ≥95%, PaO_2 ≥80 mm Hg, absence of dysrhythmias, and absence of chest pain.

- Consult with cardiologist to validate the expected patient outcomes used to determine whether or myocardial oxygen supply is sufficient.
- Review with the cardiologist the results of heart catheterization, ECG, and serum enzymes that reflect changes in myocardial oxygen supply.
- Provide small portions of easily digested low-sodium and low-saturated fat foods as prescribed.
- Limit patients with postprandial angina to smaller meals and limit activities after meals.
- Limit the patient's physical activity before manifestations of decreased myocardial oxygen supply.
- Maintain CI at 4.5 L/min/m² or greater and oxygen delivery of ≥1200 mL/min (or 600 mL/min/m² indexed for body size) to maximize oxygen supply.
- Calculate arterial oxygen delivery (DO_2), which is determined by the amount of oxygen in the blood (CaO_2) and the amount of blood delivered to the tissue (C0/CI). Report value ≤900 mL/min.
- Obtain and report hemodynamic findings that indicate decreased myocardial oxygen supply resulting from decreased coronary artery perfusion. The indicators include CAPP ≤60 mm Hg, CO ≤4 L/min, CI ≤2.7 L/min/m², DO_2 ≤900 mL/min, and DO_2I ≤500 mL/min/m². In AMI, the CAPP is especially important, since a value ≤ 40 mm

Hg can result in collapse of the coronary arteries.

- Obtain, document, and report other findings suggestive of decreased myocardial oxygen supply: HR ≥ 100 bpm, which decreases diastolic filling time; SBP 80 to 90 mm Hg; capillary refill ≥ 3 seconds; peripheral pulses $\leq 2+$; presence of dysrhythmia and chest pain.

- Continuously monitor Svo_2 to evaluate oxygen supply and demand. An $S\bar{v}o_2$ of $\leq 60\%$ can indicate decreased oxygen supply and increased oxygen demand.

- Optimize oxygen delivery by maximizing oxygen saturation through maintenance of $Pao_2 \geq 80$ mm Hg, arterial pH, and temperature.

- Optimize oxygen delivery by maximizing CO through altering HR and maintaining stroke volume to 60 to 130 mL/beat.

- Initiate continuous ECG monitoring to assess heart rate and rhythm. Document ECG rhythm strips every 2 to 4 hours in patients with dysrhythmias (see ST segment monitoring, p. 264).

- Monitor patient for chest discomfort. Should the patient experience chest discomfort, assess and report new S_3 or S_4 gallops, new or increasing crackles, and decreased activity tolerance.

- Administer prescribed oxygen 2 to 4 L/min by means of nasal cannula or mask to maintain $Pao_2 \geq 80$ mm Hg, $Sao_2 \geq 95\%$, or $Svo_2 \geq 60\%$.

- Administer prescribed IV fluids to maintain adequate hydration, $Do_2 \geq 900$ mL/min or $Do_2I \geq 500$ mL/min/m^2.

- Obtain arterial oxygen delivery (Do_2) after administration of IV fluids. Failure of the Do_2 to increase after fluid challenge with 500 to 1000 mL of colloids may indicate limited circulatory reserve capacity. Report the findings so fluid adjustments can be made.

- Administer prescribed nitrates (nitroprusside or NTG), which dilate coronary arteries leading loan increase in the supply of oxygen to the myocardium and cause ve-

nous vasodilation, which decreases the return of blood to the heart and reduces preload, ventricular size, and systolic wall tension (see Table 1–4).

- Administer prescribed positive inotrope (dobutamine) 2 μg/kg/min to maintain Do_2 ≥ 900 mL/min and $Do_2I \geq 500$ mL/min/m^2. Dobutamine improves coronary blood flow and myocardial oxygen supply over and above the increase in myocardial oxygen demand associated with the increase in inotropy (see Table 1–10).

- Obtain Do_2 after dobutamine has been administered. Failure of the Do_2 to increase after stimulation with dobutamine 10 μg/kg/min may indicate limited circulatory capacity. Report the findings so dobutamine adjustments can be made.

- Administer prescribed beta blocker (propranolol) to maintain BP within patient's normal range and HR ≤ 90 bpm (see Table 1–5).

- Administer prescribed thrombolytic therapy (streptokinase or tissue plasminogen) to maintain CAPP ≥ 60 mm Hg, CO ≥ 4 L/min, and CI ≥ 2.7 L/min/m^2 (see Table 1–8 and Thrombolytic therapy, p. 265.)

- Administer prescribed heparin or warfarin. Heparin is given after thrombolytic therapy to prevent recurring thrombus formation. Heparin is administered at 1000 U/h to maintain partial thromboplastin time at 2.0 to 2.5 times the upper limit of normal for up to 5 days. Warfarin is given for long-term post-discharge therapy (see Table 1–8)

- Administer prescribed narcotic (morphine) to maintain HR ≤ 100 bpm and reduce chest pain (see Table 1–7).

- Administer prescribed inotropic drug (dobutamine) with a vasodilating drug (nitroprusside or NTG) to maximize oxygen delivery by increasing contractility and decreasing afterload.

- Monitor patient for signs of improved oxygen delivery, which include CI 4.0 to 4.5 L/min/m^2, UO ≥ 30 mL/h or 0.5 mL/kg/h, HR ≤ 120 bpm, and mean arterial pressure (MAP) ≥ 80 mm Hg.

- Should pharmacological therapy be ineffective in increasing myocardial oxygen supply, prepare patient for PTCA insertion (see PTCA, p. 226.)
- Should PTCA and thrombolytic therapy be ineffective, prepare patient for coronary atherectomy, intracoronary stent, or CABG (see Transluminal coronary atherectomy, p. 234, Intracoronary stent, p. 237, or CABG, p. 194).
- Teach patient the importance of reporting chest pain.
- Teach patient to pace activities so as not to increase HR and subsequently decrease myocardial tissue oxygen supply.
- Teach the patient about the common side effects of vasodilators: headache, nausea, vomiting, or dizziness.
- Teach patient about the common side effects of positive inotropic agents.

Potential Complication: Increased Myocardial Oxygen Demand. Increased myocardial oxygen demand related to increased heart rate, altered contractility and increased systolic wall tension secondary to increased physical activity, increased preload or increased afterload.

Expected Patient Outcomes. Patient maintains reduced myocardial oxygen demand, as measured by oxygen extraction ratio (O_2ER) of 22% to 30%, MAP 70 to 90 mm Hg, PCWP 6 to 12 mm Hg, pulse pressure (PP) 30 to 40 mm Hg, continuous mixed venous oxygen saturation ($S\bar{v}o_2$) 60% to 80%, RPP $\leq$12,000, SVR 900 to 1200 dynes/s/cm^{-5}, SVRI 1970 to 2300 dynes/s/cm^{-5} · m^2, RVSW 10 to 15 g-m/beat, LVSW 60 to 80 g-m/beat, oxygen consumption (Vo_2) $\geq$200 or $\leq$250 mL/min, oxygen consumption index (Vo_2I) $\geq$115 or $\leq$165 mL/min/m^2, BP within patient's normal range, HR $\leq$ 100 bpm, and temperature $\leq$100°F.

- Confer with cardiologist to validate expected patient outcome parameters used to assess reduction of myocardial tissue oxygen demand resulting from adequate CO.

- Consult with dietitian about the patient's diet of small, frequent, easily digested meals and no caffeine.
- Review with cardiologist the results from cardiac scans, coronary angiogram, and ECG.
- Keep patient fasting (NPO) for the first 4 to 6 hours and then allow clear liquids for 24 hours to diminish the risk of aspiration should cardiac arrest or nausea or vomiting occur from prescribed drugs.
- After 24 hours or earlier, provide small portions of easily digested, low-sodium, low-saturated-fat foods as necessary.
- Limit physical activity to the level of activity not increasing HR and increasing myocardial oxygen demand.
- Position patient with the bed elevated 20 to 30 degrees to decrease myocardial oxygen demand.
- Promote rest by decreasing environmental stimuli, assisting with or performing personal care activities, and pacing patient activities to reduce myocardial oxygen demand.
- Provide ROM exercises, without increasing myocardial oxygen tissue demand, to maintain muscle tone and prevent deep vein thrombosis (DVT).
- Provide bed bath instead of shower for postinfarction patients. Showering may increase oxygen consumption, as evidenced by higher RPP and greater number of ST segment changes than bed baths.
- When the patient progresses to a shower, provide chair and assistance with back washing or shampooing to minimize myocardial oxygen consumption.
- Calculate arterial oxygen demand, which is the product of CO and the difference between arterial oxygen content and venous oxygen content C(a − v)o$_2$.
- Calculate oxygen utilization coefficient or oxygen extraction ratio (O_2ER) by dividing the arteriovenous oxygen content difference (C[a − v]o$_2$ by arterial oxygen content (Cao$_2$).
- Calculate the RPP by multiplying HR with SBP. This value correlates well with my-

ocardial oxygen consumption or demand (MVo_2). Report RPP $\geq 12,000$.

- Obtain Vo_2 and Vo_2I in relationship to Do_2 and Do_2I. When Vo_2 (oxygen consumption) is limited by Do_2 (oxygen delivery), the Vo_2 is thought of as being supply-dependent. The rate of oxygen consumed is limited by the rate of oxygen delivered to the tissues.

- Continuously monitor $S\bar{v}o_2$ to evaluate oxygen supply and demand. A $S\bar{v}o_2$ of $\leq 60\%$ can indicate decreased oxygen supply and increased oxygen demand.

- Monitor and report factors that may cause increased myocardial oxygen demand: hypotension, hypertension, tachycardia, increased contractility, pain, anxiety, fever, anemia, and volume depletion.

- Obtain, document, and report hemodynamic parameters that indicate increased myocardial oxygen demand resulting from decreased CO or changes in oxidative metabolism: $O_2ER \geq 25\%$, PP ≤ 30 mm Hg, RPP $\geq 12,000$, $S\bar{v}o_2 \leq 60\%$, SVR ≥ 1200 dynes/s/cm^{-5}, SVRI ≥ 2390 dynes/s/cm$^{-5} \cdot$ m^2, RVSW ≤ 10g-m/beat, LVSW ≤ 60 g-m/beat, Vo_2 ≥ 250 mL/min, and $Vo_2I \geq 165$ mL/min/m^2.

- Monitor patient's temperature, since oxygen consumption varies in proportion to body temperature. There is a 10% to 13% increase in oxygen consumption for every degree (C) in temperature above normal. Report temperature $\geq 100.8°$F.

- Obtain and report other findings suggestive of increased myocardial oxygen demand because they increase metabolic activity and subsequent myocardial work load: HR ≥ 100 bpm and BP above the patient's normal value.

- Initiate continuous ECG to assess heart rate and rhythm. Document ECG rhythm strips every 2 to 4 hours in patients with dysrhythmias.

- Administer prescribed oxygen 2 to 4 L/min by means of nasal cannula or fraction of inspired oxygen (Fio_2) $\leq 50\%$ by mask to maintain $Pao_2 \geq 80$ mm Hg and $Sao_2 \geq 95\%$.

- Monitor patient while performing orotracheal suctioning, as this activity can increase extraction of oxygen from the capillary bed (thus decreasing $S\bar{v}o_2$) as a result of pulmonary congestion.

- Administer prescribed IV fluids to maintain Do_2 and Vo_2 within normal range. Supply-dependent Vo_2 is indicated by increased $Vo_2 \geq 15$ mL/min $\cdot$ m^2 when Do_2 increases ≥ 50 mL/min/m^2 after rapid administration of fluids, such as 100 mL of 25% albumin, 500 mL of 5% albumin, 500 mL of 6% hetastarch, or 2000 mL of crystalloids.

- Administer prescribed vasodilators (nitroprusside or NTG) to decrease afterload by maintaining SVR 900 to 1200 dynes/s/cm^{-5} and SVRI 1970 to 2390 dynes/s/cm$^{-5} \cdot$ m^2. An increase in afterload of the left ventricle causes the left ventricle to develop more pressure during the systolic period, thereby increasing intramyocardial tension and oxygen demand or consumption (see Table 1–4).

- Titrate IV NTG 10 μg/min at 10-minute intervals or at preset limits to avoid hypotension (≥ 90 mm Hg systolic), tachycardia (HR increase $\leq 20\%$), or bradycardia (≥ 45 to 50 bpm).

- Encourage patients on vasodilators to change position slowly to reduce the possibility of orthostatic hypotension.

- Administer prescribed calcium channel blocker (diltiazem) to reduce myocardial oxygen consumption. Diltiazem acts as a systemic vasodilator, lowering afterload, reducing ventricular wall tension, and reducing contractility (see Table 1–6).

- Administer prescribed positive inotropes (dopamine or dobutamine) to decrease preload by maintaining PCWP ≤ 12 mm Hg. An increase preload or filling pressure in left ventricle increases tension because both internal pressure and the radius of the ventricular cavity increase with decreasing thickness. The result is increased oxygen consumption (see Table 1–10).

- Administer prescribed beta-adrenergic blockers (propranolol, metoprolol, atenolol, timolol, nadolol, or pindolol) to decrease HR and BP, thereby decreasing myocardial oxygen consumption leading to a prolonged diastolic phase (see Table 1–5).

- Administer prescribed analgesics, which help to relieve patient of pain or anxiety. The reduction in pain or anxiety decreases the release of catecholamines, which increase metabolic rate and oxygen consumption.
- Administer prescribed stool softeners to avoid straining and subsequent increase in oxygen demand.
- Teach patient to avoid behaviors that increase heart rate: excessive physical activity, straining at stool, anger, or irritability.
- Teach patient techniques to reduce myocardial tissue oxygen demand: guided imagery, meditation, or progressive relaxation.
- Teach patient to exhale with physical movement. This reduces the potential for increased intrathoracic pressure, which decreases venous return to the heart (decrease preload), and vagal stimulation, which causes a decrease in CO. When air is released, the intrathoracic pressure is decreased and preload is increased. This causes increased work load of the heart.
- Teach patient the common side effects of beta-adrenergic blockers: dizziness, fatigue, headache, or bradycardia.
- Teach the patient about the common side effects of vasodilators: headache, nausea, vomiting, or dizziness.
- Teach patient to alleviate sources of psychological stress and use progressive muscular relaxation to decrease oxygen consumption.

Potential Complication: Decreased Cardiac Output.

Decreased CO related to decreased myocardial contractility secondary to myocardial injury, reduced myocardial compliance, or loss of myocardial functional mass.

Expected Patient Outcomes. Patient maintains adequate myocardial contractility, as inferred by measuring CO 4 to 8 L/min, CI 2.5 to 4.0 L/min/m^2, ejection fraction (EF) $\geq$60%, LVSW 60 to 80 g-m/beat, left ventricular stroke work index (LVSWI) 30 to 50 g-m/beat/m^2, PCWP 6 to 12 mm Hg, RVSW 10 to 15 g-m/beat, right ventricular stroke work index (RVSWI) 7 to 12 g-m/beat/m^2, stroke volume (SV) 60 to 130 mL/beat, stroke volume index (SVI) 45 to 85 mL/m^2/beat, absence of crackles, normal heart sounds, and UO $\geq$30 mL/h or $\geq$0.5 mL/kg/h.

- Consult with physician to validate the expected patient outcomes that indicate the quality of myocardial contractility.
- Consult with the cardiologist when there is a sudden decrease in contractility as measured by decreased FCWP (preload) and SVR (afterload).
- Review with cardiologist the patient's hemodynamic parameters from catheterization that indicate decreased myocardial contractility: CO, CI, EF, LVSW, LVSWI, RVSW, RVSWI, SV, and SVI.
- Review results of 12-lead ECG.
- Limit the patient's physical activity to bed rest, thereby reducing fatigue and myocardial work load.
- Monitor patient's need for complete bed rest. Prolonged bed rest can lead to loss of blood and plasma volume, increase HR $\geq$ 15 bpm, decrease SV, and decrease CO during exercise.
- Gradually increase patient's activity after periods of bed rest.
- Obtain, document, and report hemodynamic parameters indicating critically diminished contractility: CI $\leq$2.5 L/min/m^2, EF $\leq$50%, LVSW $\leq$60 g-m/beat, LVSWI $\leq$30 g-m/beat/m^2, RVSW $\leq$10 g-m/beat, RVSWI $\leq$7 g-m/beat/m^2, SV $\leq$60 mL/beat, and SVI $\leq$45 mL/m^2/beat.
- Monitor and report changes in indicators associated with decreased CO. PCWP $\geq$12 mm Hg, pulmonary vascular congestion, hypotension, poor cerebral perfusion, or UO $\leq$30 mL/h.
- Monitor and report other clinical findings suggestive of decreased myocardial contractility: hypotension, restlessness, confusion, decreased alertness, crackles, tachycardia, decreased peripheral pulses, murmurs, pallor, mottling, cyanosis, diaphoresis, and cool skin.
- Initiate continuous ECG to assess heart rate and rhythm. Document ECG rhythm strips

every 2 to 4 hours in patients with dysrhythmias (see Dysrhythmias, p. 184 and ST segment monitoring, p. 264).

- Administer prescribed oxygen via mask or nasal cannula: Keep oxygen 2 to 4 L/min or F_{IO_2} $\leq$50% to maintain Pa_{O_2} $\geq$60 mm Hg.
- Monitor and record intake and output every 2 to 4 hours.
- Administer positive inotropes (dobutamine) to increase myocardial contractility as evidenced by CO $\geq$4 L/min, CI $\geq$2.7 L/min/m^2, LVSW $\geq$60 g-m/beat, LVSWI $\geq$30 g-m/beat/m^2, RVSW $\geq$10 g-m/beat, RVSWI $\geq$7 g-m/beat/m^2, SV $\geq$60 mL/beat, and SVI $\geq$45 mL/m^2/beat (see Table 1–10).
- Administer prescribed vasodilator (nitroprusside) to increase SV and CO. Any increase in myocardial oxygen demand resulting from increase in contractility is offset by decreases in arteriolar resistance and afterload, PCWP, and frequency of ectopic beats (see Table 1–4).
- Administer prescribed phosphodiesterase inhibitor (amrinone) to increase CO, reduce PCWP, and reduce afterload (see Table 1–10).
- Administer prescribed angiotension-converting enzyme (ACE) inhibitor, such as captopril, to increase CO by decreasing afterload secondary inhibition of vasoconstriction from angiotension II. Preload is also decreased through inhibition of sodium retention. The overall result is decrease in afterload and preload, which increases CO and reduces the work of the heart (see Table 1–10).
- If pharmacological therapy does not improve contractility, assist with the insertion of IABP (see IABP, p. 254.)
- Teach patient to avoid Valsalva's maneuver, such as straining at stool.

Potential Complication: Dysrhythmias Dysrhythmias related to increased sympathetic tone or myocardial ischemia secondary to coronary artery disease.

Expected Patient Outcomes. Patient remains in sinus rhythm, serum electrolytes within normal range, HR 60 to 100 bpm, BP within patient's normal range, and absence of pain.

- Consult with cardiologist about dysrhythmias that might occur, depending on the specific coronary artery involved and the location of the MI.
- Consult with cardiologist about the underlying causes of dysrhythmias.
- Monitor serum potassium levels that may contribute to dysrhythmias: hyperkalemia $\geq$5.5 mEq/L and hypokalemia $\leq$3.8 mEq/L.
- Review results of serial 12-lead ECG to help evaluate the location, progression, resolution of infarction and ventricular function.
- Review results of cardiac enzyme tests for resolution or extension of AMI.
- Initiate continuous ECG to assess HR and rhythm. Document ECG rhythm strips every 2 to 4 hours in patients with dysrhythmias. Measure the basic PR, QRS, and QT intervals to obtain the patient's baseline. Note ST and T wave changes that may indicate ischemia, injury, or infarction.
- Monitor and report physical signs and symptoms of dysrhythmias: abnormal HR and rhythm, palpitations, chest pain, syncope, ECG changes, and hypotension.
- Administer the prescribed oxygen 2 to 4 L/min by means of a nasal cannula or mask should the patient experience chest pain. This increases the amount of oxygen available for myocardial use.
- Measure the ECG components signifying Q wave infarctions evidenced by pathological Q waves ($\geq$0.04 s), ST segment elevation with reciprocal ST depression in the opposite leads, T wave changes positive then negative in leads facing the infarcted area.
- Measure the ECG components signifying non-Q wave infarction, revealed by ST depression and inverted T waves in leads facing the epicardial surface overlying the infarction, ST elevation and upright T waves in opposite leads.

- Measure ECG components should hypokalemia occur in conjunction with diuretic therapy: decreased amplitude and broadening of T waves, prominent U waves, and sagging ST segments.
- Measure ECG components should hyperkalemia occur in conjunction with decreased renal arterial perfusion: Peaked T waves of increased amplitude and biphasic QRS-T complexes.
- Replace potassium as needed and as prescribed (see Renal Deviations, Hypokalemia, p. 485).
- Withhold potassium, and if potassium exceeds 6.0 mEq/L administer prescribed sodium polystyrene sulfonate (Kayexalate) a sodium cycle sulfonic polystyrene exchange renin (see Renal Deviations, Hyperkalemia, p. 483).
- Monitor ECG for increase in the number of premature ventricular contractions (PVCs), noting longer or more frequent episodes of PVCs. The PVCs reflect cardiac irritability. Frequent, multiple, or multifocal PVCs can cause decrease CO and lead to ventricular tachycardia, ventricular fibrillation, or cardiac arrest.
- Monitor ECG for changes from nonsustained ($\leq$30 seconds) ventricular tachycardia to sustained ($\geq$30 seconds) of ventricular tachycardia.
- Monitor ECG for heart blocks, which can be caused by MI, decreased blood supply to the sinoatrial (SA) or AV nodes, or cardiac surgery.
- Administer prescribed antidysrhythmia agent according to the dysrhythmia's origin and potential risk to the patient (see Table 1–11, and Dysrhythmias, p. 184.)
- Should pharmacological therapy be ineffective in correcting persistent tachycardia or bradycardia; septal damage with high degree of block progression; inferior AMI with transient AV block; or persistent ectopy with compromised CO, prepare patient for pacemaker (see Pacemaker, p. 270).
- Teach patient to report an abnormal heart rate, syncope, and to describe chest pain on a scale of 1 to 10.
- Teach the patient to avoid stimulants such as tobacco, caffeine, or alcohol, which may cause dysrhythmias.
- Teach patient common side effects of prescribed dysrhythmia agents.

DISCHARGE PLANNING

The critical care nurse will provide the patient and significant other(s) with verbal or written discharge notes regarding the following subjects.

1. The signs and symptoms that warrant immediate medical attention: chest pain, shortness of breath, fatigue, syncope, or weight gain.
2. Activity schedule. A postdischarge exercise program to keep HR $\leq$100 bpm as follows: (1) first week, walk 0.25 miles within 8 to 10 minutes; (2) second week, walk 0.25 miles within 5 minutes; (3) third week, walk 0.50 miles within 15 minutes; and (4) fourth week, walk 1.0 miles within 30 minutes. Teach schedule to patient and significant other(s).
3. The ways to reduce precipitating factors (activity following a heavy meal, sexual intercourse, anger, or grief) by taking prophylactic NTG, reducing physical activity and psychologic stress resulting in chest discomfort, and countering emotional stress through progressive physical activity.
4. Informing patient and significant others about ceasing any activity that increases HR and BP or causes fatigue. These behaviors can increase myocardial tissue oxygen demand.
5. Calling for emergency medical service should post activity chest pain persist after resting for 10 minutes.
6. The names of community agencies that can enhance learning and provide support (e.g., American Heart Association).
7. A written list of side effects associated with patient's specific medication(s).
8. Written instructions on how to take warfarin (Coumadin) and potential side effects, such as bleeding.

■ CARDIOGENIC SHOCK

(For related information see Part I: Acute myocardial infarction, p. 38; Congestive heart failure, p. 87; Acute chest pain, p. 1; Dysrhythmias, p. 184. Part II: Coronary artery bypass graft, p. 194. Part III: Hemodynamic monitoring, p. 219; Percutaneous transluminal coronary angioplasty, p. 226; Coronary laser angioplasty, p. 238; Intra-aortic balloon pump, p. 254; ST segment monitoring, p. 264; Thrombolytic therapy, p. 265. See also Respiratory Deviations, Part III: Pulse oximetry, p. 426; Mechanical ventilators, p. 428. See also Behavioral Deviations, Part I: Powerlessness, p. 743.)

Diagnostic Categories and Length of Stay

DRG: 144 Other circulatory system diagnosis with complications
LOS: 5.20 days

Definition

Cardiogenic shock is a state of severe cardiac dysfunction that impairs blood flow to vital organs, causing inadequate oxygen delivery to the tissues, a shift to anaerobic metabolism, and accumulation of lactate and other anaerobic products. In this respect, cardiogenic shock becomes a complex problem characterized by systemic hypotension, arterial vasoconstriction, and impaired tissue and organ perfusion. It occurs when there is not enough functioning myocardium to support systemic perfusion.

Pathophysiology

Cardiogenic shock usually results when 40% or more of the left ventricular myocardium has ceased to function. There is severe depression of myocardial contractility and impaired ventricular compliance. This leads to decreased cardiac output (CO) and increased systemic vascular resistance (SVR) from sustained sympathetic stimulation, compromising left ventricular ejection and CO. Decreased perfusion to the skin and kidneys because of vasoconstriction and acidosis are present. In time, there is pooling of blood in the peripheral vasculature, which further decrease CO. Finally vasoconstriction impairs cellular organs, causing acute tubular necrosis, mental confusion, visceral ischemia, and necrosis, which may cause ulceration of intestinal mucosa. Furthermore, pancreatic cell ischemia and necrosis form a polypeptide (myocardial depressant factor [MOF] that causes further depression of myocardial contraction. Pulmonary parenchymal cell necrosis or ischemia releases sustained histamine, which increases pulmonary capillary permeability, intensifies ventilation–perfusion mismatch and hypoxemia, and increases interstitial edema and atelectasis. The resulting hemodynamic profile is arterial hypotension (systolic blood pressure [SBP] ≤80 mm Hg, mean arterial pressure [MAP] ≤60 mm Hg, cardiac index, CI ≤1.8 L/min/m^2, tachycardia, and pulmonary capillary wedge pressure (PCWP) ≥18 mm Hg, right ventricular stroke work (RVSW) ≤7 g-m/beat/m^2 and left ventricular stroke work (LVSW) ≤35 g-m/beat/m^2.

Nursing Assessment

PRIMARY CAUSES

- Include acute myocardial infarction, cardiac rupture, myocarditis, atrial myxoma, acute cardiac tamponade, tension pneumothorax, dysrhythmias, left ventricular aneurysm, acute mitral regurgitation, acute aortic insufficiency, dissecting aortic aneurysm, aortic or pulmonary stenosis, ruptured intraventricular septum, pump failure after cardiac surgery, dilated cardiomyopathy, and congestive heart failure.

RISK FACTORS

- History of prior MIs and hypertension.

PHYSICAL ASSESSMENT

- Inspection: Cognitive changes include altered level of consciousness, restlessness, apprehension, confusion, agitation, lethargy, or coma. Cardiac findings are palpitations or complaints of chest pain. Respiratory findings include tachypnea and dyspnea.

Peripheral hypoperfusion may be present and manifested as pale, cyanotic, or mottled skin, peripheral edema, and decreased urine volume. Fluid volume change can be reflected as distended external jugular vein.

- Palpation: The skin is cool and clammy and diaphoretic. Pulses are weak and thready.
- Auscultation: Presence of systolic pressure ≤ 90 mm Hg, tachycardia, S_3 and S_4. Pulmonary congestion is associated with crackles or wheezes, tachypnea or dyspnea.

DIAGNOSTIC TEST RESULTS

Hemodynamic Parameters. (See Table 1–1)

- Arterial-venous oxygen content difference C(a − v)o2 ≥ 6 mL/100mL, arterial oxygen content (Cao_2) ≤ 18 mL/100mL, CO ≤ 4 L/min, CI ≤ 1.8 L/min/m², ejection fraction (EF) $\leq 25\%$, pulmonary artery pressure (PAP) systolic ≥ 25 mm Hg and diastolic ≤ 15 mm Hg, PCWP ≥ 18 mm Hg, pulmonary vascular resistance (PVR) 37 to 97 dynes/s/cm^{-5}, right atrial pressure (RAP) ≥ 6 mm Hg, right ventricular pressure (RVP) systolic ≥ 25 mm Hg and diastolic ≥ 8 mm Hg, mixed venous oxygen saturation ($S\bar{v}o_2$) $\leq 60\%$, stroke volume index (SVI) ≤ 20 mL · m²/beat, SVR ≥ 1200 dynes/s/cm^{-5}, and venous oxygen content (Cvo_2) ≤ 15.5 mL/100mL.

Standard Laboratory Tests. (See Table 1–1)

- Arterial blood gases: pH ≤ 7.35, Pao_2 ≤ 60 mm Hg, and $Paco_2$ ≤ 35 mm Hg.
- Blood studies: Hemoglobin (Hgb) men 14.0 to 16.5 g/100mL and women 12 to 15 g/100mL and hematocrit (Hct) men 42 to 54 and women 38% to 46%.
- Serum chemistries: Hypokalemia ≤ 3.8 mEq/L, hyperkalemia ≥ 5.5 mEq/L, HCO_3 ≤ 22 mEq/L, blood urea nitrogen (BUN) ≥ 20 mg/dL and creatinine men ≥ 1.2 mg/dL and women ≥ 0.9 mg/dL, total serum protein 6.6 to 7.0 g/dL, serum albumin 3.3 to 4.5 g/dL, and serum osmolality 285 to 295 mOsm/kg.

- Serum enzymes: creatine kinase (CPK) ≥ 180 IU/L, CK-MB ≥ 1 IU/L, lactate dehydrogenase (LDH) men ≥ 155 units and women ≥ 131 units, LDH_2 $\geq 40\%$.

Noninvasive Cardiac Diagnostic Procedures. (See Table 1–3)

- Chest roentgenogram: Reveals cardiomegaly and pulmonary congestion.

ECG

- May reveal left ventricular hypertrophy or serial changes indicative of myocardial ischemia or necrosis or electrolyte imbalance.

MEDICAL AND SURGICAL MANAGEMENT

PHARMACOLOGY

- Positive inotropes: Dopamine (5 to 8 µg/kg/min) is given to increase contractility, heart rate (HR) and CO. Dobutamine (2.5 µg/kg/min) is given to increase CO, decrease PCWP and PVR, and redistribute CO to the coronary and skeletal muscle circulation. Combined use of dopamine and dobutamine (7.5 µg/kg/min) can be given for short term (6 to 8 hours) to increase blood pressure (BP), maintain PCWP within normal limits, lower myocardial oxygen consumption, and reduce worsening hypoxemia induced by dopamine. Amrinone (2 to 20 µg/kg/min) can be given to increase myocardial contractility, increase CO, and decrease afterload, preload, PCWP, and MAP (see Table 1–10).
- Vasodilators: Nitroprusside (0.5 to 10.0 µg/kg/min) can be given to increase CO and decrease afterload and BP. Nitroglycerin (5 µg/min, increase 5 µg every 3 to 5 minutes and titrate to desired outcome) will reduce venous return, preload, afterload, myocardial oxygen demand, PCWP, PVR, and SVR. Stroke volume is increased (see Table 1–4).
- Diuretics: Furosemide (20 to 40 mg IV undiluted over 1 to 2 minutes) or bu-

metanide (500 μg to 1 mg IV undiluted over 1 to 2 minutes and may repeat at 2 to 3 hour intervals) is given to decrease circulating volume and preload (see Table 1–13).

- Antidysrhythmia agents: Correcting dysrhythmias will decrease myocardial oxygen demand and maintain circulatory support by maintaining ventricular filling through an adequate heart rate (see Table 1–11).
- Thrombolytic agents: These are used to influence three factors that determine the progression of necrosis, such as improving collateral blood flow to decrease hypoperfusion, decrease myocardial oxygen demand, and reestablish blood flow by recannulizing the occluded coronary artery, thereby limiting the infarct size (streptokinase, tissue plasminogen, or anisoylated plasminogen streptokinase activator complex) See Table 1–8 and Thrombolytic therapy, p. 265).
- Morphine sulfate: Morphine (2 mg IV push) is used to relieve pain, promote venous pooling, and decrease dyspnea (see Table 1–7).

OXYGEN THERAPY
- Provide supplemental oxygen by means of nasal cannula, mask, high-flow rebreathing mask, intubation, or mechanical ventilation. The goal is to provide oxygenation to the tissues. Provide mechanical ventilation to improve alveolar ventilation. With mechanical ventilation, be careful not to decrease venous return and CO.

FLUID THERAPY
- Blood, plasma, colloid and crystalloid, solutions can be used to increase vascular volume and improve CO.

HEMODYNAMIC MONITORING
- Use to measure ventricular function, CO, pulmonary function, and circulating volume. Also used to evaluate the effectiveness of pharmacological interventions that decrease preload and afterload while in-

creasing contractility (see Hemodynamic monitoring, p. 219).

PERCUTANEOUS TRANSLUMINAL CORONARY ANGIOPLASTY (PTCA)
- Is used to restore adequate blood supply to the myocardium by expanding the lumen diameter of a coronary artery (see PTCA, p. 226).

INTRA-AORTIC BALLOON PUMP (IABP)
- A counterpulsation supportive device increases coronary artery perfusion by augmenting circulating blood supply, decreasing afterload, and decreasing myocardial oxygen demand, leading to improved myocardial efficiency (see IABP, p. 254).

CARDIAC ASSIST DEVICE
- The cardiac assist device is a supportive mechanical procedure that diverts blood from either the right, left, or both ventricles to an artificial pump. The device maintains systemic circulation and decreases myocardial work load so the myocardium can heal (see cardiac assist device, p. 248).

SURGICAL INTERVENTION
- Coronary Artery Bypass Graft (CABG): The surgical procedure restores adequate blood flow to the myocardium distal to coronary artery occlusion (see CABG, p. 194).

NURSING MANAGEMENT: NURSING DIAGNOSES AND COLLABORATIVE PROBLEMS

Nursing Diagnoses
Common nursing goals for patients with cardiogenic shock are to restore tissue perfusion, improve oxygenation, maintain adequate fluid volume, restore normal pattern of urinary elimination, enhance normal altered thought process, and restore a sense of control.

Altered cardiopulmonary, cerebral, renal, and peripheral tissue perfusion related to

TABLE 1–13: DIURETICS

Medication	Route/Dose	Uses and Effects	Side Effects
Distal Tubular Agents			
Chlorothiazide (Diuril)	IV/PO: 500–1000 mg/d in 1–2 doses	Management of hypertension and edema Increases excretion of sodium and water Promotes excretion of chloride, potassium, magnesium and bicarbonate Decreases renal calcium excretion	Drowsiness, lethargy, dizziness, weakness, hypotension, hypokalemia, hyperuricemia, hypoglycemia, increase of LDL cholesterol, hypercalcemia, hypomagnesemia, increase of uric acid, rash, impotence, muscle cramps, fatigue, headache, vertigo, nausea, abdominal cramps
Hydrochlorothiazide (HydroDIURIL)	PO: 25–100 mg/d in 1–2 doses; maintenance 25–100 mg/d	Management of hypertension and CHF Increases excretion of sodium and water by inhibiting sodium reabsorption in the distal tubule Promotes excretion of chloride, potassium, magnesium, and bicarbonate	See chlorothiazide
Chlorthalidone (Hygroton)	PO: Initial 25–100 mg/d; or 100 mg 3 times/wk	Management of hypertension and CHF Increases excretion of sodium and water by inhibiting sodium reabsorption in distal tubule Promotes excretion of chloride, potassium, magnesium, and bicarbonate	See chlorothiazide
Metolazone (Zaroxolyn)	PO: 2.5–5.0 mg/d single dose as extended tablet or 0.5–1.0 mg/d single dose as prompt tablet	Management of hypertension and CHF Increases excretion of sodium and water by inhibiting sodium reabsorption in distal tubule Promotes excretion of chloride, potassium, magnesium, and bicarbonate	See chlorothiazide

TABLE 1-13

TABLE 1-13

TABLE 1-13. CONTINUED

Medication	Route/Dose	Uses and Effects	Side Effects
Indapamide (Lozol)	PO: 2.5 mg/d; may increase to 5 mg/d if needed	Used to treat hypertension, edema Diuretic and direct vascular effects	Headache, dizziness, fatigue, weakness, loss of energy, muscle cramps, vertigo, blurred vision, light-headedness
Loop Diuretics			
Furosemide (Lasix)	IM or PO: 20–80 mg/d; up to 600 mg IV: 20–40 mg over 1–2 min; can be increased by 20 mg q 2 h	Inhibits reabsorption of sodium and chloride from loop of Henle and distal renal tubule; increases renal excretion of water, sodium, chloride, magnesium, hydrogen, and calcium; may cause renal and peripheral vasodilation	Headache, hearing loss, tinnitus, hypotension, metabolic alkalosis, hypovolemia, dehydration, hyponatremia, hypokalemia, hypochloremia, hypomagnesemia, hyperglycemia, rashes, nausea, vomiting, gastric burning, diarrhea, constipation, abdominal cramping
Bumetanide (Bumex)	PO: 0.5–2.0 mg/d up to 10 mg/d Intravenous: 0.5–1.0 mg may give 1–2 more doses q 2–3 hr up to 10 mg/24hr	See furosemide	See furosemide
Potassium-sparing			
Triamterene (Dyrenium)	PO: 100 mg bid for maximum of 300 mg; may decrease to 100 mg/d or qid	Used to manage edema and hypertension	Diarrhea, nausea, vomiting, headache, rash, anaphylaxis, weakness, hypotension, muscle cramps, hyperkalemia
Amiloride hydrochloride (Midamor)	PO: 5 mg/d; may increase up to 20 mg/d in 1–2 divided doses	Treatment of diuretic-induced hypokalemia Management of primary hyperaldosteronism	Headache, dizziness, confusion, drowsiness, aplastic anemia, visual disturbance, diarrhea, nausea, vomiting, thirst, dyspnea, rash
Spironolactone (Aldactone)	PO: Edema 25–200 mg/d in divided doses; continued for at least 5 days; dose adjusted to optimal response Hypertension 25–100 mg/d in single or divided doses; continued for at least 2 wk	Used to treat primary aldosteronism, essential hypertension, and refractory edema	Lethargy, confusion, fatigue, abdominal cramps, nausea, vomiting, anorexia, rash, fluid and electrolyte imbalance

TABLE 1-13

TABLE 1-13. CONTINUED

Medication	Route/Dose	Uses and Effects	Side Effects
Proximal Tubular Agents			
Acetazolamide (Diamox)	PO: 250–375 mg q AM (5 mg/kg)	Adjunct treatment of edema from CHF	Sedation, malaise, depression, fatigue, muscle weakness, flaccid paralysis, anorexia, nausea, vomiting, weight loss, thirst, diarrhea, aplastic anemia

CHF, congestive heart failure; LDL, low-density lipoprotein.

From Deglin JH, Vallerand AH, Russin MM, 1988; Govoni LE, Hayes JE, Shannon MT, et al, 1992; Loeb, S 1993; Scherer JC, 1992; Vallerand AH, Deglin JH, 1991; Kuhn M, 1992.

reduced arterial blood flow secondary to decreased myocardial contractility or vasoconstriction causing impaired cellular function of vital organs.

Expected Patient Outcomes. Patient maintains adequate tissue perfusion, as evidenced by SBP 110 to 140 mm Hg or diastolic blood pressure (DBP) 70 to 90 mm Hg (or within patient's normal range); coronary artery perfusion pressure (CAPP) 60 to 80 mm Hg; CO 4 to 8 L/min; CI 2.7 to 4.3 L/min/m^2, MAP 70 to 105 mm Hg; $S\bar{v}o_2$ 60% to 80%; HR $\leq$100 bpm; absence of dysrhythmias; absence of chest pain; PVR 155 to 255 dynes/ s/cm^{-5}, pulmonary vascular resistance index (PVRI) 200 to 450 dynes/s/cm$^{-5} \cdot$ m^2; respiratory rate (RR) 12 to 20 BPM; Pao_2 80 to 100 mm Hg; $Paco_2$ 35 to 45 mm Hg; Sao_2 $\geq$95%; absence of dyspnea; absence of rales; SVR 900 to 1200 dynes/s/cm^{-5}; systemic vascular resistance index (SVRI) 1970 to 2390 dynes/ s/cm$^{-5} \cdot$ m^2; pupils equal and normoreactive; absence of confusion and irritability; oriented to person, place, and time; normal sensorimotor function; urinary output (UO) $\geq$30 mL/h or $\geq$0.5 mL/kg/h, specific gravity 1.010 to 1.030; BUN $\leq$20 mg/dL; creatinine clearance M: 95 to 135 mL/min or W: 85 to 125 mL/min; serum creatinine 0.6 to 1.2 mg/dL; capillary refill $\leq$3 seconds; peripheral pulses; and absence of peripheral edema.

- Consult with cardiologist to validate the expected patient's outcomes that indicate adequate tissue perfusion.
- Review results from arterial blood gases, serum enzymes, and chest roentgenogram.
- Review results of 12-lead ECG to help evaluate the location, progression, resolution of infarction and ventricular function.
- Review serum electrolyte values.
- Limit physical activity to bed rest to decrease myocardial work load and myocardial oxygen demand.
- Obtain, document and report hemodynamic parameters that indicate decreased cardiopulmonary tissue perfusion: CO $\leq$4 L/min, CI $\leq$1.8 L/min/m^2, CAPP $\leq$60 mm Hg, MAP $\leq$70 mm Hg, PVR $\geq$97 dynes/s/cm^{-5} and PVRI $\geq$285 dynes/ s/cm$^{-5} \cdot$ m^2.
- Obtain, document, and report other clinical findings suggestive of decreased cardiopulmonary tissue perfusion: HR $\geq$100 bpm, dysrhythmias, chest pain, RR 12 to 20 BPM, dyspnea, and rales.
- Initiate continuous monitoring of ECG to assess HR and rhythm. Document ECG rhythm strips every 2 to 4 hours in patients with dysrhythmias (see ST segment monitoring, p. 264).
- Administer prescribed oxygen 2 to 4 L/min (24% to 36% O_2) by means of nasal cannula or fraction of inspired oxygen F_{IO_2} $\leq$50%

by mask to maintain $Pao_2 \geq 80$ mm Hg, $Sao_2 \geq 95\%$, or $S\bar{v}o_2 \geq 60\%$.

- Administer prescribed IV fluids to maintain adequate circulating volume.
- Administer prescribed morphine to relieve chest pain.
- Administer prescribed thrombolytic therapy (streptokinase, tissue plasminogen, or anisoylated plasminogen streptokinase activator complex [APSAC, Eminase]) to lyse clots within coronary artery, which increases blood flow to ischemic myocardial tissue, and to maintain CAPP ≥ 60 mm Hg, CO ≥ 4 L/min, and CI ≥ 2.7 L/min/m² (see Table 1–8 and Thrombolytic therapy, p. 265).
- Administer prescribed antidysrhythmic agents appropriate for the particular dysrhythmia resulting from decreased myocardial tissue perfusion (see Table 1–11).
- Administer positive inotropes (dopamine, dobutamine) and phosphodiesterase inhibitor (amrinone) to maintain CO ≥ 4 L/min and CI ≥ 2.7 L/min/m² (see Table 1–10).
- Should pharmacological therapy be ineffective in correcting dysrhythmias or heart block occur, prepare patient for a pacemaker (see Pacemaker, p. 270).
- Obtain, document, and report clinical findings suggestive of decreased cerebral tissue perfusion: confusion, irritability, unequal pupils, disorientation, and abnormal sensorimotor function.
- Obtain, document, and report clinical findings indicating decreased renal tissue perfusion: UO ≤ 30 mL/h or ≤ 0.5 mL/kg/h for two consecutive hours, specific gravity ≤ 1.010, and peripheral edema.
- Administer prescribed volume-reducing agents: thiazide (chlorothiazide, hydrochlorothiazide, chlorthalidone, metolazone), loop diuretics (furosemide or bumetanide), or potassium-sparing (spironolactone, amiloride, or triamterene) to maintain UO ≥ 30 mL/h or ≥ 0.5 mL/kg/h and specific gravity 1.010 to 1.030 (see Table 1–13).
- Obtain, document, and report hemodynamic parameters that indicate decreased peripheral tissue perfusion: SVR ≥ 1200 dynes/s/cm⁻⁵ and SVRI ≥ 2390 dynes/s/cm⁻⁵· m².
- Obtain, document, and report other clinical findings suggestive of decreased peripheral tissue perfusion: capillary refill ≥ 3 s, peripheral pulses $\leq +2$, and peripheral edema.
- Administer prescribed vasodilator (nitroprusside) should SVR and SVRI be elevated as a result of vasoconstriction, thereby causing increased afterload (see Table 1–4).
- Teach patient common side effects of antidysrhythmia or diuretic medications.
- Teach patient about the types of pacemakers to be used.

Impaired gas exchange related to impaired oxygen–carbon dioxide diffusion secondary to impaired pulmonary function or extravasation of intravascular fluid into the alveoli.

Expected Patient Outcomes. Patient maintains adequate oxygen gas exchange, as evidenced by arterial oxygen content (Cao_2) 18 to 20 mL/100mL, venous oxygen content (Cvo_2) 15.5 mL/100mL, $C(a - v)o_2$ 4 to 6 mL/100mL, $Paco_2$ 35 to 45 mm Hg, Pao_2 75 to 100 mm Hg, RR 12 to 20 BPM, Sao_2 95% to 97.5%, $S\bar{v}o_2$ 60% to 80%, absence of dyspnea or rales, and absence of restlessness.

- Consult with physician to validate the expected patient outcomes reflecting adequate gas exchange.
- Review results of arterial blood gases, $C(a - v)o_2$, Cao_2, Cvo_2, hemoglobin, hematocrit, and chest roentgenogram.
- Maintain bed rest, as necessaary, to reduce oxygen demand.
- Obtain, document, and report laboratory findings indicating impaired gas exchange: $Pao_2 \leq 80\%$, $Paco_2 \geq 45$ mm Hg, $Sao_2 \leq 95\%$, $Cao_2 \leq 18$ mL/100mL, $Cvo_2 \leq 15.5$ mL/100mL and $C(a - v)o_2 \leq 4$ mL/100mL.
- Obtain and report other clinical findings suggestive of impaired gas exchange: tachypnea, dyspnea, crackles, or rhonchi.

- Monitor continuous ECG to assess for the presence of dysrhythmias secondary to altered oxygenation.
- Administer low-dose morphine sulfate to promote venous pooling, decrease dyspnea, control patient's pain, and aid in reducing myocardial oxygen demand.
- Monitor transcutaneous oxygen saturation with pulse oximeter to keep $Sao_2 \geq 95\%$.
- Encourage the patient to cough, turn, and breathe deeply.
- Position patient for maximum chest excursion and comfort.
- Schedule activities or procedures to provide maximal rest, which decreases oxygen demand.
- Maintain or strengthen patient's pulmonary status through positioning, turning, chest physiotherapy, and by encouraging deep-breathing exercises.
- Auscultate the lungs every hour for the presence of abnormal or adventitious breath sounds and note the use of accessory muscles.
- Remove excess mucus and secretions from the respiratory tract following unit protocol for providing hyperventilation and supplemental oxygen before and after suctioning.
- Administer prescribed low-flow oxygen 2 to 4 L/min (24% to 35% O_2) by nasal cannula or $Fio_2 \leq 50\%$ by mask to maintain $Pao_2 \geq 80$ mm Hg, $Sao_2 \geq 95\%$, and $S\bar{v}o_2 \geq 60\%$.
- Should positioning, suctioning, and supplemental oxygen be ineffective in improving gas exchange, prepare patient for intubation and mechanical ventilation. Provide high-frequency jet ventilation (HFJV) or controlled mechanical ventilation (CMV), since the work of breathing is increased as a result of hypoxemia- or acidosis-induced hyperventilation and the perfusion of the respiratory muscle may not be sufficient to cope with the increased work. (See Respiratory Deviations: Mechanical ventilation, p. 428.)
- Monitor fluid volume status by measuring hourly intake and output and daily weight (gain of 1 kg equals 1000 mL fluid excess). Excess fluid volume can worsen extravasation of intravascular fluid into the alveoli.
- Administer prescribed diuretics to reduce circulating volume and decrease preload (see Table 1–13).

Fluid volume excess related to renal insufficiency secondary to vasoconstriction causing renal hypoperfusion.

Expected Patient Outcomes. Patient maintains adequate fluid volume, as evidenced by central venous pressure (CVP) 4 to 6 mm Hg, PCWP ≤ 18 mm Hg, HR 60 to 100 bpm, absence of jugular vein distention, BP within patient's normal range, weight within 5% of baseline, serum osmolality 285 to 295 mOsm/kg, RR 12 to 20 BPM, normal heart sounds, absence of peripheral edema, absence of crackles or rhonchi, and UO ≥ 30 mL/h or ≥ 0.5 mL/kg/h.

- Consult with cardiologist to validate the expected patient outcomes that reflect stable fluid volume.
- Consult with physician to correct underlying causes of fluid volume excess.
- Review serum electrolyte values and osmolarity to determine the need for electrolyte replacement or restriction.
- Obtain and report hemodynamic parameters that indicate fluid volume excess: CVP ≥ 8 mm Hg and PCWP ≥ 18 mm Hg.
- Obtain and report other clinical findings suggestive of fluid volume excess: pitting or dependent edema; skin pale, moist and cool to touch in edematous areas; neck vein distention; tachycardia; and S_3 and S_4.
- Monitor hourly intake and output to determine whether fluid replacement should be decreased and diuretic therapy increased.
- Monitor daily body weight and weight gain $\geq 5\%$ of baseline. It should be noted that 1kg (2.2 lb) equals 1 L fluid.
- Administer prescribed IV fluids to cover fluid loss: hypertonic intravenous solutions such as mannitol or 10% and 50% dextrose in water to increase osmotic gradient, supporting the movement of fluid from interstitial to intravascular space. Excess fluid is excreted by the kidneys.

- Monitor oral or intravenous fluid intake to document an overall decrease in extracellular fluid volume. Determine the need for fluid restriction.
- Administer prescribed diuretics to increase excretion of extra fluid and maintain UO ≥30 mL/h or ≥0.5 mL/kg/h (see Table 1–13).
- Teach patient the purpose of fluid restriction should fluid excess occur.
- Teach patient the common side effects of diuretics.

Altered urinary elimination pattern related to diminished renal function secondary to afferent arteriolar constriction secondary to increased sympathetic stimulation causing leakage of filtrate across the renal epithelium and edema.

Expected Patient Outcomes. Patient maintains adequate pattern of urinary elimination, as evidenced by UO ≥ 30 mL/h or ≥ 0.5 mL/kg/h, and specific gravity of 1.010 to 1.030, BUN 8 to 20 mg/dL, serum creatinine in men 0.8 to 1.2 mg/dL and in women 0.6 to 0.9 mg/dL, urine creatinine in men 1.0 to 1.9 g/24 h and in women 0.8 to 1.7g/24 h and creatinine clearance in men 90 mL/min/ 1.73 m² of body surface and in women 84 mL/min/1.73 m² of body surface, and electrolytes within normal range.

- Consult with physician to correct underlying causes of altered pattern of urinary elimination.
- Review BUN, serum creatinine, electrolytes, urine creatinine, and creatinine clearance.
- Monitor and report changes in urinary pattern: UO ≤30 mL/h or ≤0.5 mL/kg/h and specific gravity ≥1.030.
- Monitor intake and output every hour.
- Administer IV fluids as prescribed to maintain UO ≥30 mL/h or ≥0.5 mL/kg/h.
- Administer prescribed volume-reducing agents (furosemide and bumetanide) to maintain UO ≥30 mL/h or 0.5 mL/kg/h and specific gravity ≥1.010 (see Table 1–13).

Altered thought processes related to confusion secondary to decreased cardiac output.

Expected Patient Outcomes. Patient is alert and oriented to time, person, and place; CO 4 to 8 L/min, CI 2.7 to 4.3 L/min/m², and BP ≥90/60 mm Hg.

- Consult with physician regarding the underlying causes of the patient's altered thought process.
- Review arterial blood gas and serum electrolyte results.
- Monitor and report hemodynamic changes that could contribute to the patient's confusion: BP ≤90/60 mm Hg, COI ≤4 L/min, and CI ≤1.8 L/min/m².
- Monitor for behaviors reflective of confusion: disoriented to person, time, and place; exhibits agitation and irritability; experiences auditory, visual, and tactile hallucinations; and exhibits disoriented thought pattern.
- Listen to the patient's confusion and assist with reality orientation (time, place, and location).
- Listen to the family concerns, fears, and anxieties while encouraging interactions with the patient.
- Reduce the demand for problem solving or decision making while the patient is confused or fatigued.
- Administer prescribed oxygen 2 to 4 L/min (24% to 36 % O_2) by nasal cannula or F_{IO_2} ≤50% by mask.
- Administer prescribed positive inotropes (dopamine, dobutamine) or phosphodiesterase inhibitor (amrinone) to maintain BP ≥90 mm Hg, CO ≥ 4 L/min, and CI ≥1.8 to 2.2 L/min/m² (see Table 1–10).

Powerlessness related to the inability to control the illness experience, treatments, procedures, or life-style change.

Expected Patient Outcome. Patient gains control over some aspects of care to increase feelings of powerfulness.

- Encourage communication between the patient and health care providers.

- Explain the purpose behind supportive or diagnostic procedures and unit protocol.
- Encourage patient to ask questions.
- Allow patient to control his or her surroundings such as deciding where to put cards, drawings from children or grandchildren, or reading material.
- Provide opportunities for patients and family to participate in care, when realistic.
- Provide opportunities for control by allowing patient to make decisions about daily activities.
- Encourage patient to look at the positive aspects of the illness experience.
- Teach patient how to use guided imagery or relaxation strategies.

Collaborative Problems

Common collaborative goals in patients with cardiogenic shock are to restore myocardial oxygen supply, reduce myocardial oxygen demand, increase CO, and correct dysrhythmias.

Potential Complication: Decreased Myocardial Oxygen Supply.

Decreased myocardial oxygen supply related to reduced coronary artery perfusion secondary to tachydysrhythmias that decrease diastolic filling time or coronary artery disease.

Expected Patient Outcomes.

Patient maintains adequate myocardial oxygen supply, as evidenced by CAPP 60 to 80 mm Hg, CO 4 to 8 L/min, CI 2.7 to 4.0 L/min/m^2, oxygen delivery (Do_2) 900 to 1200 mL/min, oxygen delivery index (Do_2I) 500 to 600 mL/min/m^2, ($S\bar{v}o_2$) 60% to 80%, BP ≥90/60 mm Hg or within the patient's normal range, HR ≤90 bpm, capillary refill ≤3 seconds, Sao_2 ≥95%, Pao_2 ≥80 mm Hg, UO ≥30 mL/h or ≥0.5 mL/kg/h, specific gravity 1.010 to 1.030, absence of dysrhythmias, and absence of chest pain.

- Consult with cardiologist to validate the expected patient outcomes reflecting increased myocardial oxygen supply: CAPP, CO, CI, oxygen delivery (Do_2) and oxygen delivery index (Do_2I).

- Physician consults with cardiologist about the need for PTCA or CABG.
- Review with the cardiologist the serum enzyme values and serial ECG.
- Limit patient's physical activity before manifestations of decreased myocardial oxygen supply.
- Maintain CI at 4.5 L/min/m^2 or greater and oxygen delivery of ≥1200 mL/min (or 600 mL/min/m^2 indexed for body size) to maximize oxygen supply.
- Calculate CAPP, since a decrease leads to further myocardial ischemia and necrosis.
- Calculate Do_2 and Do_2I to evaluate the effectiveness of therapies that enhance perfusion.
- Obtain and report hemodynamic findings that indicate decreased myocardial oxygen supply as a result of decreased CAPP ≤60 mm Hg, CO ≤4 L/min, CI ≤2.7 L/min/m^2, Do_2 ≤900 mL/min and Do_2I ≤500 mL/min/m^2. In acute myocardial infarction, the CAPP is especially important, since a value ≤40 mm Hg can result in collapse of the coronary arteries.
- Obtain, document, and report other findings suggestive of decreased myocardial oxygen supply: HR ≥ 100 bpm, which decreases diastolic filling time; BP ≤90/60 mm Hg; capillary refill ≥3 seconds, peripheral pulses ≤2+; presence of dysrhythmia; and chest pain.
- Initiate continuous ECG to assess heart rate and rhythm. Document ECG rhythm strips every 2 to 4 hours in patients with dysrhythmias.
- Administer prescribed oxygen 2 to 4 L/min (24% to 36% O_2) by means of nasal cannula or Fio_2 ≤50% by mask to maintain Pao_2 ≥80 mm Hg, or Sao_2 ≥95%.
- Administer prescribed narcotic (morphine) to maintain HR ≤100 bpm and reduce chest pain.
- Administer prescribed IV fluids to maintain adequate hydration, Do_2 ≥900 mL/min or Do_2I ≥500 mL/min/m^2.
- Administer prescribed peripheral vasodilators (nitroprusside) to dilate arterial and ve-

nous vessels or nitroglycerin to decrease coronary vascular resistance. The overall goal is to maintain CAPP $\geq$60 mm Hg, CO $\geq$4L/min, CI $\geq$2.4 L/min/m^2, Do_2 $\geq$900 mL/min and Do_2I $\geq$500 mL/min/m^2 (see Table 1–4).

- Should pharmacological therapy be ineffective in increasing myocardial oxygen supply, prepare patient for PTCA (see PTCA, p. 226).
- Should pharmacological therapy and PTCA be ineffective in restoring myocardial oxygen supply, prepare patient for emergency CABG (see CABG, p. 194).
- Teach patient the importance of reporting chest pain.
- Teach patient to pace activities so not to increase HR and subsequently decrease myocardial tissue oxygen supply.
- Teach patient about the common side effects of vasodilators: headache, nausea, vomiting, or dizziness.
- Teach patient about the common side effects of positive inotropic agents.

Potential Complication: Increased Myocardial Oxygen Demand. Increased myocardial oxygen demand related to increased HR, increased preload, or increased afterload secondary to increased ventricular wall tension or vasoconstriction, which causes the failing myocardium to work harder to sustain adequate CO.

Expected Patient Outcomes. Patient maintains reduced myocardial oxygen demand, as measured by oxygen extraction ratio (O_2ER) of 25%, MAP 70 to 90 mm Hg, PCWP 6 to 12 mm Hg, pulse pressure (PP) 30 to 40 mm Hg, $S\bar{v}o_2$) 60% to 80%, rate pressure product (RPP) $\leq$12,000, SVR 900 to 1200 dynes/s/cm^{-5}, SVRI 1970 to 2300 dynes/s/cm^{-5} · m^2, right ventricular stroke work index (RVSWI) 7 to 12 g-m/beat/m^2, left ventricular stroke work index (LVSWI) 35 to 85 g-m/beat/m^2, oxygen consumption (Vo_2) $\geq$200 or $\leq$250 mL/min, oxygen consumption index (Vo_2I) $\geq$115 or $\leq$165 mL/min/m^2, BP within patient's normal range, HR $\leq$100 bpm, and temperature $\leq$100°F.

- Consult with the cardiologist to validate the expected patient outcomes that reflect decreased myocardial oxygen demand.
- Review with cardiologist the results from cardiac scans, coronary angiogram, and ECG.
- Limit physical activity to the level of activity that does not increase HR and thus increase myocardial oxygen demand.
- Position patient with the bed elevated 20 to 30 degrees to decrease myocardial oxygen demand.
- When patient progresses to a warm shower, provide chair and assistance with back washing or shampooing to minimize myocardial oxygen consumption.
- Keep patient on nothing by mouth (NPO) for the first 4 to 6 hours and then offer clear liquids for 24 hours to diminish the risk of aspiration should cardiac arrest or nausea or vomiting occur from prescribed drugs.
- After 24 hours or earlier, provide small portions of easily digested, low-sodium, low-saturated-fat foods as necessary.
- Calculate Vo_2I to evaluate the effectiveness of therapies that decrease myocardial demand.
- Estimate myocardial oxygen consumption by calculating RPP, which is determined by multiplying HR with SBP. The RRP correlates with myocardial oxygen consumption during rest and exercise.
- Obtain Vo_2 and Vo_2I in relationship to Do_2 and Do_2I. When Vo_2 (oxygen consumption) is limited by Do_2 (oxygen delivery), the Vo_2 is thought of as being supply-dependent. The rate of oxygen consumed is limited by the rate of oxygen delivered to the tissues.
- Monitor and report factors that may increase myocardial oxygen demand: hypotension, hypertension, tachycardia, increased contractility, pain, anxiety, fever, anemia, and volume depletion.
- Obtain, document, and report hemodynamic parameters that indicate increased myocardial oxygen demand as a result of decreased cardiac output: O_2ER $\geq$25%, PP $\leq$30 mm Hg, RPP $\geq$12,000, $S\bar{v}o_2$ $\leq$60%, SVR $\geq$1200 dynes/s/cm^{-5}, SVRI $\geq$2390

dynes/s/cm^{-5}/m^2, RVSWI $\leq$7 g-m/beat/m^2, LVSWI $\leq$25 g-m/beat/m^2, Vo_2 $\geq$250 mL/min, and Vo_2I $\geq$165 mL/min/m^2.

- Obtain and report other findings suggestive of increased myocardial oxygen demand because they increase metabolic activity and thus myocardial work load: HR $\geq$100 bpm, temperature $\geq$100.8°F and BP above patient's normal values.
- Initiate continuous ECG to assess HR and rhythm. Document ECG rhythm strips every 2 to 4 hours in patients with dysrhythmias.
- Administer prescribed oxygen 2 to 4 L/min (24% to 36% O$_2$) by means of nasal cannula, or Fio_2 $\leq$50% by mask to maintain Pao_2 $\geq$80 mm Hg and Sao_2 $\geq$95%.
- Administer prescribed IV fluids such as colloids should the patient be hypovolemic, with a CVP $\leq$6 mm Hg.
- Continuously monitor Svo_2, since a decreasing value $\leq$60% may indicate decreased CO and increased O$_2$ER ($\leq$25%).
- Promote rest by decreasing environmental stimuli, assisting with or performing personal care activities, and pacing patient activities to reduce myocardial oxygen demand.
- Administer prescribed direct peripheral vasodilator (nitroprusside), coronary vasodilator (nitroglycerin), or peripheral/coronary vasodilators (verapamil, nifedipine, or diltiazem) to decrease afterload by maintaining SVR 900 to 1200 dynes/s/cm^{-5} and SVRI 1970 to 2390 dynes/s/cm^{-5}/m^2. An increase in afterload of the left ventricle causes the left ventricle to develop more pressure during the systolic period, thereby increasing intramyocardial tension and oxygen consumption (see Table 1–4 and Table 1–6).
- Titrate IV nitroglycerin 10 μg/min at 10-minunte intervals or at preset limits to avoid hypotension ($\geq$90 mm Hg systolic), tachycardia (HR increase $\leq$20%), or bradycardia ($\geq$45 to 50 bpm).
- Administer prescribed positive inotropes (dopamine, dobutamine) or phosphodiesterase inhibitor (amrinone) to decrease preload by maintaining PCWP $\leq$12 mm Hg. An increased preload or filling pressure in the left ventricle increases tension because both internal pressure and the radius of the ventricular cavity increase with a decreasing thickness. The result is increased oxygen consumption (see Table 1–10).
- Teach patient to avoid behaviors that increase HR: excessive physical activity, straining at stool, anger, or irritability.
- Teach patient techniques to reduce myocardial tissue oxygen demand: guided imagery, meditation, or progressive relaxation.
- Teach patient to exhale with physical movement. This reduces the potential for increased intrathoracic pressure, which decreases venous return to the heart (decreased preload), and vagal stimulation, which causes a decrease in CO. When air is released, the intrathoracic pressure is decreased and preload is increased, causing increased work load for the heart.
- Teach patient the common side effects of beta-adrenergic blockers: dizziness, fatigue, headache, or bradycardia.
- Teach the patient about the common side effects of vasodilators: headache, nausea, vomiting, or dizziness.
- Teach patient to alleviate sources of psychological stress and use progressive muscular relaxation to decrease oxygen consumption.

Potential Complication: Decreased Cardiac Output. Decreased CO related to decreased myocardial contractility secondary to a loss of more than 40% myocardial muscle mass and decreased activator calcium to effect myocardial contraction.

Expected Patient Outcomes. Patient maintains adequate contractility, as inferred by measuring CO 4 to 8 L/min, CI 2.5 to 4.0 L/min/m^2, EF $\geq$50% to 60%, LVSW 60 to 80 g-m/beat, LVSWI 30 to 50 g-m/beat/m^2, RVSW 10 to 15 g-m/beat, RVSWI 7 to 12 g-m/beat/m^2, stroke volume (SV) 60 to 130 mL/beat, SVI 45 to 85 mL/m^2/beat, absence of crackles, normal heart sounds, and UO $\geq$30 mL/h or $\geq$0.5 mL/kg/h.

- Consult with cardiologist to validate the expected patient outcomes that indicate adequate myocardial contractility.
- Review results of chest roentgenogram and ECG.
- Restrict physical activity to bed rest in order to maintain 1.0 to 1.5 metabolic equivalents or the amount of oxygen consumed per minute at rest (approximately 3.5 to 5.0 mL/kg/min).
- Calculate LVSWI and RVSWI to infer the quality of myocardial contractility. Elevated values can indicate increased myocardial contractility, which can contribute to increased myocardial work load and increased myocardial oxygen demand or consumption.
- Obtain and report hemodynamic values indicating decreased myocardial contractility: EF $\leq$50%, CO $\leq$4 L/min, and CI $\leq$1.8 L/min/m^2, LVSW $\leq$60 g-m/beat, LVSWI $\leq$35 g-m/beat/m^2, RVSW $\leq$10 g-m/beat, RVSWI $\leq$7 g-m/beat/m^2, and SVI $\leq$35 mL/beat/m^2.
- Monitor, document, and report other clinical findings of decreased myocardial contractility: crackles, dyspnea, shortness of breath, RR $\geq$20 BPM, HR $\geq$100 bpm, chest pain, peripheral pulses $\leq$+2, capillary refill $\geq$3 seconds, BP $\leq$90/60 mm Hg, and fatigue.
- Monitor heart sounds for presence of S$_3$ and S$_4$ associated with rapid filling of noncompliant ventricle.
- Initiate continuous ECG to assess HR and rhythm. Document ECG rhythm strips every 2 to 4 hours in patients with dysrhythmias.
- Administer prescribed F$_{IO_2}$ $\leq$50% by mask or low-flow oxygen at 2 to 4 L/min (24% to 36% O$_2$) by nasal cannula to maintain Pao$_2$ $\geq$80 mm Hg or Sao$_2$ $\geq$95%.
- Administer prescribed IV fluids to maintain adequate circulatory volume as evidenced by CO $\geq$4 L/min, CI $\geq$2.7 L/min/m^2.
- Administer positive inotropes to facilitate contractility (dopamine, dobutamine) or phosphodiesterase inhibitor (amrinone) to maintain EF $\geq$50%, SV $\geq$60 mL/beat, SVI $\geq$45 mL/m^2/beat, RVSW $\geq$10 g-m/beat, RVSWI $\geq$7 g-m/beat/m^2, LVSW $\geq$60 g-m/beat, LVSWI $\geq$30 g-m/beat/m^2, CO $\geq$4 L/min, and CI $\geq$2.7 L/min/m^2 (see Table 1–10).
- Obtain and record hemodynamic data that confirms the need for IABP: hypotension (BP $\leq$90 mm Hg systolic, 60 mm Hg mean, or $\geq$30 mm Hg below previous basal levels), PCWP $\geq$16 to 18 mm Hg, and CI $\leq$2.0 L/min/m^2.
- Should pharmacological therapy be ineffective in improving myocardial contractility, assist with the initiation of IABP (see IABP, p. 254).
- Initiate continuous monitoring of IABP inflation and deflation indicators. The balloon deflates prior to systole, decreasing afterload, and inflates during diastole to promote coronary perfusion.
- Should IABP be ineffective in minimizing myocardial work load, assist in preparing patient for cardiac assist device (see cardiac assist device, p. 248).
- Teach patient to avoid Valsalva's maneuver such as straining at stool.

Potential Complication: Decreased Cardiac Output. Decreased CO related to increased left ventricular preload and afterload, secondary to impaired myocardial contractility and impaired ventricular compliance resulting from ischemia or infarction.

Expected Patient Outcomes. Patient maintains adequate left ventricular preload and afterload, as evidenced by BP $\geq$90/60 mm Hg, CO 4 to 8 L/min, CI 2.5 to 4.3 L/min/m^2, MAP 70 to 100 mm Hg, PAP systolic $\leq$25 mm Hg and diastolic $\leq$15 mm Hg, PCWP 16 to 18 mm Hg, PP 30 to 40 mm Hg, SVR 900 to 1200 dynes/s/cm^{-5}, and SVRI 1970 to 2390 dynes/s/cm^{-5}/m^2.

- Consult with cardiologist to validate the expected patient outcomes that reflect adequate left ventricular preload and afterload.
- Physician consults cardiologist about the appropriate use of IABP in patient with cardiogenic shock.

- Limit physical activity to bed rest to decrease ventricular wall tension and myocardial oxygen demand.
- Obtain, document, and report hemodynamic values that indicate increased left ventricular filling pressure or preload: PAP systolic ≥25 mm Hg and diastolic ≥15 mm Hg and PCWP ≥18 mm Hg.
- Calculate systemic vascular resistance and note trends. An increased value can reflect increased myocardial work load and myocardial oxygen demand.
- Obtain, document, and report hemodynamic values that indicate increased left ventricular afterload: MAP ≥100 mm Hg, SVR ≥1200 dynes/s/cm^{-5}, and SVRI ≥2390 dynes/s/cm^{-5}/m^2.
- Administered prescribed low-flow oxygen 2 to 4 L/min (24% to 36% O$_2$) by nasal cannula or F$_{IO_2}$ ≤ 50% by mask.
- Administer IV fluids as prescribed to maintain hydration, CO ≥4 L/min, CI ≥2.7 L/min/m^2, PCWP ≤18 mm Hg, and UO ≥30 mL/h or ≥0.5 mL/kg/h.
- Administer prescribed positive inotropes (dopamine, dobutamine) or phosphodiesterase inhibitor (amrinone) to maintain BP ≥90/60 mm Hg, CO 4 to 8 L/min, CI ≥2.7 L/min/m^2, PAP systolic ≤25 mm Hg and diastolic ≤15 mm Hg, and PCWP ≤12 mm Hg. Be cautious, as drugs may increase ventricular ectopy, size of infarction, or be ineffective if beta blockers have been administered (see Table 1–10).
- Administer vasodilators to lower systemic afterload, such as peripheral vasodilators (nitroprusside), to lower preload, such as coronary vasodilator (nitroglycerin), or peripheral/coronary vasodilators (verapamil, nifedipine, or diltiazem) to maintain BP ≥90/60 mm Hg, PP 30 to 40 mm Hg, SVR 900 to 1200 dynes/s/cm^{-5}, and SVRI 1970 to 2390 dynes/s/cm^{-5}/m^2 (see Table 1–4).
- Administer prescribed volume-reducing agents: thiazide (chlorothiazide, hydrochlorothiazide, chlorthalidone, metolazone), loop diuretics (furosemide or bumetanide) or potassium-sparing (spironolactone, amiloride or triamterene) to maintain UO ≥30

mL/h or ≥0.5 mL/kg/h and specific gravity 1.010 to 1.030 (see Table 1–13).
- Should pharmacological therapy be ineffective in reducing preload and afterload, assist with the insertion of an intra-aortic balloon pump (see IABP, p. 254).
- Teach patient the common side effects of diuretics and vasodilators.

Potential Complication: Dysrhythmias. Dysrhythmias related to compromised left ventricular function secondary to coronary artery disease or lactic acidosis.

Expected Patient Outcomes. Patient remains in sinus rhythm, serum electrolytes within normal range, HR 60 to 100 bpm and BP within patient's normal range.

- Consult with cardiologist about the underlying causes of dysrhythmias and medications used to correct them.
- Physician consults with cardiologist about the potential need for temporary or permanent pacemaker.
- Monitor serum potassium levels that may contribute to dysrhythmias: hyperkalemia ≥5.5 mEq/L and hypokalemia ≤3.8 mEq/L.
- Review results of serial 12-lead ECG to help evaluate the location, progression, resolution of infarction, and ventricular function.
- Review cardiac enzymes values for resolution or extension of acute myocardial infarction (AMI).
- Initiate continuous ECG to assess HR and rhythm. Document ECG rhythm strips every 2 to 4 hours in patients with dysrhythmias. Measure the basic PR, QRS, and QT intervals to obtain the patient's baseline (see ST segment monitoring, p. 264).
- Monitor and report physical signs and symptoms of dysrhythmias: abnormal HR and rhythm, palpitations, chest pain, syncope, ECG changes, and hypotension.
- Administer the prescribed low-flow oxygen 2 to 4 L/min (24% to 35% O$_2$) by means of a nasal cannula or F$_{IO_2}$ ≤50% by mask

should patient experience chest pain. This increases the amount of oxygen available for myocardial use.

- Measure the ECG components signifying Q wave infarctions evidenced by pathological Q waves ($\geq$0.04 s), ST segment elevation with reciprocal ST depression in the opposite leads, T wave changes positive, then negative in leads facing the infarcted area.
- Measure ECG components should hypokalemia occur in conjunction with diuretic therapy: decreased amplitude and broadening of T waves, prominent U waves, and sagging ST segments.
- Measure ECG components should hyperkalemia occur in conjunction with decreased renal arterial perfusion: peaked T waves of increased amplitude and biphasic QRS-T complexes.
- Replace potassium as needed and as prescribed. (See Renal Deviations, Hypokalemia, p. 485).
- Withhold potassium, and if potassium exceeds 6.0 mEq/L, administer prescribed sodium polystyrene sulfonate (Kayexalate), a sodium cycle sulfonic polystyrene exchange renin. (See Renal Deviations, Hyperkalemia, p. 485).
- Monitor ECG for increase in the number of premature ventricular contractions (PVCs) noting longer or more frequent episodes of PVCs. The PVCs reflect cardiac irritability. Frequent, multiple, or multifocal PVCs can cause decreased CO and lead to ventricular tachycardia, ventricular fibrillation, or cardiac arrest.
- Monitor ECG for changes from nonsustained ($\leq$30 seconds) ventricular tachycardia to sustained ($\geq$30 seconds) of ventricular tachycardia.
- Administer prescribed antidysrhythmia agents, depending upon the dysrhythmia's origin and potential risk for the patient (see Table 1–11).
- Should pharmacological therapy be ineffective in correcting persistent tachycardia or bradycardia; septal damage with high degree of block progression; inferior AMI with transient atrioventricular block; or persistent ectopy with compromised CO, prepare patient for pacemaker (see Pacemaker, p. 270).
- Teach patient to report an abnormal heart rate, syncope, or chest pain described on a scale of 1 to 10.
- Teach patient to avoid stimulants such as tobacco, caffeine, or alcohol, which may cause dysrhythmias.
- Teach patient the common side effects of antidysrhythmia medication.

DISCHARGE PLANNING

The critical care nurse will provide the patient and significant other(s) with verbal or written discharge notes regarding the following subjects:

1. The signs and symptoms that warrant immediate medical attention: chest pain, shortness of breath, fatigue, syncope, or weight gain.
2. A postdischarge exercise program to keep HR $\leq$100 bpm according to the following: (1) First week, walk 0.25 miles within 8 to 10 minutes; (2) second week, walk 0.25 miles within 5 minutes; (3) third week, walk 0.50 miles within 15 minutes; and (4) fourth week, walk 1.0 miles within 30 minutes. Teach patient and significant other(s) activity schedule.
3. The ways to reduce precipitating factors (activity following a heavy meal, sexual intercourse, anger, or grief) by taking prophylactic nitroglycerin, reducing physical activity and psychologic stress resulting in chest discomfort, and countering emotional stress by progressive physical activity.
4. Ceasing any activity that increases heart rate and blood pressure or causes fatigue. These behaviors can increase myocardial tissue oxygen demand.
5. Calling for emergency medical service if postactivity chest pain persists after resting for 10 minutes.

6. The names of community agencies that can enhance learning and provide support (e.g., American Heart Association).
7. The purpose, dosage, schedule, and side effects of medications.

■ CONGESTIVE HEART FAILURE

(For related information see Part I: Acute myocardial infarction, p. 38; Cardiogenic shock, p. 72; Acute chest pain, p. 1; Dysrhythmias, p. 184. Part II: Coronary artery bypass graft, p. 194. Part III: Percutaneous transluminal coronary angioplasty, p. 226; Coronary laser angioplasty, p. 228; Transluminal coronary atherectomy, p. 234; Intracoronary stents, p. 237; Intra-aortic balloon pump, p. 254; Thrombolytic therapy, p. 265; Hemodynamic monitoring, p. 219. See also Respiratory Deviations, Part I: Pulmonary embolism, p. 397; Pulmonary edema, p. 346. Part III: Pulse oximetry, p. 426; Mechanical ventilation, p. 428.)

Diagnostic Categories and Length of Stay
DRG: 127 Heart failure and shock
LOS: 6.0 days

Definition
Heart failure is a pathophysiological state in which an abnormality of cardiac function is responsible for the failure of the heart to pump blood at a rate adequate for the metabolic requirements of the tissue. Heart failure is considered in relation to myocardial failure and congestive heart failure. Myocardial failure is characterized by a decrease in the force and speed of muscle contractions. The decrease in heart function leads to an inability to provide enough cardiac output on demand to meet peripheral needs during exercise. Congestive heart failure (CHF) signifies systemic responses to an inadequate pump. There is enhanced sympathetic nervous activity, renal vasoconstriction, activation of the renin-angiotensin system with peripheral congestion and edema.

Pathophysiology
When CHF occurs with an increased myocardial work load, compensatory mechanisms respond to maintain adequate cardiac output. These compensatory responses consist of: (1) increased sympathetic activity, which causes an increase in the rate and force of contraction of the ventricles and vasoconstriction of the arterioles throughout the body; (2) increased activation of the renin-angiotensin-aldosterone mechanism, which augments blood volume through the aldosterone effect of sodium preservation, vasoconstriction causing increased blood pressure, increased systemic filling pressure, and venous return; the kidneys' compensation leads to enhanced preload, afterload, and contractility; (3) ventricular dilation occurs because of the increased volume of blood that enters the heart. The dilated heart requires more oxygen and blood flow, which may not be supplied by the coronary arteries; (4) myocardial hypertrophy with or without chamber dilation is a compensatory mechanism in which the heart increases its muscle mass; and (5) increased tissue oxygen extraction caused by decreased cardiac output and perfusion pressure. Left heart failure occurs when the output of the left ventricle is less than the total volume of blood received from the right side of the heart through the pulmonary circulation. The pulmonary circuit becomes congested with blood that cannot be moved forward, thereby causing decreased systemic blood pressure. Right heart failure occurs when the output of the right ventricle is less than the input from the systemic venous circuit. The systemic circuit is congested and output to the lung decreases. Other hemodynamic alterations include elevated ventricular end-diastolic pressure, pulmonary artery pressure, right ventricular pressure, right atrial pressure, central venous pressure, systemic vascular resistance, and pulmonary venous pressure. There is also decreased cardiac output, ejection fraction, tissue perfusion, renal perfusion, and renal function. Eventually the individual experiences increased pulmonary congestion.

Nursing Assessment

PRIMARY CAUSES

- Increased preload can cause CHF from volume overload, intracardiac shunt, papillary muscle dysfunction, or rupture of chordae tendineae. Decreased myocardial contractility can result from coronary artery disease, ischemia, infarction, arrhythmias, cardiomyopathy, ventricular aneurysm, myocarditis, constrictive pericarditis, or cardiac tamponade. Factors causing increased afterload that also contribute to CHF include primary or secondary hypertension, pulmonary hypertension, pulmonary embolism, aortic stenosis, or coarctation of the aorta. Finally, increased metabolic demands can cause decompensation where there is an underlying heart condition, and these include anemia, fever, septic shock, thyrotoxicosis, beriberi, Paget's disease, or arteriovenous fistulas.

RISK FACTORS

- History of prior acute myocardial infarction (AMI), coronary artery disease, hypertension, diabetes, cigarette smoking, obesity, and poor total to high-density lipoprotein (HDL) cholesterol ratio.

PHYSICAL ASSESSMENT

- Inspection: Right heart failure signs and symptoms include peripheral edema, ankle swelling, ascites, nausea, vomiting, fatigue, weakness, decreased urinary output, anorexia, dilated superficial abdominal veins, weight gain, increased jugular venous pressure, or neck vein distention. Left heart failure signs and symptoms consist of dyspnea, paroxysmal nocturnal dyspnea, orthopnea, breathlessness, tachypnea, anxiety, cyanosis or pallor, moist cough, diaphoresis, fatigue, weakness, memory loss, confusion, anorexia, or forceful and diffuse apex beat.
- Palpation: Right heart failure leads to abdominal pain, hepatomegaly, splenomegaly, cool and dry skin, diminished peripheral pulses, dependent pitting edema, or positive hepatojugular reflex. Left heart failure causes thrills, pulsus alternans, or cool and moist skin.
- Auscultation: Right-sided S_3, accentuated P_2, or murmurs signify right heart failure. Left heart failure is auscultated as tachycardia, Cheyne-Stokes, arrhythmias (tachycardia, atrial fibrillation); hypotension; decreased S_1, S_3 and S_4 gallop; or basilar crackles or wheezes.

DIAGNOSTIC TEST RESULTS

Hemodynamic Parameters. (See Table 1–9)

- Cardiac output (CO) $\leq$4 L/min/m^2, cardiac index (CI) $\leq$2.7 L/min/m^2, central venous pressure (CVP) $\geq$6 mm Hg, saturation mixed-venous oxygen (S$\bar{v}$o$_2$) $\leq$60%, pulmonary capillary wedge pressure (PCWP) $\geq$15–18 mm Hg and systemic vascular resistance (SVR) $\geq$1200 dynes/s/cm^{-5}.

Standard Laboratory Tests. (See Table 1–1)

- Arterial blood gases: Pao$_2$ $\leq$60 to 70 mm Hg, Paco$_2$ $\leq$35 mm Hg, pH $\leq$7.35, and HCO$_3$ $\leq$22 mEq/L.
- Blood studies: Hemoglobin $\leq$12 g/100mL and hematocrit $\leq$38%.
- Serum chemistry: serum albumin $\leq$3.3 g/dL as a result of decreased protein intake or proteinuria; blood urea nitrogen (BUN) $\geq$20 mg/dL and creatinine $\geq$1.2 mg/dL; or dilutional hyponatremia $\leq$130 mEq/L, hypokalemia $\leq$3.8 mEq/L, or hyperkalemia $\geq$5.5 mEq/L.
- Serum enzymes: serum glutamic-oxaloacetic transaminase (SGOT) $\geq$200 U/L, serum glutamate pyruvate transaminase (SGPT) $\geq$32 U/L, and LDH $\geq$155 U/L in hepatic congestion.
- Urinalysis: Creatinine $\geq$1.9 g/24 h, proteinuria, and high specific gravity $\geq$1.030.

Invasive Cardiac Diagnostic Procedure. (See Table 1–2)

- Cardiac scan: Technetium–99m stannous pyrophosphate imaging or thallium 201 scan documents areas of decreased myocardial perfusion, measure of ejection fraction or wall motion.

Noninvasive Cardiac Diagnostic Procedures. (See Table 1–3)

- Chest roentgenogram: In left heart failure there is cardiac enlargement, as noted by increased size of the left ventricular shadow and cardiothoracic ratio ≥0.50. The left ventricle extends past the midclavicular line and fluid effusion may be present throughout the lung fields. With right heart failure, the right ventricular shadow can be seen extending out from the right sternal border. In addition, pulmonary markings may be decreased as a result of decreased pulmonary circulation.
- M-mode echocardiogram: Systolic dysfunction manifests itself as left ventricular enlargement, poor ejection fraction (0.25%), deficient contraction of the interventricular septum (IVS) and posterior wall (PW), an increase in septal E-point separation (SEPS), and prominence of the left atrium (LA). Diastolic dysfunction is shown as normal ejection fraction (0.75%), dysfunctional ventricular filling and left ventricular hypertrophy.

ECG

- Findings include patterns of ventricular hypertrophy, myocardial ischemia, injury, or infarction. Dysrhythmias such as tachycardia, atrial fibrillation, and premature ventricular contractions also can be seen.

MEDICAL AND SURGICAL MANAGEMENT

PHARMACOLOGY

- Vasodilators: Vasodilators work by dilating the venous bed or arteriolar bed. When the venous bed is dilated, blood is pulled into the peripheral circulation, causing a reduction of left ventricular filling pressure (preload). Venodilators can enhance exercise tolerance and relieve symptoms in heart failure. Drugs in this category include isosorbide dinitrate (Isordil), erithrityl tetranitrate (Cardilate), erythritol tetranitrate (Peritrate), and nitroglycerin (see Table 1–4). Arteriolar vasodilation decrease impedance to left ventricular emptying (afterload), which improves CO, stroke volume, and tissue perfusion. Non–calcium-channel-dependent arterial vasodilators serve to increase CO and decrease SVR. Drugs in this category include hydralazine, dipyridamole, or minoxidil (see Table 1–4). Calcium channel blockers induce arterial vasodilation and subsequently reduce left ventricular afterload. These drugs include verapamil, nifedipine, and diltiazem (see Table 1–6). Second generation calcium channel blockers stimulate coronary and systemic vasodilation; however, they are less likely to produce cardiodepression. They have a greater specificity for vascular smooth muscle than for papillary muscle. These drugs include nicardipine and isradipine (see Table 1–6). While all calcium channel blockers may adversely affect the CHF patient's hemodynamic status, it is believed they may be considered for CHF patients with coexisting clinical conditions such as angina pectoris, arrhythmias, or hypertension causing left ventricular dysfunction.

  Balanced venous and arterial dilators include IV nitroprusside (0.25 μg/kg/min), which acts by dilating arteriolar beds (reduce afterload) and dilating venous beds (reduce preload). The result is a decrease in PCWP and increase in CO (see Table 1–4).
- Positive Inotropes: Inotropic agents improve contractility by improving CO and maintaining an adequate systolic blood pressure. Dopamine (2 to 5 μg/kg/min) increases stroke volume, CO, and renal blood flow, and decreases SVR. Dobutamine (2 to 5 μg/kg/min) directly increases CO, decreases left ventricular filling pressure, and indirectly decreases SVR. Optimal CO is achieved at doses of 10 to 15 μg/kg/min. Amrinone increases CO directly and indirectly, reduces left ventricular filling pres-

sure, and reduces myocardial oxygen demand and consumption (see Table 1–10).

- Diuretics: All diuretic agents block the reabsorption of sodium by renal epithelial cells and thereby diminish water reabsorption. The specific diuretic agent given is based on the location in the nephron where if exerts its primary effect. Diuretics can be categorized as distal tubular, loop, and proximal tubular agents. Distal tubular agents block only 5% to 10% of the filtered load of sodium and are minimally effective when renal dysfunction occurs. Loop diuretics block 25% of the filtered load of sodium, increase CO, and reduce preload. Proximal tubular agents inhibit hydrogen ion secretion, which reduces bicarbonate absorption, causing its excretion in urine (see Table 1–13).
- Neurohormonal agents: In heart failure, the renin-angiotensin system is activated, which causes renin release from the juxtaglomerular cells. Renin acts on angiotensinogen to form angiotensin I. Angiotensin I is converted to the potent vasoconstrictor angiotensin II by angiotensin-converting enzyme (ACE). Neurohormonal activation is decreased through use of ACE inhibitors such as captopril, enalapril, ramipril, or lisinopril (see Table 1–12).
- Morphine sulfate: Morphine is used to relieve pain, promote vasodilation, and decrease venous return, preload, and sympathetic tone, and to decrease myocardial oxygen demand or consumption.

OXYGEN THERAPY

- Supplemental oxygen is given to reduce the work load of the heart and to support cellular energy requirements.

DIET

- Restriction of dietary intake of sodium. The renin-angiotensin-aldosterone mechanism is initiated by sympathoadrenergic stimulation, which causes increased tubular reabsorption of sodium and water. In severe CHF, the body can retain 10 L of fluid and

80 g of sodium. This may require sodium restriction of 0.2 to 1.0 g/d.

HEMODYNAMIC MONITORING

- Used to measure ventricular function, CO, pulmonary function, and circulating volume. Also used to evaluate the effectiveness of pharmacological interventions that decrease preload and afterload while increasing contractility (see Hemodynamic monitoring, p. 219).

PHYSICAL ACTIVITY

- Modify activity in patients with CHF to reduce the work load demands on the heart. Isometric exercises are discouraged, since they cause an increase in blood pressure and cardiac work load.
- The metabolic equivalent (MET) can be used to determine the amount of oxygen consumed per kilogram of body weight per minute at rest. This is approximately 3.5 mL/kg/min. Level I activities use 1.0 to 1.5 MET, or approximately 3.5 to 5.2 mL/kg/min: bed rest, complete bed bath, feeding self, and turning; Level II activities use 1.5 to 2.5 MET or approximately 3.5 to 8.7 mL/kg/min: bed rest, feeding self, washing face, shave in bed, bedside commode, up in chair 20 to 30 minutes, and light recreational activity such as reading; and Level III activities use 1.5 to 3.0 MET or approximately 5.2 to 10.4 mL/kg/min: patient assists with own bath, patient stands while vital signs are taken.

INTRA-AORTIC BALLOON PUMP (IABP)

- IABP is used to temporarily support the failing heart and systemic circulation. The benefits are improved coronary artery perfusion by augmentation of arterial diastolic pressure, diminished resistance to left ventricular ejection, and a decrease in ventricular work load and myocardial oxygen demand or consumption (see IABP, p. 254).

CARDIAC ASSIST DEVICE

- Short-term mechanical support: Used as a bridge device, which temporarily assumes the function of the ventricle, in contrast to the IABP, which serves to augment CO. Ventricular assist devices can be divided into pulsatile devices (ABIOMED BVS-500), which produce systolic and diastolic flow and pressure, and centrifugal devices, which provide nonpulsatile flow that generates a steady flow with constant pressure (see Cardiac Assist device, p. 248).

- Intermediate Term Support: Provides temporary support until cardiac recovery occurs. Devices such as Novacor and HeartMate provide circulatory support for longer periods of time in transplant candidates who will not experience cardiac recovery. Both devices utilize left ventricular apical cannulation to facilitate high flow (see Cardiac assist device, p. 248).

EXTRACORPOREAL MEMBRANE OXYGENATION (EMO)

- EMO can be used during emergency situations to stabilize the cardiopulmonary system. It serves to maintain systemic blood flow, metabolic acid–base balance, and normal blood oxygen levels without the use of high inspiratory pressures or high inspired oxygen concentration (see Extracorporeal membrane oxygenation p. 437).

SURGICAL INTERVENTIONS

- Coronary Artery Bypass Graft (CABG): The candidate for CABG with depressed left ventricular function has three-vessel coronary disease, graftable coronary arteries, and the absence of biventricular failure (see CABG, p. 194).
- Heart Transplantation: A mode of treatment for patients with end-stage heart failure. Ischemic cardiomyopathy accounts for 40% to 50% of all transplants performed (see Heart transplantation, p. 211).
- Dynamic Cardiomyoplasty: Dynamic cardiomyoplasty is a new surgical technique for patients with end-stage ischemic or idiopathic cardiomyopathy. The patient's left ventricular ejection fraction is ≤40% and ≥15%. The goal is to increase ventricular ejection and decrease evolution of the un-

derlying disease process. A cardiomyostimulator is a new implantable pacemaker. The device provides short bursts of frequent stimuli, causing prolonged and more forceful contraction. The pacer senses the QRS complex and emits pulses that stimulate the thoracodorsal nerve, which causes sustained contraction of the latissimus dorsi muscle in synchrony with ventricular systole. Pulse train stimulation (PTS) transforms the fatiguable skeletal muscle into a fatigue-resistant muscle. The entire process of conditioning the latissimus dorsi takes 2 to 3 months.

NURSING MANAGEMENT: NURSING DIAGNOSES AND COLLABORATIVE PROBLEMS

Nursing Diagnoses

Common nursing goals are to improve myocardial tissue perfusion, establish effective breathing, prevent complications such as impaired skin integrity, fatigue, and activity intolerance and promote a sense of control.

Altered cardiopulmonary tissue perfusion related to reduced arterial blood flow secondary to impaired myocardial contractility.

Expected Patient Outcomes. Patient maintains adequate cardiopulmonary tissue perfusion, as evidenced by CO 4 to 8 L/min, CI 2.7 to 4.3 L/min/m^2, coronary artery perfusion pressure (CAPP) 60 to 80 mm Hg, systolic blood pressure (BP) ≥90 mm Hg, diastolic BP 60 to 90 mm Hg, PCWP ≤15 to 18 mm Hg, heart rate (HR) ≤100 bpm, absence of crackles, absence of dysrhythmias and pain, arterial blood gases within normal range, mean arterial pressure (MAP) 70 to 100 mm Hg, saturation of arterial oxygen (Sao$_2$) ≥95%, mixed venous arterial saturation (S$\bar{v}$o$_2$) 60% to 80%, and capillary refill ≤3 s.

- Consult with physician to validate the expected patient outcomes reflecting adequate cardiopulmonary tissue perfusion.
- Review results of arterial blood gases, chest roentgenogram, and ECG.

- Limit physical activity to bed rest to decrease myocardial work load and myocardial oxygen demand or consumption.
- Obtain and report hemodynamic parameters that reflect decreased cardiopulmonary tissue perfusion: CO $\leq$4 L/min, CI $\leq$2.7 L/min/m^2, CAPP $\leq$60 mm Hg, MAP $\leq$70 mm Hg, and Svo$_2$ $\leq$60%.
- Obtain and report other clinical findings that suggest decreased cardiopulmonary tissue perfusion: capillary refill $\geq$3 s, dyspnea, crackles, dysrhythmias, and chest pain.
- Administer inotropic agents (dopamine, dobutamine) to maintain CO $\geq$4 L/min, CI $\geq$2.7 L/min/m^2, CAPP $\geq$60 mm Hg, MAP $\geq$70 mm Hg, and PCWP $\leq$18 mm Hg (see Table 1–10).
- Initiate continuous monitoring of ECG to assess HR and rhythm. Document ECG rhythm strips every 2 to 4 hours in patients with dysrhythmias.
- Administer prescribed oxygen 2 to 4 L/min (24% to 36% O$_2$) by means of nasal cannula or Fio$_2$ $\leq$50% by mask to maintain in Pao$_2$ $\geq$80 mm Hg and Sao$_2$ $\geq$90%.
- Administer prescribed IV fluids to maintain adequate circulating volume.
- Teach patient to report any chest pain.
- Teach patient common side effects of inotropic agents.

Ineffective breathing pattern related to loss of alveolar elasticity secondary to vascular engorgement, restricted lung expansion, or hyperventilation.

Expected Patient Outcomes. Patient is able to maintain effective breathing pattern, as evidenced by arterial blood gases within normal range, absence of abnormal or adventitious breath sounds, respiration rate (RR) 12 to 20 BPM, and absence of dyspnea.

- Consult with physician about the underlying causes of ineffective breathing pattern.
- Consult with physician about clinical findings suggesting ineffective breathing pattern and potential need for intubation or ventilatory support.

- Review results of arterial blood gases and chest roentgenogram.
- Limit activity to bed rest and place patient in semi-Fowler's position to facilitate diaphragmatic descent during inspiration and ventilation of basilar lung areas.
- Monitor respiratory function such as RR, rhythm, and use of accessory muscles.
- Obtain and report clinical findings suggestive of ineffective breathing pattern: diminished or absent breath sounds, crackles or rhonchi, dyspnea or orthopnea.
- Encourage patient to cough and deep breathe to clear airways and enhance oxygen delivery.
- Position patient for maximal excursion and comfort.
- Initiate nasopharyngeal, oropharyngeal, or endotracheal suctioning, using unit protocol, should patient be unable to cough up excess secretions.
- Provide prescribed spirometry to enhance ventilation and effective breathing.
- Teach patient the importance of turning, deep breathing, and coughing.

High risk for impaired skin integrity related to poor nutritional state, impaired circulation, or edema.

Expected Patient Outcomes. Patient demonstrates skin integrity free of pressure ulcers or edema.

- Consult with physician and dietitian about the malnourished patient's diet: increased protein and carbohydrate intake to maintain a positive nitrogen balance.
- Review serum protein, hemoglobin, and hematocrit values.
- Provide prescribed high-protein diet.
- Observe skin for redness, blanching, edema, warmth, and diaphoresis.
- Monitor areas at risk for developing ulcers during each position change: ears, occiput, heels, sacrum, scrotum, elbows, ischium, or scapula.
- Turn patient or encourage patient to turn or shift weight every 30 minutes to 2 hours, depending on the patient's nutritional state.

- Obtain and report signs of tissue breakdown and use unit standard to treat.
- Massage around reddened or blanched areas to improve blood flow, thereby minimizing tissue hypoxia.
- Encourage patient to use range-of-motion exercises to increase blood flow to all areas.
- Use foam blocks or pillows to support the body above and below the high-risk area so it does not touch the bed surface.
- Provide prescribed alternating-pressure or eggcrate mattress or sheepskin to improve circulation and reduce skin pressure areas.
- Provide antiembolic support stockings to prevent venous stasis.
- Support feet with a footboard to prevent sliding.
- Assist patient out of bed as ordered.
- Instruct patient as to the importance of changing position while on bed rest.

Altered urinary elimination pattern related to decreased renal perfusion or altered renin-angiotensin-aldosterone mechanism secondary to decreased CO.

Expected Patient Outcomes. Patient maintains adequate pattern of urinary elimination, as evidenced by a urinary output (UO) $\geq$30 mL/h or $\geq$0.5 mL/kg/h, specific gravity 1.010 to 1.030, resolution of peripheral edema, resolution of adventitious breath sounds, absence of dyspnea, BUN 8 to 20 mg/dL, serum creatinine M: 0.8 to 1.2 mg/dL or W: 0.6 to 0.9 mg/dL, and serum electrolytes within normal range.

- Consult with cardiologist about the desired or expected urinary pattern.
- Review BUN, creatinine, serum electrolytes, and ECG.
- Obtain and report the following: UO $\leq$30 mL/h or $\leq$0.5 mL/kg/h, specific gravity $\geq$1.030, BP $\leq$90/60 mm Hg, dependent edema, crackles, dyspnea, and mental changes such as irritability or confusion.
- Monitor patient for signs and symptoms of hypokalemia: fatigue, weakness, anorexia, abdominal distention, apathy, depression, respiratory muscle weakness, respiratory muscle paralysis, hypotension, and dysrhythmias.
- Administer prescribed potassium to restore serum potassium to normal range.
- Initiate continuous ECG to assess HR and rhythm and document ECG rhythm strips every 2 to 4 hours in patients with hypokalemia-induced dysrhythmias: peaked P wave, prolonged PR intervals, flattened T wave, depressed ST segment, and U wave.
- Administer prescribed IV fluids to maintain adequate circulating volume, hydration, and UO $\geq$30 mL/h or $\geq$0.5 mL/kg/h.
- Administer ACE inhibitors (captopril, enalapril) to enhance the excretion of sodium and water, reduce preload and filling pressures, and reduce intravascular volume (see Table 1–12).
- Administer volume-reducing agents (furosemide, bumetanide) to maintain UO $\geq$30 mL/h or $\geq$0.5 mL/kg/h and specific gravity 1.010 to 1.30 (see Table 1–13).
- Should pharmacological therapy be ineffective in correcting the altered pattern of urinary elimination, prepare the patient for ultrafiltration (see Renal Deviations, Ultrafiltration, p. 505).
- Teach patient the common side effects of diuretics.

Fatigue related to increased tissue oxygen extraction secondary to decreased CO.

Expected Patient Outcomes. Patient maintains decreased tissue oxygen extraction, as evidenced by a BP $\geq$90 to 60 mm Hg or within the patient's normal range, capillary refill $\leq$3 s, arterial-venous oxygen content difference $(C[a - v]o_2)$ 4 to 6 mL/100mL, CAPP 60 to 80 mm Hg, CO 4 to 8 L/min, CI 2.7 to 4.3 L/min/m^2, oxygen delivery (Do_2) 900 to 1200 mL/min, oxygen delivery index (Do_2I) 500 to 600 mL/min/m^2, HR $\leq$90 bpm, oxygen extraction ratio (O_2ER) 25%, MAP 70 to 90 mm Hg, rate pressure product (RPP) $\leq$12,000, SVR 900–1200 dynes/s/cm^{-5}, systemic vascular resistance index (SVRI) 1970 to 2390 dynes/s/cm^{-5}/m^2, S$\bar{v}$o$_2$ of 60% to 80%, oxygen consumption (Vo$_2$) $\geq$200 or $\leq$250 mL/min, oxygen consumption index (Vo$_2$I) $\leq$115 or $\leq$165 mL/min/m^2, and hemoglobin within normal range.

- Consult with cardiologist to validate the expected patient outcomes used to evaluate the absence of fatigue and appropriate tissue oxygen extraction.
- Consult with dietitian about providing small, frequent meals to decrease energy required for digestion.
- Review arterial blood gases, hemoglobin, and Sao$_2$.
- Limit activity to bed rest should patient experience fatigue secondary to increased oxygen demand or consumption.
- Monitor and report hemodynamic parameters reflective of increased tissue oxygen extraction: C(a − v)o$_2$ $\geq$6 mL/100mL, CO $\leq$4 L/min, Do$_2$ $\leq$900 mL/min, Do$_2$I $\leq$500 mL/min/m^2, O$_2$ER $\geq$25%, Vo$_2$ $\leq$200 mL/min, Vo$_2$I $\leq$115 mL/min/m^2, SVR $\geq$1200 dynes/s/cm^{-5}, and SVRI $\geq$2390 dynes/s/cm^{-5}/m^2.
- Obtain, document, and report other clinical findings associated with increased tissue oxygen extraction: pale skin, fatigue, central cyanosis, or dyspnea.
- Administer prescribed oxygen 2 to 4 L/min (24% to 36% O$_2$) can decrease fatigue by making more oxygen available to the tissue.
- Provide frequent rest periods to conserve energy, decrease cardiac work load, and decrease oxygen demand.
- Organize care to avoid fatigue by maintaining rest periods between procedures, having patient rest before and after meals, and maintaining planned rest periods.
- Instruct patient to pace and prioritize activities: identify priorities and eliminate nonessential activity, distribute difficult tasks throughout the day, and rest before difficult activities.
- Teach patient the causes of his or her fatigue.

Activity intolerance related to weakness and fatigue secondary to loss of 25% of myocardial functional mass.

Expected Patient Outcomes. Patient maintains tolerance to increased activity, as evidenced by normal sinus rhythm, RR $\leq$24 BPM, HR $\leq$120 bpm (within 20 bpm of resting HR), BP within 20 mm Hg of patient's normal range, and absence of chest pain.

- Confer with cardiologist and cardiac rehabilitation about an individualized activity program.
- Monitor and report findings reflective of activity intolerance: chest pain, HR $\geq$120 bpm, RR $\geq$24 BPM, dysrhythmias, BP $\geq$20 mm Hg of normal range, fatigue, and dyspnea.
- Administer prescribed vasodilator, (nitroglycerin [NTG]) before activity: NTG to maintain HR $\leq$120 bpm, RR $\leq$24 BPM, BP within patient's normal range and absence of chest pain.
- Monitor patient's BP, HR, and RR before, during, and after progressive increases in physical activity.
- Provide diversional activities such as TV, radio, books to help patient cope with inactivity.
- Teach patient to monitor pulse rate while increasing activity.
- Instruct patient to report symptoms of activity intolerance: fatigue, dyspnea, or chest pain.

Powerlessness related to inability to control the illness experience, treatments, procedures, or life-style change.

Expected Patient Outcome. Patient gains control over some aspects of care to increase feelings of powerfulness.

- Encourage communication between the patient and health care providers.
- Explain the purpose behind supportive or diagnostic procedures and unit protocol.

- Encourage patient to ask questions.
- Allow patient to control his or her surroundings, such as deciding where to put cards, drawings from children or grandchildren, or reading material.
- Provide opportunities for patients and family to participate in care, when realistic.
- Provide opportunities for control by allowing patient to make decisions about daily activities.
- Encourage patient to look at the positive aspects of the illness experience.
- Teach patient how to use guided imagery or relaxation strategies.

Collaborative Problems

Common collaborative goals for patients with CHF are to reduce myocardial work load, improve myocardial contractility, improve oxygenation, and reduce peripheral fluid volume excess.

Potential Complication: Decreased Cardiac Output. Decreased CO related to diastolic dysfunction secondary to the inability of heart to relax after systole and impaired ventricular filling as a result of hypertrophied ventricular muscle.

Expected Patient Outcomes. Patient is able to maintain adequate CO, as evidenced by CVP 4 to 6 mm Hg, MAP 70 to 100 mm Hg, peripheral arterial pressure (PAP) systolic 15 to 25 mm Hg or diastolic 8 to 15 mm Hg, and PCWP $\leq$15 to 18 mm Hg.

- Consult with cardiologist to validate the expected patient outcomes that indicate adequate preload and afterload for CHF patient.
- Review chest roentgenogram, ECG, serum enzymes, and electrolytes.
- Limit physical activity to semi- to-high Fowler's position to reduce cardiac work load and maintain 1.5 to 2.5 MET or oxygen consumption at approximately 3.5 to 8.7 mL/kg/min.

- Use bedside commode as prescribed when cardiac work load can sustain 3 MET or approximately 10.4 mL/kg/min oxygen consumption.
- Provide prescribed low-sodium diet.
- Obtain and report hemodynamic parameters reflective of increased preload: MAP $\leq$70 mm Hg, CVP $\geq$6 mm Hg, PAP systolic 15 to 25 mm Hg or diastolic 8 to 15 mm Hg, and PCWP $\leq$15 to 18 mm Hg.
- Auscultate the lungs for the presence of crackles, rhonchi, or wheezes when PCWP $\geq$18 mm Hg.
- Avoid excess reduction in PCWP (preload) with diuretics, as this will compromise filling of the noncompliant left ventricle
- Administer prescribed loop diuretics (furosemide, bumetanide) to decrease PCWP $\leq$18 mm Hg.
- Monitor daily weight, intake, and output to determine if diuretics have been effective in decreasing intravascular volume and reducing preload.
- Monitor patient for side effects of diuretic therapy: fatigue, muscle cramps, hypotension, and tachycardia, hypokalemia, or hyponatremia.
- Administer prescribed IV fluids to maintain adequate circulating volume when diuretic therapy is also prescribed.
- Should diuretics be used for long-term control of heart failure, they are given with prescribed arterial and venous vasodilator ACE inhibitors (captopril, enalapril) to maintain pulse pressure (PP) 30 to 40 mm Hg, SVR $\leq$1200 dynes/s/cm^{-5}, and SVRI $\leq$2390 dynes/s/cm^{-5}/m^2 (See Table 1–13).
- Administration of inotropes (digitalis, dobutamine) and arterial vasodilators may be deleterious in patients with pure diastolic dysfunction, since these agents increase myocardial oxygen demand (MVO_2) and compromise relaxation and filling.
- Administration of vasodilators in patients with pure diastolic dysfunction reduces a normal SVR, causing hypotension and re-

flex tachycardia. This further contributes to diastolic dysfunction by reducing preload and time available for diastolic filling.

- Administer prescribed beta blockers (diltiazem, verapamil) and calcium channel blockers concurrently to decrease myocardial oxygen demand and improve relaxation. They also increase left ventricular filling and diastolic volume by decreasing HR and lengthening left ventricular diastolic filling time (see Table 1–6 and Table 1–5).
- NTG may be prescribed at doses up to 1 μg/kg/min to control preload in patients with diastolic dysfunction, while also decreasing ischemia and improving relaxation of the left ventricle. Give 0.25 μg/kg/min increments every 5 minutes up to 1 μg/kg/min, being careful not to decrease MAP so that compensatory tachycardia occurs (see Table 1–4).
- Obtain and record blood pressure and PCWP while titrating nitroglycerin or nitroprusside.
- Monitor patient for side effects of vasodilator therapy: headache, dizziness, hypotension, postural hypotension, muscle weakness or syncope.
- Should nitroprusside be ineffective in reducing filling pressure without decreasing SBP ≤90 mm Hg, add dobutamine or dopamine.
- Administer prescribed morphine to relieve pain, reduce venous return, and reduce myocardial oxygen consumption.
- Initiate continuous monitoring ECG to assess heart rate and rhythm. Document ECG rhythm strips every 2 to 4 hours in patient with dysrhythmias due to hypoxia, acidosis or electrolyte imbalance.
- Should pharmacological therapy be ineffective in reducing left ventricular afterload, prepare patient for IABP (see IABP, p. 254).
- Instruct the patient regarding the purposes of various treatments and lifestyle changes.
- Teach patient about the common side effects of afterload reducing agents.

Potential Complication: Decreased Cardiac Output. Decreased CO related to systolic dysfunction secondary to poor contractility resulting from coronary artery disease or deficit in ability of the myofibrils to shorten.

Expected Patient Outcomes. Patient maintains adequate CO, as evidenced by CO 4 to 8 L/min and CI 2.7 to 4.3 L/min/m^2, ejection fraction (EF) $\geq$ 50%, left ventricular stroke work (LVSW) 60 to 80 g-m/beat, left ventricular stroke work index (LVSWI) 30 to 50 g-m/beat/m^2, MAP 70 to 90 mm Hg, (S$\bar{v}$O$_2$) 60% to 80%, right ventricular stroke work (RVSW) 10 to 15 g-m/beat, right ventricular stroke work index (RVSWI) 7 to 12 g-m/beat/m^2, stroke volume (SV) 60 to 130 mL/beat, stroke volume index (SVI) 35 to 50 mL/beat/m^2, PP 30 to 40 mm Hg, pulmonary vascular resistance (PVR) 155 to 255 dynes/s/cm^{-5}, pulmonary vascular resistance index (PVRI) 200 to 450 dynes/s/cm^{-5}/m^2, SVR 900 to 1200 dynes/s/cm^{-5}, and SVRI 1970 to 2390 dynes/s/cm^{-5}/m^2.

- Consult with cardiologist to validate the expected patient outcomes used to evaluate adequate CO.
- Consult with cardiologist to establish a MAP parameter for hypertensive CHF patients who may require higher MAP values for perfusion to vital organs.
- Review results of echocardiography and desired hemodynamic parameters. Systolic dysfunction is defined by an EF ≤40% and a LVSWI ≤35 g-m/m^2.
- Review results of 12-lead ECG.
- Limit activity to bed rest and semi- to high Fowler's position to reduce myocardial oxygen demand.
- Provide prescribed small, frequent, easily digested meals to reduce myocardial work load and myocardial oxygen demand.
- Monitor systolic blood pressure (SBP) and MAP to determine the need for titration of IV medication. A MAP 60 to 75 mm Hg in a previously normotensive patient ensures adequate perfusion to vital organs

and is a parameter for evaluation of base therapy.

- Should CO be reduced, causing an underestimation of cuff arterial pressure, prepare patient for placement of an arterial line. This will enable accurate measuring of BP so that vasoactive drug therapy will not be prematurely discontinued.
- Obtain and report hemodynamic parameters indicating decreased CO related to systolic dysfunction: EF ≤50%, LVSW ≤60 g-m/beat, LVSWI ≤30 g-m/beat/m², MAP ≤70 mm Hg, RVSW ≤10 g-m/beat, RVSWI ≤7 g-m/beat/m², SV ≤60 mL/beat, SVI ≤35 mL/beat/m², and SVR ≥1200 dynes/s/cm⁻⁵.
- Maintain MAP 70 to 100 mm Hg to prevent myocardial ischemia. A MAP ≤60 mm Hg or SBP ≤80 mm Hg decreases coronary perfusion and blood flow, contributing to myocardial ischemia.
- Monitor patient's BP, HR, and RR before an activity, immediately upon completion of the activity, and 5 minutes after the activity's completion to determine whether metabolic demand and myocardial work load has been increased.
- Initiate continuous monitoring ECG readings to assess heart rate and rhythm. Document ECG rhythm strips every 2 to 4 hours in patients with dysrhythmias.
- Administer prescribed balanced vasodilators that affect venous and arterial beds, decreasing both filling pressures and resistance to left ventricular emptying at the same time. Nitroprusside, NTG, and amrinone are titrated to achieve a low normal SVR 900 to 950 dynes/s/cm⁻⁵ while maintaining mean arterial pressure at 60 to 70 mm Hg (see Table 1–4).
- Titrate IV nitroprusside alone or in combination with dobutamine at a rate of 0.25 μg/kg/min in increments every 10 to 15 minutes, provided mean arterial pressure is 60 to 75 mm Hg. Evaluate CI and SVR at 0.5 μg/kg/min increments (see Table 1–10).
- Titrate IV dobutamine, if prescribed, with nitroprusside for depressed LVSWI ≤35

g-m/m²/beat. Dobutamine, which is titrated first, is started at 2 μg/kg/min and titrated in 1 to 2 μg/kg/min increments every 10 to 15 minutes, provided HR ≤110 bpm. Evaluate CI and LVSWI with each 2 μg/kg/min increment of dobutamine.
- Should SVR be ≥1500 dynes/s/cm⁻⁵, nitroprusside can be added to dobutamine when LVSWI is ≥35 g-m/m²/beat or when dobutamine has been titrated to 5 μg/kg/min if LVSWI has not increased to 30 g-m/m²/beat. Note that dobutamine ≥7.5 μg/kg/min can increase myocardial oxygen demand.
- Administer prescribed IV amrinone in patient with increased SVR and reduced LVSWI and in patients with an inadequate response to dobutamine. Amrinone is initiated with a loading dose of 0.75 mg/kg over a period of 2 to 3 minutes. Continuous infusion is started at 5 μg/kg/min. Another loading dose can be initiated 30 minutes later. Evaluate CI, LVSWI, and SVR following all boluses and with each incremental change before the next dose adjustment. An effective dose is 5 to 10 μg/kg/min (see Table 1–10).
- Administer prescribed amrinone with dobutamine should CO and CI remain low. The combination gives a greater inotropic support and increases CO without increasing myocardial oxygen demand.
- Administer prescribed dobutamine or dopamine to support patient's BP when NTG is administered in doses ≥1 μg/kg/min if MAP is ≤60 to 57 mm Hg or LVSWI is compromised in the presence of adequate filling pressure (PCWP 14 to 18 mm Hg).
- Administer prescribed norepinephrine 8 to 12 μg/min should hypotension occur. Norepinephrine can be reduced by 1 to 2 μg/min increments every 5 to 10 minutes to a maintenance dose of 2 to 4 μg/min when MAP is 60 to 75 mm Hg (see Table 1–10).
- Administer prescribed loop diuretic (furosemide) in combination with renal dose dopamine (1 to 2 μg/kg/min) and IV morphine 1 to 2 mg in increment doses to reduce preload (see Table 1–13).

- Monitor transition from intravenous to oral agents in systolic dysfunction by weaning, proceeding from the inotropic agent to the vasodilator when combination therapy is used.
- During transition, administer prescribed hydralazine orally 25 mg every 6 hours while the patient is receiving dobutamine. Hydralazine is increased up to 50 to 200 mg every 6 hours, while the dobutamine infusion is reduced over 2 to 5 days (see Table 1–6).
- During transition, administer long-acting nitrates (isosorbide) 40 mg every 8 hours. This combines the arterial vasodilating effect of hydralazine with the increased venous capacitance effect of a long-acting nitrate (see Table 1–4).
- Provide an environment that fosters physical and emotional rest.
- Administer prescribed oxygen 2 to 4 L/min (24% to 36%) by nasal cannula or FiO_2 ≤50% by mask to enhance myocardial contractility by relieving hypoxia, reducing work load of the heart, and supporting cellular energy requirements.
- Administer prescribed IV fluids to maintain adequate circulating volume.
- Should pharmacological therapy be ineffective in increasing myocardial contractility, assist with IABP insertion (see IABP, p. 254).
- Should pharmacological therapy and IABP be ineffective in increasing myocardial contractility, assist with use of a cardiac assist device (see cardiac assist device, p. 248).
- Teach patient about common side effects of medications used to enhance myocardial contractility.

Potential Complication: Pulmonary Edema. Pulmonary edema related to transudation of fluid from capillaries to alveoli, increased volume in pulmonary capillary bed, and increased volume in pulmonary veins secondary to increased volume and end-diastolic left ventricular pressure or decreased emptying of the left ventricle.

Expected Patient Outcomes. Patient maintains normal intra-alveolar fluid volume, as evidenced by absence of crackles, absence of dyspnea, BP within patient's normal range, MAP 70 to 100 mm Hg; Pao_2 ≥80 mm Hg; $Paco_2$ 35 to 45 mm Hg; RR 12 to 20 BPM with normal depth; absence of dyspnea, crackles, and persistent cough; Sao_2 ≥95%; $S\bar{v}o_2$ 60% to 80%; and arterial-alveolar oxygen tension ratio ($Pao_2 - Pao_2$) of 0.75 to 0.90.

- Consult with physician to validate the nurse's established expected patient outcomes used to determine the resolution of pulmonary edema.
- Consult with physician about need for intubation or mechanical ventilation when patient doesn't respond to supplemental oxygen, diuretics, or positive inotropic agents.
- Consult with respiratory therapist about the patient's compatibility with mechanical ventilator and need for prescribed changes in tidal volume, oxygen, or positive end-expiratory pressure (PEEP).
- Review arterial blood gases and chest roentgenogram.
- Limit physical activity to chair rest or bed rest. The positions promote diuresis by recumbency-induced increase of glomerular filtration and reduction of antidiuretic hormone production. Keeping legs dependent will decrease venous return, increase venous pooling, and decrease preload.
- During periods of breathlessness, physical activity is restricted to bed rest with the head of bed elevated to allow for maximum lung expansion and legs placed in a dependent position to encourage venous pooling, which decreases venous return.
- Obtain and report the following signs and symptoms reflective of left ventricular failure and pulmonary edema: ineffective cough, dyspnea, bronchial wheezing, paroxysmal nocturnal dyspnea, orthopnea, cyanosis, pallor, confusion, pulsus alternans, S_3, S_4, and gallop rhythm.

- Obtain and report hemodynamic parameters contributing to pulmonary edema: PCWP $\geq$ 18 mm Hg.
- Continuously calculate arterial-alveolar oxygen tension ratio (PAO_2-PaO_2) as a measurement of the efficiency of gas exchange in the lungs. Report a value $\leq$ 0.75, which indicate diffusion problems.
- Administer prescribed volume-reducing agents (furosemide, bumetanide) to maintain UO $\geq$ 30 mL/h or $\geq$ 0.5 mL/kg/h, specific gravity $\leq$ 1.030, decrease neck vein distention, decrease venous return to the heart, and decrease preload.
- Administer prescribed low-dose morphine sulfate to promote decrease of venous and arterial vasoconstriction, which reduces preload and afterload; reduce edema; lessen pain; and reduce adventitious breath sounds, such as crackles.
- Administer prescribed inotropic agents (dopamine, dobutamine) to increase peripheral perfusion and enhance myocardial contractility (see Table 1–10).
- Administer peripheral vasodilator (nitroprusside) to decrease afterload (see Table 1–4).
- Initiate continuous monitoring of ECG readings to assess HR and rhythm. Document ECG rhythm strips every 2 to 4 hours.
- Monitor fluid volume status based on intake, output, specific gravity, and serum osmolality.
- Change patient's position every 2 hours. Limiting the time spent in a position that compromises oxygenation will improve PaO_2.
- Breath sounds are auscultated every 1 to 2 hours to assess for the onset or worsening of congestion by the presence of pink, frothy sputum.
- Suction patient by oropharyngeal or endotracheal tube as necessary by following the appropriate protocol of preoxygenation and postoxygenation to facilitate oxygen delivery.
- Administer prescribed supplemental oxygen 2 to 4 L/min (24% to 36% O_2) by means of nasal cannula or FIO_2 $\leq$ 50% by mask to maintain or improve oxygenation.
- While patient is receiving mechanical ventilation, monitor ventilatory settings, endotracheal tube patency, and respiratory status.
- Should pharmacological therapy be ineffective in reducing intra-alveolar edema, provide patient with mechanical ventilation to increase mean lung volume and to allow more alveoli to participate in gas exchange (see Respiratory Deviations, Part III: Mechanical ventilators, p. 428).
- Teach patient to cough, turn, and deep breathe every 1 to 2 hours if congested to clear airways and every 2 to 4 hours if not congested.

Potential Complication: Hypoxemia. Hypoxemia related to pulmonary congestion secondary to low CO (flow) syndrome.

Expected Patient Outcomes. Patient maintains adequate oxygen gas exchange, as measured by partial pressure of carbon dioxide in arterial blood ($PaCO_2$) 35 to 45 mm Hg, partial pressure of oxygen in arterial blood (PaO_2) 80 to 100 mm Hg, RR 12 to 20 BPM, oxygen saturation (SaO_2) 95.0% to 97.5%, and normal skin color.

- Consult with cardiologist to validate the expected patient outcomes used to evaluate the resolution of hypoxemia.
- Review results from arterial blood gases (PaO_2 80 to 100 mm Hg, $PaCO_2$ 35 to 45 mm Hg), and SaO_2 (95.0% to 97.5%).
- Position patient in a semi-Fowler's position to facilitate diaphragmatic movement.
- Limit patient's physical activity to bed rest or chair rest to reduce respiratory demand and decrease PaO_2 $\leq$ 80 mm Hg.
- Obtain, document and report clinical findings of hypoxemia: restlessness, confusion, irritability, anxiety hypoventilation, cyanosis, dysrhythmias, headache, angina, impaired judgment, hypotension, and tachycardia.

- Auscultate the lungs every 2 to 4 hours for crackles, rhonchi, or wheezes.
- Administer prescribed IV fluid to maintain adequate circulating volume.
- Administer prescribed low-flow oxygen 2 to 4 L/min (24% to 36% O_2) by means of nasal cannula or FIO_2 ≤50% by mask to maintain PaO_2 ≥80 mm Hg and SaO_2 ≥95%.
- Encourage use of breathing exercises to promote maximum alveolar ventilation with increased aeration to under-ventilated areas of the lungs.
- Assist patient with use of incentive spirometer to facilitate lung expansion.
- Provide nasopharyngeal or oropharyngeal suctioning as needed to remove excess secretions.
- Should supplemental oxygenation be ineffective in improving oxygenation, assist with the initiation of intubation or mechanical ventilation.
- Teach patient to use a blow bottle or incentive spirometer every hour while awake to enhance oxygen–carbon dioxide exchange.

Potential Complication: Peripheral Edema. Peripheral edema related to the accumulation of excess amounts of extracellular or intracellular fluid in peripheral tissues secondary to abnormal transcapillary fluid and protein exchange as a result of increased capillary hydrostatic pressure, decreased intravascular colloid osmotic pressure, and increased interstitial colloid osmotic pressure and lymphatic obstruction.

Expected Patient Outcomes. Patient maintains normal extracellular or intracellular fluid volume, as evidenced by capillary refill ≤3 seconds, peripheral pulses +2, absence of dependent edema, warm and dry skin, absence of weight gain, and serum protein 6.6 to 7.9 g/dL.

- Consult with physician to validate the nurse's established expected patient outcomes reflecting normal peripheral intracellular or extracellular fluid volume.

- Review results of serum protein.
- Elevate the lower extremities when sitting to enhance venous return, if not contraindicated.
- Restrict sodium intake to 2 to 3 g/d.
- Diet high in protein is given should there be a decrease in serum protein.
- Obtain and report clinical findings that indicate peripheral edema: capillary refill ≥3 s, peripheral pulses ≤+2, dependent or brawny edema, and cool and cyanotic skin.
- Report weight gain of 3 lb (6.6 kg) in 24 hours and UO ≤0.5mL/kg/h.
- Monitor extremities for peripheral edema on a scale of 1 to 4 with 4 signifying severe edema. Pitting edema is evaluated according to indentations. Mild edema shows a 1/4 inch indentation and is recorded as 1+, moderate edema can have 1/4- to 1/2-inch indentation and is recorded as a 2+, and severe edema can have 1/2- to 1-inch indentation and is recorded as 3+. Increasing dependent edema signifies increased extravascular fluid retention from systemic fluid overload.
- Administer prescribed diuretics (furosemide, bumetanide) to increase excretion of water.
- Initiate continuous monitoring of fluid balance by measuring daily weight (body weight may increase 10% before generalized edema is noted) ≥0.5 kg/d, intake, output, and specific gravity.
- Regulate prescribed IV fluids with microdrip or infusion pump to prevent sudden expansion of vascular intracellular volume.
- Provide prescribed antiembolic stockings to enhance venous return and reduce venous pooling.
- Avoid placing extremities in a dependent position for extended periods to prevent fluid stasis.
- Provide a special bed or a special mattress to prevent edematous tissue from breaking down.
- Teach patient dietary restriction of sodium and fluid intake.
- Instruct patient to do daily weight.

DISCHARGE PLANNING

The critical care nurse provides the patient and significant other(s) with verbal or written discharge notes regarding the following subjects:

1. Importance of keeping activity schedule at a comfortable and moderate pace. Should patient experience fatigue during physical activity, he or she is to stop and rest for 15 minutes before resuming activity.
2. The warning signals that necessitate stopping physical activity: chest pain, shortness of breath, dizziness, or weakness.
3. The signs of CHF that should be reported to physician: decreased activity intolerance, shortness of breath, dyspnea on exertion, paroxysmal nocturnal dyspnea, persistent cough, swelling of extremities, sudden weight gain ≥3 lb (6.6 kg) with 24 hours, and nocturia.
4. Importance of maintaining prescribed diet, fluid amounts, and need to avoid food high in sodium content.
5. Importance of daily weight at the same time and with the same amount of clothing.
6. Medication's purpose, dosage, schedule, and side effects.

■ DILATED CARDIOMYOPATHY

(For related information see Part I: Acute myocardial infarction, p. 38; Congestive heart failure, p. 87; Acute chest pain, p. 1; Acute cardiac tamponade, p. 117; Acute pericarditis, p. 123; Dysrhythmias, p. 184. Part II: Heart transplantation, p. 211. Part III: Intra-aortic balloon pump, p. 254; Hemodynamic monitoring, p. 219. See also Respiratory Deviations, Part III: Pulse oximetry, p. 426; Mechanical ventilation, p. 428. See also Behavioral Deviations, Part I, p. 725.)

Diagnostic Categories and Length of Stay

DRG: 144 Other circulatory diagnoses with complications
LOS: 5.20 days

DRG: 145 Other circulatory diagnoses without complications
LOS: 3.40 days

Definition

Dilated cardiomyopathy (DCM) is a subacute disorder of the heart muscle characterized by dilatation of the left or right ventricle, or both, with varying degrees of hypertrophy and systolic ventricular dysfunction. These changes can result in heart failure. The heart muscle is characterized by dilated, flabby, and globe-shaped heart with reduced systolic function.

Pathophysiology

In DCM, there is interference with the calcium uptake by the mitochondria of the myocardial cell, which reduces cellular contractility and impairs the pumping ability of the heart, further decreasing ejection fraction (EF). The impaired systolic ventricular function is followed by a reduction in cardiac output, a reduction in stroke volume, and an increase in left ventricular end-diastolic pressure (LVEDP). Elevated LVEDP also results in increased pressure in the left atrium, pulmonary veins, and pulmonary capillaries. Decreased stroke volume (SV) causes increased sympathetic nervous system stimulation and resulting catecholamines, which increase heart rate, contractility, and systemic vascular resistance. The greater the wall tension demand, the greater the myocardial oxygen consumption. A decreased EF means a greater volume of blood remains within the ventricle, thereby causing ventricular thrombus formation. Other changes include increased pulmonary pressure and increased venous pressure. The ventricles dilate to increase contractility. This results in an increased ventricular radius and increased ventricular wall tension and myocardial oxygen consumption.

Nursing Assessment

PRIMARY CAUSES
• The cause of DCM is largely unknown. Certain clinical conditions have been asso-

ciated with DCM, including alcohol ingestion, peripartum, viral infection, bacterial infection, hyperthyroidism, chemotherapy, and hypersensitivity to penicillin, tetracycline, and sulfonamides.

RISK FACTORS

- History of alcohol abuse and diabetes.

PHYSICAL ASSESSMENT

- Inspection: Patient experiences fatigue, dry or hacking cough with dyspnea on exertion, orthopnea, paroxysmal nocturnal dyspnea, or dyspnea at rest. Other findings include peripheral edema, cyanotic extremities, jugular vein distention, ascites, fatigue, weakness, or chest pain.
- Palpation: The extremities are cool, with diminished peripheral pulses. The apical impulse is diffuse with lateral and inferior displacement. Hepatomegaly and splenomegaly also occur.
- Auscultation: Heart sounds include soft S_1; splitting S_2, reversed by left bundle branch block, split by right bundle branch block or accentuated by pulmonary hypertension, S_3 and S_4, or apical systolic murmur of mitral insufficiency. Atrial flutter or fibrillation, hypotension, and crackles also can occur.

DIAGNOSTIC TEST RESULTS

Hemodynamic Parameters. (See Table 1–9)

- Cardiac output (CO) ≤2.5 L/min, cardiac index (CI) ≤2.0 L/min/m², EF ≤25%, left atrial pressure (LAP) 8 to 12 mm Hg, left ventricular stroke work (LVSW) ≤60 g-m/beat, left ventricular stroke work index (LVSWI) ≤30 g-m/beat/m², pulmonary artery pressure (PAP) systolic ≥25 mm Hg or diastolic ≥15 mm Hg, pulmonary capillary wedge pressure (PCWP) ≥22 mm Hg, pulmonary vascular resistance (PVR) ≥255 dynes/s/cm⁻⁵, pulmonary vascular resistance index (PVRI) ≥450 dynes/s/cm⁻⁵/m², right atrial pressure (RAP) ≥6 mm Hg, right

ventricular stroke work (RVSW) ≤10 g-m/beat, right ventricular stroke work index (RVSWI) ≤7 g-m/beat/m², SV ≤60 mL/beat, and stroke volume index (SVI) ≤33 mL/m²/beat.

Invasive Cardiac Diagnostic Procedures. (See Table 1–2)

- Cardiac scan: Thallium 201 scanning shows myocardial perfusion defect similar to those seen in patients with severe coronary artery disease.
- Endomyocardial biopsy: Can aid in identifying the type of pathological agent causing cardiomyopathy.
- Ventriculogram: Shows increased end-diastolic and end-systolic ventricular volumes, global hypokinesis, and global decrease in contractility.

Noninvasive Cardiac Diagnostic Procedures. (See Table 1–3)

- Chest roentgenogram: Increased cardiothoracic ratio (≥0.50), four-chamber enlargement, pulmonary congestion, or pleural effusion.
- Echocardiogram: In general, the test assesses the degree of left ventricular impairment and dilatation of the cardiac chamber, ventricular wall contractility, septal contractility, and valvular motion. The two-dimensional endocardiogram demonstrates global dysfunction and increased dimensions, or visualizes thrombus. The M-mode shows left ventricular enlargement with increased end-diastolic and end-systolic dimensions, together with reduced ER and fractional shortening and decreased mitral valve motion.
- Phonocardiogram: Shows evidence of S_3 to S_4 heart sounds and regurgitant atrioventricular valve murmurs, central venous to pressure (CVP) 24 to 30 mm Hg, PCWP 24 to 40 mm Hg, and systolic PAP 25 to 40 mm Hg.

ECG.

- Presence of Q waves may indicate the presence of extensive left ventricular fibrosis. ECG may also show abnormal ST segment, T wave, chamber enlargement, and axis deviation.
- Dysrhythmias consist of atrioventricular conduction disturbance, left bundle branch block, supraventricular and ventricular tachydysrhythmias, or atrial fibrillation.

MEDICAL AND SURGICAL MANAGEMENT

PHARMACOLOGY

- Vasodilators: Used to decrease filling pressure (preload) by redistributing intravascular volume from the central to the peripheral vasculature, to decrease arteriolar resistance and lessen impedance to ejection (afterload), and to decrease pulmonary congestion by redistributing venous volume (see Table 1–4).
- Angiotensin-converting Enzyme (ACE) Inhibitors: Include captopril or enalapril to decrease preload and afterload (See Table 1–12).
- Inotropic Agents: Amrinone, dopamine, dobutamine, or digoxin are used to enhance myocardial contractility, to increase CO, and increase coronary blood flow (see Table 1–10).
- Diuretics: Used to reduce excessive edema without causing hypovolemia (see Table 1–13).
- Antidysrhythmia Agents: Used to control dysrhythmias (see Table 1–11).
- Calcium Channel Blockers: Used to produce vasodilation and decrease myocardial work load (see Table 1–6).
- Anticoagulants: Used to prevent thrombosis or embolization resulting from atrial fibrillation (see Table 1–8).

DIET

- Restriction of sodium should fluid retention occur.

PHYSICAL ACTIVITY

- Limited to bed rest or modified bed rest to decrease myocardial oxygen demand. Eventually activity is based upon the patient's history, physical findings, chest roentgenogram, and exercise capacity.

OXYGEN THERAPY

- Supplemental oxygen is given to maintain saturation of arterial oxygen (SaO_2) $\geq 95\%$ and pressure of arterial oxygen (PaO_2) ≥ 80 mm Hg.

INTRA-AORTIC BALLOON PUMP (IABP)

- IABP is used to temporarily support the failing heart and systemic circulation. The benefits are improved coronary artery perfusion by augmentation of arterial diastolic pressure, diminished resistance to left ventricular ejection, and a decrease in ventricular work load and myocardial oxygen demand or consumption (see IABP, p. 254).

SURGICAL INTERVENTION.

- Heart Transplantation: A mode of treatment of patients with end-stage heart failure. Ischemic cardiomegaly accounts for 40% to 50% of all transplants performed (see Heart transplantation, p. 211).

NURSING MANAGEMENT: NURSING DIAGNOSES AND COLLABORATIVE PROBLEMS

Nursing Diagnoses

Common nursing goals in patients with dilated cardiomyopathy are to reduce pain, improve oxygenation, reduce excess fluid volume, enhance urinary elimination, prevent complications such as activity intolerance, and encourage appropriate individual coping.

Pain related to impaired systolic function.

Expected Patient Outcomes. Patient experiences relief of chest pain, as evidenced by absence of verbalization of pain, heart rate

(HR) 60 to 100 bpm, and absence of ST and T wave changes.

- Consult with cardiologist about ECG changes seen in patients with DCM.
- Obtain and review results of 12-lead ECG.
- Limit physical activity to bed rest while patient is experiencing chest pain in order to reduce myocardial oxygen demand.
- Obtain, document, and report patient's description of chest pain including location, radiation, duration, intensity, quality, and precipitating factors.
- Continuously monitor ECG every 2 to 4 hours to assess heart rate, ST and T wave changes, and presence of dysrhythmias.
- During the pain episode, assess the HR and rhythm, blood pressure (BP), and skin for the presence of pallor, cyanosis, and diaphoresis.
- Remain with patient while he or she experiences chest pain. Anxiety associated with pain can increase sympathetic nervous system stimulation, which causes an increase in catecholamines. Catecholamines increase the HR, which can decrease diastolic filling time and coronary artery perfusion and increase risk of pain.
- Administer prescribed oxygen at 2 to 4 L/min by means of nasal cannula or mask to enhance oxygenation.
- Administer prescribed IV morphine sulfate in 2 mg increments every 5 minutes to relieve chest pain (see Table 1–7).
- Administer prescribed IV nitroglycerin (NTG), infusion 5 μg/min to maintain systolic blood pressure (SBP) $\geq$90 mm Hg, decrease preload (PCWP), and decrease afterload (systemic vascular resistance [SVR]). Sublingual NTG can be given as one tablet every 5 minutes three times (see Table 1–4).
- During each titration of NTG, monitor patient's BP and resolution of chest pain. Should SBP $\leq$90 mm Hg occur, decrease the flow rate to a predetermined rate. If patient's SBP is $\leq$80 mm Hg, or diaphoresis, tachydysrhythmias, or bradydysrhythmias

occur, stop the infusion and consult with physician for further direction.
- Administer prescribed beta blockers (propranolol) to decrease myocardial oxygen demand (see Table 1–5).
- Assist patient with activities of daily living to reduce pain caused by increased myocardial oxygen demand.
- Teach patient to describe pain using a scale of 1 to 10, with 10 being severe pain.
- Teach patient to use stress reduction techniques of mediation or progressive relaxation.

Impaired gas exchange related to pulmonary congestion secondary to impaired contractile function and increased left ventricular end-diastolic volume causing increased pressure in the left atrium, pulmonary veins, and pulmonary capillaries.

Expected Patient Outcomes. Patient maintains adequate gas exchange, as evidenced by PCWP 6 to 12 mm Hg, Pao$_2$ 80 to 100 mm Hg, Sao$_2$ $\geq$ 95%, respiration rate (RR)12 to 20 BPM, absence of cyanosis, mixed venous oxygen saturation S$\bar{v}$o$_2$ 60% to 80%, and absence of adventitious lung sounds.

- Review arterial blood gases and chest roentgenogram.
- Position patient to maximize optimal gas exchange and chest excursion. Evaluate the response to positional change with pulse oximetry (Spo$_2$) and S$\bar{v}$o$_2$.
- Obtain and report hemodynamic parameters that indicate impaired gas exchange resulting from increased pulmonary pressures: Pulmonary artery diastolic (PAD) $\geq$15 mm Hg, pulmonary artery systolic (PAS) $\geq$30 mm Hg, and PCWP $\geq$12 to 15 mm Hg.
- Continuously monitor oxygenation with S$\bar{v}$o$_2$ and report value $\leq$60%. The S$\bar{v}$o$_2$ may fall when oxygen supply (Do$_2$) decreases or when oxygen demand (Vo$_2$) increases. The latter may occur with pain, fever, anxiety, shivering, physical activity, or increased work of breathing.

- Monitor and report clinical findings associated with impaired gas exchange: tachypnea, crackles, cyanosis, dyspnea, restlessness, and use of accessory muscles.
- Continuously monitor ECG every 2 to 4 hours to assess HR and dysrhythmias resulting from hypoxemia.
- Encourage patient to cough, turn, deep breathe to reduce risk of atelectasis when on bed rest.
- Encourage patient to use incentive spirometer to facilitate lung expansion and gas exchange.
- Calculate arterial-alveolar oxygen tension ratio (Pao_2 − Pao_2) ratio as an index of gas exchange efficiency. A value ≤0.75 may indicate ventilation-perfusion inequalities or a diffusion problem.
- Administer prescribed oxygen 2 to 4 L/min to maintain Pao_2 ≥80 mm Hg and Sao_2 ≥95%.
- Administer prescribed low-dose morphine sulfate to promote venous pooling and decrease dyspnea.
- Administer prescribed diuretics to reduce circulatory volume (see Table 1–13).
- Teach patient to cough, deep breathe, and turn frequently.

Fluid volume excess related to increased right ventricular end-diastolic pressure (RVEDP) secondary to decreased myocardial contractility or compromised regulatory mechanism.

Expected Patient Outcomes. Patient maintains adequate fluid volume status, as evidenced by PCWP 6 to 12 mm Hg, PAS 15 to 30 mm Hg and PAD 5 to 15 mm Hg, RAP 4 to 6 mm Hg, CVP 2 to 6 mm Hg, urinary output (UO) ≥30 mL/h or ≥0.5mL/kg/h, absence of peripheral edema, flat neck veins, and absence of crackles.

- Review results of blood urea nitrogen (BUN) and creatinine to evaluate renal function.
- Obtain and report hemodynamic parameters that indicate excess fluid volume: PAS ≥30 mm Hg, PAD ≥15 mm Hg, PCWP ≥12 mm Hg, and CVP ≥6 mm Hg.
- Monitor and report other clinical findings that suggest fluid volume excess: jugular vein distention, peripheral edema, tachycardia, S_3, crackles, or rapid weight gain (0.5 to 1.0 kg/d).
- Monitor intake and output to evaluate patients fluid status.
- Administer prescribed IV fluids to maintain adequate circulating volume.
- Administer prescribed diuretics to remove excess fluid volume and maintain UO ≥30 mL/h or ≥0.5 mL/kg/h (see Table 1–13).

Activity intolerance related to chest pain, fatigue, and dyspnea secondary to increased myocardial oxygen demand.

Expected Patient Outcomes. Patient maintains adequate cardiac tolerance to increased activity, as evidenced by normal sinus rhythm, RR ≤24 BPM, HR ≤120 bpm (within 20 bpm of resting HR), BP within 20 mm Hg of patient's normal range, peripheral pulses +2, capillary refill ≤3 seconds, and absence of chest pain.

- Confer with cardiologist and cardiac rehabilitation about an individualized activity program.
- Consult with physical therapy for exercise training before and after discharge.
- Initiate a schedule of activities that includes bed to chair for at least 20 minutes three times a day to prevent further deconditioning.
- Develop progressive activity regimen with patient and physical therapist, occupational therapy, and significant others in order to increase patient's functional capacity.
- Monitor and report findings reflective of activity intolerance: chest pain, HR ≥120 bpm, RR ≥24 BPM, shortness of breath, dysrhythmias, BP ≥20 mm Hg of normal range, fatigue, and dyspnea.
- Monitor patient's BP, HR, and RR before, during, and after progressive increases in physical activity.

- Monitor continuous ECG to assess HR and rhythm before, during, and after incremental increases in activity. Document rhythm every 2 to 4 hours in patient with dysrhythmias.
- Encourage flexion and extension of extremities while in bed 15 times each day.
- Encourage patient to deep breathe four times a day for 15 breaths and to change position from side to side.
- Implement passive and active range of motion (ROM) exercises to maintain muscle tone.
- Organize nursing care so patient will have uninterrupted rest periods.
- Provide diversional activities such as TV, radio, books to help patient cope with inactivity.
- Administer prescribed vasodilator (nitroglycerin NTG) before activity: NTG to maintain HR ≤120 bpm, RR ≤ 24 BPM, BP within patient's normal range, and absence of chest pain (see Table 1–4).
- Teach patient to monitor pulse rate while increasing activity.
- Teach patient ways to conserve energy.

Urinary elimination, altered pattern of related to increased sympathetic nervous system stimulation secondary to decreased CO.

Expected Patient Outcomes. Patient maintains adequate pattern of urinary elimination, as evidenced by BUN 8 to 20 mg/dL, serum creatinine M: 0.8 to 1.2 mg/dL or W: 0.6 to 0.9 mg/dL, serum electrolytes within normal range, UO ≥30 mL/h or ≥0.5 mL/kg/h, specific gravity 1.010 to 1.030, and resolved peripheral edema.

- Review results of BUN, creatinine, and serum electrolytes for renal function. A BUN ≥20 and creatinine ≥1.5 suggest renal impairment.
- Assess, document, and report findings reflective of an altered pattern of UO: UO ≤30 mL/h or ≤0.5 mL/kg/h, specific gravity ≤1.010, increased body weight, and peripheral edema.

- Monitor daily weight, intake, and output.
- Monitor continuous ECG to assess HR and rhythm. Document ECG rhythm strips every 4 hours in patients with hypokalemia-induced dysrhythmias.
- Administer prescribed IV fluids to maintain adequate hydration, UO ≥30 mL/h or ≥0.5 mL/kg/h and specific gravity 1.010 to 1.030.
- Administer volume-reducing agents: furosemide or bumetanide to maintain stable body weight, decrease peripheral edema, UO ≥30 mL/h or ≥0.5 mL/kg/h and specific gravity 1.010 to 1.030 (see Table 1–13).
- Administer prescribed potassium to correct hypokalemia.
- Teach patient the common side effects of diuretics: weakness or hypokalemia.

Coping, ineffective individual related to depression secondary to the illness and life-style changes.

Expected Patient Outcomes. Patient verbalizes feelings related to the current illness experience, identifies coping pattern and consequences of coping behaviors, and makes decisions about changes in life-style.

- Confer with physician about patient's depression and need for a psychiatric consultation.
- Listen to patient's verbalization of sadness, loneliness, worry, fear, vague confusion, helplessness, and hopelessness, all of which indicate depression.
- Monitor for depression-related behaviors: fatigue, constipation or diarrhea, anorexia, headache, dry mouth, stiffness, dizziness, numbness, and frequent crying episodes.
- Evaluate with the patient how cardiomyopathy can contribute to depression by causing sudden changes in life pattern, depleting economic resources, or impacting on support systems.
- Determine with patient the onset of depressive feelings and symptoms and their relationship to the illness and life changes.
- Help the patient to identify problems that he or she cannot control directly and how to

use guided imagery, meditation, or progressive relaxation to relieve stress.

- Assist the family to cope with the patient's feelings of depression.
- Identify ways patient can maintain modified activity within the scope of gradually increasing activity intolerance.
- Teach patient to perform activities that can enhance self-esteem: personal grooming, reading, or writing letters.

Collaborative Problems

Common collaborative goals in patients with DCM are to increase cardiac output, reduce myocardial oxygen demand, correct dysrhythmias and prevent thromboembolism.

Potential Complication: Decreased Cardiac Output.

Decreased CO related to increased preload secondary to impaired systolic function.

Expected Patient Outcomes. Patient maintains adequate preload, as evidenced by normal BP ≥90 mm Hg; CO is 2.5 to 3.0 L/min and CI 2.0 to 2.5 L/min/m²; CVP ≤24 mm Hg with care not to lower CVP so that intravascular volume is depleted, thereby diminishing left ventricular ejection; LAP 8 to 12 mm Hg; PAP systolic 15 to 25 mm Hg or diastolic 8 to 15 mm Hg; PCWP ≤18 mm Hg; RAP 4 to 6 mm Hg; right ventricular pressure (RVP) systolic 15 to 25 mm Hg or diastolic 0 to 8 mm Hg; neck veins not distended; specific gravity 1.010 to 1.030; warm and dry skin; resolution of peripheral edema; peripheral pulses +2; capillary refill ≤3 seconds; HR ≤100 bpm; and UO ≥30 mL/h or ≥0.5 mL/kg/h.

- Consult with cardiologist to validate expected patient outcomes used to evaluate preload.
- Review results from ventriculogram, thallous chloride TP 201 scan, endomyocardial biopsy, chest roentgenogram, ECG, and echocardiogram.
- Limit physical activity to high Fowler's position with legs dependent, if severely dyspneic, to decrease venous return, increase venous pooling, and decrease preload.
- Elevate the edematous extremity, if not contraindicated by heart failure.
- Obtain and report hemodynamic parameters reflective altered preload: BP ≤90/60 mm Hg, CO ≤2.5 L/min, CI ≤2.0 L/min/m², CVP ≥24 mm Hg, LAP ≥12 mm Hg, PAP systolic ≥25 mm Hg or diastolic ≥15 mm Hg, PCWP ≥22 mm Hg, RAP ≥6 mm Hg, and RVP systolic ≥25 mm Hg or diastolic ≥8 mm Hg.
- Assess, document, and report the following: palpable shift to the left in the point of maximal impulse (PMI), right ventricular heave, S_3 indicating a high ventricular filling pressure, S_4 caused by decreased ventricular compliance, summation gallop, jugular venous distention with a prominent "a" wave, S_3 gallop, dependent peripheral edema, ascites, hepatomegaly, and positive hepatojugular reflux.
- Monitor continuous ECG to assess heart rate and rhythm. Document ECG rhythm strips every 2 to 4 hours in patients with dysrhythmias.
- Limit fluid intake to 1000 L/d.
- Monitor daily weight, intake, and output to evaluate fluid balance.
- Administer prescribed IV fluids to maintain hydration, UO ≥30 mL/h or ≥0.5 mL/kg/h, and specific gravity 1.010 to 1.030.
- Administer prescribed vasodilator (NTG or nitroprusside). NTG infusion is started at 5 μg/min to maintain SBP ≥90 mm Hg and increase dose every 5 to 10 minutes by 5 to 10 μg/min. NTG is used as a venous dilator, which reduces preload as measured by CVP ≤24 mm Hg and PCWP ≤18 mm Hg. Should nitroprusside infusion be used, titrate 0.5 to 10.0 μg/kg/min to maintain SBP at 100 to 120 mm Hg. Nitroprusside is not to exceed 10 μg/kg/min. The goal is to keep PCWP at 18 to 22 mm Hg to stretch dilated ventricles and achieve acceptable outputs and PAP systolic 25 to 40 mm Hg.
- Should SVR be high but PCWP be within the patient's normal limits, the nurse can

maintain NTG infusion and slowly increase the nitroprusside infusion (see Table 1–4).

- Administer ACE inhibitors (captopril, enalapril) to block the renin-angiotensin-aldosterone mechanism and subsequently maintain UO ≥30mL/h or ≥0.5mL/kg/h, specific gravity 1.010 to 1.030, BP within patient's normal range, and mean arterial pressure (MAP) 70 to 90 mm Hg (see Table 1–12).
- Should SVR be within the patient's normal limits but PCWP be high, the NTG infusion can be slowly increased while maintaining the nitroprusside infusion.
- Instruct patient regarding diagnostic procedures, treatments, and need for limited physical activity.
- Teach patient common side effects of vasodilators: headache, nausea, vomiting, or dizziness.
- Teach patient common side effects of diuretics: weakness and fatigue.
- Instruct patient how to use diversional activities to reduce stress and subsequent catecholamine release: meditation and guided imagery.

Potential Complication: Decreased Cardiac Output.

Decreased CO related to decreased myocardial contractility secondary to impaired pumping ability of the heart, interference with calcium uptake by the mitochondra of the myocardial cells, or reduced number of functional myocytes, which reduces the degree of myofibril shortening.

Expected Patient Outcomes. Patient maintains adequate contractility, as inferred by CO 2.5 to 3.0 L/min, CI 2.0 to 2.5 L/min/m^2, EF ≥25%, LVSW 60 to 80 g-m/beat, LVSWI 35 to 85 g-m/beat/m^2, PCWP 4 to 12 mm Hg, MAP 70 to 90 mm Hg, RVSW 10 to 15 g-m/beat, right ventricular stroke work index (RVSWI) 7 to 12 g-m/beat/m^2, SV 60 to 130 mL/beat, SVI 35 to 50 mL/beat/m^2, UO ≥30 mL/h or ≥0.5 mL/kg/h, normal heart sounds, HR ≤100 bpm, RR 12 to 20 BPM, BP ≥90/60 mm Hg, absence of chest pain, capil-

lary refill ≤3 seconds, Pao$_2$ ≥80 mm Hg, Sao$_2$ ≥95%, and absence of fatigue.

- Confer with cardiologist about the hemodynamic parameters used to measure left ventricular preload: CO 2.5 to 3.0 L/min, CI 2.0 to 2.5 L/min/m^2, and EF ≤25%, all of which are lower than for other patients, yet are considered normal in DCM.
- Consult with cardiologist to validate expected patient outcomes used to determine whether myocardial contractility is sufficient.
- Review results from chest roentgenogram, ventriculogram, or echocardiogram, if available.
- Obtain and report hemodynamic values reflective of decreased myocardial contractility indicated by: EF ≥25%, CO ≤2.5 L/min, CI ≤2.0 L/min/m^2, LVSW ≤60 g-m/beat, LVSWI ≤35 g-m/beat/m^2, MAP ≤70 mm Hg, RVSW ≤10 g-m/beat, RVSWI ≤7 g-m/beat/m^2, SV ≤60 mL/beat, and SVI ≤45 mL/beat/m^2.
- Obtain, document, and report other clinical findings associated with decreased myocardial contractility: a shift to the left in the point of maximal impulse, S$_3$ resulting from high ventricular filling pressure, S$_4$ resulting from decreased ventricular compliance, PCWP ≥22 mm Hg, a summation gallop, tachycardia, pulsus alternans, hypotension, fatigue, and activity intolerance.
- Monitor continuous ECG to assess HR and rhythm. Document ECG rhythm strips every 2 to 4 hours in patients with nonspecific ST and T wave changes and increase in QRS voltage in precordial leads with a decrease in standard leads.
- Measure LVSWI and SVI against PCWP at regular intervals to follow trends in left ventricular function.
- Monitor patient's BP, HR, and RR before an activity, immediately upon completion of the activity, and 5 minutes after the activity's completion to determine whether metabolic demand and myocardial work load has been increased.

- Limit activity to bed rest or semi- to high-Fowler's position to reduce myocardial oxygen demand.
- Provide an environment that fosters physical and emotional rest.
- Administer oxygen 2 to 4 L/min by means of nasal cannula or FIO_2 at 50% by mask to enhance myocardial contractility by relieving hypoxia, reducing work load of the heart, supporting cellular energy requirements, and maintaining PaO_2 ≥80 mm Hg or SaO_2 ≥95%.
- Administer prescribed IV fluids to maintain adequate hydration, capillary refill ≥3 seconds, and UO ≥30 mL/h or ≥0.5 mL/kg/h.
- Administer prescribed inotropic agents, such as dopamine, at a dose 0.5 μg/kg/min or phosphodiesterase inhibitors, such as amrinone, at a dose of IV bolus 0.75 mg/kg over 2 to 3 minutes followed by a titrating dose at 5 to 10 μg/kg/min, not to exceed 10 mg/kg in a 24-hour period. The goals is to maintain CO 2.5 to 3.0 L/min and CI 2.0 to 2.5 L/min/m², EF ≥25%, LVSW 60 to 80 g-m/beat, LVSWI 30 to 50 g-m/beat/m², MAP 70 to 90 mm Hg, RVSW 10 to 15 g-m/beat, RVSWI 7 to 12 g-m/beat/m², SV 60 to 130 mL/beat, and SVI 35 to 50 mL/beat/m² (see Table 1–10).
- Administer peripheral vasodilators (nitroprusside) or coronary vasodilator (NTG) to enhance coronary perfusion, MAP 70 to 90 mm Hg, CO ≥2.5 L/min, and CI 2.0 L/min/m² (see Table 1–4).
- When the SVR is ≥1200 dynes/s/cm⁻⁵ but the PCWP is within patient's normal limit, maintain NTG infusion and slowly increase nitroprusside infusion.
- When the SVR is 900 to 1200 dynes/s/cm⁻⁵ but the PCWP is ≥22 mm Hg slowly increase the NTG infusion and maintain the nitroprusside infusion.
- Should pharmacological therapy be ineffective in increasing myocardial contractility, assist with IABP insertion (see IABP, p. 254).
- Should pharmacological therapy and IABP be ineffective in increasing myocardial con-

tractility, assist with use of a cardiac assist device (see Cardiac assist device, p. 248).
- Should pharmacological therapy be ineffective in sustaining myocardial contractility and patient's condition deteriorate, prepare for possible heart transplantation (see Heart transplantation, p. 211).
- Teach patient how to use stress reduction techniques, such as guided imagery, meditation, progressive relaxation, and music.
- Instruct patient as to the diagnostic procedures and treatments that may ultimately require more invasive procedures or heart transplantation.

Potential Complication: Increased Myocardial Oxygen Demand. Increased myocardial oxygen demand related to increased myocardial work load secondary to increased HR, contractility, or wall tension.

Expected Patient Outcomes. Patient maintains reduced myocardial oxygen demand, as evidenced by arteriovenous oxygen content difference $(C[a-v]O_2)$ 4 to 6 mL/100mL, oxygen utilization coefficient or oxygen extraction ratio (O_2ER) 25%, MAP 70 to 90 mm Hg, rate pressure product (RPP) ≤12,000, VO_2 ≥200 or ≤250 mL/min, oxygen consumption index (VO_2I) ≥115 or ≤165 mL/min/m², and mixed venous oxygen saturation $(S\bar{v}O_2)$ 60% to 80%.

- Confer with cardiologist to validate expected patient outcomes used to measure reduced myocardial oxygen demand.
- Position patient in Fowler's, semi-Fowler's position, or on complete bed rest to minimize myocardial tissue oxygen demand or work load.
- Limit physical activity to bed rest to decrease myocardial oxygen demand.
- Reduce myocardial oxygen demand by decreasing anxiety, provide a liquid diet in the acute phase, decrease pain, and provide uninterrupted rest periods.
- Evaluate the use of a bedpan, bedside commode, bathroom privileges, bed bath, or

shower based on the activity's effect on oxygen demand.

- Monitor and report hemodynamic values reflective of increased myocardial tissue oxygen demand: $C(a-v)o_2 \geq 6$ mL/100mL, $O_2ER \geq 25\%$, $RPP \geq 12,000$, $S\bar{v}o_2 \leq 60\%$, $SW \leq 45$ mL/beat/m^2, $Vo_2 \geq 250$ mL/min, and $Vo_2I \geq 165$ mL/min/m^2.
- Monitor continuous $S\bar{v}o_2$, which reflects the ability of the body to satisfy tissue oxygen demand, and SVR, which reflects the force (demand) the heart must perform to achieve CO.
- When patient gradually increases physical activity, assess and report findings reflective of increased myocardial oxygen consumption: chest pain, fatigue, and dyspnea.
- Monitor HR, as tachycardia will increase myocardial work load and myocardial oxygen consumption (MVo_2) .
- Administer prescribed oxygen 2 to 4 L/min by nasal cannula or Fio_2 at 50% by mask to increase oxygen supply and restore arterial oxygen saturation to normal limits.
- Administer vasodilators (NTG or nitroprusside) to decrease SVR and the resistance against which the heart must pump. This will decrease myocardial oxygen demand (see Table 1–4).
- Administer beta-adrenergic blockers (propranolol) to reduce the disparity between myocardial oxygen demand and supply (see Table 1–5).
- Administer positive inotropic agent (dobutamine, dopamine) to maintain Vo_2 200 to 250 mL/min, and Vo_2I 115 to 165 mL/min/m^2 (see Table 1–10).
- Inform patient that increased physical activity, increased HR, straining while having a stool, suctioning, or moods such as irritability, anxiety, or nervousness can increase myocardial oxygen demand.

Potential Complication: Dysrhythmias. Dysrhythmias related to increased catecholamines secondary to increased sympathetic nervous system stimulation.

Expected Patient Outcomes. Patient remains in sinus rhythm, serum electrolytes within normal range, HR 60 to 100 bpm, and absence of chest pain.

- Consult with cardiologist about dysrhythmias associated with DCM.
- Review results of serial ECG to help evaluate location, prognosis, and ventricular function.
- Initiate continuous ECG to assess HR and rhythm. Document ECG rhythm strips every 2 to 4 hours in patients with dysrhythmias.
- Monitor and report physical signs and symptoms dysrhythmias: abnormal HR and rhythm, palpitations, chest pain, syncope, and hypotension.
- Administer the prescribed oxygen 2 to 4 L/min by means of a nasal cannula or mask should patient experience chest pain.
- Administer prescribed IV fluids to maintain adequate circulating volume.
- Administer prescribed antidysrhythmiac agents according to the dysrhythmia's origin and potential risk to patient (see Table 1–11 and Dysrhythmias, p. 184).
- Teach patient to report an abnormal HR, syncope, or describe chest pain on a scale of 1 to 10.
- Teach patient common side effects of prescribed dysrhythmia agents.
- Teach patient meditation, progressive relaxation, or other stress reduction techniques to reduce patient's response to stress and heighten patient's sense of control.

Potential Complication: Thromboembolism. Thromboembolism related to retention of blood in the apical portion of the left ventricle, causing atrial and ventricular thrombus formation secondary to increased end-systolic volume resulting from decreased EF.

Expected Patient Outcomes. Patient maintains absence of thromboembolism, as evidenced by peripheral pulses +2, absence of leg pain, absence of pleuritic pain, normal peripheral skin color, HR ≤100 bpm, RR 12 to 20 BPM, absence of crackles and shortness of breath, Pa_{O_2} ≥80 mm Hg, capillary refill ≤3 seconds, and Sa_{O_2} ≥95%.

- Consult with physician about the use of antiembolic stockings or sequential pressure device.
- Review results of coagulation studies.
- Review serial arterial blood gases: Pa_{O_2} ≤60 mm Hg, Pa_{CO_2} ≤35 mm Hg, pH ≥7.45, and increased $P_{A_{O_2}} - Pa_{O_2}$ ≥15 mm Hg.
- Elevate the affected extremity, if not contraindicated, to reduce interstitial swelling by enhancing venous return.
- Obtain and report clinical findings suggesting thromboembolism: peripheral pulses ≤+2, capillary refill ≥3 seconds, leg pain, cyanosis, dyspnea, RR ≥24 BPM, HR ≥100 bpm, and absence of pleuritic pain.
- Assess, document, and report findings reflective of impaired pulmonary circulation: Sa_{O_2} ≤95%, shortness of breath, tachycardia, and chest pain.
- Assess, document, and report findings reflective of impaired peripheral circulation: diminished or absent peripheral pulses, cool extremity, mottling or cyanotic extremity, increased extremity girth, leg pain, or Homan's sign.
- Monitor and report signs of systemic embolism, including a change in the color, temperature, or girth of an extremity; a positive Homan's sign; and, complaints of tenderness.
- Initiate continuous monitoring of ECG to assess HR and rhythm. Note changes that could suggest pulmonary embolism: right-axis deviation, ST segment depression in V_1 to V_4, new right bundle branch block, and tachycardia rhythm.
- Continuously monitor oxygen saturation with pulse oximetry (Sp_{O_2}). Monitor patient activities and interventions that might affect oxygen saturation.
- Assist patient to a position that promotes chest expansion and ease of breathing.

- Encourage patient to perform ROM exercises or isotonic leg exercises to promote venous return.
- Apply antiembolic stockings to reduce risk of thrombosis.
- Initiate use of sequential pressure device, if not contraindicated.
- Administer oxygen 2 to 4 L by means of nasal cannula or $F_{I_{O_2}}$ at 50% by mask to maintain Pa_{O_2} ≥80 mm Hg or Sa_{O_2} ≥95%.
- Administer prescribed IV fluids to maintain adequate hydration, UO ≥ 30 mL/h or ≥0.5 mL/kg/h and specific gravity 1.010 to 1.030.
- Administer anticoagulants (heparin, warfarin) to prevent extension of the thromboembolism. An initial bolus of heparin, 5000 to 10,000 U, may be required, followed by a continuous infusion at rate of 1000 U/h (see Table 1–8).
- Administer analgesics or narcotics to relieve pain.
- Instruct patient receiving anticoagulation therapy to report any bleeding such as hematuria, bleeding gums, ecchymoses, petechiae, or epistaxia.
- Instruct patient to report any chest pain or peripheral pain.
- Teach patient to reduce risk factors associated with thromboembolism by doing ROM exercises to extremities when appropriate.

DISCHARGE PLANNING
The critical care nurse provides the patient and significant other(s) with verbal or written discharge notes regarding the following subjects:

1. Signs and symptoms that require immediate medical attention: fatigue, shortness of breath, activity intolerance, tachycardia, tachypnea, and weight gain ≥2.3 to 3.0 L/d over 2 consecutive days.
2. Medication's name, purpose, dosage, schedule, and side effects.
3. Need to keep follow-up appointments.
4. Names of community agencies such as American Heart Association.

■ HYPERTROPHIC CARDIOMYOPATHY

(For related information see Part I: Acute myocardial infarction, p. 38; Congestive heart failure, p. 87; Acute chest pain, p. 1; Acute cardiac tamponade, p. 117; Acute pericarditis, p. 123; Dysrhythmias, p. 184. Part II: Heart transplantation, p. 211. Part III: Hemodynamic monitoring, p. 219; Intra-aortic balloon pump, p. 254. See also Respiratory Deviations, Part III: Pulse oximetry, p. 426; Mechanical ventilation, p. 428.)

Diagnostic Categories and Length of Stay

DRG: 144 Other circulatory diagnoses with complications
LOS: 5.60 days
DRG: 145 Other circulatory diagnoses without complications
LOS: 3.50 days

Definition

Hypertrophic cardiomyopathy (HCM) is a disease of unknown etiology. It is characterized by a hypertrophied, nondilated ventricle, in the absence of a cardiac or systemic disease that could lead to left ventricular hypertrophy. HCM is also called idiopathic hypertrophic subaortic stenosis (IHSS).

Pathophysiology

In HCM, there are disorganization of ventricular septal myocardial fiber, a symmetric septal hypertrophy, diffuse ventricular hypertrophy that reduces the size of the left and right ventricular cavities, and dilated atria. Secondary abnormalities associated with HCM consist of a fibrous plaque in the mural endocardium of the outflow portions of the septum; a decrease in ventricular cavity size or lack of ventricular dilatation secondary to hypertrophy of the septum and the left ventricular walls (LVFW) inability to distend outward; anterior and posterior mitral valve thickening in response to the small ventricular cavity; and left atrial dilatation in response to the increased ventricular filling pressure. As the papillary muscle contracts, the anterior mitral valve leaflet is pulled forward toward the hypertrophied ventricular septum, causing a reduction in end-systolic ventricular volume and left ventricular outflow tract obstruction (LVOTO). The result is increased left ventricular end-diastolic pressure or PCWP ≥ 22 mm Hg.

Nursing Assessment

PRIMARY CAUSES

- HCM is usually genetically transmitted by an autosomal dominant gene. Adrenergic catecholamines lead to increased circulating levels in utero and fetal receptor hypersensitivity. Cytosolic calcium overload causes abnormal membrane permeability or ischemia. Abnormal adenosine metabolism may cause impaired receptor function. Structural abnormalities include catenoid shape of septum and primary myocardial hypertrophy.

RISK FACTORS

- Family history of autosomal dominant pattern of transmission with the risk of offspring inheriting the disorder is 25% to 50%.

PHYSICAL ASSESSMENT

- Inspection: Presented as dyspnea on exertion, syncope, chest pain, palpitations, dizziness, jugular venous pulse with large a wave, dysrhythmias.
- Palpation: Systolic thrill in lower chest, presystolic apical impulse, and left atrial pulse.
- Auscultation: Normal S_1 preceded by a loud S_4, S_2 split physiologically and harsh, crescendo–decrescendo systolic murmur.

DIAGNOSTIC TEST RESULTS

Invasive Cardiac Diagnostic Procedures. (See Table 1–2)

- Cardiac catheterization: A systolic gradient found during catheter pull-back between the middle and basal regions of the left ventricle, impaired diastolic compliance, mitral valve irregularities, or LVOTO. There is also spade-shaped or slipper-foot contour of the left ventricle.

- Endomyocardial Biopsy: Biopsy of the left ventricular muscle helps to diagnose HCM.
- Ventriculogram: A small or normal-sized left ventricular cavity, hypercontractile left ventricle, and asymmetric septal hypertrophy (ASH).

Noninvasive Cardiac Diagnostic Procedures. (See Table 1–3)

- Chest roentgenogram: Reveals mild to moderate enlargement of the cardiac silhouette, rounded left ventricular contour, and enlarged left atrium and left ventricle.
- Echocardiography: The M-mode shows asymmetrical septal hypertrophy, systolic anterior motion of the mitral valve, and early systolic closure of the aortic valve. Two-dimensional may show three different sites of outflow tract narrowing. The sites include classic narrowing between the basal septum and the mitral valve leaflet; narrowing between the upper third of the ventricular septum and the distal free edge of the mitral valve; and midventricular narrowing between the midseptum and the papillary muscle. Doppler echocardiography provides information about the pressure and velocities of abnormal blood flow in the cardiac chamber and great vessels.
- Cardiac scan: Gated blood-pool scanning is used to differentiate HCM from other cardiomyopathies.

ECG

- Reveals hypertrophy and atrial abnormalities noted as increased QRS voltage and depressed T wave of left ventricular hypertrophy. Other findings include atrial fibrillation, ventricular premature beats, conduction defects, and left axis deviation.

MEDICAL AND SURGICAL MANAGEMENT

PHARMACOLOGY

- Beta-adrenergic blocking agents: The advantages in using beta blockers, such as pro-pranolol hydrochloride, include decreased heart rate response to exercise; decreased outflow gradient; relief of angina by a decrease in myocardial oxygen demand; improved diastolic left ventricular filling; antiarrhythmic effect; and decreased left ventricular work (see Table 1–5).

- Calcium channel blockers: Verapamil, nifedipine, or diltiazem are used only in patients who fail to respond to beta blockers. There may be a subset of patients who will undergo hemodynamic deterioration when the systemic blood pressure is decreased by the vasodilatory effect of calcium channel blockers. With hemodynamic deterioration, the outflow gradient and left ventricular end-diastolic pressure (LVEDP) may increase (see Table 1–6).
- Antidysrhythmic agents: Amiodarone may be used to convert or prevent supraventricular or ventricular tachydysrhythmias. The drug also can promote electrical stability of the myocardium. Other antidysrhythmia agents may need to be used (see Table 1–11).
- Antibiotics: Antibiotic prophylaxis can be used when bacterial endocarditis occurs in patients with LVOTO.
- Anticoagulants: Used to prevent thrombus formation, especially in patients with atrial fibrillation (see Table 1–8).

HEMODYNAMIC MONITORING
- Used to determine the effectiveness of therapeutic interventions.

PHYSICAL ACTIVITY
- Limit physical activity in patients with LVOTO by avoiding strenuous exercise and rapid rising to a standing position.

SURGICAL INTERVENTION
- Myectomy: Used to resect muscle in severely symptomatic patients who are unresponsive to medical therapy.
- Transaortic Ventriculomyotomy: Procedures used to relieve outflow obstruction.

NURSING MANAGEMENT: NURSING DIAGNOSES AND COLLABORATIVE PROBLEMS

Nursing Diagnoses

Common nursing goals in patients with HCM are to restore tissue perfusion, maintain effective breathing pattern, and reduce anxiety,

Altered cardiopulmonary tissue perfusion related to compression of coronary arteries or abnormal diastolic relaxation secondary to left ventricular failure.

Expected Patient Outcomes. Patient maintains adequate cardiopulmonary tissue perfusion, as evidenced by blood pressure (BP) $\geq$90/60 mm Hg or within patient's normal range; coronary artery perfusion pressure (CAPP) 60% to 80%; cardiac output (CO) $\geq$2.5 to 3.0 L/min; cardiac index (CI) $\geq$2.7 L/min/m^2, ejection fraction (EF) $\geq$60% or greater; pulse pressure (PP) 30 to 40 mm Hg; alveolar-arterial oxygen gradient (PAO_2 $-$ Pao_2) $\leq$15 mm Hg (room air) or 10 to 65 mm Hg (100% O_2); arterial-alveolar oxygen tension ratio (P[a/A]o_2) 0.75 to 0.90; arteriovenous oxygen content difference (C[a$-$v]o_2) 4 to 6 mL/100mL; mean arterial pressure (MAP) 70 to 100 mm Hg; peripheral pulses $+$2; heart rate (HR) $\leq$100 bpm; capillary refill $\leq$3 seconds; absence of dysrhythmias; absence of dyspnea; absence of syncope; respiratory rate (RR) 12 to 20 BPM; and absence of chest pain.

- Consult with cardiologist to validate expected patient outcomes used to measure adequate cardiopulmonary tissue perfusion.
- Review results of cardiac catheterization and ECG.
- Obtain and report hemodynamic changes that reflect decreased cardiopulmonary tissue perfusion: C0 $\leq$2.5 L/min, CI $\leq$2.7 L/min/m^2, and EF $\leq$60%.
- Monitor and report other clinical findings suggesting decreased cardiopulmonary tissue perfusion: dysrhythmias, syncope, palpitations, dyspnea, tachycardia, tachypnea,

capillary refill $\geq$3 seconds, and peripheral pulses $\leq$$+$2.
- Continuously monitor ECG to assess HR and rhythm. Document ECG rhythm strips every 2 to 4 hours in patients with dysrhythmias.
- Initiate monitoring of CAPP every 1 to 2 hours while cardiopulmonary tissue perfusion is compromised and hemodynamic monitoring is available.
- Obtain and record PP since, a PP 40 mm Hg may reflect increased stroke volume associated with HCM and decreased peripheral resistance.
- Calculate and report C[a$-$v]O_2 $\geq$6 mL/100 mL, which reflects inadequate cardiovascular function.
- Administer prescribed IV fluids to maintain adequate circulating volume, urinary output (UO) $\geq$30 mL/h or $\geq$0.5 mL/kg/h and specific gravity 1.010 to 1.030.
- Provide prescribed oxygen 2 to 4 L/min by means of nasal cannula or FIO_2 at 50% by mask to maintain arterial oxygen saturation (Sao_2) $\geq$95%.
- Administer prescribed beta-adrenergic blocking agents (propranolol) to relieve angina caused by a decrease in myocardial oxygen demand, improve left ventricular filling and decrease left ventricular work.

Ineffective breathing pattern related to dyspnea secondary to elevated LVEDP resulting from poor left ventricular compliance.

Expected Patient Outcomes. Patient maintains effective breathing pattern, as evidenced by C(a$-$v)o_2 4 to 6 mL/100mL; pulmonary capillary wedge pressure (PCWP) $\leq$22 mm Hg; arterial oxygen pressure (Pao_2) $\geq$80 mm Hg; Sao_2 $\geq$95%, RR 12 to 20 BPM; HR $\leq$100 bpm; absence of crackles, rhonchi, or wheezes; and absence of cyanosis.

- Consult with physician to validate expected patient outcomes used to assess effective breathing pattern.
- Review chest roentgenogram and arterial blood gas results.

- Place in semi-Fowler's or high Fowler's position to reduce venous return and enhance lung expansion only when it is believed the treatment will not increase LVOTO.
- Obtain and report hemodynamic parameters reflective of ineffective breathing pattern resulting from increased PCWP ≥22 mm Hg.
- Obtain, document, and report the following changes reflective of increased PCWP: dyspnea, crackles, cyanosis, RR ≥20 BPM, Pao_2 ≤80 mm Hg, Sao_2 ≤95%, and $C(a-v)o_2$ ≥6 mL/100 mL.
- Auscultate lungs for the presence of crackles, rhonchi, or wheezes.
- Provide prescribed oxygen at 2 to 4 L/min by nasal cannula or mask to maintain Pao_2 ≥80 mm Hg and Sao_2 ≥95%.
- Administer prescribed IV fluids to maintain adequate hydration.
- Teach patient to cough, turn, and deep breathe to facilitate effective breathing pattern.
- Instruct patient how to reduce stress by using guided imagery or meditation.

Anxiety related to angina or syncope secondary to HCM.

Expected Patient Outcomes. Patient is free of the signs of harmful anxiety, as evidenced by HR ≤100 bpm, RR ≤20 BPM, BP within patient's normal range, and absence of diaphoresis, irritability, restlessness, or fatigue.

- Review results of 12-lead ECG and compare with baseline ECG for changes reflecting ischemia.
- Discuss with patient the reasons behind angina or syncope in relationship to HCM.
- Stay with patient experiencing angina.
- Provide prescribed oxygen 2 to 4 L/min by nasal cannula or mask.
- Monitor and report clinical findings suggesting anxiety: increased HR, elevated BP, fatigue, increased respiratory rate, diaphoresis, palpitation, and restlessness.
- Teach patient progressive muscle relaxation technique, which may reduce anxiety and relax chest muscle.

- Instruct patient to take deep breaths as a technique to reduce anxiety.

Collaborative Problems

Common collaborative goals in patients with HCM are to enhance CO, reduce angina, and correct dysrhythmias.

Potential Complication: Decreased Cardiac Output. Decreased CO related to impaired diastolic filling of the left ventricle secondary to a decrease in compliance and prolonged relaxation period.

Expected Patient Outcomes. Patient maintains adequate CO, as evidenced by PCWP ≤18 mm Hg, HR ≤100 bpm, absence of dyspnea on exertion, absence of chest pain, CAPP 60 to 80 mm Hg, arterial oxygen delivery (Do_2) 900 to 1200 mL/min, and arterial oxygen delivery index (Do_2I) 500 to 600 mL/min.

- Consult with physician to validate expected patient outcomes that reflect decreased CO related to impaired diastolic compliance (filling).
- Review result of cardiac catheterization, echocardiogram, and ventriculogram.
- Obtain and report hemodynamic parameters that suggest decreased CO related to impaired diastolic filling: CAPP ≤60 mm Hg and PCWP ≥18 mm Hg.
- Obtain and report other clinical findings suggesting decreased CO related to impaired diastolic filling: dyspnea, chest pain, or tachycardia.
- Continuously monitor ECG to assess HR and rhythm. Document rhythm strips every 2 to 4 hours in patients with dysrhythmias.
- Administer beta-adrenergic blocking agent (propranolol) to decrease HR during exercise, improve diastolic left ventricular filling and decreased left ventricular work (see Table 1–5).
- Should pharmacological therapy be ineffective, prepare patient for surgery, such as myectomy.

- Teach patient to use relaxation technique to reduce HR, thereby maintaining oxygen supply.

Potential Complication: Decreased Cardiac Output.

Decreased CO related to altered systolic function secondary to LVOTO.

- Consult with physician to validate expected patient outcomes used to assess adequate CO and systolic function.
- Review results of echocardiogram and heart catheterization
- Limit physical activity to bed rest when LVOTO is accentuated to lessen angina and decrease myocardial oxygen demand.
- Avoid having patient rapidly assume an upright position, since this will increase LVOTO.
- Position patient in a Trendelenburg position to decrease LVOTO.
- Auscultate heart and report harsh, crescendo–decrescendo systolic murmur.
- Calculate oxygen consumption (Vo_2) and oxygen consumption index (Vo_2I) in patients with hemodynamic monitoring and report $Vo_2 \leq 200$ mL/min and $Vo_2I \leq 115$ mL/min/m^2.
- Monitor and report findings reflective of HCM: dyspnea on exertion, angina, and syncope.
- Administer prescribed oxygen 2 to 4 L/min by nasal cannula or mask.
- Administer prescribed IV fluids to maintain adequate circulating volume and avoid dehydration, which will increase LVOTO.
- Administer prescribed beta-adrenergic blocking agent (propranolol) to decrease outflow gradient and decrease in myocardial oxygen demand (see Table 1–5).
- Administer prescribed calcium channel blocking agents only as a second line drug of choice should beta-adrenergic blockers fail to control symptoms.
- Avoid using positive inotropes, vasodilators, or diuretics, as these drugs can increase LVOTO.
- Should pharmacological management be ineffective in reducing LVOTO (50 mm Hg), prepare patient for transaortic ventriculomyotomy.
- Teach patient to avoid Valsalva's maneuver, which can increase LVOTO.
- Teach patient to report any chest pain.

Potential Complication: Angina.

Angina related to abnormal diastolic filling resulting in an imbalance of oxygen supply and demand secondary to a noncompliant or thickened ventrical or LVOTO.

Expected Patient Outcomes. Patient verbalizes relief of chest pain and absence of ST-T wave changes on ECG.

- Review results of 12-lead ECG.
- After exercise, patient may experience angina resulting from a sudden decrease in BP and venous return, which decreases stroke volume; therefore, limit activity to bed rest and keep patient in supine position or semi-Fowler's to decrease myocardial demand.
- Continuously monitor ECG to assess HR, rhythm, and ST and T wave changes.
- Should angina occur, immediately monitor and report changes in HR, BP, and ECG.
- Assist patient to avoid situations that increase LVOTO: exercise, stress, Valsalva's maneuver, or dehydration.
- Stay with patient experiencing angina and provide a calm environment.
- Provide prescribed supplemental oxygen at 2 to 4 L/min by nasal cannula or mask to maintain or improve oxygenation.
- Administer prescribed IV fluids to maintain adequate circulating volume.
- Administer prescribed morphine sulfate (IV push in 2 mg increments every 5 minutes) to relieve chest discomfort.
- Avoid using nitroglycerin, since the drug may aggravate angina in HCM patients.
- Instruct patient to inform health care team when pain occurs.

Potential Complication: Dysrhythmias.

Dysrhythmias related to left ventricular hypertrophy secondary to HCM.

Expected Patient Outcomes. Patient's rhythm remains in sinus rhythm, serum electrolytes within normal range, HR ≤100 bpm, BP within patient's normal range, and absence of palpitations.

- Consult with cardiologist about dysrhythmias that could occur with HCM, such as supraventricular or ventricular tachycardia.
- Review results of 12-lead ECG and serum electrolytes.
- Monitor continuous ECG to assess HR and rhythm. Document ECG rhythm strips every 2 to 4 hours in patients with supraventricular tachycardia (SVT) or ventricular tachycardia (VT).
- Should dysrhythmias occur, monitor and report BP ≤90/60 mm Hg, CO ≤2.5 L/min, capillary refill ≥3 seconds, thready peripheral pulses, dizziness, or chest pain.
- Administer prescribed FIO_2 at 50% or oxygen 2 to 4 L/min by means of nasal cannula or mask.
- Administer prescribed IV fluids to maintain adequate hydration.
- Administer prescribed antidysrhythmic agents such as amiodarone to abolish SVT and VT in HCM patients.
- Instruct patient to report any chest pain or palpitations.
- Teach patient common side effects of antidysrhythmia medication.

DISCHARGE PLANNING

The critical care nurse provides the patient and significant other(s) with verbal or written discharge notes regarding the following subjects:

1. Signs and symptoms that require immediate medical attention: fatigue, shortness of breath, activity intolerance, tachycardia, tachypnea, and weight gain ≥2.3 to 3.0 L/day for 2 consecutive days.
2. Medication's name, purpose, dosage, schedule, and side effects.
3. Need to keep follow-up appointments.
4. Names of community agencies such as American Heart Association.

■ ACUTE CARDIAC TAMPONADE

(For related information see Part I: Acute myocardial infarction, p. 38; Congestive heart failure, p. 87; Acute chest pain, p. 1; Acute pericarditis, p. 123; Dysrhythmias, p. 184. Part III: Hemodynamic monitoring, p. 219. See also Respiratory Deviations, Part III: Pulse oximetry, p. 426.)

Diagnostic Category and Length of Stay

DRG: 144 Other circulatory system diagnoses with complications
LOS: 5.20 days
DRG: 144 Other circulatory system diagnoses without complications
LOS: 3.40 days

Definition

Acute cardiac tamponade is the accumulation of fluid within the inelastic pericardial sac. There is impaired hemodynamic functioning resulting from increased intrapericardial pressure that overcomes normal compensatory mechanisms. Hemodynamic changes include impaired cardiac output, reduced stroke volume, and epicardial coronary artery compression.

Pathophysiology

The pericardium normally contains 10 to 50 mL of serous-type fluid, which is drained by lymphatics into the mediastinum and right heart cavities. Intrapericardial pressure usually equals intrapleural pressure and is slightly lower than right and left ventricular end-diastolic pressures. Thus a pressure gradient that allows the heart to fill is maintained between the chambers of the heart and the pericardium. In acute cardiac tamponade, there is increased intrapericardial fluid and intrapericardial pressure, which causes compression of the heart and prevents the ventricles from completely filling during diastole. In acute cardiac tamponade, as much as 50 to 2500 mL fluid can accumulate in the pericardial sac. Because the right atrium and ventricle have the lowest diastolic pressure, they are the first structures to be compressed. Impairment of cardiac function occurs when the intrapericardial pressure increases, resulting in an impairment of ventricular filling during diastole. Stroke volume and cardiac output are reduced. The body compensates through adrenergic stimulation, which increases heart rate; systemic and pulmonary venous pressure increases in order to improve ventricular filling; adrenergic stimulation increases ejection fraction; and increase in peripheral resistance serves to support arterial blood pressure. Normal pressure in the pericardial space is −2 to −4 mm Hg, which is less than ventricular diastolic pressure (4 mm Hg in the right ventricle, 8 mm Hg in the left ventricle) and equal to pleural pressure. Intrapericardial pressure may rise to as high as 20 to 30 mm Hg. As fluid accumulates in the pericardial space, intrapericardial pressure and right ventricular diastolic pressure rise together to the level of left ventricular diastolic pressure. As a result, all intracardiac pressures during diastole are then equal to the intrapericardial pressure. This is called diastolic pressure plateau.

Nursing Assessment

PRIMARY CAUSES

- Viral and bacterial infections and neoplastic invasion of the myocardium pericardium cause acute cardiac tamponade. Cardiopulmonary mechanisms include chest trauma, chest radiation, pericarditis, heart surgery, aneurysm, coronary angiography, insertion and removal of pacing wires, rupture of heart after infarction, aortic dissection, insertion of central venous catheter, and anticoagulant treatment. Finally, collagen disease such as rheumatoid arthritis and systemic lupus erythematosus can lead to acute cardiac tamponade. Other causes include hypothyroidism, renal failure, and coagulation disorders.

RISK FACTORS

- History of acute myocardial infarction or recent cardiac trauma.

PHYSICAL ASSESSMENT

- Inspection: Patient experiences tachypnea, dyspnea, orthopnea, chest pain, shortness of breath, or cough. Skin is pale, cyanotic, or diaphoretic. Patient may also experience confusion, apprehension, restlessness, jugular vein distenion, pulsus paradoxus of ≥10 mm Hg, hepatojugular reflux, Kussmaul's sign, ascites, or increased abdominal girth.
- Palpation: Peripheral pulses are thready or absent with point of maximal impulse (PMI) absent. Skin is cool, pale, and disaphoretic and there is peripheral edema.
- Auscultation: The S_1 and S_2 heart sounds are muffled because the heart is surrounded by fluid. Other findings include pericardial rub, tachycardia, and hypotension.

DIAGNOSTIC TEST RESULTS

Hemodynamic Parameters. (See Table 1–9)

- Increased intrapericardial pressure (IPP), increased systemic vascular resistance (SVR), increased central venous pressure (CVP), increased left atrial pressure (LAP), increased pulmonary artery systolic pressure (PAS), increased pulmonary artery diastolic pressure (PAD), increased right ventricular end-diastolic pressure (RVEDP), increased left ventricular end-diastolic pressure (LVEDP), and decreased cardiac output (CO).

Invasive Cardiac Diagnostic Procedures. (See Table 1–2)

- Cardiac catheterization: Reveals equal right and left heart pressures and increased thickness of the pericardial shadow.

Noninvasive Cardiac Diagnostic Procedures. (See Table 1–3)

- Chest roentgenogram: Reveals enlarged cardiac silhouette, globular shape of heart, widened mediastinum, pleural fields, and superior vena cava with normal lung fields.
- Echocardiogram: Shows inadequate ventricular filling (diastolic collapse of the right

ventricle); variations in ventricular dimensions during the respiratory cycle and in the direction and rate of movement of the aortic and mitral valves and the septum. Also shows effusion, since as little as 15 mL of fluid in the pericardial sac can be determined.

ECG

- Changes may include decreased voltage of QRS complex and T wave, and ST segments can be elevated in leads I, II, AVL, and AVF and depressed in AVR. Electrical alternans is manifested on ECG as an alteration in the direction and amplitude of the QRS and T wave with every other beat.

MEDICAL AND SURGICAL MANAGEMENT

PHARMACOLOGY

- Inotropic agents: Used to increase heart rate, myocardial contractility, and stroke volume while decreasing the SVR. Drugs used are dopamine, amrinone, norepinephrine, epinephrine, and isoproterenol (see Table 1–10).

PERICARDIOCENTESIS

- The procedure is used to aspirate fluid from the pericardial sac by inserting a needle into the sac, using a subxyphoid or left parasternal approach. Continued drainage can be accomplished by inserting a drainage catheter, thereby decreasing the necessity for repeated pericardiocentesis.

FLUID THERAPY

- Fluid resuscitation with whole blood, colloid or crystalloid, can be used to improve fluid volume and CO.

OXYGEN THERAPY

- Supplemental oxygen is used to improve tissue oxygenation, maintain cardiopulmonary function, and achieve comfort.

HEMODYNAMIC MONITORING

- Used to assess changes associated with resistance to right heart filling and decreased CO. Increased CVP can occur when resis-

tance to right ventricular filling is due to increased IPP. Likewise, CO can decrease as filling of the heart decreases. Left heart filling pressures can be monitored by pulmonary artery wedge pressure.

SURGICAL INTERVENTIONS

- Pericardial window: In this intervention, a subxyphoid approach is used. An incision is made vertically over the xiphoid process and the tip of the process is removed. The pericardium is visualized and incised. A chest tube may be inserted to drain the pericardial fluid in patients whose pericardium shows cardiac tamponade.
- Pericardectomy: This is excision of part of the pericardium.
- Pericardiotomy: This is incision of the pericardium.

NURSING MANAGEMENT: COLLABORATIVE PROBLEMS AND NURSING DIAGNOSES

Nursing Diagnoses

Common nursing goals in patients with acute cardiac tamponade are to enhance tissue perfusion, provide oxygenation, reduce risk of infection, minimize pain, and reduce anxiety. **Altered cardiopulmonary, peripheral, cerebral, and renal tissue perfusion** related to compromised arterial and venous perfusion secondary to compression of the myocardium by pericardial fluid and increased IPP.

Expected Patient Outcomes. Patient maintains adequate tissue perfusion, as evidence by (BP) within patient's normal range, CO 4 to 8 L/min, cardiac index (CI) 2.7 to 4.3 L/min/m², coronary artery perfusion pressure (CAPP) 60 to 80 mm Hg, mean arterial perfusion (MAP) 70 to 90 mm Hg, saturation of arterial oxygen (Sao₂) ≥95%, heart rate (HR) ≤100 bpm, absence of chest pain, normal lung sounds, warm and dry skin, normal heart sounds, capillary refill ≤3 seconds, peripheral pulses +2, absence of confusion, equal and normoreactive pupils, normal sensorimotor function, arterial oxygen pressure (Pao₂) ≥80 mm Hg, arterial carbon dioxide pressure ($Paco_2$) 35 to 45 mm Hg, arterial oxygen saturation (Sao_2) $\geq$95%, respiratory rate (RR) 12 to 20 BPM, urinary output (UO) $\geq$30 mL/h or $\geq$0.5 mL/kg/h, and specific gravity 1.010 to 1.030.

- Consult with cardiologist to validate expected patient outcomes used to evaluate adequate tissue perfusion.
- Review results of ECG, echocardiogram, chest roentgenogram, and arterial blood gas measurement.
- Restrict physical activity to bed rest with head of bed elevated to decrease myocardial tissue oxygen demand should there be decreased myocardial tissue perfusion.
- Obtain and report hemodynamic parameters reflective of decreased myocardial tissue perfusion when CO is decreased: CAPP $\leq$60 mm Hg, CO $\leq$4 L/min, and CI $\leq$2.7 L/min/m^2.
- Monitor, document, and report other clinical findings suggestive of decreased myocardial tissue perfusion: chest pain, capillary refill $\geq$3 seconds, pallor, diaphoresis, crackles, shortness of breath, HR $\geq$100 bpm, or BP $\leq$90 mm Hg.
- Assess, document, and report findings reflective of decreased pulmonary tissue perfusion: Pao_2 $\leq$80 mm Hg, $Paco_2$ $\geq$45 mm Hg, Sao_2 $\leq$95%, mottled or cyanotic skin, shortness of breath, dyspnea, RR $\geq$20 BPM, and crackles.
- Encourage patient to deep breathe and cough every 2 hours.
- Assess, document, and report clinical findings indicating decreased cerebral tissue perfusion: confusion, disorientation to time and place, pupils unequal, and sensorimotor dysfunction.
- Assess, document, and report clinical findings indicating decreased peripheral tissue perfusion: capillary refill $\geq$3 seconds; peripheral pulses weak or absent; skin cool, clammy, and cyanotic; and BP 90/60 mm Hg.
- Monitor, document, and report clinical findings reflecting decreased renal tissue perfusion: UO $\leq$30 mL/h or $\leq$0.5 mL/kg/h,

specific gravity 1.010 to 1.030, and peripheral edema.

- Monitor intake, output, and specific gravity every 1 to 2 hours should UO be $\leq$30 mL/h. Note that diuretics will decrease volume and further impair ventricular filling.
- Administer prescribed oxygen 2 to 4 L/min or Fio_2 $\leq$50% by means of nasal cannula or mask to maintain Sao_2 $\geq$95%.
- Should oxygenation not improve arterial blood gas readings, prepare patient for intubation and mechanical ventilation.
- Administer prescribed blood products, colloids or crystalloids, to maintain adequate hydration, UO $\geq$30 mL/h or $\geq$0.5 mL/kg/h and specific gravity 1.010 to 1.030.
- Administer positive inotropes (dopamine or dobutamine) to maintain MAP 70 to 90 mm Hg, HR $\leq$100 bpm, BP within patient's normal range, and UO $\geq$30 mL/h.
- Teach patient to report the presence of chest pain.

Impaired gas exchange related to compromised cardiopulmonary perfusion secondary to restriction of ventricular diastolic filling and increased LVEDP resulting from the accumulation of fluid in the pericardial sac.

Expected Patient Outcomes. Patient maintains adequate gas exchange, as evidenced by Pao_2 $\geq$70 mm Hg, $Paco_2$ 35 to 45 mm Hg, pH 7.35 to 7.45, absence of cyanosis, Sao_2 $\geq$95 mm Hg, RR 12 to 20 BPM, absence of crackles, HR $\leq$100 bpm, absence of dyspnea and restlessness.

- Consult with cardiologist to validate expected patient outcomes used to assess gas exchange.
- Review results of chest roentgenogram and arterial blood gas measurement.
- Monitor clinical indicators of respiratory status: RR and depth, use of accessory muscles, symmetry of chest movement, skin color, and lung sounds.
- Report clinical findings associated with impaired gas exchange: tachypnea, cyanosis,

tachycardia, dyspnea, restlessness, and use of accessory muscles.

- Administer prescribed oxygen 2 to 4 L/min by nasal cannula or mask to maintain adequate oxygenation.
- Provide calm, relaxed environment while the patient is dyspneic and restless.

High risk for infection related to invasive procedures secondary to pericardiocentesis.

Expected Patient Outcomes. Patient is free of infection, as evidenced by temperature within normal limits; HR ≤100 bpm; absence of purulent drainage; or absence of edema, redness, or tenderness around the catheter site.

- Consult with dietitian about the patient's nutritional status and need to provide adequate protein and caloric intake for healing.
- Review complete blood count (CBC) results and negative cultures.
- Assess all invasive lines or catheters for signs of redness, swelling, tenderness, or drainage.
- Monitor and report temperature ≥100.8°F and HR ≥100 bpm.
- Maintain aseptic technique for all invasive devices, changing sites, dressings, tubings, and solutions per unit standard.
- Administer prescribed antibiotics should an infection occur (Table 1–14).
- Teach patient to report any tenderness, redness, or drainage from invasive lines or catheter sites.

Pain related to dyspnea or pericardial inflammation.

Expected Patient Outcome. Patient verbalizes the reduction or absence of pain.

- Help patient to identify the position of optimal comfort. Pain may be reduced by sitting in an upright position or leaning forward. The latter can reduce tension in the inflamed pericardial sac.
- Monitor output from the pericardial catheter and evaluate effect on pain reduction.

- Reassure patient that pain will subside when the intrapericardial fluid is removed.
- Document patient's description of pain, frequency of occurrence, response to reduction, and vital signs before and after medication.
- Administer prescribed oxygen 2 to 4 L/min by nasal cannula or mask.
- Administer prescribed nonsteroidal anti-inflammatory agents (salicylates or indomethacin) to reduce inflammation of the pericardial sac.
- Teach patient to report any chest pain following pericardiocentesis.

Anxiety related to pain, invasive procedures, or separation from significant others.

Expected Patient Outcomes. Patient does not appear anxious, BP within normal range for patient, HR ≤100 bpm, RR 12 to 20 BPM, and posture and facial expression relaxed.

- Listen to patient's verbalization of concern or fear.
- Explain diagnostic procedures and treatments.
- Evaluate patient's need for pain medication.
- Provide diversional activities to reduce stress: meditation, relaxation, reading, watching TV, or listening to music.
- Encourage patient and significant others to ask questions and to express concerns and fears.
- Prepare patient for possible surgery.
- Administer prescribed analgesics to maintain HR ≤100 bpm, RR 12 to 20 BPM, and resolve chest pain.

Collaborative Problems

Common collaborative goals in patients with acute cardiac tamponade are to increase CO and reduce excess fluid accumulation around the heart.

Potential Complication: Decreased Cardiac Output. Decreased CO related to impaired ventricular filling secondary to increased IPP.

TABLE 1-14

TABLE 1–14. ANTIBIOTICS

Medication	Route/Dose	Uses and Effects	Side Effects
Amphotericin B (Fungizone)	IV test dose 1 mg dissolved in 20 mL of D$_5$W by slow infusion over 1–30 min to reduce risk of anaphylactic reaction IV initial dose 250 μg/kg/d infused over 4–6 h Adjusted daily in increments of 250 μg/kg/d or faster if tolerated, up to 1.0 mg/kg/d or 1.5 mg/kg/d qid; maximum daily dosage of 1.5 mg/kg should not be exceeded PO: 50 mg/d except in severe infections	Treatment of active, progressive potentially fatal fungal infections	Headache, muscle pain, weakness, vertigo, hypotension, diarrhea, nausea, fever, chills, nephrotoxicity, anorexia, weight loss, CHF
Ampicillin (Polycillin)	IV/IM: systemic infections 250–2000 mg q 6 h PO: 25–500 mg q 6 h	Broad-spectrum antibiotic for respiratory infections, genitourinary infections, and endocarditis Prophylaxis for bacterial infections	Seizures, rashes, urticaria, hemolytic anemia, nausea, vomiting, diarrhea, allergic reaction
Cefazolin sodium (Ancef)	IV/IM: Severe infection 250–2000 mg q 8 h, up to 2000 mg q 4 h for a maximum of 12 g/d Surgical prophylaxis 1–2 g 30–60 min before surgery, then q 8 h for 24 h	Treatment of endocarditis Perioperative prophylaxis in patients undergoing procedures with high risk of infection, such as open heart surgery	Diarrhea, anorexia, abdominal cramps, rashes, anaphylaxis, fever, nephrotoxicity
Trimethoprim and sulfa-methoxazole (co-trimoxazole) (Bactrim)	PO: 160 mg trimethoprim (TPM)/800 mg SMZ q 12 h	Treatment of endocarditis Rheumatic fever prophylaxis	Headache, fatigue, depression, nausea, vomiting, rashes, aplastic anemia, leukopenia, phlebitis at IV site
Erythromycin stearate (Erythrocin); estolate; ethyl-succinate	IV: 1–4 g/d in divided doses q 6 h, or continuous infusion PO: Base, estolate, stearate 250–500 mg q 6 h; ethylsuccinate 400–800 mg q 6–8 h	Treatment of streptococcal infection Endocarditis prophylaxis	Nausea, vomiting, rashes, dizziness, headache, tremors, tachycardia, fever, chills, chest discomfort, dyspnea, hyperventilation, hypotension, palpitation, tachycardia
Gentamycin (Garamycin)	IV/IM: 3–5 mg/kg/d in divided doses q 8 h	Treatment of endocarditis, skin, soft tissue	Ototoxicity, nephrotoxicity, enhanced neuromuscular blockade, infection
Nafcillin sodium (Unipen)	IV/IM: 500–2000 mg q 4–6 h up to 12 g/d PO: 25–1000 mg q 4–6 h	Treatment of endocarditis and septicemia	Urticaria, rash, nausea, anaphylaxis, vomiting, diarrhea, allergic reaction

TABLE 1-14

TABLE 1-14. CONTINUED

Medication	Route/Dose	Uses and Effects	Side Effects
Oxacillin sodium (Bactocill)	IV/IM: 500–2000 mg q 4–6 h up to 12 g/d Oral: 250–1000 mg q 4–6 h	Treatment of endocarditis and septicemia	Nausea, vomiting, rashes, diarrhea, anaphylaxis, interstitial nephritis, allergic reactions
Penicillin G potassium (Pfizerpen)	IV/IM: 1.2–24 million U, divided q 4 h PO: 1.6–3.2 million U divided q 8 h	Treatment of rheumatic heart disease, streptococcal infections, and endocarditis	Electrolyte imbalance, systemic anaphylaxis, fever, malaise, skin rashes, urticaria, injection site reactions, nausea, or vomiting
Streptomycin sulfate	IM: Enterococcal endocarditis 1 g q 12 h for 2 wk, then 500 mg q 12 h for 4 wk Streptococcal endocarditis 1 g q 12 h for 1 wk, then 500 mg q 12 h for 1 wk	Treatment of streptococcal or enterococcal endocarditis	Ototoxicity, nephrotoxicity, enhanced neuromuscular blockade
Vancomycin (Vancocin)	IV: Systemic infection 500 mg q 6 h or 1 g q 12 h Endocarditis prophylaxis in penicillin-allergic patients 1 g single dose 1 h preprocedure	Treatment of endocarditis and staphylococcal infection	Ototoxicity, hypotension, nausea, vomiting, nephrotoxicity, rashes, phlebitis, anaphylaxis

CHF, congestive heart failure; IM, intramuscular; IV, intravenous; PO, by mouth.

From Govoni LE, Hayes JE, 1992; Loeb S, 1993; Payne JL, 1992; Vallerand AH, Deglin JH, 1991.

Expected Patient Outcomes. Patient maintains adequate CO as evidenced by CO 4 to 8 L/min, CI 2.7 to 4.3 L/min/m^2, CVP 2 to 6 mm Hg, ejection fraction (EF) $\geq$50% to 60%, IPP $\leq$2 to 4 mm Hg, MAP 70 to 90 mm Hg, pulmonary artery pressure (PAP) systolic 15 to 25 mm Hg or diastolic 8 to 15 mm Hg, pulmonary capillary wedge pressure (PCWP) 6 to 12 mm Hg, pulse pressure (PP) $\geq$30 mm Hg, right atrial pressure (RAP) 4 to 6 mm Hg, right ventricular pressure (RVP) systolic 15 to 25 mm Hg or diastolic 0 to 8 mm Hg, stroke volume (SV) 60 to 130 mL/beat, stroke volume index (SVI) 45 to 85 g-m/beat/m^2, SVR 900 to 1200 dynes/s/cm^{-5}, SVRI 1970 to 2390 dynes/s/cm^{-5}/m^2, UO $\geq$30 mL/h or $\geq$0.5 mL/kg/h, absence of pulsus paradoxus, absence of neck vein distention, normal heart sounds, HR $\leq$100 bpm, RR 12 to 20 BPM, and normal skin color.

- Confer with cardiologist to validate expected patient outcomes used to assess adequate CO.
- Review results of 12-lead ECG, chest roentgenogram, and echocardiogram.
- Review results of intracardiac pressures: cardiac transmural pressure (TMP=cavity pressure minus pericardial pressure), which increases as IPP decreases.
- Position dyspneic acute cardiac tamponade patient in a high Fowler's position, if hemodynamically stable. This allows accumulated blood in pericardial sac to be dependent, thereby causing less compression on the lungs. A high Fowler's position also helps to decrease venous return.
- Obtain and report clinical findings reflective of acute cardiac tamponade: Beck's triad or cardiac compression triad, which consists of decreasing arterial pressure,

rising venous pressure, and a small, quiet heart.

- Obtain and report other clinical findings associated with acute cardiac tamponade: a systolic-to-diastolic gradient (pulse pressure) ≤ 30 mm Hg; neck vein distention; bluish discoloration of the skin in the upper chest or face; and Kussmaul's sign, which is present when the patient is lying with head of bed at a 60-degree angle and the neck veins distend on inspiration, indicating increased LAP.
- Obtain and report hemodynamic parameters reflective of decreased CO caused by increased IPP: CO ≤ 4 L/min, CI ≤ 2.7 L/min/m^2, CVP ≥ 6 mm Hg, MAP ≤ 70 mm Hg, PAP systolic ≥ 25 mm Hg or diastolic ≥ 15 mm Hg, PCWP ≥ 12 mm Hg, RAP ≥ 6 mm Hg, RVP systolic ≥ 25 mm Hg or diastolic ≥ 8 mm Hg, SV ≤ 60 mL/beat, SVI ≤ 45 g-m/beat/m^2, SVR ≥ 1200 dynes/s/cm^{-5}, and SVRI ≥ 2390 dynes/s/cm^{-5}/m^2.
- Obtain and report the presence of pulsus paradoxus (via arterial tracing or during normal BP reading), which is a fall of more than 10 mm Hg peak systolic pressure during inspiration. Monitor BP every 5 to 15 minutes during acute phase of acute cardiac tamponade. The BP cuff is inflated 20 to 30 mm Hg higher than the systolic pressure while the patient is breathing normally. The difference in millimeters of mercury between the first Korotkoff's sounds heard and the continuous Korotkoff's sounds is the pulsus paradoxus. With the arterial line, the height of the wave for (pressure) will decrease during inspiration. The difference between the pressure during expiration and inspiration is the amount of paradoxus.
- Calculate and report hemodynamic parameters suggesting increased IPP: MAP ≤ 70 mm Hg, SVR ≥ 1200 dynes/s/cm^{-5}, and PP ≤ 30 mm Hg.
- Assess, document, and report the parameters reflecting the need for intrapericardial fluid removal: CVP ≥ 20 cm H$_2$O, pulse paradoxus ≥ 20 mm Hg, and pulse pressure ≤ 20 mm Hg.

- Monitor continuous ECG to assess HR and rhythm. Document ECG rhythm strips every 4 hours if acute cardiac tamponade is suspected: electrical alternans, which is alternating large and small QRS complexes or altered direction of the complexes; low voltage; and flat or inverted T waves; or sinus tachycardia.
- Evaluate the results of Keck's tamponade score system in postoperative coronary artery bypass graft patients: serum creatinine ≥ 1.6, cumulative chest tube drainage ≥ 1400 mL, pressure plateau for a 2-hour period, mediastinal widening on radiograph; or Beck's triad: arterial hypotension, muffled heart sounds, and elevated CVP.
- Monitor daily weight, intake, and output, since a decrease in UO ≤ 30 mL/h or ≤ 0.5 mL/kg/h may indicate reduced renal perfusion secondary to decreased SV.
- Administer prescribed IV fluids such as blood products, colloids or crystalloids, which increase ventricular filling pressure and temporarily maintain increased SV.
- Administer prescribed F$_{IO_2}$ at 50% by mask or oxygen 2 to 4 L/min by nasal cannula to increase arterial oxygen saturation and improve oxygen delivery to the tissues.
- Administer prescribed volume-reducing agents (furosemide or bumetanide) to maintain CVP 2 to 6 mm Hg or 5 to 12 cm H$_2$O, UO ≥ 30 mL/h or ≥ 0.5 mL/kg/h, resolved neck vein distention, specific gravity 1.010 to 1.030 (see Table 1–13).
- Assist with pericardiocentesis with venous pressure ≥ 10 mm Hg, pulsus paradoxus ≥ 20 mm Hg, and pulse pressure ≤ 20 mm Hg.
- Monitor patient's respiratory status and HR during procedure and report change in ECG (elevated ST, ventricular fibrillation, premature atrial contraction (PAC), or pneumothorax.
- Should pericardiocentesis not relieve the IPP, prepare patient for pericardial window surgery to drain fluid via an interpericardial catheter placed along the anterior wall of the pericardial cavity. The catheter extends from

the window to the skin surface and is anchored to the skin near the xiphoid process. The catheter is connected to a closed drainage bottle with underwater seal, interpericardial catheter connected to a closed drainage bottle with underwater seal: the subxiphoid approach or the left parasternal approach via the left fourth and fifth intercostal space. Removal of 20 to 50 mL of fluid will increase BP and CO.

- Instruct patient in the purpose behind pericardiocentesis or, if necessary, pericardial window surgery.
- Teach patient common side effects of positive inotropes and diuretics.

Potential Complication: Pericardial Effusion. Pleural effusion related to excess fluid accumulation around the heart secondary to acute cardiac tamponade.

Expected Patient Outcomes. Patient is free of excess pericardial fluid accumulation, as evidenced by normal heart sounds; absence of dyspnea, anxiety, or restlessness; and absence of pericardial rub.

- Monitor and report muffled S_1 and S_2 heart sounds heard over the base of the heart while patient is leaning forward.
- Obtain and report other clinical findings that may indicate pericardial effusion: quiet precordium, PMI not palpable, pericardial rub, dyspnea, anxiety, and restlessness.
- Administer prescribed IV fluid to maintain adequate circulatory volume.
- Assist with pericardiocentesis.

DISCHARGE PLANNING

The critical care nurse provides the patient and significant other(s) with verbal or written discharge notes regarding the following subjects:

1. Dates of follow-up appointments.
2. Signs and symptoms requiring immediate medical attention: chest pain for pericar-

dial friction rub, anxiety, restlessness, hypotension, or shortness of breath.
3. Activity schedule, which is reduced for 1 to 2 weeks then increased. A postdischarge exercise program to keep HR ≤ 100 bpm according to the following: (1) First week, walk 0.25 miles within 8 to 10 minutes; (2) second week, walk 0.25 miles within 5 minutes; (3) third week, walk 0.50 miles within 15 minutes; and (4) fourth week, walk 1.0 miles within 30 minutes.
4. Medications including purpose, dosage, schedule, or side effects.

■ ACUTE PERICARDITIS

(For related information see Part I: Acute myocardial infarction, p. 38; Congestive heart failure, p. 87; Acute chest pain, p. 1; Acute cardiac tamponade, p. 117; Dysrhythmias, p. 184. Part III: Hemodynamic monitoring, p. 219. See also Respiratory Deviations, Part III: Pulse oximetry, p. 426.)

Diagnostic Category and Length of Stay
DRG: 144 Other circulatory diagnoses with complications
LOS: 5.20 days
DRG: 145 Other circulatory diagnoses without complications
LOS: 3.40 days

Definition
Acute pericarditis is the inflammation of the pericardium, the fibrous tissue surrounding the heart. The pericardium is a protective layer. Inflammation of the pericardium leads to friction between the pericardium and myocardium.

Pathophysiology
In acute pericarditis, there is infiltration of polymorphonuclear leukocytes into the pericardium, increased pericardial vascularity, and fibrinous deposits on and possibly be-

tween the pericardial membranes. The inflammatory process may extend beyond the pericardium into the epicardium and the adjacent pleura. Serous exudation may cause the occurrence of pleural effusion. Early acute pericarditis is characterized by fibrin deposition and possible pericardial effusion. Chronic inflammation progresses to fibrous scarring and pericardial thickening with effusion obliterating the pericardial sac. In time, dense calcium deposits may contribute to pericardial thickening and noncompliance. Pericarditis can alter myocardial contractility and elevation and equilibration of the right and left heart filling pressures.

Nursing Assessment

PRIMARY CAUSES
- Causes include myocardial and pericardial injury such as myocardial infarction, cardiac surgery, chest trauma, and anticoagulant therapy; viral, bacterial, fungal, and parasitic infections; connective tissue disorders such as rheumatoid arthritis, systemic lupus erythematosus, acute rheumatic fever, and scleroderma. The renal cause is uremia. Neoplastic disease, such as lymphoma, leukemia, or disease secondary to lung and breast cancer can cause acute pericarditis. Irradiation is also a factor causing acute pericarditis. Lastly, drugs such as procainamide, hydralazine, isoniazid, diphenylhydantoin, penicillin, minoxidil, phenylbutazone, or anthracycline neoplastic agents may induce acute pericarditis.

RISK FACTORS
- History of infections during the previous 4 weeks, recent fatigue, weight loss, fever, chills and use of immunosuppressive drugs since these predispose to microbial invasion.

PHYSICAL ASSESSMENT
- Inspection: Chest pain is located as sharp, dull, aching and is located in the retrosternal or left precordial regions. The pain may radiate to or be confined to the neck, back, epigastrium, or right chest. Dyspnea occurs as a result of the need to splint chest to reduce precordial discomfort. Other associated symptoms may include fever, cough, neck vein distention, weight loss, fatigue, pallor, or sputum production.
- Palpation: A precordial rub may be palpable, producing a thrill along the middle to lower middle sternal border.
- Auscultation: A precordial friction rub occurs with an atrial systolic (presystolic), a ventricular systolic, and an early diastolic component. Crackles may also occur. Blood pressure may reveal a pulsus paradoxus ≥ 10 mm Hg.

DIAGNOSTIC TEST RESULTS

Hemodynamic Parameters. (See Table 1–9)

- Central venous pressure increased, equilibration of right and left end-diastolic pressures; right atrial pressure (RAP) shows "M" or "W" pattern resulting from an X descent with a prominent early diastolic Y descent and increases as clinically manifested by Kussmaul's sign; right ventricular pressure (RVP) shows a dip–plateau contour in which dip corresponds to the rapid early diastolic filling and plateau corresponds to the mid and late diastolic period, where there is restriction of cardiac volume expansion. Other findings include elevated pulmonary artery pressure (PAP) and pulmonary capillary wedge pressure (PCWP). As effusion increases there can be a reduction in cardiac output.

Standard Laboratory Tests. (See Table 1–1)

- Blood studies: The white blood count (WBC) is $\geq 10,000$ to $20,000/\mu L$ with an elevated sedimentation rate.
- Immunodiagnostic studies: Antistreptolysin O (ASO) titer increases when pericarditis is due to immunological problem.
- Serum enzymes: Small increases creatine kinase (CK-MB).

Invasive Cardiac Diagnostic Procedures. (See Table 1–2)

- Angiography: In lateral border of the right atrium is straight, pericardial thickening and left anterior descending coronary artery within the cardiac silhouette.
- Cardiac catheterization: Diastolic expansion of both ventricles is affected equally, elevated diastolic pressure, ventricular pressure curves show a characteristic "square root" sign, a and v waves are usually equal, x and y descents are quick and prominent, moderately elevated PAP, low or decreased cardiac index, and normal intracardiac pressure.

Noninvasive Cardiac Diagnostic Procedures. (See Table 1–3)

- Chest roentgenogram: The cardiac silhouette may be normal but can show globular enlargement if there is pericardial effusion ($\geq$250 mL of fluid).
- Computed tomography: Can be used to evaluate pericardial thickening and effusion.
- Echocardiogram: Effusion as small as 15 mL can be identified. Pericardial fluid appears as an echo-free space between the anterior wall of the right ventricle and the chest wall and the posterior left ventricle wall and the posterior parietal pericardium.

ECG
- Stage I: Concave upward ST segment in leads I, II, aVL, aVF, and V_3 to V_6; ST segment depression in aVR and V_1; T waves upright in leads showing ST segment elevation; PR segment depression. Stage II: Transitional phase in which ST segment returns to baseline followed by progressive flattening, eventual inversion of those T waves formerly upright, and PR segment depression. Stage III: T wave inversion in most leads. Stage IV: Return to ECG findings present before the development of pericarditis. Other findings include atrial fibrillation, paroxysmal supraventricular tachycardia, or sinus tachycardia.

MEDICAL AND SURGICAL MANAGEMENT

PHARMACOLOGY
- Nonsteroidal anti-inflammatory drugs (NSAIDs): Agents such as aspirin (650 mg every 3 to 4 hours), indomethacin (25 to 75 mg qid), or ibuprofen are used to relieve discomfort and reduce inflammation.
- Steroids: Prednisone (60 to 80 mg every day for 5 to 7 days) may be given if the symptoms continue unresolved from NSAID therapy (Table 1–15).
- Azathioprine: May be used if acute pericarditis recurs despite pharmacological therapy. The recurrence is possible due to an immune response to a previous precordial injury (see Table 1–15).

PHYSICAL ACTIVITY
- Bed rest: Activity is limited to sitting up and leaning forward in an attempt to reduce chest pain.

HEMODYNAMIC MONITORING
- Monitor changes in cardiac index (CI), cardiac output (CO), central venous pressure (CVP), PAP, and PCWP.

PERICARDIOCENTESIS
- The procedure consists of aspirating fluid from the pericardial sac by inserting a needle into the sac using a subxyphoid or left parasternal approach. Insertion of a drainage catheter allows continued drainage, thereby decreasing the necessity for repeated pericardiocentesis.

SURGICAL INTERVENTIONS
- Pericardectomy: This is the excision of part of the pericardium.

NURSING MANAGEMENT: NURSING DIAGNOSES AND COLLABORATIVE PROBLEMS

Nursing Diagnoses
Common nursing goals for patients with acute pericarditis are to reduce chest pain,

enhance oxygenation, restore activity tolerance, and reduce anxiety.

Pain related to inflammation of the pericardium secondary to stretching of the pericardial sac resulting from increased intrapericardial fluid.

Expected Patient Outcomes. Patient verbalizes pain relief and breathes with ease.

- Consult with cardiologist about providing analgesics to reduce patient's chest pain.
- Assist patient with relief of pain by encouraging shallow breathing, sitting upright, and leaning forward.
- Observe, document, and report clinical findings indicating acute pericarditis: chest pain described as sharp, dull, and aching and localized to the retrospinal or left precordial region, dyspnea, fever, cough, sputum production, weight gain, BP ≤90/60 mm Hg, and capillary refill ≤3 seconds.
- Monitor for the presence of pericardial friction rub by examining patient in supine position, in left lateral decubitus position, and sitting up, while holding inspiration and expiration.
- Obtain temperature every 4 hours or as indicated when patient is febrile.
- Monitor continuous ECG to assess heart rate and rhythm. Document ECG rhythm strips every 2 to 4 hours in patients with dysrhythmias. ST segments will return to baseline within 7 days, followed by T wave inversion 1 to 2 weeks from the beginning of chest pain.
- Administer prescribed oxygen 2 to 4 L/min by means of nasal cannula or mask.
- Administer prescribed NSAIDs (ibuprofen or indomethacin) to relieve chest pain (see Table 1–7).
- Administer the prescribed corticosteroidal therapy should NSAIDs be ineffective in reducing inflammation and pain (see Table 1–15).
- Teach patient which factors aggravate pericardial pain, such as assuming a prone position, muscle movement, inspiration, laughter, coughing, or left lateral position.

Ineffective breathing pattern related to guarding secondary to chest pain.

Expected Patient Outcomes. Patient maintains effective breathing pattern, as evidenced by respiratory rate (RR) 12 to 20 BPM, absence of dyspnea, resolution of chest pain, arterial blood gases within normal range, and arterial oxygen saturation (Sao_2) ≥95%.

- Review arterial blood gas and Sao_2 readings.
- Raise head of bed so patient is able to lean forward in order to relieve the pericardial pain.
- Evaluate the intensity and location of chest pain.
- Monitor and report chest pain, guarding respirations, and RR ≥20 BPM.
- Support patient's chest by splinting with pillows to facilitate coughing and deep breathing.
- Promote pulmonary hygiene to prevent the potential for atelectasis.
- Encourage patient to breathe shallowly while experiencing chest pain.
- Auscultate chest for RR, rhythm, and presence of pericardial friction rub.
- Encourage patient to use incentive spirometry excursions every 2 to 4 hours when pericardial pain subsides.
- Provide prescribed oxygen 2 to 4 L/min by means nasal cannula or mask to maintain arterial oxygen pressure (Pao_2) ≥80 mm Hg and Sao_2 ≥95%.
- Administer prescribed NSAIDs (ibuprofen or indomethacin) to relieve chest pain.
- Instruct patient to report any chest pain when patient turns, coughs or breathes deeply.

Activity intolerance related to fatigue, weakness, or chest pain secondary to decreased CO.

Expected Patient Outcomes. Patient is able to tolerate increased activity, as evidenced by

TABLE 1-15

TABLE 1–15. IMMUNOSUPPRESSIVE AGENTS

Medications	Route/Dose	Uses and Effects	Side Effects
Corticosteroids			
Prednisone (Deltasone)	PO: Maintenance 5–15 mg/d Rejection 1–3 mg/d Following rejection episode tapered to 0.5 mg/kg	Suppresses bone marrow production of monocytes and B lymphocytes, decreasing number of cells available for immune protection Blocks release of IL-1 by macrophages Reduces production of activated helper T cells and cytotoxic T cells Interferes with production of immunoglobulins, (e.g., IgG, IgA, IgM) by inhibition of plasma cell synthesis of antibodies Impairs phagocytes	Mood swings, increased appetite, weight gain, glucose intolerance, hypernatremia, fluid retention, acne, hirsutism, ulcers, potential for infection
Prednisolone (Cortalone)	IV: 2–30 mg q 12 h; doses up to 400 mg/d IM: 2–30 mg q 12 h; doses up to 400 mg/d PO: 5–60 mg/d as single or divided doses	Suppresses bone marrow production of monocytes and B lymphocytes, decreasing number of cells available for immune protection Blocks release of IL-1 by macrophages Reduces production of activated helper T cells and cytotoxic T cells Interferes with production of immunoglobulins (e.g., IgG, IgA, IgM) by inhibition of plasma cell synthesis of antibodies Impairs phagocytes	Hirsutism, hypotension, sensitivity to heat
Cytotoxic Agents			
Azathioprine (Imuran)	IV/PO: Initial 3–5 mg/kg/d; maintenance 1–2 mg/kg/d	Interferes with nucleic acid synthesis and inhibits cell division of immunoblastic cells, especially lymphocytes Inhibits B cell activity Inhibits antigen receptor sites on T cells Affects other rapidly dividing cells, including lymphoid cells, bone marrow, skin, and cells in GI tract	Vomiting, nausea, diarrhea, anorexia, skin eruptions, secondary infection, hepatotoxicity, dysphagia, muscle twitching

TABLE 1-15

TABLE 1-15. CONTINUED

Medications	Route/Dose	Uses and Effects	Side Effects
Cyclophos- phamide (Cytoxan)	IV: Induction 40–50 mg/kg (1.5–1.8 g/m²) in doses divided over 2–5 d; to 100 mg/kg Maintenance 10–15 mg/kg (350–550 mg/m²) q 7–10 d or 3–5 mg/kg twice/wk (110–185 mg/m²) PO: Induction 1–5 mg/kg/d Maintenance 1–5 mg/kg/d	Interferes with nucleic acid synthesis and inhibits cell division of immunoblastic cells, especially lymphocytes Inhibits antigen receptor sites on T cells Affects other rapidly dividing cells, including lymphoid cells, bone marrow, skin, and cells in GI tract Inhibits B-cell activity	Nausea, vomiting, anorexia, hepatotoxicity, diarrhea, nephrotoxicity, hyperkalemia, weight gain, weight loss, dizziness, fatigue, facial flushing, pulmonary edema
Antimetabolites			
Methotrexate sodium (Rheumatrex)	IV/IM: 10–25 mg/wk until adequate response is achieved PO: 2.5 mg/d or 5 d, followed by 2-d rest period	Inhibition of folic acid synthesis Inhibits rapidly proliferating cells in S phase Suppresses both cell-mediated and humoral immunity, as well as inflammation	Pruritus, hepatotoxicity, nausea, vomiting, diarrhea, headache, blurred vision, aphasia, confusion, tremors, malaise, fatigue, fever, chills, hematuria
Cyclosporine (Sandimmune)	IV: Initial 5–6 mg/kg/d; infused in NS or 5% dextrose over 2–6 h or as a continuous (24 h) infusion PO: First dose before transplant 15 mg/kg/d for 1–2 wk; taper by 5% weekly to maintenance dose of 5–10 mg/kg/d	Interferes with secretion of IL-2 by T lymphocytes Inhibits T cell proliferation Inhibits T-cell-mediated immune response	Hypertension, hirsutism, bruising, tinnitus, ototoxicity, visual disturbances, diarrhea, nausea, vomiting, anorexia, gastritis, tremor, convulsion, headache, paresthesia, hyperesthesia, flushing, urinary retention, muscle and joint pain, leg cramps, edema, weight loss
Antilymphocyte ALG, ATG	IV: Before transplant 10–15 mg/kg for 5–10 d Rejection 10–15 mg/kg for 10–14 d	ATG acts specifically against T cells, is preferred over ALG, which coats lymphocytes in general Removes active lymphocytes from spleen, lymph nodes, and reticuloendothelial system Interferes with cell-mediated rejection by decreasing number of active cells Inhibits maturation and differentiation of T cells	Fever, chills, pain in chest or back, shortness of breath, hypotension, nausea, vomiting, malaise, anemia

TABLE 1-15. CONTINUED

TABLE 1-15

Medications	Route/Dose	Uses and Effects	Side Effects
Murine Monoclonal Antibody			
Muromonab-CD3 (OKT3)	IV: 5 mg for 10–14 days	Treatment of rejection	Chills, fever, tightness of chest, wheezing, shortness of breath, diarrhea, nausea, vomiting, hypotension, tachycardia
		Depresses T-cell function by removing most cytoxic T cells from circulation	
		Renders remaining T cells unresponsive to antigenic stimulation	
FK 506	IV/PO: 0.15 mg/kg	Prevents the activity of T cells in response to foreign tissue	Headache, nausea, tremors, itching, abdominal pain

GI, gastrointestinal; IL, interleukin; IM, intramuscular; IV, intravenous; NS, normal saline; PO, by mouth.

From Deglin JH, Vallerand AH, Russin MM, 1988; Govoni LE, Hayes JE, Shannon MT, et al, 1992; Loeb S, 1993; Scherer JC, 1992; Vallerand AH, Deglin JH, 1991.

heart rate (HR) ≤20 bpm over patient's resting HR, peak systolic blood pressure (BP) ≤20 mm Hg over patient's resting systolic BP, mixed venous oxygen saturation (S$\bar{v}$o$_2$) ≥60%, RR ≤24 BPM, absence of chest pain, absence of crackles, and normal sinus rhythm.

- Consult with cardiologist to validate expected patient outcomes used to evaluate effective breathing pattern.
- Consult with cardiac rehabilitation to individualize patient's activity program.
- Monitor and report findings reflective of activity intolerance: RR ≥20 BPM; HR ≥20 bpm over resting heart rate; systolic BP decreased below resting level; pallor or cyanosis; cool, moist skin; S$\bar{v}$o$_2$ ≤60%; and complaints of dyspnea, shortness of breath, dizziness, weakness, or fatigue.
- Provide rest periods before, during, and after progressive increase in activity.
- Monitor patient's HR, rhythm, BP, RR, skin color, and temperature after acitivity. Recheck after a 10-minute rest period.
- Teach patient to report worsening dyspnea, shortness of breath, dizziness, or weakness.
- Teach patient to perform different activities more slowly or for a shorter period of time until the inflammatory process is corrected.

Anxiety related to pain or potential need for invasive procedures.

Expected Patient Outcome. Patient exhibits reduced anxious behavior.

- Provide emotional support by remaining with anxious patient and encouraging communication with the critical care nurse or significant other.
- Maintain a calm environment, since anxiety causes a release of catecholamines from the sympathetic nervous system, which increase BP, HR, and afterload and activates the renin-angiotensin system.
- Explain procedures and treatments to patient.
- Reassure patient about the causes of acute pericarditis and treatments.

Collaborative Problems

Common collaborative goals for patients with acute myocarditis are to increase CO, correct dysrhythmias, and maintain acid–base balance.

Potential Complication: Decreased Cardiac Output. Decreased CO related to restriction of ventricular filling or loss of atrial kick secondary to the accumulation of pericardial fluid.

Expected Patient Outcomes. Patient maintains adequate CO, as evidenced by CO 4 to 8 L/min, CI 2.7 to 4.3 L/min/m², CVP 2 to 6 mm Hg, mean arterial pressure (MAP) 70 to 100 mm Hg, PAP systolic 15 to 25 mm Hg or diastolic 8 to 15 mm Hg, PCWP 6 to 12 mm Hg, RAP 4 to 6 mm Hg, RVP systolic 15 to 25 mm Hg or diastolic 0 to 8 mm Hg, BP ≥90/60 mm Hg, capillary refill ≤3 seconds, peripheral pulses +2, flat neck veins, urinary output (UO) ≥30 mL/h or ≥0.5 mL/kg/h, normothermia, absence of dyspnea, normal sinus rhythm, HR ≤100 bpm, RR 12 to 20 BPM, Pao_2 ≥80 mm Hg, and Sao_2 ≥95%.

- Consult with cardiologist to validate expected patient outcomes used to evaluate effective CO.
- Review results from ECG, chest roentgenogram, and echocardiogram.
- Review results of sedimentation rate, WBC, serum enzymes, and immunodiagnostic studies.
- Limit physical activity to bed rest while patient is experiencing chest pain. Raise head of bed so patient is able to lean forward. This relieves the pericardial pain.
- Monitor and report hemodynamic parameters reflective of decreased CO: CO ≤4 L/min, CI ≤2.7 L/min/m², CVP ≥6 mm Hg, MAP ≤70 mm Hg, PAP systolic ≥25 mm Hg or diastolic ≥15 mm Hg, PCWP ≥12 mm Hg, RAP ≥6 mm Hg, RVP systolic ≥25 mm Hg or diastolic ≥8 mm Hg.
- Obtain, document, and report other clinical findings associated with decreased CO resulting from acute pericarditis: chest pain described as sharp, dull, and aching and localized to the retrospinal or left precordial region, dyspnea, fever, cough, sputum production, weight gain, BP ≤90/60 mm Hg, and capillary refill ≤3 seconds.
- Obtain, document, and report the presence of pulsus paradoxus: The amplitude is decreased with inspiration and returns to full amplitude on expiration; the amplitude of the pulse may be detected by BP cuff. Pulses paradoxus exists when BP sounds are ≥10 mm Hg apart: An abnormal inspiratory drop in systemic blood pressure greater than 15 mm Hg.
- Monitor patient for the presence of pericardial effusion, which can decrease CO: dull ache or pressure within the chest, dyspnea, tachypnea, dysphagia, cough, hoarseness, hiccups, and nausea.
- Monitor continuous ECG to assess HR and rhythm. Document ECG rhythm strips every 2 to 4 hours in patients with dysrhythmias.
- Auscultate chest for the presence of pericardial friction rub, which is heard as a scratching, grating, high-pitched sound, is triphasic with an atrial systolic (presystolic), a ventricular systolic, and an early diastolic component.
- Assist with pericardiocentesis to remove excess pericardial fluid.
- Should pericardiocentesis be ineffective, prepare patient for pericardiectomy to relieve the restriction and prevent cardiac compression.
- Administer prescribed IV fluids, such as colloids or crystalloids, to avoid overdistention of the thin-walled right ventricle and maintain PCWP 6 to 12 mm Hg and CVP 2 to 6 mm Hg.
- Administer prescribed Fio_2 at 50% and oxygen 2 to 4 L/min by means of nasal cannula or mask.
- Administer prescribed NSAIDs (aspirin, ibuprofen, or indomethacin) to manage patient's pain.
- Administer prescribed corticosteroids (prednisone or prednisolone) to decrease pericardial sac inflammation (see Table 1–15).
- Administer prescribed positive inotropes (dobutamine or dopamine) to maintain CO ≤4 L/min, CI ≤2.7 L/min/m², CVP 2 to 6 mm Hg, MAP 70 to 100 mm Hg, PAP systolic 15 to 25 mm Hg or diastolic 8 to 15 mm Hg, PCWP 6 to 12 mm Hg, RAP 4 to 6 mm Hg, and RVP systolic 15 to 25 mm Hg or diastolic 0 to 8 mm Hg (see Table 1–10).

- Administer prescribed volume-reducing agents (furosemide or bumetanide) to maintain CO $\geq$4 L/min, CI $\geq$2.7 to 4.3 L/min/m^2, UO $\geq$30 mL/h or $\geq$0.5 mL/kg/h, and specific gravity 1.010 to 1.030 (see Table 1–13).
- Should acute pericarditis recur as a result of an immune response from a previous pericardial injury, administer prescribed cytotoxic agents such as azathioprine.
- Instruct patient to reduce pericardial pain by not lying down, turning in bed, coughing, or deep breathing.

Potential Complication: Dysrhythmias. Dysrhythmias related to inflammatory process and accumulation of pericardial fluid secondary to acute pericarditis.

Expected Patient Outcomes. Patient remains in sinus rhythm, HR 60 to 100 bpm, and is free of chest pain.

- Review ECG with cardiologist to determine which of the four stages applies to patient.
- Monitor continuous ECG to assess HR and rhythm. Document ECG rhythm strips every 2 to 4 hours in patients with dysrhythmias.
- Maintain a calm environment to reduce release of catecholamines from the sympathetic nervous system and subsequent tachycardia. Tachycardia increases myocardial oxygen consumption, decreases filling time, and decreases coronary artery perfusion.
- Administer prescribed IV fluids to maintain adequate circulatory volume.
- Administer prescribed antidysrhythmia drugs to reduce sinoatrial nodal irritation resulting from the inflammatory process (see Table 1–11).

Potential Complication: Respiratory Alkalosis. Respiratory alkalosis related to hyperventilation or dyspnea secondary to compression of adjacent bronchi and lung parenchyma by a large pericardial effusion.

Expected Patient Outcomes. Patient maintains adequate gas exchange, as evidenced by Pao$_2$ $\geq$80 mm Hg, arterial carbon dioxide pressure (Paco$_2$) 35 to 45 mm Hg, HCO$_3$ 22 to 26 mEq/L, Sao$_2$ $\geq$95%, RR 12 to 20 BPM, HR $\leq$100 bpm, absence of shortness of breath and dyspnea, and serum electrolytes within normal limits.

- Review arterial blood gas, and serum electrolyte readings and chest roentgenogram.
- Obtain and report clinical findings reflective of respiratory alkalosis: lightheadedness, numbness, tingling of digits and toes, muscle weakness, seizure, altered consciousness, Paco$_2$ $\leq$35 mm Hg, HCO$_3$ $\leq$22 mm Hg, and potassium $\leq$3.8 mEq/L.
- Auscultate lungs for rate, rhythm, and presence of crackles, rhonchi, or wheezes.
- Monitor continuous ECG to assess HR and rhythm. Document ECG rhythm strips every 2 to 4 hours in patients with tachycardia, atrial fibrillation, and occasional ventricular dysrhythmias.
- Calm anxious patient to decrease hyperventilation.
- Administer IV fluids to maintain adequate hydration or electrolytes.
- Administer prescribed antidysrhythmia agents (see Table 1–11).
- Teach patient how to breathe in a paper bag to relieve symptoms of respiratory alkalosis.
- Teach patient strategies to reduce stress and control respirations: guided imagery, progressive relaxation, or meditation.

DISCHARGE PLANNING
The critical care nurse provides patient and significant other(s) with verbal or written discharge notes regarding the following subjects:

1. Medications including purpose, dosage, schedule, and side effects.
2. Significance of reporting any episodes of chest pain, fever, fatigue, and difficult respiration to physician.
3. Need to avoid persons with infections or experiencing upper respiratory infection.

4. Activity schedule, which is reduced for 1 to 2 weeks, then increased. A postdischarge exercise program to keep HR ≤100 bpm according to the following: (1) First week, walk 0.25 miles within 8 to 10 minutes; (2) second week, walk 0.25 miles within 5 minutes; (3) third week, walk 0.50 miles within 15 minutes; and (4) fourth week, walk 1.0 miles within 30 minutes.

■ ACUTE INFECTIVE ENDOCARDITIS

(For related information see Part I: Congestive heart failure, p. 87; Cardiogenic shock, p. 72; Valvular heart disease, p. 153; Dysrhythmias, p. 184. Part II: Valve surgery, p. 203; Part III: Hemodynamic monitoring, p. 219; Percutaneous aortic valvuloplasty, p. 243. See also Respiratory Deviations, Part I: Pulmonary embolism, p. 397; Pulmonary infarction, p. 404; and Renal Deviations, Part I: Acute renal failure, p. 459).

Diagnostic Category and Length of Stay
DRG: 126 Acute and subacute endocarditis
LOS: 16.30 days

Definition
Acute infectious endocarditis (AIE) is a bacterial, fungal, or rickettsial infection of the endocardial surface of the heart. AIE is caused by an inflammatory lesion found in collagen vascular diseases or rheumatic fever in an infectious process.

Pathophysiology
In endocarditis there is injury to the endothelial structures, presence of a microbial infection, and alteration in blood velocity. During the initial stages of valvulitis, there is inflammation, edema of the valve leaflets, formation of tiny beadlike vegetative growths (verrucae), and platelet aggregation and fibrin deposition along the edges of the valves. The leaflets of the affected valves adhere to one another, causing fusion of the commissures. In addition, there is also shortening, fibrosis, and fusion of the chordae tendineae. There are changes in blood flowing from a high- to low-pressure zone through a narrowed orifice. This causes a consistent distribution of pathogens beyond the low-pressure area. In the later stages, granulation tissue develops and fibrotic changes occur, leading to fibrosis and thickening, with the valve's leaflets becoming calcified. The overall pathological changes lead to stenosis, regurgitation, or combined stenosis and regurgitation of the involved valves.

Nursing Assessment

PRIMARY CAUSES
- Microorganisms such as gram-positive cocci, staphylococci, gram-positive bacilli, gram-negative cocci, gram-negative bacilli, and fungi can cause AIE. Intravascular foreign bodies can be introduced through intravenous catheters, intra-arterial catheters, dialysis shunts, hyperalimentation catheters, and pacemakers. A range of valvular diseases such as heart disease, congenital heart disease, mitral valve prolapse, Marfan's syndrome, idiopathic hypertrophic subaortic stenosis, degenerative heart disease, and syphilic aortic disease can contribute to AIE. Cardiac and prosthetic valve surgery or prosthetic aortic grafts may cause AIE. Other causes are alcoholism, immunosuppression, or burns.

RISK FACTORS
- History of diabetes mellitus or carcinoma and life-style factors, such as IV drug abuse.

PHYSICAL ASSESSMENT
- Inspection: Findings such as fever, chills, diaphoresis; fatigue, malaise, easy fatigability; weight loss, anorexia; jaundice of skin and sclera; neck vein distention, ascites, or hematuria. Osler's nodes, which are transient, raised, painful, erythematous nodules over tips of fingers or toes. Janeway lesions are nonpainful, flat, ery-

thematous lesions of thenar and hypothenar eminences of the hands and soles of feet that blanch with pressure and elevation of extremities. Roth's spots are white-centered, round or oval hemorrhagic spots in the retina; petechiae are located on mucous membranes of mouth, conjunctiva, anterior chest, and neck, wrists, and ankles. Splinter hemorrhages are linear black streaks on the distal third of the fingernails or toenails.

- Palpation: Splenomegaly, abdominal pain, or decreased or no pulses in cold limbs.
- Percussion: Dullness in lower half of sternum.
- Auscultation: Tachycardia, hypotension, systolic murmur of mitral insufficiency, or early diastolic decrescendo murmur of aortic incompetence, pericardial friction rub, S_3 or S_4, and crackles or rales.

DIAGNOSTIC TEST RESULTS.

Hemodynamic Parameters. (See Table 1–9)

- Reduced cardiac output and stroke volume. Elevated pulmonary capillary wedge pressure (PCWP), central venous pressure (CVP), peripheral arterial pressure (PAP), and right atrial pressure (RAP).

Standard Laboratory Tests. (See Table 1–1)

- Blood cultures: Positive for gram-negative bacilli, streptococci, or cocci; gram-positive cocci, staphylococci, and gram-positive bacilli.
- Blood studies: Reduced hemoglobin, elevated erythrocyte sedimentation rate (ESR), white blood cell count (WBC) $\geq 25,000/\mu L$, presence of rheumatoid factor, appearance of a C-reactive protein (CRP) and antistreptolysin O titer (ASOT) after the streptococcal infection.
- Serum enzymes: Elevated creatine kinase (CK-MB), lactic dehydrogenase isoenzyme cardiac (LD-1), and serum glutamic-oxaloacetic transaminase (SGOT) should acute myocardial infarction occur from embolization of vegetation.

- Urinalysis: May reveal microscopic hematuria.

Noninvasive Cardiac Diagnostic Procedures. (See Table 1–3)

- Chest roentgenogram: Reveals cardiac chamber enlargement and the presence of pulmonary venous congestion or pulmonary hypertension.
- Echocardiogram: Assists in identification of vegetation with intramyocardial abscess and destruction of valvular supporting structures and valvular tissue, which result in valvular incompetence.

ECG

- Nonspecific: The changes include premature ventricular contractions, T wave abnormalities, and various levels of intraventricular conduction defects.

MEDICAL AND SURGICAL MANAGEMENT

PHARMACOLOGY

- Antimicrobial therapy: In acute endocarditis, antibiotic therapy is started immediately and therapy is adjusted once the causative agent is identified. Antibiotic prophylaxis is given before any procedure such as dental surgery, minor skin surgery, genitourinary procedures, or operations involving a contaminated field (see Table 1–14).
- Anticoagulation: Used in patients undergoing prosthetic valve surgery to prevent valve thrombosis and peripheral thromboembolism (see Table 1–8).
- Vasodilators: Nitroglycerin is used if congestive heart failure develops and to decrease reduction of circulating volume (see Table 1–4).
- Positive inotropes: Digoxin, dobutamine, or amrinone are used to enhance myocardial contractility and cardiac output (see Table 1–10).
- Diuretics: Furosemide or bumetanide are used to reduce circulating volume (see Table 1–5).

PHYSICAL ACTIVITY

- Bed rest initially to reduce myocardial work.

OXYGEN THERAPY

- Administer FIO_2 ≤50% by mask to maintain arterial oxygen pressure (PaO_2) ≥60 mm Hg and arterial oxygen saturation (SaO_2) ≥95%.

SURGICAL INTERVENTION

- Prosthetic valve replacement: The goals of surgical intervention are to remove all infected tissue, restore valve function through valve replacement, and correct any mechanical or structural defects such as fistulas, conduction abnormalities, septal perforations, or aneurysms (see Valve surgery, p. 203).

NURSING MANAGEMENT: NURSING DIAGNOSES AND COLLABORATIVE PROBLEMS

Nursing Diagnoses

Common nursing goals for patients with acute infective endocarditis are to restore myocardial tissue perfusion, maintain normothermia, facilitate adequate gas exchange, prevent or correct infection, prevent injury, and encourage effective individual coping.

Altered myocardial tissue perfusion related to reduced coronary artery perfusion secondary to decreased cardiac output or vegetative embolization.

Expected Patient Outcomes. Patient maintains adequate myocardial tissue perfusion, as evidenced by a blood pressure (BP) ≥90 to 60 mm Hg or within the patient's normal range, capillary refill ≤3 seconds, coronary artery perfusion pressure (CAPP) 60 to 80 mm Hg, cardiac output (CO) 4 to 8 L/min, cardiac index (CI) 2.7 to 4.3 L/min/m^2, heart rate (HR) ≤100 bpm, mean arterial pressure (MAP) 70 to 100 mm Hg, mixed venous oxygen saturation ($S\bar{v}O_2$) of 60% to 80%, and SaO_2 ≥95 mm Hg.

- Consult with cardiologist to validate expected patient outcomes used to evaluate effective myocardial tissue perfusion.
- Review the results of echocardiogram, ECG, and serum enzymes to note changes associated with decreased myocardial tissue perfusion.
- Obtain, document, and report hemodynamic values reflective of reduced myocardial tissue perfusion: CAPP ≤60 mm Hg, CO ≤4 L/min, CI ≤2.7 L/min/m^2, $S\bar{v}O_2$ ≤60%.
- Monitor continuous ECG to assess HR and rhythm. Document ECG rhythm strips every 2 to 4 hours in patients with dysrhythmias.
- Monitor BP capillary refill and HR. A slow HR increases diastolic filling time, which extends the time during which oxygenated blood is available to the coronary vasculature.
- Monitor patient for chest discomfort. Should patient experience chest discomfort, assess and report new S_3 or S_4 gallops, new or increasing crackles, and decreased activity tolerance.
- Monitor intake and output every hour and report urinary output (UO) ≤30 mL/h.
- Administer prescribed oxygen 2 to 4 L/min via nasal cannula or mask to increase oxygen supply and restore arterial oxygen saturation to within normal limits.
- Administer prescribed IV fluids to maintain adequate circulating volume and hydration.
- Administer prescribed positive inotropes (dopamine or dobutamine) and phosphodiesterase inhibitor (amrinone) to maintain CO ≥4 L/min, CI ≥2.7 L/min/m^2, $S\bar{v}O_2$ ≥60% (see Table 1–10).
- Instruct patient to report presence of chest pain, indicating decreased myocardial tissue perfusion.

Thermoregulation, ineffective related to infection secondary to prolonged administration of antibiotics.

Expected Patient Outcomes. Patient maintains effective thermoregulation, as evidenced by temperature $\leq 100°F$, MAP ≥ 70 mm Hg, UO ≥ 30 mL/h or ≥ 0.5 mL/kg/h and specific gravity 1.010 to 1.030, negative blood cultures, WBC $\leq 11,000/\mu l$ HR ≤ 100 bpm, respiratory rate (RR) 12 to 20 BPM, absence of chills, and urinalysis normal.

- Review results of blood cultures and WBC.
- Monitor and report the presence of triad supporting diagnosis of acute infectious endocarditis: fever, malaise, and murmur.
- Document the course of fever in staphylococcis-related AIE, since an acute fulminant infectious process causes high temperature elevation with spikes and shaky chills.
- Document the course of fever in streptococcis-related AIE, since a subacute infectious process causes moderate temperature elevation, no chills, fatigability, weight loss, anorexia, and night sweats.
- Measure temperature every 1 to 4 hours while patient is febrile.
- Obtain blood cultures per agency standards when temperature spikes in order to identify organisms and maintain drug adequacy.
- Monitor daily weight, intake, and urinary output for color, amount, and presence of odor.
- Change tubing, collection containers, peripheral lines, central lines, or catheters every 48 to 72 hours per agency or unit standards.
- Administer prescribed IV fluids to maintain adequate hydration, MAP 70 to 100 mm Hg, UO ≥ 30 mL/kg or ≥ 0.5 mL/kg/h and specific gravity 1.010 to 1.030.
- Administer antibiotics as prescribed: penicillin, streptomycin, gentamicin, nafcillin, vancomycin, ampicillin, amphotericin B, cotrimoxazole, or cefazolin (see Table 1–14).
- Should antibiotics and antipyretics be ineffective in reducing elevated temperature, provide cooling measures as prescibed.
- Instruct patient regarding the need for prophylactic antibiotics and, if necessary, continued home treatment with antibiotics.
- Teach patient to report signs and symptoms of infection: redness, tenderness or swelling around a catheter site, or temperature $\geq 100°F$.

Impaired gas exchange related to decreased alveolar–capillary diffusion of oxygen as a result of pulmonary congestion.

Expected Patient Outcomes. Patient maintains adequate gas exchange, as evidenced by PaO_2 ≥ 80 mm Hg, arterial carbon dioxide pressure $(PaCO_2)$ 35 to 45 mm Hg, SaO_2 95 to 99%, RR ≤ 20 BPM, $S\bar{v}O_2$ 60% to 80%, HR ≤ 100 bpm, absence of cyanosis, and resolution of adventitious breath sounds.

- Review chest roentgenogram red blood count (RBC), and arterial blood gas results reflecting impaired gas exchange.
- Place patient in semi-high Fowler's position to facilitate lung expansion.
- Monitor clinical indicators of respiratory status: rate, depth, symmetry of chest excursion, presence of cyanosis, or presence of adventitious breath sounds.
- Auscultate the lungs every 2 hours and report the presence of crackles, rhonchi, or wheezing.
- Evaluate oxygenation with oximetry or $S\bar{v}O_2$ to determine oxygen supply and demand. SaO_2 and $S\bar{v}O_2$ decrease when there is increased metabolic demand or when extraction of oxygen exceeds oxygen delivery.
- Observe patient's skin for presence of pallor suggesting impaired oxygenation.
- Obtain and report the following changes suggestive of impaired gas exchange: PaO_2 ≤ 70 mm Hg, $PaCO_2$ ≥ 45 mm Hg, SaO_2 $\leq 95\%$, $S\bar{v}O_2$ $\leq 60\%$ mm Hg, RR ≥ 20 BPM, cyanosis, and crackles.
- Assess, document, and report findings reflecting hypoxemia: dyspnea, cyanosis, restlessness, confusion, anxiety, delirium, tachypnea, tachycardia, hypertension, dysrhythmias, and tremors.
- Schedule incentive spirometry every 2 to 4 hours to prevent atelectasis.
- Encourage patient to cough and deep breathe every 2 to 4 hours to enhance lung expansion.

- Administer prescribed oxygen at 2 to 4 L/min by means of nasal cannula or mask to maintain $PaO_2 \geq 80$ mm Hg.
- Encourage patient to turn, cough, and deep breathe in order to reduce the risk of atelectasis or alveolar congestion from stasis.

High risk of infection related to invasive procedures secondary to inadequate defense as a result of antibiotic therapy.

Expected Patient Outcomes. Patient is free of infection as evidenced by absence of redness, swelling, tenderness, or discharge from invasive procedure sites.

- Review results of WBC, wound culture, and blood cultures.
- Report the presence of redness, swelling, tenderness, or discharge from dressing or invasive sites.
- Obtain culture from wound or catheter sites.
- Inspect urine for evidence of infection such as casts, cloudiness, or foul odor.
- Monitor temperature every 2 to 4 hours when patient is febrile.
- Use strict aseptic technique when changing a dressing or caring for site of all invasive monitoring devices and IV tubing.
- Administer prescribed IV antibiotics and obtain serum antibiotic peak and trough level to determine their effectiveness (see Table 1–14).
- Instruct patient to report presence of redness or tenderness around catheter or tubing insertion sites.

High risk for injury related to side effects from antibiotic therapy.

Expected Patient Outcome. Patient is free of side effects from antibiotic therapy.

- Consult with pharmacist about potential side effects associated with antibiotic therapy in AIE patient.
- Document and report the presence of drug toxicity: vertigo, tinnitus, and visual disturbances.

- Instruct patient to report any auditory changes that may reflect potential hearing loss associated with antibiotic therapy.
- Instruct patient to report loss of appetite, nausea, or vomiting associated with antibiotic therapy.

Ineffective individual coping related to depression secondary to prolonged hospitalization.

Expected Patient Outcomes. Patient is able to verbalize when feeling depressed, initiates measures to decrease feelings of depression, and uses appropriate coping mechanisms in controlling depression.

- Assist patient to facilitate realistic appraisal of role changes.
- Assist patient to establish realistic goals, knowing that small accomplishments can enhance positive feelings of the future.
- Encourage patient to describe the illness, treatment, or prognosis.
- Encourage patient to participate in self care.
- Provide patient with personal space in the technical environment.

Collaborative Problems

Common collaborative goals in patients with AIE are to increase CO, correct dysrhythmias, and prevent thromboembolism.

Potential Complication: Decreased Cardiac Output. Decreased CO related to incompetent valves secondary to stenosis or insufficiency.

Expected Patient Outcomes. Patient maintains adequate CO, as evidenced by CO 4 to 8 L/min, CI 2.7 to 4.3 L/min/m^2, CVP 2 to 6 mm Hg, left atrial pressure (LAP) 8 to 12 mm Hg, MAP 70 to 100 mm Hg, PAP systolic 15 to 25 mm Hg or diastolic 8 to 15 mm Hg, PCWP ≤ 12 mm Hg, RAP 4 to 6 mm Hg, right ventricular pressure (RVP) systolic 15 to 25 mm Hg or diastolic 0 to 8 mm Hg, HR $\leq$ 100 bpm, BP $\geq$90/60 mm Hg, UO $\geq$30 mL/h or $\geq$0.5 mL/kg/h, specific gravity 1.010 to 1.030, hemoglobin within normal limits, absence of S_3

or S_4 heart sounds, flat neck veins, absence of peripheral edema, peripheral pulses +2, and capillary refill ≤3 seconds.

- Consult with cardiologist to validate patient's expected patient outcomes used to determine whether CO is sufficient.
- Review results of echocardiogram, ECG, and blood studies.
- Limit activity to bed rest to decrease venous return and myocardial work load.
- Obtain and report hemodynamic parameters reflective of decreased left ventricular CO: CO≤4 L/min, CI ≤2.7 L/min/m², PAP systolic ≥25 mm Hg or diastolic ≥15 mm Hg, PCWP ≥12 mm Hg, and LAP ≥12 mm Hg.
- Assess, document, and report other findings suggestive of decreased left ventricular CO: HR ≥100 bpm, RR ≥20 BPM, presence of S_3 or S_4 heart sounds, crackles, dyspnea, tachypnea, digital clubbing, BP ≤90/60 mm Hg, capillary refill ≥3 seconds, and diminished peripheral pulses.
- Monitor and report the presence of the diagnostic trend of AIE: fever, anemia, and murmur.
- Monitor and report hemodynamic parameters reflective of decreased right ventricular CO: CVP ≥6 mm Hg, RAP ≥6 mm Hg, and RVP systolic ≥25 mm Hg or diastolic ≥8 mm Hg.
- Obtain, document, and report findings suggestive of decreased right ventricular CO: CVP≥6 mm Hg, distended neck veins, positive hepatojugular reflex, peripheral edema, jaundice, and ascites.
- Monitor ECG for changes reflective of right atrial enlargement: P pulmonale in leads II, III, aVF, and V_1. P wave is ≥2.5 mm voltage; and right ventricular enlargement R voltage increased in V_1 and V_2, S voltage increased in V_5 and V_6.
- Monitor heart sounds for murmur every 2 to 4 hours for pulmonic stenosis: systolic blowing murmur at second intercostal space (ICS), left sternal border (LSB), and may radiate to the neck; and heart sounds for murmur indicating pulmonic insufficiency: diastolic murmur at second ICS, LSB that starts later and is lower-pitched than an aortic murmur.
- Monitor heart sounds for murmur every 2 to 4 hours indicative of tricuspid stenosis: diastolic murmur at fourth ICS; and heart sounds for murmur indicating tricuspid insufficiency: pansystolic murmur at fourth ICS, LSB that increases in intensity with inspiration.
- Monitor hemodynamic changes associated with decreased CO related to aortic stenosis or insufficiency: increased left ventricular pressure, increased pulmonary artery end-diastolic pressure (PAEDP), decreased CO, decreased aortic pressure, and increased systolic pressure; and to mitral stenosis or insufficiency: increased mean PAP, giant v waves in pulmonary artery and occlusive tracing, increased systolic PAP.
- Monitor heart sounds for murmurs every 2 to 4 hours indicating aortic stenosis: systolic, blowing murmur at second ICS, right sternal border (RSB) may radiate to the neck; and for heart sounds indicating aortic insufficiency: diastolic blowing murmur at second ICS, RSB and beginning immediately with S_2.
- Monitor heart sounds for murmurs every 2 to 4 hours indicating mitral stenosis: long, loud diastolic murmur at fifth ICS; S_1 is loud and there is opening snap with S_2; mitral insufficiency: systolic murmur at fifth ICS, midclavicular line.
- Monitor ECG for changes reflective of left atrial enlargement: P wave is M-shaped with a duration ≥0.1 second found in leads II, III, aVF, and V_1; and of left ventricular enlargement: R voltage increases V_4 to V_6, R in any V lead ≥25 mm, S voltage increases in V_1 and V_2.
- Monitor and record daily weight, intake, and output to determine if patient is adequately hydrated or needs diuretic therapy.
- Administer prescribed FIO_2 at 50% or oxygen 2 to 4 L/min by means of nasal cannula or mask.

- Administer prescribed IV fluids to maintain hydration, UO $\geq$30 mL/h or $\geq$0.5 mL/kg/h and specific gravity 1.010 to 1.030.
- Administer volume-reducing agents (furosemide or bumetanide) to maintain MAP 70 to 90 mm Hg, UO $\geq$30 mL/h or 0.5 mL/kg/h and specific gravity 1.010 to 1.030 (see Table 1–13).
- Administer positive inotropes (dopamine, dobutamine, or amrinone) to enhance CO and contractility (see Table 1–10).
- Should pharmacological therapy be ineffective, prepare the patient for valve replacement (see Valve surgery, p. 203.)

Potential Complication: Dysrhythmias. Dysrhythmias related to focal lesions in the conduction pathway secondary to vegetation formation.

Expected Patient Outcomes. Patient remains in sinus rhythm, serum electrolytes within normal, HR $\leq$100 bpm, and BP within patient's normal range.

- Consult with cardiologist about possible dysrhythmias associated with AIE should right or left atrial or ventricular enlargement occur: bundle branch block, premature ventricular contraction, paroxysmal atrial tachycardia, supraventricular tachycardia, atrial fibrillation, or atrial flutter.
- Monitor continuous ECG to assess HR and rhythm. Document ECG strips every 2 to 4 hours in patient with dysrhythmias associated with right or left atrial or ventricular enlargement.
- Monitor patient for physical signs and symptoms of dysrhythmias: abnormal HR and rhythm, palpitations, chest pain, syncope, ECG changes, and hypotension.
- Administer prescribed oxygen 2 to 4 L/min by means of a nasal cannula or mask.
- Administer prescribed IV fluids to maintain hydration, UO $\geq$30 mL/h or 0.5 mL/kg/h and specific gravity 1.010 to 1.030.
- Administer prescribed antidysrhythmia agents to correct dysrhythmias (see Table 1–11).

- Administer prescribed antibiotic (erythromycin) should patient be allergic to penicillin.
- Administer prescribed vancomycin or erythromycin for higher-risk patients who have prosthetic heart valve and are allergic to penicillin (see Table 1–14).
- Should pharmacological therapy and resolution of AIE be ineffective in correcting bundle branch block, prepare patient for pacemaker insertion (see Pacemaker, p. 270.)

Potential Complication: Thromboembolism. Thromboembolism related to fragmentation of vegetation growth secondary to blood passing through the valve orifice.

Expected Patient Outcomes. Patient is free of or shows resolution of systemic embolism, affected organs show normal function, and extremities have adequate perfusion.

- Consult with cardiologist about use of anti-embolic stockings or sequential pressure device to enhance venous return, reduce venous stasis, and prevent thromboembolis.
- Review arterial blood gas and complete blood count results (CBC).
- Provide range of motion (ROM) exercises and frequent change of position to decrease risk of thrombus formation.
- Check patient for calf tenderness, swelling, or tenderness, which can indicate thrombus formation.
- Monitor skin color and temperature of extremities, pulses, and capillary refill for development of peripheral emboli.
- Obtain and report changes suggestive of pulmonary emboli associated with right-sided AIE: shortness of breath, tachypnea, dyspnea, diaphoresis, cyanosis, crackles, increased intensity of P_2, fixed splitting of S_2, murmur heard over lung field pleural friction rub.
- Obtain and report findings suggestive of peripheral emboli associated with left-sided AIE: Homan's sign, peripheral pulse $\leq$+2, swelling, erythema, coolness, and decreased capillary refill.

- Monitor and report findings suggestive of cerebral emboli associated with left-sided AIE: confusion, sensorimotor changes, sudden blindness, or cognitive changes.
- Monitor and report findings suggestive of renal emboli-induced glomerulonephritis caused by left-sided AIE: U0 $\leq$30 mL/h or $\leq$0.5 mL/kg/h.
- Obtain and report findings reflecting acute myocardial infarction from left-sided AIE: chest pain, diaphoresis, shortness of breath, pallor, nausea, vomiting, BP $\leq$90/60 mm Hg, and HR $\geq$120 bpm.
- Apply antiembolic stockings to prevent venous stasis.
- Administer prescribed oxygen (2 to 4 L/min) by means of nasal cannula or mask to resolve dyspnea, tachypnea, or to maintain Pao_2 $\geq$80 mm Hg and Sao_2 $\geq$95%.
- Administer prescribed IV fluids to maintain adequate hydration, UO $\geq$30 mL/h or $\geq$0.5 mL/kg/h and specific gravity 1.010 to 1.030.
- Administer antibiotics to correct *Staphylococcus aureus*–induced native valve endocarditis (nafcillin or oxacillin) or to correct *Streptococcus*-induced acute infectious endocarditis (aqueous penicillin and/or streptomycin) (see Table 1–14).
- Administer prescribed heparin to resolve and prevent further thrombus formation (see Table 1–8).
- Administer prescribed narcotic or analgesics to relieve pain.

DISCHARGE PLANNING

The critical care nurse provides patient and significant other(s) with verbal or written discharge notes regarding the following subjects:

1. Importance of learning that patients with acquired heart disease are at risk for developing AIE.
2. Risk of AIE increases after traumatic procedures to mucosal surface.
3. Using prophylactic antibiotics before traumatic procedures such as dental procedures.
4. Importance of continuing to take antibiotics as ordered or until discontinued.

5. Importance of ongoing outpatient care.
6. Medication's purpose, dosage, schedule, and side effects.
7. Importance of reporting symptoms to physician: fatigue, fever, chills, and weight loss.

■ ACUTE HYPERTENSIVE CRISIS

(For related information see Part I: Acute myocardial infarction, p. 38; Congestive heart failure, p. 87; Dysrhythmias, p. 184. Part III: Hemodynamic monitoring, p. 219. See also Neurological Deviations, Part I: Cerebrovascular accident, p. 630. Renal Deviations, Part I: Acute renal failure, p. 459.)

Diagnostic Category and Length of Stay
DRG: 134 Hypertension
LOS: 3.90 days

Definition
Acute hypertensive crisis is an abnormal elevation of systolic pressure (SBP) $\geq$140 to 200 mm Hg and diastolic pressure (DBP) $\geq$120 mm Hg. The mean arterial pressure is $\geq$150 mm Hg. Patients usually require immediate intervention in the reduction of blood pressure. There are two types of hypertensive crisis. A hypertensive emergency is the presentation of a patient with a diastolic blood pressure 120 mm Hg with evidence of end-organ damage that is new or progressive and is associated with complications. It can develop within hours to days, and the blood pressure must be reduced within minutes to an hour to reduce the risk of complication or progressive end-organ damage. When the DBP is 120 to 140 mm Hg, hypertensive urgency develops over days to weeks, with marked elevation of DBP 100 to 120 mm Hg without clinical manifestation of end-organ damage.

Pathophysiology
Usually two or three mechanisms of hypertension coexist. The mechanisms consist of autoregulation, fluid overload, vasoconstric-

tion, humoral factors, the renin-angiotension-aldosterone system, kinins, and catecholamines. Four factors are responsible for autoregulation: (1) myogenic response in the smooth muscle of precapillary small vessels can increase; (2) metabolic response can dilate vessels when tissues are deprived of essential nutrients; (3) interstitial hydrostatic pressure can cause fluid shifts in response to changes in capillary pressure; (4) blood viscosity can increase vascular resistance by increasing pressure and by fluid transducing from blood. Besides the slow autoregulatory process that converts fluid excess in high resistance, hypertension and subsequent fluid overload can cause acute hypertensive crisis. Vasoconstriction is initiated by an increase in calcium within the smooth muscle cell. Humoral factors alter vascular tone. Humoral control involves renin-angiotensin, prostaglandin, and kallikrein-kinin. Renin forms angiotensin I, which is converted into a powerful vasoconstrictor, angiotensin II. Angiotensin II causes vasoconstriction in the arterioles, which leads to an increase in peripheral resistance and blood pressure. Prostaglandin contributes to the control of extravascular fluid volume, vascular tone, renal circulation homeostasis, sodium balance, and renin release. Bradykinin, a component of the kallikrein-kinin system, is a potent stimulus for prostaglandin generation. Bradykinin causes arterial vasodilation and hypotension, venoconstriction, natriuresis, and diuresis. Aldosterone causes the kidneys to retain salt and water through the action of antidiuretic hormone (ADH), leading to an increase in arterial pressure. Cerebral blood flow is maintained at a mean arterial pressure (MAP) of 120 to 180 mm Hg. When MAP drops below the lower limit of autoregulation, cerebral ischemia occurs. Over time, autoregulation diminishes and arteriolar fibrinoid necrosis occurs, leading to end-organ ischemia and damage. The ischemia causes the release of more vasoactive substances, initiating further vasoconstriction and myointimal proliferation. Target-organ damage is manifested as vascular destruction, which is fibrinoid necrosis of small artrioles and proliferative endoarteritis of entire arteriolar wall. Eventually there is swelling, loss of structural integrity, and altering focal dilatation and constriction of blood vessels, most prominently renal arterioles.

Nursing Assessment

PRIMARY CAUSES

- General noncompliance or inadequate treatment in chronic hypertension; ingestion of drugs such as cocaine, phencycladine (PCP), amphetamines, diet pills, monoamine oxidase (MAO) inhibitor with tyramine; withdrawal of therapy; preeclampsia or eclampsia; renovascular hypertension; head trauma or spinal cord syndrome; vasculitis or collagen vascular diseases; and pheochromocytoma or renin-secretory tumor.
- Hypertensive urgencies are hypertension (HTN) associated with coronary artery disease, accelerated and malignant HTN, severe HTN in the kidney transplant patient, postoperative HTN, uncontrolled HTN in the patient who requires emergency surgery.
- Hypertensive emergencies are involved in HTN encephalopathy, acute aortic dissection, pulmonary edema, pheochromocytoma crisis, MAO inhibitors, intracranial hemorrhage, or eclampsia.

RISK FACTORS

- Family history of HTN or coronary artery disease; other conditions, such as hyperlipidemia, elevated triglycerides and cholesterol levels, or diabetes mellitus; life-style factors such as cigarette smoking, obesity, stress, and alcohol intake.

PHYSICAL ASSESSMENT

- Inspection: Occipital or anterior headache, dizziness, fatigue, nocturia, forgetfulness, irritability, confusion, agitation, convulsion, blurred vision, ataxia, epistaxis, distended neck veins, nausea, vomiting, neck stiffness, pallor, diasphoresis, chest pain or visual tortuosity, reduced visual acuity, or papilledema.

- Palpation: Femoral pulse delay, left ventricular heave, apical impulse felt at anterior axillary line, and pulsus alternans.
- Auscultation: Elevated DBP ≥125 to 140 mm Hg, S_4, accentuated aortic component S_2, abdominal or flank bruit (renal artery stenosis), tachycardia, or bradycardia.

DIAGNOSTIC TEST RESULTS

Standard Laboratory Tests. (See Table 1–1)

- Blood studies: Complete blood count (CBC) may reveal microangiopathic hemolytic anemia with red cell fragmentation and decreased hemoglobin.
- Serum chemistry: Elevated blood urea-nitrogen (BUN), creatinine, thyroid hormones, cholesterol, triglycerides, sodium, and bicarbonate.
- Urinalysis: Proteinuria, hematuria, low fixed specific gravity, presence of granular or red cell casts. Elevated catecholamine metabolites (VMA), aldosterone, and urine steroids.

Noninvasive Cardiac Diagnostic Procedures. (See Table 1–3)

- Chest roentgenogram: Shows notching of the ribs or abnormalities of the thoracic aorta in the region of the arch; widened mediastinum is suggestive of aortic dissection; or descending thoracic aorta may be due to coarctation of the aorta as a cause of HTN. There is also increased cardiothoracic ratio.
- Echocardiogram: Shows left ventricular hypertrophy and left ventricular wall thickness with or without increasing chamber size.
- CT scan: May reveal widespread areas of diminished density in white matter and represent focal collection of edema fluid.

ECG

- Left ventricular hypertrophy is indicated by increased voltage in the left ventricle precordial leads (V_3 and V_6). T wave inversion or ST segment elevation can indicate ischemic changes.

MEDICAL AND SURGICAL MANAGEMENT

PHARMACOLOGY

- Diuretics: Diuretics are used to increase urine volume, inhibit tubular reabsorption of sodium and chloride, decrease peripheral vascular resistance, reduce venous filling pressure, reduce cardiac output, and reduce blood pressure. Diuretic categories consist of thiazide, loop, and potassium-sparing (see Table 1–13).
- Beta-adrenergic blockers: They cause antihypertensive effects by decreasing cardiac output. The cardioselective agents metoprolol, acebutolol, atenolol, betaxolol are preferable for treating hypertensive patients with obstructive pulmonary disease. Nonselective agents carteolol, nadolol, penbutolol, pindolol, propranolol and timolol may tend to cause complications in patients with underlying pulmonary disease. The choice among beta-adrenergic blockers is determined by the existence of co-illness such as diabetes, congestive heart failure, peripheral vascular disease, angina pectoris, or obstructive pulmonary disease (see Table 1–5).
- Calcium channel blockers: The primary antihypertensive mechanisms of calcium channel blockers is vasodilation. The drugs (diltiazem, nicardipine, nifedipine, and verapamil) relax smooth muscle including vascular smooth muscle (see Table 1–6).
- Angiotension converting enzymes (ACE) inhibitors: ACE inhibitors are used as initial therapy for HTN. Blood pressure is decreased by blocking the activation of angiotensin and the production of aldosterone. ACE inhibitors include captopril, enalapril, lisinopril, benazepril, quinapril, fosinophil, and ramipril (see Table 1–12).
- Vasodilators: Vasodilators are used to alter tone in the arterial or venous side of the circulation, or they may have a balanced effect. Direct-acting vasodilators include hydralazine, diazoxide, and minoxidil. Their direct arterial effect lowers blood pressure by decreasing peripheral vascular resistance. Sodium nitroprusside and nitroglycerin are

mixed arterial and venous vasodilators. Sodium nitroprusside has a direct effect on arterial and venous vascular smooth muscle. It is useful for rapid reduction of blood pressure in hypertensive emergencies. Nitroglycerin has a prominent venodilating effect and is useful for treating hypertension associated with pulmonary congestion (see Table 1–4).

- Central-acting alpha adrenergic agonists: Central agonists lower blood pressure by stimulating inhibitor alpha-adrenergic receptors in the central nervous system. There is inhibition of peripheral sympathetic activity and peripheral vasodilation, resulting in reducing blood pressure. Central agonists include methyldopa, clonidine, guanbenz, and guanfacine (Table 1–16).
- Peripherally acting antiadrenergics: Used to affect the release of catecholamines, such as norepinephrine, from peripheral sites. The drugs used consist of guanethidine, guanadrel, and reserpine (see Table 1–16).

PHYSICAL ACTIVITY

- Patient is encouraged to participate in reasonable exercise program under medical supervision. The exercise program is either walking or a more vigorous program such as jogging, bicycling, or swimming.

DIET

- Salt restriction: A goal is moderate sodium restriction of 90 mEq per day.
- Weight reduction: With weight loss there can be a decrease or blood pressure accompanied by decreases in plasma renin activity and plasma aldosterone level.

NURSING MANAGEMENT: NURSING DIAGNOSES AND COLLABORATIVE PROBLEMS

Common nursing goals for patients with acute hypertensive crisis are to enhance tissue perfusion, restore fluid balance, reduce pain, provide information about HTN, and encourage compliance.

Nursing Diagnoses

Altered cardiopulmonary, cerebral, and renal tissue perfusion related to arterial blood flow disruption secondary to vasoconstriction or arteriosclerosis.

Expected Patient Outcomes. Patient maintains adequate tissue perfusion, as evidenced by SBP 110 to 140 mm Hg or DBP 70 to 90 mm Hg (or within patient's normal range); coronary artery perfusion pressure (CAPP) 60 to 80 mm Hg; cardiac output (CO) 4 to 8 L/min; cardiac index (CI) 2.7 to 4.3 L/min/m^2; MAP 70 to 100 mm Hg; peripheral vascular resistance (PVR) 155 to 255 dynes/s/cm^{-5}; peripheral vascular resistance index (PVRI) 200 to 450 dynes/s/cm^{-5}/m^2; mixed venous oxygen saturation (S$\bar{v}o_2$) 60% to 80%; systemic vascular resistance (SVR) 900 to 1200 dynes/s/cm^{-5}; systemic vascular resistance index (SVRI) 1970 to 2390 dynes/s/cm^{-5}/m^2; capillary refill $\leq$3 seconds; warm skin; absence of cyanosis; equal and normoreactive pupils; oriented to person, place, and time; normal sensorimotor function; arterial oxygen pressure (Pao$_2$) 80 to 100 mm Hg; arterial carbon dioxide pressure (Paco$_2$) 35 to 45 mm Hg; arterial oxygen saturation (Sao$_2$) $\geq$95%; absence of rales; urinary output (UO) $\geq$30 mL/min, specific gravity 1.010 to 1.030; BUN $\leq$20 mg/dL; creatinine clearance M: 95 to 135 mL/min or W: 85 to 125 mL/min; and serum creatinine 0.6 to 1.2 mg/dL.

- Consult with cardiologist to validate expected patient outcomes used to evaluate cardiopulmonary, cerebral, and renal tissue perfusion.
- Review arterial blood gas, BUN, serum creatinine, creatinine clearance, chest roentgenogram, and ECG results.
- Limit activity to bed rest in renin-mediated hypertensive patients, since walking may increase serum catecholamines and renin.
- Monitor and report hemodynamic parameters reflecting altered tissue perfusion: CAPP $\leq$60 mm Hg, CO $\leq$4 L/min, CI $\leq$2.7

L/min/m^2, PVR $\geq$255 dynes/s/cm^{-5}, PVRI $\geq$450 dynes/s/cm^{-5}/m^2, and S$\bar{v}$o$_2$ $\leq$60%.

- Monitor clinical indicators of neurological status every 2 hours: level of consciousness, pupils equal and normoreactive, sensori-motor function, reflexes, and vital signs.

- Monitor every 2 to 4 hours while DBP $\geq$120 mm Hg and report for changes reflecting altered cerebral tissue perfusion: occipital headache, fatigue, weakness, irritability, forgetfulness, confusion, blurred vision, and papilledema.

- Monitor daily weight for gain or loss $\geq$1 kg (2 lb).

- Monitor and report changes suggestive of altered renal perfusion: weight gain $\geq$2 lb (1kg)/day, UO $\leq$30 mL/h or $\leq$0.5 mL/kg/h, specific gravity $\leq$1.010, peripheral edema, BUN $\geq$20 mg/dL, serum creatinine $\geq$1.2 mg/dL, and creatinine clearance M: $\leq$95 mL/min or W: $\leq$85 mL/min.

- Auscultate lungs and report respiratory rate (RR) $\geq$20 BPM, crackles, or dyspnea.

- Monitor patient every 2 to 4 hours while DBP $\geq$120 mm Hg and report findings suggestive of altered cardiopulmonary tissue perfusion: CAPP $\leq$60 mm Hg, CO $\leq$4 L/min, CI $\leq$2.7 L/min/m^2, PVR $\geq$255 dynes/s/cm^{-5}, PVRI $\geq$450 dynes/s/cm^{-5}/m^2, S$\bar{v}$o$_2$ $\leq$60%, Pao$_2$ $\leq$80 mm Hg, Paco$_2$ $\geq$45 mm Hg, and Sao$_2$ $\leq$95%.

- Monitor and report clinical findings suggestive of altered peripheral tissue perfusion: capillary refill $\geq$3 seconds, peripheral pulses $\leq$+2, cool skin, and cyanotic extremities.

- Monitor continuous ECG to assess heart rate and rhythm. Document ECG rhythm strips every 2 to 4 hours in patients with dysrhythmias.

- Administer prescribed F$_{IO_2}$ at 50% or oxygen 2 to 4 L/min by nasal cannula or mask to maintain Pao$_2$ $\geq$80 mm Hg, Sao$_2$ $\geq$95%, and S$\bar{v}$o$_2$ $\geq$60%.

- Administer prescribed IV fluids to maintain hydration, UO $\geq$30 mL/h or $\geq$0.5 mL/kg/h, and specific gravity 1.010 to 1.030.

- Administer prescribed volume-reducing agents: thiazide (chlorothiazide, hydrochlorothiazide, chlorthalidone, metolazone), loop diuretics (furosemide or bumetanide), or potassium-sparing (spironolactone, amiloride, or triamterene) to maintain UO $\geq$30 mL/h or $\geq$0.5 mL/kg/h; specific gravity 1.010 to 1.030; DBP 70 to 90 mm Hg; MAP 70 to 90 mm Hg; peripheral pulses +2; capillary refill $\leq$3 seconds; and BUN, serum creatinine, and creatinine clearance within normal range (see Table 1–13).

- Administer prescribed ACE inhibitors (captopril or enalapril) or vasodilators (nitroglycerin or nitroprusside) to maintain SBP $\leq$140 mm Hg, DBP $\leq$90 mm Hg, PVR 155 to 255 dynes/s/cm^{-5}, PVRI 200 to 450 dynes/s/cm^{-5}/m^2, SVR 900 to 1200 dynes/s/cm^{-5}, SVRI 1979 to 2390 dynes/s/cm^{-5}/m^2, UO $\geq$30 mL/h or 0.5 mL/kg/h, specific gravity 1.010 to 1.030, and peripheral pulses +2 (see Table 1–12).

- Administer beta-adrenergic blockers to maintain DBP 70 to 90 mm Hg (see Table 1–5).

- Administer calcium channel blockers (verapamil, nifedipine, or diltiazem) to maintain CAPP 60 to 80 mm Hg, Sao$_2$ $\geq$95%, SBP 110 to 140 mm Hg or DBP 70 to 90 mm Hg, MAP 70 to 90 mm Hg, and S$\bar{v}$o$_2$ 60% to 80% (see Table 1–6).

- Teach patient common side effects of diuretics.

Fluid volume excess related to sodium and fluid retention secondary to release of aldosterone.

Expected Patient Outcomes. Patient maintains adequate fluid volume, as evidenced by absence of peripheral edema, CVP 2 to 6 mm Hg, UO $\geq$30 mL/min or $\geq$0.5 mL/kg/h, specific gravity 1.010 to 1.030, absence of crackles, absence of cyanosis, resolution of neck vein distention, arterial blood gases within normal range, serum electrolytes within normal range, hematocrit M: 42% to 54% and W: 38% to 46%.

TABLE 1–16. ANTIHYPERTENSIVE AGENTS

Medication	Route/Dose	Uses and Effects
Centrally Acting Alpha-Adrenergic Agonists		
Clonidine (Capapres-TTS)	PO: 0.2–1.2 mg/d	Management of hypertension Decreases systemic vascular resistance Decreases cardiac output Decreases HR Decreases plasma renin activity Decreases BP
Methyldopa (Aldomet)	PO: 250–1000 mg q 6 h	Management of hypertension Decreases BP Decreases systemic vascular resistance Slows HR Maintains cardiac output Decreases renal vascular resistance
Guanabenz acetate (Wytensin)	PO: Initial, 8–23 mg/d; 4 mg bid, may increase q 1–2 wk in 4–8 mg increments (range 8–16 mg/d; not to exceed 32 mg/d)	Management of hypertension Stimulates CNS alpha-adrenergic receptors resulting in decreased sympathetic outflow Decreases peripheral resistance Slightly increases HR No change in cardiac output
Guanfacine hydrochloride (Tenex)	PO: Initial 1–3 mg/d at bedtime; may be increased if necessary at 3–4 wk intervals up to 3 mg/d	Management of hypertension in conjunction with thiazide diuretics Stimulates CNS alpha-adrenergic receptors, resulting in decreased sympathetic outflow Decreases peripheral vascular resistance
Peripherally Acting Alpha-Adrenergic Blockers		
Terazosin hydrochloride (Hytrin)	PO: Initial, 1 mg/d, then slowly increase up to 5 mg/d; may be single dose or in 2 divided doses, not to exceed 20 mg/d	Management of hypertension Dilates both arteries and veins by blocking postsynaptic alpha$_1$-adrenergic receptors
Doxazosin mesylate (Cardura)	PO: Initial dose 1 mg, then 2–16 mg/d as a single dose	Blocks postsynaptic alpha-adrenergic receptors, resulting in arterial and venous dilation

TABLE 1-16

Preparation/Administration	Side Effects	Nursing Implications
Administration: Gradually reduce drug over 2–4 d to avoid severe hypertension	Drowsiness, nervousness, depression, dry mouth, constipation, bradycardia, palpitations, rash, sodium retention, weight gain, anorexia, malaise, nausea, vomiting, insomnia, impotence, urinary retention	Rebound may be seen during abrupt withdrawal Monitor drug's effectiveness by evaluating BP and pulse rate Monitor site of transdermal patch for dermatitis
	Drowsiness, dizziness, weakness, nasal congestion, blurred vision, dry eyes, dyspnea, chest pain, bradycardia, arrhythmias, palpitations, hypotension, diarrhea, nausea, vomiting, impotence, rashes, backache, sedation, dry mouth, urinary frequency, pruritus	Monitor drug's effectiveness through BP, HR, ECG Weigh patient daily, since sodium and water retention may occur Monitor CBC before and during therapy
	Drowsiness, weakness, fatigue, dizziness, headache, tinnitus, dyspnea, bradycardia, palpitations, dry mouth, constipation, abdominal pain, nausea or impotence	Abrupt withdrawal may result in excessive elevation of BP caused by an increased release of catecholamines
	Drowsiness, weakness, fatigue, dizziness, headache, tinnitus, dyspnea, bradycardia, palpitations, dry mouth, constipation, abdominal pain, nausea, impotence	See guanabenz
	Dizziness, nervousness, weakness, headache, palpitations, hypotension, tachycardia, nasal congestion, blurred vision, peripheral edema, fever, nausea, vomiting, diarrhea, dry mouth, abdominal pain, weight gain, dyspnea	Monitor BP and HR to check drug's effectiveness and presence of orthostatic hypotension
	Dizziness, vertigo, headache, drowsiness, fatigue, syncope, orthostatic hypotension, edema, palpitations, tachycardia, rash, pruritus, muscle weakness	Initial dose is given at bedtime; advise patient to remain recumbent for 3 h

TABLE 1-16

TABLE 1–16: CONTINUED

Medication	Route/Dose	Uses and Effects
Prazosin hydrochloride (Minipress)	Initial dose 1 mg, then 6–15 mg/d in 2–3 divided doses	See doxazosin

Peripherally Acting Antiadrenergics

Medication	Route/Dose	Uses and Effects
Guanethidine monosulfate (Ismelin)	PO: 10 mg/d initially; may be increased every 5–7 days by 10–12.5 mg/d. Usual maintenance dose is 25–50 mg/d	Management of hypertension Prevents release of norepinephrine from adrenergic nerve endings in response to sympathetic stimulation
Guanadrel sulfate (Hylorel)	PO: Initial 5 mg bid, may increase weekly by 10–40 mg/d Usual dose is 20–75 mg/d given in 2 divided doses, up to 400–600 mg/d	Management of hypertension Prevents release of norepinephrine from adrenergic nerve endings and adrenal medulla in response to sympathetic stimulation Decreases vasoconstriction
Reserpine	PO: 1–0.25 mg/d	Management of hypertension Depletes stores of norepinephrine and inhibits uptake in postganglionic adrenergic nerve endings

Other Medications

See Table 1–4
    Hydralazine hydrochloride (Apresoline Hydrochloride)
    Nitroprusside (Nipride)
    Nitroglycerin

See Table 1–5
    Labetalol hydrochloride (Normodyne)
    Esmolol (Brevibloc)

See Table 1–6
    Nicardipine hydrochloride (Cardene)
    Nifedipine (Procardia)
    Minoxidil (Loniten)

See Table 1–12
    Captopril (Capoten)

BP, blood pressure; CBC, complete blood count; CNS, central nervous system; ECG, electrocardiogram; GI, gastrointestinal; HR, heart rate; PO, by mouth.

From Deglin JH, Vallerand AH, Russin MM, 1988; Govoni LE, Hayes JE, Shannon MT, et al, 1992; Loeb S, 1993; Scherer JC, 1992; Vallerand AH, Deglin JH, 1991; Deglin JH, Deglin SG, 1992.

TABLE 1-16

Preparation/Administration	Side Effects	Nursing Implications
	Dizziness, vertigo, headache, drowsiness, fatigue, syncope, orthostatic hypotension, edema, palpitations, tachycardia, rash, pruritus, muscle weakness	See doxazosin
	Drowsiness, fatigue, confusion, headache, dizziness, fainting, nasal stuffiness, chest pain, palpitations, visual disturbance, shortness of breath, orthostatic hypotension, diarrhea, gas pain, constipation, anorexia, nausea, leg cramps, diarrhea, sexual dysfunction	Monitor BP, since catecholamines and BP-lowering effect are prolonged May require concurrent diuretic therapy
	Drowsiness, fatigue, confusion, headache, pheochromocytoma, dizziness, fainting, nasal stuffiness, chest pain, palpitations, visual disturbance, shortness of breath, orthostatic hypotension, diarrhea, gas pain, constipation, anorexia, nausea, leg cramps, diarrhea, sexual dysfunction, dry mouth, thirst, abdominal distress, nocturia	Monitor BP, since catecholamines and BP-lowering effect are prolonged May require concurrent diuretic therapy
	Drowsiness, fatigue, lethargy, depression, acute headache, nasal stuffiness, bradycardia, diarrhea, dry mouth, nausea, vomiting, GI bleeding, impotence, dizziness, tremors, convulsions, flushing, blurred vision, pruritus, muscle aches, dull sensorium	Monitor HR, since bradycardia can occur

- Consult with cardiologist about the need for a low-sodium diet of ≤90 mEq/day or a 2-g sodium diet.
- Consult with dietitian about patient's dietary needs in relation to either a low-calorie or low-sodium diet.
- Review arterial blood gas, serum electrolyte, and hematocrit results.
- Auscultate lungs for crackles every 4 hours in patients with peripheral edema, weight gain ≥1 kg/day, or neck vein distention.
- Assess extremities for presence of peripheral edema or distended neck veins resulting from dependent venous pooling or venostasis.
- Monitor daily weight and output. Report weight gain ≥1 kg/day, UO ≤30 mL/h or ≤0.5 mL/kg/h.
- Encourage patient to alternate horizontal rest (legs elevated) with vertical activity (standing) if not contraindicated.
- Administer prescribed IV fluids to maintain hydration, UO ≥30 mL/h or ≥0.5 mL/kg/h, and specific gravity 1.010.
- Administer prescribed alpha-adrenergic inhibitor in sodium-mediated HTN (prazosin or phentolamine) or central alpha-adrenergic inhibitors in sodium-mediated HTN (clonidine or methyldopa) to maintain DBP 70 to 90 mm Hg and MAP 70 to 90 mm Hg.
- Administer prescribed calcium channel blockers (nifedipine, verapamil, or diltiazem) in sodium-mediated HTN to cause peripheral and coronary arterial vasodilation (see Table 1–6).
- Administer prescribed volume-reducing agents in sodium-mediated HTN (thiazides such as chlorothiazide, hydrochlorothiazide, chlorthalidone, metolazone, indapamide; potassium-sparing agents such as amiloride, spironolactone or triamterene; or loop diuretics like furosemide) to maintain UO ≥30 mL/h, resolution of neck vein distention, and peripheral edema, and resolve crackles (see Table 1–13).
- Instruct patient as to the need for dietary sodium restriction and medication compliance.
- Teach patient common side effects of diuretics.

Pain related to headache secondary to cerebral edema.

Expected Patient Outcome. Patient experiences absence or decrease in verbalized pain.

- Elevate head of bed to reduce discomfort caused by cerebral edema.
- Maintain bed rest or limit activity while DBP ≥120 mm Hg and patient experiencing a headache.
- Monitor patient for headache pain while SBP ≥140 to 160 mm Hg and DBP ≥120 mm Hg and encourage patient to rate pain from 0 (no pain) to 10 (severe pain).
- Monitor patient for situations contributing to headache.
- Report the presence of epistaxis. Should epistaxis occur, record SBP and DBP and apply pressure over distal third of nose. This will compress the capillaries and may reduce the bleeding.
- Should epistaxis continue, assist with nasal packing. Provide frequent mouth care since nasal packing may require mouth breathing and subsequent drying of the mucous membranes.
- Eliminate or minimize vasoconstricting activities that may contribute to headaches: stress or smoking.
- Provide atmosphere conducive to stress reduction and limit visitors as appropriate.
- Provide rest periods.
- Maintain a quiet, low-lighted environment while patient is hypertensive.
- Administer prescribed analgesics to reduce headache-related pain.
- Teach patient to eliminate or minimize vasoconstricting activities (stress or smoking) that may aggravate headache.
- Instruct patient to avoid Valsalva's maneuver, which might increase blood pressure (BP).
- Teach patient stress-reducing techniques: Guided imagery, meditation, or relaxation exercises.

Knowledge deficit concerning the disease process, its consequences, and treatment related to lack of interest, fatigue, or lack of effective teaching.

Expected Patient Outcomes. Patient is able to describe the disease process, causes of HTN, and procedures for hypertensive control.

- Consult with cardiologist about the type and assessment of information to be shared with patient and significant other(s).
- Develop and individualize a teaching plan that covers anatomy and physiology of the arterial system, causes of HTN, pathophysiological effects of HTN, and treatment used to reduced HTN.
- Evaluate and report factors contributing to patient's knowledge deficit such as emotional readiness for learning, level of knowledge, ability to understand, support systems, and health beliefs.
- Teach patient to avoid standing still for any length of time, since vasodilation of the leg vessels causes blood pooling, leading to syncope or weakness.
- Teach patient to increase large muscle activity or lie down if hypotensive effect occurs.
- Instruct patient to report symptoms of chest pain, palpitation, dizziness, and headache.
- Teach patient the common side effects of antihypertensive medications such as lightheadedness, lethargy, or orthostatic hypotension.
- Teach patient the relationship between smoking, excess alcohol consumption, high-calorie or high-sodium diet, and stress to hypertension.
- Teach patient to take own BP and report changes above or below a preset number.

Noncompliance related to inability to follow treatment regimens or knowledge deficit.

Expected Patient Outcomes. Patient assumes responsibility for self-care and develops an attitude that contributes to adherence and to control of high BP.

- Assist patient to develop a self-care program: monitor own sodium intake, BP, and response to medication therapy.

- Evaluate patient's compliance with medication, diet, weight, exercise, stress reduction, smoking, and alcohol regimens.
- Assist patient to establish hypertensive control goals: weight reduction and gradual increase in exercises.
- Encourage patient to express concerns of self-care needs.
- Provide patient with written instructions as to how to take medications, side effects and goals of therapy.
- Teach patient how to measure and record BP.
- Teach patient the importance of not discontinuing medication and keeping follow-up appointments.

Collaborative Problem
A common collaborative goal for patients with acute hypertensive crisis is to increase CO.

Potential Complication: Decreased Cardiac Output. Decreased CO related to increased left ventricular afterload secondary to structural changes of chronic hypertension and to acute functional vasoconstricting forces.

Expected Patient Outcomes. Patient maintains adequate CO as evidenced by CO 4 to 8 L/min, CI 2.7 to 4.3 L/min/m^2, MAP 70 to 100 mm Hg, pulse pressure (PP) 30 to 40 mm Hg, SVR 900 to 1200 dynes/s/cm^{-5}, SVRI 1970 to 2390 dynes/s/cm^{-5}/m^2, capillary refill ≤ 3 seconds, SBP ≤ 140 mm Hg or DBP ≤ 100 mm Hg, UO ≥ 30 mL/h or ≥ 0.5 mL/kg/h, specific gravity 1.010 to 1.030, and peripheral pulses +2.

- Consult with cardiologist about DBP measurements requiring pharmacological therapy (mild HTN 90 to 104 mm Hg, moderate HTN 105 to 114 mm Hg, accelerated HTN 120 to 130 mm Hg, and malignant HTN ≥ 140 mm Hg) and the desired hemodynamic parameters.
- Consult with dietitian about the low-sodium diet that includes the patient's personal and cultural preferences and use of seasonal variations.

- Review results of BUN, creatinine, serum sodium, ECG, echocardiogram, and chest roentgenogram for changes supporting the presence of HTN.
- Limit physical activity to bed rest when patient experiences DBP ≥130 mm Hg, headache, dizziness, blurred vision, or chest pain.
- Encourage patient to rest periodically during the day and after meals to decrease myocardial oxygen demand.
- When SBP and DBP are stable, ambulate to tolerance.
- Maintain low-calorie and low-sodium diet as prescribed.
- Monitor BP and MAP every 1 to 5 minutes during titration of antihypertensive agents to maintain SBP ≤140 to 160 mm Hg, DBP ≤90 mm Hg, and MAP ≤110 mm Hg.
- Obtain and report hemodynamic parameters reflecting increased left ventricular afterload: SVR ≥1200 dynes/s/cm^{-5}, SVRI ≥2390 dynes/s/cm^{-5}/m^2, and PP ≤30 mm Hg.
- Obtain and report clinical signs and symptoms of accelerated HTN: DBP ≥120 mm Hg, retinopathy with exudates, retinal hemorrhages, headache, restlessness, epistaxis, tachycardia, crackles, S$_3$ and S$_4$.
- Monitor and report clinical signs and symptoms of malignant HTN: DBP ≥140 mm Hg, papilledema of optic disk, retinopathy, headache, blurred vision, dyspnea, and chest pain.
- Monitor for side effects associated with beta-adrenergic inhibiting agents: drowsiness, depression, hypotension, fluid retention, hypoglycemia, blurred vision, diarrhea, and weight gain.
- Monitor daily weight, intake, and output to maintain balanced hydration.
- Restrict fluids as ordered.
- Maintain progressive ambulation: elevate head of bed slowly, then take BP, progress to dangling for 10 minutes if BP is stable, take BP while sitting up, and have patient stand at bedside and take BP.

- Observe for orthostatic hypotension: pallor, diaphoresis, fainting, or loss of consciousness.
- Assist patient and significant other(s) in constructing a convenient schedule for taking medications.
- Administer prescribed IV fluids to maintain adequate hydration and UO ≥30 mL/h.
- Administer beta-adrenergic blockers (propranolol, metoprolol, atenolol, nadolol, timolol, acebutolol, labetalol, or pindolol); central alpha receptor receptors (clonidine or methyldopa); alpha receptor blocker (prazosin); and peripheral neural inhibitors (guanethidine and reserpine) to maintain SBP ≤140 mm Hg, DBP ≤90 mm Hg, MAP 70 to 100 mm Hg, and capillary refill ≤3 seconds (see Table 1–5).
- Administer vasodilator ACE inhibitors (captopril or enalapril) or peripheral vasodilators (hydralazine, minoxidil, or nitroprusside) to maintain SBP ≤140 mm Hg, DBP ≤90 mm Hg, SVR 900 to 1200 dynes/s/cm^{-5}, SVRI 1979 to 2390 dynes/s/cm^{-5}/m^2, UO ≥30 mL/h or 0.5 mL/kg/h, specific gravity 1.010 to 1.030, and peripheral pulses +2 (see Table 1–5).
- Teach patient to avoid foods high in sodium: milk products, processed food, prepared foods, canned or foreign foods, and fast foods.
- Teach patient the importance of taking the antidysrrhythmia medications without interruption unless indicated by the physician.
- Teach patient the importance of reducing other risk factors besides salt in the diet: cessation of smoking, moderation in alcohol consumption, use of dynamic exercise such as swimming or bicycling, and use of stress reduction techniques.
- Teach patient the common side effects of antihypertensive medications.

DISCHARGE PLANNING

The critical care nurse provides patient and significant other(s) with verbal or written discharge notes regarding the following subjects:

1. Symptoms of reoccurrence and need to report them to physician: headache, dizziness, faintness, nausea, and vomiting.
2. Importance of daily weight taking and reporting gains of $\geq$2 to 3 lb (1 to 1.5 kg)/d.
3. Importance of planned daily exercise program and rest periods throughout the day.
4. Taking and recording BP, as demonstrated to patient and significant other(s).
5. Medication, purpose, dosage, schedule, and side effects.
6. Limitation of smoking, caffeinated coffee or tea, and alcohol.
7. Importance of learning how to take own BP.

■ VALVULAR HEART DISEASE

(For related information see Part I: Congestive heart failure, p. 87; Dysrhythmias, p. 184. Part II: Valve surgery, p. 203; Part III: Percutaneous aortic valvuloplasty, p. 243; Hemodynamic monitoring, p. 219; Pacemakers, p. 270. See also Respiratory Deviations, Part I: Pulmonary edema, p. 346, Pulmonary embolism, p. 397.)

Diagnostic Category and Length of Stay
DRG: 135 Cardiac congenital and valvular disorders age $\geq$17 with complications
LOS: 4.90 days
DRG: 136 Cardiac congenital and valvular disorders age $\geq$17 without complications
LOS: 3.20 days

Definition
Valvular heart disease is categorized into two functional types, regurgitation and stenosis. Regurgitation (insufficiency) is blood flowing backward across the valve. Eventually effective forward blood flow may diminish while blood volume and pressure behind the valve increase. Stenosis is a narrowing of the valve and impedance of forward blood flow. Effective forward blood flow then requires greater pressure to open the valve and move the blood volume.

Pathophysiology
Mitral regurgitation results from a malfunction of the valve components (leaflets, annulus, chordae tendineae, and papillary muscles). In mitral regurgitation, there is bidirectional blood flow, with blood flowing from the left atrium into the left ventricle during diastole and blood flowing back from the left ventricle into the left atrium during systole. Left atrial pressure increases, causing left atrial hypertrophy and dilatation. The left ventricle also hypertrophies and dilates in an attempt to maintain systolic pressures and effective stroke volumes through the aortic valve. The patient also experiences atrial fibrillation, thrombus formation, decreased cardiac output, increased heart rate, and increased systemic vascular resistance. In mitral stenosis, nodules develop along the edges of the leaflets at the commissures and within the leaflets; fusion of the commissures and thickened, stiff leaflets, calcification of the leaflets, and eventually commissure adhesions are common. The normal orifice is 4 to 6 cm^2, with symptoms occurring when the orifice is 1 to 2 cm^2. At this time, left atrial blood volume and pressures are elevated, leading to left atrial hypertrophy, atrial fibrillation, and poor blood flow, causing atrial thrombus. Subsequently, the blood volume and pressures occur in the pulmonary capillaries and arteries. Perivascular and perialveolar transudates stiffen the lung and can lead to pulmonary edema. Eventually the pulmonary vascular system becomes hypertrophic, which contributes to increased right ventricular afterload and right ventricular hypertrophy.

Aortic regurgitation causes increased left ventricular volume as a result of systemic blood flowing back into the left ventricle during diastole, left ventricular dilatation, and increased wall tension. Eventually the ventricle hypertrophies and thickens. Vasodilation decreases diastolic pressure, while tachycardia decreases diastolic time. The result is decreased coronary perfusion. As pulmonary capillary wedge pressure (PCWP) increases, the mitral valve closes prematurely, causing blood volume to increase in the left atrium and subsequent left atrial pressure. Increases in pulmonary venous volume and pressure are followed by increase in pulmonary capillary, pulmonary artery, right ventricular, and right ventricular pressures.

In aortic stenosis, the valve is calcified, causing a decrease in the valve's mobility and orifice size. Initially the left ventricle compensates by hypertrophying from the increased systolic pressures. Hypertrophy elevates left ventricular end-diastolic pressure (LVEDP), which increases the work of the left atrium. As stenosis continues, the left ventricle begins to fail and dilate. This causes a decrease in stroke volume and increased left ventricular volume and pressure. The continued strain in the left atrium leads to backward failure. The latter causes increases in left atrial volume and pressure, pulmonary venous pressure, pulmonary capillary pressure, and arterial pressure.

Blood flows from the right ventricle to the right atrium during systole in tricuspid regurgitation. With increased right atrial volume, there is increased right atrial pressure, right atrial hypertrophy, and right atrial dilatation. Furthermore, there is increased central venous volume and pressure, peripheral edema, fluid weight gain, hepatomegaly, ascites, and intestinal vein distention. There is also decreased right ventricular output through the pulmonary system, causing decreased left ventricular output; the right ventricule dilates to accommodate the greater diastolic volume, and right ventricular hypertrophy results.

Tricuspid stenosis leads to the accumulation of blood in the right atrium, increased volume and pressure causing dilatation and hypertrophy of the right atrium, dilatation of the veins entering the veins because of the volume of blood backing into the system, increased pressure in the liver and spleen, causing engorgement and peripheral edema, and decreased right ventricular filling volumes, leading to reduced cardiac output.

Pulmonic regurgitation leads to blood flowing from the pulmonary artery into the right ventricle during diastole. Should pulmonary artery pressure be elevated, the right ventricular volume and pressure also increase. Increased right atrial volume and pressure may cause right atrial hypertrophy and increased atrial venous pressure. Pulmonic stenosis causes obstruction to right ventricular systolic ejection. This results in elevated right ventricular volume and pressure, elevated right atrial volume and pressure, and reduced right ventricle stroke volume.

Nursing Assessment

PRIMARY CAUSES

- *Aortic stenosis* is caused by endocarditis, rheumatic inflammation, idiopathic calcification, or congenital stenosis. *Aortic regurgitation* can be attributed to deceleration blunt chest trauma, syphilis, Marfan's syndrome, osteogenesis, rheumatic heart disease, arthritic disease, infectious endocarditis, aortic valve sclerosis, aortic aneurysm, calcification, dysfunction of an aortic valve prosthesis, and senile dilation of the annulus. *Mitral stenosis* results from rheumatic heart disease, tumors, left atrial ball-valve thrombus, bacterial vegetation, or calcification. *Mitral regurgitation* is due to coronary heart disease, acute bacterial endocarditis, mitral valve prolapse, dilation of the left ventricle distorting the annulus, calcification, trauma, dysfunction of a mitral valve prosthesis, myoxomatous changes in the leaflets, lupus erythematosus, cardiomyopathies, left ventricular failure, and Hurler's syndrome. *Pulmonic stenosis* is caused by rheumatic fever, whereas regurgitation is attributed to factors associated with pulmonary hypertension. *Pulmonic regurgitation* is due to pulmonary hypertension or rheumatic endocarditis. *Tricuspid stenosis* is due to rheumatic disease. *Tricuspid regurgitation* is due to congenital malformation of the valve or the absence of one of the leaflets.

PHYSICAL ASSESSMENT

Aortic Stenosis
- Inspection: Effort syncope, angina pectoris, dyspnea, orthopnea, paroxysmal nocturnal dyspnea, atrial fibrillation, fatigue, or cough.
- Palpation: Point maximal impulse (PMI) is exaggerated, presystolic heave and systolic thrill at the second intercostal space.
- Auscultation: Blood pressure (BP) is normal; pulse pressure decreases to 30 mm Hg in severe disease; aortic ejection click; a high-pitched sound heard best along left sternal border; harsh, high pitched systolic murmur that is crescendo–decrescendo in nature); soft S_1, crackles; low systolic BP (SBP); normal diastolic BP (DBP); diminished or absent aortic S_2, S_3; and S_4 gallop.

Aortic Regurgitation
- Inspection: Diaphoresis at night; headache; palpitation; dyspnea; cough; orthopnea; paroxysmal nocturnal dypsnea; peripheral edema or ascites or Quincke's sign (visible capillary pulsation of nail bed when fingertip is pressed); DeMussel's sign of head bobbing, neck pain, and visible arterial pulsation of neck, bounding with rapid rise and fall.
- Palpation: Capillary beds flush during systole and pale in diastole, water hammer pulse (rapid upstroke and then disappears quickly), PMI shifted to left, and diastolic thrill at suprasternal notch.
- Auscultation: A blowing, high-pitched decrescendo diastolic murmur at second intercostal space; systolic ejection murmur radiating to the carotid may be heard if the valve is distended or the aorta is dilated; second diastolic murmur heard at apex and a low-pitched, rumbling sound that is mid-diastolic, holodiastolic, or presystolic (Austin Flint murmur); widened pulse pressure; hypertension; tachycardia; S_3, S_4 and Hill's sign (popliteal BP is higher than brachial BP by 40 mm Hg); increased SBP; low DBP; and brisk sounds called pistol-shot over the femoral artery.

Mitral Stenosis
- Inspection: Dyspnea, orthopnea, paroxysmal nocturnal dyspnea, hemoptysis, chest pain, palpitations, peripheral cyanosis, fatigue, ascites, distended jugular neck veins, chronic cough, dysphagia, and hoarseness.
- Palpation: Hepatomegaly, peripheral dependent edema, left upper quadrant fullness, abdominal enlargement, cold extremities, and apical impulse may include a tapping vibration of S_1.
- Auscultation: Murmur is early to mid-diastolic; low-pitched rumbling sound heard at the apex; opening snap prior to the murmur; a high-pitched sound follows S_2; tachypnea; tachycardia; wheezes and crackles.

Mitral Regurgitation
- Inspection: Exertional dyspnea, weakness, dyspnea, paroxysmal nocturnal dyspnea, dysphagia, distended neck veins, orthopnea, palpitations, fatigue, exhaustion, dysrhythmia (atrial fibrillation and tachycardia), chest pain, diaphoresis, cyanosis, or confusion.
- Palpation: Hepatomegaly, peripheral edema, PMI is laterally displaced, systolic thrill, and peripheral edema.
- Auscultation: Blowing, high-pitched pansystolic murmur, systolic thrill over the left sternal border at third intercostal space, S_2 may be widely split, S_1 diminished, S_3 widely split, S_3 gallop, and tachycardia.

Tricuspid Stenosis
- Inspection: Positive hepatojugular reflex and diastolic hepatic pulsation in right flank.
- Palpation: Pulsations at the lower right sternal border as a result of right atrial hypertrophy, or diastolic thrill at the lower left sternal border during inspiration.
- Auscultation: Accentuated S_4; murmur is rumbling, low-pitched, decrescendo diastolic sound at the left sternal border in

fourth intercostal space or lower; and opening snap at the left sternal border of the fourth intercostal space.

Tricuspid Regurgitation
- Inspection: Positive hepatojugular reflex, jugular venous distention with observable liver pulsation, peripheral edema, anorexia, weight loss, pulsation of lower left sternal border with right ventricular hypertrophy, and pulsation of right sternal border with right atrial hypertrophy.
- Palpation: Hepatomegaly and edema.
- Auscultation: Pansystolic murmur heard at the left sternal border in the fourth intercostal space; and S_3 murmur is a blowing, high-pitched systolic sound heard at the lower left sternal border or xyphoid area, enhanced by inspiration, lying down, or exercise.

Pulmonic Stenosis
- Inspection: A round or triangular face, distended neck veins or large jugular vein waves, and a left parasternal lift.
- Palpation: A left parasternal or subxyphoid pulsation caused by right ventricule hypertrophy, thrill at the second intercostal space at the left sternal border, hepatomegaly, hepatojugular reflex, and peripheral edema.
- Auscultation: S_2 split on exhalation and widens during inspiration; ejection click at second intercostal space at left sternal border as the stenotic valve snaps open; murmur is a harsh, crescendo–decrescendo, systolic sound heard in the second intercostal space at the left sternal border.

Pulmonic Regurgitation
- Palpation: Pulsation at lower left sternal border characteristic of right ventricular hypertrophy, systolic pulsation, systolic thrill or diastolic thrill of an enlarged pulmonary artery at the second intercostal space of the left sternal border.
- Auscultation: Loud S_2 that is widely split, S_3 and S_4 at fourth intercostal space at the lower left sternal border, pulmonary artery ejection click may precede the murmur.

DIAGNOSTIC TEST RESULTS

Aortic Stenosis

Hemodynamic Parameters. (See Table 1–9)
- Elevated central venous pressure (CVP) reveals prominent a, c, and v waves, PCWP, pulmonary artery systolic (PAS) pressure, pulmonary artery diastolic pressure (PAD), and pulmonary vascular resistance (PVR).

Standard Laboratory Tests. (See Table 1–1)
- Blood studies: Reduced red blood count (RBC) and red blood cell indices show normocytic, normochromic red cells.

Invasive Cardiac Diagnostic Procedures. (See Table 1–2).
- Cardiac catheterization: Used to measure left ventricular and aortic pressures. Also can determine the gradient, systolic blood flow, and valve orifice area.

Noninvasive Cardiac Diagnostic Procedures. (See Table 1–3).
- Chest roentgenogram: Reveals characteristics of left ventricular failure, left ventricular dilation, left atrial dilation, and pulmonary congestion or edema. The calcified valve or dilated aorta caused by the ejection of ventricular systole is visualized.
- Echocardiogram: M-mode echocardiogram shows aortic cusp thickness, movement, left ventricular diameter, and wall thickness. Two-dimensional echocardiogram reveals the number, thickness, shape, movement, and calcification of the aortic cusps. In addition, left ventricular function is also evaluated.
- Radionuclide imaging: Used to document ventricular function, myocardial perfusion, and left ventricular ejection fraction.

ECG
- Large S waves in V_1 and V_2 leads, large R waves in V_4 to V_6 with depressed ST seg-

ment and inverted T waves reflecting left ventricular strain. Left atrial hypertrophy is demonstrated by P wave ending negatively in V_1. In addition, left axis deviation, left anterior hemiblock, and right or left bundle branch block.

Aortic Regurgitation

Invasive Cardiac Diagnostic Procedure. (See Table 1–2)

- Cardiac catheterization: Used to visualize the aorta for dilation and lesions and to determine the degree of regurgitation. Also measures left ventricular pressures, cardiac output, ejection fraction, and regurgitation fraction. In addition, left ventricular wall motion is recorded while coronary arteries are visualized.

Noninvasive Cardiac Diagnostic Procedures. (See Table 1–3)

- Chest roentgenogram: Reveals left ventricular hypertrophy reflective of chronic aortic regurgitation. Also shows dilation of the ascending aorta, left atrial enlargement, and pulmonary congestion.
- Echocardiography: Reveals characteristics of chronic aortic regurgitation including aortic valve leaflet movement, thickness, and vegetation. In addition, left ventricular diameter and wall thickness and motion can be evaluated. Tracking of the left ventricular end-systolic diameter is used to determine when surgery should occur. Fluttering of the anterior or posterior mitral valve leaflet or the ventricular septum during systole as a result of the regurgitant blood flow can be revealed.
- Phonocardiogram: Used to detect acute aortic regurgitation when tachycardia alters the sounds and shortens diastole. In chronic aortic regurgitation, the Austin Flint murmur can be recorded.
- Graded exercise studies: Used to evaluate patient's activity tolerance.

ECG

- Shows left ventricular hypertrophy, left atrial hypertrophy, and atrial fibrillation, or may have septal Q wave in V_5 and V_6.

Mitral Stenosis

Hemodynamic Parameters. (See Table 1–9)

- Elevated left atrial pressure (LAP) with an exaggerated a wave and a slow y descent and right atrial pressure (RAP). Cardiac output is normal until the orifice is ≤ 1 cm^2.

Standard Laboratory Tests. (See Table 1–1)

- Blood studies: Increased red blood cell destruction occurs across the stenotic valve.
- Serum chemistry: Elevated liver enzymes when right ventricular failure occurs.

Invasive Cardiac Diagnostic Procedures. (See Table 1–2)

- Cardiac catheterization: Shows systolic pressure gradient between the left ventricle and aorta (≥ 50 mm Hg) with decreased valve orifice (1.5 cm). The cardiac output may be normal or low. There can also be increased LAP, increased right ventricular pressure (RVP) and RAP when right ventricle failure occurs, and increased PCWP.

Noninvasive Cardiac Diagnostic Procedures. (See Table 1–3)

- Chest roentgenogram: Reveals left atrium is enlarged, which can elevate the left mainstem bronchus; elevated pulmonary pressures causing redistribution of blood flow to the upper lobes of the lung, Kerley's B lines in the lung fields, and enlargement of the pulmonary arteries and right ventricle; and calcification of the mitral valve.
- Echocardiogram: M-mode echocardiography can reveal the thick leaflets and their limited or abnormal movement and can document the rate of diastolic closure of the mitral valve leaflet or annulus calcification,

leaflet vegetation, atrial thrombus, and left atrial, left ventricular, and right ventricular size. Two-dimensional echocardiogram can be used to determine the size of the mitral valve orifice.

- Phonocardiogram: Used to clarify S_2 and the timing of the opening snap. As pulmonary hypertension develops, phonocardiogram reveals the increased intensity of the pulmonic component of S_2.
- Radionuclide imaging: Used to calculate ejection fraction and to evaluate left ventricular function.
- Graded exercise studies: Used to show patient's activity tolerance and to document dysrhythmias.

Invasive Cardiac Diagnostic Procedures. (See Table 1–2).

ECG

- Shows wide (≥ 0.12 seconds) notched P waves in leads II, III, and aVF or biphasic P waves, with the second portion negative, in V_1, which is characteristic of left atrial hypertrophy. Right ventricular hypertrophy can cause a right axis deviation and R waves in V_3.

Mitral Regurgitation

Hemodynamic Parameters. (See Table 1–9)

- Cardiac output is low. There is elevated LAP, PCWP (≥ 25 to 35 mm Hg), PVR, and CVP.

Standard Laboratory Tests. (See Table 1–1)

- Blood studies: Elevated white blood cell count, neutrophils, band neutrophils, and lymphocytes.
- Serium enzymes: Should mitral regurgitation complicate a myocardial infarction, there may be elevated creatinine kinase (CK), CPK-MB bands, or lactic dehydrogenase (LDH) $\geq LDH_2$.

Invasive Cardiac Diagnostic Procedure. (See Table 1–2)

- Cardiac catheterization: Provides measurement for determining left ventricular function and left ventricular mass and stress. It is also used to determine intracardiac pressure and a regurgitation fraction. The fraction is the ratio of blood volume regurgitated into the left atrium during systole to the total volume of blood ejected into both the left atrium and aorta by the left ventricule during systole. Mild mitral regurgitation is 1 to 2+ on a scale of 4; pulmonary artery wedge pressure (PAWP) ≤ 12 mm Hg at rest and exercise; and ejection fraction is $\geq 55\%$. Moderate mitral regurgitation of +3 signifies marked dilatation of left atrium and ventricle, increased PCWP at rest, and slightly decreased ejection fraction. Chronic mitral regurgitation of 4+ signifies gross dilatation of the left atrium and ventricle, increased PCWP at rest, and ejection fraction of 0.6 or greater.

Noninvasive Cardiac Diagnostic Procedures. (See Table 1–3)

- Chest roentgenogram: Left ventricular and left atrial enlargement may be seen in chronic mitral regurgitation; there is calcification of the annulus; left main-stem bronchus may be elevated by the enlarged left atrium.
- Echocardiogram: Can be used to identify the etiology of the regurgitation. With chronic mitral regurgitation there is enlargement of the left ventricle, enlarged left atrium, and increased wall motion of these chambers. The jet of blood regurgitated to the atrium, mitral valve leaflet thickening, and annulus calcification may be shown. The test can also be used to identify an enlarged left ventricle or atrium when it is present, increased systolic wall motion, or the causes of acute regurgitation.

- Graded exercise studies: Used to evaluate functional cardiac reserve in chronic mitral regurgitation.
- Phonocardiogram: Used to demonstrate the diminished first heart sound and accentuation of the murmur with increased afterload and to graph the murmur. With chronic mitral regurgitation, the phonocardiogram shows a high frequency, pansystolic murmur, third heart sound, and a mid-diastolic component.
- Radionuclide scanning: Used to identify ejection fraction, diastolic and systolic ventricular volumes, and left ventricular function.

ECG

- P wave may widen and notch with atrial hypertrophy. Increased amplitude or wide QRS and wide T wave are characteristic of left ventricular hypertrophy.

Tricuspid Stenosis

Hemodynamic Parameters. (See Table 1–9)

- Central venous wave forms correspond with jugular vein pulsation noted during inspiration, elevated CVP, and reduced cardiac index.

Standard Laboratory Tests. (See Table 1–1)

- Blood culture: May be positive in presence of an active infectious process.

Invasive Cardiac Diagnostic Procedures. (See Table 1–2)

- Cardiac catheterization: Used to simultaneously measure pressure in the right atrium and ventricle to confirm a gradient.

Noninvasive Cardiac Diagnostic Procedures. (See Table 1–3)

- Chest roentgenogram: Used to demonstrate right atrial or superior vena cava enlargement.
- Echocardiogram: M-mode used to demonstrate atrial thrombus, leaflet vegetation, calcification, and atrial and ventricular size. Two-dimensional echocardiogram is used to document the size of the tricuspid valve orifice.
- Phonocardiogram: Used to record the component of the S_1, S_2, and opening snap.

ECG

- Reveals prolonged PR interval and tall peaked P wave.

Tricuspid Regurgitation

Hemodynamic Parameters. (See Table 1–9)

- CVP wave form correlates with jugular vein pulsation and is elevated. The cardiac index is reduced.

Standard Laboratory Tests. (See Table 1–1)

- Blood culture: Results are positive in presence of an infection process.

Invasive Cardiac Diagnostic Procedures. (See Table 1–2)

- Cardiac catheterization: Used to obtain wave form and measures intracardiac pressures. An indicator-dilution curve helps to diagnose tricuspid regurgitation.

Noninvasive Cardiac Diagnostic Procedure. (See Table 1–3)

- Chest roentgenogram: Reveals right atrial, right ventricle, or superior vena cava enlargement. In addition, the azygous vein may be distended and pleural effusion may be seen.
- Echocardiogram: M-mode is used to document right atrial and ventricular size, septal movement, vegetation, and systole leaflet movement. Two-dimensional echocardiogram is used to identify vegetation and, with an intravenous contrast agent, shows blood flow back and forth across the valve.
- Phonocardiogram: Reveals components of S_1 and murmur.

ECG

- Reveals axis deviation to the right, right ventricular hypertrophy confirmed by voltage criteria, and right atrial enlargement conformed by Q wave in V_1.

Pulmonic Stenosis

Hemodynamic Parameter (See Table 1–9)

- CVP or RAP are elevated.

Invasive Cardiac Diagnostic Procedure. (See Table 1–2)

- Cardiac catheterization: Using the right heart, the severity and location of the pulmonic stenosis can be determined. In addition, CVP, RAP, and RVP are evaluated.

Noninvasive Cardiac Diagnostic Procedures. (See Table 1–3)

- Chest roentgenogram: Reveals enlargement of the pulmonary artery and left branch.
- Echocardiogram: M-mode demonstrates atrial contractions and ventricular size and wall motion. Two-dimensional echocardiogram reveals the shape, thickness, and movement of the pulmonic valve leaflets. In addition, vegetation, stenosis, ventricular size, and wall motion can be identified and determined.
- Phonocardiogram: Used to differentiate the aortic and pulmonic components of S_2 from the murmur and ejection click.

ECG

- Reveals ventricular hypertrophy with incomplete or complete right bundle branch block (RBBB), and right axis deviation. Right atrial enlargement may be seen by upright P waves in V_1.

Pulmonic Regurgitation

Hemodynamic Parameters. (See Table 1–9).

- RAP, RVP and CVP elevated.

Invasive Cardiac Diagnostic Procedures. (See Table 1–2)

- Cardiac catheterization: Used to measure pressure gradient or record regurgitation of a contrast material from the pulmonary artery into the right ventricle.

Noninvasive Cardiac Diagnostic Procedures. (See Table 1–3)

- Chest roentgenogram: Reveals enlargement of the pulmonary artery in pulmonic regurgitation without pulmonary hypertension. Shows enlarged pulmonary artery, right atrium, and right ventricle in pulmonic regurgitation patients with pulmonary hypertension.
- Echocardiogram: Used to show leaflet movement, vegetation, ventricular enlargement, or hypertrophy using M mode or two-dimensional echocardiogram.

ECG

- Reveals rSr of rsR in leads V_1 and V_2 in pulmonary regurgitation patients without pulmonary hypertension. Other findings include right ventricular hypertrophy or RBBB in pulmonary regurgitation patients with pulmonary hypertension.

MEDICAL AND SURGICAL MANAGEMENT

PHARMACOLOGY

- Diuretics: Diuretics such as chlorothiazide, chlorthalidone, or furosemide are given when left ventricular failure (aortic regurgitation or stenosis) and right ventricular failure (tricuspid regurgitation or stenosis) occur (see Table 1–13).
- Vasodilators: Nitrates (nitroglycerin), nitroprusside, hydralazine (Apresoline), prazosin (Minipress) or captopril (Capoten) are used to decrease afterload, which decreases regurgitation and increases aortic flow and combines with decreasing preload to minimize left ventricular volumes and the size of the mitral orifice (see Table 1–4).

- Antiobiotics: Infection process can be treated with penicillin, sulfadiazine, or erythromycin. Antibiotic prophylaxis for infection, surgery, or any instrumentation procedure consists of amoxicillin (3.0 g orally 1 hour before procedure and 1.5 g 6 hours after the initial dose, ampicillin, vancomycin, clindamycin, or gentamicin (see Table 1–14).
- Antidysrhythmics: Digitalis, quinidine, propranolol, or calcium channel blockers are used to treat atrial fibrillation (see Table 1–11 and Table 1–6).
- Anticoagulation agents: Anticoagulation with warfarin is given 2 to 3 weeks prior to cardioversion for long-standing atrial fibrillation that could cause systemic emboli. In addition low blood flow in the right ventricle may predispose prosthesis to thrombus (see Table 1–8).
- Positive inotropes: Digoxin, dobutamine, and dopamine are used to augment myocardial contractility and reduce pulmonary congestion.

DIET
- Restrict dietary sodium intake to reduce right ventricular failure and symptoms of venous congestion.

PHYSICAL ACTIVITY
- Limit activity to reduce dyspnea and other respiratory symptoms associated with mitral stenosis. With aortic regurgitation, isometric exercises are avoided because they can increase diastolic pressure and accentuate the regurgitation.

FLUID THERAPY
- Limit of fluid intake to reduce symptoms of venous congestion.

PERCUTANEOUS BALLOON VALVULOPLASTY
- Percutaneous balloon valvuloplasty (PBV) is a nonsurgical treatment for patients experiencing aortic or mitral stenosis. In aortic stenosis, the balloon causes valvular dilata-

tion through fracture of the calcifications, either nodules on the valvular cusps; commissural separation; leaflet stretching or tearing; or annulus rupture. The goal is to increase the valve orifice area and decrease the transvalvular gradient. With mitral valvuloplasty, the balloon separates the fixed commissures (see PBV, p. 243).

CARDIOVERSION
- Cardioversion may be helpful to restore normal sinus rhythm in patients with atrial fibrillation.

INTRA-AORTIC BALLOON PUMP
- Intra-aortic balloon pump (IABP) can be used in patients with decompensated aortic stenosis. The benefit is augmentation of the diastolic coronary filling pressure when left ventricular systolic pressure is not decreased. IABP is not used in patient with aortic regurgitation, since the pump can increase diastolic pressure and accentuate the regurgitation (see IABP, p. 254).

SURGICAL INTERVENTION
- Commissurotomy: Closed commissurotomy for mitral stenosis uses one or two balloons, finger or mechanical dilation. Closed commissurotomy is performed with the aid of a transventricular dilator. The procedure does not require cardiopulmonary bypass. Open commissurotomy is performed to remove an atrial thrombus, to perform amputation of left atrial appendage to reduce the risk of thrombus formation, for removal of fused chordae, split of scarred papillary muscle, and removal of calcium deposits from the leaflets and annulus. In general, a commissurotomy corrects fixed or calcified commissures by splitting the commissures open to within 2 to 3 mm of the annulus.
- Valve replacement: Prosthetic heart valves are classified as mechanical (caged-ball, tilting disk, or bileaflet) and tissue (homeograft, xenograft, heterograft, or allograft) valves (see Valve surgery, p. 203).

NURSING MANAGEMENT: NURSING DIAGNOSES AND COLLABORATIVE PROBLEMS

Nursing Diagnoses

Common nursing goals in patients with valvular heart disease are to increase cerebral tissue perfusion, enhance activity tolerance, prevent injury, promote oxygenation, reduce pain, and prevent infection.

Altered cerebral tissue perfusion related to thromboembolism secondary to aortic stenosis or insufficiency causing stasis of blood in the left ventricle.

Expected Patient Outcomes. Patient maintains adequate cerebral tissue perfusion, as evidenced by cardiac output (CO) 4 to 8 L/min, cardiac index (CI) 2.7 to 4.3 L/min/m²; mean arterial pressure (MAP) 70 to 100 mm Hg; SBP 110 to 140 mm Hg or DBP 70 to 90 mm Hg; equal and normoreactive pupils; oriented to person, place, and time; and normal sensorimotor function.

- Consult with cardiologist about potential pulmonary or systemic embolization from mural thrombi developing in the atrium as blood moves across the valve or atrial fibrillation occurs.
- Consult with physician about the type and duration of activity restriction.
- Perform passive range of motion (ROM) exercises to all extremities daily to prevent venous pooling.
- Monitor patient's neurological status every 1 to 2 hours as an indicator of cerebral blood flow.
- Obtain and report findings reflective of altered cerebral tissue perfusion: occipital headache, irritability, forgetfulness, confusion, sensorimotor dysfunction, and blurred vision.
- Obtain and report hemodynamic parameters contributing to decreased cerebral tissue perfusion: CO ≤4 L/min, CI ≤2.7 L/min/m², MAP ≤70 mm Hg, and heart rate (HR) ≥100 bpm.

- Monitor continuous ECG to assess HR and rhythm. Document ECG rhythm strips every 2 to 4 hours in patients with dysrhythmias.
- Measure and record intake and output to determine patient's level of hydration or need for additional diuretic therapy.
- Administer prescribed IV fluids to maintain adequate hydration and MAP 70 to 100 mm Hg.
- Administer prescribed oxygen 2 to 4 L/min by means of nasal cannula or mask to maintain appropriate oxygenation.
- Administer prescribed prophylactic anticoagulants should the patient experience atrial fibrillation and require cardioversion.
- Administer prescribed antidysrhythmic agents (quinidine, procainamide, or disopyramide) to manage atrial and ventricular premature beats, tachycardia, atrial flutter, or atrial fibrillation. Be cautious, since myocardial depressant's or peripheral vasodilator's effect may be enhanced if used in conjunction with drugs possessing similar properties (see Table 1–11).
- Instruct patient about the importance of continuing anticoagulant therapy until changed or discontinued by the physician.

Activity intolerance related to insufficient oxygen supply, dyspnea, or fatigue secondary to altered hemodynamics.

Expected Patient Outcomes. Patient maintains activity tolerance, as evidenced by HR ≤120 bpm (within 20 bpm of resting HR); respiratory rate (RR) ≤24 BPM; BP within 20 mm Hg of patient's normal range; and absence of chest pain, shortness of breath, or dyspnea.

- Consult with cardiologist to validate expected patient outcomes used to evaluate patient's tolerance to gradual increases in physical activity.
- Consult with cardiologist and rehabilitation specialist to individualize patient's exercise and daily activity program.
- Monitor patient's cardiac tolerance of gradual but progressive increase in physi-

cal activity: RR ≤24 BPM; HR ≤120 bpm, which is within 20 bpm of resting HR; BP within 20 mm Hg of patient's normal range; absence of dyspnea; and absence of chest pain.

- Document and report clinical findings that suggest activity intolerance: angina, fatigue, tachypnea, shortness of breath, dizziness, HR ≥120 bpm, and dysrhythmias.
- Assist patient to complete activities of daily living that do not lead to exercise increase in HR, BP, or RR.
- Provide adequate rest periods for patient between therapeutic care activities.
- Plan and implement incremental increases in activity such as assisted ROM while on bed rest.
- Encourage patient to rest or decrease level of activity if the signs or symptoms of exercise intolerance are present.
- Develop a plan that helps patient achieve desired activities.
- Encourage patient to use relaxation technique and deep breathing to decrease oxygen demand.
- Administer prescribed oxygen 2 to 4 L/min before and after progressive increases in physical activity.
- Teach patient about signs of activity intolerance: fatigue, HR ≥120 bpm, RR ≥24 BPM, and shortness of breath.
- Teach patient to consult with physician before changing physical activity schedule after discharge.

High risk for injury related to risk of bleeding secondary to anticoagulation therapy.

Expected Patient Outcomes. Patient is free of symptoms of bleeding as evidenced by BP within patient's normal range, HR ≤100 bpm, CO 4 to 8 L/min, CI 2.7 to 4.3 L/min/m^2, CVP 4 to 6 mm Hg, RAP ≥4 mm Hg, urinary output (UO) ≥30 mL/h, and absence of bleeding from catheter or tubing sites.

- Consult with cardiologist about results of clotting studies and need to decrease patient's anticoagulation therapy.

- Review and report changes in clotting studies such as prolonged prothrombin time (PT), partial thromboplastin time (PTT), and activated partial thromboplastin time (APTT) and reduced platelet count.
- Obtain and report hemodynamic changes suggesting hypovolemia resulting from blood loss: CO ≤4 L/min, CI ≤2.7 L/min/m^2, CVP ≤4 mm Hg, and RAP ≤4 mm Hg.
- Obtain and report other clinical findings associated with hypovolemia resulting from blood loss: hypotension, tachycardia, MAP ≤70 mm Hg, and UO ≤30 mL/h.
- Monitor catheter sites for bleeding.
- Administer prescribed IV fluids to maintain adequate hydration and hemodynamic stability.
- Should bleeding occur, administer prescribed packed RBCs to replace blood volume.
- Administer prescribed platelets, fresh frozen plasma, cryoprecipitate to replace clotting factors and blood volume if necessary.
- Instruct patient to report any bleeding from nose, gums, or around catheter insertion sites.

Impaired gas exchange related to pulmonary congestion secondary to incompetent aortic or mitral valve.

Expected Patient Outcome. Patient maintains adequate gas exchange, as evidenced by RR ≤24 BPM, arterial blood gases within normal range, PCWP 6 to 12 mm Hg, CO 4 to 8 L/min, CI 2.7 to 4.3 L/min/m^2, arterial oxygen saturation (Sao$_2$) ≥95%, mixed venous oxygen saturation (S$\bar{v}$o$_2$) 60% to 80%, absence of cyanosis, absence of crackles or wheezes, HR ≤100 bpm, and absence of dyspnea or shortness of breath.

- Consult with cardiologist to validate expected patient outcomes used to determine whether gas exchange is sufficient.
- Review results of chest roentgenogram, Sao$_2$, and arterial blood gases.
- Obtain and report hemodynamic findings that might influence gas exchange: CO ≤4L/min, CI ≤2.7 L/min/m^2, PCWP ≥12 mm Hg, and S$\bar{v}$o$_2$ ≤60%.

- Obtain and report factors that negatively affect oxygen delivery: $SaO_2 \leq 95\%$, hemoglobin ≤ 15 g, or CO ≤ 4 L/min.
- Monitor $S\bar{v}O_2$ to determine if oxygen demand is exceeding oxygen supply. A reduced $S\bar{v}O_2$ ($\leq 60\%$) indicates that oxygen demand (VO_2) exceeds oxygen supply (DO_2) and that oxygen supply needs to be increased by increasing CO, hemoglobin, or SaO_2 and that oxygen demands need to be reduced.
- Auscultate patient's lungs every 1 to 2 hours while crackles or wheezes are present.
- Encourage patient to reduce stress through relaxation techniques or deep-breathing maneuvers to reduce oxygen demand.
- Evaluate hemoglobin in relation to blood loss, since hemorrhage results in acute hemoglobin loss, thereby threatening oxygen supply, not only by decreasing hemoglobin but also by decreasing CO as preload deficits accrue. In this case, $S\bar{v}O_2$ is a more sensitive indicator of occult bleeding than changes in HR, pulse pressure (PP), CVP, or PCWP.
- Administer prescribed oxygen 2 to 4 L/min by means of nasal cannula or $FIO_2 \leq 50\%$ by mask to increase oxygen supply.

Pain related to decreased coronary artery perfusion or dysrhythmias.

Expected Patient Outcome. Patient acknowledges being pain free.

- Limit patient's physical activity to bed rest during pain to reduce oxygen demand.
- Obtain, document, and report patient's description of chest pain including location, radiation, duration, intensity, quality, and precipitating factors.
- Monitor continuous ECG to assess HR and rhythm. Document ECG rhythm strips every 2 to 4 hours in patients with atrial fibrillation.
- Administer prescribed antidysrhythmia agents (digitalis, propranolol, or quinidine) (see Table 1–11).
- Administer prescribed analgesics to relieve pain and reduce oxygen demand.

- Administer prescribed nitrates to decrease coronary vascular resistance and increase coronary blood flow (see Table 1–4).
- Instruct patient to describe pain using a scale of 1 to 10, with 10 being severe pain.
- Instruct the patient to report increased or decreased chest pain immediately.
- Instruct patient in the use of alternative pain relief measures: relaxation, repositioning, guided imagery, and distraction.

High risk for infection related to valvular irregularities or invasive techniques.

Expected Patient Outcomes. Patient will be free of infection, as evidenced by normothermia; white blood count (WBC) $\leq 11,000/\mu L$; negative cultures; HR ≤ 100 bpm; absence of redness, swelling, tenderness, or drainage from insertion sites.

- Review results of WBC and cultures.
- Ensure strict aseptic technique of insertion site care of all invasive monitoring devices and IV lines. Change tubing, collection containers, and peripheral needles and catheters every 48 to 72 hours per agency protocol.
- Obtain and report elevated temperature and redness, swelling, tenderness, or drainage from catheter sites.
- Monitor intake and output to determine whether fluid volume should be increased or diuretic therapy decreased.
- Administer prescribed IV fluids to maintain adequate hydration.
- Should infection occur, administer prescribed antibiotics (see Table 1–14).
- Teach patient to report tenderness, swelling, or drainage from invasive monitoring devices or IV lines.

Collaborative Problems

Common collaborative goals in patients with valvular heart disease are to increase CO or correct dysrhythmias.

Potential Complication: Cardiac Output Altered. Decreased CO related to increased preload and after-load secondary to valvular regurgitation or stenosis.

Expected Patient Outcomes. Patient maintains adequate CO, as evidenced by CO 4 to 8 L/min, CI 2.7 to 4.3 L/min/m^2, LAP 8 to 12 mm Hg, MAP 70 to 100 mm Hg, pulmonary artery pressure (PAP) systolic 15 to 25 mm Hg or diastolic 8 to 15 mm Hg, PCWP 6 to 12 mm Hg, RAP 4 to 6 mm Hg, right ventricular systolic pressure (RVSP) 20 to 25 mm Hg or diastolic (RVDP) 4 to 6 mm Hg, PVR 155 to 255 dynes/s/cm^{-5}, pulmonary vascular resistance index (PVRI) 200 to 450 dynes/s/cm^{-5}/m^2, systemic vascular resistance (SVR) 900 to 1200 dynes/s/cm^{-5}, systemic vascular resistance index (SVRI) 1970 to 2390 dynes/s/cm^{-5}/m^2, SBP $\leq$140 mm Hg or DBP $\geq$30 mm Hg, peripheral pulses +2, resolution of neck vein distention, absence of peripheral edema, capillary refill $\leq$3 seconds, and UO $\geq$30 mL/h.

- Consult with cardiologist to validate expected patient outcomes used to assess adequate CO.
- Consult with cardiologist about indicators for aortic valve replacement: evidence of left ventricular hypertrophy documented in chest roentgenogram and ECG; SBP$\geq$140 mm Hg or more with a DBP $\leq$30 mm Hg or less; and evidence of left ventricular dysfunction at rest or exercise.
- Consult with cardiologist regarding when surgery is required for acute mitral regurgitation: 3 to 4+ on a scale of 1 to 4, CO 1.5 L/min/m2 or greater, and an ejection fraction (EF) $\geq$35%.
- Consult with dietitian about providing a prescribed low-sodium diet that includes the patient's preferences.
- Review results from ECG, echocardiogram, chest roentgenogram, cardiac scans, and cardiac catheterization.
- Limit physical activity to reduce myocardial demand or fatigue while patient's SBP is $\geq$140 mm Hg and DBP $\leq$30 mm Hg.
- Limit activity to bed rest. Avoid elevating the supine patient's legs, since pulmonary pressure may increase leading to further orthopnea or dyspnea.
- Obtain and report hemodynamic parameters reflecting increased left ventricular preload: CO $\leq$4 L/min, CI $\leq$2.7 L/min/m^2, LAP $\geq$12 mm Hg, PAP systolic $\geq$25 mm Hg or diastolic $\geq$15 mm Hg, PCWP $\geq$12 mm Hg, SBP $\geq$130 m Hg or DBP $\leq$30 mm Hg, RAP $\geq$6 mm Hg, RVSP $\geq$25 mm Hg, and RVDP $\geq$6 mm Hg.
- Assess, document, and report findings suggestive of increased left ventricular preload secondary to aortic regurgitation: diaphoresis, flushing, diastolic thrill palpable at the left lower sternal border, apical impulse displaced laterally, S$_3$ gallop, throbbing in neck, tachycardia, palpitations, dizziness, fatigue, exertional dyspnea, orthopnea, nocturnal dyspnea, and Quincke's sign.
- Assess, document, and report findings reflective of increased left ventricular preload secondary to mitral regurgitation: exertional dyspnea, palpitations, fatigue, pansystolic murmur, splitting of S$_3$, and S$_3$ gallop.
- Obtain and report hemodynamic parameters reflective of increased right ventricular preload secondary to pulmonic or tricuspid regurgitation: CVP $\geq$6 mm Hg, RAP $\geq$6 mm Hg, and RVSP $\geq$25 mm Hg or RVDP $\geq$8 mm Hg.
- Obtain and report hemodynamic parameters reflective of increased left ventricular afterload secondary to aortic stenosis: CO $\leq$4 L/min, CI $\leq$2.7 L/min/m^2, PP $\leq$30 mm Hg, PAP systolic $\geq$25 mm Hg or diastolic $\geq$15 mm Hg, PCWP $\geq$12 mm Hg, SVR $\geq$1200 dynes/s/cm^{-5} and SVRI $\geq$2390 dynes/s/cm^{-5}/m^2.
- Monitor, document, and report other findings suggesting aortic stenosis: syncope, chest pain, dyspnea, systolic murmur, an ejection click, absent aortic S$_2$, and S$_4$ gallop.
- Obtain and report hemodynamic parameters reflecting increased right ventricular afterload secondary to pulmonary stenosis: PAP systolic $\geq$25 mm Hg or diastolic $\geq$15 mm Hg, PVR $\geq$255 dynes/s/cm^{-5} and PVRI $\geq$450 dynes/s/cm^{-5}/m^2.

- Assess, document, and report other findings suggestive of pulmonary stenosis: dyspnea, dizziness or faintness on exertion, palpitations, chest pain, split S_2, S_4, harsh systolic diamond-shaped ejection murmur in upper left sternal border, and systolic thrill in second intercostal space.
- Assess, document, and report other findings reflective of pulmonic regurgitation: early diastolic decrescendo murmur.
- Assess, document, and report other findings suggestive of tricuspid regurgitation: hepatomegaly, ascites, peripheral edema, hepatojugular reflux, jugular venous distention, observable systolic pulsation, and pansystolic murmur at left sternal border or the fourth intercostal space.
- Monitor peripheral skin color for cyanosis or peripheral pulses $\leq +2$ indicating reduced CO across the stenotic aortic valve.
- Monitor continuous ECG to assess HR and rhythm. Document ECG rhythm strips every 2 to 4 hours in patients with dysrhythmias such as atrial fibrillation, bradydysrhythmias, or supraventricular tachydysrhythmias.
- Auscultate breath sounds every 4 hours for presence of crackles or rhonchi.
- Monitor daily weight, intake, and output to ensure fluid balance.
- Assess skin for mottling, cyanosis, and presence of edema.
- Monitor BP every 1 to 2 hours in patient with severe aortic regurgitation: SBP may be 60 mm Hg higher in the legs than in the arms (Hill's sign), which is due to an acceleration of the normal BP response in the lower extremities.
- Perform passive ROM exercises to extremities four times a day to avoid venous stasis and maintain muscle tone.
- Administer F_{IO_2} at 50% or oxygen 2 to 4 L/min by means of nasal cannula or mask.
- Administer IV fluids to maintain adequate hydration, UO ≥ 30 mL/h or ≥ 0.5 mL/kg/h and specific gravity 1.010 to 1.030.
- Administer prescribed antibiotics such as penicillin V, streptomycin, or ampicillin.
- Administer volume-reducing agents such as furosemide or bumetanide to maintain UO ≥ 30 mL/h or ≥ 0.5 mL/kg/h and specific gravity 1.010 to 1.030.
- Administer prescribed volume-reducing agents (furosemide or bumetanide) to maintain SVR 900 to 1200 dynes/s/cm^{-5}, and SVRI 1970 to 2390 dynes/s/cm^{-5}/m^2.
- Administer prescribed digoxin to maintain CO 4 to 8 L/min, CI 2.7 to 4.3 L/min/m^2, MAP 70 to 100 mm Hg, PAP systolic 15 to 25 mm Hg or diastolic 8 to 15 mm Hg, and PCWP 6 to 12 mm Hg.
- Administer prescribed vasodilator (nitroprusside) to maintain SBP ≤ 140 mm Hg or DBP ≥ 30 mm Hg.
- Should pharmacological therapy be ineffective in decreasing preload or afterload, prepare patient for percutaneous balloon valvuloplasty (see PBV, p. 243.)
- Should percutaneous balloon valvuloplasty be ineffective or inappropriate, prepare patient for valve replacement (see Valve surgery, p. 203.)
- Instruct patient as to the relationship between valvular dysfunction, signs and symptoms, and treatments.
- Provide patient with postoperative information and self-care activities.
- Teach patient to report any episodes of syncope and to note circumstances in which syncope occurs.

Potential Complication: Dysrhythmias. Dysrhythmias related to left atrial hypertrophy secondary to mitral stenosis.

Expected Patient Outcomes. Patient remains in sinus rhythm, HR ≤ 100 bpm, BP within patient's normal range, and absence of chest pain.

- Consult with cardiologist about dysrhythmias that might occur with mitral stenosis.
- Consult with cardiologist about the underlying cause of dysrhythmias and antidysrhythmia agents used to correct it.
- Review results of ECG.
- Initiate continuous ECG to assess HR and rhythm. Document ECG rhythm strips every 2 to 4 hours in patients with dysrhythmias.

- Monitor and report physical signs and symptoms of dysrhythmias: abnormal HR and rhythm, palpitations, chest pain, syncope, ECG changes, and hypotension.
- Administer prescribed IV fluids to maintain adequate hydration.
- Administer prescribed oxygen 2 to 4 L/min by nasal cannula of $FIO_2 \leq 50\%$ by mask to maintain appropriate oxygenation.
- Administer prescribed antidysrhythmia agent to correct atrial fibrillation and slow ventricular response (digoxin, propanolol, or quinidine) (see Table 1–11).
- Administer prescribed anticoagulation agents 2 to 3 weeks prior to elective cardioversion for long-standing atrial fibrillation or with unresolved atrial fibrillation (see Table 1–8).
- Should pharmacological therapy be ineffective in correcting atrial fibrillation, prepare patient for cardioversion. Cardioversion can be used for atrial fibrillation of sudden onset or in situations of mild regurgitation or atrial hypertrophy. Also indicated when there is the loss of the atrial kick, which decreases CO.
- Teach patient to report an abnormal heart rate, syncope, or describe chest pain on a scale of 1 to 10.

Potential Complication: Thromboembolism. Thromboembolism related to stagnated blood in the left atrium secondary to atrial dilatation caused by mitral valve disease.

Expected Patient Outcome. Patient is free of thromboembolism.

- Consult with cardiologist about physical activity should thromboembolism occur.
- Review results of coagulation studies such as PT, PTT, ACT and platelet count and arterial blood gas measurement.
- Limit patient's physical activity to bed rest until the thromboembolic event is corrected.
- Monitor and report clinical findings associated with thrombophlebitis: heat and erythema of calf or thigh, increased circumference of calf or thigh, tenderness or pain in extremity, or pain in the calf area with dorsiflexion.
- Change patient's position every 2 hours to prevent venous pooling.
- Maintain adequate hydration 2 to 3 L/day, if appropriate, to prevent dehydration and concomitant increase in blood viscosity, which may promote thrombus formation.
- Apply antiembolic hose as prescribed.
- Maintain rest of affected extremity, keeping extremity in a neutral or elevated position as prescribed.
- Administer prescribed oxygen 2 to 4 L/min by nasal cannula or mask to maintain adequate oxygenation.
- Administer prescribed anticoagulants (see Table 1–8).
- Teach patient to report shortness of breath, dyspnea, tachypnea, or calf tenderness.

DISCHARGE PLANNING

The critical care nurse provides patient and significant other(s) with verbal or written discharge notes regarding the following subjects:

1. Medications, purpose, dosage, schedule, and side effects.
2. Importance of reporting signs and symptoms of heart failure to physician: increased fatigue, tachypnea, orthopnea, or cough.
3. Importance of reporting to physician events that predispose patient to bacteremia: dental gum manipulation, drainage of abscess, gynecologic procedure, or genitourinary procedure.
4. Need to avoid fatigue, to plan rest periods before and after activity.
5. Importance of taking prophylactic antibiotic therapy.
6. Importance in keeping up ongoing outpatient care.

■ CARDIAC TRAUMA

(For related information see Part I: Acute cardiac tamponade, p. 117; Congestive heart failure, p. 87; Cardiogenic shock, p. 72; Shock, p. 174; Dysrhythmias, p. 184. Part III:

Intra-aortic balloon pump, p. 254; Hemodynamic monitoring, p. 219; Pacemakers, p. 270. See also Respiratory Deviations Part I: Acute respiratory distress syndrome, p. 327; Pulmonary edema, p. 346; Pulmonary embolism, p. 397; Respiratory acidosis, p. 412; and Respiratory Deviations, Part III: Intravascular oxygenator, p. 442.)

Diagnostic Category and Length of Stay

DRG: 144 Other circulatory system diagnoses with complications
LOS: 5.20 days
DRG: 145 Other circulatory system diagnoses without complications
LOS: 3.40 days

Definition

Trauma is an injury resulting from external forces. Injury occurs when energy is dissipated or transferred to body tissues. Cardiac trauma occurs from damage caused by penetrating or nonpenetrating (blunt) injuries to the heart. With both types of trauma, there may be injury to the pericardium, myocardium, coronary arteries, cardiac valves or their supporting structures, atrial or ventricular septum, or the great vessels.

Pathophysiology

Blunt cardiac trauma results from physical forces that act externally on the body. There can be two responses. The first is myocardial concussion, a less severe injury, which nevertheless produces clinical manifestations of cardiac trauma. The second is myocardial contusion, which may cause cellular necrosis of the myocardium. The following are five mechanisms that produce myocardial injury: (1) an impact of a force directly against the chest; (2) a decelerative force, where the body stops suddenly but the internal organs continue in a forward motion; (3) a compressive force against the chest on either side; (4) the compression of the abdomen or lower extremities, displacing blood and abdominal contents upward; (5) or concussive forces that

interfere with the cardiac rhythm. Blunt trauma can cause cardiac tamponade or aortic rupture or cardiac rupture.

Penetrating cardiac trauma occurs after a pericardial injury, vessel injury, or cardiac chamber injury. A penetrating injury to the pericardium leads to the accumulation of fluid in the pericardial sac, or cardiac tamponade. Great-vessel injuries include those of the inferior and superior vena cava, brachiocephalic and subclavian vessels, carotid arteries, and pulmonary arteries. Aortic rupture can be caused by a rapid deceleration or acceleration injury (steering wheel impact), resulting in the application of differential forces to intrathoracic structures. Other causes of aortic rupture include puncture from ribs and vertebrae. The right ventricle is most commonly affected by stab wounds because of its anterior position in the thorax.

Nursing Assessment

PRIMARY CAUSES

- Blunt cardiac trauma includes pericardial injury such as hemorrhagic pericarditis, pericardial laceration, tamponade, constrictive pericarditis, and intrapericardial diaphragmatic hernia. Myocardial injury involves contusion, ischemic infarction, myocardial hematoma, myocardial rupture, and aneurysm. Endocardial injury can occur. Other mechanisms include atrioventricular and semilunar injury, intimal tear or thrombosis or laceration of the coronary arteries, and damage to the aortic and pulmonary artery involving rupture or aneurysm.
- Penetrating cardiac trauma occurs from wounds of knives, ice picks, glass, wooden splinters, or bullets.

PHYSICAL ASSESSMENT

Blunt Cardiac Trauma

- Inspection: Bruises on chest; jugular vein distention; cyanosis of upper torso, face, neck, and arms; pulsus paradoxus; and confusion.

- Palpation: Dyskinetic segment palpable if an entire thickness of myocardium has been contused; systolic, diastolic, or continuous thrills; apex impalpable with pericardial fluid accumulation; rapid, weak peripheral pulses.
- Auscultation: Tachycardia, hypotension, triphasic friction rub, intrascapular systolic murmur (hematoma in thoracic aorta).

Penetrating Cardiac Trauma

- Inspection: Weakness, shortness of breath, diaphoresis, cool and clammy skin, anxiousness, restlessness.
- Palpation: Rapid, weak peripheral pulses.
- Auscultation: Hypotension and tachycardia.

DIAGNOSTIC TEST RESULTS

Blunt Cardiac Trauma

Standard Laboratory Tests. (See Table 1–1)

- Blood studies: Reduced hemoglobin and hematocrit. Elevated white blood count (WBC) should infection develop.
- Cardiac enzymes: Elevated creatine kinase-MB (CK-MB)

Invasive Cardiac Diagnostic Procedure. (See Table 1–2)

- Coronary arteriography: Defines coronary arterial lesions and quantifies structural cardiac lesions.

Noninvasive Cardiac Diagnostic Procedures. (See Table 1–3)

- Cardiac scan: Technetium 99m pyrophosphate images the myocardial contusion. Thallium 201 imaging permits differentiation between myocardial ischemia (decreased blood flow) and myocardial contusion. Resting radionuclide angiography delineates wall motion abnormalities, distinguishes right and left ventricular contusion, and ejection fraction from right and left ventricle.
- Chest roentgenogram: Detects pericardial effusion such as a separation between the parietal pericardial shadow and a lucent line of epicardial fat, water-bottle cardiac silhouette, or enlargement of the azygous and superior vena caval shadows; cardiomegaly; rupture of the atrial or ventricular septum.
- Echocardiogram: Two-dimensional findings include: pericardial effusion, myocardial thinning, segmented wall motion abnormalities, structural complications, distinction of right from left ventricular injury or of right ventricular contusion from cardiac tamponade. Doppler echocardiography detects valvular regurgitation and intracardiac shunts.
- Multiple gated acquisition (MUGA) scan: Can reveal decreased ability of the heart to pump effectively when myocardial contusion is present.

ECG

- Shows T wave flattening or inversion in one or more leads, ST segment depression, Q wave, prolongation of QT internals, and conduction abnormalities.

Penetrating Cardiac Trauma

Noninvasive Cardiac Diagnostic Procedure. (See Table 1–3)

- Chest roentgenogram: Presence of a missile, widening mediastinum; obliteration of the aortic knob; and space between the pulmonary artery and aorta with aortic rupture.
- Echocardiogram: Penetrating injuries to the valves and septal or wall motion abnormalities.

ECG

- ST segment elevation, T waves flattened or inverted.

MEDICAL AND SURGICAL MANAGEMENT

PHARMACOLOGY

- Positive inotropes: Dopamine or dobutamine is used to enhance cardiac contractility and cardiac output (see Table 1–10).
- Vasodilators: Nitroprusside is used to decrease preload and afterload, thereby pre-

venting complete disruption of the involved vessel (see Table 1–4).

- Antidysrhythmia agents: Used to treat cardiac dysrhythmias, if necessary, caused by myocardial contusion (see Table 1–11).
- Antibiotics: Used to control infection that occurs in response to contamination from a penetrating injury (see Table 1–14).

FLUID THERAPY

- Volume resuscitation is directed to replace blood loss from the intravascular space and fluid loss from the extravascular space. Colloids are maintained in the intravascular space because of their oncotic properties. Crystalloids replace losses in the extravascular space. If signs of class I (750 mL blood loss) or class II (750 to 1500 mL blood loss) are present, crystalloid solution is rapidly infused at a rate of 3 mL/1mL of blood loss. Plasma expanders such as hetastarch can be used to augment crystalloids in patients who do not show improvement with crystalloids. With class III (1500 to 2000 mL blood loss) or class IV (≥2000 mL blood loss), crystalloids plus blood are administered. Blood products are replaced 1 mL for each 1 mL of blood loss to maintain a hemoglobin concentration above 10 to 12 g/100 mL and a hematocrit of 30%.

PHYSICAL ACTIVITY

- Activity is restricted to bed rest.

HEMODYNAMIC MONITORING

- Used to monitor changes in central venous pressure (CVP), mean arterial pressure (MAP), pulmonary capillary wedge pressure (PCWP), pulmonary artery pressure (PAP), cardiac output (CO), and cardiac index (CI).

PNEUMATIC ANTISHOCK GARMET (PASG)

- PASG is a pneumatic counterpulsation device that is used to control hemorrhage by tamponading intra-abdominal, pelvic, and lower-extremity bleeding. The PASG in-

creases vascular resistance and prevents further blood loss into the abdomen and legs.

SURGICAL INTERVENTION

- Surgical intervention is used to correct vessel injury to cardiac chamber injury.

NURSING MANAGEMENT: NURSING DIAGNOSES AND COLLABORATIVE PROBLEMS

Nursing Diagnoses

Common nursing goals in patients with cardiac trauma are to enhance tissue perfusion, correct fluid volume deficit, prevent infection, maintain tissue integrity, and reduce pain.

Altered cardiopulmonary, cerebral, and renal tissue perfusion related to arterial blood flow disruption secondary to decreased myocardial contractility.

Expected Patient Outcomes. Patient maintains adequate tissue perfusion, as evidenced by blood pressure (BP) ≥90 mm Hg; heart rate (HR) ≤100 bpm; respiratory rate (RR) ≤24 BPM; coronary artery perfusion pressure (CAPP) 60 to 80 mm Hg; CO 4 to 8 L/min; CI 2.7 to 4.3 L/min/m^2; MAP 70 to 100 mm Hg; normal sinus rhythm; absence of neck vein distention; pulmonary vascular resistance (PVR) 155 to 255 dynes/s/cm^{-5}; pulmonary vascular resistance index (PVRI) 200 to 450 dynes/s/cm^{-5}/m^2; mixed venous oxygen saturation (S$\bar{v}$o$_2$) 60% to 80%; systemic vascular resistance (SVR) 900 to 1200 dynes/s/cm^{-5}; systemic vascular resistance index (SVRI) 1970 to 2390 dynes/s/cm^{-5}/m^2; peripheral pulses +2; capillary refill ≤3 seconds; equal and normoreactive pupils; oriented to person, place, and time; normal sensorimotor function; arterial oxygen pressure (Pao$_2$) 80 to 100 mm Hg; arterial carbon dioxide pressure (Paco$_2$) 35 to 45 mm Hg; arterial oxygen saturation (Sao$_2$) ≥95%; absence of crackles; urinary output (UO) ≥30 mL/h; specific gravity 1.010 to 1.030; blood urea nitrogen (BUN) ≤20 mg/dL; creatinine clearance M:

95 to 135 mL/min or W: 85 to 125 mL/min; and serum creatinine 0.6 to 1.2 mg/dL.

- Consult with cardiologist to validate expected patient outcomes used to evaluate tissue perfusion.
- Review results from arterial blood gas measurement, BUN, serum creatinine, creatinine clearance, chest roentgenogram, and ECG.
- Limit activity to bed rest in order to decrease oxygen demand.
- Monitor and report hemodynamic parameters reflecting altered cardiopulmonary tissue perfusion: CAPP $\leq$60 mm Hg, CO $\leq$4 L/min, CI $\leq$2.7 L/min/m^2, PVR $\geq$255 dynes/s/cm^{-5}, PVRI $\geq$450 dynes/s/cm^{-5}/m^2, SVR $\geq$1200 dynes/s/cm^{-5}, SVRI $\geq$2390 dynes/s/cm^{-5}/m^2 , and S$\bar{v}o_2$ $\geq$60%.
- Obtain and report other clinical findings associated with altered cardiopulmonary tissue perfusion: crackles, cyanosis, capillary refill $\geq$3 seconds, peripheral pulses $\leq$+2, neck vein distention, dysrhythmias, hypotension, tachycardia, tachypnea, or chest pain.
- Monitor clinical indicators of neurological status every 2 hrs: level of consciousness, pupillary size and normoreaction, sensorimotor function, and vital signs.
- Monitor every 2 to 4 hours and report for changes reflecting altered cerebral tissue perfusion: pupils unequal, abnormal sensorimotor function, fatigue, weakness, irritability, forgetfulness, or confusion.
- Monitor daily weight for weight gain or loss $\geq$1 kg or 2 pounds.
- Obtain and report changes suggestive of altered renal perfusion: weight gain, UO $\leq$30 mL/h or $\leq$0.5 mL/kg/h, specific gravity $\leq$1.010, peripheral edema, BUN $\geq$20 mg/dL, serum creatinine $\geq$1.2 mg/dL, and creatinine clearance M: $\leq$95 mL/min or W $\leq$85 mL/min.
- Obtain and report other clinical findings associated with altered renal tissue perfusion: UO $\leq$30 mL/h, specific gravity $\leq$1.010, peripheral edema, and neck vein distention.
- Auscultate lungs and report RR $\geq$20 BPM, crackles, or dyspnea.

- Monitor continuous ECG to assess HR and rhythm. Document ECG rhythm strips every 2 to 4 hours in patients with dysrhythmias.
- Administer prescribed Fio_2 at 50% by mask oxygen 2 to 4 L/min by nasal cannula to maintain Pao_2 $\geq$80 mm Hg, Sao_2 $\geq$95%, and S$\bar{v}o_2$ $\geq$60%.
- Administer prescribed IV fluids to maintain hydration, UO $\geq$30 mL/h or $\geq$0.5 mL/gk/h, specific gravity 1.010 to 1.030, and BP $\geq$90 mm Hg.
- Administer prescribed volume-reducing agents: thiazide (chlorothiazide, hydrochlorothiazide, chlorthalidine, metolazone), loop (furosemide or bumetanide), or potassium-sparing (spironolactone, amiloride, or triamterene) diuretics to maintain UO $\geq$30 mL/h or $\geq$0.5 mL/kg/h; specific gravity 1.010 to 1.030; BP$\geq$90 mm Hg; MAP 70 to 90 mm Hg; peripheral pulses +2; capillary refill $\leq$3 seconds; and BUN, serum creatinine, and creatinine clearance within normal range (see Table 1–13).
- Administer prescribed antidysrhythmia agents appropriate for the particular dysrhythmia caused by myocardial contusion (see Table 1–11).
- Should pharmacological therapy be ineffective or heart block occur, prepare patient for a temporary pacemaker (see Pacemakers, p. 270.)
- Should critically altered hemodynamic stability occur from ruptured valve, torn papillary muscle, or torn intraventricular septum, prepare patient for emergency surgical repair.
- Teach patient common side effects of antidysrhythmia medication.
- Teach patient about the type of pacemaker to be used.

High risk for infection related to contaminated foreign object or invasive procedures secondary to trauma tissue injury.

Expected Patient Outcomes. Patient is free of infection, as evidenced by temperature within normal limits; HR $\leq$100 bpm; absence of purulent drainage or absence of edema, redness, or tenderness around the puncture, abscess, or catheter site.

- Consult with dietitian about patient's nutritional status and need to provide adequate protein and caloric intake for healing.
- Review complete blood count (CBC) results and cultures.
- Obtain and report hemodynamic parameters that may reflect systemic infection: reduced CVP, PAP, PCWP, CO, CI, SVR, and SVRI.
- Assess all invasive lines or catheters for signs of redness, swelling, tenderness, or drainage.
- Monitor and report temperature every 1 hour while patient is febrile.
- Maintain aseptic technique for all invasive devices, changing sites, dressings, tubings, and solutions per policy schedule in order to reduce bacterial introduction into an already compromised trauma patient.
- Administered prescribed oxygen 2 to 4 L/min by nasal cannula or FIO_2 ≤50% by mask to maintain adequate oxygenation.
- Administer prescribed IV fluids to avoid overhydration with a balanced electrolyte solution to maintain tissue perfusion.
- Administer prescribed antibiotics to reduce circulating endotoxins (see Table 1–14).
- Teach patient to report any tenderness, redness, or drainage from invasive lines or catheter sites.

Fluid volume deficit related to blood loss secondary to vessel injury or cardiac chamber injury as a result of penetrating cardiac trauma.

Expected Patient Outcomes. Patient maintains adequate fluid volume, as evidenced by BP within patient's normal range, CVP 2 to 6 mm Hg, PAP 15 to 25 or 8 to 15 mm Hg, CO 4 to 8 L/min, CI 2.7 to 4.3 L/min/m², MAP 70 to 100 mm Hg, PCWP 6 to 12 mm Hg, peripheral pulses +2, capillary refill ≤3 seconds, normal skin turgor, absence of external bleeding, hemoglobin and hematocrit within patient's normal range, and UO ≥30 mL/h.

- Consult with cardiologist to validate expected patient outcomes used to evaluate adequate fluid volume.
- Review results from hemoglobin, hematocrit, platelet count, WBC, arterial blood gas and serum electrolyte measurement.
- Assess arterial blood pressure, HR, and RR frequently to determine trends in volume status. Hypotension in blunt trauma is due to distant blood loss and not from a primary cardiac injury; hypotension in penetrating cardiac trauma can signify direct injury to myocardium or great vessels.
- Obtain and report hemodynamic parameters reflective of fluid volume loss as a result of bleeding: CO ≤4 L/min, CI ≤2.7 L/min/m², CVP ≤2 mm Hg, MAP ≤70 mm Hg, PAP systolic ≤15 mm Hg or diastolic ≤8 mm Hg, and PCWP ≤6 mm Hg.
- Control external bleeding by applying direct pressure to the site.
- Apply PASG, if necessary, to provide peripheral resistance, perform arterial tamponade, and promote shunting of blood to vital organs.
- Should PASG be used, monitor patient's response: BP, trouser pressure, and ventilatory response.
- Monitor IV fluid therapy in relationship to BP and HR: Failure of systemic BP to increase and HR to decrease after multiple incremental boluses may reflect continued rapid hemorrhage or cardiac failure.
- Measure daily weight, intake, and output to evaluate fluid balance.
- Evaluate patient for bleeding from wound, drainage, or dressing every 15 minutes or until bleeding subsides or surgery corrects problem.
- Reduce patient's anxiety through reassurance, support, and explanations.
- Administer isotonic crystalloid solution as the initial infusion solution in penetrating cardiac injuries: IV fluid is delivered in increments of approximately 10% of patient's calculated intravascular volume (500 mL) and infused rapidly over 5 to 10 minutes. Administer 3 mL/1 mL of blood loss. Mul-

tiple incremental boluses of IV fluid are administered to produce a systemic BP ≥90 mm Hg, MAP 70 to 90 mm Hg, HR ≤100 bpm, CVP 2 to 6 mm Hg, CO 4 to 8 L/min, CI 2.7 to 4.3 L/min/m², and UO ≥30 mL/h or 0.5 mL/kg/h.
- Administer prescribed blood products 1 mL/1 mL of blood loss.

Impaired tissue integrity, related to integumentary or subcutaneous tissue trauma secondary to penetrating cardiac trauma.

Expected Patient Outcomes. Patient maintains tissue integrity, as evidenced by normal temperature; absence of edema; absence of reddened skin; peripheral pulses +2; capillary refill ≤3 seconds; is warm, dry, and smooth skin; $S\bar{v}o_2$ 60 to 80%; BP within patient's normal range; normothermia; and MAP 70 to 90 mm Hg.

- Confer with patient's cardiologist or trauma team physician as to the degree of tissue injury and expected healing time.
- Consult with dietitian about providing patient with sufficient protein or carbohydrate to facilitate tissue healing.
- Review results from hematocrit, hemoglobin, WBC, and cultures.
- Limit activity to bed rest while integumentary and subcutaneous tissues repair themselves.
- Assess skin for color, edema, and evidence of tissue regeneration.
- Obtain temperature every 1 to 2 hours while patient is febrile and while skin shows signs of inflammation or swelling at the catheter, abrasion, or puncture site.
- Cleanse and irrigate all open wounds following agency protocol to remove debris and decrease bacteria that causes infection.
- Cover open wounds with sterile dressings to monitor sterile environment. Note the amount, color and consistency of drainage from wound(s).
- Cover sucking wounds with impregnated (petroleum jelly) gauze to restore skin integrity and reduce further chest wall injury.

- Obtain culture of any drainage from the abrasion of puncture site.
- Administer prescribed IV fluids to maintain adequate hydration and UO ≥30 mL/h.
- Administer prescribed antibiotics based on the type of cardiac traumatic injury and results of culture and sensitivity test.
- Instruct patient as to the relationship between cardiac injury and tissue trauma.

Pain related to myocardial contusion or penetrating wound.

Expected Patient Outcome. Patient experiences a decrease or absence in precordial chest pain.

- Place patient in a comfortable position with head of bed elevated 30 to 45 degrees.
- Assess and document the location, type, severity, and duration of patient's pain, using a scale of 0 (no pain) to 10 (severe pain).
- Monitor cardiac rhythm during chest pain for changes in configuration of PR, QRS, ST, and T segment or dysrhythmias.
- Provide chest splinting to damaged bony structures in order to lessen pain and encourage lung expansion while encouraging patient to cough and deep breathe.
- Administer morphine sulfate to patient who is not hypotensive to relieve chest discomfort (see Table 1–17).
- Instruct patient to immediately report chest pain.
- Instruct patient to report posttraumatic pericarditis, which may occur after the injury or months later: fever, diaphoresis, and precordial chest pain.

Collaborative Problems
A common collaborative goal in patients with cardiac trauma is to correct dysrhythmias.

Potential Complication: Dysrhythmias. Dysrhythmias related to myocardial contusion secondary to blunt cardiac trauma.

Expected Patient Outcomes. Patient maintains regular sinus rhythm once the source of trauma is corrected, HR ≤100 bpm, and BP within patient's normal range.

- Confer with trauma team physician regarding the expected dysrhythmia associated with myocardial contusion or penetrating cardiac injury.
- Review results of 12-lead ECG.
- Monitor continuous ECG for HR and rhythm. Document ECG rhythm strips every 2 to 4 hours in patients with sinus tachycardia, heart block, and ventricular dysrhythmias.
- Measure ECG components signifying cardiac contusion: ST changes, T wave changes, and prolonged QT interval suggestive of myocardial ischemia.
- Administer prescribed F_{IO_2} at 50% or oxygen 2 to 4 L/min by means of nasal cannula or mask.
- Administer prescribed IV fluids to maintain adequate hydration.
- Administer prescribed antidysrhythmia agents that accelerate repolarization, thereby shortening the action potential duration (lidocaine or tocainide) to manage automatic reentrant ventricular dysrhythmias. Be cautious, as these drugs might potentiate myocardial depression (see Table 1–11).
- Administer prescribed narcotic (morphine) to relieve pain caused by reduced myocardial oxygen supply or increased myocardial oxygen demand from dysrhythmia.
- Should pharmacological therapy be ineffective or patient develop heart block, prepare patient for temporary pacemaker (see Pacemakers, p. 270).

(For additional collaborative problem, see Acute cardiac tamponade: **Potential complication: Decreased Cardiac Output** related to intrapericardial pressure, p. 270).

DISCHARGE PLANNING
The critical care nurse provides patient and significant other(s) with verbal or written discharge notes regarding the following subjects:

1. Need to report any chest pain to physician.
2. Medication purpose, dosage, schedule, or side effects.

■ SHOCK

(For related information see Part I: Cardiogenic shock, p. 72; Cardiac tamponade, p. 117; Dysrhythmias, p. 184. Part II: Coronary artery bypass graft, p. 194. Part III: Cardiac assist device, p. 248; Intra-aortic balloon pump, p. 254; Hemodynamic monitoring, p. 219. See also Respiratory Deviations, Part I: Acute respiratory distress syndrome, p. 327. Renal Deviations, Part I: Acute renal failure, p. 459. Multisystem Deviations, Part I: Disseminated intravascular coagulation, p. 751; Sepsis, p. 772.)

Diagnostic Category and Length of Stay
DRG: 127 Heart failure and shock
LOS: 6.0 days

Definition
Shock is an acute clinical state of reduced tissue perfusion and inadequate effective circulating intravascular blood volume. At the cellular level there is nutritional insufficiency that occurs as a result of inadequate tissue perfusion. In shock there is a systemic imbalance between oxygen supply and oxygen demand.

Pathophysiology
In general, shock occurs when there is an inadequate cardiac output as a result of the heart's inability to pump effectively or when there is a decrease in the venous return to the heart resulting from decreased circulating blood volume or from peripheral vasodilation. Specifically there is poor perfusion, anaerobic metabolism, and release of mediators that damage tissue. The resulting vasoconstrictive response to shock and the subsequent increase in vascular permeability lead to the loss of intravascular volume. Cardiac function is compromised by reduced oxygen delivery together with an increased oxygen demand secondary to increased sympathetic tone and tachycardia. The three phases of shock are nonprogressive, progressive, and irreversible. In the *nonprogressive phase,* tissue perfusion is altered. Compensatory mechanisms are

stimulated to prevent tissue loss and restore homeostasis. The compensatory mechanisms consist of aldosterone secretion, sodium and water retention, increased blood pressure (BP), increased heart rate (HR), increased respiratory rate (RR), increased glycolysis, decreased urinary output (UO), decreased perfusion to internal organs, cool skin, and diaphoresis. In the *progressive phase* there is low blood flow, poor tissue perfusion, inadequate oxygen delivery, and increased end products of metabolic wastes. The *irreversible phase* occurs when there is decreased oxygen supply in proportion to oxygen demand, increased accumulation of metabolic wastes, increased progress of multisystem organ failure, and increased tissue damage.

Nursing Assessment

PRIMARY CAUSES

- Hypovolemic shock state: The fluid volume in the circulation has decreased as a result of loss of blood volume loss or intravascular fluid loss from the skin, loss of fluid from persistent vomiting or diarrhea, or loss of fluid from the intravascular compartment to interstitial spaces. The size of the intravascular compartment has increased in proportion to the fluid volume, which occurs with hemorrhage, diarrhea, fistula, dehydration, burns, third spacing, tubular damage, diabetes insipidus, spinal cord injury, severe allergic reaction, gram-positive bacteria, gram-negative bacteria, fungi, viruses, or acute pancreatitis.
- Distributive (Transport) shock state: There is a decreased supply of hemoglobin to carry oxygen to the tissues. Transport shock can occur with anemia, hemorrhage, or carbon monoxide poisoning.
- Obstructive shock state: This occurs as a result of a mechanical barrier to blood flow that blocks oxygen delivery to the tissues. It is associated with pulmonary thromboembolism, tension pneumothorax, aortic dissection, or pericardiac tamponade.
- Cardiogenic shock state: This clinical condition is produced when the right or left ventricle fails. Cardiogenic shock state includes left ventricular failure, acute mitral regurgitation, ventricular septal defect, and right ventricular infarction (see Cardiogenic shock, p. 72).

RISK FACTORS

- History of drug reactions, chronic disease, immune diseases, alcohol abuse, or malnutrition.

PHYSICAL ASSESSMENT

Hypovolemic Shock

- Inspection: Syncope, vertigo, restlessness, anxiety, flat neck veins, weakness, collapsed peripheral veins, altered levels of mental state, pale skin, thirst, and hypothermia.
- Palpation: Skin cool and clammy.
- Auscultation: Tachycardia, hypotension, and tachypnea.

Cardiogenic Shock

- Inspection: Restlessness, anxiety, agitation, apathy, lethargy, orthopnea, skin pale, thirst, nausea, or vomiting.
- Palpation: Skin cool and clammy, weak and thready pulse.
- Auscultation: Crackles, S_3, S_4, tachypnea, or tachycardia.

Septic Shock

- Inspection: Anxious, skin flushed, decreased level of consciousness, hyperthermia, or pale skin.
- Palpation: Skin warm and full bounding pulses.
- Auscultation: Tachycardia, tachypnea, crackles, and wheezes.

DIAGNOSTIC TEST RESULTS.

Hypovolemic Shock

Hemodynamic Parameters. (See Table 1–2)

- Cardiac index (CI) ≤ 2.0 L/min/m^2 (which is lower than normal of 2.7 L/min/m^2);

mixed venous oxygen saturation S̄v̄o₂ ≤60%; mean arterial pressure (MAP) ≤80 mm Hg; and reduced peripheral artery pressure (PAP), central venous pressure (CVP), and pulmonary capillary wedge pressure (PCWP).

Standard Laboratory Tests. (See Table 1–1)

- Serum chemistries: Lactate dehydrogenase (LDH) ≥2 mmol/L, elevated creatinine, and elevated blood urea nitrogen (BUN).
- Urinalysis: Low urine sodium ≤20 mEq/L.

Septic Shock

Hemodynamic Parameters. (See Table 1–9)

- CI ≤2.2 L/min/m², systemic vascular resistance (SVR) ≥1300 dynes/s/cm⁻⁵, PCWP ≥18 mm Hg, and pulse pressure narrowed in hypodynamic septic shock.

Standard Laboratory Tests. (See Table 1–1)

- Serum chemistries: Elevated serum LDH.
- Blood studies: Positive blood cultures and elevated white blood count (WBC).

Cardiogenic Shock

Hemodynamic Parameters. (See Table 1–9)

- CI ≤1.8L/min/m², PCWP ≥18 mm Hg, narrowed pulse pressure (PP), SVR ≥1200 dynes/s/cm⁻⁵, and CVP ≥15 mm Hg. Patient also experiences reduced stroke index, reduced left ventricular stroke work (LVSW), and reduced ejection fraction (EF).

Standard Laboratory Tests. (See Table 1–1)

- Serum chemistries: Elevated creatinine and BUN.
- Serum enzymes: Increased serum glutamic-oxaloacetic transaminase (SGOT), serum glutamate pyruvate transaminase (SGPT), LDH, and creatine kinase (CK).

MEDICAL AND SURGICAL MANAGEMENT

PHARMACOLOGY

- Vasopressors and inotropes: Dopamine increases cardiac contractility and dilates renal and mesenteric vessels to assist in improving blood flow to them despite the low cardiac output. Dobutamine enhances contractility and is used in managing cardiogenic and distributive shock. Isoproterenol enhances contractility and is useful in treating bradycardia and elevated pulmonary vascular resistance because it can lower resistance. A disadvantage of the drug is that it may create supraventricular and ventricular tachyarrhythmia or extension of myocardial infarction in cardiogenic shock. Amrinone inhibits the enzyme phosphodiesterase, thereby enhancing the availability of adenosine monophosphate (AMP) and subsequently contractility (see Table 1–10).
- Vasodilators: Vasodilators dilate veins and arterioles. Dilatation of veins and venules leads to an increase in venous capacitance, decrease in preload, and decrease in pulmonary congestion. Dilating the arterioles lowers SVR, which decreases impedance to left ventricular ejection. The overall goal is to reduce myocardial oxygen consumption. Vasodilators are not always used in hypovolemic shock but can be used to decrease SVR (afterload) and preload. They are useful in cardiogenic and septic shock (see Table 1–4).
- Antidysrhythmia agents: Used to treat bradycardia, atrial fibrillation, flutter, tachycardia, and ventricular tachycardia (see Table 1–11).
- Corticosteroids: Used to reduce cellular permeability, interfere with leukocyte degranulation, and prostaglandin (see Table 1–15, p. 129).
- Diuretics: Diuretics such as furosemide, bumetadine, or ethacrynic acid are useful in maintaining patency of the renal tubules, reducing preload, and diminishing pulmonary congestion. Mannitol can be used in the pressure of normovolemia and ade-

quate left ventricular function (see Table 1–13).

- Naloxone (Narcan): This is a controversial drug in the treatment of shock. The drug is believed to reverse the hypotension in hypovolemic, endotoxemic, and spinal shock resulting from endorphins and other endogenous products.
- Diphenhydramine (Benadryl): Can be used in patient with hyperdynamic septic shock; can block histamine release.
- Antibiotics: Used in septic shock when the infectious organisms are identified.
- Heparin: Low-dose heparin may be necessary should disseminated intravascular coagulation occur in septic shock, deep venous thrombosis, pulmonary embolism, or other arterial thrombus (see Table 1–8)

FLUID THERAPY

- Crystalloids: Crystalloids are used to expand both the intravascular and interstitial components: crystalloid solution consisting of 0.9% normal saline to increase intravascular volume when extracellular fluid volume expansion is desired; lactated Ringer's solution to provide volume replacement and to buffer acidosis in treating hypovolemic shock; and dextrose in water (D_5W) to increase fluid volume in hypovolemic shock or severe dehydration.
- Colloids: Colloids determine the oncotic or colloidal osmotic pressure that maintains the balance of water between the interstitial space and the intravascular space. Colloid solutions include albumin 5% to 25% to increase the plasma colloid osmotic pressure and plasma volume; hetastarch to increase BP, cardiac output, and tissue perfusion; and dextran to rapidly expand volume.
- Blood and blood products: Whole blood is used in hemorrhagic hypovolemic shock when hemoglobin is ≤12 g/100 mL and hematocrit is ≤30%. Packed red cells are used as replacement agents when the hematocrit is ≤30% and the red cell mass needs to be increased to improve the oxygen-carrying capacity of the blood. Fresh frozen plasma is used when partial thromboplastin time (PTT) as a measure of intrinsic pathway and prothrombin time (PT) as a measure of extrinsic pathway are abnormal. Cryoprecipitate is administered to control coagulopathies.

PNEUMATIC ANTISHOCK GARMENT (PASG)

- The device is used to increase arterial pressure by compressing vascular beds by means of the inflatable layers, thereby increasing SVR and compression also redistributing blood flow from the peripheral circulation, making it available for the perfusion of vital organs.

OXYGEN THERAPY

- Supplemental oxygen through intubation or ventilatory support may be required should oxygenation status deteriorate (see Respiratory Deviations, Mechanical ventilation, p. 428).

HEMODYNAMIC MONITORING

- Hemodynamic monitoring allows repeated measurement of cardiac output and vascular resistance as a guide to fluid management. It also permits measurement of oxygen supply and oxygen demand by means of $S\bar{v}O_2$.

INTRA-AORTIC BALLOON PUMP (IABP)

- Inflation allows blood to be pumped retrograde into the aortic root. The result is increased coronary artery blood supply and oxygenation. Deflation of the balloon before systolic ejection creates as negative intra-aortic pressure and decreases afterload. The IABP is used in patients with cardiogenic and septic shock (see IABP, p. 254).

CARDIAC ASSIST DEVICE

- The device bypasses the ventricle and requires no ventricular contraction. It is used on patients with end-stage cardiac disease who are awaiting transplantation. (see cardiac assist device, p. 248).

NURSING MANAGEMENT: NURSING DIAGNOSES AND COLLABORATIVE PROBLEMS

Nursing Diagnoses

Common nursing goals in patients with shock are to promote oxygenation, restore tissue perfusion, maintain adequate fluid volume, promote effective thermoregulation, encourage appropriate cognitive function, and reduce anxiety.

Impaired gas exchange related to intraalveolar congestion secondary to left ventricular dysfunction or increased pulmonary vascular resistance.

Expected Patient Outcomes.

Patient will maintain adequate gas exchange, as evidenced by arterial oxygen pressure (Pao_2) ≥80 mm Hg, arterial carbon dioxide pressure ($Paco_2$) 35 to 45 mm Hg, $S\bar{v}o_2$ 60% to 80%, arterial oxygen saturation (Sao_2) ≥95%, RR 12 to 20 BPM, HR ≤100 bpm, absence of cyanosis, resolution of crackles, absence of restlessness, capillary refill ≤3 seconds, hemoglobin 12 to 16.5 g/100mL, hematocrit 38% to 54%, and arterial-venous oxygen content difference ($C[a - v]o_2$) 4 to 6 mL/100mL.

- Consult with trauma physician to validate expected patient outcomes used to determine whether or not gas exchange is sufficient.
- Consult with physician and respiratory therapist about the need to adjust the ventilation for the best positive end-expiratory pressure (PEEP). This is the pressure that achieves the best Sao_2 without decreasing the $S\bar{v}o_2$.
- Consult with physician about criteria used to determine if mechanical ventilation is necessary: minute ventilation ≤6 to 8 L/min or ≥15 L/min, vital capacity ≤10 to 12 mL/kg, $Paco_2$ ≥45 mm Hg in metabolic acidosis or ≥50 to 55 mm Hg with normal bicarbonate, Pao_2 ≤60 mm Hg on 40% oxygen or Pao_2 ≤200 mm Hg on 100% oxygen, RR ≥35 BPM, and increased ventilatory effort.

- Review results of chest roentgenogram, arterial blood gas, hemoglobin, and hematocrit measurement.
- Limit physical activity to bed rest and semi-Fowler's (20 to 30 degree) position, if not contraindicated, to decrease oxygen consumption and enhance lung expansion by allowing the diaphragm to fall and the chest to expand.
- Continuously monitor oxygen status with pulse oximetry (Spo_2) and pulmonary artery systolic pressure.
- Obtain and report findings reflective of impaired gas exchange: tachypnea, dyspnea, crackles, confusion, restlessness, irritability, Pao_2 ≤80 mm Hg, PAP systolic ≥25 mm Hg or diastolic ≥15 mm Hg, PCWP ≥12 mm Hg, $S\bar{v}o_2$ ≤60%, and Sao_2 ≤95%.
- Auscultate lungs every 1 to 2 hours for the presence of crackles, rhonchi, or wheezes.
- Perform orotracheal or endotracheal suction following hospital standards to remove excess secretions. Suction for no longer than 15 seconds so as not to reduce oxygen supply.
- Obtain Sao_2 and $S\bar{v}o_2$ before suctioning to assess oxygen supply and demand status.
- Using unit protocol, hyperoxygenate (100%) or hyperinflate (with several breaths with the tidal volume setting on the ventilator or ambu bag) before and after suctioning to protect patient from suction-induced hypoxemia or increased oxygen demand as a result of agitation or coughing.
- Monitor for dysrhythmias or changes in BP that may signify $S\bar{v}o_2$ ≤40% resulting from suctioning.
- Monitor $S\bar{v}o_2$ during weaning, since a decrease in $S\bar{v}o_2$ can indicate a deterioration in Sao_2 and Pao_2 or an increase in the work of breathing from increased carbon dioxide.
- Continuously monitor $S\bar{v}o_2$ and ventilation after a position change or any change in ventilator settings or oxygen administration.
- Obtain and document indicators of improved oxygen delivery: CI 4 to 4.5 L/min/m², UO ≥30 mL/h, HR ≤120 bpm, and MAP ≥80 mm Hg.

- Minimize oxygen demand by decreasing anxiety, fever, shivering, and pain.
- Position patient to maintain airway patency, chest excursion and comfort.
- Encourage patient to deep breathe and cough q 1 to 2 h.
- Provide prescribed FIO_2 at 50% or oxygen 2 to 4 L/min by means of mask or nasal cannula to maintain PaO_2 ≥80 mm Hg, $S\bar{v}O_2$ ≥60% and SaO_2 ≥95%.
- Administer prescribed IV fluids such as whole blood, packed red cells, crystalloids or colloids to maintain adequate circulating volume.
- Administer neuromuscular blocking agent, pavulon, to decrease oxygen consumption of voluntary muscles while patient is receiving mechanical ventilatory support.
- Administer prescribed volume reducing agents such as furosemide or bumetanide to maintain UO ≥30 mL/hr or ≥0.5 mL/kg/hr and specific gravity 1.010 to 1.030 (See Table 1–10, p. 50).
- Administer prescribed analgesics to maintain RR ≤20 BPM, HR ≤100 bpm, BP within patient's normal limits and reduce chest pain.
- Instruct the patient to report the presence of pain.
- Instruct the patient on the use of alternative pain relief measures: Relaxation, repositioning, guided imagery and distraction.

Altered tissue perfusion related to abnormal distribution of intravascular blood volume secondary to massive vasodilation as a result of infection or septicemia.

Expected Patient Outcomes. Patient maintains adequate tissue perfusion, as evidenced by BP ≥90 mm Hg; HR ≤100 bpm; RR ≤24 BPM; $C(a - v)O_2$ 4 to 6 mL/min; coronary artery perfusion pressure (CAPP) 60 to 80 mm Hg, cardiac output (CO) 4 to 8 L/min; CI 2.7 to 4.3 L/min/m^2; CVP 4 to 6 mm Hg; MAP 70 to 90 mm Hg; normal sinus rhythm; absence of neck vein distention; PCWP 6 to 12 mm Hg; pulmonary vascular resistance (PVR) 155 to 255 dynes/s/cm^{-5}; pulmonary vascular resistance index (PVRI) 200 to 450 dynes/s/cm^{-5}/m^2; $S\bar{v}O_2$ 60% to 80%; SVR 900 to 1200 dynes/s/cm^{-5}; systemic vascular resistance index (SVRI) 1970 to 2390 dynes/s/cm^{-5}/m^2; skin warm and dry; good skin turgor; peripheral pulses ≤+2; capillary refill ≤3 seconds; equal and normoreactive pupils; oriented to person, place, and time; normal sensorimotor function; PaO_2 80 to 100 mm Hg; $PaCO_2$ 35 to 45 mm Hg; SaO_2 ≥95%; $S\bar{v}O_2$ ≥60%; oxygen consumption index (VO_2I) ≥115 mL/min/m^2; oxygen extraction ratio (O_2ER) 25%; or oxygen delivery index (DO_2I) ≥500 mL/min/m^2; absence of crackles; UO ≥30 mL/h; and specific gravity 1.010 to 1.030.

- Consult with physician to validate patient's expected outcomes used to determine whether tissue perfusion is adequate.
- Review results of blood cultures, WBC, hemoglobin, and hematocrit.
- Obtain and report clinical findings indicating hyperdynamic stage of sepsis: reduced SVR ≤900 dynes/s/cm^{-5}, SVRI ≤1970 dynes/s/cm^{-5}/m^2, CO ≥4 L/min, systolic BP ≤90 mm Hg, warm and flushed skin, and hyperthermia.
- Obtain and report clinical findings indicating hypodynamic stage of sepsis: SVR ≥1200 dynes/s/cm^{-5}, SVRI ≥2390 dynes/s/cm^{-5}/m^2, CO ≤4 L/min, CI ≤2.7 L/min/m^2, hypotension, cool and clammy skin, and hypothermia.
- Calculate and report DO_2I ≤500 mL/min/m^2, VO_2I ≤115 mL/min/m^2, and O_2ER ≥35% suggesting inadequate oxygen delivery and increased oxygen demand.
- Continuously monitor $S\bar{v}O_2$, SaO_2, hemoglobin, and CO as indications of oxygen supply and oxygen demand.
- Calculate and report $C(a - v)O_2$ ≥6 mL/100 mL, which can indicate increased oxygen uptake at the tissue level and reduced CO.
- Initiate continuous ECG monitoring to assess HR and rhythm. Document ECG

rhythm strips every 2 to 4 hours in patients with dysrhythmias.

- Administer prescribed oxygen 2 to 4 L/min or FIO_2 ≤50% to enhance oxygen supply.
- Administer prescribed IV fluids such as colloids or crystalloids to maintain adequate preload (PCWP 6 to 12 mm Hg).
- Administer prescribed vasodilators (nitroprusside or nitroglycerin) as an adjunct agent in decreasing increased SVR and preload (see Table 1–4).
- Administer prescribed corticosteroids in the early stages of septic shock (see Table 1–15).
- Administer prescribed broad-spectrum antibiotic therapy to correct infection (see Table 1–14).
- Administer prescribed antidysrhythmia agents to correct dysrhythmias associated with acidosis or hypoxemia.

Fluid volume deficit related to increase vasodilation secondary to abnormal distribution of intravascular volume.

Expected Patient Outcomes. Patient maintains adequate fluid volume, as evidenced by balanced intake and output, body weight within 5% of baseline, CO ≥4 L/min, CI ≥2.7 L/min/m², CVP 2 to 6 mm Hg, PCWP 6 to 12 mm Hg, right atrial pressure (RAP) 4 to 6 mm Hg, HR ≤100 bpm, MAP 70 to 100 mm Hg, UO ≥30 mL/h, normal skin turgor, peripheral pulses +2, capillary refill ≤3 seconds, BP within patient's normal range, electrolytes and hematocrit within normal limits.

- Consult with physician to validate expected patient outcomes used to determine whether fluid volume is adequate.
- Review electrolytes and hematocrit.
- Position patient with head of bed elevated 20 to 30 degrees to facilitate breathing and comfort.
- Place hypovolemic patient, in Trendelenburg position, if not contraindicated, until volume replacement has been achieved.
- Obtain and report hemodynamic parameters associated with fluid volume deficit: CO ≤4 L/min, CI ≤2.7 L/min/m², CVP ≤2 mm Hg, PCWP ≤6 mm Hg, and RAP ≤4 mm Hg.
- Obtain and report other clinical indicators of fluid volume deficit: hypotension, poor skin turgor, tachycardia, peripheral pulses ≤+2, and capillary refill ≥3 seconds.
- Monitor and record intake, hourly urinary output, nasogastric output, and specific gravity. Report UO ≤30 mL/h.
- Administer prescribed IV fluids to restore or maintain tissue perfusion and adequate hydration.

Ineffective thermoregulation related to infecting pathogens.

Expected Patient Outcomes. Patient maintains effective thermoregulation, as evidenced by temperature 36.5°C to 38°C, absence of shivering, and absence of diaphoresis.

- Review results of blood or wound cultures and WBC.
- Continuously monitor and report core temperature: ≥38.5°C (101°F) suggesting sepsis or 33.6°C (96°F) suggesting hypovolemic shock.
- Obtain and report other clinical findings associated with infection: shivering, chills, or diaphoresis.
- Measure the temperature gradient between the ventral surface of the great toe and ambient room temperature. Patient with toe minus ambient room temperature gradient ≥4°C has a higher probability of surviving shock than patient with a gradient ≤3°C for 12 hours.
- Apply tepid sponge bath or a cooling blanket, as indicated, during hyperthermia episode.
- Administer prescribed antipyretic agents to reduce temperature.
- Administer prescribed antibiotics to eliminate infection.

Anxiety related to hemorrhage or potential loss resulting from injury.

Expected Patient Outcome. Patient exhibits a decrease in anxiety by verbalizing needs and fears.

- Provide a calm and reassuring environment.
- Encourage patient to describe his or her own anxiety and coping pattern.
- Remove excess stimulation that can make patient anxious, thereby increasing oxygen demand.
- Explain the purpose behind invasive procedures and treatment.
- Observe for the signs and symptoms of anxiety: restlessness, agitation, diaphoresis, tachycardia, tachypnea, palpitations, and verbalization of fears.
- Provide patient with positive feedback of reinforcement to enhance feelings of self-confidence.
- Involve patient in decision making, regarding care when appropriate.
- Teach patient to use alternative anxiety-reducing measures: progressive relaxation, repositioning, guided imagery, and distraction.

Collaborative Problems

Common collaborative goals in patients with shock are to correct hypovolemia, increase cardiac output and reduce abnormal distribution of intravascular volume.

Potential Complication: Hypovolemic Shock. Hypovolemic shock related to insufficient blood volume to fill the intravascular space secondary to penetrating injuries.

Expected Patient Outcomes. Patient maintains normal fluid volume, as evidenced by BP within normal range, CO 4 to 8 L/min, CI 2.7 to 4.3 L/min/m², CVP 2 to 6 mm Hg, MAP 70 to 90 mm Hg, PAP systolic 15 to 25 mm Hg and PAP diastolic 8 to 15 mm Hg, PCWP 4 to 12 mm Hg, RAP 4 to 6 mm Hg, stroke volume (SV) 60 to 130 mL/beat, PP 30 to 40 mm Hg, $S\bar{v}O_2$ ≥60%, SaO_2 ≥90%, HR ≤100 bpm, UO ≥0.5 mL/kg/h, skin turgor good, capillary refill ≤3 seconds, peripheral pulses +2, and skin warm and dry.

- Consult with physician to validate expected patient outcomes that determine whether circulating intravascular volume is sufficient.

- Consult with cardiologist regarding the desired type and amount of fluid replacement.
- Review the results of CBC, serum electrolyte levels, arterial blood gas measurements, urinalysis, ECG, and chest roentgenogram.
- Monitor the amount and type of fluid loss such as blood loss, profuse vomiting, or diarrhea.
- Monitor fluid intake and output: emesis, diarrhea, or urinary (≥0.5 mL/kg/h).
- Obtain and report hemodynamic parameters suggestive of decreased intravascular fluid volume: CVP ≤2 mm Hg, CO ≤4 L/min, CI 2.7 L/min/m², PCWP ≤6 mm Hg, PAP systolic ≤15 mm Hg and diastolic ≤8 mm Hg, PP ≤30 mm Hg, SVR ≥1200 dynes/s/cm⁻⁵ and $S\bar{v}O_2$ ≤60%.
- Obtain and report signs and symptoms of minimal fluid volume loss: slight tachycardia; normal supine BP; positive postural vital signs (systolic BP decrease ≥ 10 mm Hg or pulse increase ≥20 bpm); capillary refill time ≥3 seconds; UO ≥30 mL/h; cool, pale skin or arms and legs; and anxious mental status.
- Obtain and report signs and symptoms of moderate fluid volume loss: rapid, thready pulse; supine hypotension; cool truncal skin; UO 10 to 30 mL/h; severe thirst; and restlessness, confusion, or irritability.
- Obtain and report signs and symptoms of severe volume loss: marked tachycardia; hypotension; weak or absent peripheral pulses; cold, mottled or cyanotic skin; UO ≤10 mL/h; and unconsciousness.
- Apply direct and continuous pressure to active external bleeding sites.
- Continuously monitor $S\bar{v}O_2$, SaO_2, hemoglobin, and CO. Hemorrhage causes an acute loss of hemoglobin, which threatens oxygen supply. An $S\bar{v}O_2$ ≤60% can be an indicator of an acute decrease in oxygen supply resulting from occult bleeding.
- Monitor patient's fluid intake and output: emesis, nasogastric tube drainage, diarrhea, or urinary (≥5 mL/kg/h).
- Continuously monitor ECG to assess HR and rhythm. Document ECG rhythm strips

every hour until hypovolemic shock is corrected.

- Administer prescribed oxygen by mask or intubation to maintain adequate oxygenation.
- Administer IV fluids as prescribed: isotones such as saline (0.9% NaCl in water), Ringer's solution and lactated Ringer's solution, hypotonic fluids such as 0.45% NaCl or water, D_5W water; or hypertonic fluid such as mannitol, hypertonic saline (3% and 5% NaCl in water), and 50% dextrose to maintain BP within patient's normal range, MAP 70 to 90 mm Hg, UO ≥30 mL/h, and adequate hydration.
- Administer blood or blood products as prescribed: whole blood to restore the hemoglobin to a minimum level of 12.5 to 14 g/100 and to maintain the hematocrit above 30% packed red blood cells to improve the oxygen-carrying capacity of the blood; fresh frozen plasma to provide plasma proteins and clotting factors; plasma protein fraction to provide albumin, alpha and beta globulins, and sodium chloride; albumin to expand the plasma volume (5% albumin equals 50 g of albumin per liter or 25% solution contains 250 g of albumin per liter) to maintain CO 4 to 8 L/min and CI ≥2.7 to 4.3 L/min/m².
- Administer plasma expanders as prescribed: hetastarch to expand plasma volume, dextran used to draw water into the vascular compartment, and mannitol to raise intravascular volume, to reduce interstitial and intracellular edema, and to promote osmotic diuresis of UO ≥30 mL/h.
- Administer crystalloids as prescribed: normal saline or 0.5% NaCl in water to replace body fluid, Ringer's solution as 0.9% NaCl in water to replace body fluid loss, lactated Ringer's solution, one-half normal saline used to increase the plasma volume and decrease blood viscosity; or D_5W.
- Assist with use of PASG to redistribute blood flow for the peripheral circulation to perfuse vital organs.
- Assist with the insertion of chest tube should a penetrating chest trauma con-

tribute to hypovolemic shock (See Respiratory Deviations Chest drainage, p. 434).

Potential Complication: Decreased Cardiac Output.

Decreased CO related to decreased preload or contractility secondary to reduced intravascular fluid volume or myocardial damage.

Expected Patient Outcomes. Patient will maintain adequate CO, as evidenced by BP within normal range, CO 4 to 8 L/min, CI 2.7 to 4.3 L/min/m², CVP 2 to 6 mm Hg, MAP 70 to 90 mm Hg, PAP systolic 15 to 25 mm Hg and PAP diastolic 8 to 15 mm Hg, PCWP 4 to 12 mm Hg, $S\bar{v}o_2$ ≥60%, Sao_2 ≥90%, HR ≤100 bpm, UO ≥0.5 mL/kg/h, BP within normal limits, PCWP ≤24 mm Hg, SVR 900 to 1200 dynes/s/cm⁻⁵, absence of dysrhythmias, peripheral pulses +2, capillary refill ≤3 seconds, and skin warm and dry.

- Consult with physician to validate expected patient outcomes used to evaluate whether CO is sufficient.
- Limit physical activity to bed rest to reduce oxygen demand.
- Obtain and report hemodynamic parameters that suggest decreased preload as a result of reduced intravascular fluid volume or decreased contractility resulting from myocardial damage: CO ≤4 L/min, CI ≤2.7 L/min/m², PCWP ≥18 mm Hg, SVR ≥1200 dynes/s/cm⁻⁵, and $S\bar{v}o_2$ ≤60%.
- Obtain and report other clinical findings associated with decreased CO: HR ≥100 bpm, hypotension, skin cool and clammy, peripheral pulses ≤ +2, MAP ≤70 mm Hg, capillary refill ≥3 seconds, and dysrhythmias.
- Monitor intake, output, specific gravity, and daily weight to determine hydration status. Report UO ≤30 mL/h.
- Continuously monitor Sao_2, hemoglobin, and CO in relation to $S\bar{v}o_2$ to determine whether an imbalance exists between oxygen supply and oxygen demand.
- Administer prescribed IV fluids to maintain adequate circulating volume.

- Administer prescribed oxygen via mask to maintain adequate oxygen delivery.
- Should oxygenation be ineffective, prepare patient for intubation and mechanical ventilatory support to maintain arterial blood gases within normal range.
- Administer prescribed inotropes (dobutamine, dopamine, or amrinone) to maintain CO $\geq$4 L/min and CI $\geq$2.7 L/min/m^2.

Potential Complication: Distributive Shock. Distributive shock related to the abnormal distribution of intravascular volume secondary to massive vasodilation caused by microorganisms and their by-products (sepsis), loss of vasomotor tone (neurogenic), or vasodilation and increased capillary permeability with loss of fluid into the interstitial space caused by antigen-antibody reaction (anaphylaxis).

Expected Patient Outcomes. Patient maintains adequate distributive volume, as evidenced by CO 4 to 8 L/min; CI 2.7 to 4.3 L/min/m^2; CVP 2 to 4 mm Hg; PP 30 to 30 mm Hg; SVR 900 to 1200 dynes/s/cm^{-5}; SVRI 1970 to 2390 dynes/s/cm^{-5}/m^2; BP $\geq$ 90/60 mm Hg; HR $\geq$60 bpm; RR $\leq$20 BPM; UO $\geq$30 mL/h or $\geq$0.5 mL/kg/h; absence of adventitious breath sounds; absence of edema; HR $\leq$100 bpm; normal sinus rhythm; resolution of pitting edema; resolution of laryngeal edema, bronchospasm, wheezes, or respiratory distress; peripheral pulses +2; temperature within normal range; skin warm and dry; capillary refill $\leq$3 seconds, Pao$_2$ $\geq$80 mm Hg, Paco$_2$ 35 to 45 mm Hg, or Sao$_2$ $\geq$95%.

- Consult with physician to validate expected patient outcomes used to determine whether the distribution of intravascular volume is sufficient.
- Review the results of urinalysis, CBC, and ECG.
- Limit physical activity to bed rest until patient's sympathetic innervation is stable or patient adjusts to the changes in vasomotor tone.

- Obtain and report hemodynamic parameters reflecting neurogenic shock: BP $\leq$90/60 mm Hg, CO $\leq$4 L/min, CI $\leq$2.7 L/min/m^2, CVP $\leq$2 mm Hg, SVR $\leq$900 dynes/s/cm^{-5}, SVRI $\leq$1970 dynes/s/cm^{-5}/m^2, pulse pressure $\leq$30 mm Hg, peripheral pulses $\leq$+2, or capillary refill $\geq$3 seconds.
- Elevate the lower extremities to decrease venous pooling, increase venous return, increase CO, and increase tissue perfusion.
- Apply antiembolic stockings to decrease venous pooling, increase venous return, and decrease venous stasis.
- Monitor HR since bradycardia, characteristic of spinal shock, occurs as a result to unopposed parasympathetic innervation to the heart by means of the vagus nerve.
- Monitor patient's extremities for the presence of signs vasodilation, which include warmth, dry skin, and decreased body temperature.
- Obtain and report findings reflecting decreased intravascular fluid volume secondary to anaphylactic shock: stridor, wheezing, RR $\geq$20 BPM, HR $\geq$100 bpm, BP $\leq$90/60 mm Hg, seizure, disorientation, confusion, nausea, vomiting, anxiety, abdominal pain, and warm and moist skin.
- Place patient in an upright position to allow for chest wall expansion, diaphragmatic excursion, and use of accessory muscles.
- Assess BP and HR, since increased BP and decreased HR can be indicative of adequate circulating volume and CO.
- Implement measures to relieve itching (urticaria) and maintain skin integrity by applying cold compresses to the affected area and instructing patient to avoid scratching.
- Obtain and report findings indicative of hyperdynamic (warm) septic shock: CO normal to increased; SVR $\leq$900 dynes/s/cm^{-5}; MAP $\leq$60 mm Hg; HR $\geq$100 bpm; RR $\geq$20 BPM; UO $\leq$30 mL/h or $\leq$0.5 mL/kg/h; hyperthermia; chills; warm, flushed skin; confusion; restlessness; disorientation; crackles; Pao$_2$ $\leq$80 mm Hg and Sao$_2$ $\leq$95%.
- Monitor and report findings reflective of hypodynamic (cold) septic shock: CO

≤ 4 L/min; CI ≤ 2.7 L/min/m^2; SVR ≥ 1200 dynes/s/cm^{-5}, SVRI ≥ 2390 dynes/s/cm^{-5}/m^2, BP $\leq 90/60$ mm Hg; HR ≥ 100 bpm; peripheral pulses $\leq +2$; skin cold, clammy, and pale; and hypothermia.

- Monitor all catheter sites or wounds for redness, tenderness, drainage or swelling.
- Administer prescribed oxygen 2 to 4 L/min by means of nasal cannula or mask to maintain Pao$_2$ ≥ 80 mm Hg and Sao$_2$ $\geq 95\%$.
- Administer prescribed IV fluids of lactated Ringer's to maintain BP $\geq 90/60$ mm Hg, MAP 70 to 90 mm Hg, UO ≥ 30 mL/h or ≥ 0.5 mL/kg/h, and specific gravity 1.010 to 1.030.
- Adminster prescribed positive inotropes and vasopressors such as dopamine or dobutamine to maintain MAP 70 to 90 mm Hg, SVR ≥ 900 dynes/s/cm^{-5} and SVRI ≥ 1970 dynes/s/cm^{-5}/m^2 (see Table 1–10).
- Administer prescribed subcutaneous injection of epinephrine to control bronchospasm and improve ventilation.
- Administer corticosteroids such as prednisone during the early phase of shock to stabilize lysosomal membrane (see Table 1–15).
- Administer prescribed antibiotics determined by cultures of drainage from lungs, urinary tract, or catheters (see Table 1–14).
- Instruct patient to avoid exposure to allergies that trigger the onset of allergic reaction.

DISCHARGE PLANNING

The critical care nurse provides patient and significant other(s) with verbal or written discharge notes regarding the following subjects:

- Discussion of medications, purpose, dosage, schedule and side effects.
- Importance of reporting signs and symptoms of heart failure, associated with cardiogenic shock, to physician: increased fatigue, dyspnea and activity intolerance.
- Importance of ongoing follow-up care and keeping appointments.

■ DYSRHYTHMIAS

(For related information see Part III: Automatic implantable cardioverter-defibrillator, p. 260; Hemodynamic monitoring, p. 219; Pacemakers, p. 270; and ST segment monitoring, p. 264).

Diagnostic Categories and Length of Stay

DRG: 138 Cardiac arrhythmia and conduction disorders with complications
LOS: 4.50 days
DRG: 139 Cardiac arrhythmia and conduction disorders without complications
LOS: 3.10 days

Definition

Cardiac dysrhythmias are abnormal rhythms of the heart's electrical system. They result from either abnormal impulse initiation, abnormal impulse conduction, or both mechanisms operating together. Dysrhythmias can originate in any part of the conduction system: sinus node, atria, atrioventricular (AV) node, bundle branches, and ventricles.

Pathophysiology

Cardiac dysrhythmias result from abnormal impulse initiation, abnormal impulse conduction, or both mechanisms operating together. Abnormal impulse initiation occurs because of a change in the flow of ions across the cardiac cell membrane, which causes either abnormal automaticity or triggered activity. Impulse initiation can be shifted from the sinus node to other parts of the heart if the rate of the sinoatrial (SA) node falls below a subsidiary pacemaker or if the rate of a subsidiary pacemaker exceeds the SA node (atrial or ventricular myocardial cells). Factors that allow a subsidiary pacemaker to assume control of the heart include increased vagal influences, drugs, or disease of the sinus node.

Abnormal impulse conduction can lead to block or reentry. *Decremental conduction* refers to the progressive decrease in conduction velocity of an impulse as it travels through a region of the myocardium. The failure of conduction can occur in the sinus node, causing sinus exit block; in the AV node causing AV blocks; or in the bundle branches, causing bundle branch block. *Reentry* means that an impulse can travel through an area of myocardium, depolarize it, and then reenter that same area to depolarize it again. Reentry occurs as a result of an area of slow conduction and an area of undirectional block.

Abnormal repolarization that is prolonged can cause ventricular dysrhythmias and risk of sudden death. Prolonged ventricular repolarization leads to disproportionately prolonged refractory periods in some regions of the ventricles, whereas other regions repolarize earlier. Disparity in refractoriness within the ventricles leads to areas of slow conduction and unidirectional block, causing reentry and possible sustained ventricular activity.

Nursing Assessment

PRIMARY CAUSES

Sinus Node Dysrhythmias

- Sinus bradycardia: Can be a response to vagal stimulation from carotid sinus massage, ocular pressure, or vomiting. Diseases that may cause sinus bradycardia include inferior wall myocardial infarction, uremia, myxedema, hypothyroidism, hyperkalemia, increased intracranial pressure, glaucoma, or obstructive jaundice. Drugs causing sinus bradycardia are methyldopa, reserpine, digitalis, beta blockers, and calcium channel blockers.
- Sinus tachycardia: Underlying clinical situations causing sinus tachycardia include fever, blood loss, congestive heart failure, shock, acute rheumatic fever, pulmonary embolism, acute myocardial infarction (AMI), hyperthyroidism, or anemia. Sinus tachycardia can be a compensatory response to decreased cardiac output. Drugs contributing to sinus tachycardia include atropine, isoproterenol, epinephrine, dopamine, dobu-

tamine, norepinephrine, or nitroprusside. Other causes include emotional stress, exercise, fever, and pain.
- Sinus arrhythmia: Sinus arrhythmia can occur as a normal response associated with phases of respiration or increased intracranial pressure. Drugs contributing to sinus arrhythmia include digitalis and morphine.
- Sinus arrest: Sinus arrest is due to vagal stimulation, carotid sinus sensitivity and interrupted blood flow to sinus node as a result of AMI, carotid stimulation of the patient with digitalis intoxication, acute myocarditis, coronary artery disease, and acute infection. Drugs causing sinus arrest include digitalis, beta blockers, and calcium channel blockers.

Atrial Dysrhythmias

- Premature atrial contraction (PAC): PAC can be caused by excess alcohol, caffeine, nicotine, congestive heart failure, pulmonary disease, AMI, atrial dilatation or hypertrophy resulting from mitral stenosis, hypoxia, digitalis toxicity, or anxiety. Also related to emotional stress are fatigue and heart disease.
- Wandering atrial pacemaker (WAP): WAP can be caused by increased vagal stimulation slowing the sinus pacemaker or enhancing the atrial or junctional pacemaker cells.
- Atrial tachycardia: This can occur in healthy individuals and in those with heart disease. Other causes include rheumatic heart disease, coronary heart disease, AMI, or digitalis intoxicity.
- Multifocal atrial tachycardia: The rhythm disturbance occurs in acutely ill elderly patients with acute and chronic lung disease, hypertension, or valvular heart disease.
- Atrial flutter: Causes of atrial flutter include rheumatic heart disease, mitral stenosis, hypertensive heart disease, pericarditis, cardiomyopathy, acute or chronic cor pulmonale, atherosclerotic heart disease, thyrotoxicosis, congestive heart failure, and AMI.

• Atrial fibrillation: Atrial fibrillation is seen in patients with atherosclerotic or rheumatic heart disease, mitral disease, hypertensive heart disease, congestive heart failure, pulmonary disease, AMI, and following coronary artery bypass surgery. Less common causes include cardiomyopathy, acute myocarditis, acute pericarditis, or chest trauma.

AV Junctional Dysrhythmias

• Premature junctional contraction (PJC): PJC can be caused by coronary artery disease, rheumatic fever, inferior wall AMI, caffeine, anxiety, or digitalis.
• Paroxysmal AV junctional tachycardia: Can be caused by inferior wall myocardial infarction, coronary artery disease, hypertension, rheumatic heart disease, hyperthyroidism, or digitalis toxicity.
• AV junctional dysrhythmias: Common causes are digitalis intoxication, AMI, intracardiac surgery, or myocarditis.
• Atrial fusion complexes: Causes are those of the atrial ectopic beat or rhythm.
• Atrial parasystole: A common cause is myocardial infarction.

Atrial Ventricular Conduction (Block) Dysrhythmias

• First degree AV block: First degree AV block is caused by coronary artery disease, rheumatic heart disease, or drugs such as digitalis, beta blockers, and calcium channel blockers.
• Mobitz type I second degree AV block, or Wenckebach: Causes of this block include inferior wall myocardial infarction, coronary artery disease, aortic valve disease, mitral valve prolapse, or atrial septal defects. Drugs contributing to type I second degree AV block are digitalis, beta blockers, and calcium channel blockers.
• Mobitz type II second degree AV block: This block occurs in rheumatic heart disease, coronary artery disease, and acute anterior wall MI.
• Third degree AV block (complete block): Third degree AV block is due to coronary

artery disease, AMI, open heart surgery, and digitalis toxicity.

Ventricular Dysrhythmias

• Premature ventricular contraction (PVC): PVCs are caused by hypoxia, myocardial ischemia, AMI, hypokalemia, acidosis, digitalis, caffeine, heavy smoking, and emotional stress. Drugs include epinephrine, isoproterenol, or aminophylline.
• Ventricular tachycardia (VT): Caused by hypoxia, myocardial ischemia, AMI, hypertension, rheumatic heart disease, cardiomyopathy, congestive heart failure (CHF), mitral valve prolapse hypokalemia, acidosis, and digitalis toxicity.
• Ventricular flutter: Can be caused by AMI; myocardial ischemia; frequent, paired, or multifocal PVCs in the setting of AMI.
• Ventricular fibrillation: Caused by severe heart disease, AMI, or digitalis toxicity.
• Accelerated idioventricular rhythm: Can occur in patients with acute inferior or anterior myocardial infarction, hypertension, rheumatic heart disease, or congenital heart disease.
• Ventricular fusion complex: The cause is that of the ventricular ectopic beat of rhythm.

AV Conduction Dysrhythmias

• Advanced AV block: Caused by electrolyte imbalance, acute infection, acute inferior MI, acute anterior myocardial infarction, and drug intoxication (digitalis, propranolol, or guanethidine).

Ventricular Conduction Abnormalities

• Right bundle branch block: Can appear in patients with coronary artery disease, hypertension, cardiac tumors, cardiosurgery, rheumatic heart disease, acute pericarditis, trauma, and CHF.
• Left bundle branch block: Causes include hypertension heart disease, aortic stenosis, cardiomyopathy, ischemic heart disease, aortic stenosis, and AMI.
• Left posterior hemiblock: Can be caused by chronic obstructive lung disease, right ven-

tricular enlargement, and lateral wall myocardial infarction.
- Trifascicular block: Can be caused by coronary artery disease, Lenegre's disease, or Lev's disease.
- Wolff-Parkinson-White syndrome (WPN): Can occur in young adults and can be associated with paroxysmal supraventricular tachycardia (PSVT) as a result of a circus movement or atrial fibrillation.

PHYSICAL ASSESSMENT
- Inspection: Faintness, dizziness, syncope, shortness of breath, fatigue, chest pain, momentary loss of consciousness, activity intolerance, confusion, nausea, anxiety, and restlessness.
- Palpation: Irregular or absent pulses.
- Auscultation: Palpitations, tachypnea, tachycardia, and pulse deficit.

DIAGNOSTIC TEST RESULTS

Standard Laboratory Tests. (See Table 1–1)

- Arterial blood gases: Reduced PaO_2 resulting from hypoxia.
- Blood studies: CBC may demonstrate infectious process that caused myocardial irritability and dysrhythmia.
- Serum chemistry: Elevated cholesterol and triglycerides. Reduced potassium level can contribute to dysrhythmias.
- Serum enzymes: Elevated creatine kinase (CK) and lactate dehydrogenase (LDH) in myocardial injury.

Invasive Cardiac Diagnostic Tests. (See Table 1–2)

- Electrophysiologic study (EPS): The test determines the origin of dysrhythmias, records activity of the conduction system, and effectiveness of drug therapy.

Noninvasive Cardiac Diagnostic Test. (See Table 1–3)

- Chest roentgenogram: Shows enlarged cardiac shadow as a result of myocardial failure.

- Graded exercise test (stress test): The patient's ECG and BP are taken while patient walks on a treadmill. Myocardial work load is also assessed at this time. The test continues until patient achieves a target heart rate (HR) or signs of dysrhythmia occur.

ECG

Sinus Node Dysrhythmias
- Sinus bradycardia.
  - Rhythm: Regular.
  - Rate: ≤60 bpm.
  - P wave: Normal configuration and precedes each QRS.
  - PR interval: Normal 0.12 to 0.20 second.
  - QRS complex: Normal 0.04 to 0.10 second.
- Sinus tachycardia.
  - Rhythm: Regular.
  - Rate: 100 bpm.
  - P waves: Normal configuration and precede each QRS.
  - PR interval: Normal 0.12 to 0.20 second.
  - QRS complex: Normal 0.04 to 0.10 second.
- Sinus arrhythmia.
  - Rhythm: Irregular.
  - Rate: Varies with respirations.
  - P wave: Normal configuration and precedes each QRS.
  - PR interval: Normal 0.12 to 0.20 second.
  - QRS complex: Normal 0.04 to 0.10 second.
- Sinus arrest.
  - Rhythm: Irregular during period of arrest.
  - Rate: 60 to 90 bpm.
  - P wave: Absent during period of arrest and same shape during regular rhythm.
  - PR interval: Absent during period of arrest.
  - QRS complex: Absent during period of arrest.

Atrial Dysrhythmias
- Premature atrial contraction.
  - Rhythm: Irregular in presence of PACs.
  - Rate: That of the underlying rhythm.

- P wave: Premature P wave is distorted, may be found in preceding T wave, and precedes QRS.
- PR interval: Normal.
- QRS complex: May be normal, wide, or absent.
- Wandering atrial pacemaker.
  - Rhythm: Slightly irregular.
  - Rate: Normal ≤60 bpm.
  - P wave: May vary slightly or markedly; positive in lead II and inverted in aVR.
  - PR interval: Within normal limits and relatively constant.
  - QRS Complex: Normal.
- Atrial tachycardia.
  - Rhythm: Regular.
  - Rate: 160 to 250 bpm.
  - P wave: May be difficult to see but superimposed in the preceding QRS complex, ST segment, T wave or U wave.
- Multifocal atrial tachycardia.
  - Rhythm: Irregular.
  - Rate: 100 to 250 bpm.
  - P wave: Variable.
  - PR interval: Varying interval.
- Atrial flutter.
  - Rhythm: Atrial regular while ventricular rhythm depends on the AV conduction pattern.
  - Rate: Atrial rate is 250 to 350 bpm while ventricular rate is 100 to 150 bpm.
  - P wave: Absent; rhythm shows F waves in sawtooth shape.
  - PR interval: 0.26 to 0.46 second.
  - QRS complex: Usually normal, 0.06 to 0.10 second.
- Atrial fibrillation.
  - Rhythm: Irregular.
  - Rate: Uncontrolled 110 to 180 bpm; controlled 70 to 80 bpm.
  - P wave: Absent; rhythm shows F waves seen as undulation.
  - PR interval: Unmeasurable.
  - QRS complex: Usually normal, 0.06 to 0.10 second.
- Paroxysmal atrial tachycardia.
  - Rhythm: Regular.
  - Rate: 150 to 200 bpm.

- P wave: Normal or buried in QRS. T wave may or may not be visible.
- PR interval: Usually normal, 0.12 to 0.20 second.
- QRS complex: Usually normal, 0.06 to 0.10 second.

AV Junction Dysrhythmias

- Junctional premature contraction.
  - Rhythm: Regular except for occurrence of premature beat.
  - Rate: 60 to 100 bpm or whatever the rate of the base rhythm.
  - P wave: May occur before, during, or after QRS complex.
  - PR interval: Short, 0.10 or less when P wave preceded the QRS.
  - QRS complex: Usually normal.
- Paroxysmal AV junctional tachycardia.
  - Rhythm: Regular.
  - Rate: 140 to 250 bpm.
  - P wave: Configuration varies, depending on the site of activation from the atria.
  - QRS complex: Normal or aberrant, depending on the status of the ventricular conduction system.
- Junctional tachycardia.
  - Rhythm: Regular.
  - Rate: 100 to 130 bpm.
  - P wave: Precedes or follows QRS.
  - PR interval: Not applicable.
  - QRS complex: Usually normal, 0.06 to 0.10 second.
- Atrial fusion complex.
  - Rhythm: Regular.
  - Rate: That of the underlying rhythm.
  - P wave: P wave of the fusion beat is sometimes isoelectric or intermediate between the P waves of the fusing impulses.
  - PR interval: The PR interval of the fusion beat is the same as that of the sinus rhythm.
  - QRS complex: That of the underlying rhythm.
- Atrial parasystole.
  - Rhythm: Irregular, because of premature atrial beats.
  - Rate: That of the underlying rhythm.
  - PR interval: Normal.

- QRS complex: Normal.
- First degree atrioventricular block.
  - Rhythm: Regular.
  - Rate: Usually 60 to 100 bpm.
  - P wave: Normal, precedes every QRS.
  - PR interval: Prolonged above 0.20 second.
  - QRS complex: Usually normal, 0.06 to 0.10 second.
- Mobitz type I second degree AV block.
  - Rhythm: Irregular.
  - Rate: Atrial regular and ventricular varies according to degree of block.
  - P wave: Normal; some P waves are not conducted.
  - PR interval: Progressively lengthening ≥0.28 second until one P wave is blocked.
  - QRS complex: 0.06 to 0.10 second.
- Mobitz type II second degree AV block.
  - Rhythm: Irregular.
  - Rate: Atrial 60 to 90 bpm; ventricular rate will vary accordingly to degree of block.
  - P wave: Usually regular and precedes each QRS; periodically a P wave will not follow a QRS complex.
  - PR interval: Normal; some P waves are not conducted.
  - QRS complex: Wide and distorted.
- Third degree heart block
  - Rhythm: Regular.
  - Rate: Atrial rate is normal; ventricular rate ≤58 bpm.
  - P wave: Normal but dissociated from QRS complex.
  - PR interval: No consistent PR interval.
  - QRS complex: Normal if impulse originates from bifurcation of bundle of His, ≥0.12 second.

Ventricular Dysrhythmias

- Premature ventricular contraction.
  - Rhythm: Irregular.
  - Rate: That of the underlying rhythm.
  - P wave: No P wave associated with PVC.
  - PR interval: That of the underlying rhythm.
  - QRS complex: Wide and bizarre, lasting longer than 0.12 second.
- Ventricular tachycardia

- Rhythm: Usually regular.
- Rate: 100 to 170 bpm.
- P wave: Absent, may be retrograde to atria.
- PR interval: Not applicable.
- QRS complex: Wide and bizarre in configuration, lasting longer than 0.12 to 0.14 second.
- Ventricular flutter
  - Rhythm: Regular or irregular.
  - Rate: Ventricular rate 150 to 300 bpm.
  - P wave: None seen.
  - PR interval: Not applicable.
  - QRS complex: Wide and regular.
- Ventricular fibrillation.
  - Rhythm: Irregular.
  - Rate: Not applicable.
  - P wave: None seen.
  - PR interval: Not applicable.
  - QRS complex: Not applicable.
- Accelerated ventricular rhythm.
  - Rhythm: Usually regular.
  - Rate: 40 to 100 bpm.
  - P wave: May be seen but at a slower rate than the ventricular focus and dissociated from QRS.
  - PR interval: Not applicable.
  - QRS complex: ≥0.12 to 0.4 second.
- Ventricular fusion complex.
  - Rhythm: Regular.
  - Rate: That of the underlying rhythm.
  - PR interval: PR interval of the fusion beat may be the same as or shorter than that of the sinus rhythm but not ≥0.06 second.
  - QRS: Normal in the underlying rhythm.
- Ventricular Conduction Dysrhythmias (Blocks).
  - Right bundle branch block.
    - Rhythm: Normal.
    - Rate: Normal.
    - PR interval: Normal.
    - QRS complex: 0.12 second or greater; classical pattern in V_1 is rSR.
  - Left bundle branch block.
    - Rhythm: Normal.
    - Rate: Normal.
    - P wave: Normal.
    - PR interval: Normal.
    - QRS complex: 0.12 second or greater.

- Trifascicular block.
  - Rhythm: That of the underlying rhythm.
  - Rate: That of the underlying rhythm.
  - P wave: Normal or that of the underlying rhythm.
  - PR interval: That of the underlying rhythm.
  - QRS complex: Broad.
- Wolff-Parkinson-White syndrome (WPN)
  - Rhythm: Regular.
  - Rate: Normal.
  - PR interval: ≤0.12 second.
  - QRS complex: ≥0.11 second, broad.

MEDICAL AND SURGICAL MANAGEMENT

PHARMACOLOGY
- Sodium channel and conduction blockers: Used to decrease automaticity of ventricular conduction, delay ventricular repolarization, decrease conduction velocity, increase conduction through AV node, and suppress ventricular automaticity. Class IA drugs (quinidine, procainamide hydrochloride, and disopyramide) decrease depolarization and prolong repolarization. Class IB drugs (lidocaine, mexiletine, aprindine, phenytoin, tocainide) decrease depolarization and shorten repolarization. Class IC drugs (encainide, flecainide, propafenone, indecainide) decrease depolarization with little effect or repolarization (see Table 1–11).
- Beta blockers: Class II used to slow sinus automaticity, slow conduction via AV node, and shorten the action potential of Purkinje's fibers. Drugs used include propranolol, acebutolol, metoprolol, pindolol, nadolol, atenolol, or timolol (see Table 1–5).
- Potassium channel blockers: Class III drugs used to increase action potential and refractory period of Purkinje's fibers, increase ventricular fibrillation threshold, and suppress reentrant dysrhythmias. Drugs used include amiodarone and bretylium (see Table 1–11).
- Calcium channel blockers: Class IV drugs used to depress automaticity in the SA and AV nodes and reduce conduction via the

AV node. Drugs used include diltiazem, nifedipine, or verapamil (see Table 1–6).
- Unclassified: Adenosine is used to create a transient block in the atrioventricular node, thereby terminating paroxysmal supraventricular tachycardia through interruption of the reentrant circuit.

S-T SEGMENT MONITORING
- Continuous ST segment monitoring: Can be used to identify transient and sustained ischemia or sudden reocclusion in high-risk patients. The ST segment in the surface ECG changes within seconds of coronary artery occlusion. It provides a means for determining a patient's ability to tolerate activity such as suctioning or eating (see S-T segment monitoring, p. 264).

AUTOMATIC IMPLANTABLE CARDIOVERTER-DEFIBRILLATOR (AICD)
- The AICD is used to detect VT or ventricular fibrillation (VF) and deliver a shock synchronously for VT or asynchronously for VF if it cannot be synchronized. The AICD is activated by sensing a rapid HR or a rapid HR and a rhythm with a wide QRS complex (see AICD, p. 260).

PACEMAKERS
- A temporary or permanent pacemaker is used to provide an artificial stimulus to the myocardium when the heart is unable to initiate an impulse or the conduction system is defective. Pacing mode can be asynchronous, involving an impulse that is generated at a fixed rate regardless of patient's rhythm, or synchronous, involving an impulse generated on demand or need (see Pacemakers, p. 270).

NURSING MANAGEMENT: NURSING DIAGNOSES AND COLLABORATIVE PROBLEMS

Nursing Diagnoses
Common nursing goals in patients with dysrhythmias are to increase tissue perfusion, en-

able a sense of power, and provide knowledge.

Altered tissue perfusion related to abnormal heart rate in disturbance in the conduction of an impulse secondary to myocardial damage.

Expected Patient Outcomes. Patient maintains adequate tissue perfusion, as evidenced by warm skin, absence of cyanosis, capillary refill ≤3 seconds, peripheral pulses +2, (BP) within patient's normal range, mean arterial pressure (MAP) 70 to 100 mm Hg, absence of confusion or restlessness, absence of chest pain, HR ≤100 bpm, respiratory rate (RR) ≤24 BPM, urinary output (UO) ≥30 mL/h or ≥0.5 mL/kg/h, and absence of dysrhythmias.

- Consult with cardiologist to validate expected patient outcomes used to evaluate adequate tissue perfusion.
- Review results of ECG, chest roentgenogram, and serum enzymes.
- Monitor and report clinical findings suggesting decreased peripheral tissue perfusion: skin cold and pale or cyanotic, capillary refill ≥3 seconds, and peripheral pulses ≤+2.
- Obtain and report clinical findings suggesting altered cerebral tissue perfusion: confusion or restlessness.
- Obtain and report clinical indicators of altered cardiovascular tissue perfusion: HR ≤100 bpm, dysrhythmias, chest pain, BP ≤90/60 mm Hg, MAP 70 mm Hg, and RR ≥24 BPM.
- Continuously monitor ECG to assess HR and rhythm. Document ECG rhythm strips every 2 to 4 hours or more frequently in patients with dysrhythmias.
- Continuously monitor ST segment, if equipment available, to determine change in myocardial oxygen supply and demand.
- Provide a quiet and relaxed environment, which will decrease the release of catecholamines that can increase myocardial oxygen demand.
- Administer prescribed oxygen 2 to 4 L/min by nasal cannula or mask to promote adequate oxygenation.

- Administer prescribed class I, II, III, or IV antidysrhythmic agents to suppress dysrhythmias, relieve symptoms, and reduce the risk of sudden death (see Table 1–11).
- Administer prescribed analgesia or narcotics to relieve chest pain (see Table 1–7).
- Should ventricular tachycardia or fibrillation occur, initiate unit protocols, standing orders, or advanced cardiac life support (ACLS) algorithms or prepare patient for defibrillation to reestablish normal sinus rhythm.
- Teach patient to report the presence of chest pain.

Powerlessness related to loss of physiological control over dysrhythmia and dependency on medications.

Expected Patient Outcome. Patient verbalizes and demonstrates it control by adhering to treatments and procedures.

- Increase physical activity slowly and monitor patient's response.
- Explain procedures and events in order to decrease anxiety and increase in sense of control.
- Identify positive body responses to treatment or procedure.
- Listen to patient's concerns regarding potential dependency on antidysrhythmia medications.
- Assist patient to achieve environmental control by allowing family members to remain at patient's bedside, by explaining the purpose behind equipment, and by explaining the relationship dysrhythmias and medications.
- Provide decisional control as to where patient would like to place get-well cards, when to ambulate, when to bathe, or which diversional activities to begin.
- Instruct patient as to control strategies to facilitate positive health behavior: taking medications, temporarily limiting physical activity, altering dietary regimen, ceasing smoking, and gradually increasing exercise after discharge.

- Teach patient common side effects of anti-dysrhythmia drugs.

Knowledge deficit related to the disease process causing dysrhythmias and treatment modalities.

Expected Patient Outcomes. Patient demonstrates increased understanding of the disease process and self-care management.

- Reinforce or clarify the physician's explanations of rhythm disturbances and associated symptoms.
- Explain the purpose of treatment and equipment.
- Teach patient how to take his or her pulse.
- Teach patient dietary restriction as prescribed and the need to avoid stimulating foods, such as caffeine, or nicotine.
- Teach patient the name, dosage, time of administration, purpose, and side effects of antidysrhythmic agents.
- Teach patient the need to exercise as tolerated or as prescribed.

Collaborative Problems

Common collaborative goals in patients with dysrhythmias are to increase cardiac output and maintain oxygen supply/demand balance.

Potential Complication: Decreased Cardiac Output.

Decreased cardiac output related to arterial heart rate, secondary to conduction changes or dysrhythmias.

Expected Patient Outcomes. Patient maintains adequate cardiac output (CO), as evidenced by CO 4 to 8 L/min; cardiac index (CI) 2.7 to 4.3 L/min/m^2; central venous pressure (CVP) 2 to 6 mm Hg; left atrial pressure (LAP) 8 to 12 mm Hg; MAP 70 to 100 mm Hg; peripheral arterial pressure (PAP) systolic 15 to 25 mm Hg or diastolic 8 to 15 mm Hg; pulmonary capillary wedge pressure (PCWP) 6 to 12 mm Hg; right atrial pressure (RAP) 4 to 6 mm Hg; RR 12 to 20 BPM; HR 60 to 100 bpm; BP $\geq$90/60 mm Hg; normal sinus rhythm on ECG; peripheral pulses +2; absence of syn-cope, dizziness, dyspnea, orthopnea, restlessness, and shortness of breath; UO $\geq$30 mL/h or $\geq$0.5 mL/kg/h; arterial oxygen pressure (PaO$_2$) 80 to 100 mm Hg; arterial oxygen saturation (SaO$_2$) $\geq$95%; and absence of chest pain.

- Consult with cardiologist to validate expected patient outcomes used to evaluate the presence of decreased CO.
- Consult with cardiologist about patient's specific dysrhythmia, its cause and treatment.
- Review results of 12-lead ECG and serum electrolyte valves.
- Limit activity to bed rest while patient is experiencing HR $\geq$100 bpm or ventricular dysrhythmia, which might cause lightheadedness, dizziness, syncope, or increased myocardial oxygen demand.
- Obtain and report hemodynamic parameters reflecting decreased CO resulting from an atrial or ventricular rate $\leq$60 bpm or atrial or ventricular rate $\geq$100 bpm: CO $\leq$4 L/min, CI $\leq$2.7 L/min/m^2, CVP $\geq$6 mm Hg, LAP $\geq$12 mm Hg, PCWP $\geq$12 mm Hg, and RAP $\geq$6 mm Hg.
- Assess, document, and report clinical findings associated with decreased CO as a result of altered atrial or ventricular rates: faintness, dizziness, syncope, chest discomfort, tachypnea, tachycardia, capillary refill $\geq$3 seconds, and hypotension.
- Monitor continuous ECG to assess HR and rhythm. Document ECG rhythm strips every 2 to 4 hours in patients with dysrhythmias or change in dysrhythmia.
- Document and report the absence of atrial contraction (atrial kick) in rhythms such as atrial fibrillation that can result in decreased ventricular filling.
- Continuously monitor ST segment for ischemic myocardium. The lead combination of V$_1$, lead I plus II, III, or avF can be used. In addition a lead combination including V$_1$ lead I and lead aVF can also be helpful (see ST segment monitoring, p. 264).
- Provide reassurance and support to patient and significant other(s) while experiencing dysrhythmias and administering treatment.

- Monitor BP and apical rate in patients experiencing dysrhythmias.
- Measure intake and output to maintain adequate fluid balance.
- Administer prescribed oxygen 2 to 4 L/min by means of nasal cannula or mask to maintain $PaO_2 \geq 80$ mm Hg and $SaO_2 \geq 95\%$.
- Administer prescribed IV fluids to maintain hydration, CVP 2 to 6 mm Hg, and UO ≥ 30 mL/h or ≥ 0.5 mL/kg/h.
- Administer prescribed class I, II, III, and IV antidysrhythmic agents to suppress or correct dysrhythmia.
- Should pharmacological therapy be ineffective in managing tachy- or bradydysrhythmias, prepare patient for cardioversion or carotid sinus massage.
- Should pharmacological therapy be ineffective in managing progressive heart block, prepare patient for pacemaker (see Pacemaker, p. 270).
- Should pharmacological therapy be ineffective in managing life-threatening dysrhythmias, prepare patient for defibrillation, which initiates complete depolarization and encourages SA node to reestablish normal sinus rhythm.
- Should sudden cardiac death or syncope caused by ventricular tachycardia or ventricular fibrillation be a concern, prepare patient for an AICD (see AICD, p. 260).
- Teach patient the common side effects of antidysrhythmia agents.

Potential Complication: Imbalanced Oxygen Supply or Demand.
Imbalanced oxygen supply or demand related to abnormal impulse initiation and abnormal impulse conduction secondary to coronary artery disease.

Expected Patient Outcomes. Patient maintains decreased myocardial oxygen demand, as evidenced by coronary artery perfusion pressure (CAPP) 60 to 80 mmHg, CO 4 to 7 L/min, CI 2.7 to 4.3 L/min/m², oxygen delivery (DO_2) 900 to 1200 mL/min, oxygen delivery index (DO_2I) 500 to 600 mL/min/m², MAP 70 to 90 mm Hg, oxygen extraction ratio (O_2ER) 25%, rate pressure product (RPP) $\leq 12,000$, mixed venous oxygen saturation ($S\bar{v}O_2$) 60% to 80%, oxygen demand (VO_2) 200 to 250 mL/min, oxygen demand index (VO_2I) 115 to 165 mL/min/m², BP $\geq 90/60$ mm Hg, HR ≤ 100 bpm, absence of pain, serum electrolytes and enzymes within normal limits, SaO_2 95.0% to 97.5%, arterial-venous oxygen content difference ($C[a - v]O_2$) 4 to 6 mL/100 mL, hemoglobin within normal limits, normal sinus rhythm, peripheral pulses +2, capillary refill ≤ 3 seconds, and absence of cyanosis.

- Confer with cardiologist to validate expected patient outcomes used to determine whether oxygen supply and demand are balanced.
- Review results of 12-lead ECG, serum enzymes, serum electrolytes, and.
- Limit physical activity to bed rest while patient is experiencing HR ≥ 100 bpm or ventricular dysrhythmia, which might cause light-headedness, dizziness, syncope or increased myocardial oxygen demand.
- Give low-sodium and low-saturated fat diet as prescribed.
- Obtain and report hemodynamic parameters reflecting oxygen supply and demand imbalance: CAPP ≤ 60 mm Hg, CO ≤ 4 L/min, CI ≤ 2.7 L/min/m², DO_2 ≤ 900 mL/min, DO_2I ≤ 500 mL/min/m², MAP ≤ 70 mm Hg, O_2ER $\geq 25\%$, RPP $\geq 12,000$, $S\bar{v}O_2$ $\leq 60\%$, VO_2 ≤ 200 mL/min and VO_2I ≤ 115 mL/min/m².
- Assess, document, and report other clinical findings indicating altered oxygen supply or demand: HR ≥ 100 bpm, BP $\leq 90/60$ mm Hg, capillary refill ≥ 3 seconds, chest pain, peripheral pulses $\leq +2$, diaphoresis, and pallor or cyanosis.
- Continuously monitor $S\bar{v}O_2$ to determine whether oxygen demand exceeds oxygen supply. An increase in oxygen demand (VO_2 ≤ 900 mL/min) and $S\bar{v}O_2$ $\leq 60\%$.
- Report a $S\bar{v}O_2$ ≤ 60, since this indicates a need to increase oxygen supply by increasing CO, hemoglobin, or SaO_2 and a need to decrease oxygen demand.
- Monitor $S\bar{v}O_2$ while providing nursing care activities such as turning, bathing, linen

change, or suctioning to determine whether oxygen demand is pushing the patient beyond physiological limits. A $S\bar{v}o_2 \leq 60\%$ should cause the nurse to consider the increase in oxygen demand that accompanies the above nursing care activities.

- Should $S\bar{v}o_2 \leq 50\%$, oxygen delivery (Do_2) is marginal for patient's oxygen demand. Nursing care activities such as turning, bathing, linen change, or suction can further increase the oxygen demand as well as reduce CO or Sao_2.
- Monitor continuous ECG to assess HR and rhythm. Document ECG rhythm strips every 2 to 4 hours or more frequently in patients with dysrhythmias.
- Continuously monitor ST segment for deviations suggesting a current of injury associated with myocardial oxygen supply and demand imbalance (see ST segment monitoring, p. 264).
- Obtain drug levels to verify toxicity (digitalis, quinidine, or procainamide) that can cause dysrhythmias.
- Provide a quiet and relaxed environment to decrease the release of catecholamines that stimulate sympathetic nervous system, vasoconstriction, and increase myocardial work load.
- Administer prescribed oxygen 2 to 4 L/min by means of nasal cannula or mask to maintain $Pao_2 \geq 80$ mm Hg and $Sao_2 \geq 95\%$.
- Administer prescribed IV fluids to maintain hydration, CVP 2 to 6 mm Hg, and UO ≥ 30 mL/h or ≥ 0.5 mL/kg/h.
- Administer prescribed positive inotropes (dopamine or dobutamine) to increase CO ≥ 4 L/min. Should oxygen delivery be low (CO ≤ 1.6 L/min), it may limit the tissue consumption of oxygen to amounts less than the tissue demand (see Table 1–10).
- Administer prescribed dysrhythmia drugs to maintain normal sinus rhythm (see Table 1–11).
- Administer prescribed analgesic or narcotic for chest pain.
- Instruct patient to use stress-reducing techniques to decrease HR: relaxation, meditation, or guided imagery.
- Instruct patient as to the purpose of treatment and medication.

DISCHARGE PLANNING

The critical care nurse provides patient and significant other(s) with verbal or written discharge notes regarding the following subjects:

1. Discussion of medications, purpose, dosage, schedule, and side effects.
2. Instructions to patient and significant other(s) on how to take and record pulse rate and to notify physician if heart rate is lower or higher than prescribed rates.
3. Names of community agencies such as American Heart Association.
4. Importance of ongoing follow-up care and keeping appointments.

PART II: SURGICAL CORRECTIONS AND NURSING MANAGEMENT

■ CORONARY ARTERY BYPASS GRAFT

(For related information see Part I: Acute myocardial infarction, p. 38, Cardiogenic shock, p. 72; Dysrhythmias, p. 184. Part III: Percutaneous transluminal coronary angioplasty, p. 226; Cardiac assist device, p. 248; Intra-aortic balloon pump, p. 254; Hemodynamic monitoring, p. 219. Respiratory Deviations, Part I: Acute pulmonary edema, p. 346; Pulmonary embolism, p. 397. Part III: Mechanical ventilation, p. 428; Chest drainage, p. 434.)

Diagnostic Category and Length of Stay
DRG: 106 Coronary bypass with cardiac catheterization
LOS: 13.60 days
DRG: 107 Coronary bypass without cardiac catheterization
LOS: 11.30 days

Definition

Coronary artery bypass grafting (CABG) is a surgical procedure in which a blood vessel (saphenous vein or internal mammary artery) is anastomosed to a coronary artery distal to the point of occlusion. The overall goal for performing surgical revascularization or aortocoronary bypass grafting is to restore adequate blood flow or blood supply to the myocardium.

Patient Selection

INDICATIONS. CABG is performed to relieve angina and preserve myocardial function. Bypass surgery can also be used to prevent myocardial infarction in patients for whom angioplasty or fibrinolytic therapy is ineffective or contraindicated. There are three indicators for the use of CABG surgery: (1) chronic, stable angina with a 75% stenosis of the left main coronary artery, (2) a proximal lesion of the anterior descending artery coexisting with stenosis of another vessel, or (3) three-vessel disease and left ventricular dysfunction. Surgery should not be performed on only one vessel unless it is the left main coronary artery or there is obstruction of a high-grade proximal left anterior descending coronary artery. Additional indicators are patients with high-risk clinical characteristics, such as ischemic heart failure with cardiogenic shock, history of hypertension and myocardial infarction, or ST segment depression in a resting ECG. Chronic unstable angina pectoris, left main coronary artery occlusion, triple-vessel coronary artery disease, unstable angina pectoris, intractable ventricular irritability, left ventricular failure, and percutaneous transluminal coronary angioplasty (PTCA) failure.

CONTRAINDICATIONS. A CABG is contraindicated in patients with bleeding disorders, acute cerebrovascular accident, cardiomyopathy, severe congestive heart failure, recent myocardial infarction, high left ventricular end-diastolic pressure, aortic root anomalies, severe aortic sclerosis, or inadequate ejection fraction (EF). Patients with an EF of 30% to 35% are poor risks and those with an EF of 20% to 25% are inoperable. Technical constraints such as small, narrowed, atheromatous coronary vessels ($\leq$1.0 to 1.5 mm in diameter) accompanied by diffuse distal disease and poor collateralization may not permit bypass grafting. Other contraindications include lack of a conduit or suitable graft material with severe systemic vascular disease; left ventricular (LV) dysfunction (LVEF $\leq$20%) accompanied by cardiomegaly or increased LV end-diastolic volume increase the risk of surgical mortality; and preexisting pulmonary disease, renal insufficiency, and carotid disease.

Procedure

TECHNIQUE. The CABG operation involves the construction of new conduits between the aorta or other major arteries and segments of the coronary arteries beyond the stenosed lesions. The goal is to enhance myocardial blood flow. The vein most frequently used is the aortocoronary greater or lesser saphenous. The saphenous veins are used as free grafts, anastomosed proximately to the ascending aorta and distally to one or more coronary arteries. The internal mammary artery (IMA) is left attached to its origin from the left subclavian artery, mobilized from the chest wall, and anastomosed to the left anterior descending coronary artery. The IMA has qualities that make it immune to the three biological modes of graft failure affecting venous conduits, namely, early thrombus, intermediate subintimal fibrosis, and late atherosclerosis. The right gastroepiploic artery (RGEA), a branch of the gastroduodenal artery, supplying the greater curvature of the stomach, is capable of reaching the posterior and lateral surfaces of the heart. The inferior epigastric artery (IEA) has been used in areas vascularized by branches of the right coronary artery and is used in patients in whom it is difficult to obtain enough conduit.

EQUIPMENT. The heart-lung machine.

Complications

- Hemorrhage, thromboembolism, pulmonary edema, acute cardiac dysrhythmia, atelectasis, infection, postpericardiotomy syndrome, acute myocardial infarction, and acute renal failure.

MEDICAL AND SURGICAL MANAGEMENT

PHARMACOLOGY

- Combined inotropes and vasodilators: Dobutamine is indicated in patients with a low cardiac output state (LCOS) in the absence of severe hypotension because of its vasodilating properties. Amrinone is indicated for LCOS in patients with adequate blood pressure. Enoximone is a new phosphodiesterase inhibitor undergoing clinical investigation. When used in patients with impaired ventricular function, cardiac index (CI) increased 4% to 41%, systemic vascular resistance (SVR) decreased 8% to 38%, and heart rate (HR) showed little effect (see Table 1–10; Table 1–4).
- Combined inotropes and vasopressors: Dopamine at low doses results in vasodilation of renal and mesenteric arteries leading to increased urine output with little cardiac or blood pressure effect. Epinephrine and norepinephrine are used for severe LCOS that is unresponsive to other agents (see Table 1–10; Table 1–4).

HEMODYNAMIC MONITORING

- Used to determine the type and dose of drug to be administered in CABG patient with impaired cardiac function. The hemodynamic profile reveals impaired cardiac ejection, low cardiac output, low CI, and elevated SVR (see Hemodynamic monitoring, p. 219).

INTRA-AORTIC BALLOON PUMP

- Intra-aortic balloon pump (IABP) can be used before induction of anesthesia in patients with severe coronary artery stenosis when significant areas of the myocardium are in jeopardy. IABP can also be used for patients experiencing difficulty weaning from the cardiopulmonary bypass machine when a modest increase in cardiac output is necessary to wean from full cardiac support and to permit time for recovery from transient myocardial depression (see IABP, p. 254).

CARDIAC ASSIST DEVICE

- A cardiac assist device is capable of assuming 100% of the cardiac pumping function. The mechanical assist device is intended for temporary support of a failing ventricle that does not respond to IABP and pharmacological therapy. The cardiac assist device is used in postcardiotomy patients when they develop cardiogenic shock on attempts at weaning from cardiopulmonary bypass despite maximal pharmacological therapy and a IABP (see cardiac assist device, p. 248).

NURSING MANAGEMENT: NURSING DIAGNOSES AND COLLABORATIVE PROBLEMS

Nursing Diagnoses

Common nursing goals in patients undergoing CABG are to prevent injury, prevent infection, promote adequate fluid volume, improve gas exchange, provide normothermia, and minimize fear.

Injury, high risk for related to postcardiotomy syndrome secondary to autoimmune response against the pericardial tissue or trauma of surgery.

Expected Patient Outcomes. Patient exhibits absence of postpericardiotomy syndrome (PPS), as evidenced by resolution of pericardial and pleuritic pain, temperature $\leq 100°F$, absence of friction rub, and normal sinus rhythm.

- Confer with cardiologist as to expected findings associated with PPS: pericardial pain and severe pleuric pain.
- Review 12-lead ECG for changes suggesting PPS: Concave ST segment elevation in early stage of acute pericarditis noted in lead I, II, aVL, aVF, and V_1 to V_6; as ST seg-

ment returns to baseline, T waves begin to dimple and then invert; PR depression for atrial inflammation; a slight decrease in the voltage of the T wave and QRS complex with normal P wave voltage.
- Review chest roentgenogram findings: Blunting of the costophrenic cardiac silhouette if pericardial effusion is present.
- Review echocardiography findings: Can detect much smaller volumes of fluid than larger amount seen on chest film.
- Review serum chemistry results: Cardiac enzyme levels increased, white blood count (WBC) increased without a left shift, and elevated erythrocyte sedimentation rate.
- Encourage passive and active leg exercises to enhance venous flow.
- Limit physical activity while patient experiences pericardial pain or pleuritic pain.
- Position patient to relieve pain: Elevate head of bed and provide a pillow and table upon which the patient can lean.
- Wrap a pillow around the patient's chest and support patient from behind with nurse's arms to enhance alveolar ventilation without unnecessary pain.
- Obtain and report clinical indicators of PPS: pain, fever, and friction rub.
- Monitor and report patient's description of pain with PPS: sharp, shooting, or stabbing. The presence of dull, deep pain may occur as a result of extensibility of the pericardiac sac. The pain is located in precordial or retrosternal area.
- Monitor temperature: An elevation may occur as an intermittent spike or may appear to be a continuation of the postoperative fever.
- Auscultate the heart for the presence of pericardial friction rub: triphasic with atrial or presystolic, ventricular systolic, and early systolic components; ventricular systolic rub is loudest because the heart exhibits the greatest motion during ventricular systole.
- Continuously monitor ECG for HR and rhythm. Supraventricular tachycardia may occur as a result of sympathetic stimulation of the heart caused by anxiety or cardiac irritability from inflammation or effusion.

- Encourage family to verbalize their concerns should patient remain hospitalized for prolonged period of time.
- Administer anti-inflammatory and antipyretic medication (indomethacin) to reduce tissue inflammation.
- Administer analgesics to reduce pericardial pain.
- Teach patient to cough effectively to maximize ventilation and minimize pain and energy expenditure.
- Instruct patient regarding relaxation technique.
- Instruct patient that PPS is a short-term problem.

Infection, high risk for related to interruption or integrity of skin, invasive monitoring, or long surgical time.

Expected Patient Outcomes. Patient is free of infection, as evidenced by temperature within normal range; absence of redness, drainage, swelling, or tenderness at catheter site or incision; WBC $\leq 10,000/\mu L$ and negative cultures.

- Review results from WBC and cultures.
- Monitor temperature every 1 to 2 hours while patient is febrile.
- Assess the incision or intravascular lines for swelling, redness, tenderness, or drainage.
- Evaluate patient for signs of systemic infection: chills, fever, diaphoresis, altered level of consciousness (LOC), warm peripheral skin, increased WBC, or positive cultures.
- Change IV every 48 hours, arterial pressure line every 4 days, central pressure line every 3 to 4 days, and dressing as ordered or according to unit standard.
- Culture any drainage from wound.
- Maintain aseptic technique when changing dressings, lines, or tubes.
- Administer prescribed IV fluid to maintain adequate hydration.
- Administer prescribed antipyretics for elevated temperature.
- Administer prescribed antibiotics depending upon results of cultures (see Table 1–14).

Fluid volume deficit related to bleeding secondary to coagulopathy associated with cardiopulmonary bypass, hemorrhage, or inadequate heparin reversal from a vessel or suture line within the chest.

Expected Patient Outcomes. Patient maintains adequate fluid volume, as evidenced by cardiac output (CO) 4 to 8 L/min and CI 2.7 to 4.3 L/min/m², central venous pressure (CVP) 2 to 6 mm Hg, left atrial pressure (LAP) 8 to 12 mm Hg, mean arterial pressure (MAP) 70 to 90 mm Hg, pulmonary artery pressure (PAP) systolic 15 to 25 mm Hg or diastolic 8 to 15 mm Hg, pulmonary capillary wedge pressure (PCWP) 6 to 12 mm Hg, right atrial pressure (RAP) 4 to 6 mm Hg, chest tube drainage ≤100 mL/h, capillary refill ≤3 seconds, peripheral pulses +2, urinary output (UO) ≥30 mL/h, blood pressure (BP) within patient's normal range, coagulation tests within normal range, and serum electrolytes within normal range.

- Consult with cardiologist to validate expected patient outcomes used to evaluate whether fluid volume is adequate.
- Review serum electrolytes, hematocrit, hemoglobin, and coagulation studies such as prothrombin time, partial thromboplastin time, fibrinogen split product levels, complete blood cell count, and platelet count.
- Encourage patient to eat prescribed diet of clear liquids to regular diet and restrict sodium to 2 g.
- Obtain and report hemodynamic parameters reflecting decreased fluid volume: BP ≤90/60 mm Hg, CO ≤4 L/min, CI ≤2.7 L/min/m², CVP ≤2 mm Hg, LAP ≤8 mm Hg, MAP ≤70 mm Hg, PAP systolic ≤15 mm Hg or diastolic ≤8 mm Hg, PCWP ≤6 mm Hg, or RAP ≤4 mm Hg.
- Evaluate indicators of fluid status every 1 to 2 hours until the desired hemodynamics are achieved: peripheral pulses +2, capillary refill ≤3 seconds, and UO ≥30 mL/h.
- Monitor the amount of postoperative bleeding to determine the need for volume replacement. Bleeding at a rate of 3

mL/kg/min or more requires therapy beyond volume replacement.
- Observe for signs of dehydration: dry mucous membranes, dry coated tongue, thirst, tachycardia, UO ≤30 mL/h, hypotension, and peripheral veins filling ≥3 seconds.
- Obtain daily weights, since patient may retain fluid if fluid intake is greater than output. Daily weight is a reliable indicator of hydration status (2.2 pounds equals 1 liter of fluid).
- During rewarming assess LAP, MAP, PAP, and RAP every 5 minutes, then every 30 to 60 minutes.
- Obtain and report intake and output from chest tube output ≥100 mL/h for the first 4 hours, UO ≥120 mL/h, and drainage from nasogastric tube ≥50 mL/h.
- Check all pressure line connectors to prevent accidental blood loss.
- Monitor dressings over chest tube and incision for bleeding.
- Administer prescribed crystalloid solutions such as Ringer's lactate; colloid solutions such as albumin or hetastarch; blood or blood products if the hematocrit is low; platelets, fresh frozen plasma, or fresh whole blood is used to replace coagulation factors.
- Administer prescribed protamine sulfate fresh frozen plasma (FFP), platelets, or specific deficient coagulation factors such as cryoprecipitate to reverse the coagulopathy and reduce bleeding.

Impaired gas exchange related to anesthesia, atelectasis, interstitial pulmonary congestion secondary to pulmonary capillary leak syndrome or cardiopulmonary bypass.

Expected Patient Outcome. Patient maintains adequate gas exchange, as evidenced by difference between arterial and venous oxygen concentration (C[a−v]o₂) 4 to 6 mL/100mL, oxygen utilization coefficient (o₂ER) 25%, arterial oxygen partial pressure (Pao₂) ≥80 mm Hg, arterial carbon dioxide partial pressure (Paco₂) 35 to 45 mm Hg, arterial oxygen saturation (Sao₂) 95% to 97.5%, mixed venous oxygen saturation (Sv̄o₂) 60% to

80%, respiratory rate (RR) 12 to 20 BPM, ventilation-perfusion ratio 0.08 to 1.0, absence of cyanosis, and resolution of crackles.

- Review chest roentgenogram and arterial blood gas results.
- Monitor respirations: rate, depth, symmetry of chest excursions after anesthesia.
- Support patient's chest or incision with a pillow when encouraging deep breathing.
- Monitor ventilation($\dot{V}$)-perfusion(Q) ratio: Changes in chest wall and diaphragm from anesthesia can lead to low $\dot{V}/\dot{Q} \leq 1.0$ resulting in a widened alveolar-arterial oxygen difference.
- Evaluate and report physiological shunt (Qs/Qt) $\geq 8\%$, which can signify lung dysfunction, such as atelectasis or pulmonary edema.
- Evaluate patient for pleuritic chest pain or distant heart sounds: Internal mammary artery bypass patients have more pulmonary problems, since they develop pleural effusion secondary to pleural trauma or hemorrhage.
- Auscultate lungs for changes in breath sounds: Atelectasis is worse in the left than right lower lobe because of retraction of left lower lobe during surgery, postoperative gastric distention, or transient paresis of the left hemidiaphragm from hypothermic injury to the phrenic nerve.
- Provide prescribed mechanical ventilation to facilitate lung expansion and minimize atelectasis until blood gases are within normal range and patient is alert.
- Evaluate patient's weaning process from mechanical ventilation: vital capacity ≥ 10 mL/kg of body weight, alertness, adequacy of pulmonary gas exchange, CO 4 to 8 L/min, Sao$_2$ $\geq 95\%$, Pao$_2$ ≥ 80 mm Hg, and S$\bar{v}$o$_2$ $\geq 60\%$.
- Monitor arterial blood gases and vital signs while patient is being weaned from mechanical ventilation.
- Suction patient by endotracheal tube, using unit standards, when crackles are auscultated. Oxygenate 1 to 2 minutes before and after procedure. Assess and record dysrhythmias during the procedure.

- Assist patient to cough and deep breathe every 1 to 2 hours to remove upper airway mucus.
- Assist patient with weaning from mechanical ventilation by encouraging to relax.
- Assist and encourage patient to use insensitive spirometry when extubated.
- Administer prescribed inspired oxygen fraction (Fio$_2$) $\leq 50\%$ to maintain Pao$_2$ ≥ 80 mm Hg, Sao$_2$ $\geq 95\%$, and S$\bar{v}$o$_2$ $\geq 60\%$.
- Administer analgesics to lessen pain and enhance deep breathing.
- Instruct patient how to cough and deep breathe while minimizing incisional pain.
- Teach patient relaxation techniques while being weaned from ventilator.

Hypothermia related to prolonged cooling secondary to cardiopulmonary bypass.

Expected Patient Outcome. Patient's temperature returns to normal.

- Obtain and report findings reflective of postcardiotomy hypothermia: cool, pale skin; shivering; confusion; drowsiness; restlessness; tachycardia; increased CO; increased MAP; and decreased RR.
- Observe patient for cardiovascular physiological consequences of hypothermia: myocardial depression, ventricular dysrhythmias, increased blood viscosity, atropine-resistant bradycardia, reduced effective blood volume, and elevated pulmonary-systemic vascular resistance.
- Monitor and report the presence of shivering, which is the body's attempt to generate heat.
- Continuously monitor S$\bar{v}$o$_2$ since shivering, from hypothermia, can increase oxygen demand and decrease S$\bar{v}$o$_2$ $\leq 60\%$.
- Provide frequent temperature monitoring of the degree of hypothermia and the rate of temperature decreases, which are important in assessing and managing hypothermia.
- Initiate fluid circulating blanket as a rewarming technique.
- Evaluate the drop between the completion of cardiopulmonary bypass (37°C) and

admission to critical care (34°C and 36.5°C), which can be 2° to 3°C.

- Continuously monitor temperature to avoid rapid rewarming. Rapid rewarming can cause an increase in the metabolic rate and oxygen demand of body tissues, which contribute to rewarming acidosis caused by the release of accumulated acids and metabolites with peripheral vascular vasodilation.

- Observe the rewarming process and the use of vasodilating drugs, since both can produce significant vasodilation (rewarming shock), which results in a decrease in SVR and systemic BP.

- Monitor skin for warmth, color, and presence of edema.

- Monitor arterial BP and MAP: BP may decrease as a result of peripheral vasodilation from rewarming.

- Administer prescribed vasodilators (nitroprusside or phentolamine) to promote gradual rewarming through vasodilatation (see Table 1–4).

- Administer prescribed morphine sulfate and meperidine to suppress shivering (see Table 1–7).

- Instruct patient that temperature will gradually return to normal.

Fear related to critical care environment, invasive procedure, or incisional pain.

Expected Patient Outcome. Patient able to discuss fear or concerns.

- Provide rest periods, since sleep deprivation can contribute to fear.

- Give patient positive reinforcement about physical accomplishments.

- Explain conditions and postoperative procedures by identifying how they will help patient progress.

- Allow patient to participate in care as appropriate in order to give positive feedback that he or she is making progress.

- Schedule patient's day so that periods of rest and relaxation can be alternated with nursing care activities.

- Include patient in planning for and carrying out care, which will reduce feelings of depression and loss of control.

- Provide a relaxed environment and meaningful conversation while performing nursing activities.

- Explain the purpose of procedures and care activities to be accomplished. This will decrease fear of the unknown.

- Allow the family to visit as much as possible according to unit protocol.

- Listen to patient's discussion of fear of surgery, loss of control, alteration in body image or pain.

- Reassure patient that invasive lines are temporary and will be removed.

- Support the family during the early phase after surgery.

- Instruct patient as to events occurring during surgery and immediately after surgery.

- Explain to patient that incision is smaller than the dressing.

Collaborative Problems

Common collaborative goals in patients undergoing CABG are to increase cardiac output, prevent hypovolemia and correct dysrhythmias.

Potential Complication: Decreased Cardiac Output. Decreased CO related to altered preload and afterload secondary to postcardiotomy myocardial depression.

Expected Patient Outcomes. Patient maintains adequate cardiac output, as evidenced by CO 4 to 8 L/min, CI 2.7 to 4.3 L/min/m², MAP 70 to 90 mm Hg, PAP systolic 15 to 25 mm Hg or diastolic 8 to 15 mm Hg, PCWP 6 to 12 mm Hg, pulse pressure (PP) 30 to 40 mm Hg, RAP 4 to 6 mm Hg, RVP systolic 15 to 25 mm Hg or diastolic 0 to 8 mm Hg, S$\bar{v}o_2$ 60% to 80%, SVR 900 to 1200 dynes/s/cm^{-5}, systemic vascular resistance index (SVRI) 1970 to 2390 dynes/s/cm^{-5}/m², UO ≥30 mL/h or ≥0.5 mL/kg/h, specific gravity 1.010 to 1.030, BP within the patient's normal range,

HR ≤100 bpm, capillary refill ≤3 seconds, or peripheral pulses +2.

- Consult with cardiologist to validate expected patient outcomes used to evaluate whether CO is effective.
- Limit physical activity to a position of comfort so as not to accidentally remove chest tubes.
- Dangle, as prescribed, first postoperative day and then advance to chair if stable.
- Obtain and report hemodynamic parameters reflecting a low CO state: CO ≤4 L/min, CI ≤2.7 L/min/m^2, MAP ≤70 mm Hg, PAP systolic ≥25 mm Hg or diastolic ≥15 mm Hg, PCWP ≤6 mm Hg, PP ≤30 mm Hg, S$\bar{\text{v}}$o$_2$ ≤60%, SVR ≥1200 dynes/s/cm^{-5}, and SVRI ≥2390 dynes/s/cm^{-5}/m^2.
- Obtain, document, and report other clinical findings associated with decreased CO: cool, pale, or mottled skin; weak peripheral pulses; capillary refill ≥3 seconds; and UO ≤30 mL/h or 0.5 mL/kg/h.
- Monitor patient for postoperative situation that may cause increased SVR: hypothermia, anxiety and pain resulting from the release of endogenous catecholamines.
- Observe patient for postoperative situations that may cause decrease in CO: decreased contractility, decreased HR, and dysrhythmias.
- Monitor continuous ECG to assess HR and rhythm. Document ECG rhythm strips every 2 to 4 hours in patients with dysrhythmias.
- Monitor BP, apical pulse, and peripheral pulse every 15 to 30 minutes for 2 hours then every hour as ordered and report systolic BP (SBP) drop 20 mm Hg or SBP ≤80 or ≥100, diastolic BP (DBP) ≥100 mm Hg, decreased amplitude in pulses, and HR ≤60 or ≥100 bpm.
- Evaluate patient for the presence of pain and anxiety stress response caused by the release of epinephrine and norepinephrine, which increases afterload.
- Monitor patient's temperature, as hypothermia causes vasoconstriction and subsequent increased afterload.

- Administer prescribed blood, crystalloids, or colloid fluid replacement to maintain LAP 15 mm Hg and RAP 18 mm Hg, which are higher than normal, to optimize CO.
- Administer prescribed oxygen 2 to 4 L/min or F$_{\text{I}}$o$_2$ ≤50% by means of nasal cannula or mask to maintain S$\bar{\text{v}}$o$_2$ 60% to 80%.
- Administer prescribed combined inotropes and vasodilator drip (dobutamine or amrinone) to increase myocardial contractility and decrease vascular resistance (see Table 1–10).
- Administer prescribed combined inotropic and vasopressor drugs (dopamine, epinephrine, or norepinephrine) to cause vasodilation of renal and mesenteric arteries resulting in UO ≥30 mL/h with enhanced CO or BP (see Table 1–4).
- Administer prescribed morphine to reduce pain.
- Should pharmacological therapy be ineffective in correcting increased left ventricular afterload, prepare patient for IABP (see IABP, p. 254.)
- Teach patient about postoperative care that might create discomfort such as suctioning, coughing, or deep breathing.
- Instruct patient to report chest pain.
- Teach patient common side effects of medication: hypotension, dysrhythmias, or dyspnea.

Potential Complication: Hypovolemia. Hypovolemia related to insufficient blood within the cardiac chamber or intravascular space to completely fill secondary to reduced diastolic filling, diuresis, or third spacing.

Expected Patient Outcomes. Patient maintains adequate volume, as evidenced by CO 4 to 8 L/min, CI 2.7 to 4.3 L/min/m^2, MAP 70 to 90 mm Hg, PAP systolic 15 to 25 mm Hg or diastolic 8 to 15 mm Hg, PCWP 6 to 12 mm Hg, RAP 4 to 6 mm Hg, S$\bar{\text{v}}$o$_2$ 60% to 80%, SVR 900 to 1200 dynes/s/cm^{-5}, SVRI 1970 to 2390 dynes/s/cm^{-5}/m^2, absence of dysrhythmias, hemoglobin and hematocrit within normal limits, UO ≥30 mL/h or ≥0.5 mL/kg/h, specific gravity 1.010 to 1.030, BP within the patient's normal range, HR ≤100 bpm, capillary refill ≤3 seconds, or peripheral pulses +2.

- Consult with cardiologist to validate expected patient outcomes used to evaluate whether volume is adequate.
- Consult with cardiologist about the predictors of blood loss during the first 4 hours after surgery. The predictors include length of time on cardiopulmonary bypass (CPB) and the hematocrit at 2 hours after completion of CPB.
- Review results of ECG, hemoglobin, hematocrit, and transesophageal echocardiogram, which can delineate the volume of the ventricle at end diastole and the function of the valves and myocardium.
- Obtain and report hemodynamic parameters suggesting hypovolemia after bypass surgery: PCWP ≤15 mm Hg, RAP ≤8 mm Hg, CI ≤2 L/min/m², and SVR ≥1200 dynes/s/cm^{-5}.
- Obtain and report other clinical findings of hypovolemia: UO ≤30 mL/h; hypotension; diaphoresis; cool, pale skin; HR ≥100 bpm; peripheral pulses ≤+2; flat neck veins; capillary refill ≥3 seconds; fatigue; weakness; thirst; or poor skin turgor.
- Observe and report factors that contribute to hypovolemia after cardiac surgery, including blood volume loss as a result of diuresis, third spacing, or bleeding and reduced diastolic filling resulting from positive end-expiratory pressure, venous return obstruction, vasodilatation, or dysrhythmias.
- Monitor potassium level during induced diuresis and replace to keep the serum potassium 4.0 to 5.0 mmol/L to reduce the risk of ventricular dysrhythmias.
- Monitor intake, output, and daily weight to evaluate the loss of third space fluid. One liter of fluid is equal to 1 kg of weight.
- Monitor patient for the presence of edema suggesting third spacing.
- Administer prescribed crystalloids after cardiac surgery. Potassium is also added to 5% dextrose in water, normal saline, or 5% lac-

tated Ringer's solution to replace urine and chest tube drainage. Colloids do not pull additional fluid into the intravascular space.

- Administer prescribed colloid solution, which increases the intravascular colloid osmotic pressure, which pulls fluid from the interstitium into the intravascular space. A solution of 25% albumin can expand blood volume; 100 mL of 25% albumin moves 350 mL of fluid from the interstitium into the circulation.
- Administer prescribed synthetic colloid (hetastarch) if necessary, because it stays in the intravascular space for 24 hours.
- Administer prescribed packed erythrocytes should the hematocrit feel to ≤30%, contributing to limited oxygen-carrying capacity. Each unit of erythrocytes can increase the hematocrit by 3%.
- Should other disturbances in coagulation occur, administer packed FFP, platelet concentration, coagulation factor concentration, or cryoprecipitate.

Potential Complication: Dysrhythmia. Dysrhythmia related to intra-operative trauma, secondary to cardiopulmonary bypass.

Expected Patient Outcomes. Patient maintains normal sinus rhythm, MAP 70 to 90 mm Hg, HR ≤100 bpm, BP within patient's normal range, and serum electrolytes within normal range.

- Review serum enzyme and serum electrolyte values.
- Review 12-lead ECG for conduction disturbance or supraventricular and ventricular arrhythmias.
- Monitor continuous ECG to assess HR and rhythm. Document ECG rhythm strip every 2 to 4 hours or more frequently in patients with atrial fibrillation, supraventricular, or ventricular dysrhythmias.
- Monitor and report findings that suggest patient is not tolerating the dysrhythmias: palpitations, chest pain, syncope, and hypotension.
- Measure ECG components should hypokalemia occur in conjunction with di-

uretic therapy: decreased amplitude and broadening of T waves, prominent U waves, and sagging ST segment.

- Administer prescribed IV fluids to maintain hydration, replace electrolytes and maintain UO $\geq$30 mL/h or $\geq$0.5 mL/kg/h.
- Should atrial flutter occur, prepare patient for rapid atrial pacing, if necessary, for 30 seconds or until the atrial ECG complex changes from a negative to a positive deflection in lead II.
- Administer prescribed digitalis should atrial fibrillation's ventricular response exceed 110 bpm.
- Administer prescribed procainamide or digoxin when atrial flutter ceases after atrial pacing.
- Administer prescribed procainamide or lidocaine to treat premature ventricular beats more than 6 bpm, coupled premature ventricular contractions (VPCs), or run of ventricular tachycardia.
- Should dysrhythmias be caused by hypokalemia, administer prescribed potassium according to agency standards.
- Should antidysrhythmia agents be ineffective or conduction blocks occur, prepare patient for a pacemaker (see Pacemaker, p. 270.)
- Teach patient the common side effects of antidysrhythmia agents.

DISCHARGE PLANNING

The critical care nurse provides patient and significant other(s) with verbal or written discharge notes regarding the following subjects:

1. Medication's purpose, dosage, schedule, and side effects.
2. Need to avoid fatigue and sitting for long periods of time.
3. Possible contraindication of sexual activity for 2 to 4 weeks and need to check with physician when permissible to resume.
4. Need to record and report shortness of breath, fatigue, swelling of hands or legs, or nausea during or 24 hours after exercises.
5. Importance of keeping outpatient appointments.
6. Names of community agencies or support groups such as American Heart Association or Mended Hearts.

■ VALVE SURGERY

(For related information see Part I: Acute infectious endocarditis, p. 134; Shock, p. 174; Dysrhythmias, p. 184. Part III: Percutaneous aortic valvuloplasty, p. 243; Intra-aortic balloon pump, p. 254; Hemodynamic monitoring, p. 219; Neurological Deviations, Part I: Cerebrovascular accident, p. 607. Respiratory Deviations, Part I: Pulmonary embolism, p. 397. Part III: Mechanical ventilation, p. 428; Chest drainage, p. 434).

Diagnostic Category and Length of Stay
DRG: 104 Cardiac valve procedure with cardiac catheterization
LOS: 18.10 days
DRG: 105 Cardiac valve procedure without cardiac catheterization
LOS: 12.70 days

Definition
Valvular reconstruction is used to repair diseased valves by means of splitting of fused leaflets (commissurotomy), repair or reconstruction of the valve (valvuloplasty), or repair or reconstruction of the annulus of the valve (annuloplasty). Surgical repair permits the patient to keep the native valve for several years, thereby avoiding complications associated with prosthetic valves. Valvular surgery is the replacement of a degenerating heart valve with either a mechanical or tissue prosthetic device.

Patient Selection

INDICATIONS. Aortic stenosis, aortic regurgitation, mitral stenosis, and mitral regurgitation.

CONTRAINDICATIONS. Bleeding tendencies.

Procedure

TECHNIQUE. Open commissurotomy involves an incision of the left atrium and cardiopulmonary bypass. The surgical techniques involve a median sternotomy and cooling the heart. The aorta is cross-clamped; multidose, hypothermic potassium cardioplegia is used to protect the heart; and the left atrium is open and examined for thrombi. Incisions are made into the anterior lateral and posterior medial commissures. Should the chordae and papillary muscle be fused, they can be separated by a sharp incision. Closed commissurotomy does not require bypass. In closed commissurotomy, a surgeon's finger and later a dilator is introduced through the stenotic mitral valve to open the fused or immobile leaflets. Annuloplasty uses a single, semicircular suture (purse-string suture); depending on how tightly the stitch is tied, this will purse the annulus to the desired size. It will only reduce the overall valvular orifice.

The surgical technique for valvular replacement is similar to that for commissurotomy. Prosthetic heart valves are divided into two categories: The first category, mechanical valves, consists of caged-ball, caged-disk, or tilting disk valves. The caged-ball valve consists of a ball housed in a cage, which is attached to a sewing ring. As a pressure gradient develops, the ball moves forward in the cage and the valve opens. Caged-disk valves consist of a sewing ring with an attached cage that houses a movable silicone disk. The disk sits in the sewing ring when the valve is closed and drops into the cage as blood flows through the open valve. The tilting disk valve rests against the sewing ring when the valve is closed. When the valve opens, the disk tilts at an angle that allows a semicentral flow of blood through the orifice. The second category, tissue or biological valves, consists of porcine or bovine heterografts and homografts. The porcine heterograft is mounted in a cloth-covered stent, sewing ring, or steel alloy. The valve is made from excised pig aortic valves. The bovine heterograft is made from calf pericardium cut into three leaflets

and mounted into a stent. The homograft is a human heart valve that has been extracted from a donated heart. Homograft valves have been associated with less degenerative valve failure and calcification.

PROSTHESIS. Mechanical valves include caged-ball, tilting disk and bileaflet. The most widely used porcine valves are the Hancock/Vaser and the Carpenter-Edwards prothesis. Both heterograft valves are made from excised pig valves and are mounted on stents to support the valve leaflets. The Ionescu-Shiley bioprosthesis is a bovine heterograft made from calf pericardium. The pericardial tissue is molded into three leaflets and mounted on a Dacron-covered titanium stent. Homografts are obtained from organ donors, treated with antibiotic solution, and cryopreserved at temperatures as low as 4°C.

Complications
- Thromboembolism, prosthetic malfunction, paravalvular leaks, hemolysis, hemolytic anemia, and prosthetic valve endocarditis.

MEDICAL AND SURGICAL MANAGEMENT

PHARMACOLOGY
- Anticoagulation therapy: Warfarin is used to maintain a moderate anticoagulation effect (prothrombin time ratio 1.5) in patient with mechanical cardiac valves. It can offer equal protection to that of a higher anticoagulation effect with a lower risk for bleeding. Some advocate the use of only antiplatelet medication, such as aspirin or dipyridamole.
- Antibiotics: Antibiotic prophylaxis in patients undergoing valvular surgery decreases the risk of endocarditis. Antibiotics are also given for dental, oral respiratory tract, gastrointestinal, and genitourinary tract procedures.

FLUID THERAPY
- Administer crystalloids, colloids, or blood products based on patient's particular volume need.

NURSING MANAGEMENT: NURSING DIAGNOSES AND COLLABORATIVE PROBLEMS

Nursing Diagnoses

Common nursing goals in patients undergoing valve surgery are to maintain adequate fluid volume, enhance tissue perfusion, promote effective breathing pattern, relieve pain, reduce anxiety, and provide knowledge.

Fluid volume deficit related to hypovolemia or bleeding secondary to intraoperative heparization, leaking or bleeding from suture line.

Expected Patient Outcomes. Patient maintains adequate fluid volume, as evidenced by cardio output (CO) 4 to 8 L/min, cardiac index (CI) 2.7 to 4.3 L/min/m², central venous pressure (CVP) 2 to 6 mm Hg, left atrial pressure (LAP) 8 to 12 mm Hg, mean arterial pressure (MAP) 70 to 100 mm Hg, pulmonary artery pressure (PAP) systolic 15 to 25 mm Hg or diastolic 8 to 15 mm Hg, pulmonary capillary wedge pressure (PCWP) 6 to 12 mm Hg, right atrial pressure (RAP) 4 to 6 mm Hg, chest tube drainage ≤100 mL/h, capillary refill ≤3 seconds, peripheral pulses +2, urinary output (UO) ≥30 mL/h, blood pressure (BP) within patient's normal range, coagulation tests within normal range, and serum electrolytes within normal range.

- Consult with cardiologist to validate expected patient outcomes used to evaluate the adequacy of fluid volume.
- Review serum electrolyte, hematocrit, hemoglobin values; coagulation studies such as prothrombin time, partial thromboplastin time, fibrinogen degradation product levels, and platelet count.
- Obtain and report hemodynamic parameters reflecting decreased fluid volume: BP ≤90/60 mm Hg, CO ≤4 L/min, CI ≤2.7 L/min/m², CVP ≤2 mm Hg, LAP ≤8 mm Hg, MAP ≤70 mm Hg, PAP systolic ≤15 mm Hg or diastolic ≤8 mm Hg, PCWP ≤6 mm Hg, or RAP ≤4 mm Hg.
- Evaluate indicators of fluid status every 1 to 2 hours until the desired hemodynamics are achieved: peripheral pulses +2, capillary refill ≤3 seconds, and UO ≥30 mL/h.
- Rewarm patient gradually to avoid peripheral vasodilation, which increases intravascular compartment and can contribute to inadequate circulating volume.
- Monitor daily weight and report weight gain ≥2 lb (1kg)/d.
- Obtain and report intake and output from chest tube ≥100 mL/h, urine output ≥120 mL/h, and drainage from nasogastric tube ≥50 mL/h.
- Monitor dressings over chest tube every hour and chest drainage every 15 minutes for quality, rate of drainage, and consistency.
- Administer prescribed crystalloid solutions such as Ringer's lactate; colloid solutions such as albumin or hetastarch; blood or blood products if the hematocrit is low; platelets, fresh frozen plasma, or fresh whole blood is used to replace coagulation factors and maintain CO 4 to 8 L/min, CI 2.7 to 4.3 L/min/m², CVP 2 to 6 mm Hg, LAP 8 to 12 mm Hg, MAP 70 to 100 mm Hg, BP within normal range, and UO 30 mL/h or ≥0.5 mL/kg/h.
- Administrate cryoprecipitate when fibrinogen or factors I or VIII are needed.
- Administer prescribed fraction inspired oxygen (FIO₂) ≤ 50% or oxygen 2 to 4 L/min by means of nasal cannula of mask to maintain adequate oxygenation.

Altered cerebral tissue perfusion related to decreased CO secondary to mechanical valve prosthesis, atrial fibrillation, and inadequate coagulation.

Expected Patient Outcomes. Patient maintains adequate cerebral tissue perfusion, as evidenced by equal and normoreactive pupils; oriented to time, place, and location; normal sensorimotor function; MAP 70 to 100 mm Hg; BP within patient's normal range; heart rate (HR) ≤100 bpm; normal cardiac rhythm; and coagulation studies within normal range.

- Review results of ECG and coagulation profile.

- Monitor and report hemodynamic parameters reflecting altered cerebral tissue perfusion: CO $\leq$4 L/min, CI $\leq$2.7 L/min/m^2, and MAP $\leq$70 mm Hg.
- Monitor and report findings reflecting altered cerebral tissue perfusion: irritability, forgetfulness, confusion, sensorimotor dysfunction, unequal pupils, and HR $\geq$100 bpm.
- Monitor continuous ECG to assess HR and rhythm. Document ECG rhythm strips every 2 to 4 hours in patient with dysrhythmias.
- Monitor ECG for the determinant of atrial fibrillation: irregular rhythm, atrial rate $\geq$350, ventricular rate variable, no P wave, fibrillatory waves creating a wavy or undulating border, no PR interval, and QRS 0.10 seconds.
- Administer prescribed IV fluids to maintain adequate circulating volume.
- Administer prescribed blood products to replace lost coagulation factors and maintain optimum oxygen-carrying capacity.
- Administer prescribed antidysrhythmia agents to correct atrial fibrillation (see Table 1–11).
- Administer prescribed anticoagulant to minimize clot formation on prosthetic valve.
- Should pharmacological therapy be ineffective, prepare patient for cardioversion.

Ineffective breathing pattern related to atelectasis secondary to decrease in chest wall compliance resulting from general anesthesia or thoracic incisional pain.

Expected Patient Outcomes. Patient maintains effective breathing pattern, as evidenced by respiratory rate (RR) $\leq$24 BPM; HR $\leq$100 bpm; skin color normal; blood gases within normal range; symmetrical chest movement; absence of crackles; absence of pain; and absence of dyspnea, shortness of breath, and restlessness.

- Collaborate with physician on the application of pressure mechanical ventilation or the use of a ventilator that will not increase the work of breathing, such as intermittent

mandatory ventilation (IMV) or synchronized IMV.
- Review chest roentgenogram and arterial blood gas values.
- Position patient in semi-Fowler's position for best use of ventilatory muscles and to facilitate diaphragmatic descent.
- Place patient in a position of comfort to facilitate effective lung expansion.
- Monitor and report clinical findings suggesting ineffective breathing pattern: RR $\geq$24 BPM, HR $\geq$100 bpm, cyanosis, diaphoresis, dyspnea, shortness of breath, restlessness, asymmetrical chest excursion, and crackles.
- Administer prescribed oxygen 2 to 4 L/min or FIO_2 $\leq$50% to maintain partial pressure of arterial oxygen (PaO_2) 95 mm Hg.
- Administer prescribed analgesics or narcotics to reduce thoracic pain.
- Teach patient to take deep breaths to reduce the risk of atelectasis.

Impaired gas exchange related to atelectasis secondary to intraoperative ventilation at high oxygen levels, decrease in chest wall compliance, or decrease in functional residual capacity (FRC).

Expected Patient Outcomes. Patient maintains adequate gas exchange, as evidenced by arterial blood gases within normal range, arterial-venous oxygen content difference ($C[a-v]O_2$) 4 to 6 mL/100 mL, CO 4 to 8 L/min, CI 2.7 to 4.3 L/min/m^2, arterial oxygen saturation (SaO_2) 95%, mixed venous oxygen saturation ($S\bar{v}O_2$) 60% to 80%, RR $\leq$24 BPM, physiological shunt (Qs/Qt) 0% to 8%, dynamic compliance 35 to 55 mL/cm H_2O, static compliance 50 to 100 mL/cm H_2O, absence of cyanosis, absence of crackles, symmetrical chest movement, and absence of dyspnea.

- Collaborate with physician on expected patient outcomes used to validate adequate gas exchange.
- Review chest roentgenogram and arterial blood gas values.

- Elevate the head of bed to promote diaphragmatic excursion.
- Obtain and report Qs/Qt ≥8%, indicating lung dysfunction such as atelectasis leading to ineffective oxygenation.
- Obtain and report hemodynamic parameters associated with impaired gas exchange: C0 ≤4 L/min, CI ≤2.7 L/min/m², and S$\bar{v}$o$_2$ ≤60%.
- Obtain and report C(a−v)o2 ≥6 mL/100 mL, which reflects inadequate cardiovascular function.
- Evaluate and report dynamic compliance (Cdyn) ≤35 mL/cm H$_2$0, signifying reduced compliance, and static compliance (Cstat) ≤50 mL/cm H$_2$0, signifying lung stiffness.
- Obtain and report clinical findings suggesting impaired gas exchange: RR ≥24 BPM, HR ≥100 bpm, dyspnea, restlessness, use of accessory muscles, and fatigue.
- Institute measures to mobilize and remove secretions as well as open closed alveoli. Turn and position patient every 2 hours and use endotracheal suctioning as necessary, followed by manual hyperinflation of the lungs.
- Encourage progressive ambulation after removal of the endotracheal tube and pulmonary artery catheter.
- Administer prescribed pain medications to decrease splinting and hypoventilation.
- Teach patient to use a pillow to support the incisional area to increase comfort during deep breathing, coughing, and movement. This will improve alveolar ventilation.

Pain related to coronary artery vasospasm or sternal incision.

Expected Patient Outcomes. Patient verbalizes that pain is reduced to a tolerable level or is removed, pain rating on a scale of 1 to 10 is lower, and BP within patient's normal range.

- Review results of ECG.
- Explain the factors responsible for pain production.
- Obtain and report clinical findings associated with coronary artery vasospasm: hypotension, atrioventricular block, and ventricular tachycardia.
- Continuously monitor ECG to assess HR and rhythm. Document ECG rhythm strips every 2 to 4 hours in patient with dysrhythmias.
- Continuously monitor ST segment for elevation, which suggests coronary artery vasospasm and altered oxygen delivery (see ST segment monitoring, p. 264).
- Perform rehabilitation exercises or activity such as turning, deep breathing, or ambulating shortly before peak of drug effect, since this is optimal time for the patient to increase activity with minimal risk of increasing pain.
- Administer prescribed analgesic or narcotic to break the pain cycle without altering the level of consciousness or vital signs.
- Monitor patient for indicators of undertreatment of pain: verbalization that pain is not relieved, restlessness, sleeplessness, irritability, anxiety, and decreased activity level.
- Monitor patient for indications of overtreatment: hypotension, bradycardia, RR ≤10 BPM, or excessive sedation.
- Establish optimal analgesic dose that brings optimal pain relief.
- Teach patient to report the presence of chest or sternal pain.
- Teach patient alternative strategies to reduce pain: progressive muscle relaxation, meditation, or guided imagery.

Anxiety related to pain or feeling of helplessness regarding the prognosis of events or routines.

Expected Patient Outcomes. Patient's anxiety is reduced or absent, as evidenced by verbalization of a decrease in anxiety and verbalization of effective ways to dealing with anxiety.

- Place patient in a position of comfort to relieve anxiety associated with discomfort.
- Should patient be intubated, explain why he or she is unable to talk.
- Provide patient with a writing pad and pen to develop a mode of communication.

- Encourage patient to communicate sources of anxiety.
- Monitor patient for nonverbal cues of pain: facial grimacing, stiffness, or reluctance to move in bed and splinting of body parts.
- Encourage patient to participate in care by making decisions, in order to minimize feelings of helplessness and loss of control.
- Communicate signs of progress to patient.
- Administer prescribed antianxiety medications.
- Instruct patient to report when anxious feelings occur.

Knowledge deficit about cardiac surgery, postoperative care, risk factors, or return to work related to lack of information, cognitive limitation, or misunderstanding.

Expected Patient Outcomes. Patient is able to describe the surgery, risk factors, perform physical care, and discuss activity goals.

- Consult with cardiologist about the amount of information to be included in patient's teaching plan.
- Consult with cardiac rehabilitation about developing an individualized exercise activity program.
- Teach patient about taking prescribed prophylactic antibiotics during dental cleaning or surgical procedures.
- Teach patient what to expect during the days following surgery.
- Teach patient about the common side effects of antibiotics and anticoagulants.
- Teach patient about any postoperative dietary restrictions such as low-sodium or low-fat diet.
- Instruct patient about the need for anticoagulant therapy should thromboembolism or atrial fibrillation occur.
- Instruct patient as to dietary modifications.
- Instruct patient how to gradually increase physical activity.

Collaborative Problems

Common collaborative goals in patients undergoing valve surgery are to increase cardiac output and correct dysrhythmias.

Potential Complication: Decreased Cardiac Output. Decreased CO related to inadequate valve seating secondary to suture displacement causing loss of adherence between the valve ring and the annulus.

Expected Patient Outcomes. Patient maintains adequate valve replacement and subsequent CO, as evidenced by CO 4 to 8 L/min, CI 2.7 to 4.3 L/min/m^2, CVP 2 to 6 mm Hg, LAP 8 to 12 mm Hg, MAP 70 to 90 mm Hg, PAP systolic 15 to 25 mm Hg or diastolic 8 to 15 mm Hg, PCWP 6 to 12 mm Hg, Pao$_2$ $\geq$80 mm Hg, Sao$_2$ $\geq$95%, S$\bar{\text{v}}$o$_2$ 60% to 80%, UO $\geq$30 mL/h, capillary refill $\leq$3 seconds, peripheral pulses +2, resolution of crackles, and resolution of peripheral edema.

- Collaborate with physician to establish expected patient outcomes used to validate adequate CO or postoperative valvular replacement.
- Consult with cardiologist about expected valve sounds: mechanical valve reveals opening and closing with clicks. Heterograft and homograft produce no clicks.
- Review results of ECG.
- Obtain and report hemodynamic parameters suggestive of decreased CO from inadequate valve seating: CO $\leq$4 L/min and CI $\leq$2.7 L/min/m^2.
- Obtain, document, and report signs and symptoms of mitral regurgitation in patient with inadequate mitral valve seating: palpitations, fatigue, dysrhythmias, diaphoresis, cyanosis, confusion, peripheral edema, systolic thrill, pansystolic murmur, S$_2$ widely split, and S$_3$ gallop.
- Obtain, document, and report signs and symptoms of aortic regurgitation reflecting inadequate aortic valve seating: diaphoresis; headache; peripheral edema; Quincke's sign (capillary pulsation representing peripheral vasodilation, observed as alternating flushing and paling of the nail beds or legs); Hill's sign; Traube's sign (pistol-shot sounds heard over the femoral arteries); Duroziez's sign (systolic and diastolic murmurs heard with slight compression proxi-

mally and distally); a blowing, high-pitched diastolic decrescendo murmur; S_3; and S_4.

- Monitor BP every 1 to 2 hours in patient with severe aortic regurgitation: systolic BP (SBP) may be 60 mm Hg higher in the legs than in the arms (Hill's sign), which is due to an acceleration of the normal BP response in the lower extremities.
- Monitor continuous ECG to assess rate and rhythm. Document ECG rhythm strips every 2 to 4 hours in patients with dysrhythmias such as atrial fibrillation, bradydysrhythmias, or supraventricular tachydysrhythmias.
- Auscultate the lungs every 1 to 2 hours for the presence of crackles or rhonchi, indicating intra-alveolar congestion resulting from inadequate mitral or aortic valve seating.
- Should inadequate valve seating compromise CO, prepare patient for aortic or mitral valve repair or replacement.
- Administer prescribed IV fluids to maintain adequate hydration and UO $\geq$30 mL/h.
- Administer prescribed oxygen 2 to 4 L/min by means of intubation in early postoperative period, nasal cannula, or mask or to maintain PaO_2 $\geq$80 mm Hg, SaO_2 $\geq$95%, and $S\bar{v}O_2$ 60% to 80%.
- Administer volume-reducing agents such as furosemide or bumetanide to maintain UO $\geq$30 mL/h, resolve peripheral edema and resolve crackles (see Table 1–13).
- Administer prescribed inotropes to maintain CO 4 to 8 L/min, CI 2.7 to 4.3 L/min/m², PAP systolic 15 to 25 mm Hg or diastolic 8 to 15 mm Hg, and PCWP 6 to 12 mm Hg (see Table 1–10).
- Inform patient about the complication and need for surgical correction.

Potential Complication: Decreased Cardiac Output. Decreased CO related to altered preload, afterload, and contractility secondary to transient biventricular dysfunction after cardiopulmonary bypass.

Expected Patient Outcomes. Patient maintains adequate CO, as evidenced by CO 4 to 8 L/min, CI 2.7 to 4.3 L/min/m², coronary artery perfusion pressure (CAPP) 60 to 80 mm Hg, MAP 70 to 90 mm Hg, PAP systolic 15 to 25 mm Hg or diastolic 8 to 15 mm Hg, PCWP 6 to 12 mm Hg, pulse pressure (PP) 30 to 40 mm Hg, RAP 4 to 6 mm Hg, right ventricular pressure (RVP) systolic 15 to 25 mm Hg or diastolic 0 to 8 mm Hg, $S\bar{v}O_2$ 60% to 80%, systemic vascular resistance (SVR) 900 to 1200 dynes/s/cm⁻⁵, systemic vascular resistance index (SVRI) 1970 to 2390 dynes/s/cm⁻⁵·m², UO $\geq$30 mL/h or $\geq$0.5 mL/kg/h, specific gravity 1.010 to 1.030, BP within the patient's normal range, HR $\leq$100 bpm, capillary refill $\leq$3 seconds, or peripheral pulses +2.

- Collaborate with cardiologist to validate expected patient outcomes used to evaluate adequate CO.
- Collaborate with cardiologist as to the causes of transient biventricular dysfunction after cardiopulmonary bypass (CPB): preexisting ventricular dysfunction, microembolism to the subendocardia, inadequate cardioplegic protection, premature or uneven rewarming, elevation in pulmonary vascular resistance and SVR, or ischemic ventricular injury.
- Provide complete bed rest to decrease metabolic demand and oxygen demand.
- Obtain and report hemodynamic parameters suggesting decreased CO: CO $\leq$4 L/min, CI $\leq$2.7 L/min/m², MAP $\leq$70 mm Hg, PAP systolic $\geq$25 mm Hg or diastolic $\geq$15 mm Hg, PCWP $\geq$15 mm Hg, $S\bar{v}O_2$ $\leq$60%, SVR $\geq$1200 dynes/s/cm⁻⁵, and SVRI $\geq$2390 dynes/s/cm⁻⁵/m².
- Monitor, document, and report other clinical findings associated with decreased CO: cool, pale, or mottled skin; peripheral pulses $\leq$+2; capillary refill $\geq$3 seconds; HR $\geq$100 bpm; RR $\geq$24 BPM; MAP $\leq$70 mm Hg; and UO $\leq$30 mL/h or 0.5 mL/kg/h.
- Continuously monitor $S\bar{v}O_2$ to determine whether oxygen supply (DO_2) and oxygen demand (VO_2) are balanced at the time of nursing activities. Monitoring $S\bar{v}O_2$ can be a means of determining how to protect patient from oxygen demands of turning and

whether the turn affected patient's oxygen supply or demand tolerance.

- Administer prescribed IV fluids to maintain adequate circulating volume.
- Administer prescribed vasodilators to keep SBP ≥90 mm Hg, PCWP ≤ 15 mm Hg, pulmonary artery diastolic pressure (PADP) ≤15 mm Hg, and SVR ≤1200 dynes/s/cm^{-5} (see Table 1–4).
- Administer prescribed inotropes to keep CO ≥4 L/min and CI ≥2.7 L/min/m^2.
- Should pharmacological therapy be ineffective in increasing CO, prepare patient for an intra-aortic balloon pump (IABP) (see IABP, p. 254).
- Should pharmacological therapy and IABP be ineffective in increasing CI associated with transient bioventricular dysfunction, prepare patient for cardiac assist device (see cardiac assist device, p. 248).
- Teach patient relaxation exercises such as progressive muscle relaxation, meditation, or guided imagery to reduce anxiety, thereby limiting catecholamine release.

Potential Complication: Dysrhythmias. Dysrhythmias related to operative factors secondary to cardiopulmonary bypass.

Expected Patient Outcome. Patient is free of conduction defects or ventricular dysrhythmias.

- Collaborate with cardiologist as to the operative factors that contribute to postoperative supraventricular tachydysrhythmias, premature ventricular contraction (PVC), or bradydysrhythmias: premature myocardial rewarming, electromechanical atrial activity during anoxic states, hypoxemia, hypotension, increased sympathetic stimulation, fluid shifts, metabolic imbalances, or irritation from prosthetic valves.
- Position patient with supraventriculartachydysrhythmias supine to increase preload.
- Obtain and report clinical findings associated with supraventricular tachycardia: sudden drop in BP, atrial or ventricular rate ≥100 bpm, UO ≤30 mL/h, decreased mentation, chest pain, and dyspnea.
- Obtain and report clinical findings associated with ventricular tachycardia: sudden drop in BP, syncope, loss of consciousness, faint or absent peripheral pulses.
- Continuously monitor and report pre-ventricular tachycardia dysrhythmias: ≥6 PVC/min, multifocal PVC, R on T phenomenon, couplets, bursts of ventricular tachycardia, bigeminy, or trigeminy.
- Obtain and evaluate apical-radial pulse to identify deficits indicating nonperfused beats. Evaluate amplitude of peripheral pulses to determine perfusion to extremities.
- Administer prescribed IV fluids and potassium to maintain adequacy circulating volume and potassium within normal range.
- Administer prescribed oxygen by means of intubation, nasal prongs, nasal cannula, or mask to maintain Pao$_2$ 95 mm Hg.
- Administer prescribed supraventricular antidysrhythmia agents such as verapamil, quinidine, procainamide, propranolol, digoxin, or phenylephrine.
- Should pulseless ventricular tachycardia occur, prepare patient for defibrillation.
- Should sporadic ventricular dysrhythmias progress to ventricular tachycardia or ventricular fibrillation, prepare patient for implementation of synchronized cardioversion.
- Should bradydysrhythmias be attributed to injury of the conduction system, prepare patient for temporary atrial or ventricular pacing.
- If bradydysrhythmias lead to the loss of the atrial conduction to CO, prepare patient for temporary atrioventricular sequential pacing.

DISCHARGE PLANNING

The critical care nurse provides patient and significant other(s) with verbal or written discharge notes regarding the following subjects:

1. Medication's purpose, dosage, schedule, and side effects.

2. Importance of taking anticoagulant medications as prescribed.
3. Importance of keeping outpatient appointments.
4. Maintaining an activity schedule as ordered (see Acute myocardial infarction,
   Discharge planning, p. 71).

■ HEART TRANSPLANTATION

(For related information see Part I: Conges-
tive heart failure, p. 87; Dysrhythmias, p. 184.
Part III: Intra-aortic balloon pump, p. 254;
Cardiac assist device, p. 248; Hemodynamic
monitoring, p. 219; Pacemakers, p. 270. Res-
piratory Deviations, Part I: Acute pulmonary
edema, p. 346; Pulmonary embolism, p. 397;
Pneumonia, p. 375. Anxiety, p. 725; Body im-
age disturbance, p. 730; Ineffective individual
coping, depression, p. 733; Fear, p. 740; Pain,
p. 742; Powerlessness, p. 743; Sleep pattern
disturbance, sleep deprivation, p. 746. Part
III: Pulse oximetry, p. 426; Mechanical venti-
lation, p. 428; Chest drainage, p. 434; Renal
Deviations. Part I: Acute renal failure, p. 459;
Psychosocial Deviations, Part I, p. 725.)

Diagnostic Category and Length of Stay
DRG: 103 Heart transplantation
LOS: 25.2 days

Definition
Heart transplantation is a treatment for end-
stage heart disease. Heart transplantation is
the surgical removal of a diseased heart and
the transfer of a donor heart from an individual who matches the patient's tissue type.

Patient Selection

INDICATIONS. In general the patient must have
end-stage heart failure not amenable to further medical or surgical intervention. Such a
patient is unable to carry on many physical
activities without discomfort. The patient is
usually younger than 55, psychologically stable, compliant, reliable, and able to understand the procedure and risks involved.

CONTRAINDICATIONS. Patients who are unable to tolerate immunosuppressive agents,
who are older than 55 years, who have irreversible renal and hepatic failure, or who
have an active infection are not candidates.
Bleeding disorders such as peptic ulcer or
bleeding diathesis are contraindicated. The
insulin-dependent diabetic patient is prone to
poor wound healing and prone to myocardial
infarction. Patients with malignant, peripheral, or cerebrovascular disease will have limited long-term survival. Severe pulmonary
vascular hypertension is a contraindication
because a normal transplanted right ventricle
will fail when faced with increased work
load. Finally, patients who have a history of
substance abuse and noncompliance with a
medical regimen, disruption of work, and
poor family relationships are poor candidates
for heart transplantation.

Procedure

TECHNIQUE. There are two approaches to
heart transplantation. The first is heterotopic
heart transplantation. It involves the anastomosis of the donor's heart to the recipient's
heart in such a way that the donor's heart is
placed in a right-sided position. The second
technique is an orthotopic procedure. In this
procedure, the recipient's heart is excised, retaining the left and right posterior atrial walls,
inferior and superior vena cava, and pulmonary veins. The donor's left atrium is sutured to the posterior wall of the recipient's
remnant left atrium and atrial septum. The
right atrial walls are then sutured in place. Finally, anastomoses of the aorta and pulmonary vessels complete the transplantation
procedure. The donor pulmonary artery and
aorta are anastomosed to the recipient vessels. Upon completion of the procedure,
temporary epicardial atrial and, frequently,
ventricular pacing wires are placed.

DONOR-RECIPIENT. There are several factors
that are important in matching the donor heart
to the recipient. The donor's and recipient's

blood group must be compatible to prevent acute rejection and ultimate loss of the organ. The patient's body size and weight should be within a 20% to 30% range difference with that of the donor. The heart itself must be of comparable size to be able to meet the hemodynamic demands of the recipient. Finally, the cytotoxicity of a potential recipient is determined preoperatively by means of a panel for reactive antibodies (PRA). The PRA measures the presence of recipient cytotoxic antibodies against a panel of lymphocyte antigens present in a randomly selected population. A PRA ≥5% to 10% requires crossmatching of the recipient's serum and specific donor lymphocytes to reduce the potential for hyperactive rejection after transplantation.

Complications

- Acute rejection may occur any time after the fourth or fifth postoperative day. With acute rejection, infiltration by mononuclear cells and edematous changes occur, with possible myocyte necrosis. Chronic rejection occurs over a wide span of time (months to years). Fibrous and scar tissue can form in the transplanted organ and vasculature.
- Other complications include congestive heart failure, hemorrhage, ECG abnormality, infection, acute renal failure, or graft atherosclerosis.

MEDICAL AND SURGICAL MANAGEMENT

PHARMACOLOGY

- Immunosuppressive therapy: Cyclosporine is a fungal metabolite that blocks the activation of interleukin-2 (IL-2) and other lymphokine genes required for the proliferation of T cells. Azathioprine is an antimetabolite that blocks DNA synthesis required for T-cell production by inhibiting gene replication and T-cell activation. Corticosteroids block T-cell proliferation through their ability to block activation of the IL-2 genes. Monoclonal antibody (OKT3) is used to destroy cells expressing the T3 antigen and

produces antigenic modulation of the returning T cells. With modulation, the target antigens are removed, thereby leaving the rest of the T cell undisturbed. Anti-human thymocyte globulin (ATG) combines with the T cell to either destroy it or render it immunologically inactive. Rabbit antithymocyte globulin (RATG) can be indicated for primary suppression of host immune response in organ transplant recipients. RATG use is limited only to certain institutions (see Table 1–15).
- Dopamine: Used to enhance myocardial contractility, thereby increasing cardiac output and renal perfusion (see Table 1–10).
- Nitroprusside: Used to maintain MAP between 65 mm Hg and 85 mm Hg (see Table 1–4).

FLUID THERAPY

- Nomal saline, plasma expanders, or blood products are given to maintain central venous pressure 8 mm Hg to 12 mm Hg.

DIET

- High-calorie diet to achieve weight gain.
- High-protein intake to promote wound healing and replenish body protein store.

PHYSICAL ACTIVITY

- Conditioning exercises commence when patient is able to sit in a chair at the bedside. Low-level exercise is begun at an oxygen consumption range of 5 to 9 mg/kg/min with extremity and shoulder flexion, extension, and abductor exercises. When appropriate, the intensity and duration are progressed to an oxygen consumption range of 9 to 14 mg/kg/min.

PACEMAKER

- Temporary or permanent pacemakers may be required in patients with sinus node dysfunction resulting from injury during procurement, surgery, or distortion of the atria with transplantation or acquired as the result of cardiac rejection.

NURSING MANAGEMENT: NURSING DIAGNOSES AND COLLABORATIVE PROBLEMS

Nursing Diagnoses

Common nursing goals for patients undergoing heart transplantation are to prevent infection, maintain nutritional balance, promote gas exchange, enhance urinary output, maintain adequate fluid volume, support skin integrity, encourage feelings of control, and encourage effective coping.

Infection, high risk for related to impaired wound healing secondary to malnutrition or immunosuppressive agents.

Expected Patient Outcomes. Patient experiences absence of infection, as evidenced by normal temperature; white blood count (WBC) ≤11,000/μL; absence of adventitious lung sounds; negative cultures; and absence of redness, swelling, tenderness, or drainage from wound or catheter site.

- Consult with dietitian to individualize a dietary program that includes patient's prescribed diet while incorporating personal preferences.
- Review results of complete blood count (CBC), hemoglobin, hematocrit, and cultures.
- Limit physical activity to bed rest while patient is febrile.
- Restrict fresh unpeeled fruits and vegetables for 6 to 8 weeks after transplantation because of the presence of gram-negative bacteria.
- Change all IV solutions, tubings, stopcocks, and any heparin-locked lines using protocol (every 24 to 48 hours).
- Provide pulmonary care such as inspirometers, deep breathing, coughing, and promote early mobility to reduce risk of atelectasis and of pulmonary infection.
- Monitor and report findings indicating infection: temperature ≥37.5°C; WBC ≥11,000/μL; positive blood, urine, or wound cultures; presence of redness, swelling, erythema, and wound drainage at the IV site;

discharge from chest tube site or Foley catheter; HR ≥100 bpm; and cloudy urine.
- Maintain isolation protocols and isolation technique for all visitors and staff entering patient's room to reduce the risk of infection.
- Monitor continuous ECG to assess heart rate and rhythm. Document ECG rhythm strips every 4 hours in patients with voltage alterations of dysrhythmias.
- Use strict sterile technique when changing dressing, lines, tubes, or pacemaker wire exit site.
- Monitor all wounds, IV, and pacemaker wire sites daily for drainage, redness, swelling, or heat.
- Obtain culture of any suspicious drainage.
- Obtain temperature every 2 to 4 hours in febrile patient. Corticosteroid therapy reduces normal basal and maximal body temperature. A temperature ≥37°C can indicate presence of a systemic infection.
- Maintain protective isolation for patient receiving immunosuppressive agents.
- Monitor urinary output for color, clearance, odor, and specific gravity.
- Prepare patient for possible surgical debridement if mediastinitis or sternal wound infection occur.
- Administer prescribed IV fluids to maintain adequate hydration, urinary output (UO) ≥30 mL/h or ≥0.5 mL/kg/h, specific gravity 1.010 to 1.030, peripheral pulses +2, and capillary refill ≤3 seconds.
- Administer prescribed antibiotics based on results of cultures.
- Instruct patient to report any drainage or discomfort around incision or catheter sites.

Altered nutrition: Less than body requirements related to malnourished preoperative state and side effects of immunosuppressive therapy.

Expected Patient Outcomes. Patient shows appropriate weight gain and increases nutritional intake.

- Consult with dietitian for calorie count and evaluation of patient's dietary needs.
- Consult with physician about possible indicators for hyperalimentation and supplemental Intralipid intake.
- Consult with dietitian to determine fat requirements. Some fat must be provided to prevent essential fatty acid deficiency, but excess fat may be as harmful as excess carbohydrates. Fat emulsions can affect the immune system in patients already immunosuppressed by interfering with neutrophilic function and by interfering with the reticuloendothelial system.
- Monitor patient for semistarvation process should respiratory failure or wound infection occur. These patients are unable to take in sufficient protein and calories to meet hypermetabolic requirements.
- Observe patient for clinical findings suggesting complications from overfeeding: hypercapnia, increased metabolic rate, increased carbon dioxide production, respiratory acidosis, inability to wean from the respirator, and refeeding edema.
- Promote foods high in protein and carbohydrate to achieve weight gain and replenish body protein stores.
- Encourage patient to identify beverage that best disguises the taste of cyclosporine. The most frequent choices are low-fat chocolate milk, orange juice, and cranberry juice.
- Determine patient's carbohydrate needs by establishing energy needs: multiply the body weight in kilograms by 25 to 35 kilocalories to approximate daily caloric requirements. A 70-kg man would require between 1750 to 2450 kcal/d.
- Determine patient's energy needs using indirect calorimetry, if available, to measure oxygen and carbon dioxide volumes (V_{O_2}, V_{CO_2}).
- Provide prescribed protein intake 0.8 to 1.0 g/kg of body weight/d.
- Use sterile technique in changing dressings over central venous pressure (CVP) lines. Because of access to superior vena cava by the subclavian vein, or proximity to the endotracheal tube in the neck (if used), patient at risk for cross-contamination.
- Administer intravenous or enteral hyperalimentation to malnourished patient to improve respiratory muscle strength and body cell mass.
- Administer prescribed IV fluids to maintain adequate hydration in patients receiving fat. Fat is more calorically dense than other nutrients provided to supplement diet for a fluid-restricted patient.
- Administer prescribed parenteral nutrition of 20% fat emulsions or 15% amino acid solution via central venous route as appropriate for patient's nutritional status.

Impaired gas exchange related to interstitial and intra-alveolar fluid congestion secondary to increased alveolar-capillary permeability.

Expected Patient Outcomes. Patient maintains adequate gas exchange, as evidenced by arterial oxygen partial pressure (Pa_{O_2}) ≥ 80 mm Hg, arterial carbon dioxide partial pressure (Pa_{CO_2}) 35 to 45 mm Hg, arteriovenous oxygen content difference ($C(a-v)_{O_2}$) 4 to 6 mL/100mL, arterial oxygen saturation (Sa_{O_2}) $\geq 95\%$, mixed venous oxygen saturation ($S\bar{v}_{O_2}$) ≥ 60 mm Hg, resolution of crackles, skin warm and dry, absence of cyanosis, respiratory rate (RR) 12 to 20 BPM, and heart rate (HR) ≤ 100 bpm.

- Review results of ECG, arterial blood gas measurement, or chest roentgenogram.
- Limit physical activity to bed rest while patient has chest tube, and place patient in a position that enhances chest tube drainage.
- Obtain and report findings reflecting impaired gas exchange: Pa_{O_2} ≤ 70 mm Hg, Pa_{CO_2} ≥ 45 mm Hg, Sa_{O_2} $\leq 95\%$, $S\bar{v}_{O_2}$ ≤ 60 mm Hg, $C(a-v)_{O_2}$ ≥ 6 mL/100 mL, crackles, cyanosis, HR ≥ 100 bpm, and RR ≥ 20 BPM.
- Auscultate the lungs every 1 to 2 hours for crackles, rhonchi, or wheezes.
- Monitor drainage from chest tube ≤ 50 mL/h.

- Monitor skin for the presence of cyanosis.
- Encourage patient to cough and deep breathe to mobilize and clear pulmonary secretions, which may predispose to infection.
- Suction using aseptic technique to avoid pulmonary infection.
- Administer prescribed oxygen 2 to 4 L/min by means of nasal cannula or fraction of inspired oxygen (FIO_2) $\leq$50% by mask to maintain Pao_2 $\geq$80 mm Hg and Sao_2 $\geq$95%.
- Administer prescribed IV fluids to maintain adequate hydration and UO $\geq$30 mL/h or $\geq$0.5 mL/kg/h.
- Administer prescribed antibiotics as needed or based upon results of cultures.
- Teach patient the importance of diaphragmatic excursion and coughing to enhance gas exchange and prevent atelectasis.

Altered urinary pattern related to decreased cardiac output secondary to preoperative cardiac failure.

Expected Patient Outcomes. Patient maintains adequate urinary pattern, as evidenced by UO $\geq$30 mL/h or $\geq$0.5 mL/kg/h; specific gravity 1.010 to 1.030; absence of edema; and serum creatinine, urine creatinine, and blood urea nitrogen (BUN) within normal range.

- Consult with physician about reducing or delaying administration of cyclosporine in patients with elevated serum creatinine and BUN.
- Review results of serum creatinine and urine creatinine clearance.
- Obtain and report clinical findings suggesting altered renal pattern: UO $\leq$30 mL/h or $\leq$0.5 mL/kg/h, specific gravity 1.010, weight gain, and peripheral edema.
- Monitor intake, output, and specific gravity every 2 hours in patients with elevated serum creatinine and UO $\leq$30 mL/h.
- Administer prescribed dopamine to maintain renal perfusion.
- Administer prescribed IV fluids to maintain adequate circulating volume without causing fluid overload.

Fluid volume deficit related to postoperative bleeding secondary to clotting deficiencies associated with hepatic dysfunction.

Expected Patient Outcomes. Patient maintains adequate fluid volume, as evidenced by cardiac output (CO) 4 to 8 L/min; cardiac index (CI) 2.7 to 4.3 L/min/m²; CVP 2 to 4 mm Hg; UO $\geq$30 mL/h; absence of bleeding; HR $\leq$100 bpm; blood pressure (BP) within patient's normal range; skin turgor normal; absence of cyanosis; and coagulation tests, hemoglobin, and hematocrit within normal range.

- Review results of coagulation tests, hemoglobin, and hematocrit.
- Obtain and report hemodynamic parameters associated with decreased fluid volume: CO $\leq$4 L/min, CI $\leq$2.7 L/min/m², and CVP $\leq$2 mm Hg.
- Obtain and report other clinical findings associated with decreased fluid volume: HR $\geq$100 bpm, RR $\geq$24 BPM, hypotension, skin cool and pale, and UO $\leq$30 mL/h.
- Monitor and report bleeding from dressing, catheter sites, or chest tube in excess of 100 mL/h.
- Assist with prescribed autotransfusion to replace blood.
- Evaluate patient for vitamin K deficiency, which can contribute to postoperative bleeding.
- Should vitamin K be deficient preoperatively, administer prescribed vitamin K.
- Administer prescribed fresh frozen plasma to restore coagulation factors.
- Should additional blood replacement be required, consider patient's cytomegalovirus titer. If the titer is negative, patient receives only blood that also has a negative cytomegalovirus titer to avoid the possibility of an opportunistic infection.

High risk for impaired skin integrity related to immunosuppressive drug therapy.

Expected Patient Outcomes. Patient's skin is free of abrasions and incision heals normally.

- Encourage patient to change position frequently to relieve pressure points and provide comfort.
- Provide moisture to prevent dryness of skin in patients who receive corticosteroid and azathioprine therapy. These patients may develop thin and fragile skin.
- Should patient be malnourished, provide a foam pad on the bed to protect fragile skin areas over bony prominences.
- Keep the incision clean by using sterile technique while changing dressings.
- Inspect skin and oral mucous membrane daily for signs of injury. Skin lesions can be a source of potential infection.
- Teach patient how to monitor the condition of skin and report lesions that do not heal well or become infected.

Powerlessness related to loss of control over the disease, surgical procedure, treatment, or life-style changes.

Expected Patient Outcome. Patient verbalizes and demonstrates control over following postoperative therapy and home care.

- Encourage patient to ask questions about postoperative regimen including physical activity and medications.
- Encourage patient to participate in postoperative care, thereby achieving a sense of personal control.
- Help patient to participate in decisions about self-care, such as when to cough, turn, deep breathe, and ambulate.
- Encourage the use of diversional activities such as reading, talking, watching TV, or listening to the radio.
- Personalize patient's environment to give a sense of personal control.
- Assist patient to redefine the illness situation by identifying its positive aspects.
- Teach patient stress-reducing activities: progressive relaxation, medication, or guided imagery.

Coping, ineffective individual related to depression in response to identifiable stressors, such as operative risks, life long use of immunosuppressive drugs, or body-image changes.

Expected Patient Outcomes. Patient verbalizes feelings related to emotional state, identifies coping patterns, identifies personal strengths, and makes decisions and follows them through with appropriate actions.

- Assist patient to identify causative and contributing factors of depression: negative self-concept, inadequate problem solving, sudden change in life pattern, recent change in health state, or inadequate support systems.
- Encourage patient to identify the onset of depressive feelings and their origin so origin can be evaluated or changed.
- Provide support to patient and family by giving reassurance that their feelings are understandable.
- Provide a positive view of self: provide meaningful communication, facilitate realistic appraisal of role changes, enhance decision-making control, foster accomplishment of specific tasks, and encourage a positive self-concept.
- Provide a positive view of experiences: create a personal space in a technical environment, encourage participation in care, identify positive changes in patient's physical status, encourage discussion of the illness experience, and facilitate knowledge of risk factors.
- Provide a positive view of future: facilitate establishment of realistic goals, assist with role transition, facilitate patient's acceptance of the future, and facilitate family's acceptance of the future.

Collaborative Problems

Common collaborative goals in patients undergoing heart transplantation are to prevent immunodeficiency, increase cardiac output and correct dysrhythmias.

Potential Complication: Immunodeficiency. Immunodeficiency related to presence of a foreign antigen secondary to rejection or immunosuppressive agents.

Expected Patient Outcomes. Patient maintains adequate immune system, as evidenced by WBC ≤11,000 µL/dL and normothermia.

- Review 12-lead ECG voltage, chest roentgenogram, endocardiography, creatine kinase isoenzyme level and endomyocardial biopsy to determine rejection.
- Limit physical activity to bed rest while patient is showing signs of heart rejection.
- Monitor and report signs and symptoms reflecting rejection: decreasing voltage in ECG; atrial and ventricular gallop; pericardial friction rub; atrial and ventricular dysrhythmias; tachycardia; fever; malaise and fatigue; and jugular vein distention.
- Obtain temperature every 1 hour while patient is febrile.
- Auscultate lung and heart sounds every 4 hours or more frequently for crackles, rhonchi, or wheezes.
- Maintain isolation protocol and monitor isolation techniques of staff and visitors entering patient's room.
- Change all IV solutions, tubing, stopcocks, and heparin-locked lines daily using agency standards.
- Provide rest periods.
- Administer immunosuppressive agents to alter either the cellular immune response or humoral immune response: cyclosporine, ATG, azathioprine, corticosteroids, or OKT_3.
- Instruct patient to report feelings of fatigue or malaise, which can warn of rejection.
- Instruct patient as to the seriousness of taking immunosuppressive agents.
- Teach patient the purpose behind postoperative endomyocardial biopsy within the first 7 days following transplantation. Cyclosporine can mask signs and symptoms of rejection until the problem is severe.

Potential Complication: Decreased Cardiac Output. Decreased cardiac output related to myocardial dysfunction and heart denervation secondary to a global ischemic injury of the myocardium and increased right ventricular afterload.

Expected Patient Outcomes. Patient maintains adequate cardiac output, as evidenced by BP within patient's normal limits, coronary artery perfusion pressure (CAPP) 60 to 80 mm Hg, CO 4 to 8 L/min, CI 2.7 to 4.3 L/min/m², CVP 2 to 6 mm Hg, ejection fraction (EF) ≥50%, left atrial pressure (LAP) 8 to 12 mm Hg, mean arterial pressure (MAP) 70 to 90 mm Hg, pulmonary capillary wedge pressure (PCWP) 6 to 12 mm Hg, pulmonary vascular resistance (PVR) 155 to 255 dynes/s/cm⁻⁵, pulmonary vascular resistance index (PVRI) 200 to 450 dynes/s/cm⁻⁵/m², right atrial pressure (RAP) 4 to 6 mm Hg, stroke volume (SV) 60 to 130 mL/beat, stroke volume index (SVI) 33 to 47 mL/m²/beat, $S\bar{v}o_2$ 60% to 80%, systemic vascular resistance (SVR) 900 to 1200 dynes/s/cm⁻⁵, systemic vascular resistance index (SVRI) 1970 to 2390 dynes/s/cm⁻⁵/m², no fever, absence of infection, and UO ≥30mL/h.

- Collaborate with cardiologist to validate expected patient outcomes used to evaluate whether cardiac output is adequate.
- Review results of chest roentgenogram, ECG, echocardiography, cardiac catheterization, and radionuclide imaging.
- Review results of endomyocardial biopsy (EMB) when rejection is suspected as origin of low cardiac output.
- Limit physical activity to bed rest and turn patient to optimize chest tube drainage and prevent accumulation of blood in the pericardial sac.
- Obtain and report hemodynamic parameters reflecting decreased cardiac output caused by myocardial dysfunction: CO ≤4 L/min, CI ≤2.7 L/min/m², CVP ≥6 mm Hg, EF ≤50%, LAP ≥12 mm Hg, MAP ≤70 mm Hg, PCWP ≥12 mm Hg, PVR ≥97 dynes/s/cm⁻⁵, PVRI ≥285 dynes/s/cm⁻⁵/m², RAP ≥6 mm Hg, SV ≤60 mL/beat, SVI ≤33

mL/m^2/beat, SVR ≥1200 dynes/s/cm^{-5}, SVRI ≥2390 dynes/s/cm^{-5}/m^2.

- Obtain, document, and report other findings indicating decreased cardiac output caused by myocardial dysfunction: HR ≤100 bpm; loss of sinus rhythm may be considered bradycardia for the immediate postoperative transplant; peripheral pulses ≤+2; capillary refill ≥3 seconds; distended neck vein; and peripheral edema.
- Monitor patient's volume status: intake, peripheral pulses +2, capillary refill ≤3 seconds, CVP 2 to 6 mm Hg, UO ≥30 mL/h or ≥0.5 mL/kg/h and specific gravity 1.010 to 1.030.
- Monitor continuous ECG to assess HR and rhythm. Document ECG rhythm strips every 2 to 4 hours in patients with dysrhythmias.
- Measure ECG components, as there are two sources of sinoatrial (SA) node stimulation. The native atria retain autonomic innervation so they can respond to sympathetic or parasympathetic stimuli. The donor SA node is unaffected by autonomic nervous stimulation or recipient SA node activity as it initiates the impulse that results in ventricular depolarization and contraction. The dissociation of the two SA nodes is reflected as the recipient P wave, which occurs independent of the donor P wave and QRS complex.
- Monitor tolerance to increased physical activity in the patient with a denervated heart. In early exercise the HR is unchanged. CO will increase as a result of preload augmented with increased venous return because of muscular activity. After several minutes of exercise, CO output will increase because of increased plasma catecholamines.
- Provide rewarming after surgery to decrease peripheral vasoconstriction and hypothermia.
- Administer prescribed blood products, colloid or crystalloid fluids to maintain adequate hydration: CVP 2 to 6 mm Hg and UO ≥30 mL/h.
- Notify physician should hypotension not respond to volume therapy or CVP be ≤2 mm

Hg. This may indicate the need for further inotropic therapy to increase contractility.

- Administer prescribed oxygen 2 to 4 L/min by means of nasal cannula, or fraction of inspired oxygen (F$_{IO_2}$) ≤50% by mask to maintain Pao$_2$ ≥80 mm Hg, Sao$_2$ ≥95%, or S$\bar{v}$o$_2$ ≥60%.
- Administer prescribed positive inotropes (dopamine or dobutamine) to maintain CO ≥4 L/min and CI ≥2.7 L/min/m^2 (see Table 1–10).
- Should pharmacological therapy be ineffective in increasing CO, prepare patient for intra-aortic balloon pump or cardiac assist device (see IABP, p. 254 or Cardiac assist device, p. 248.)

Potential Complication: Dysrhythmias. Dysrhythmias related to transection of the sympathetic and parasympathetic innervation secondary to the removal of the donor heart.

Expected Patient Outcome. Patient maintains rhythm appropriate for heart transplantation.

- Review results of postoperative ECG.
- Monitor continuous ECG to assess HR and rhythm. Document ECG rhythm strips every 2 to 4 hours in patients with dysrhythmias.
- Measure ECG components, as there are two sources of SA node stimulation. The native atria retain autonomic innervation, so they can respond to sympathetic or parasympathetic stimuli. The donor SA node is unaffected by autonomic nervous stimulation or recipient SA node activity as it initiates the impulse that results in ventricular depolarization and contraction. The dissociation of the two SA nodes is reflected as the recipient P wave, which occurs independent of the donor P wave and QRS complex.
- Monitor ECG and report the development of junctional rhythm, which results in bradycardia or hypotension. This is due to myocardial edema around the SA node.
- Obtain and report hemodynamic parameters reflecting changes in preload (PCWP ≥12 mm Hg), or afterload (SVR ≥1200

dynes/s/cm^{-5}), which may lead to hemodynamic instability.

- Obtain and report characteristics of the nonrejecting transplanted heart: donor HR at rest is increased and gradually increases with exercise to an average rate of 90 to 110 bpm. Recipient HR is low normal and increases with exercise to an average of 60 to 80 bpm. Arterial BP is normal at rest and increases with exercise as a result of increased SVR. Finally CO at rest is low normal and increases with exercise.
- Administer prescribed isoproterenol to increase the HR.
- Should pharmacological therapy be ineffective in increasing HR, prepare patient for temporary pacing.
- Should bradycardia be unresponsive to pharmacological therapy, prepare patient for atrial pacing.
- Administer prescribed IV fluids to maintain adequate circulating volume, since a denervated heart depends on a large SV to stretch myocardial fibers.
- Teach patient to take pulse before, during, and after exercises.

DISCHARGE PLANNING

The critical care nurse provides patient and significant other(s) with verbal or written discharge notes regarding the following subjects:

1. Medication's purpose, dosage, schedule, and side effects.
2. Instructions and guidelines pertaining to medication administration, diet, exercise, and self-monitoring technique for complications.
3. Any dietary restrictions such as low-sodium and low-saturated fat diet.
4. Physical activity program developed in consultation with cardiac rehabilitation and patient's cardiologist.
5. Need to report signs and symptoms of rejection to physician: fever, malaise, and fatigue.
6. Importance of keeping follow-up appointments and biopsy for approximately 6 weeks.

7. Importance of reporting any signs of infection.
8. Significance of continuing immunosuppressant therapy.

....

PART III: SUPPORTIVE PROCEDURES AND NURSING MANAGEMENT

....

■ HEMODYNAMIC MONITORING

(For related information see Part I: Acute myocardial infarction, p. 38; Acute chest pain, p. 1; Dysrhythmias, p. 184. Respiratory Deviations, Part I: Pulmonary embolism, p. 397. Multisystem Deviations, Part I: Sepsis, p. 772.)

Diagnostic Category and Length of Stay
None applicable.

Definition
Hemodynamic monitoring (HM) is the measurement of hemodynamic status, which provides qualitative information about intravascular volume, intracardiac pressure, blood flow, and oxygen consumption and delivery parameters. The performance of the heart as a pump is reflected by the cardiac output (CO), which is the amount of blood ejected from the heart per unit of time and is the product of stroke volume (SV) and heart rate (HR).

CARDIAC OUTPUT. CO refers to the rate at which blood is ejected by the heart and is expressed in liters per minute. Measurement of blood flow from one ventricle can be assumed to be the same for the other ventricle. CO measurement is a reflection of the systolic performance of the ventricle. To compare individual differences in CO in relation to body size, cardiac index (CI) is measured. Reduced CO values can be due to inadequate left ventricular filling or inadequate ventricular ejection. Elevated CO values at rest occur in hyperdynamic states, such as hyperthyroidism or early in the course of severe vasodilating conditions associated with sepsis or anaphylaxis.

STROKE VOLUME. The SV is the volume of blood ejected from the ventricle with each contraction. The three determinants of SV are preload, afterload, and myocardial contractility.

Preload. Preload is the amount of diastolic volume as the distending force that stretches the ventricles just before electrical excitation and contraction. The force of myocardial contraction is a function of initial myocardial muscle fiber length. The more the fibers are stretched, the more forcefully they contract. The length-tension relationship of cardiac muscle is known as Starling's law of the heart. The law states that an increase in left ventricular end-diastolic volume leads to increased pressure, with a subsequent increase in blood volume ejected during the contraction. Excessive stretch or volume can cause reduced contractility. Preload is used clinically as an index of ventricular volume and reflects ventricular end-diastolic pressure, or venous return to the heart.

Factors that increase preload include volume gain (excess intravenous fluid, blood products, and renal failure); Trendelenburg position; venous constriction (hypothermia or drugs such as epinephrine, norepinephrine, dopamine, or phenylephrine) and shock; or HR (bradycardia). Factors that decrease preload include volume loss (hemorrhage, diuresis, diaphoresis, vomiting, diarrhea, or third spacing); orthostatic hypotension; venous dilatation (hyperthermia, drugs such as nitroglycerin, nitroprusside, amrinone, calcium channel blockers) and shock; and HR (tachycardia).

There are clinical indicators used to measure preload. Right ventriclar diastolic (filling) pressure (RVEDP) is reflected by central venous pressure (CVP) and right atrial pressure (RAP). Left ventricular diastolic (filling) pressure (LVEDP) is reflected by left atrial pressure (LAP), pulmonary artery diastolic (PADP) and pulmonary capillary wedge pressure (PCWP).

Afterload. Afterload refers to the load the heart muscle must overcome to eject blood during contraction. Afterload is largely determined by aortic end-diastolic pressure, aortic distensibility, and peripheral vascular resistance. The heart's ability to contract is influenced by the amount of active pressure above the preload it must generate. With a smaller afterload, the heart is able to contract more rapidly. Likewise, against a large afterload, contraction is slower. This is referred to as the force-velocity relationship. A higher afterload requires greater myocardial work load, increased oxygen consumption, and decreased coronary blood flow. Factors that increase afterload are volume loss, arterial constriction caused by drugs (epinephrine, norepinephrine, dopamine, and phenylephrine) and shock, and atherosclerosis. Factors that decrease afterload are arterial dilatation caused by drugs (nitroprusside, nitroglycerin, amrinone, and calcium channel blockers) and shock.

There are clinical indicators used to measure afterload. Right ventricular afterload is evaluated by calculating pulmonary vascular resistance (PVR) and pulmonary vascular resistance index (PVRI). Left ventricular afterload is evaluated by calculating systemic vascular resistance (SVR) and systemic vascular resistance index (SVRI).

Contractility. Contractility is the intrinsic ability of the heart muscle to shorten or develop tension, both independent of variations in preload, and afterload.

Factors that increase contractility are increased preload, increased afterload, positive inotropes (beta stimulants and amrinone), oxygen supply (aerobic metabolism), and ≤40% loss of functional myocardium. Factors that decrease contractility are decreased preload, decreased afterload, negative inotropes (beta blockers or calcium antagonists), ionic environment (hyponatremia and hyperkalemia), oxygen supply (anaerobic metabolism), and $\geq 40\%$ loss of functional myocardium. Contractility cannot be evaluated directly. Inferences can be made about myocardial contractility from the following indicators: CI, ejection fraction (EF), left ventricular stroke work (LVSW), left ventricular stroke work index (LVSWI), right ventricular stroke work (RVSW), right ventricular stroke work index (RVSWI), stroke volume index (SVI), stroke work (SW), and stroke work index (SWI).

HEART RATE. The HR is the number of beats or contractions per minute and is controlled by the parasympathetic and sympathetic branches of the autonomic nervous system. Sympathetic stimulation causes an increased HR, whereas parasympathetic stimulation, dominant in the resting state, causes decreased HR. Increased HR with a constant SV causes increased CO. Tachycardia is associated with decreased CO, as diastolic time is shortened, leading to reduced coronary perfusion and ventricular filling time. Likewise, bradycardia decreases CO because of longer ventricular filling time, unless SV increases.

There are two approaches to hemodynamic monitoring. The first (indirect or noninvasive) method of hemodynamic monitoring includes measuring of arterial pressure by blood pressure (BP) cuff or Doppler test and measuring of CO by an echo Doppler device. Direct, or invasive, methods include pulmonary artery pressure monitoring, intra-arterial pressure monitoring, CVP monitoring, and LAP monitoring.

PULMONARY ARTERY PRESSURE (PAP) MONITORING. The multiple lumens of the pulmonary artery catheter provide a means to physiologically assess the intracardiac pressures. Assessment data obtained from the monitoring device include: CO, mixed venous oxygen saturation ($S\bar{v}o_2$), PAP, pul-

monary artery wedge pressure, PVR, PVRI, SVR, SVRI, SVI, left ventricular stroke volume index, and right ventricular stroke volume index.

Mixed venous oxygen saturation ($S\bar{v}o_2$). $S\bar{v}o_2$ reflects the balance between oxygen supply (Do_2) and demand (Vo_2). The $S\bar{v}o_2$ can also be measured continuously with a special pulmonary arterial (PA) catheter (Oximetrex).

Pulmonary artery pressure (PAP). The PA pressure wave form is divided into three phases: systolic, diastolic, and mean. The systolic phase signifies the rapid blood flow from the right ventricle into the PA. The PA systolic pressure normally is equal to right ventricular systolic pressure. The systolic peak of the PA pressure occurs after the QRS complex on the ECG. PADP is measured at the nadir immediately before systole. Causes of increased PAP values include volume overload, pulmonary hypertension or embolism, ventricular septal defect, left heart dysfunction (mitral stenosis or insufficiency, decreased left ventricular compliance or left ventricular failure), cardiac tamponade, constrictive pericarditis, pulmonary parenchymal disease, and positive-pressure breathing. Causes of decreased PAP values include hypovolemia, right ventricular failure, pulmonic stenosis, and shock.

Pulmonary capillary wedge pressure (PCWP, PAWP). The first positive deflection in the PAWP wave form is the A wave, which reflects left atrial contraction and corresponds to the PR interval on the ECG. The V wave represents bulging of the mitral valve during left ventricular systole and passive left atrial filling. The peak of the V wave occurs during the TP interval on the ECG. The mean PAWP can be measured at the end-expiration bisecting the A and V waves.

Causes of increased PCWP values include volume overload, pulmonary edema, left heart dysfunction, left ventricular failure, mitral stenosis or insufficiency, decreased left ventricular compliance, pulmonary embolism, chronic pulmonary obstructive disease, acute respiratory distress syndrome, hypoxemia, sepsis, cardiac tamponade, constrictive pericarditis, and positive-pressure breathing (IPEEP). Causes of decreased PCWP values are hypovolemia, shock, right ventricular failure, pulmonary stenosis, and pulmonary embolism.

Pulmonary vascular resistance (PVR). The PVR represents the resistance against which the right ventricle must pump to eject its volume. The resistance is created by the pulmonary arteries and arterioles.

Factors that increase PVR include mitral or aortic valve disease, left ventricular heart failure, hypoxia, chronic obstructive pulmonary disease, or pulmonary embolism. PVRI is a measure of PVR adjusted for body size.

Systemic vascular resistance (SVR). The SVR represents the resistance against which the left ventricle must pump to eject its volume. The resistance is created by the systemic arteries and arterioles.

Stroke volume index (SVI). SVI is the SV indexed to body surface area.

Left ventricular stroke work index (LVSWI). The LVSWI is the amount of work the left ventricle performs with each heartbeat.

Right ventricular stroke work index (RVSWI). The RVSWI is the amount of work the right ventricle does with each heartbeat.

CENTRAL VENOUS PRESSURE (CVP) MONITORING. The CVP measures the pressure within the superior vena cava, which represents the pressure in the right atrium. CVP is an important determinant of both venous return and CO. CVP is assessed to determine changes in right ventricular function and the adequacy of vascular volume. CVP decreases with bleeding, dehydration, drug-induced vasodilation, or vigorous diuresis. Increased CVP occurs with ventricular fail-

ure, acute cardiac tamponade, vasoconstriction, tricuspid stenosis or regurgitation, overtransfusion, or overhydration.

Right atrial pressure (RAP). The RAP is demonstrated by three positive deflections. The A wave reflects right atrial contraction (follows P wave on the ECG tracing); X descent follows the A wave and represents atrial relaxation; and C reflects positive deflection and results from tricuspid valve closure (follows QRS complex on the ECG).

Right ventricular pressure (RVP). The RVP reflects the pulsatile, pumping nature of the ventricle with a rapid rise to systolic pressure and a drop to a near zero during diastole. RVP is measured during catheter insertion only. The right ventricular systolic pressure is indirectly monitored via the PA systolic pressure, which should be the same as the peak right ventricular systolic pressure in the absence of pulmonary stenosis. Right ventricular systolic pressure is elevated in pulmonary hypertension, ventricular septal defects (VSD), and in pulmonary stenosis. Right ventricular diastolic pressure is elevated with right ventricular failure, acute cardiac tamponade, or constrictive pericarditis.

LEFT ATRIAL PRESSURE (LAP) MONITORING. The LAP is a direct measure of LVEDP and monitoring may be indicated in cardiac surgery or coronary artery bypass patients with significant pulmonary hypertension.

INTRA-ARTERIAL PRESSURE MONITORING. Intra-arterial pressure monitoring provides a continuous measurement of four parameters: systolic, diastolic, and mean arterial pressure and pulse pressure.

Systolic blood pressure (SBP). The SBP reflects the peak pressure generated by the left ventricle. It also reflects the compliance of the large arteries, the total peripheral resistance. SBP is a clinical indicator of the amount of work the left ventricle generates during systole. The SBP is determined by vascular tone, stroke volume, and peripheral resistance.

Diastolic blood pressure (DBP). The DBP represents the runoff of blood into the arterial system. It is determined by volume of blood in the arterial system, elasticity of the arterial system, and peripheral resistance. Coronary artery perfusion occurs during diastole so the slower the HR the longer the diastolic period, and the greater the fall in the diastolic pressure.

Mean arterial pressure (MAP). MAP refers to the average pressure in the arterial system during systole and diastole. The MAP reflects the driving or perfusion pressure and is determined by the volume of blood flow in the arterial system (CO) and the elasticity or resistance of the vessels (SVR). The MAP determines tissue perfusion. The myocardium of the left ventricle, which receives most of its blood flow during diastole, requires an arterial driving pressure of 60 to 80 mm Hg to maintain perfusion to the coronary arteries. When MAP decreases, coronary blood flow decreases.

Pulse pressure (PP). PP reflects SV and arterial compliance. Widened PP is associated with a decrease in peripheral resistance or increased SV. Narrowed PP is associated with an increase in peripheral resistance or decreased SV.

Patient Selection

INDICATIONS
- PAP monitoring: Indications for use of PAP monitoring include acute myocardial infarction complicated by left ventricular failure or cardiogenic shock; cardiogenic or noncardiogenic pulmonary edema; diagnosis and treatment of acute respiratory distress syndrome; vasoactive pharmacological support; perioperative fluid imbalance; acute respiratory failure in patients with chronic obstructive pulmonary disease; and septic and hypovolemic shock.
- CVP monitoring: Monitoring CVP is useful in patients with active bleeding, recent surgery, acute trauma, and heart transplantation.
- LAP monitoring: Indicated in cardiac surgical patients with critical pulmonary hypertension.
- Intra-arterial pressure monitoring: Intra-arterial pressure monitoring is indicated for critically ill patients with hypertension, hypotension, fluctuation in BP, arteriolar vasoconstriction or vasodilatation, or for frequent drawing of blood samples. Patients in shock states such as hypovolemic, cardiogenic, or septic can also be monitored.

CONTRAINDICATIONS. Recurrent sepsis or a hypercoagulable state.

Procedure

TECHNIQUE

PAP monitoring. Insertion of the radiopaque PA catheter is performed, with or without fluoroscopy, by means of percutaneous cannulation. The access sites most commonly used are the subclavian and jugular veins. The quadruple-lumen catheter is passed through a catheter sheath introducer to prevent damage to the balloon tip. The balloon is inflated in the right atrium and the catheter is carried by the blood flow into either the right or left division of the right or left PA. The catheter stops in the pulmonary vessel the same size as the inflated balloon. This is the PA wedge position, which can be measured when the balloon is inflated. The balloon is left in the deflated position except when obtaining a PAWP to prevent pulmonary tissue necrosis.

CVP monitoring. A CVP catheter can be inserted into the internal or external jugular, subclavian, or antecubital vein. CVP can be measured with a water manometer or with an electronic transducer in conjunction with PAP monitoring.

LAP monitoring. The LAP catheter is inserted into the left atrium during cardiac surgery and brought through the chest wall. Because patient is at risk for air or tissue emboli, an in-line air filter is added to the flush system to reduce the risk. The LAP wave form consists of an A wave (atrial systole), a C wave (valvular closure), and a V wave (signifying ventricular systole).

Intra-arterial pressure monitoring. Sites for intra-arterial catheterization include the radial, brachial, femoral, and dorsalis pedis arteries. The radial artery is most commonly used because it is readily accessible and collateral circulation of the hand distal to the site of cannulation is normally adequate.

The arterial wave form appears on the bedside monitor so that SBP, DBP, and MAP can be continuously observed. A normal arterial wave form consists of a sharp ascent during systole with a gradual descent during diastole. The downstroke has a dicrotic notch, indicating closure of the aortic value. The ascent during systole correlates with the QRS complex in the ECG. The dicrotic notch correlates with the T wave. Clinical conditions that influence arterial wave forms include hypertension, certain drugs, CO, and SVR. Mechanical factors that affect the wave form include overdamping, reflected as smaller wave forms than usual with a slow rise and decreased or absent dicrotic notch; catheter whip, shown as an erratic wave form; no wave form; or inability to obtain a wedge reading.

EQUIPMENT

PAP monitoring. Quadruple-lumen thermodilution catheter. One lumen terminates in the right atrium and is used for measuring RAP and CO. A second lumen terminates in the PA and is used for measuring PAP. The third terminates in the PA and is used to measure PCWP by inflating the balloon-tipped port with up to 1.5 milliliters of air. There is an additional proximal port that can be used to administer fluids and medications. The $S\bar{v}o_2$ thermodilution catheter includes the features of the triple lumen. The fiberoptic filament transmits light of selected wavelengths through the PA catheter and out through the

catheter tip in the PA. A second fiberoptic filament transmits the light back to a photodetector on the optical module. The venous saturation is displayed at a bedside module. The blood sample for calibrating the $S\bar{v}o_2$ catheter is obtained through the PA port. The system contains a transducer, an amplifier, and a display screen.

CVP monitoring. Consists of water manometer with a pressure transducer.

LAP monitoring. The system consists of a transducer, in-line air filter, and amplifier.

Intra-arterial pressure monitoring. There are five components that make up the direct intra-arterial pressure monitoring system: catheter, pressure tubing, intravenous solution, transducer, and a monitor.

Complications
- PAP monitoring. Some complications include infection, PA rupture, pulmonary thromboembolism, pulmonary infarction, dysrhythmias, bacteremic infective endocarditis, valve rupture, and air embolism. Mechanical complications are catheter kinking and intracardiac irritability.
- CVP monitoring: Complications consist of localized infection, atrial or ventricular dysrhythmias, right ventricular perforation, laceration of the vein, hydrothorax, brachial plexus injury, dysrhythmias, emboli, thrombophlebitis, hematoma at the insertion site, and pneumothorax.
- LAP monitoring: The patient is at risk for air or tissue emboli.
- Intra-arterial pressure monitoring: Complications include air embolism or sepsis.

NURSING MANAGEMENT: NURSING DIAGNOSES AND COLLABORATIVE PROBLEMS

Nursing Diagnoses
Common nursing goals for patients with hemodynamic monitoring are to maintain tissue perfusion, prevent infection, and prevent injury.

Altered peripheral and cardiopulmonary tissue perfusion related to interrupted blood flow secondary to PA catheter compromising circulation as a result of migration of PA catheter into a wedge position, local vascular thrombus, or overwedging of balloon.

Expected Patient Outcomes. Patient maintains adequate peripheral and cardiopulmonary tissue perfusion, as evidenced by normal PA wave form, respiratory rate (RR) 12 to 20 BPM, absence of dyspnea or tachypnea, regular sinus rhythm, absence of hemoptysis, absence of pleuritic chest pain, and normal skin color in digit distal to intra-arterial cannulation.

- Review results of chest roentgenogram for catheter placement.
- Monitor the cannulated extremity every hour for color, temperature, capillary refill, sensation, and blanching.
- Obtain, document, and report clinical findings reflecting decreased peripheral tissue perfusion resulting from obstructed intra-arterial catheter: numbness and absence of pulses in distal extremity, coolness, pallor or cyanosis of extremity, and capillary refill ≥3 seconds.
- Monitor PA wave form continuously and report if the wave form decreases and appears flattened. This can indicate a leak in the system, a loose or cracked transducer dome, stopcock turned wrong way, catheter tip occluded, or inadequate pressure in pressure bag.
- Check to be sure balloon is deflated except when measuring PCWP. Be cautious, as prolonged or frequent measurements can traumatize the vessel wall. Always allow passive deflation of the balloon and do not remove air with a syringe. Notify cardiologist should PA wave form remain in the wedge position after balloon deflation.
- Monitor clinical conditions where PADP may exceed PCWP by 5 mm Hg: hypoxia, acidosis, pulmonary emboli, lung disease, and pulmonary hypertension.

- Monitor PAP and PCWP at end-exhalation in presence of respiratory variations.
- Monitor changes in PA wave form when patient moves, turns, sits at side of bed, sits in a chair.
- Monitor and record indirect arterial pressure every 4 hours.
- Cleanse catheter insertion site and apply iodophor ointment or new sterile dressing, using unit standard.
- Administer prescribed analgesics to relieve pain.
- Should flushing lines not correct altered wave-form configuration or restore peripheral perfusion, prepare patient for discontinuation of the pressure line.
- Administer prescribed lidocaine, using unit standard, for patient with ventricular irritability.
- Instruct patient to report any pain in extremity distal to catheter insertion.

Infection, high risk for related to multiple lines or insertion site.

Expected Patient Outcomes. Patient is free of infection, as evidenced by normothermia; white blood count (WBC) ≤11,000 μL; negative cultures; absence of redness, tenderness, swelling, or drainage at catheter insertion site.

- Review results of WBC and cultures.
- Monitor temperature every 1 to 2 hours in patients who are febrile.
- Monitor catheter insertion site for redness.
- Obtain culture of any drainage from catheter insertion site.
- Apply povidine-iodine and alcohol to the catheter insertion site daily or use unit protocol.
- Change dressing per unit standard using aseptic technique.
- Change IV fluid, tubing, stopcocks, and disposable transducer every 48 to 72 hours as per unit standard.
- Flush arterial system with normal saline, not glucose. Glucose solution may promote growth of bacteria.

- Place sterile caps over the openings of the stopcocks.
- Instruct patient to report any tenderness at the insertion site.

Injury, high risk for related to intimal trauma or ventricular irritability from PA line secondary to arterial line.

Expected Patient Outcomes. Patient has no complications from intra-arterial, PA, or CVP catheter insertion, as evidenced by BP ≥90/60 mm Hg, HR ≤100 bpm, RR 12 to 20 BPM, normal sinus rhythm, partial pressure of arterial oxygen (Pao_2) ≥80 mm Hg, arterial oxygen saturation (Sao_2) ≥95%, absence of crackles, and absence of chest pain.

- Review results of chest roentgenogram and ECG.
- Obtain and report clinical findings suggestive of vessel intimal trauma: BP ≤90/60 mm Hg, HR ≥100 bpm, RR≥20 BPM, diminished or absent breath sounds, muffled heart sounds, or pulsus paradoxus.
- Monitor continuous ECG to assess HR and rhythm. Document ECG rhythm strips every 2 to 4 hours in patient with dysrhythmia.
- Restrain patient, if necessary, since a restless or confused patient may accidentally remove the catheter or disconnect the tubing.
- Administer prescribed oxygen 2 to 4 L/min by means of nasal cannula or mask to maintain Pao_2 ≥80 mm Hg and Sao_2 ≥95%.
- Administer prescribed prophylactic lidocaine to patients at risk for ventricular dysrhythmia: electrolyte imbalance, acidosis, or myocardial ischemia.
- Administer prescribed analgesics or narcotic to relieve pain.
- Instruct patient to report any pain at the catheter site.

■ PERCUTANEOUS TRANSLUMINAL CORONARY ANGIOPLASTY

(For related information see Part I: Acute myocardial infarction, p. 38; Acute chest pain, *p. 1; Acute cardiac tamponade, p. 117; Shock, p. 174; Dysrhythmias, p. 184. Part III: Coronary laser angioplasty, p. 228; Cardiac assist device, p. 248; Intra-aortic balloon pump, p. 254; Hemodynamic monitoring, p. 219.)*

Diagnostic Category and Length of Stay
DRG: 112 Percutaneous cardiovascular procedure
LOS: 4.80 days

Definition
Percutaneous transluminal coronary angioplasty (PTCA) is used to reestablish adequate blood supply to the myocardium by restoring the lumen diameter of a coronary artery using a balloon-tipped catheter, which is guided under fluoroscopy with a contrast medium. The PTCA is an effective method for improving symptoms and correcting the metabolic, hemodynamic, and functional consequences of myocardial ischemia in selected patients.

Patient Selection

INDICATIONS. PTCA is a treatment for occlusive coronary artery disease before myocardial infarction occurs and is an alternative to coronary artery bypass surgery. PTCA is also a viable treatment option for obstruction of grafted vessels. Other clinical indicators for PTCA are: single-vessel or multiple-vessel disease associated with recent onset of angina and clinical signs of ischemia with subtotal lesions not located at the orifice or bifurcation of a coronary artery. PTCA can also be used in conjunction with thrombolytic therapy in patients with angina of less than 6 hours and ECG evidence of evolving transmural myocardial infarction.

CONTRAINDICATIONS. PTCA is contraindicated in patients with severe diffuse coronary atherosclerosis. Other contraindications include the presence of central (aortic, iliac, etc.) and peripheral atherosclerosis because of the necessity to cannulate the femoral artery and pass a catheter into the aorta.

Procedure

TECHNIQUE. The PTCA involves the introduction of a guiding catheter and a double-lumen dilatation catheter into either the femoral or the brachial artery. The catheter is advanced to the affected coronary artery. Once the lesion is crossed, the balloon is inflated. This compresses the atherosclerotic plaque in an effort to increase the lumen diameter. Continuous pressure monitoring reveals blockage of the coronary artery and allows measurement of the pressure gradient across the lesion. Balloon inflations are repeated at intervals until reduction in the pressure gradient is ≤ 16 mm Hg. The patient receives intravenous heparin during the procedure. Intracoronary thrombolytic therapy may be administered to treat acute thrombosis formation local to the involved vessel.

Complications

Dysrhythmias; bleeding or hematoma; acute coronary occlusion; acute myocardial infarction; tear of the coronary vessel wall; dissection of coronary, aortic, iliac, or femoral arteries; inability to dilate the stenosis; embolization of the plaque fragment; hypersensitivity to the contrast medium; acute cardiac tamponade; cerebrovascular accident; and compromise of peripheral circulation.

NURSING MANAGEMENT: NURSING DIAGNOSES AND COLLABORATIVE PROBLEMS

Nursing Diagnoses

Common nursing goals for patients undergoing PTCA are to foster tissue perfusion, maintain adequate fluid volume, and relieve pain.

Altered peripheral tissue perfusion related to invasive sheath secondary to cannulation of femoral artery.

Expected Patient Outcomes. Patient maintains adequate peripheral tissue perfusion, as evidenced by absence of peripheral cyanosis, warm skin, resolution of peripheral edema, peripheral pulses +2, absence of pain at the insertion site, and capillary refill ≥ 3 seconds.

- Consult with physician should patient experience a loss of or change in the quality of peripheral pulses.
- Review coagulation studies and complete blood count (CBC).
- Limit activity to bed rest and place patient in reverse Trendelenburg position to promotion of blood flow to lower extremities. Be careful not to bend groin with sheath.
- Immobilize the cannulated extremity for 6 hours or until the sheath is removed.
- Monitor bilateral pedal pulse quality every 30 minutes four times, then every hour for 6 hours after the sheath has been removed.
- Assess extremity distal to the catheter insertion for findings reflective of decreased peripheral tissue perfusion: peripheral pulses $\leq +2$, skin color mottled or cyanotic, extremity cool, capillary refill ≥ 3 seconds, and sensorimotor change such as numbness or tingling in the extremity.
- Inspect sheath site for evidence of external or subcutaneous bleeding, redness, swelling, or irritation.
- Monitor catheter site for evidence of bleeding.
- Assist with the removal of the sheath by preparing the access site per protocol (local anesthesia, povidone-iodine preparation and suture removal).
- Remove catheter and apply direct pressure until hemostasis is achieved.
- Apply a pressure dressing, once the site is stable, and monitor the site plus peripheral pulses for quality.
- Monitor sheath patency and evaluate the effectiveness of continuous prescribed infusion into the involved vessel to maintain sheath patency.
- Administer prescribed anticoagulants.
- Instruct patient to report any bleeding from catheter site.
- Instruct patient to report numbness or pain, tingling or numbness, coolness, pallor or cyanosis in the affected extremity.

Fluid volume deficit related to bleeding secondary to injury of the cannulated femoral artery or concomitant anticoagulation.

Expected Patient Outcomes. Patient maintains normal volume status: Skin turgor normal; intake equal to output; cardiac output (CO) 4 to 8 L/min; cardiac index (CI) 2.7 to 4.3 L/min/m²; central venous pressure (CVP) 2 to 6 mm Hg; heart rate (HR) ≤100 bpm; urinary output (UO) ≥30 mL/h or ≥0.5 mL/kg/h; specific gravity 1.010 to 1.030; blood urea nitrogen (BUN) ≤20 mg/dL; serum electrolytes, serum creatinine, and coagulation profile within normal limits.

- Review serum creatinine, BUN, serum electrolytes, and coagulation profile.
- Monitor intake and output for 24 hours: UO ≥125 mL/h may be due to osmotic diuresis from contrast dye.
- Monitor for signs and symptoms of hypovolemia: dizziness, fatigue, anorexia, nausea, vomiting, weakness, thirst, confusion, or constipation.
- Monitor the patient for fluid volume deficit: CO ≤4 L/min, CI ≤2.7 L/min/m², CVP ≤2 mm Hg, orthostatic hypotension, increased HR, decreased UO, poor skin turgor, flat neck veins, increased temperature, and weight loss.
- Obtain and report findings that may signify femoral or iliac dissection: retroperitoneal ecchymosis or flank pain.
- Assess femoral insertion site every 15 to 30 minutes for oozing and hematoma formation.
- Administer prescribed IV fluids to maintain adequate hydration, CVP 2 to 6 mm Hg, UO ≥30 mL/h or ≥0.5 mL/kg/h, and specific gravity 0.010 to 1.030.
- Instruct patient to report any warmth in the groin or leg or sharp flank pain, reflecting blood flow from the cannula.

Pain related to hematoma formation at the percutaneous access site.

Expected Patient Outcome. Patient is free of pain.

- Review results of coagulation profile.
- Evaluate the patient's comfort every 1 to 2 hours for 12 to 24 hours.
- Should pain develop at the groin access site, assess for hematoma formation.
- Apply pressure dressing on the access site should a hematoma form.
- Administer prescribed analgesia for groin pain.

DISCHARGE PLANNING
The critical care nurse provides patient and significant other(s) with verbal or written discharge notes regarding the following subjects:

1. Need to report any discomfort in the cannulated extremity that might be postprocedure vasospasm.
2. Medications' purpose, dosage, schedule, and side effects.
3. Importance of reporting any chest pain to physician.

■ CORONARY LASER ANGIOPLASTY

(For related information see Part I: Acute myocardial infarction, p. 38; Acute chest pain, p. 1; Acute cardiac tamponade, p. 117; Shock, p. 174; Dysrhythmias, p. 184. Part III: Percutaneous transluminal coronary angioplasty, p. 226; Cardiac assist device, p. 248; Intraaortic balloon pump, p. 254; Hemodynamic monitoring, p. 219.)

Diagnostic Category and Length of Stay
DRG: 112 Percutaneous cardiovascular procedure
LOS: 4.80 days

Definition
Laser-assisted balloon angioplasty is an adjunct to percutaneous transluminal coronary angioplasty (PTCA) and coronary bypass surgery in the revascularization of

occluded vessels. Laser energy is used to ablate tissue and remove atheroma from the diseased arteries.

Patient Selection

INDICATIONS. Coronary laser angioplasty is used to open coronary atherosclerotic plaque obstruction and is based on the ability to transmit the laser through an optical fiber, to direct it precisely, and to use it for tissue photocoagulation. The coronary obstruction is vaporized and stenotic vessel widened as during PTCA.

CONTRAINDICATIONS. The contraindications for coronary laser angioplasty are the same as for PTCA.

Procedure

TECHNIQUE. The technique of laser angioplasty is similar to that of PTCA. When the access to the arterial system has been achieved, a flexible catheter is positioned at the site of the coronary occlusion. Rather than a balloon that is inflated, a laser beam is directed at the plaque until circulation is restored distal to the occlusion.

There are three laser techniques: laser angioplasty, laser-assisted balloon angioplasty, and thermal laser welding balloon angioplasty. Laser angioplasty is a technique in which free-beam or direct laser energy is used to remove atherosclerotic material from the lumen of a vessel. Laser energy only is used to create a hemodynamically improved luminal area. The degree of laser penetration of atherosclerotic plaque depends on the beam focus, the total energy delivered, duration of exposure, and density and absorptive characteristics of the atherosclerotic tissue. Laser-assisted balloon angioplasty involves laser energy in its free-beam format or indirectly in a hot-tip catheter. The laser makes a small opening through an arterial obstruction, which then allows for the passage of a guide wire

and placement of a balloon. The balloon is inflated the same as in PTCA. Thermal welding balloon angioplasty applies laser energy that radiates from the interior of the balloon and causes fusion of disrupted tissue elements. When the balloon deflates, a smooth lumen, the same size and shape as the balloon, is created. Laser recanalization of obstructed vessels can be approached in two ways: (1) Laser energy is passed through a semiflexible laser fiber using a percutaneous transluminal approach. (2) Direct laser application is used in laser-assisted endarterectomy.

EQUIPMENT. The laser catheter consists of an optical fiber attached to a mitral cap with a central extruding guide-wire tip. The common lasers are argon, carbon dioxide, and synthetic neodynium: yttrium-aluminum-garnet laser (Nd:YAG). Newer lasers undergoing investigation are excimer laser and SMART lasers. Finally, laser probes are used to control the laser beam that removes the sphere of plaque. They consist of a contact laser probe and spectraprobe.

Complications

Because high energy is directed at a vessel wall, perforation of the artery can occur during the procedure. There may be difficulty in resecting a significant volume of atherosclerotic plaque. Long-term complications include aneurysm formation, accelerated atherosclerosis, and intimal hyperplasia. Other complications include reocclusion of the vessel, coronary artery vasospasm, reperfusion dysrhythmias, or embolization.

NURSING MANAGEMENT: NURSING DIAGNOSES AND COLLABORATIVE PROBLEMS

Nursing Diagnoses

Common nursing goals for patients undergoing coronary laser angioplasty are to facilitate tissue perfusion and reduce fear.

Altered peripheral tissue perfusion related to obstruction in the limb distal to the site of vessel cannulation secondary to cannulation or embolization.

Expected Patient Outcomes. Patient maintains adequate peripheral tissue perfusion, as evidenced by cardiac output (CO) 4 to 8 L/min, peripheral pulses +2, capillary refill ≤3 seconds, absence of peripheral cyanosis or pallor distal to cannulation site, absence of extremity swelling, absence of extremity pain, and urinary output (UO) ≥30 mL/h or ≥0.5 mL/kg/h.

• Consult with cardiologist to validate expected patient outcomes used to evaluate whether peripheral tissue perfusion is adequate.
• Monitor cannulated extremity every 15 minutes and compare to other extremity: peripheral pulses, extremity color and warmth, extremity girth, presence of tenderness, and capillary refill.
• Obtain, document, and report clinical findings associated with decreased peripheral tissue perfusion: peripheral pulses ≤+2 or absent in the cannulated extremity, peripheral cyanosis or pallor distal to the cannulation site, capillary refill ≥3 seconds, cool skin, and increased girth of the cannulated extremity as a result of swelling, and presence of tenderness.
• Monitor the catheterization site for bleeding.
• Apply pressure to the catheterization site should bleeding occur and keep the limb immobilized until physician orders discontinuation.
• Change dressing using aseptic technique following agency standard.
• Administer prescribed anticoagulants, if not contraindicated, to enhance peripheral tissue perfusion.
• Instruct patient to report discomfort in the limb distal to the site of vessel cannulation.

Fear related to laser therapy and possibility of complications requiring surgery.

Expected Patient Outcome. Patient verbalizes concerns and fear regarding laser therapy.

• Confer with cardiologist regarding patient's fear and concerns.
• Assess factors contributing to patient's fear: unfamiliar environment, life-style changes, and biological changes.
• Reduce or eliminate factors contributing to patient's fear by orienting patient to the critical care environment, avoiding painful stimuli, removing threatening stimuli, and encouraging gradual mastery of tasks such as moving the once-tender extremity.
• Encourage patient to express feelings of hopelessness should a complication such as bleeding from the cannulation site or obstruction of the vessel distal to the cannulation occur.
• Encourage patient to confront the fear and use coping strategies to reduce fear should coronary laser angioplasty be ineffective.
• Teach patient stress-reduction techniques should there be extremity tenderness: progressive relaxation, meditation, or guided imagery.

Collaborative Problems

Common collaborative goals for patients undergoing coronary laser angioplasty are to increase CO and correct dysrhythmias.

Potential Complication: Decreased Cardiac Output. Decreased cardiac output related to complication of invasive procedure or bleeding as a result of anticoagulation.

Expected Patient Outcomes. Patient maintains adequate CO, as evidenced by coronary artery perfusion pressure (CAPP) 60 to 80 mm Hg, CO 4 to 8 L/min, cardiac index (CI) 2.7 to 4.3 L/min/m^2, central venous pressure (CVP) 2 to 6 mm Hg, mean arterial pressure (MAP) 70 to 100 mm Hg, pulmonary artery pressure (PAP) systolic 15 to 25 mm Hg or diastolic 8 to 15 mm Hg, pulmonary capillary wedge pressure (PCWP) 6 to 12 mm Hg, right atrial pressure (RAP) 4 to 6 mm Hg, mixed venous oxygen saturation (S$\bar{v}$o$_2$) 60% to 80%, blood pressure (BP) within patient's normal range, heart rate (HR) ≤100 bpm, UO

≥30 mL/h or 0.5 mL/Kg/h, normal sinus rhythm, serum enzymes within normal limits, peripheral pulses 2+, capillary refill ≤3 seconds, and absence of bleeding.

- Consult with cardiologist to validate expected patient outcomes used to evaluate whether CO is adequate.
- Review results of heart catheterization, coronary arteriogram, ECG, blood urea nitrogen (BUN), creatinine, serum electrolyte measurements, complete blood count (CBC), coagulation profile, or echocardiogram.
- Obtain and measure serum enzyme creatine kinase (CK-MB) after coronary laser angioplasty to evaluate altered myocardial tissue perfusion as a result of coronary artery obstruction.
- Limit activity immediately after angioplasty until limitation discontinued by physician.
- Obtain and report hemodynamic parameters reflecting decreased CO: CAPP ≤60 mm Hg, CO ≤4L/min, CI ≤2.7 L/min/m², CVP ≥6 mm Hg, MAP ≤70 mm Hg, PAP systolic ≥25 mm Hg or diastolic ≥15 mm Hg, PCWP ≥12 mm Hg, RAP ≥6 mm Hg, and S$\bar{v}o_2$ ≤60%.
- Assess, document, and report other findings suggestive of decreased CO related to bleeding: BP ≤90/60 mm Hg, HR ≥100 bpm, UO ≤30 mL/h or ≤0.5 mL/kg/h, peripheral pulses ≤+2, and capillary refill ≥3 seconds.
- Monitor patient continuously for bleeding at sheath insertion site, gums, or IV sites.
- Monitor continuous ECG to assess HR and rhythm. Document ECG rhythm strips every 2 to 4 hours in patients with dysrhythmias.
- Discontinue prescribed heparin and antiplatelet drugs should bleeding occur.
- Monitor daily weight, intake, specific gravity, and UO.
- Administer prescribed IV fluids to maintain adequate hydration, MAP 70 to 90 mm Hg, CVP 2 to 6 mm Hg, UO ≥30 mL/h or ≥0.5 mL/kg/h, or specific gravity 1.010 to 1.030.
- Administer prescribed oxygen 2 to 4 L/min by means of nasal cannula or mask to maintain Pao₂ ≥80 mm Hg.

- Should pharmacological therapy be ineffective and debris embolization critically impair CO, prepare patient for emergency coronary artery bypass graft (CABG) (see CABG, p. 194).
- Instruct patient to report any bleeding.

Potential Complication: Dysrhythmias. Dysrhythmias related to reperfusion.

Expected Patient Outcome. Patient is free of dysrhythmias.

- Review results of 12-lead ECG.
- Monitor continuous ECG to assess HR and rhythm. Document ECG rhythm strips every 2 to 4 hours in patients with dysrhythmias.
- Obtain and report re-stenosis dysrhythmias such as bradycardia, heart block, ventricular ectopy, tachycardia, or accelerated idioventricular rhythm.
- Obtain and report clinical findings associated with reperfusion dysrhythmias: HR ≤60 bpm or ≥100 bpm and SBP ≤90 mm Hg, changes in sensorium, cool and pale skin, and diaphoresis.
- Administer prescribed low-flow oxygen 2 to 4 L/min by nasal cannula or mask to maintain tissue oxygenation.
- Administer prescribed atropine should bradycardia develop.

■ PERCUTANEOUS LASER MYOPLASTY

(For related information see Part I: Acute myocardial infarction, p. 38; Acute chest pain, p. 1; Acute cardiac tamponade, p. 123; Hypertrophic cardiomyopathy, p. 112; Shock, p. 174; and Dysrhythmias, p. 184. Part III: Percutaneous transluminal coronary angioplasty, p. 226, Cardiac assist device, p. 248, Intra-aortic balloon pump, p. 254, Hemodynamic monitoring, p. 219.)

Diagnostic Category and Length of Stay
DRG 112: Percutaneous cardiovascular procedure
LOS: 4.80 days

Definition

Percutaneous laser myoplasty is a new treatment approach for obstructive hypertrophic cardiomyopathy. While experimental, it can be used in nonsurgical patients. The procedure can result in reduced intraventricular septal wall contractility and thickness, and increased systolic left ventricular outflow tract dimensions. The patient can experience several outcomes such as a decrease in gradient, systolic obstruction and symptoms.

Patient Selection

INDICATIONS. Percutaneous laser myoplasty is used in patients who are refractory to medical therapy, have persistent symptoms, are a poor surgical risk, or desire an alternative therapy to surgery.

CONTRAINDICATIONS. None known.

Procedure

TECHNIQUE. A Nd: YGA (Neodynmium, yttrium-aluminum-garnet) laser can be used to create a well defined myocardial trough with the laser energy. The myoplasty catheter is advanced through the guidewire catheter and situated in the left ventricular myocardium. A pressure gradient (difference in pressure above and below the area of hypertrophy) is measured by simultaneously recording the central arterial pressure and the pressure in the ventricle below the area of hypertrophy.

EQUIPMENT. A Nd: YGA catheter, a temporary transvenous pacing wire (because the septum becomes the focus area for the laser therapy placing the patient at risk for developing a heart block) and a pulmonary artery thermodilution catheter.

Complications

Because high energy is directed at the septum, perforation of the septum, perforation of the myocardium, dysrhythmia, and bleeding may occur.

NURSING MANAGEMENT: NURSING DIAGNOSES AND COLLABORATIVE PROBLEMS

Common nursing goals in patients undergoing percutaneous laser myoplasty are to reduce anxiety.

Anxiety related to laser therapy and potential complications associated with the procedure.

Expected Patient Outcome. Patient verbalizes concerns and benefits of laser therapy.

- Confer with cardiologist regarding patient's anxious behaviors regarding laser therapy.
- Assess patient's understanding of the procedure and clarify misconceptions.
- Monitor the patient for signs and symptoms of anxiety including increased heart rate, increased blood pressure, nervousness and tearfulness.
- Encourage patient to express feelings of hopelessness should a complication such as bleeding from the cannulation site or dysrhythmia occur.
- Explain the rationale for preoperative testing and postoperative procedures.
- Encourage patient to confront the fear and use coping strategies to reduce fear should coronary laser angioplasty be ineffective.
- Instruct patient as to stress reduction techniques should there be extremity tenderness: progressive relaxation, meditation, or guided imagery.

Collaborative Problems

Common collaborative goals in patients undergoing percutaneous laser myoplasty are to increase cardiac output and correct dysrhythmias.

Potential Complication: Decreased Cardiac Output. Decreased cardiac output related to perforation of myocardium or bleeding due to anticoagulation.

Expected Patient Outcomes. Patient maintains adequate cardiac output, as evidenced by CAPP 60 to 80 mm Hg CO 4 to 8 L/min, CI 2.7 to 4.3 L/min/m^2, CVP 2 to 6 mm Hg, MAP

70 to 100 mm Hg, PAP systolic 15 to 25 mm Hg or diastolic 8 to 15 mm Hg, PCWP 6 to 12 mm Hg, RAP 4 to 6 mm Hg, SṽO₂ 60% to 80%, BP within patient's normal range, HR ≤100 bpm, UO ≥30 mL/hr or 0.5 mL/Kg/hr, normal sinus rhythm, serum enzymes within normal limits, peripheral pulses 2+, capillary refill ≤3 seconds and absence of bleeding.

- Consult with cardiologist to validate expected patient outcomes used to evaluate whether or not cardiac output is adequate.
- Review results of heart catheterization, coronary arteriogram, ECG, BUN, creatinine, serum electrolytes, CBC, coagulation profile, or echocardiogram.
- Assess for signs and symptoms of septal rupture: shortness of breath, hypoxemia, holosystolic murmur, hypotension and cyanosis.
- Limit activity immediately after angioplasty until discontinued by patient's physician.
- Obtain and report hemodynamic parameters reflecting decreased cardiac output: CAPP ≤60 mm Hg, CO ≤ 4L/min, CI ≤2.7 L/min/m², CVP ≥6 mm Hg, MAP ≤70 mm Hg, PAP systolic ≥25 mm Hg or diastolic ≥15 mm Hg, PCWP ≥12 mm Hg, RAP ≥6 mm Hg, and SṽO₂ ≤60%.
- Assess, document and report other findings suggestive of decreased cardiac output related to bleeding: BP ≤90/60 mm Hg, HR ≥100 bpm, UO ≤30 mL/h or ≤0.5 mL/kg/h, peripheral pulses ≤+2, and capillary refill ≥3 sec.
- Monitor patient continuously for bleeding at sheath insertion site, gums or IV sites.
- Monitor continuous ECG to assess heart rate and rhythm. Document ECG rhythm strips every 2 to 4 hours in patients with dysrhythmias.
- Discontinue prescribed heparin and antiplatelet drugs should bleeding occur.
- Monitor daily weight, intake, specific gravity and urinary output.
- Administer prescribed IV fluids to maintain adequate hydration, MAP 70 to 90 mm Hg, CVP 2 to 6 mm HG, UO ≥30 mL/h or ≥0.5 mL/kg/h or specific gravity 1.010 to 1.030.

- Administer prescribed oxygen 2 to 4 L/min by means of nasal cannula or mask to maintain Pao² ≥80 mm Hg.
- Should septal rupture occur, prepare the patient for Intra-aortic balloon pump (see IABP, p. 254).
- Instruct patient to report any bleeding.

Potential Complication: Dysrhythmias. Dysrhythmias related to damage of the atrial-ventricular node secondary to injury of the septum.

Expected Patient Outcome. Patient is free of dysrhythmias.

- Review results of 12-lead ECG.
- Monitor continuous ECG to assess heart rate and rhythm. Document ECG rhythm strips every 2 to 4 hours in patients with dysrhythmias.
- Obtain and report dysrhythmias such as heart block or ventricular ectopy.
- Obtain and report clinical findings associated with reperfusion dysrhythmias: HR ≤60 bpm or ≥100 bpm and SBP ≤90 mm Hg, changes in sensorium, cool and pale skin, and diaphoresis.
- Administer prescribed low flow oxygen 2 to 4 L/min by nasal cannula or mask to maintain tissue oxygenation.
- Administer prescribed antidysrhythmia agents (see Table 1–12, p. 60).
- Monitor the effectiveness of pacemaker activity should heart block occur.
- Report dysrhythmias that initiate pacemaker activity.
- Teach the patient the possible reasons for atrial-ventricular (A-V) dysrhythmia because of the proximity of the A-V node to the myoplasty trough.

DISCHARGE PLANNING
The critical care nurse provides the patient and significant other(s) with verbal or written discharge notes regarding the following areas:

1. Importance of reporting any chest pain to physician.

2. Importance of keeping outpatient appointment.
3. Discuss medication's purpose, schedule or side effects should any be prescribed.

■ TRANSLUMINAL CORONARY ATHERECTOMY

(For related information see Part I: Acute chest pain, p. 1; Acute myocardial infarction, p. 38; Acute cardiac tamponade, p. 117; Shock, p. 174; Dysrhythmias, p. 184. Part II: Coronary artery bypass graft, p. 194. Part III: Percutaneous transluminal coronary angioplasty, p. 226; Hemodynamic monitoring, p. 219.)

Diagnostic Category and Length of Stay
DRG: 112 Percutaneous cardiovascular procedure
LOS: 4.80 days

Definition
Transluminal coronary atherectomy employs of a catheter similar to that in percutaneous transluminal coronary angioplasty (PTCA) under direct fluoroscopy to remove an atheromatous plaque with either a rotating cutter blade system or a high-speed rotary device. The device is positioned toward the lesion and the plaque is shaved away.

Patient Selection

INDICATIONS. The lesion should be accessible in the proximal or midleft anterior descending (LAD) coronary artery or be a proximal lesion of the left circumflex coronary artery. The patient should be a candidate for coronary artery bypass graft (CABG), a single-vessel lesion, discrete subtotal stenotic lesion, and with a stenosis of a vessel that has previously undergone PTCA. A vessel's size should be 3.0 to 3.5 mm in diameter and ≤10 mm in length.

CONTRAINDICATIONS. The procedure is contraindicated in patients with a left coronary artery lesion, a calcified aorta, tortuous coronary vessel, or patient who is not in good condition for CABG.

Procedure

TECHNIQUE. The atherectomy catheter is inserted under direct fluoroscopy. A percutaneous femoral approach is used. A guide catheter is advanced with an introducer and once it's in place, the atherectomy device is advanced. The rotating cutter blade system shears layers of the atheromatous plaque. Several cuts may be needed to remove the plaque. The high-speed rotary device pulverizes the atheromatous plaque. The lesion is removed via a suction device, which prevents embolization. The procedure may be used in conjunction with PTCA before or after the atherectomy. The sheath is left in place in the femoral artery until removed by the physician.

EQUIPMENT. There are four types of atherectomy devices. The first, the Simpson atherectomy catheter, is a double-lumen catheter with a rotating cutting blade. The second, the Auth atherectomy catheter, is a single-lumen catheter with a rotating abrasive tip that is a diamond-coated brass burr. The third device, the Kensey catheter, has a single lumen with a rotating metallic cam at the distal tip. The device uses fluid under pressure and projects a fine jet spray that is directed against the artery wall. Finally, the transluminal extraction catheter has a motorized stainless steel cutting head mounted on a flexible torque tube with a moveable guide wire and vacuum to retrieve the atheromatous fragments. The latter two devices are experimental.

Complications
Complications consist of inability to cross the lesion with the catheter, dissection of the

coronary artery, perforation of the vessel, distal embolization, spasm, acute thrombolytic occlusion, hypotension, ischemia, hemorrhage, infection, acute myocardial infarction, and dysrhythmias.

NURSING MANAGEMENT: NURSING DIAGNOSES AND COLLABORATIVE PROBLEMS

Nursing Diagnoses

Common nursing goals for patients undergoing transluminal coronary atherectomy are to increase cardiopulmonary tissue perfusion, maintain fluid volume, reduce anxiety, and relieve pain.

Altered cardiopulmonary tissue perfusion related to acute dissection of the coronary artery.

Expected Patient Outcomes. Patient maintains adequate cardiopulmonary tissue perfusion, as evidenced by coronary artery perfusion pressure (CAPP) 60 to 80 mm Hg, mean arterial pressure (MAP) 70 to 100 mm Hg, blood pressure (BP) within patient's normal range, heart rate (HR) $\leq$100 bpm, mixed venous oxygen saturation ($S\bar{v}o_2$) 60% to 80%, warm skin, absence of cyanosis, and absence of chest pain.

- Obtain and report clinical findings suggesting altered cardiopulmonary tissue perfusion: hypotension, tachycardia, cool and pale skin, and chest pain.
- Monitor and report CAPP $\leq$60 mm Hg and $S\bar{v}o_2$ $\leq$60%, which indicates reduced coronary artery perfusion and decreased oxygen supply.
- Monitor continuous ECG to assess heart rate and rhythm. Document ECG rhythm strips every 2 to 4 hours in patients with dysrhythmias.
- Administer prescribed oxygen 2 to 4 L/min by nasal cannula or mask to provide oxygenation.

- Administer prescribed IV fluids to maintain adequate circulatory volume.
- Should acute dissection of the coronary artery occur, provide postoperative CABG care (see CABG, p. 194).

Fluid volume deficit, high risk for related to bleeding secondary to perforation of the vessel or vascular injury at the cannulation site.

Expected Patient Outcomes. Patient maintains adequate fluid volume, as evidenced by absence of bleeding at the insertion site, intact cannulated vessel, peripheral pulses +2, capillary refill $\leq$3 seconds, and coagulation studies within normal range.

- Consult with cardiologist about when the sheath will be removed.
- Review results of coagulation studies.
- Restrict patient to bed rest with the affected groin area strengthened so not to bend the sheath until it is removed or until physician orders increased activity.
- Obtain and report findings reflecting fluid volume deficit: BP$\leq$90/60 mm Hg, heart rate (HR) $\geq$100 bpm, peripheral pulses $\leq$+2, and cool and clammy extremity.
- Monitor the cannulation site every 15 minutes for 1 to 2 hours for bleeding.
- Should bleeding occur from the cannulation site, apply pressure and report finding to cardiologist.
- Monitor continuous ECG to assess HR and rhythm. Document ECG rhythm strips every 4 hours if patient develops chest pain or dysrhythmia after the procedure.
- When sheath is removed, apply pressure to the insertion site for at least 30 minutes to decrease bleeding.
- Monitor pulses distal to the site at frequent intervals.
- Observe the color and temperature of the involved extremity.
- Should bleeding occur, consult with the physician about temporarily discontinuing anticoagulation.

- Apply pressure to insertion site should bleeding occur.
- Administer prescribed IV fluids to maintain adequate hydration and urinary output (UO)≥ 30 mL/h.
- Instruct patient to report and bleeding at the insertion site.

Anxiety related to the atherectomy procedure and future implications regarding potential re-stenosis of the treated coronary artery.

Expected Patient Outcomes. Patient experiences reduced anxious behavior and expression of anxiety.

- Encourage patient to verbalize fear and anxieties about the need for further invasive treatments such as PTCA or CABG.
- Answer questions about postoperative care and need to keep the cannulated extremity immobilized until the sheath is removed.
- Provide support regarding the new technologies and allow patient to talk with others who have experienced the same procedure.
- Instruct patient to report any discomfort at the cannulation site.
- Teach patient stress-reducing techniques: progressive relaxation, meditation, or guided imagery.

Pain related to coronary atherectomy or acute myocardial infarction.

Expected Patient Outcome. Patient experiences minimal discomfort.

- Should chest pain occur, obtain an ECG immediately and notify physician.
- Place the cannulated extremity in a position of comfort for patient.
- Encourage patient to verbalize discomfort after the procedure.
- Note the duration, location, gravity, and radiation of chest pain.
- Monitor and report chest pain, diaphoresis, shortness of breath, nausea, HR ≥100 bpm, and RR ≥20 BPM indicating acute myocardial infarction.

- Monitor and report extremity tenderness, peripheral pulses ≤+2, pallor or cyanosis in cannulated extremity, capillary refill ≥3 seconds, and swelling in the cannulated extremity, indicating cannulated vessel injury.
- Administer prescribed analgesics to relieve pain.
- Instruct patient to report chest pain.

(For additional nursing diagnoses see Coronary laser angioplasty: **Altered peripheral tissue perfusion,** *p. 322.)*

Collaborative Problems

Common collaborative goals for patients undergoing transluminal coronary atherectomy are to increase cardiac output and correct dysrhythmias.

Potential Complication: Decreased Cardiac Output. Decreased cardiac output related to myocardial injury secondary to dissection of the coronary artery.

Expected Patient Outcomes. Patient maintains adequate CO, as evidenced by CAPP 60 to 80 mm Hg, cardiac output (CO) 4 to 8 L/min, cardiac index (CI) 2.7 to 4.3 L/min/m^2, mean arterial pressure (MAP) 70 to 100 mm Hg, absence of chest pain, BP within the patient's normal range, HR ≤100 bpm, respiratory rate (RR) 12 to 20 BPM, capillary refill ≤3 seconds, peripheral pulses +2, regular sinus rhythm.

- Consult with cardiologist to validate expected patient outcomes used to evaluate CO.
- Consult with cardiologist about criteria used to evaluate a successful procedure: a reduction of stenosis of 20%, residual stenosis ≤50%, successful tissue removal, and no major complications of acute myocardial infarction, CABG, or death.
- Obtain and report hemodynamic parameters indicating decreased CO: CAPP ≤60 mm Hg, CO ≤ 4L/min, CI ≤2.7 L/min/m^2, and MAP ≤70 mm Hg.

- Monitor BP, HR, and RR every 15 minutes for 1 to 2 hours, then every 2 to 4 hours while patient experiences chest pain.
- Obtain, document, and report other findings reflecting decreased CO: peripheral pulses $\leq +2$; capillary refill ≥ 3 seconds; HR ≥ 100 bpm; RR ≥ 20 BPM; cool, clammy skin; diaphoresis; and chest pain.
- Monitor continuous ECG to assess HR and rhythm. Document ECG rhythm strips every 1 to 2 hours in patients with chest pain and dysrhythmias associated with coronary occlusion during or after coronary atherectomy.
- Evaluate the cannulation site for evidence of bleeding or tenderness.
- Administer prescribed oxygen 2 to 4 L/min by means of nasal cannula or mask to relieve chest pain and maintain arterial oxygen saturation (Sao_2) $\geq 95\%$.
- Administer prescribed IV fluids to maintain adequate circulating volume.
- Administer prescribed analgesics to relieve pain.
- Administer prescribed antidysrhythmia agents to correct dysrhythmias (see Table 1–11).
- Administer prescribed inotropes (dopamine or dobutamine) to maintain adequate CO (see Table 1–10).
- Should coronary atherectomy be ineffective in removing the atheromatous plaque or complications occur, prepare patient for CABG (see CABG, p. 194).
- Instruct patient to report any chest pain (chest pain could indicate acute closure of the coronary artery).
- Instruct patient as to life-style changes that can reduce the potential for re-stenosis: smoking cessation; low-fat, low-cholesterol diet; stress reduction; and exercise.

Potential Complication: Dysrhythmias. Dysrhythmias related to decreased coronary perfusion secondary to damaged vessel.

Expected Patient Outcome. Patient maintains regular sinus rhythm.

- Monitor continuous ECG to assess HR and rhythm. Document ECG rhythm strips every 1 to 2 hours in patients with chest pain and dysrhythmias associated with coronary occlusion during or after coronary atherectomy.
- Obtain and report clinical findings that may be associated with dysrhythmias: hypotension, tachycardia, shortness of breath, lightheadedness, fatigue, and chest pain.
- Administer prescribed oxygen 2 to 4 L/min by nasal cannula or mask to oxygenate tissue.
- Administer prescribed IV fluids to maintain adequate circulating volume and serve as a port for antidysrhythmia agents.
- Administer prescribed antidysrhythmia agents to correct dysrhythmias (see Table 1–11).
- Should pharmacological therapy be ineffective in correcting dysrhythmias, prepare patient for pacemaker (see Pacemakers, p. 270).

DISCHARGE PLANNING
The critical care nurse provides patient and significant other(s) with verbal or written discharge notes regarding the following subjects:

1. Implications of reporting any chest pain to physician.
2. Any prescribed medication's purpose, dosage, schedule, or side effects.

■ INTRACORONARY STENT

(For related information see Part I: Acute chest pain, p. 1; Acute myocardial infarction, p. 38; Shock, p. 174; Dysrhythmias, p. 184. Part II: Coronary artery bypass graft, p. 194. Part III: Percutaneous transluminal coronary angioplasty, p. 226; Hemodynamic monitoring, p. 219.)

Diagnostic Category and Length of Stay
DRG: 112 Percutaneous cardiovascular procedure
LOS: 4.80 days

Definition

The intracoronary stent is a wire device designed to support the coronary artery and prevent acute stenosis after percutaneous transluminal coronary angioplasty (PTCA). The intracoronary stent is used to oppose recoil of elastic vascular stenosis after balloon angioplasty has failed to do so, and it provides a framework or scaffold for arterial lesions that may dissect or embolize after balloon angioplasty.

Patient Selection

INDICATIONS. Intracoronary stent may be used in patients with a high (20% to 40%) vessel reocclusion rate after PTCA.

CONTRAINDICATIONS. None.

Procedure

TECHNIQUE. The delivery system by means of a standard balloon positions the stent at the lesion site, where it is released. The stent expands and improves the vessel's intraluminal diameter. In general, the intracoronary stent is compressed to a small diameter in a delivery catheter. There are three approaches to providing intracoronary stents. The first, a spring-loaded stent, is a stainless steel device of small diameter that opens inside the target vessel when the catheter or containing sleeve is released. The specific diameter achieved after release is the result of an equilibrium between the elastic recoil of the vessel wall and the elasticity of the stent after expansion. The second, the thermal memory stent, is a thermally expandable coil made of nickel that is able to alter its configuration when it comes in contact with warm blood or saline. Last, the balloon-expandable stent is placed over any balloon delivery system. The stent is a stainless steel tube with its walls etched into multiple rows of staggered rectangles. The stent is expanded after delivery to the site by expanding the balloon, which embeds the

stent the vessel wall. When the balloon is deflated and removed, the stent remains in place, holding the vessel open.

EQUIPMENT. The three types of stents, the spring-loaded, thermal memory, and balloon-expandable stent are described above.

Complications

Complications of intracoronary stents are bleeding, acute chest pain, dysrhythmias, or embolus or claudication.

NURSING MANAGEMENT: NURSING DIAGNOSES AND COLLABORATIVE PROBLEMS

Nursing Diagnoses

A common nursing goal for patients undergoing intracoronary stent is to maintain tissue perfusion.

Altered cardiopulmonary and peripheral tissue perfusion related to coronary artery spasm, thrombi, dissection of the lumen, acute cardiac tamponade, or bleeding at the cannulation site secondary to traumatic procedure.

Expected Patient Outcomes. Patient maintains adequate myocardial tissue perfusion, as evidenced by coronary artery perfusion pressure (CAPP) 60 to 80 mm Hg, arteriovenous oxygen content difference ($C[a-v]o_2$) 4 to 6 mL/100mL, oxygen supply (Do_2) 900 to 1200 mL/min, oxygen supply index (Do_2I) 500 to 600 mL/min/m^2, mean arterial pressure (MAP) 70 to 100 mm Hg, oxygen utilization coefficient (O_2ER)25%, arterial oxygen saturation (Sao_2) $\geq$95%, rate pressure product (RPP) $\leq$12,000, mixed venous oxygen saturation ($S\bar{v}o_2$) 60% to 80%, heart rate (HR) $\leq$100 bpm, systemic vascular resistance (SVR) 900 to 1200 dynes/s/cm^{-5}, (SVRI) 1970 to 2390 dynes/s/cm^{-5}/m^2, absence of peripheral edema, absence of mottling or cyanosis, skin warm, systemic vascular resistance capillary refill index $\leq$3 seconds, and peripheral pulses +2 in both extremities.

- Consult with cardiologist to validate expected patient outcomes used to evaluate cardiopulmonary and peripheral tissue perfusion.
- Confer with cardiologist as to the specific intracoronary stent used: Spring-loaded stents may have a tendency to underexpand, leading to migration or thrombus, whereas overexpansion leads to thrombus and excessive intimal proliferation.
- Consult with cardiologist about precatheterization preparation: aspirin, dipyridamole, or nifedipine; 1 L low-molecular weight Dextran 2 hours before stenting; nitroglycerin drip and typed blood in the event emergency surgery is required.
- Confer with cardiologist as to the potential for bleeding based on events occurring during intracoronary stenting.
- Review test results: hemoglobin, hematocrit, coagulation profile, and coronary angiography.
- Review results of coronary angiography and coronary arteriography.
- Restrict physical activity to bed rest to decrease myocardial tissue oxygen demand should there be decreased myocardial tissue perfusion.
- Obtain and report hemodynamic parameters reflective of altered cardiopulmonary tissue perfusion: $C(a-v)o_2 \geq 6$ mL/100mL, CAPP ≤ 60 mm Hg, $Do_2 \leq 900$ mL/min, $Do_2I \leq 500$ mL/min/m^2, MAP ≤ 70 mm Hg, $O_2ER \geq 25\%$, RPP $\geq 12,000$, and $S\bar{v}o_2 \leq 60\%$.
- Obtain, document, and report other findings suggestive of decreased myocardial tissue perfusion: chest pain, capillary refill ≥ 3 seconds, pallor, diaphoresis, BP ≤ 90 mm Hg, or diaphoresis.
- Obtain, document, and report findings reflective of acute cardiac tamponade: Beck's triad (arterial hypotension, muffled heart sound, and increased central venous pressure); a systolic-to-diastolic gradient (pulse pressure [PP]) ≤ 30 mm Hg; neck vein distention; bluish discoloration of the skin in the upper chest or face; and Kussmaul's sign, which is present when patient is lying with head of bed at a 60-degree angle and the neck veins distend on inspiration, indicating increased left atrial pressure (LAP).
- Obtain and report the presence of pulsus paradoxus, which occurs in cardiac tamponade: a decline of systolic arterial pressure with normal inspiration that is absent if patient's pressure is ≤ 50 mm Hg. During inspiration, the diaphragm descends and exerts traction on the fluid-filled pericardial sac. The movement restricts left ventricular function, which decreases systolic blood pressure and stroke volume.
- Obtain, document, and report parameters reflecting the need for intrapericardial fluid removal: central venous pressure (CVP) ≥ 20 cm H$_2$O, pulsus paradoxus ≥ 20 mm Hg, and PP ≤ 20 mm Hg.
- Monitor continuous ECG to assess HR and rhythm. Document ECG rhythm strips every 2 to 4 hours if acute cardiac tamponade is suspected: observe for changes such as electrical alternans, which is alternating large and small QRS complexes or altered direction of the complexes, low voltage, and flat or inverted T waves or sinus tachycardia.
- Monitor perfusion indicators in the affected limb: peripheral pulses, temperature, skin color, and sensation every 30 minutes four times, then every 2 hours.
- Obtain and report findings reflecting decreased peripheral tissue perfusion resulting from embolus or claudication: cool, mottled skin; peripheral pulses in cannulated limb $\leq 2+$; numbness of the cannulated limb; and decreased motility of toes in the cannulated limb.
- Monitor catheter site for signs of external or subclavian bleeding: swelling, tenderness, or blood on dressing.
- Position sandbag on insertion site until discontinued by physician.

- Maintain immobilization of the involved limb until discontinued by physician.
- Administer prescribed IV fluid such as blood products, colloids, or crystalloids to increase cardiac output (CO) $\geq$4 L/min, cardiac index (CI) $\geq$2.7 L/min/m^2, and urinary output (UO) $\geq$30 mL/h or $\geq$0.5 mL/kg/h after intrapericardial pressure is reduced.
- Administer prescribed oxygen 2 to 4 L/min by means of nasal cannula or mask or fraction of inspired oxygen (FIO$_2$) $\leq$50% to maintain SaO$_2$ $\geq$95%.
- Assist with pericardiocentesis to aspirate excess pericardial fluid from the pericardium by the subxiphoid or left parasternal approach: monitor ECG for elevated ST and PR segment, premature atrial contraction (PAC), or premature ventricular contraction (PVC).
- Administer positive inotropes (dopamine or dobutamine) to maintain MAP 70 to 90 mm Hg, HR $\leq$100 bpm, BP within patient's normal range, and UO $\geq$30 mL/h (see Table 1–10).
- Administer prescribed anticoagulant, if not contraindicated, when decreased peripheral tissue perfusion is caused by embolism (see Table 1–8).
- Teach patient to report the presence of chest pain.
- Instruct patient to report any numbness, tingling, or pain in the affected limb.
- Instruct patient to keep the sandbag in place until discontinued.

DISCHARGE PLANNING

The critical care nurse provides patient and significant other(s) with verbal or written discharge notes regarding the following subjects:

1. Importance of reporting any chest pain to physician.
2. Importance of keeping outpatient appointments.
3. Any prescribed medications' purpose, dosage, schedule, and side effects.

■ CARDIOPULMONARY BYPASS SURGERY

(For related information see Part I: Acute chest pain, p. 1; Acute myocardial infarction, p. 38; Acute cardiac tamponade, p. 117; Shock, p. 174; Dysrhythmias, p. 184. Part III: Coronary laser angioplasty, p. 226; Cardiac assist device, p. 248; Intra-aortic balloon pump, p. 254; Hemodynamic monitoring, p. 219.)

Diagnostic Category and Length of Stay
DRG: 112 Percutaneous cardiovascular procedure
LOS: 4.80 days

Definition
Cardiopulmonary bypass (CPB) is a method by which venous blood is diverted from the arrested heart's right atrium to pass through either a membrane or a bubble oxygenator. The CPBS is intended to decrease myocardial work while providing systemic hemodynamic support.

Patient Selection

INDICATIONS. Patients who might benefit from CPB surgery are those: at risk for coronary angioplasty as a prophylactic measure to provide hemodynamic stability; with left ventricular dysfunction and ejection fraction of $\leq$25%, who are at high risk for percutaneous transluminal coronary angioplasty (PTCA) because they can't tolerate minimal balloon inflation; who require dilation of a lesion in the vessel that supplies most of the functional left ventricle; with presence of myocardial ischemia with episodes of unstable angina or a positive stress test; in advanced age; with a history of previous open heart surgery; with diabetes; with pulmonary or renal dysfunction; with cardiogenic shock associated with acute myocardial infarction or cardiac arrest. Other indicators for CPBS are high-risk valvuloplasty candidates; patients with high risk of atherectomy; or presence of massive pulmonary embolism.

CONTRAINDICATIONS. Patients who have severe peripheral vascular disease, increased risk of severe bleeding, and those over the age of 75 who have undergone CPBS.

Procedure

TECHNIQUE. CPBS is performed in the cardiac catheterization laboratory using fluoroscopy. Cannulas are placed in the femoral artery and femoral vein. The venous cannula is positioned with the tip of the catheter just above the junction of the inferior vena cava and the right atrium. The arterial and venous cannulas are connected to the CPBS system. The support machine used for cardiopulmonary bypass consists of the following: compact system with hollow-fiber membrane oxygenation, water-based heat exchanger, and temperature controller. Oxygen-deficient blood is aspirated into the venous cannula, circulated to the water-based heat exchanger, and circulated to the central core of the oxygenator. Once gas exchange occurs, the oxygenated blood returns to the patient via the left femoral artery. Depending on the size of the cannula, flow rate can vary from 2 to 6 L/min. The angioplasty is achieved via sheaths placed in the opposite femoral system. During PTCA, the CPBS flow rate can be adjusted. An increase in the flow rate will decrease myocardial oxygen demand by reducing preload.

EQUIPMENT. Compact system with a hollow-fiber membrane oxygenator, water-based heat exchanger, temperature controller, priming solutions, and cannulas.

Complications

PCBS complications consist of asymptomatic vessel closure following angioplasty, femoral artery, or femoral nerve trauma; cannulation site infection and necrosis; thrombophlebitis; hematoma; embolism; post PTCA myocardial ischemia or infarction; and cardiac arrest.

NURSING MANAGEMENT: NURSING DIAGNOSES AND COLLABORATIVE PROBLEMS

Nursing Diagnoses

Common nursing goals in patients undergoing CPBS are to maintain tissue perfusion, maintain fluid volume, enhance physical mobility, and reduce pain.

Altered tissue perfusion related to thromboembolism or hematoma secondary to cannulation or arterial or venous sheath.

Expected Patient Outcomes. Patient maintains adequate tissue perfusion, as evidenced by peripheral pulses +2, capillary refill ≤3 seconds, mixed venous oxygen saturation ($S\bar{v}o_2$) 60% to 80%, warm skin, absence of pallor or cyanosis, normal sensory motor function, and absence of edema.

- Review results of coagulation studies.
- Monitor tibial pulses every 30 minutes using a Doppler while the CPBS cannulas are clamped and left in place. Report any decrease in the quality of pulses.
- Monitor leg temperatures and color to determine whether peripheral tissue perfusion is adequate.
- Assist physician with the removal of bypass cannulas after 4 to 6 hours based upon the following indicators: partial thromboplastin time (PTT) ≤120 seconds, activated clotting time (ACT) ≤240 seconds or after last dose of heparin.
- Once the cannulas are removed and a compression device (C-clamp applied), assess pedal circulation and lower extremity circulation every 30 minutes for 2 hours, then hourly.
- Monitor continuous $S\bar{v}o_2$ and report finding ≤60%, which can indicate decrease in tissue oxygenation.
- Evaluate and report loss of motion and sensory function during and after C-clamp application.
- Instruct patient to report any lower-extremity sensory-motor changes, which can result from femoral nerve weakness from C-clamp.

Fluid volume deficit related to bleeding secondary to anticoagulant therapy.

Expected Patient Outcomes. Patient maintains adequate fluid volume, as evidenced by cardiac output (CO) 4 to 8 L/min, cardiac index (CI) 2.7 to 4.3 L/min/m², central venous pressure (CVP) 2 to 6 mm Hg, blood pressure (BP) within normal range, mean arterial pressure (MAP) 70 to 100 mm Hg, heart rate (HR) ≤100 bpm, pulmonary capillary wedge pressure (PCWP) 6 to 12 mm Hg, absence of bleeding from cannula, and urinary output (UO) ≥30 mL/h or ≥0.5 mL/kg/h.

- Review results of coagulation profile.
- Obtain and report hemodynamic parameters indicating decreased fluid volume: CO ≤4 L/min, CI ≤2.7 L/min/m², CVP ≤2 mm Hg, and PCWP ≤6 mm Hg.
- Monitor and report other clinical findings indicating fluid volume deficit: hypotension, tachycardia, UO ≤30 mL/h and bleeding from cannula sites.
- When cannulas are removed, apply manual pressure for 20 to 30 minutes.
- Place a C-clamp over the site where manual compression is most effective in preventing bleeding. The C-clamp compression device can be adjusted to apply pressure over a vascular site with the use of a circulation disk.
- Monitor C-clamp in place for 90 minutes, then released in increments of 1 to 2 mm every 20 to 30 minutes as long as no bleeding or oozing occurs.
- Maintain C-clamp in the same position.
- Measure the circumference hourly in order to assess for occult bleeding.
- Should bleeding occur, remove C-clamp, apply manual pressure until the bleeding ceases, and reposition C-clamp.
- Once C-clamp is removed, monitor pedal pulses and BP every 30 minutes for 2 hours, then hourly for 2 hours, then every 2 hours for 2 hours, then every 4 hours. Report peripheral pulses ≤+2, pain in leg or groin, change in temperature, or change in color or extremity.

- Continuously monitor BP with an arterial line and report BP ≤90/60 mm Hg.
- Monitor UO for amount and presence of hematuria.
- Apply a 5-lb sandbag over the cannula removal site at the groin for 6 hours.
- Administer prescribed IV fluids and blood transfusion to maintain adequate circulating volume.
- Administer prescribed autologous transfusion of blood volume for the CPBS system to maintain adequate blood volume and pressure.
- Administer prescribed heparin after the sheath is removed to prevent clot formation (see Table 1–8).

Pain related to immobilization or femoral nerve trauma.

Expected Patient Outcome. Patient verbalizes minimal pain.

- Provide alternative stress reduction strategies, since patient must remain in a supine position with minimal mobility of the affected extremity for prolonged time: progressive relaxation, meditation, or guided imagery.
- Provide air mattress or egg-crate mattress to facilitate comfort.
- Facilitate movement of the nonaffected leg and other extremity with passive and active range of motion.
- Encourage family member to apply firm manual pressure to the lower back.
- Administer prescribed analgesia to reduce discomfort.
- Instruct patient to report changes of sensation in lower leg.

Impaired physical mobility related to cannulation and need to prevent bleeding complication.

Expected Patient Outcome. Patient's physical mobility returns to normal after cannulas are removed.

- Keep head of bed at 30 degrees or less to prevent bending at the groin site.

- Immobilize the leg loosely to the foot of the bed to prevent abduction of the knee.
- Provide a knee immobilizer to keep the extremity straight so not to bed the cannula.
- Provide diversional activities while patient remains supine on bed rest for 6 hours after cannula removal and cessation of bleeding at the groin site.

Collaborative Problem
A common collaborative goal for patients with PCBS is to increase CO.

Potential Complication: Decreased Cardiac Output.
Decreased CO related to myocardial ischemia secondary to restenosis.

Expected Patient Outcomes. Patient maintains adequate CO, as evidenced by coronary artery perfusion pressure (CAPP) 60 to 80 mm Hg, CO 4 to 8 L/min, CI 2.7 to 4.3 L/min/m^2, PCWP 6 to 12 mm Hg, S$\bar{v}o_2$ ≤60%, BP within patient's normal range, MAP 70 to 100 mm Hg, HR ≤100 bpm, capillary refill ≤3 seconds, absence of dysrhythmias, absence of chest pain, and warm and dry skin.

- Review results of ECG and serum enzymes.
- Obtain and report hemodynamic parameters reflecting decreased CO: CAPP ≤60 mm Hg, CO ≤4 L/min, CI ≤2.7 L/min/m^2, CVP ≤2 mm Hg, PCWP ≥16 mm Hg, and S$\bar{v}o_2$ ≤60%.
- Obtain and report other clinical findings suggesting decreased CO: hypotension, tachycardia, dysrhythmias, capillary refill ≥3 seconds, diaphoresis, cyanotic skin, and chest pain.
- Continuously monitor ECG to assess HR and rhythm. Document rhythm strips every 2 to 4 hours in patients with dysrhythmia.
- Administer prescribed oxygen 2 to 4 L/min by nasal cannula or mask to provide oxygenation.
- Administer prescribed IV fluids to maintain adequate circulating volume.
- Administer prescribed inotropes such as dopamine, dobutamine, or amrinone to en-

hance CO to ≥4 L/min and CI ≥2.7 L/min/m^2.
- Administer prescribed antidysrhythmia agents.
- Instruct patient to report any chest pain.

DISCHARGE PLANNING
The critical care nurse provides patient and significant other(s) with verbal or written discharge notes regarding the following subjects:

1. Report any discomfort in the cannulated extremity that might be postprocedure vasospasm.
2. Medication's purpose, dosage, schedule, and side effects.
3. Importance of reporting any chest pain to physician.

■ PERCUTANEOUS BALLOON VALVULOPLASTY

(For related information see Part I: Acute chest pain, p. 1; Acute myocardial infarction, p. 38; and Acute cardiac tamponade, p. 117; Dysrhythmias, p. 184. Part II: Valve surgery, p. 203. Part III: Intra-aortic balloon pump, p. 226; Hemodynamic monitoring, p. 219. Respiratory Deviations, Part I: Pulmonary embolism, p. 397.)

Diagnostic Category and Length of Stay
DRG: 112 Percutaneous cardiovascular procedure
LOS: 4.80 days

Definition
Percutaneous balloon valvuloplasty (PTBV) is the dilation of a stenotic cardiac valve by means of a balloon-tipped catheter that is introduced into the valve and inflated. The purpose of percutaneous valvuloplasty (PTBV) is to restore normal blood flow through a previously stenotic cardiac valve. With balloon PTBV, the stenotic cardiac valve is dilated by means of a balloon-tipped catheter introduced into the valve and inflated.

Patient Selection

INDICATIONS. Aortic valvuloplasty is performed as a short-term palliation of symptoms in patients unable to undergo surgical aortic valve replacement; as a bridge to valve replacement in patients with poor left ventricular function; or in patients with aortic stenosis who requires urgent bowel surgery or repair of abdominal aortic aneurysm, for whom PV will allow tolerance of anesthesia. Mitral valvuloplasty is used in patients with noncalcified mitral stenosis, especially pregnant women, and as palliative treatment for patients with calcific disease who are not surgical candidates.

CONTRAINDICATIONS. Significant valvular regurgitation or left atrial thrombus in patients with mitral stenosis.

Procedure

TECHNIQUE. Aortic valvuloplasty uses a dilating balloon catheter, which is inserted into the femoral or brachial artery and advanced retrograde across the aortic valve. Once in position, the balloon is then inflated around the orifice of the stenotic aortic valve. Valvular dilation leads to fracture of the calcified nodules or frame of the valvular cusps, commissural separation, leaflet stretching, or annulus rupture. The overall goal is to increase the valve opening and to decrease the existing transvalvular gradient. Mitral valvuloplasty also uses a dilating balloon catheter, which is inserted antegrade into the right heart and advanced transseptally across the right atrium into the left atrium. Once across the mitral valve, the balloon is inflated.

EQUIPMENT. Percutaneous balloon catheter and fluoroscopy.

Complications

Complications consist of ventricular perforation, acute aortic insufficiency, acute valvular regurgitation, acute myocardial infarction, re-stenosis, cerebrovascular accident, acute cardiac tamponade, emboli, vascular trauma, severe hypotension, or death.

NURSING MANAGEMENT: NURSING DIAGNOSES AND COLLABORATIVE PROBLEMS

Nursing Diagnoses

Common nursing goals in patients undergoing PTBV are to reduce risk of vascular trauma, provide progressive physical mobility, and prevent fluid volume deficit.

High risk for vascular trauma related to the use of a large balloon catheter secondary to valvuloplasty.

Expected Patient Outcomes. Patient experiences no vascular trauma, as evidenced by absence of bleeding, swelling, or hematoma, peripheral pulses +2, capillary refill ≤3 seconds, absence of mottling or cyanosis in cannulated limb, absence of tenderness distal to cannulation site, and warm and dry skin.

- Consult with cardiologist about criteria used to validate successful procedure in mitral valvuloplasty: a 75% to 100% increase in the valve orifice size with a reduction in the transvalvular gradient to ≤10 mm Hg.
- Consult with cardiologist about criteria used to validate successful procedure in aortic valvuloplasty: the valve area increases to 1.0 cm² or more or the gradient across the aortic valve is decreased 50% or more.
- Review coagulation studies.
- Limit activity to supine position with the cannulated extremity immobilized until ordered discontinued by the physician.
- Palpation or auscultation with a Doppler, if necessary, of peripheral pulses. Absent peripheral pulses in the cannulated limb indicates thrombus or occluded vessel from vascular trauma.
- Obtain, document, and report findings suggestive of peripheral vascular trauma: swelling, hematoma, or tenderness at can-

nulation site, peripheral pulses ≤+2, capillary refill ≥3 seconds, mottled or cyanotic extremity, skin cool and pain distal to the catheter site.

- Assess for pain every 1 to 2 hours for 12 to 24 hours. Should pain develop in the groin access site, evaluate for local hematoma formation.
- Place a 5-lb sandbag over the cannulation site after PTBV and after the sheath has been removed.
- Administer prescribed analgesics or narcotic to relieve pain.
- Administer prescribed anticoagulants should vascular trauma be due to thromboembolism.
- Teach patient to report any tingling or numbness in the cannulated extremity.

Impaired physical mobility related to arterial and venous sheath placement, hematoma, or bleeding.

Expected Patient Outcome. Patient regains mobility when the sheath is removed.

- Confer with cardiologist as to any deviation from unit protocol regarding immobilization of the affected limb.
- Limit physical activity to bed rest to decrease bleeding from the cannulation site and to keep the groin with sheath straight.
- Head of bed may be elevated 15 to 20 degrees to prevent dislodgment of the groin access.
- Obtain, document, and report findings reflective of impaired physical mobility: pain in the cannulated limb, peripheral pulses ≤+2 in cannulated limb, capillary refill ≥3 seconds, and numbness in the cannulated limb.
- Once the 5-lb sandbag has been removed from the groin area, place patient in a comfortable position.
- Provide range of motion (ROM) of the unaffected extremity.
- Provide diversional activities while patient is immobilized: reading, watching TV, or listening to the radio.

- Monitor sensorimotor function should patient experience decreased peripheral tissue perfusion.
- Administer prescribed narcotic or analgesic to relieve pain.
- Teach patient reasons for immobilizing the affected extremity.
- Teach patient to report any pain, tingling, or numbness in the affected limb.

Fluid volume deficit related to bleeding or hypovolemia secondary to vascular injury, abnormal coagulation studies, or decreased postprocedure hydration.

Expected Patient Outcomes. Patient maintains adequate fluid volume, as evidenced by hemoglobin ≥12 g/dL (female) or 14 g/dL (male), hematocrit ≥37% (female) or ≥40% (male), partial thromboplastin time (PTT) 30 to 40 s, serum electrolytes within normal range, urinary output (UO) ≥30 mL/h or ≥0.5 mL/kg/h, heart rate (HR) ≤100 bpm, blood pressure (BP) ≥90/60 mm Hg, peripheral pulse +2, and mean arterial pressure (MAP) 70 to 90 mm Hg.

- Review electrolyte, hemoglobin, hematocrit, and coagulation studies results and compare to preprocedure baseline.
- Obtain, document, and report clinical findings associated with fluid volume deficit: UO ≤30 mL/h, poor skin turgor, specific gravity ≤1.010, BP ≤90/60 mm Hg, and elevated hematocrit.
- Monitor catheter site for bleeding every 15 minutes for first 2 to 4 hours, then hourly should patient experience hypovolemia.
- Monitor intake and output every 1 to 2 hours, as diuresis may occur when there is improved valvular function.
- Administer prescribed oxygen 2 to 4 L/min by means of nasal cannula or mask to provide oxygenation.
- Administer prescribed IV fluids such as blood products, colloids, or crystalloids, if necessary, to maintain adequate hydration, UO ≥30 mL/h or ≥0.5 mL/kg/h, specific

gravity 1.010 to 1.030, and MAP 70 to 100 mm Hg.

- Instruct patient to report any bleeding at the catheter insertion site.

Collaborative Problems

Common collaborative goal in patients undergoing PTBV are to increase cardiac output and correct dysrhythmias.

Potential Complication: Decreased Cardiac Output.

Decreased cardiac output related to increased intrapericardial pressure secondary to potential cardiac tamponade from perforation with a guide wire or catheter.

Expected Patient Outcomes. Patient maintains adequate intrapericardial pressure, as evidenced by cardiac output (CO) 4 to 8 L/min, cardiac index (CI) 2.7 to 4.3 L/min/m^2, central venous pressure (CVP) 2 to 6 mm Hg, ejection fraction (EF) $\geq$50%, intrapericardial pressure (IPP) $\leq$2 to 4 mm Hg, MAP 70 to 100 mm Hg, pulmonary artery pressure (PAP) systolic 15 to 25 mm Hg or diastolic 8 to 15 mm Hg, pulmonary capillary wedge pressure (PCWP) 6 to 12 mm Hg, pulse pressure (PP) $\geq$30 mm Hg, right atrial pressure (RAP) 4 to 6 mm Hg, right ventricular pressure (RVP) systolic 15 to 25 mm Hg or diastolic 0 to 8 mm Hg, stroke volume (SV) 60 to 130 mL/beat, stroke volume index (SVI) 40 to 80 g-m/beat/m^2, systemic vascular resistance (SVR) 900 to 1200 dynes/s/cm^{-5}, systemic vascular resistance index (SVRI) 1970 to 2390 dynes/s/cm^{-5}/m^2, UO $\geq$30 mL/h or $\geq$0.5 mL/kg/h, no pulsus paradoxus, no neck vein distention, normal heart sounds, HR $\leq$100 bpm, RR 12 to 20 BPM, and skin color normal.

- Confer with cardiologist to validate expected patient outcomes used to assess adequate CO.
- Review results of ECG, chest roentgenogram, and echocardiogram.
- Review results of intracardiac pressure measurements: cardiac transmural pressure

(TMP equals cavity pressure minus pericardial pressure), which increases as IPP decreases.

- Position dyspneic acute cardiac tamponade patient in a high Fowler's position, if hemodynamically stable. This allows accumulated blood in pericardial sac to be dependent, thereby causing less compression on the lungs. A high Fowler's position also helps to decrease venous return.
- Obtain and report clinical findings reflective of acute cardiac tamponade: Beck's or cardiac compression triad, which includes decreasing arterial pressure, rising venous pressure, and a small, quiet heart.
- Obtain and report other clinical findings associated with acute cardiac tamponade: a systolic-to-diastolic gradient (pulse pressure) $\leq$30 mm Hg, neck vein distention, bluish discoloration of the skin in the upper chest or face, and Kussmaul's sign, which is present when patient is lying with head of bed at a 60 degree angle and the neck veins distend on inspiration, indicating increased left atrial pressure (LAP).
- Obtain and report hemodynamic parameters reflective of decreased CO caused by increased IPP: CO $\leq$4 L/min, CI $\leq$2.7 L/min/m^2, CVP $\geq$6 mm Hg, MAP $\leq$70 mm Hg, PAP systolic $\geq$25 mm Hg or diastolic $\geq$15 mm Hg, PCWP $\geq$12 mm Hg, RAP $\geq$6 mm Hg, RVP systolic $\geq$25 mm Hg or diastolic $\geq$8 mm Hg, SV $\leq$60 mL/beat, SVI $\leq$40 g-m/beat/m^2, SVR $\geq$1200 dynes/s/cm^{-5}, and SVRI $\geq$2390 dynes/s/cm^{-5}/m^2.
- Report the presence of pulsus paradoxus (via arterial tracing or during normal BP reading), which is a fall of more than 10 mm Hg peak systolic pressure during inspiration. Monitor BP every 5 to 15 minutes during acute phase of acute cardiac tamponade. The BP cuff is inflated 20 to 30 mm Hg more than the systolic pressure while patient is breathing normally, The difference in millimeters of mercury between the first Korotkoff's sounds heard and the continuous Kortkoff's

sounds is the pulsus paradoxus. With the arterial line, the height of the wave for (pressure) will decrease during inspiration. The difference between the pressure during expiration and inspiration is the amount of pulsus paradoxus.

- Calculate and report hemodynamic parameters suggesting increased IPP: MAP ≤ 70 mm Hg, SVR ≥ 1200 dynes/s/cm^{-5}, and PP ≤ 30 mm Hg.
- Assess, document, and report the parameters reflecting the need for intrapericardial fluid removal: CVP ≥ 20 cm H$_2$0, pulse paradoxus ≥ 20 mm Hg, and PP ≤ 20 mm Hg.
- Monitor continuous ECG to assess HR and rhythm. Document ECG rhythm strips every 4 hours if acute cardiac tamponade is suspected: report electrical alternans, which is alternating large and small QRS complexes or altered direction of the complexes, low voltage, and flat or inverted T waves or sinus tachycardia.
- Evaluate the results of Keck's tamponade score system in postoperative coronary artery bypass graft (CABG) patients: Postoperative serum creatinine ≥ 1.6, postoperative cumulative chest tube drainage ≥ 1400 mL, pressure plateau for a 2-hour period, mediastinal widening on radiograph; or Beck's triad: arterial hypotension, muffled heart sounds, and elevated CVP.
- Monitor daily weight, intake, and output, since a decrease in UO ≤ 30 mL/h or ≤ 0.5 mL/kg/h may indicate reduced renal perfusion secondary to decreased SV.
- Administer prescribed IV fluids such as blood products, colloids, or crystalloids, which increase ventricular filling pressure and temporarily maintain an increased SV.
- Administer prescribed inspired oxygen fraction (FIO$_2$) at 50% by mask or oxygen 2 to 4 L/min by nasal cannula to increase arterial oxygen saturation and improve oxygen delivery to the tissues.
- Administer prescribed volume-reducing agents (furosemide or bumetanide) to maintain CVP 2 to 6 mm Hg or 5 to 12 cm H$_2$O,

UO ≥ 30 mL/h or ≥ 0.5 mL/kg/h, resolved neck vein distention, specific gravity 1.010 to 1.030.
- Assist with pericardiocentesis when venous pressure is ≥ 10 mm Hg, pulsus paradoxus ≥ 20 mm Hg, and pulse pressure ≤ 20 mm Hg.
- Monitor patient's respiratory status and HR during procedure and report change in ECG (elevated ST, ventricular fibrillation, premature atrial contraction (PAC), or pneumothorax.
- Should pericardiocentesis not relieve the IPP, prepare patient for pericardial window surgery to drain fluid via an interpericardial catheter connected to a closed drainage bottle with underwater seal; using the subxiphoid approach or the left parasternal approach via the left fourth and fifth intercostal space. Removal of 20 to 50 mL of fluid will increase BP and CO.
- Teach patient the purpose behind pericardiocentesis or pericardial window surgery, if necessary.
- Teach patient common side effects of positive inotropes and diuretics.

Potential Complication: Dysrhythmias. Dysrhythmias related to mechanical irritation of the myocardium secondary to the guide wire position in the left ventricle.

Expected Patient Outcomes. Patient maintains in sinus rhythm, serum electrolytes are within normal range, UO ≥ 30 mL/h, HR ≥ 100 bpm, and BP within patient's normal range.

- Confer with physician as to the expected dysrhythmia related to mechanical irritation.
- Review results from 12-lead ECG: atrial fibrillation, bundle branch block, bradydysrhythmia, ventricular tachycardia, or ventricular fibrillation.
- Monitor continuous ECG to assess HR and rhythm. Document ECG rhythm strips every 2 to 4 hours in patients with dysrhythmias.

- Monitor for physical signs and symptoms of dysrhythmias: abnormal HR and rhythm, palpitations, chest pain, syncope, ECG changes, and hypotension.
- Administer the prescribed oxygen 2 to 4 L/min by means of a nasal cannula or mask.
- Administer prescribed IV fluids to maintain hydration and UO $\geq$ 30 mL/h or $\geq$0.5 mL/kg/h.
- Administer prescribed antidysrhythmic agents to correct dysrhythmias (see Table 1–11).
- Should pharmacological therapy be ineffective to correct persistent tachycardia or bradycardia, septal damage with high degree of block progression, inferior acute myocardial infarction with transient atrioventricular block, or persistent ectopy with compromised CO, prepare patient for pacemaker (see pacemaker, p. 270.)
- Assist with the treatment of heart block: external pacemaker or temporary pacemaker.

DISCHARGE PLANNING

The critical care nurse provides patient and significant other(s) with verbal or written discharge notes regarding the following subjects:

1. Importance of reporting any chest pain to physician.
2. Importance of keeping outpatient appointments.
3. Any prescribed medication's purpose, dosage, schedule, and side effects.

■ CARDIAC ASSIST DEVICE

(For related information see Part III: Intra-aortic balloon pump, p. 254; Hemodynamic monitoring, p. 219. Respiratory Deviations, Part III: Mechanical ventilation, p. 428; Chest drainage, p. 434.)

Diagnostic Category and Length of Stay
DRG: 110 Major cardiovascular procedure with complications
LOS: 10.30 days

DRG: 111 Major cardiovascular procedures without complications
LOS: 7.50 days

Definition
The cardiac assist device is a roller or pneumatic device to maintain systemic circulation and improve tissue perfusion in patients with severe ventricular dysfunction while allowing the ventricle(s) to recover. The cardiac assist device can assist a single ventricle (VAD) or both ventricles at the same time. The temporary device decreases left ventricular work demand, reduces oxygen demand, increases blood flow to meet the body's metabolic need, and decreases preload.

Patient Selection

INDICATIONS. The cardiac assist device is used in patients who have a potentially reversible heart condition and those who cannot be weaned from cardiopulmonary bypass following an uneventful surgery. In addition, patients with severe myocardial dysfunction and right ventricular failure (RVF) secondary to an acute right ventricular infarct that continues despite aggressive medical treatment may require a cardiac assist device. Other patients who can benefit from such a device are those awaiting cardiac transplantation, those with ejection fraction $\leq$25%, and those whose target vessels support more than half of their viable myocardium. Finally, patients with low output syndrome after vardiotomy may benefit from a cardiac assist device. Hemodynamic criteria include: cardiac index (CI) $\leq$1.8 L/min/m^2, pulmonary artery wedge pressure (PAWP) $\geq$25 mm Hg, systolic blood pressure (SBP) $\leq$80 mm Hg despite maximal medical therapy including intra-aortic balloon pump (IABP).

CONTRAINDICATIONS. If the patient's body surface area is less than 1.0 m^2, the devices are too large to be implanted or the cannula placement would be too difficult. A concurrent illness such as chronic renal failure, cerebrovascular disease, pulmonary disease, or hepatic disease would preclude the use of the cardiac assist device. Finally, patients with metastatic cancer or significant blood dyscrasias are not good candidates for cardiac assist devices.

Procedure

TECHNIQUE. A cardiac assist device requires surgical implantation of a cannula by means of a median sternotomy or thoracotomy incision. The cannula is connected to the device. The right ventricular assist device (RVAD) diverts blood around the right ventricle (RV) through a cannula placed in the right atrium (RA) for outflow of blood and a cannula placed in the pulmonary artery (PA) for the return of blood. In cannulation with a left ventricular assist device (LVAD), blood is removed from the left atrium and returned to the system circulation by means of the aorta.

EQUIPMENT. There are six different types of cardiac assist devices. The first, the centrifugal VAD, uses centrifugal force to propel blood through nonocclusive pump heads. Kinetic energy is added to blood contained within the VAD by rotating it at high speeds. Blood flows into the pump head, where blades rotate, causing the return of blood through a cannula. Available centrifugal pumps are the Biomedicus centrifugal VAD pump and the Sarns centrifugal VAD.

The second, the Thoratec ventricular assist device, is a pneumatically activated prosthetic ventricle that the device alternately compresses and evacuates air behind the blood-pumping sac. This provides a pulsatile stroke volume of 65 mL. Blood is diverted from the failing ventricle via air inflow cannula to the assist device. Blood is then pumped back through the aorta or pulmonary artery via air outflow cannula. This ensures systemic or pulmonary perfusion despite severe ventricular dysfunction.

The third device is the Thermo Cardiosystems Left Ventricular Assist or HeartMate.

The device is a pneumatically driven, implantable blood pump with an external console. It consists of an air chamber and a blood chamber. Compressed air from the console is alternately forced into the air chamber, which in turn causes movement of the pusher plate and diaphragm, generating the pump systole. The stroke volume of the pump is 83 mL with a rate range of 40 to 140 bpm.

The fourth, Hemopump temporary cardiac assist system, turns at high speeds, draws blood from the left ventricle, through a silicone cannula, and propels it into the systemic circulation. The pump generates 0.5 to 3.5 L/min of nonpulsatile continuous flow. The goals of the Hemopump assist device are to reduce ventricular preload, afterload, and wall stress. This leads to reduced myocardial oxygen consumption.

The fifth, Novacor left ventricular assist system (VAS) is an electrically driven pump that provides temporary circulatory support for patient with heart failure. A cannula in the left ventricular apex is attached to a conduit which diverts blood flow to the pump. Bioprosthetic valves are placed at the inflow and outflow site of the pump to maintain unidirectional blood flow. Blood is returned to systemic circulation through a second conduit anastomased to the ascending aorta. The left ventricule is directly decompressed and serves as a low pressure filling chamber for the implanted systemic pump. A pressure gradient of 10 mm Hg is required to fill the pump.

Lastly, in the total artificial heart (TAH), each ventricle contains four independent polyurethane diaphragms that separate air space from the blood-occupying space. As air is intermittently pulsed in and out through the artificial ventricles, the diaphragm synchronously expands and deflates allowing for blood filling in diastole and forward ejection in systole. The TAH is based on a principle of partial fill and full ejection. Partial filling allows the device to operate on the Starling curve and necessitates less manipulation of drive parameters. Likewise, full ejection ensures that all blood entering the TAH is completely ejected during systole. This allows for adequate filling in the diastolic phase.

Complications

Thromboembolism, acute respiratory distress syndrome, neurologic deficits such as transient ischemic attacks or cerebrovascular accidents, hemolysis, mechanical failure, infection, bleeding, sepsis, biventricular failure, acute renal failure, or multiorgan failure.

NURSING MANAGEMENT: NURSING DIAGNOSES AND COLLABORATIVE PROBLEMS

Common nursing goals for patients with cardiac assist devices are to increase peripheral tissue perfusion, correct infection, restore fluid volume, maintain oxygenation, and support physical mobility.

Nursing Diagnoses

Altered peripheral tissue perfusion related to thromboembolism or vasoconstriction secondary to ineffective ventricular assistance.

Expected Patient Outcomes. Patient maintains adequate peripheral tissue perfusion, as evidenced by peripheral pulses +2; capillary refill ≤ 3 seconds; systemic vascular resistance (SVR) 900 to 1200 dynes/s/cm^{-5}; systemic vascular resistance index (SVRI) 1970 to 2390 dynes/s/cm^{-5}/m^2; urinary output (UO) ≥ 30 mL/h or ≥ 0.5 mL/kg/h; skin pink and warm; device maintains adequate flow for tissue perfusion; and coagulation studies, hemoglobin, and hematocrit are within normal range.

- Confer with the cardiologist as to the expected coagulation profile for patient.
- Confer with perfusionist as to the desired cardiac assist device flow rate to maintain tissue perfusion.
- Review results of hemoglobin, hematocrit, and coagulation studies.
- Obtain and report hemodynamic parameters predisposing patient to decreased peripheral tissue perfusion: SVR ≥ 1200 dynes/s/cm^{-5} and SVRI dynes/s/cm^{-5}/m^2.

- Obtain, document, and report other clinical findings suggesting decreased peripheral tissue perfusion related to thrombus or vasoconstriction: absent peripheral pulses, cool and clammy skin, cyanotic nail beds, capillary refill ≥ 3 seconds, and hypertension.
- Should IABP be used, assess and report decreased or absent peripheral pulses in the cannulated extremity; tenderness or swelling in the cannulated extremity; and cool, clammy and cyanotic skin in the cannulated extremity.
- Obtain, document, and report clinical findings indicating pulmonary embolism: dyspnea, tachypnea, restlessness, anxiety, palpitations, syncope, respiratory rate (RR ≥ 20 BPM), heart rate (HR) ≥ 100 bpm, crackles, decreased chest excursion for splinting, S$_3$, S$_4$ gallop rhythm, diaphoresis, and cyanosis.
- Assist the perfusionist in monitoring the number of revolutions per minute in the device. An increase in the number of revolutions per minute may indicate thrombus formation in the pump head or tubing. Report any changes immediately.
- Monitor cardiac assist device flow ≥ 3 L/min; complete filling and emptying can prevent thrombus formation.
- Administer prescribed fraction of inspired oxygen (F$_{IO_2}$) by endotracheal tube or oxygen 2 to 4 L/min by means of nasal cannula or mask to maintain tissue oxygenation.
- Administer prescribed IV fluids to maintain hydration and UO ≥ 30 mL/h.
- Administer prescribed anticoagulants (heparin) based on pump flow: no heparin if flow is ≥ 3 L/min; constant heparin infusion if flow 2 to 3 L/min and activated clotting time (ACT) is 100 to 200 seconds; full heparization to an ACT of 480 seconds and flow of 1.5 L/min; heparization to ACT 480 seconds before weaning from cardiac assist device (see Table 1–8).
- Instruct patient to report any sudden shortness of breath or angina attributed to pulmonary emboli.

High risk for infection related to inadequate primary defenses secondary to multiple lines or tubes.

Expected Patient Outcomes. Patient experiences no infection, as evidenced by normothermia; absence of drainage, swelling or tenderness around incision or tubes; white blood count (WBC) ≤11,000/μL; no signs of sepsis and negative culture.

- Review results of WBC and cultures.
- Provide nutritional intake via total parenteral nutrition to maintain 1 to 5 g protein/kg/d and calorie intake of 100 cal/kg/d.
- Assess and report any drainage, swelling, redness, or tenderness around catheter cannulation site.
- Monitor temperature every 2 to 4 hours in patients who are febrile.
- Obtain and report hemodynamic parameters suggestive of sepsis: cardiac output (CO) ≤4 L/min, CI ≤2.7 L/min/m², pulmonary capillary wedge pressure (PCWP) ≤6 mm Hg, SVR ≤900 dynes/s/cm⁻⁵, and SVRI ≥2390 dynes/s/cm⁻⁵/m².
- Culture suspected abnormal drainage, secretions, urine, and blood.
- Use strict aseptic technique when suctioning, changing dressings, manipulating invasive lines, or changing VAD lines or pump head.
- Provide protective isolation for patient with elevated WBC and temperature.
- Place patient in reverse isolation.
- Administer prescribed IV fluids to maintain hydration and UO ≥30 mL/h.
- Administer prescribed thermally controlled blanket to decrease temperature and myocardial work load.
- Administer prescribed antipyretics to reduce temperature.
- Administer prescribed antibiotics depending upon cultures (see Table 1–14).

Fluid volume deficit related to postoperative bleeding or hypovolemia secondary to abnormal coagulation studies or traumatization from cardiac assist device.

Expected Patient Outcomes. Patient maintains adequate fluid volume, as evidenced by CO 4 to 8 L/min, CI 2.7 to 4.3 L/min/m², central venous pressure (CVP) 2 to 6 mm Hg, left atrial pressure (LAP) ≥20 mm Hg, mean arterial pressure (MAP) ≥70 mm Hg, right atrial pressure (RAP) ≥20 mm Hg, blood pressure (BP) within patient's normal range, HR 60 to 100 bpm, peripheral pulses +2, absence of bleeding from incision, UO ≥30 mL/h or 0.5 mL/Kg/h, specific gravity 1.010 to 1.030, chest tube bleeding ≤50 to 100 mL/h, normal skin turgor, hematocrit and coagulation studies within normal range.

- Consult with cardiologist to validate expected patient outcomes used to measure adequate fluid volume.
- Review complete daily hematologic profile: complete blood count (CBC), prothrombin time, partial thromboplastin time, activated clotting time (ACT), reticulocyte count, fibrinogen, and fibrin split products.
- Review results of plasma hemoglobin level, since ≥40 mg/dL indicates the presence of hemolysis.
- Observe for bleeding from any source such as chest tube, urine, or stool.
- Observe dressing site for bleeding.
- Obtain and report hemodynamic parameters reflecting decreased fluid volume: CO ≤4 L/min, CI ≤2.7 L/min/m², CVP ≤2 mm Hg, LAP ≤8 mm Hg, MAP ≤70 mm Hg, and RAP ≤4 mm Hg.
- Obtain, document, and report other findings indicating decreased fluid volume related to bleeding: BP ≤90/60 mm Hg; HR ≥100 bpm; pallor; peripheral pulses ≤+2; cool, clammy skin; and UO ≤30 mL/h.
- Monitor chest tube drainage every 30 to 60 minutes.
- Report chest tube drainage ≥200 mL/h for 2 consecutive hours after clotting factors have been restored.
- Provide autotransfusion of chest tube drainage whether immediately after collection or after additional washing procedure is carried out following unit standard.

- Keep an extra set of cardiac assist device tubing and clamps at the bedside.
- Administer prescribed low-molecular-weight dextran (25 mL/h) to limit embolic complication.
- Administer prescribed anticoagulation (heparin) once chest tube drainage is ≤100 mL/h for 2 to 3 hours to maintain ACT between 140 to 150 seconds.
- Administer prescribed alternative regimens, which include dextran at 25 mL/h for 1 to 2 days followed by heparin or dipyridamole 100 mg three times daily plus warfarin to maintain prothrombin time (PT) at 20% to 30%.
- Administer prescribed platelets should bleeding be excessive and platelet dysfunction occur.
- Should chest tube drainage be ≥200 mL/h for 2 consecutive hours after clotting factors have been established, prepare patient for reexplorative surgery.
- Instruct patient to report any bleeding.

Impaired gas exchange related to surgical trauma or multiple cannulation secondary to cardiac assist device instrumentation.

Expected Patient Outcomes. Patient maintains adequate gas exchange, as evidenced by arterial blood gases and hemoglobin within normal range, RR 12 to 20 BPM, absence of adventitious breath sounds, absence of cyanosis, mixed venous oxygen saturation ($S\bar{v}o_2$) 60% to 80%, arterial oxygen partial pressure (Pao_2) ≥80 mm Hg, difference in arterial and venous oxygen concentration ($C[a-v]o_2$) 4 to 6 mL/100mL, arterial oxygen saturation (Sao_2) 95.0% to 97.5%, and UO ≥30 mL/h or ≥0.5 mL/kg/h.

- Review results of chest roentgenogram, hemoglobin, and arterial blood gas measurement.
- Limit physical activity to coughing, turning, and deep breathing every 1 to 2 hours while avoiding dislodging cannula.
- Obtain, document, and report findings reflecting impaired gas exchange: RR ≥20

BPM, HR ≥100 bpm, cyanosis, rales, dyspnea, $C(a-v)o_2$ ≥6 mL/100mL, Pao_2 ≤60 mm Hg, Sao_2 ≤95%, and confusion.
- Assist patient to rotate position so the cardiac assist device cannula will not be dislodged.
- Auscultate lung sounds for the presence of crackles, rhonchi, or wheezes.
- With patient intubated and ventilated, follow unit protocol for ventilator checks and arterial blood gas and Svo_2 measurement.
- Instill saline and suction every 2 hours or as needed, following unit standards.
- Wean from ventilator as ordered, following unit standard.
- Extubate as ordered when hemodynamics stabilize, anesthesia effects subside, and arterial blood gases are adequate. This is usually within 48 hours after insertion.
- Administer prescribed sedatives to decrease work of breathing and oxygen demand.

Collaborative Problems

A common collaborative goal for patients with cardiac assist devices is to increase CO.

Potential Complication: Decreased Cardiac Output. Decreased cardiac output related to mechanical failure or myocardial dysfunction secondary to cardiac assist device.

Expected Patient Outcomes. Patient maintains adequate CO, as evidenced by CO 4 to 8 L/min, CI 2.7 to 4.3 L/min/m², CVP 6 to 12 mm Hg, LAP 8 to 12 mm Hg, MAP 70 to 100 mm Hg, pulmonary artery pressure (PAP) systolic 15 to 25 mm Hg or diastolic 8 to 15 mm Hg, PCWP 6 to 12 mm Hg, RAP 4 to 6 mm Hg, $S\bar{v}o_2$ 60% to 80%, pulmonary vascular resistance (PVR) 155 to 255 dynes/s/cm⁻⁵, pulmonary vascular resistance index (PVRI) 200 to 450 dynes/s/cm⁻⁵/m², SVR 900 to 1200 dynes/s/cm⁻⁵, SVRI 1970 to 2390 dynes/s/cm⁻⁵/m², HR 60 to 100 bpm, UO ≥30 mL/h or 0.5 mL/kg/h, skin warm and dry, absence of cyanosis, absence of angina, Pao_2 80 to 100 mm Hg, blood urea nitrogen (BUN) 10 to 20 mg/dL, serum electrolytes within normal range, and creatinine M: 0.8 to 1.2 mg/dL and F: 0.6 to 0.9 mg/dL.

- Confer with cardiologist to validate expected patient outcomes used to determine adequate CO.
- Confer with cardiologist about the expected VAD flow, which can never be more than the flow returning to it. Maintain flow between 2.2 L/min/m² or 2 to 4 L/min and pressure in right or left atrium at 5 to 15 mm Hg.
- Review BUN, creatinine, and serum electrolyte values.
- Review results of echocardiogram, which is done 24 hours after VAD support to assess ventricular contraction and ejection fraction.
- Limit physical activity to bed rest to avoid dislodging or kinking cannula.
- Monitor criteria indicating the need for cardiac assist device: CI ≤2 L/min/m², SBP ≤90 mm Hg, UO ≤20 mL/h, SVR ≥2100 dynes/s/cm⁻⁵, blood lactate level ≥0.2 mmol/L, and LAP or RAP ≥20 mm Hg.
- Maintain VAD flow rate at 2 to 4 L/min, since higher flow rates may cause poor ventricular filling, collapse of the atrium around the cannula and tubing, vibration or "chatter," indicating the need to decrease VAD flow rate.
- Monitor indicators of adequate perfusion: skin warm, pink, and dry; UO ≥30 mL/h or ≥0.5 mL/kg/h; BP within normal range; capillary refill ≤3 seconds; normal sinus rhythm; peripheral pulses +2; and normal sensorimotor function.
- Obtain and report hemodynamic parameters reflecting impaired CO: CO ≤4 L/min, CI ≤2.7 L/min/m², CVP ≥6 mm Hg, LAP ≥20 mm Hg, MAP ≤70 mm Hg, PCWP ≥12 mm Hg, PVR ≥255 dynes/s/cm⁻⁵, RAP ≥20 mm Hg, SVR ≥1200 dynes/s/cm⁻⁵, and SVRI ≥2390 dynes/s/cm⁻⁵/m².
- Obtain, document, and report other clinical findings suggesting decreased CO or poor cardiac assist device function: UO ≤30 mL/h or ≤0.5 mL/kg/h, capillary refill ≥3 seconds, peripheral pulses ≤+2, and dysrhythmias.
- Monitor arterial pressure wave form for documentation of dicrotic notch for LVAD patient and PA dicrotic notch for RVAD patient.
- Maintain RAP and LAP at 5 to 15 mm Hg by adjusting flow rate and volume infusion according to unit standards or orders to provide sufficient ventricular assist output.
- Report ventricular assist flow ≤2 to 4 L/min or within ordered parameters, even with adequate volume infusion. This can indicate heart failure. Hemodynamic indicators of left ventricular failure are CI ≤1.8 L/min/m², SBP ≤90 mm Hg, UO ≤20 mL/h, MAP ≤60 mm Hg, SVR ≥2100 dynes/s/cm⁻⁵, and LAP ≥25 mm Hg. Right ventricular failure indicators include CI ≤1.8 L/min/m², SBP ≤90 mm Hg, and a LAP ≤15 mm Hg despite volume loading.
- Assess and document patient's progress through low VAD flow (500 mL/min) weaning for up to 5 minutes following unit standards: LAP, MAP, RAP, skin color, and respiratory effort. If patient is stable after 5 minutes, mixed venous blood gases and CO are measured to assess intrinsic cardiac function. The weaning process is limited to 5 minutes to prevent thrombus formation.
- Monitor cardiac rhythm for alteration, especially in the heart transplant patient: The transplanted heart lacks neural feedback to assist it in adapting to hemodynamic stresses and, as a result, is dependent on adequate preload and circulating catecholamines to increase HR and contractility.
- Monitor intake and output: UO ≥30 mL/h or ≥0.5 mL/kg/h and chest tube drainage ≤100 mL/h.
- Administer prescribed IV fluids to maintain adequate hydration, MAP 70 to 90 mm Hg, RAP ≥6 mm Hg, and LAP ≥8 mm Hg.
- Administer prescribed fraction of inspired oxygen (FIO_2) at 50% by use of endotracheal tube or oxygen 2 to 4 L/min by means

of nasal cannula or mask to provide tissue oxygenation.

- Administer prescribed peripheral vasodilators (hydralazine, minoxidil, or nitroprusside) or coronary vasodilator (nitroglycerin) to maintain PVR 155 to 255 dynes/s/cm^{-5} and PVRI 200 to 450 dynes/s/cm^{-5}·m^2 (see Table 1–4).
- Administer prescribed angiotensin converting enzyme (ACE) inhibitors (captopril or enalapril) should right ventricular afterload indicators (PVR and PVRI) and left ventricular afterload indicators (SVR and SVRI) be critically high (see Table 1–12).
- Prepare patient for weaning once anticoagulation parameters have been established.
- Should patient tolerate repeated weaning testing and cardiac function be adequate, the cardiac assist device is decreased to no less than 1.5 L/min. The flow is maintained until the device is removed.
- Administer immunosuppressive agents in heart transplantation patients on cardiac assist device: cyclosporine, prednisone, and azathioprine (see Table 1–15).
- Instruct patient to report any acute chest pain.
- Instruct patient as to the purpose behind the cardiac assist device and its relationship to ventricular function or heart transplantation.
- Teach patient and family the purposes behind various noninvasive and invasive treatments.

(For additional nursing diagnoses, see Heart transplantation: **Coping, ineffective individual,** p. 216; Percutaneous balloon valvulplasty, **Impaired physical mobility,** p. 245.)

DISCHARGE PLANNING

The critical care nurse will provide patient and significant other(s) with verbal or written discharge notes regarding the following subjects:

1. Any prescribed medication's purpose, dosage, schedule, or side effects.

2. Importance of following diet or activity program as prescribed.
3. Importance of keeping follow-up appointments.
4. Reporting any chest pain to physician.

■ INTRA-AORTIC BALLOON COUNTERPULSATION

(For related information, see Part I: Acute myocardial infarction, p. 38; Valvular heart disease, p. 203; Dysrhythmias, p. 184. Part III: Cardiac assist device, p. 167; Hemodynamic monitoring, p. 219. See also Respiratory Deviations, Part I: Pulmonary embolism, p. 397. See Neurological Deviations, Part I: Cerebrovascular accident, p. 630. See Multisystem Deviations, Part I: Disseminated intravascular coagulopathy, p. 751; Sepsis, p. 772. See Psychosocial Deviations, Part I: Anxiety, p. 725; Denial, ineffective, p. 737; Pain, p. 742; Sensory/perceptual alterations: sensory overload, p. 745.)

Diagnostic Category and Length of Stay
DRG: 112 Percutaneous cardiovascular procedures
LOS: 4.20 days

Definition
Counterpulsation is the term that describes balloon inflation in diastole and deflation during isometric contraction or early systole. The intra-aortic balloon is an inflatable plastic device mounted on a vascular catheter that is usually inserted percutaneously through the common femoral artery. Intra-aortic balloon counterpulsation (IABC) an intraaortic balloon pump (IABP) is a mechanical aid to the circulatory function of the heart, which provides internal counterpulsation. The overall goal of IABC is to optimize myocardial oxygen balance and improve perfusion of the dysfunctional heart.

Patient Selection

INDICATIONS. IABC is used in patients with preinfarction angina, acute myocardial infarction, cardiogenic shock, refractory ventricular dysrhythmias related to ischemia, severe mitral regurgitation, low cardiac output syndrome, and septic shock. Surgical indications for IABC include prospective open heart surgery or cardiac transplantation, intraoperative open heart surgery, weaning from cardiopulmonary bypass, or after open heart surgery.

CONTRAINDICATIONS. Absolute contraindications to IABC are aortic aneurysm, bypass grafting of the aorta to peripheral vessels, and aortic insufficiency. Relative contraindications include peripheral or central atherosclerosis, age, severe left ventricular dysfunction, chronic end-stage heart disease, dissecting aorta or thoracic aneurysm, multisystem failure, chronic or debilitating disease, bleeding disorders, or history of embolic phenomena.

Procedure

TECHNIQUE. IABC is initiated by insertion of a distensible polyurethane, nonthrombogenic balloon (40 mL) in the patient's descending thoracic aorta. The balloon is passed retrogradely to a position just below the left subclavian artery but above the renal arteries. There are two approaches for initiating IABC. The first is a surgical technique that requires a femoral arteriotomy, which is performed in the operating room. The second, the percutaneous insertion technique, is performed at the bedside with or without fluoroscopy. The prewrapped balloon is placed into the left common femoral artery by means of a large-lumen introducer sheath. The catheter is then threaded into the thoracic descending aorta just below the left subclavian artery. Once the balloon is in place, as determined by fluoroscopy or roentgenography, it is filled with helium gas. The helium is shifted from the balloon pump console into the balloon catheter, escapes through the pores, and inflates the balloon. Inflation occurs immediately upon onset of diastole. Deflation occurs during isometric contraction or early systole. The balloon is phasically pulsed counter to the patient's cardiac cycle.

The balloon can inflate and deflate with each ejection (1:1 frequency), with every other ejection (1:2) or every third ejection (1:3). Counterpulsation is timed to inflate at the beginning of diastole and deflate prior to the next systolic ejection. The patient's R wave is used to signal the beginning of systole. The timing of inflation must be precisely coordinated with mechanical cardiac events to optimize the effects of counterpulsation. A continuous arterial wave form is used for minute adjustments in balloon inflation and deflation. Inflation occurs at the dicrotic notch, which reflects closure of the aortic valve. Deflation occurs prior to the next upstroke of the systolic wave.

During diastolic augmentation, blood situated in the aorta is forced back into the aortic arch, increasing the pressure with which the coronary arteries are perfused. Diastolic augmentation of coronary perfusion offsets the imbalance between oxygen supply and demand. During deflation of the balloon, before systole, diastolic unloading occurs. Blood is redistributed away from the aortic root, which decreases the pressure against which the left ventricle must work. The result is decreased myocardial oxygen demand. As the myocardium heals, the frequency of counterpulsation is decreased to 1:2 and then to 1:3. Once the patient has remained stable for 24 hours, after 2 to 4 days, and stable hemodynamic parameters have been achieved, the intra-aortic balloon pump is removed.

EQUIPMENT. A polyurethane balloon receptacle, a pneumatic drive system, console, helium gas, and fluoroscopy.

Complications

Mechanical complications include vascular occlusion, aortic wall damage, balloon rupture, catheter migration, or gas embolization. Physiological complications include thrombus, embolus, hematological problems, or infection.

NURSING MANAGEMENT: NURSING DIAGNOSES AND COLLABORATIVE PROBLEMS

Nursing Diagnoses

Common nursing goals for patients with IABC are to increase tissue perfusion, maintain tissue integrity, maintain fluid volume, minimize pain, reduce anxiety, and encourage feelings of control or powerfulness.

Altered cardiopulmonary and peripheral tissue perfusion related to catheter migration or emboli phenomena secondary to IABC.

Expected Patient Outcomes. Patient maintains adequate cardiopulmonary and peripheral tissue perfusion; as evidenced by coronary artery pressure (CAPP) 60 to 80 mm Hg; cardiac output (CO) 4 to 8 L/min; blood pressure (BP) within patient's normal range; mean arterial pressure (MAP) 70 to 100 mm Hg; absence of chest pain; capillary refill ≤3 seconds; peripheral pulses +2; skin warm and dry; absence of redness, swelling, tenderness, or drainage at IABC cannulation site, systemic vascular resistance (SVR) 900 to 1200 dynes/s/cm^{-5}, systemic vascular resistance index (SVRI) 1970 to 2390 dynes/s/cm^{-5}/m^2, blood pressure (BP) within patient's normal range; coagulation studies, hemoglobin, and hematocrit within normal range.

- Consult with cardiologist to validate expected patient outcomes used to evaluate whether tissue perfusion is adequate.
- Review results of coagulation studies, hemoglobin, and hematocrit.
- Limit physical activity to bed rest while maintaining head of bed at a 15 degree position.

- Obtain and report CAPP 60 mm Hg, BP ≤90/60 mm Hg, and MAP ≤70 mm Hg.
- Obtain and report clinical findings associated with decreased cardiopulmonary tissue perfusion: tachycardia, hypotension, tachypnea, chest pain, and cyanosis.
- Perform an Allen test on hand that contains indwelling radial artery catheter. Patient makes a fist while the nurse manually compresses the ulnar artery. The nurse maintains compression on ulnar artery while patient opens his or her fist. The hand should flush and resume pink color immediately if blood perfusion through the radial artery is adequate.
- Maintain cannulated extremity in a straight position to avoid decreasing blood flow through the cannula.
- Monitor femoral, posterior tibial, and dorsalis pedis pulses before pump insertion and then afterwards every 15 to 30 minutes (four times), then every 1 to 2 hours. Monitor color and temperature of affected extremity every 30 minutes and ability to move toes of affected extremity.
- Monitor the cannulated extremity for decreased perfusion. Report clinical findings of decreased peripheral perfusion: pallor, coolness, and decreased capillary refill of nail bed; decrease in or absence of peripheral pulses; or ischemia evidenced by local pain, tingling, or numbness.
- Assess the insertion site for bleeding, phlebitis, or infection.
- Monitor pulses distal to the cannulation site.
- Maintain continuous inflation and deflation of balloon to minimize the possibility of thrombus formation.
- Encourage patient to do ankle flexion and extension every 1 to 2 hours. Exercise of calf muscles tends to minimize venous stasis and possible deep venous thrombosis.
- Check dressing and assess drainage amount and color. Change dressing using unit standards.
- Administer prescribed oxygen 2 to 4 L/min by nasal cannula or mask to maintain oxygenation.

- Administer prescribed IV fluids to reduce risk of thrombus formation.
- Administer prescribed low-molecular-weight dextran to limit embolic complication.
- Administer anticoagulant (heparin) to decrease thrombin formation (see Table 1–8).
- Instruct patient as to the reasons for keeping the affected extremity immobilized.
- Instruct patient to report any extremity pain or claudication.

High risk for impaired tissue integrity related to compartment syndrome secondary to IABC.

Expected Patient Outcomes. Patient maintains tissue integrity, as evidenced by absence of throbbing sensation in calf of leg with balloon insertion, absence of calf pain with dorsal foot flexion, normal sensation in lower leg, and no sign of pallor when feet are elevated 45 degrees.

- Review results of creatine kinase (CK) measurement; is elevated (1000 to 5000 IU), it is an index of muscle ischemia.
- Review myoglobinuria value which is elevated 3 hours after circulation is restored.
- Monitor and report loss of lower leg sensation or paresthesia, which may progress to hypoesthesia.
- Assist with the insertion of a needle or catheter into the suspect compartment, allowing direct pressure measurement to confirm the diagnosis of compartment syndrome. The normal tissue pressure measure is 0 to 12 mm Hg.
- Evaluate lower limb sensation or pressure in patients who experience no changes in pulse status.
- Monitor patient for the presence of complications: persistent hyperesthesia, motor weakness, infection of the bone and soft tissue, and renal failure.
- Should compartment syndrome occur, prepare patient for a fasciotomy to relieve pressure.

- Instruct patient to report any changes in lower limb sensation.

High risk for fluid volume deficit related to bleeding secondary to anticoagulation therapy.

Expected Patient Outcomes. Patient maintains adequate fluid volume, as evidenced by absence of bleeding and normal coagulation profile.

- Review results of coagulation profile and hematocrit.
- Monitor and report bleeding at insertion site, gums, mucous membranes, urine, or stool.
- Test gastrointestinal drainage and stool daily for blood.
- Temporarily discontinue prescribed anticoagulation therapy until bleeding subsides.
- Teach patient to report any bleeding from insertion site or gums.

Pain related to intra-aortic balloon catheter insertion.

Expected Patient Outcome. Patient's discomfort is minimal.

- Inspect balloon insertion site for signs of infection that might contribute to pain.
- Immobilize or stabilize the cannulated leg to prevent movement of balloon catheter within femoral artery and nerve irritation.
- Provide patient with a quiet environment and uninterrupted time to facilitate sleep.
- Administer prescribed analgesics to reduce discomfort.
- Instruct patient to report any pain in the cannulated leg on a scale of 1 to 10.

Anxiety related to the need for mechanical circulatory support and the possibility of weaning difficulties.

Expected Patient Outcomes. Patient experiences reduced appearance of anxiety and verbalizes concerns and understanding of IABC.

- Assess patient's perception of threat or physiological factors that may prolong use of intra-aortic balloon pump.
- Prevent anxiety from escalating by providing reassurance and comfort and give brief, factual information about the IABC and weaning process.
- Encourage patient to verbalize concerns and fears regarding the invasive procedure.
- Provide patient with diversional activities during confinement to bed rest.
- Explain all aspects of the treatment or care to patients and significant other(s).

Powerlessness related to loss of control over physiological and environmental factors.

Expected Patient Outcome. Patient's feelings of powerlessness are minimized.

- Orient patient to the balloon pump, noise from the pump, and reasons why physiological parameters are continually monitored.
- Explore the purpose behind the alarm system that monitors balloon pump function.
- Should a long-leg knee brace be used to immobilize the leg with the intra-aortic balloon cannula, allow patient to control tightness of velcro straps and when brace is used.
- Encourage patient to participate in self-care, as appropriate.
- Ask if patient has questions or needs additional information.
- Encourage patient to tell nurse what could be done to make him or her more comfortable.

Collaborative Problems

Common collaborative goals for patients with IABC are to increase CO, maintain oxygen supply and demand, and balance and correct dysrhythmias.

Potential Complications: Decreased Cardiac Output. Decreased cardiac output related to impaired myocardial contractility secondary to myocardial ischemia or left ventricular failure.

Expected Patient Outcomes. Patient maintains adequate CO, as inferred by CO 4 to 8 L/min, cardiac index (CI) 2.5 to 4.3 L/min/m², central venous pressure (CVP) 6 to 12 mm Hg, left ventricular stroke work (LVSW) 60 to 80 g-m/beat, left ventricular stroke work index (LVSWI) 30 to 50 g-m/beat/m², right ventricular stroke work (RVSW) 10 to 15 g-m/beat, and right ventricular stroke work index (RVSWI) 7 to 12 g-m/beat/m².

- Consult with cardiologist to validate expected patient outcomes used to evaluate adequate CO.
- Confer with cardiologist as to desired counterpulsation and augmentation frequency and schedule.
- Review results of ECG, blood urea nitrogen (BUN), and serum creatinine.
- Limit patient movement to supine position with head of bed at 45 degrees and never raise head ≥45 degrees.
- Obtain and report hemodynamic parameters indicating myocardial contractility: LVSW ≤60 g-m/beat; LVSWI ≤30 g-m/beat/m²; RVSW ≤10 g-m/beat; RVSWI ≤7 g-m/beat/m², and stroke work index (SWI) ≤40 g-m/beat/m².
- Obtain, document, and report other findings indicating decreased CO: heart rate (HR) ≥100 bpm; peripheral pulses ≤+2; capillary refill ≥3 seconds; urinary output (UO) ≤30 mL/h; hypotension; diaphoresis; restlessness; decreased alertness; and cool, clammy, cyanotic skin.
- Monitor timing of balloon inflation. It should occur just before (50 milliseconds) dicrotic notch of arterial wave form is generated by peripheral arterial catheter or occur at peak systole (120 milliseconds) of arterial wave form generated by femoral arterial catheter.
- Monitor timing of balloon deflation. It should achieve reduction of aortic end-diastolic pressure and assisted peak systolic

pressure and drop in aortic end-diastolic pressure be 5 to 10 mm Hg.

- Evaluate calibration and timing of balloon inflation and deflation every hour or as necessary.
- Monitor balloon markers on console every 15 to 30 minutes. Balloon inflation marker should be synchronized on T wave during inflation and after P wave during deflation.
- Monitor continuous ECG to assess HR and rhythm. Document ECG rhythm strips every 2 to 4 hours in patients on intra-aortic balloon pump with atrial fibrillation, premature ventricular contraction, or ventricular dysrhythmia.
- Auscultate lung sounds every 1 to 2 hours while on mechanical ventilator, then every 4 to 6 hours when off ventilatory support.
- Administer prescribed oxygen 2 to 4 L/min by means of nasal cannula or mask. Fraction of inspired oxygen (FIO_2) can be $\leq 50\%$ administered by means of endotracheal tube while patient on mechanical ventilation. The goal of both approaches is to maintain arterial oxygen partial pressure (PaO_2) 80 to 100 mm Hg, arterial oxygen saturation (SaO_2) $\geq 95\%$ and mixed venous oxygen saturation ($S\bar{v}O_2$) 60% to 80% mm Hg.
- Administer prescribed IV fluids to maintain adequate hydration, UO ≥ 30 mL/h or 0.5 mL/kg/h.
- Administer prescribed inotropes such as dopamine, dobutamine, and amrinone to maintain CO ≥ 4 L/min and CI ≥ 2.7 L/min/m^2.
- Administer volume-reducing agents (furosemide or bumetanide) to maintain UO ≥ 30 mL/h or ≥ 0.5 mL/kg/h, specific gravity 1.010 to 1.030, and pulmonary capillary wedge pressure (PCWP) ≤ 12 mm Hg.
- Administer the prescribed analgesics to relieve discomfort.
- Should patient's HR be ≥ 150 bpm, it may be necessary to change balloon pump frequency to 1:2, as prescribed or according to unit standards. Evaluate timing every 4 hours and whenever patient's HR changes by plus or minus 10 bpm or a significant change in hemodynamic status is noted.

- Instruct patient to report any angina.
- Teach patient alternative coping strategies: progressive relaxation, guided imagery, or meditation.
- Provide patient with information regarding the purpose of IABC on afterload reduction.

Potential Complication: Imbalanced Oxygen Supply and Demand. Imbalanced oxygen supply and demand related to incorrectly timed IABC or dysrhythmias secondary to balloon pump malfunction.

Expected Patient Outcomes. Patient maintains balanced oxygen supply and oxygen demand, as evidenced by SaO_2 95%, hemoglobin within normal limits, $S\bar{v}O_2$ 60% to 80%, difference between arterial and venous oxygen concentrations ($C[a-v]O_2$) 4 to 6 mL/100 mL, oxygen extraction ratio (O_2ER) 25%, oxygen diffusing capacity (DO_2) 900 to 1200 mL/min, oxygen diffusion capacity index (DO_2I) 500 to 600 mL/min/m^2, oxygen consumption (VO_2) 200 to 250 mL/min, oxygen consumption index (VO_2I) 115 to 165 mL/min/m^2, absence of chest pain, absence of dysrhythmias, and HR ≤ 100 bpm.

- Consult with physician to validate expected patient outcomes used to evaluate oxygen supply and demand balance.
- Review results of hemoglobin test.
- Review with cardiologist the determinants of myocardial oxygen supply: patency of coronary arteries, diastolic perfusion gradient (aortic diastolic pressure minus left ventricular end-diastolic pressure), and the diastolic pressure time index.
- Monitor diastolic pressure time index (DPTI) and tension time index (TTI) to determine balloon counterpulsation's effect on myocardial oxygen supply and indicators of adequate left ventricular subendocardial blood flow. Bedside-monitoring software makes this evaluation possible.
- Determine the adequacy of subendocardial perfusion by calculating myocardial supply: demand ratio, which is the ratio of DPTI divided by the systolic pressure TTI.

The DPTI describes pressure–time events during diastole and estimates diastolic and subendocardial blood flow.

- Evaluate DPTI in conjunction with IABC inflation. DPTI increases with IABC because of an increase in diastolic BP and a decrease in end-diastolic pressure.
- Estimate TTI in relationship to the balloon deflation. TTI decreases with balloon deflation as a result of a decrease in systolic BP.
- Evaluate DPTI: TTI, which provides an accurate estimate of the adequacy of oxygen delivery to the myocardium. This is expressed as the endocardial viability ratio (EVR): EVR = DPTI (oxygen supply): TTI (oxygen). A EVR of 1.0 signifies oxygen supply and demand balance.
- Obtain and report indicators of oxygen supply and demand imbalance: $C(a-v)O_2$ ≥6 mL/100 mL, O_2ER ≥25%, VO_2 ≤200 mL/min, VO_2I ≤115 mL/min/m², DO_2≤900 mL/min, and DO_2I ≤500 mL/min/m².
- Obtain and report $S\bar{v}O_2$ ≤60%, which can signify that oxygen demand exceeds supply.
- Obtain and report clinical findings that may indicate decreased oxygen supply: chest pain, dysrhythmias, and cyanosis.
- Monitor $S\bar{v}O_2$ before suctioning or turning patient. Suctioning or turning a patient with $S\bar{v}O_2$ ≤60% can further increase oxygen demand and reduce CO or SaO_2. A falling $S\bar{v}O_2$ during care can therefore mean that the demands of care have exceeded the patient's oxygen supply.
- Administer prescribed FIO_2 ≤40% to increase oxygen supply.
- Administer IV fluids to maintain adequate circulating volume.

Potential Complication: Dysrhythmias. Dysrhythmias related to coronary artery spasm or mechanical dysfunction secondary to IABC.

Expected Patient Outcomes. Patient maintains regular sinus rhythm, HR ≤100 bpm, BP within patient's normal range, and serum electrolytes within normal range.

- Review results of 12-lead ECG for dysrhythmias: balloon pump automatically deflates when short intervals occur; when premature beat is close to preceding beat, counterpulsation will occur but with reduced efficiency.
- Review results of serum electrolytes.
- Monitor continuous ECG to assess HR and rhythm. Document ECG rhythm strips every 2 to 4 hours in patients with atrial fibrillation, premature ventricular contraction, or ventricular dysrhythmia.
- Monitor cardiac rhythm continually, noting any alteration in PQRST configuration and interval time.
- Administer prescribed oxygen 2 to 4 L/min by means of nasal cannula or mask.
- Administer prescribed IV fluids to maintain hydration.
- Administer prescribed antidysrhythmia agents (see Table 1–11).
- Use manufacturer-recommended trigger mode during dysrhythmias.
- Instruct patient to report any angina.
- Instruct patient as to the purpose and common side effects of dysrhythmia medications.

DISCHARGE PLANNING

The critical care nurse will provide patient and significant other(s) with verbal or written discharge notes regarding the following subjects:

1. Importance of reporting any pain in the cannulated extremity which might be due to vasospasm.
2. Importance of reporting any chest pain to physician.

■ AUTOMATIC IMPLANTABLE CARDIOVERTER-DEFIBRILLATOR

(For related information see Part I: Acute cardiac tamponade, p. 117; Dysrhythmias, p. 184. Part III: Hemodynamic monitoring, p. 219; Pacemakers, p. 270. Respiratory De-

viatis, Part I: Pulmonary embolism, p. 397.
Multisystem Deviations, Part I: Sepsis, p. 772.)

Diagnostic Category and Length of Stay

DRG: 117 Cardiac pacemaker revision except device replacement
LOS: 3.70 days

Definition

The automatic implantable cardioverter-defibrillator (AICD) provides for immediate termination of ventricular fibrillation (VF) and ventricular tachycardia (VT) in patients in whom these dysrhythmias cannot be controlled by pharmacological or surgical therapies. The device is designed to continuously monitor cardiac activity and treat tachyarrhythmia with countershocks delivered through surgically implanted electrodes around the heart.

Patient Selection

INDICATIONS. AICD is indicated for those patients who have survived at least one episode of cardiac arrest caused by hemodynamically unstable tachyarrhythmia not associated with acute myocardial infarction; with absence of previous arrest; or who have experienced recurrent tachycarrhythmias and can be induced into sustained hypotensive VT or VF.

CONTRAINDICATIONS. Patients who require multiple shocks for VT or VF during a brief period will have premature battery depletion. Unsustained VT can trigger the AICD, causing shocks in spite of spontaneous conversion. Patients with uncontrolled congestive heart failure are not candidates because AICD will not necessarily prolong their lives. A history of noncompliance to medical treatment is also a contraindication.

Procedure

TECHNIQUE. The surgical approaches to AICD are median sternotomy, lateral thorocotomy, using the subxiphoid and subcostal approaches. Electrodes are placed epicardially (ventricle), endocardially (ventricle), and within the superior vena cava. These leads are passed through the diaphragm to the abdomen and a battery-powered defibrillator is placed on the abdomen. The AICD is activated by sensing a rapid heart rate or a rapid heart rate combined with a rhythm with a wide QRS complex. Usually the QRS must be greater than 150 milliseconds in duration to satisfy the probability density function (PDF). The PDF prevents inappropriate shocks for narrow QRS complex tachycardias, such as atrial fibrillation. Once a tachycardia that competes with the programmed rate or the rate combined with the PDF is detected, the device generates and delivers a shock. Six cutoff rate settings are available, ranging from 126 to 208 bpm. The cutoff rates exceed the maximal exercise heart rate. This is less than the rate of the patient's VT.

After lead positioning and before placement of the pulse generator, defibrillation levels are determined intraoperatively by use of an external cardioverter-defibrillator unit. The unit delivers a wave form identical to that of the AICD. Once the leads are implanted, a pocket is created for the generator in the subcutaneous tissue of the mid left abdomen. The pulse generator can deliver up to four discharges for one triggering event. The unit requires 5 to 30 seconds to identify a dysrhythmia, plus 5 to 15 seconds to charge the output capacities to fire.

The AICD has several modes: active, inactive, and standby. In the active mode, the unit is able to sense dysrhythmias and deliver shocks. In the inactive mode, the unit is unable to sense dysrhythmias and deliver shocks. It is inactivated after 30 seconds of magnet placement. Finally, the standby mode is used during electrophysiological testing when the magnet has not been removed. The advantage of the standby mode is that dysrhythmia-induction techniques, such as rapid ventricular pacing, will not be sensed. However, when the magnet is removed, the unit reverts to the active mode.

EQUIPMENT. The AICD system consists of a pulse generator, which contains a lithium-powered battery, and capacitors to store the generated charge and sensing leads. The defibrillator patches are titanium mesh with a silicone rubber coating. The patches are attached to the inner or outer aspect of the pericardium, while the rate- and morphology-sensing leads are placed on the epicardium.

Complications

Surgical complications consist of congestive heart failure, acute cardiac tamponade, pneumothorax, pleural effusion, pulmonary embolism, dysrhythmias, bleeding, acceleration of VT, and generator pocket infection. Component failures include a shock if there is insufficient energy, loss of sensing, loss of discharge capability, or total premature unit failure; all lead to nonconversion of the tachydysrhythmia. Lead-related complications involve lead fracture, lead connection breakage, and migration of the superior vena cava leads from their original position. Antidysrhythmia medication can change the appearance or rate of the dysrhythmias or interfere with the defibrillator's threshold.

NURSING MANAGEMENT: NURSING DIAGNOSES AND COLLABORATIVE PROBLEMS

Nursing Diagnoses

Common nursing goals for patients with AICD are to improve oxygenation, prevent infection, promote physical mobility, and reduce pain.

Impaired gas exchange related to hypoventilation, atelectasis, or retained secretions secondary to postanesthesia sedation.

Expected Patient Outcomes. Patient maintains adequate gas exchange, as evidenced by partial pressure of arterial oxygen (PaO_2) ≥ 80 mm Hg; partial pressure of arterial carbon dioxide ($PaCO_2$) 35 to 45 mm Hg; arterial oxygen saturation (SaO_2) $\geq 95\%$; mixed venous oxygen saturation ($S\bar{v}O_2$) 60% to 80%; heart rate

(HR) ≤ 100 bpm; respiratory rate (RR) 12 to 20 BPM; urinary output (UO) ≥ 30 mL/h; absence of dyspnea, crackles, and cyanosis.

- Consult with cardiologist to determine the specific AICD mode used.
- Review results of ECG, chest-roentgenogram and arterial blood gas measurement.
- Elevated head of bed 45 to 60 degrees while patient awake to expand lungs.
- Obtain and report clinical findings associated with impaired gas exchange: RR ≥ 20 BPM, HR ≥ 100 bpm, dyspnea, cyanosis, or crackles.
- Auscultate heart sounds. The absence of friction rub signifies that heart has adapted to the epicardial patches.
- Auscultate the lungs every 4 hours for the presence of crackles, rhonchi, or wheezes.
- Encourage patient to use incentive spirometry every 2 hours after being extubated.
- Assist patient with splinting incision with hand or pillow to promote optimal excursion.
- Assist patient to turn, cough, and deep breathe every 2 to 4 hours while splinting chest.
- Wean and extubate from ventilator, when patient is alert, hemodynamically stable, and arterial blood gases are within normal range.
- Monitor chest tube drainage and report ≥ 50 to 100 mL/h for 2 consecutive hours.
- Assist physician with chest tube removal, using unit standard, when drainage is ≤ 50 mL/h and arterial blood gases are within normal range.
- Administer oxygen by mask or nasal cannula after extubation to maintain PaO_2 ≥ 80 mm Hg, SaO_2 $\geq 95\%$, and $S\bar{v}O_2$ $\geq 60\%$
- Administer prescribed IV fluids to maintain adequate hydration and UO ≥ 30 mL/h.
- Administer analgesics or narcotic to relieve pain.

Infection, high risk for related to invasive procedures, indwelling catheter, or incision secondary to AICD.

Expected Patient Outcomes. Patient is free of infection, as evidenced by absence of incisional redness, swelling, tenderness; white blood count (WBC) $\leq 11,000/\mu L$; negative cultures; normothermia; and no drainage from incision.

- Confer with cardiologist about the need for additional cultures.
- Review results from CBC and cultures.
- Administer prescribed 2000-calorie diet.
- Monitor incision site and report redness, swelling, tenderness, warmth, or drainage.
- Obtain culture of drainage from pocket or catheter site.
- Monitor temperature every 4 hours in febrile patients and report changes ≥101.5°F.
- Cleanse incision every shift using aseptic technique with half-strength hydrogen peroxide and sterile 4 × 4 dressing. Apply povodine-iodine and 4 × 4 or follow unit standard.
- Assess abdominal pocket and surrounding tissue for fluid and evidence of bleeding.
- Administer prescribed IV fluids to maintain adequate hydration.
- Administer prescribed antibiotics to control infection, based on the results of cultures.
- Instruct patient to report any incisional pain.
- Teach patient signs and symptoms of infection at the incision site.

Impaired physical mobility related to discomfort secondary to AICD surgery.

Expected Patient Outcome. Patient is able to gradually increase ambulation without discomfort or fatigue.

- Consult with cardiac rehabilitation department to individualize an activity program for AICD patient.
- Physical activity 12 to 24 hours postoperation: allow patient to sit at side of bed.
- Physical activity 24 to 48 hours postoperation: allow patient out of bed to chair, three times a day if hemodynamically stable.
- Physical activity after 48 hours: assist patient to ambulate three times a day and gradually increase the distance.
- Provide rest period immediately after increased physical mobility.

- Monitor continuous ECG to assess HR and rhythm. Document ECG rhythm strips every 2 to 4 hours in patient with dysrhythmia.
- Should generator discharge during increased physical mobility, monitor patient's rhythm and response.
- Obtain, document, and report signs and symptoms during generator discharge: dizziness, loss of consciousness, and diffuse muscle contraction.
- Administer analgesics to reduce pain prior to increasing physical mobility.
- Instruct patient how to safely increase physical mobility.

Pain related to AICD surgery.

Expected Patient Outcome. Patient is free of pain and is able to perform activities of daily living.

- Consult with cardiologist about the type of incision used (thoracotomy, subxiphoid, or sternotomy) and whether any wire fractured during surgery.
- Review results of chest roentgenogram should AICD wire fracture occur.
- Assess patient for clinical evidence of pain: facial grimace, splinting, HR ≥100 bpm, RR ≥20 BPM, and shallow respirations.
- Organize nursing care to take place 30 minutes after prescribed analgesic has been administered.
- Monitor and report pain associated with AICD wire fracture: pain along path of wires radiating from subclavian area to abdomen.
- Administer prescribed analgesic to relieve pain.
- Instruct patient to report chest or abdominal pain indicating AICD complication.

DISCHARGE PLANNING

The critical care nurse will provide patient and significant other(s) with verbal or written discharge notes regarding the following subjects:

1. Need for a continuous ambulatory electrocardiogram recording immediately

after generator discharge to monitor the unit's function.

2. Importance of maintaining clinic visits to check the device's status. Nonprogrammable units need to be followed every 2 months for the first year, then monthly. Programmable units are checked every 2 months until explantation.

3. Importance of maintaining a method of recording events after a shock: number of shocks, symptoms before and after, time of each shock, activity at the time of shock, and actions taken.

4. Importance of avoiding situations causing electromagnetic interference.

5. How to use the magnet in order to inactivate the AICD when instructed to do so by a cardiologist or during emergency medical service. Both patient and significant other need to be taught this information.

6. How to observe for and prevent skin breakdown, because the generator unit or leads passing over the left clavicle may cause tissue erosion.

7. Need to avoid wearing a tight belt or clothing over the generator or leads.

8. Prohibition against continuing to drive an automobile, operate dangerous machinery, or swim, because of risk of recurrent cardiac arrest.

9. That shocks can result from benign dysrhythmias, skeletal muscle electrical potentials, or unit malfunction.

10. Need for patient and significant other to consult American Heart Association so family can learn cardiopulmonary resuscitation (CPR) while patient is taught cough CPR.

11. Need to keep follow-up appointments every 2 months to check the battery.

12. Need to wear a Medic-Alert bracelet designating patient as having an AICD.

■ ST SEGMENT MONITORING

(For related information see Part I: Acute chest pain, p. 1; Acute myocardial infarction, p. 38).

Diagnostic Category and Length of Stay

None applicable.

Definition

ST segment monitoring provides a bedside diagnosis of myocardial ischemia or infarction and a means for gauging a patient's ability to tolerate activity or procedures. Continuous ST segment monitoring can assist in the identification of ischemic and other ST-related changes at the time they occur.

Patient Selection

INDICATIONS. Indications for ST segment monitoring include patients with known suspected coronary artery disease (CAD) or other ischemic myocardial disease; patients with diagnosis of reperfusion or reocclusion during and following thrombolytic therapy; intraoperative and postoperative patients with cardiac and other high-risk surgical procedures; patients after percutaneous transluminal coronary angiography; and, patients with chest, head, or vascular trauma.

CONTRAINDICATIONS. There are no contraindications.

Procedure

TECHNIQUE. Software in bedside monitors analyzes the ST segment for changes and displays the changes in a variety of ways. Depending on the hardware, ST analysis can be displayed continuously or displayed only on command. The ST segment represents early repolarization. It is measured from the end of the S wave (at the J-point) to the beginning of the T wave. If myocardial oxygen supply is insufficient, the ST segment deviates from baseline. The ST changes are observed in the lead or leads that reflect electrical activity from the ischemia area of myocardium. Bedside ST segment monitors analyze a precordial lead and up to three limb leads. The precordial lead V_1 is used because it can aid in diagnosing cardiac rhythms with a wide QRS complex. The limb leads used are III and aVF. The final choice depends upon the lead with the greatest QRS axis (aVF). Should placement of electrode in the V_1 location be impossible, the dual lead choice of V_6 plus II or V_6 plus aVF can be used. An ST segment deviation of greater than 1 mm is considered significant.

EQUIPMENT. Computer capable of monitoring and analyzing two, three, or four leads; and software.

NURSING MANAGEMENT: NURSING DIAGNOSES AND COLLABORATIVE PROBLEMS

Nursing Diagnoses
Common nursing goals for patients with ST segment monitoring are to provide knowledge about the technique and reduce anxiety.

Knowledge deficit related to the ST segment monitoring's purpose and need for continuous evaluation.

Expected Patient Outcome. Patient will be able to discuss the purpose of ST segment monitoring.

- Explain that by continuing monitoring ST segment, the nurse can determine how the patient is tolerating suctioning, turning, eating, or using a bedside commode. Should ST segment elevation occur during these nursing care activities, they can be interrupted or postponed to reverse the ischemia event or initiate treatment.
- Explain that ST segment monitoring during thrombolytic therapy allows determination of reperfusion. The ST segment returns to a baseline and is an indicator of successful treatment.
- Teach patient the purpose of ST segment monitoring, including the need for a bedside monitor and continuous or demand assessment, depending upon the program.

- Teach patient to report any chest pain, as ST segment changes can be recorded if the program shows ST segment analysis on command.

Anxiety related to the need for continuing ST segment display and analysis.

Expected Patient Outcome. Patient is able to verbalize anxiety.

- Reassure patient that ST segment monitoring helps to decide how he or she tolerates nursing care activities.
- Encourage patient to share concerns about the additional piece of technology attached to his or her body.
- Answer patient's questions about why ST segment monitoring is important.
- Provide positive feedback when no significant ST segment changes have occurred during rest, nursing care, or progressive exercises.
- Teach patient progressive relaxation, meditation, or guided imagery should ST segment changes occur, causing cessation of nursing care activities or initiation of treatments.

■ THROMBOLYTIC THERAPY

(For related information see Part I: Acute myocardial infarction, p. 38; Acute chest pain, p. 1; Cardiogenic shock, p. 72; Dysrhythmias, p. 184. Part II: Coronary artery bypass graft, p. 194, Part III: Percutaneous transluminal coronary angioplasty, p. 226; ST segment monitoring, p. 228; Hemodynamic monitoring, p. 219.)

Diagnostic Category and Length of Stay
None applicable.

Definition
Thrombolytic therapy increases myocardial perfusion and limits myocardial damage by dissolution of clot in the involved coronary artery. Thrombolytic agents act as plasminogen activators and have an affinity for circu-

lating plasminogen (not clot-specific) or fibrin-bound plasminogen (clot specific). Thrombolytic agents activate the conversion of plasminogen to plasmin, the enzyme that breaks down or lyses a thrombus.

Patient Selection

INDICATIONS. Patients who will benefit from thrombolytic therapy are those with confirmation of an acute myocardial infarction by chest pain and ECG changes. The chest pain is of sudden onset; is severe substernally; may radiate to neck, jaw, or arms; and is unrelieved by sublingual nitroglycerin. The ECG changes include ST segment elevation of 1 mm or more in at least two contiguous leads, T wave inversion, and significant Q waves (0.04 wide, $\geq$25% height of R wave in a given lead).

CONTRAINDICATIONS. Absolute contraindications include active internal bleeding; recent intracranial, intraspinal, or intraocular trauma; neoplasms or aneurysms; severe, uncontrolled hypertension; or severe blood dyscrasia. Relative contraindications include minor trauma; major surgery or biopsy within the past 10 days; prior cerebrovascular accident; subacute bacterial endocarditis; or acute pericarditis.

Procedure

TECHNIQUE. IV lines are used: one heparin lock for blood sampling and two large-bore IV catheters for thrombolytic drugs and IV fluid administration. There are three types of thrombolytic agents. Streptokinase (SK), which is clot-specific (activates systemic fibrinolysis), may be administered twice within 24 hours. The dosage is 1.5 million U over 60 minutes or an intracoronary 25,000 to 50,000 U bolus, followed by a 2000 to 4000 U/min infusion. Tissue plasminogen activator (t-PA) (Activase) is clot-specific. The recommended dosage is 100 mg IV, begun as a 10-mg bolus, then a continuous infusion of 50 mg for 1 hour, then 20 mg for 2 hours. Anisoylated plasminogen streptokinase activator complex (APSAC) (Eminase) is nonselective for fibrin; thus systemic fibrinolysis is stimulated. The recommended dose is 30 UIV over 2 to 5 minutes.

EQUIPMENT. A heparin lock for blood sampling, two large-bore IV catheters for thrombolytic drug, IV fluid administration, and thrombolytic agent.

Complications

The complications associated with thrombolytic therapy include bleeding; reocclusion, reinfarction, and reperfusion dysrhythmias; or allergic response.

NURSING MANAGEMENT: NURSING DIAGNOSES AND COLLABORATIVE PROBLEMS

Nursing Diagnoses

Altered myocardial tissue perfusion related to reocclusion of the affected artery after successful thrombolysis.

Expected Patient Outcomes. Patient maintains adequate myocardial tissue perfusion, as evidenced by coronary artery perfusion pressure (CAPP) 60 to 80 mm Hg, cardiac output (CO) 4 to 8 L/min, cardiac index (CI) 2.7 to 4.3 L/min/m^2, mean arterial pressure (MAP) 70 to 100 mm Hg, pulmonary artery pressure (PAP) systolic 15 to 25 mm Hg or diastolic 8 to 15 mm Hg, pulmonary capillary wedge pressure (PCWP) 6 to 12 mm Hg, mixed venous oxygen saturation ($S\bar{v}o_2$) 60% to 80%, absence of chest pain, evolution of ECG infarct pattern without evidence of new injury, blood pressure (BP) within patient's normal range, heart rate (HR) $\leq$100 bpm, skin cool and diaphoretic, capillary refill $\leq$3 seconds, and peripheral pulses +2.

- Consult with cardiologist to validate expected patient outcomes used to evaluate whether myocardial tissue perfusion is effective.

- Confer with cardiologist about potential re-occlusion or rethrombosis of the involved artery within the first 24 to 48 hours.
- Review results of ECG for the presence of ST segment elevation in same leads seen with primary infarction.
- Review serum enzyme values. Approximately 80% of the enzymes within the necrotic tissues wash out during reperfusion. There is an abrupt rise in serum creatine kinase (CK) and CK-MB.
- Limit physical activity to bed rest so as to reduce myocardial oxygen demand.
- Obtain and report hemodynamic parameters reflecting decreased myocardial tissue perfusion: CO $\leq$4 L/min, CI $\leq$2.7 L/min/m^2, MAP $\leq$70 mm Hg, BP $\leq$90/60 mm Hg, PAP systolic $\geq$25 mm Hg or diastolic $\geq$15 mm Hg, and PCWP $\geq$12 mm Hg.
- Monitor patient for the three indicators of reperfusion: resolution of chest pain, resolution of ST segment elevation, and appearance of reperfusion dysrhythmias.
- Assess, document, and report clinical findings of reocclusion: diaphoresis, chest pain, pallor, dyspnea, HR $\geq$100 bpm, and dysrhythmia.
- Monitor continuous ECG to assess HR and rhythm. Document ECG rhythm strips every 2 to 4 hours in patients with dysrhythmias.
- Obtain, document, and report clinical findings occurring with dysrhythmias: palpitations, dizziness, light-headedness, and syncope.
- Administer prescribed oxygen 2 to 4 L/min by means of nasal cannula or mask.
- Administer prescribed IV fluids to maintain hydration, MAP 70 to 100 mm Hg and CO $\geq$4 L/min.
- Readminister thrombolytic therapy: 50 to 60 mg of t-PA infused over a 1-hour period; or, if occlusion occurs more than 6 hours later, a full course of t-PA is administered (see Table 1–8).
- Administer beta-blocking agents (propranolol and metoprolol) to decrease the myocardial demand for oxygen (see Table 1–5).

- Administer prescribed aspirin or heparin in addition to thrombolytic therapy. Heparin can be started immediately after SK, 4 to 8 hours after APSAC, and after the first hour of t-PA infusion to prevent reocclusion of the coronary artery.
- Should thrombolytic recanalization be ineffective in increasing coronary artery or myocardial tissue perfusion, prepare patient for percutaneous transluminal coronary angioplasty (PTCA) (see PTCA, p. 226.)
- Should patient's condition deteriorate, prepare patient for coronary artery bypass graft (CABG) (see CABG, p. 194).
- Instruct patient to report acute chest pain.
- Instruct patient as to the reason for readministration of thrombolytic therapy or need for more invasive procedures.

High risk for fluid volume deficit related to bleeding secondary to manipulation of the clotting cascade or thrombolytic therapy.

Expected Patient Outcomes. Patient maintains adequate fluid volume, as evidenced by hematocrit and coagulation studies within normal range; BP within patient's normal range; urinary output (UO) $\geq$30 mL/h or 0.5 mL/Kg/h; HR $\leq$100 bpm; absence of hematoma; absence of blood from invasive lines; capillary refill $\leq$3 seconds; peripheral pulses +2; normoreactive pupils; and absence of headache, dizziness, or confusion.

- Confer with cardiologist to validate expected patient outcomes used to evaluate fluid volume after thrombolytic therapy.
- Review results of hemoglobin, hematocrit, and coagulation studies.
- Limit physical activity to bed rest to avoid movement of the extremity and dislodgment of a newly formed clot.
- Assess level of consciousness, pupils, sensorimotor function, peripheral pulses, capillary refill, guaiac results of secretions and excretions every 4 hours to detect bleeding complication.
- Obtain and report clinical findings of intracranial bleeding: altered level of conscious-

ness, abnormal sensorimotor function, speech changes, vision disturbances, and headache.

- Monitor and report retroperitoneal ecchymosis and severe lower back pain, since catheterization by means of the femoral artery can lead to iliac or femoral dissection.
- Observe oral, nasal, gastrointestinal, or genitourinary bleeding as well as oozing from puncture sites.
- Evaluate urine and stool for signs of occult bleeding every shift for the first 72 hours.
- Monitor BP and HR every 15 to 30 minutes until stable, then every 24 hours to detect bleeding.
- Maintain alignment of the extremity used in the procedure and apply 5- to 10-lb sandbag over the site to promote hemostasis.
- Administer prescribed IV fluids and plasma expanders to maintain adequate hydration, CO ≥4 L/min and UO ≥30 mL/h.
- Administer prescribed blood products containing clotting factors to supplement clotting cycle.
- Administer prescribed heparin drip to maintain partial thromboplastin time (PTT) at one and a half to two times control level or according to unit standard.
- Discontinue prescribed anticoagulant therapy and thrombolytic therapy, as ordered, should bleeding occur.
- Teach patient to avoid activities that could predispose to bleeding or bruising: shaving, venipuncture, vigorous teeth brushing, or noninvasive BP cuff.

High risk for injury, related to allergic reaction secondary to antigen-antibody response to SK or t-PA.

Expected Patient Outcomes. Patient has no symptoms of allergic response, as evidenced by RR 12 to 20 BPM; HR ≤100 bpm; BP within patient's normal range; skin pink and dry; and absence of itching and musculoskeletal pain, headache, or dyspnea; normothermia; and UO ≥30 mL/h.

- Inquire if patient has experienced a previous streptococcal infection, which may produce an allergic response; in addition, the antibodies formed in the bloodstream would inactivate SK, thereby reducing its effectiveness to lyse the intracoronary thrombus. Report response to physician.
- Assess BP, temperature, HR, and skin color during the first 48 to 72 hours for an allergic reaction.
- Monitor and report clinical findings associated with allergic reaction: hypotension, urticaria, itching, fever, headache, muscular pain, tachycardia, dyspnea, or bronchospasm.
- Apply heat or cold to skin irritation.
- Administer IV fluids to maintain adequate circulating volume.
- Administer prescribed corticosteroids and diphenhydramine should allergic response occur.
- Instruct patient to report any itching, flushed sensation, nausea, malaise, or difficulty breathing.

COLLABORATIVE PROBLEMS

Common collaborative goals for patients receiving thrombolytic therapy are to increase CO and correct dysrhythmias.

Potential Complications: Decreased Cardiac Output. Decreased CO related to myocardial damage secondary to reocclusion of the affected artery.

Expected Patient Outcomes. Patient maintains adequate CO, as evidenced by CO 4 to 8 L/min, CI 2.7 to 4.3 L/min/m², central venous pressure (CVP) 2 to 6 mm Hg, CAPP 60 to 80 mm Hg, normal sinus rhythm, absence of chest pain, skin warm and dry, peripheral pulses +2, capillary refill ≤3 seconds, BP within normal range, and MAP 70 to 100 mm Hg.

- Review results of ECG and serum enzyme values. With reocclusion and possible acute myocardial infarction, CK and CK-MB peak at 24 to 30 hours; early reperfusion with thrombolytic agents causes a higher and earlier rise in CK, peaking at 10 to 12 hours.

- Administer prescribed oxygen 2 to 4 L/min by mask to increase myocardial oxygen supply.
- Administer prescribed IV fluids to maintain adequate circulating volume.
- Administer prescribed inotropes (dopamine, dobutamine, or amrinone) to increase CO $\geq$4 L/min and CI $\geq$2.7 L/min/m^2.
- Administer prescribed vasodilators (nitroglycerin) to increase CAPP.
- Prepare patient for reapplication of thrombolytic therapy should reocclusion occur.
- Obtain and report hemodynamic parameters indicating decreased CO: CO $\leq$4 L/min, CI $\leq$2.7 L/min/m^2, and CAPP $\leq$60 mm Hg.
- Obtain and report clinical findings of reocclusion: chest pain, diaphoresis, dysrhythmias, and nausea.
- Continuously monitor ECG to assess HR and rhythm. Document rhythm strips every 2 to 4 hours or as needed should patient experience dysrhythmias.

Potential Complication: Dysrhythmia. Dysrhythmia related to reestablishment of blood flow to ischemic myocardium secondary to thrombolytic therapy.

Expected Patient Outcomes. Patient maintains regular sinus rhythm, CO 4 to 8 L/min, HR $\leq$100 bpm, RR 12 to 20 BPM, BP within patient's normal range, CAPP 60 to 80 mm Hg, MAP 70 to 100 mm Hg, absence of chest pain, and serum enzymes normal for post-thrombolytic therapy washout of enzymes from necrotic tissue.

- Confer with cardiologist about the potential for reperfusion dysrhythmias.
- Review results of 12-lead ECG and serum enzyme values.
- Limit activity to bed rest until reperfusion indicates successful thrombolytic recannalization: absence of chest pain, CAPP 60 to 80 mm Hg, and MAP 70 to 100 mm Hg.
- Limit physical activity to bed rest to reduce myocardial oxygen demand.

- Obtain and report hemodynamic parameters associated with dysrhythmias: CAPP $\leq$60 mm Hg, CO $\leq$4 L/min, and MAP $\leq$70 mm Hg.
- Obtain and report reperfusion dysrhythmias resulting from release of oxygen free radicals plus increased automaticity: rapid, abrupt onset of accelerated idioventricular rhythm (AIVR) with more than three premature ventricular depolarizations at less than 120 bpm; development of malignant ventricular dysrhythmias.
- Monitor and report other dysrhythmias signifying transient changes in atrioventricular conduction with development of an intraventricular block or reversal of a new-onset atrioventricular conduction defect.
- Obtain, document, and report clinical findings associated with dysrhythmias: chest pain, light-headedness, palpitation, dizziness, nausea, shortness of breath, RR $\geq$20 BPM, diaphoresis, and BP $\leq$90/60 mm Hg.
- Monitor continuous ECG to assess HR and rhythm. Document ECG rhythm strips for the indicators of reperfusion: normalization of ST segment within a 30 to 180-millisecond time span. Report no improvement in ST segment, which indicates myocardial reperfusion has not been achieved.
- Continuously monitor the ECG lead that displays the greatest ST segment elevation (see ST segment monitoring, p. 264).
- Reassure patient that reperfusion dysrhythmia occurs frequently after successful thrombolysis.
- Administer prescribed oxygen 2 to 4 L/min by means of nasal cannula or mask.
- Administer prescribed IV fluids to maintain hydration, MAP 70 to 100 mm Hg, and CO $\geq$4 L/min.
- Administer prescribed lidocaine infusion, 1 mg/kg bolus, according to unit standard to manage ventricular ectopy, ventricular tachycardia, and ventricular fibrillation.
- Administer prescribed drugs used in life-threatening dysrhythmias: epinephrine is indicated in cardiac arrest secondary to ventricular fibrillation, pulseless ventricu-

lar tachycardia, asystole, or electromechanical dissociation. Atropine is indicated in excessive vagus-induced bradycardia.

- Administer prescribed low-dose atropine (0.5 mg) with intravenous fluid administration should bradycardia occur as a result of vagal stimulation caused by reperfusion of the inferior or posterior ventricular wall.
- Should myocardial reperfusion be ineffective, prepare patient for additional thrombolytic therapy.
- Instruct patient as to the reasons behind dysrhythmias and their treatment.

DISCHARGE PLANNING
The critical care nurse will provide patient and significant other(s) with verbal or written discharge notes regarding the following subjects:

1. Need to follow instructions for taking anticoagulation therapy.
2. Importance of keeping appointments and follow-up laboratory coagulation studies.
3. Importance of reporting and excessive bleeding to physician.

■ CARDIAC PACEMAKERS

(For related information see Part I: Acute myocardial infarction, p. 38; Acute chest pain, p. 1; Acute cardiac tamponade, p. 117; Shock, p. 174. Part III: Automatic implantable cardioverter-defibrillator, p. 260; Hemodynamic monitoring, p. 219. Multisystem Deviations, Part I: Sepsis, p. 772.)

Diagnostic Category and Length of Stay
DRG: 115 Permanent cardiac pacemaker implant with acute myocardial infarction, heart failure, or shock
LOS: 11.90 days
DRG: 116 Permanent cardiac pacemaker implant without acute myocardial infarction, heart failure, or shock.
LOS: 5.70 days

Definition
Cardiac pacing is the delivery of an electrical stimulus to the heart to initiate a contraction. The cardiac pacemaker is a device that provides an artificial electric stimulus to the heart muscle when either the impulse initiation or the intrinsic conduction system is defective. Both temporary and permanent pacemaker units are used.

Patient Selection

INDICATIONS. Dysrhythmias that may require pacing include Mobitz type II atrioventricular (AV) heart block, complete heart block, sick sinus syndrome, bradydysrhythmias, tachydysrhythmias, and intermittent ventricular tachycardia unresponsive to drug therapy. Artificial pacing is indicated in patients in whom there is a failure of the conduction system to transmit impulses from the sinus node to the ventricles, to generate an impulse spontaneously, or to maintain primary control of the pacing function of the heart. Pathophysiological conditions that may impair cardiac conduction include acute myocardial infarction, myocardial ischemia, autonomic nervous system failure, and electrolyte imbalance. Iatrogenic reasons for pacemaker insertion include drug toxicity and cardiac surgery or ablation.

CONTRAINDICATIONS. None

TECHNIQUE. Artificial pacemakers can be used temporarily or on a permanent basis. Methods of temporary pacing are external (transthoracic), epicardial (transthoracic), and endocardial (transvenous). *Transient external pacing* is used in emergency settings for treatment of cardiac arrest complicated by asystole, severe symptomatic bradycardia, or overdrive for tachyarrhythmias until temporary or permanent pacing can be instituted. This noninvasive pacing delivers electricity from an external power source through large electrodes attached to the patient's chest. *Transthoracic pacing* is used in emergencies and involves either threading a myocardial pacing wire through a percutaneous cardiac needle or inserting a catheter by means of an introducer through the chest wall into the right ventricular myocardium. The needle or introducer is removed, leaving the electrode in place. The terminal positive and negative electrodes are attached to a pulse generator. *Epicardial pacing* is used after cardiac surgery should the patient develop dysrhythmias or critically diminished cardiac output. One or two pacing electrodes are sutured through the epicardial surface of the atrium. An electrode can also be placed on the right ventricle in anticipation of AV block. The terminals of the catheter(s) are brought through the chest wall and sutured to the skin. Atrial pacing wires are usually located in the right subcostal area and ventricle wires in the left subcostal area. The exposed wire tips are insulated with nonconductive clear tape. An external power source is available should asynchronous or fixed-mode pacing be required. *Transvenous (endocardial) pacing* involves threading an electrode catheter through a vein, into the right atrium or right ventricle, and attaching the terminal positive and negative poles to an external pulse generator. Veins used are the brachial, femoral, subclavian, or external or internal jugular.

The methods of permanent pacing are epicardial and transvenous. The *epicardial* approach involves a left anterior thoracotomy. Pacing electrodes are sutured into the exterior surface of the right or left ventricle or the atria. The pacing lead(s) are threaded through a connecting subcutaneous tunnel and attached to the pulse generator. The pulse generator is placed in a surgically created pocket. The two approaches are the left antethoracic pocket or the abdominal wall above or below the waist. With the *transvenous* approach, the electrode is threaded through a cutdown into the cephalic vein or by a percutaneous cannulation into the subclavian or internal or external jugular vein.

The modes of artificial pacing include fixed-rate, demand, AV sequential, atrial synchronous ventricular demand, and universal (DDD mode). The *fixed-rate pacemaker* delivers a pacing stimulus to the heart at a preset fixed rate regardless of the occurrence of spontaneous myocardial depolarization. The asynchronous mode is used to induce competition to interrupt, block, and cardiovert both atrial and ventricular tachyarrhythmias. The *demand pacemaker* delivers a pacing stimulus only when the heart's own pacemaker fails to function at a predetermined rate. The pacing stimuli will either be inhibited or triggered into the QRS complex when the intrinsic pacemaker functions. The *AV sequential (dual chamber) pacemaker* delivers a pacing stimulus to both the atrium and ventricle in proper sequence with sufficient AV delay to permit adequate ventricular filling. The *atrial synchronous ventricular demand pacemaker* has sensing in both the atrium and ventricle, but pacing occurs only in the ventricles. The atrial sensing electrode perceives the patient's own atrial depolarization, waits for a preset interval, and then triggers the ventricular pacemaker to fire. The *universal (DDD mode) pacemaker* utilizes sensing and pacing in both chambers. The two modes of pacing achieve both synchrony (DVI mode) and rate variability (VDD mode).

EQUIPMENT. Equipment consists of a pulse generator (pacer box), catheter with electrodes (lead wires), and bridging cable.

Complications

External transthoracic pacing complications consist of pain with impulse delivery, skin burns, muscular twitching, failure to capture, or failure to sense. Complications for epicardial pacing include dislodgment of a lead, microshock, acute cardiac tamponade, infection, failure to capture, or failure to sense. Finally, endocardial (transvenous pacing) complications are due to perforation of chamber or septum, infection, embolism, abdominal twitching, hiccups, failure to capture, or failure to sense.

NURSING MANAGEMENT: NURSING DIAGNOSES AND COLLABORATIVE PROBLEMS

Nursing Diagnoses
Common nursing goals for patients with a pacemaker are to prevent infection, reduce discomfort, alleviate anxiety, and foster positive self concept.

High risk of infection related to surgical site.

Expected Patient Outcomes. Patient is free of infection, as evidenced by normothermia, white blood count (WBC) ≤11,000/µL; lack of redness, swelling, tenderness, or drainage from surgical site; and negative cultures.

- Review results of WBC with differential, sedimentation rate, and wound drainage culture.
- Monitor and report abnormal drainage, redness, induration, swelling, localized heat, or increased tenderness.
- Assess patient for feeling of malaise resulting from basic metabolites from bacteria and injured tissues that enter the lymphatic drainage.
- Monitor temperature every 4 hours and as necessary.
- Promote rest by spacing activities such as procedures, exercise, and family visits to reduce fatigue and lower basal metabolic rate.
- Encourage fluid intake, if not contraindicated, to replace intravascular volume lost secondary to fever or perspiration.
- Keep surgical site clean and dry with dry sterile occlusive dressing, which will aid healing by absorbing any drainage oozing from the incision.
- Change dressing using strict aseptic technique according to unit protocol.
- Administer IV fluids to maintain adequate hydration.
- Administer prescribed antibiotics based on cultures.

- Instruct patient to report any increased tenderness at the surgical site.

Pain related to musculoskeletal contractions and required current for threshold.

Expected Patient Outcomes. Patient does not appear anxious and experiences little discomfort.

- Evaluate patient's anxiety level, as it may affect the degree of tolerance and perceived discomfort during pacing.
- Reposition the pacing electrode over intact skin to increase patient's comfort and tolerance of the procedure.
- Administer prescribed analgesics or narcotics to lessen discomfort and apprehension.
- Instruct patient to report any stinging or burning sensation directly under the pacing electrode.

Anxiety related to the procedure or dependency on a pacemaker.

Expected Patient Outcome. Patient exhibits reduced anxious behavior.

- Encourage patient to relax, since fear may increase the degree of discomfort experienced during transcutaneous pacing.
- Provide patient with explanations regarding the purpose, appearance, and function of the transcutaneous pacemaker.
- Minimize movement of the affected shoulder to minimize stimuli to sensory nerve endings and decrease pain.
- Elevate the affected area by keeping head of bed 20 degrees or higher or having patient sit in chair. Pain is less intense if swelling is decreased and gravity promotes lymphatic drainage.
- Prepare family and patient for the eventual placement of a transvenous or permanent pacemaker for long-term management of the illness.
- Encourage patient to ask questions about the procedure in relationship to the pacing device.

Self concept disturbance related to dependency on a pacemaker or disfigurement.

Expected Patient Outcome. Patient verbalizes acceptance of the pacemaker as a part of his or her body.

- Evaluate patient's level of comfort with the pacemaker by determining if there is any difficulty accepting a continual reminder of a cardiac condition.
- Encourage patient to share concerns about the pacemaker, such as fear of malfunction, loss of control or independence, and cosmetic appearance.
- Refer patient and family to a support group, if necessary.
- Provide patient with written information about the pacemaker.
- Teach patients that their concerns are not unique but are shared by other patients with pacemakers.
- Teach patient about the benefits of the pacemaker.

Collaborative Problems

Common collaborative goals for patients with pacemakers are to increase cardiac output and correct dysrhythmias.

Potential Complication: Decreased Cardiac Output. Decreased cardiac output related to loss of AV synchrony or inappropriate sensing secondary to pacemaker malfunction.

Expected Patient Outcomes. Patient maintains adequate cardiac output, as evidenced by pacemaker sensing spontaneous myocardial depolarization.

- Review results of ECG, chest roentgenogram, and echocardiogram.
- Limit physical activity to bed rest to decrease myocardial work load, decrease intrapericardial pressure, and increase coronary artery perfusion.
- Monitor continuous ECG rhythm for competition between paced complexes and the heart's intrinsic rhythm. Report malfunc-

tion findings on ECG: pacing artifacts that follow too closely behind spontaneous QRS complexes, or R on T phenomenon.
- Should R on T phenomenon be attributed to inadequate wave amplitude (or height of the P or R wave), increase the sensitivity by moving the sensitivity dial toward its lowest sensitivity. Report continued phenomenon, since other causes could be lead displacement or fracture, pulse generator failure, or electromagnetic interference (EMI)-precipitated asynchronous pacing.
- Monitor ECG for presence of oversensing from inappropriate sensing of extraneous electrical signals, causing unnecessary triggering or inhibiting of stimulus output. This is noted on ECG by presence of tall, peaked T waves or unexplained pauses in the ECG tracing caused by EMI.
- Should oversensing occur, move the sensitivity dial, as ordered, toward 20 mV.
- If an external pacemaker is used, check all electrodes for adequate surface contact and connection between the generator and patient.
- Should there be faulty sensing mechanisms in the circuitry or a faulty battery pack, change the pulse generator or batteries.
- Monitor continuous ECG rhythm for improper sensing, which is seen as the pacer spike following during a vulnerable period of the T wave. Report and check that pacer is in demand mode, not fixed-rate; increase sensitivity of pulse generator; reposition patient; and record ECG to determine catheter position.
- Should EMI occur, remove all potential sources of interference from the room.
- Should sympathetic hypotension occur as a result of a slow rate, increase pacemaker rate.

Potential Complication: Dysrhythmias. Dysrhythmias related to failure of pacer to capture appropriately secondary to pacemaker malfunction or lead displacement.

Expected Patient Outcomes. Patient maintains appropriate pacing, as evidenced by blood pressure (BP) ≥90/60 mm Hg; cardiac output (CO) 4 to 8 L/min; cardiac index (CI) 2.7 to 4.3 L/min/m^2; mean arterial perfusion (MAP) 70 to 100 mm Hg; absence of crackles; capillary refill ≤3 seconds; peripheral pulses +2; resolution of neck vein distention; ECG rhythm shows proper pacing; urinary output (UO) ≥30 mL/h or ≥0.5 mL/kg/h; and absence of fainting, vertigo, or fatigue.

- Consult with cardiologist to validate the method and mode of artificial pacing used in patient.
- Consult with cardiologist to validate the pacemaker's sensing ability, capture frequency, threshold, current setting, and mode.
- Review results of 12-lead ECG and chest roentgenogram.
- Monitor ECG for presence of pacing artifact that is not followed by QRS complex or, if pacing is atrial, not followed by P wave. Report and check the pulse generator to determine threshold (increase voltage in generator by 1 to 2 mA) and to determine if one connection between catheter and pulse generator are intact.
- Reposition patient if the pacemaker fails to capture appropriately. Move arm if the catheter is in the antecubital area or turn on either side for establishment of better catheter contact with the endocardium.
- Monitor and record stimulation threshold every 8 hours or more frequently if necessary, and monitor sensitivity threshold a minimum of once every 24 hours.
- Attach a monitor rhythm strip at least every 4 hours. Measure rate and automatic interval to confirm that the pacer is functioning properly.
- Obtain and report hemodynamic parameters reflecting decreased CO resulting from dysrhythmias: CO ≤4 L/min, CI ≤2.7 L/min/m^2, and MAP ≤70 mm Hg.
- Obtain, document, and report clinical findings associated with dysrhythmias caused by pacemaker dysfunction: Hypotension, capillary refill ≥3 seconds, peripheral pulses ≤+2, pallor or cyanosis, bradycar-

dia, fatigue, shortness of breath, and UO ≤30 mL/h.
- Obtain, document, and report clinical findings indicating catheter dislodgment: changes in QRS configuration, loss of artifact on ECG, failure to sense, hiccups, or muscle twitching in chest or abdomen.
- Monitor pacemaker system through strip analysis every shift, including: integrity of lead connections, battery, power generator, and pacer settings.
- Administer prescribed oxygen 2 to 4 L/min by means of nasal cannula or mask to maintain partial pressure of arterial oxygen (Pao$_2$) ≥80 mm Hg and arterial oxygen saturation (Sao$_2$) ≥95%.
- Administer prescribed IV fluids to maintain hydration and UO ≥30 mL/h or ≥0.5 mL/kg/h.

DISCHARGE PLANNING

The critical care nurse will provide patient and significant other(s) with verbal or written discharge notes regarding the following subjects:

1. The need for patients with a temporary pacemaker to avoid use of electrical equipment such as shaver.
2. The need to seek medical care should such pacemaker failures occur as sustained dysrhythmia or failure to pace.
3. Referral to a community organization, to learn more about pacemakers, such as the American Heart Association
4. The need to keep appointments so pacemaker stimulation threshold can be checked.
5. The need during the first 2 months to avoid full range of arm motion, heavy lifting, or active sports that could cause bleeding in the pacemaker pocket, lead displacement, or disruption in the integrity of the incision.
6. Freedom after 2 months to perform any activity not contraindicated.
7. The need to monitor for infection, pain, and environmental safety hazards.
8. Ability to use electrical tools, toothbrushes, and hair dryers if not held right

next to the pacemaker, which could create electrical signals that interfere with the pacemaker.

9. Information about the use of transtelephonic monitor. The receiver is in the hospital or doctor's office. The patient calls at a predetermined interval to evaluate pacer function.

SELECTED BIBLIOGRAPHY

Abraham T. Arrhythmogenic mechanisms. *AACN Clin Issues Crit Care Nurs.* 1992;3:157–165.

Ahrens T. Changing perspectives in the assessment of oxygenation. *Crit Care Nurse.* 1993;13(4): 78–83.

Albert N. Laser angioplasty and intracoronary stents: going beyond the balloon. *AACN Clin Issues Crit Care Nurs.* 1994;5:15–20.

Aretz HT, Martinelli MA. Intraluminal ultrasound guidance of transverse laser coronary atherectomy. *Int J Card Imaging.* 1989;4:153–157.

Arteaga WJ, Drew BJ. Device therapy for ventricular tachycardia or fibrillation: the implantable cardioverter defibrillator and antitachycardia pacing. *Crit Care Nurs Q.* 1991;14:60–71.

Awdi-Abou N. Thermo cardiosystems left ventricular assist device as a bridge to cardiac transplant. *AACN Clin Issues Crit Care Nurs.* 1991;2:345–551.

Barbiere CC, Liberatore K. Automated external defibrillators: an update of additions to the ACLS algorithms. *Crit Care Nurse.* 1992;12(5): 17–20.

Barbiere CC, Liberatore K. From emergent transvenous pacemaker to permanent implant. *Crit Care Nurse* 1993;13(2):39–44.

Barden C, Austin JH, Burgman V, Wood MK. Balloon aortic valvuloplasty: nursing care implications. *Crit Care Nurse.* 1990;10(6):22–30.

Barden C, Lee R. Update on ventricular assist device. *AACN Clin Issues Crit Care Nurs.* 1990;1:13–27.

Barden RM. Patients with hypertension. In: Clochesy JM, Breu C, Cardin S, et al, eds. *Crit Care Nurs.* Philadelphia, Pa: WB Saunders Co, 1993:462–484.

Bavin TK. Nursing considerations for patients requiring cardiopulmonary support. *AACN Clin Issues Crit Care Nurs.* 1991;2:501–514.

Bell NM. Clinical significance of ST-Segment monitoring. *Crit Care Nurs Clin North Am.* 1992;4:313–323.

Berron K. Role of the ventricular assist device in acute myocardial infarction. *Crit Care Nurs Q.* 1989;12:25–37.

Bopp-Laurent D. Heart failure. In: Woods SL, Froelicher S, eds. *Cardiac Nursing.* 3rd ed. Philadelphia, Pa: JB Lippincott Co, 1995: 561–569.

Bopp-Laurent D. Pathophysiology of heart failure. In: Woods SL, Froelicher S, eds. *Cardiac Nursing,* 3rd ed. Philadelphia, Pa: JB Lippincott Co; 1995:220–227.

Bopp-Laurent D. Cardiomyopathies and myocarditis. In: Woods SL, Froelicher S, eds. *Cardiac Nursing,* 3rd ed. Philadelphia, Pa: JB Lippincott Co; 1995:924–930.

Bortone A, Hess OM, Chiddo A, et al. Functional and structural abnormalities in patients with dilated cardiomyopathy. *Am J Cardiol.* 1989;14: 613–623.

Brannon PH, Johnson R. The internal cardioverter defibrillation: Patient-family teaching. *Crit Care Nurse.* 1992;19:41–46.

Briones TL. Tissue-plasminogen activation: nursing implications. *Dimensions Crit Care Nurs.* 1989;8:200–209.

Bullock BL, Rosendahl PP. *Pathophysiology: Adaptations and Alterations in Function.* 3rd ed. Philadelphia, Pa: JB Lippincott Co; 1992.

Bustin B. Hemodynamic Monitoring for Critical Care. Norwalk, Conn: Appleton-Century-Crofts, 1986.

Cardin S. Patients with cardiomyopathy. In: Clochesy JM, Breu C, Cardin S, et al, eds. *Crit Care Nurs.* Philadelphia, Pa: WB Saunders Co; 1993:356–369.

Casey PE. Pathophysiology of dilated cardiomyopathy: nursing implications. *J Cardiovasc Nurs.* 1987;2:1–12.

Christopherson DJ, Froelicher ES. In: Woods SL, Froelicher S, eds. *Cardiac Nursing,* 3rd ed. Philadelphia, Pa: JB Lippincott Co; 1995: 934–942.

Cicciu-Vitello J, Eagan JS. Data acquisition from the cardiovascular system. In: Kinney MR, Packa DR, Dunbar SB, eds. *AACN'S Clinical Reference for Critical Care Nursing,* 3rd ed. St. Louis, Mo: Mosby-Year Book; 1993:471–507.

Cicciu-Vitello J, Morrissey AM. Coronary artery disease. In: Kinney MR, Packa DR, Dunbar SB, eds. *AACN'S Clinical Reference for Critical Care Nursing,* 3rd ed. St. Louis, Mo: Mosby-Year Book; 1993:509–570.

Cicciu-Vitello J, Johantgen M. Cardiomyopathy. In: Kinney MR, Packa DR, Dunbar SB, eds. *AACN'S Clinical Reference for Critical Care Nursing,* 3rd ed. St. Louis, Mo: Mosby-Year Book; 1993:571–582.

Cicciu-Vitello J, Lapsley DP. Valvular heart disease. In: Kinney MR, Packa DR, Dunbar SB, eds. *AACN'S Clinical Reference for Critical Care Nursing,* 3rd ed. St. Louis, Mo: Mosby-Year Book; 1993:583–606.

Clark BK. Beta-adrenergic blocking agents: their current status. *AACN Clin Issues Crit Care Nurs.* 1992;3:447–460.

Clements JV. Sympathomimetics, inotropics and vasodilators. *AACN Clin Issues Crit Care Nurs.* 1992;3:395–408.

Coleman B, Lavieri MC, Gross S. Patients undergoing cardiac surgery. In: Clochesy JM, Breu C, Cardin S, et al, eds. *Crit Care Nurs.* Philadelphia, Pa: WB Saunders Co; 1993:385–436.

Coombs VJ, Black L, Townsend SN. Myocardial reperfusion injury: the critical challenge. *Crit Care Nurs Clin North Am.* 1992;4:339–346.

Cone M, Hoffman M, Jessen D, et al. Cardiopulmonary support in the intensive care unit. *Am J Crit Care.* 1992;1:98–108.

Constancia PE. The Ross procedure: aortic valve replacement using autologous pulmonary valve. *Crit Care Nurs Clin North Am.* 1991;3:717–722.

Cross JA. Pharmacologic management of heart failure. Positive inotropic agents. *Crit Care Nurs Clin North Am.* 1993;5:589–597.

Cunny J, Enger EL. Medical management of chronic heart failure: direct-acting vasodilators and diuretic agents. *Crit Care Nurs Clin North Am.* 1993;5:575–587.

Daily EK. Percutaneous balloon valvuloplasty in adult patients with valvular heart disease. *Crit Care Nurs Clin North Am.* 1989;1:339–357.

Deglin JH, Deglin SG. Hypertensive: current trends and choices in pharmacotherapeutics. *AACN Clin Issues Crit Care Nurs.* 1992;3:507–526.

Deglin JH, Vallerand AH, Russin MM. *Davis's Drug Guide for Nurses,* 3rd ed. Philadelphia, Pa: FA Davis Co; 1995.

Dimengo JM. Dynamic cardiomyoplasty and its use in patients with congestive heart fail-

ure. *Crit Care Nurs Clin North Am.* 1993;5:627–633.

Dixon JF, Farris C. The ABIOMED BVS 5000 system. *AACN Clin Issues Crit Care Nurs.* 1991;2:552–561.

Dix-Sheldon DK. Pharmacologic management of myocardial ischemia. *J Cardiovasc Nurs.* 1989;3(4):17–30.

Dolan JT. *Critical Care Nursing: Clinical Management Through the Nursing Process.* Philadelphia, Pa: FA Davis Co; 1991.

Dossey BM, Guzzetta CE, Kenner CV. *Critical Care Nursing Body—Mind—Spirit,* 3rd ed. Philadelphia, Pa: JB Lippincott Co; 1992.

Dressler DK. Transplantation in end-stage heart failure. *Crit Care Nurs Clin North Am.* 1993;5:635–648.

Drew BJ, Tisdale LA. ST-segment monitoring for coronary artery occlusion following thrombolytic therapy and coronary angioplasty: identification of optimal bedside monitoring leads. *Am J Crit Care.* 1993;2:280–292.

Drew BS. Bedside electrocardiogram monitoring. *AACN Clin Issues Crit Care Nurs.* 1993;4(1):25–33.

Dunbar LM. Emergency room management of congestive heart failure. *Hosp Pract.* 1990;25 (suppl): 7–14.

Enfanto P, Pickett S, Pieczek A, et al. Percutaneous laser myoplasty; nursing care implications. *Crit Care Nurse.* 1994;14:94–101.

Epstein CD, Henning RJ. Oxygen transport variables in the identification and treatment of tissue hypoxia. *Heart Lung.* 1993;22:328–347.

Estes ME. Management of the cardiac tamponade patient: a nursing framework. *Crit Care Nurse.* 1985;5(5):17–26.

Fabiszewski R, Volosin KJ. Refusal of implantable cardioverter defibrillator generator replacement: the nurse's role. *Focus Crit Care.* 1992;19(2):97–100.

Fischbach F. *A Manual of Laboratory Diagnostic Tests,* 4th ed. Philadelphia, Pa: JB Lippincott Co; 1992.

Fitzgerald CA. Current perspectives in prosthetic heart valves and valve repair. *AACN Clin Issues Crit Care Nurs.* 1993;4:228–243.

Fleg JL, Gavras IH, Langford HG, et al. Fine points of hypertensive therapy. *Patient Care* 1990;24(3):171–197.

Fleury J, Murdaugh C. Patients with coronary artery disease. In: Clochesy JM, Breu C, Cardin

S, et al, eds. *Crit Care Nurs.* Philadelphia, Pa: WB Saunders Co; 1993:257–301.

Flynn JB, Bruce NP. Introduction to Critical Care Skills. St. Louis, Mo: Mosby-Year Book, 1993.

Ford RD. *Diagnostic Tests Handbook.* Springhouse, Pa: Springhouse Corp; 1987.

Franey-Halfman M, Coburn C. Techniques in cardiac care: lasers, stents, and atherectomy devices. *AACN Clin Issues Crit Care Nurs.* 1990;1:87–109.

Franey-Halfman M, Levine, S. Intracoronary stents. *Crit Care Nurs Clin North Am.* 1989;1: 327–337.

Franey-Halfman M, Tukan T, Bergstrom D, et al. Using stents in the coronary circulation: a nursing perspective. *Focus Crit Care.* 1991;18: 132–142.

Fuentes F. Cardiomyopathies and specific myocardial diseases. In: Weeks, LC. ed. *Advanced Cardiovascular Nursing*; Boston, Mass: Blackwell Scientific Publications; 1986: 177–187.

Funk M. Epidemiology of heart failure. *Crit Care Nurs Clin North Am.* 1993;5:569–573.

Furst E. Automatic implantable cardioverter-defibrillator, *J Cardiovasc Nurs.* 1988;3(1): 77–81.

Gardner PE. Pulmonary artery pressure monitoring (1993). *AACN Clin Issues Crit Care Nurs.* 1993;4:98–119.

Gillespie DJ, Didier EP, Rehder K. Ventilation-perfusion distribution after aortic valve replacement. *Crit Care Med.* 1990;18:136–140.

Goodkind J, Coombs V, Golobic R. Excimer laser angioplasty. *Heart Lung.* 1993;22:26–35.

Govoni LE, Hayes JE, Shannon MT, et al. *Drugs and Nursing Implications,* 8th ed. Norwalk, Conn: Appleton & Lange; 1995.

Grady K, Nordin-Costanzo MR. Myocarditis: review of a clinical enigma. *Heart Lung.* 1989;18:347–353.

Granger CB, Califf RM, Topol EJ. Thrombolytic therapy for acute myocardial infarction. *Drugs.* 1992;44:293–325.

Hall LT. Endovascular surgery: an overview. *Prog Cardiovasc Nurs.* 1990;5(2):43–49.

Hanisch PJ. Identification and treatment of AMI by electrocardiographic site classification. *Focus Crit Care.* 1991;18:480–488.

Haskin JB. Pacemakers. In: Woods SL, Froelicher S, eds. *Cardiac Nursing*, 3rd ed. Philadelphia, Pa: JB Lippincott Co; 1989:766–804.

Hickey CS, Baas LS. Temporary cardiac pacing. *AACN Clin Issues Crit Care Nurs.* 1991;2: 107–117.

Holloway NM. Shock. Critical Care Plans. Springhouse, Pa: Springhouse Corp; 1989: 173–190.

Holt SK, Sparger G. Nursing management of the patient with thoracic, abdominal, and orthopedic trauma. In: Dolan JT, eds. *Critical Care Nursing Clinical Management Through the Nursing Process.* Philadelphia, Pa: FA Davis Co; 1991:1317–1341.

Hudgins C, Sorenson G. Directional coronary atherectomy: a new treatment for coronary artery disease. *Crit Care Nurs.* 1994;14(1): 61–66.

Jacobson C. Mechanisms of arrhythmia formation. *Crit Care Nurs Q.* 1991;14(2):1–9.

Johnson KL. Shock states. In: Kidd PS, Wagner KD, eds. *High Acuity Nursing.* Norwalk, Conn: Appleton & Lange; 1992:175–195.

Joiner GA, Kolodychuk GR. Neoplastic cardiac tamponade. *Crit Care Nurs.* 1991;2(2):50–58.

Kellic KA. Diuretics. *AACN Clin Issues Crit Care Nurs.* 1992;3:472–442.

Kennedy GT. Acute congestive heart failure: pharmacologic intervention. *Crit Care Nurs Clin North Am.* 1992;4:365–375.

Kidd PS, Wagner KD. Shock. In: Kidd PS, Wagner KD, eds. *High Acuity Nursing.* Norwalk: Conn: Appleton & Lange; 1992:

Kubo SH. Neurohormonal activity in congestive heart failure. *Crit Care Med.* 1990;18:539–544.

Kuhn M. Nitrates. *AACN Clin Issues Crit Care Nurs.* 1992;3:409–422.

Kuhn M. Angiotensin-converting enzyme inhibitors. *AACN Clin Issues Crit Care Nurs.* 1992;3:461–471.

Lancaster LE. Immunogenetic basis of tissue and organ transplantation and rejection. *Crit Care Nurs Clin North Am.* 1992;4:1–24.

Lee TH, Ting HH, Shammash JB, et al. Long-term survival of emergency department patients with acute chest pain. *Am J Cardiol.* 1992;69: 145–150.

Ley SJ. The thoracic ventricular assist device: nursing guidelines. *AACN Clin Issues Crit Care Nurs.* 1991;2:529–544.

Ley SJ. Myocardial depression after cardiac surgery: pharmacologic and mechanical support. *AACN Clin Issues Crit Care Nurs.* 1993; 4:293–308.

Loeb S. Nurse's Handbook of Drug Therapy. Springhouse, Pa: Springhouse Corp, 1993.

McErlean ES. Dual-chamber pacing. *AACN Clin Issues Crit Care Nurs.* 1992;2:126–131.

McErlean ES, Cross JA, Booth JE. Percutaneous cardiopulmonary bypass support: a new approach to high-risk angioplasty. *Crit Care Clin North Am.* 1992;4:358–364.

Manion PA. Temporary epicardial pacing in the postoperative cardiac surgical patients. *Crit Care Nurs.* 1993;13(2):30–38.

Maseri A. Clinical syndromes of angina pectoris. *Hosp Pract.* 1989;24(3):65–80.

Mattioni TA. Long-term prognosis after myocardial infarction. *Postgrad Med.* 1992;92(8): 107–114.

Menzel CK. The electrocardiogram during myocardial infarction. *AACN Clin Issues Crit Care Nurs.* 1992;3:190–202.

Menzel CK. ECG interpretation. In: Clochesy JM, Breu C, Cardin S, et al, eds. *Crit Care Nurs.* Philadelphia, Pa: WB Saunders Co; 1993: 117–121.

Mest-Kronick C. Postpericardiotomy syndrome: etiology, manifestations and interventions. *Heart Lung.* 1989;18:192–197.

Michaelson CR. *Congestive Heart Failure.* St. Louis, Mo: CV Mosby; 1983.

Miracle VA. Coronary atherectomy. *Crit Care Nurse.* 1992;12(3):41–48.

Morton PG. Rate-responsive cardiac pacemakers. *AACN Clin Issues Crit Care Nurs.* 1991;2: 140–149.

Moser DK. Pharmacologic management of heart failure: neurohormonal agents. *Crit Care Nurs Clin North Am.* 1993;5:599–608.

Moser SA, Crawford D, Thomas A. Automatic implantable cardioverter debribrillations. *Crit Care Nurse.* 1993;13(2):62–71.

Muirhead J. Constrictive pericarditis. *Prog Cardiovasc Nurs.* 1988;3(4):122–127.

Muirhead J. Pericardial disease. In: Woods SL, Froelicher S, eds. *Cardiac Nursing,* 3rd ed. Philadelphia, Pa: JB Lippincott Co; 1995: 913–922.

Muirhead J. Heart and heart-lung transplantation. *Crit Care Nurs Clin North Am.* 1992;4:97–109.

Murphy LM, Conforti CG. Nutritional support of the cardiopulmonary patient. *Crit Care Nurs Clin North Am.* 1993;5:57–64.

Norris SO. Managing low cardiac output states: maintaining volume after cardiac surgery. *AACN Clin Issues Crit Care Nurs.* 1993;4: 309–319.

Ohler L, Fleagle DJ, Lee BI. Aortic valvuloplasty: medical and critical care nursing perspectives. *Focus Crit Care.* 1989;16:275–287.

Osguthorpe SG. Hypothermia and rewarming after cardiac surgery. *AACN Clin Issues Crit Care Nurs.* 1993;4:276–292.

Ostrow CL. Thrombolytics. *AACN Clin Issues Crit Care Nurs.* 1992;3:424–434.

Payne JL. Immune modification and complications of immunosuppression. *Crit Care Clin North Am.* 1992;4:43–61.

Pedersen A, Groves JL, Coleman RB, et al. Intramuscular administration of RATG in the heart transplant patient. *Crit Care Nurs.* 1993;13(1): 22–31.

Peterson K, Brown MM. Extracorporeal membrane oxygenation in adults: a nursing challenge. *Focus Crit Care.* 1990;17:40–49.

Pierce CD. Transcutaneous cardiac pacing expanding clinical applications. *Crit Care Nurs Clin North Am.* 1989;1:423–435.

Purcell JA. Cardiac electrical activity. In: Kinney MR, Packa DR, Dunbar SB, eds, *AACN's Clinical Reference for Critical Care Nursing,* 3rd ed. St. Louis, Mo: Mosby-Year Book; 1993: –2713.

Quaal SJ. *Cardiac Mechanical Assistance Beyond Balloon Pumping.* St. Louis, Mo: Mosby-Year Book, 1993.

Quaal SJ. Centrifugal ventricular assist devices. *AACN Clin Issues Crit Care Nurs.* 1991;2: 515–526.

Quaal SJ. *Comprehensive Intraaortic Balloon Counterpulsation.* St. Louis, Mo: Mosby-Year Book, 1993.

Rafalowski M. Cardiac valve replacement: the homograft. *Focus Crit Care.* 1990;17:111–114.

Randall EM. Recognizing cardiac tamponade. *J Cardiovasc Nurs.* 1989;3(3):42–51.

Rice V. Shock, a clinical syndrome: an update. Part I, an overview of shock. *Crit Care Nurs.* 1991;11(4):20–27.

Rice V. Shock, a clinical syndrome: an update. Part 2, the stages of shock. *Crit Care Nurs.* 1991;11(5):74–82.

Rice V. Shock, a clinical syndrome: an update. Part 3, therapeutic management. *Crit Care Nurs.* 1991;11(6):34–39.

Rice V. Shock, a clinical syndrome: an update. Part 4, nursing care of the shock patient. *Crit Care Nurs.* 1991;11(7):28–40.

Riegel B. Patients with MI. In: Clochesy JM, Breu C, Cardin S, et al, eds. *Crit Care Nurs.* Philadelphia, Pa: WB Saunders Co; 1993: 320–322.

Roberts SL. *Congestive heart failure. Physiological concepts and the critically ill patient.* Englewood Cliffs, NJ; Prentice Hall; 1985:1–54. [out of print]

Roberts SL. *Cardiogenic shock. Physiological concepts and the critically ill patient.* Englewood Cliffs, NJ: Prentice-Hall; 1985:55–100. [out of print]

Roberts SL. *Cardiac tamponade. Physiological concepts and the critically ill patient.* Englewood Cliffs, NJ: Prentice-Hall; 1985:101–133. [out of print]

Roberts SL. Cognitive model of depression and the myocardial infarction patient. *Prog Cardiovasc Nurs.* 1989;4(2):61–70.

Rosborough D. Surgical myocardial revascularization in the 1990's. *AACN Clin Issues Crit Care Nurs.* 1993;4:219–227.

Rountree D. The hemopump temporary cardiac assist system. *AACN Clin Issues Crit Care Nurs.* 1991;2:562–574.

Rountree DW, Rutan PM, McClure A. The HEMOPUMP cardiac assist system: nursing care of the patient. *Crit Care Nurs.* 1991;11(4):46–57.

Ruzevich S. Heart assist devices: state of the art. *Crit Care Nurs Clin North Am.* 1991;3:723–732.

Schakenback LH. Patients with valvular disease. In: Clochesy JM, Breu C, Cardin S, et al, eds. *Crit Care Nurs.* Philadelphia, Pa: WB Saunders Co; 1993:320–322.

Scherer JC. *Nurse's Drug Manual,* 4th ed. Philadelphia, Pa; JB Lippincott Co; 1992.

Schoenbaum MP, Drew BJ. Proarrhythmia: mechanisms, evaluation and treatment. *Crit Care Nurs Q.* 1991;14(2):10–18.

Shekleton ME, Litwack K. *Critical Care Nursing of the Surgical Patient.* Philadelphia, Pa: WB Saunders Co; 1991.

Shinn JA. Novacor left ventricular assist system. *AACN Clin Issues in Crit Care Nurs.* 1991;2: 575–586.

Shinn JA. Cardiac transplantation. In: Woods SL, Froelicher S, eds. *Cardiac Nursing,* 3rd ed. Philadelphia, Pa: JB Lippincott Co; 1995: 585–600.

Smith-Roman P. Pacing for tachydysrhythmias. *AACN Clin Issues Crit Care Nurs* 1991;2: 132–139.

Smith RG, Cleavinger M. Current perspectives on the use of circulatory assist devices. *AACN Clin Issues Crit Care Nurs.* 1991;2:488–499.

Sokolow M, Mellroy MB, Cheitlin MD. *Clinical Cardiology,* 5th ed. Norwalk, Conn: Appleton & Lange, 1990.

Sollek MV, Lee KA. High blood pressure. In: Woods SL, Froelicher S, eds. *Cardiac Nursing,* 3rd ed. Philadelphia, Pa: JB Lippincott Co; 1989:814–852.

Sparger G, Shea-Sanning S, Selfridge J. Patients with trauma. In: Clochesy JM, Breu C, Cardin S, et al. eds. *Crit Care Nurs.* Philadelphia, Pa: WB Saunders Co; 1993:1219–1244.

Stewart SL, O'Sullivan CO, Vitello-Cicciu J, et al. Cardiac surgery. In: Kinney MR, Packa DR, Dunbar SB, eds. *AACN'S Clinical Reference for Critical Care Nursing,* 3rd ed. St. Louis, Mo: Mosby-Year Book; 1993:635–657.

Stier F. Antidysrhythmic agents. *AACN Clin Issues Crit Care Nurs.* 1992;3:483–493.

Stillwell SB. *Mosby's Critical Care Nursing Reference.* St. Louis, Mo: Mosby-Year Book; 1992.

Suhl J. Patients with shock. In: Clochesy JM, Breu C, Cardin S, et al, eds. *Crit Care Nurs.* Philadelphia, Pa: WB Saunders Co; 1993: 1258–1270.

Swearingen P, Keen JH. *Manual of Critical Care,* 2nd ed. St. Louis, Mo: Mosby-Year Book; 1992.

Tisdale LA, Drew BJ. ST segment monitoring in myocardial ischemia. *AACN Clin Issues Crit Care.* 1993;4:34–43.

Turk M. Acute pericarditis in the postmyocardial infarction patient. *Crit Care Nurs Q.* 1989; 12(3):34–38.

Turner JT. Cardiovascular trauma. *Nurs Clin North Am.* 1990;25:119–130.

Vallerand AH, Deglin JH. *Drug Guide for Critical Care and Emergency Nursing.* Philadelphia, Pa: FA Davis Co; 1991.

Vaska PL. Common infections in heart transplant patients. *Am J Crit Care.* 1993;2(2):145–156.

Waggoner PC. Transcutaneous cardiac pacing. *AACN Clin Issues Crit Care Nurs.* 1991;2: 118–125.

Waggoner PC. Mechanical interventions after acute myocardial infarction: impact on patient outcome. *Crit Care Nurs Clin North Am.* ;4:359–364.

Wallace PL. Nursing management of the patient with heart failure. In: Dolan JT, eds. *Critical Care Nursing Clinical Management Through the Nursing Process.* Philadelphia, Pa: FA Davis Co; 1991:923–956.

Weiner B. Thrombolytic agents in critical care. *Crit Care Nurs Clin North Am.* 1993;5: 355–366.

Whalen DA, Izzi G. Pharmacologic treatment of acute congestive heart failure resulting from LV systolic or diastolic dysfunction. *Crit Care Nurs Clin North Am.* 1992;5: 261–269.

Whipple JK, Bringa-Medicus MA, Schimel BA, et al. Selected vasoactive drugs: a readily available chart reference. *Crit Care Nurs.* 1992; 12(1):23–29.

White P. Calcium channel blockers. *AACN Clin Issues Crit Care Nurs.* 1992;3:437–446.

Whitman GR. Shock. In: Kinney MR, Packa DR, Dunbar SB, eds. *AACN's Clinical Reference for Critical Care Nursing,* 3rd ed. St. Louis, Mo: Mosby-Year Book. 1993;133–172.

Wojciechowicz V. Pericardial window surgery for cardiac tamponade. *Crit Care Nurs.* 1985;5(5): 28–33.

Wojner AW. Assessing the five points of the intra-aortic balloon pump waveform. *Crit Care Nurs.* 1994;14(3):48–52.

Woods SL, Osguthorpe S. Cardiac output determination. *AACN Clin Issues Crit Care Nurs.* 1993; 4(1):81–97.

Workman LM. Anticoagulants and thrombolytics: what's the difference. *AACN Clin Issues Crit Care Nurs.* 1994;5:26–35.

Vascular Deviations

■ ABDOMINAL AORTIC ANEURYSM

For related information see Cardiac Deviations, Part 1: Acute myocardial infarction, p. 38; Shock, p. 178; Dysrhythmias, p. 184. Part III: Hemodynamic monitoring, p. 219. Part I: Hypertensive crisis, p. 141; Deep vein thrombosis, p. 304. Part II: Aneurysmectomy, p. 316).

Diagnostic Category and Length of Stay
DRG: 132 Atherosclerosis with complications
LOS: 4.00 days
DRG: 133 Atherosclerosis without complications
LOS: 3.00 days

Definition
An aneurysm is an irreversible dilatation of an artery secondary to a localized weakness of an arterial wall that may predispose the artery to thrombosis, distal embolization, or rupture. An abdominal aneurysm is the dilatation or ballooning of the abdominal aorta from localized weakness and stretching of the arterial wall. Abdominal aortic aneurysms are atherosclerotic and arise at a level below the branches of the renal arteries. The ballooning may be small and localized or large and diffuse. The aneurysm can extend to and include the iliac arteries.

Pathophysiology
With atherosclerosis there can be widening of the aortic wall resulting from destruction of the media, the middle layer containing elastic fibers. The primary defect is a loss of elasticity within the medial layer of the aorta. The elastic tissue becomes fragmented, with smooth muscle cell loss and medial necrosis. The loss of elasticity leads to increased tension within the vessel wall. The increased wall tension weakens the arterial wall and causes more segmented widening. Blood flow becomes turbulent, placing more stress on an already weakened arterial wall. The gradual weakening of the media plus hemodynamic forces may cause thickening of the vasa vasorum.

Nursing Assessment

PRIMARY CAUSES

Atherosclerosis and nonatherogenic mechanisms, such as prevention of collagen cross-linking (copper or amino acid deficiency), disrupted collagen (collagenase, protease), syphilis, arteritis, poststenotic dilatation, or recessive chromosomal mutation. Other causes include malnutrition or trauma from surgical procedures.

RISK FACTORS

- Family history of atherosclerosis or other conditions such as hyperlipidemia, hypertension, diabetes, or cigarette smoking.

PHYSICAL ASSESSMENT

- Inspection: Widened midline pulsation proximal to the umbilicus; back pain radiating to lower back, groin, or leg accompanied by abdominal pain; peripheral skin color normal or cyanotic; or gastrointestinal disturbances (constipation) if aneurysm presses on duodenum; abdominal fullness; or lower extremity edema.
- Palpation: Aortic aneurysm originates below the renal arteries and common iliac aneurysms; the peripheral pulses normal or diminished. There is also tenderness on palpation of the abdominal aorta.
- Auscultation: Thigh blood pressure less than arm blood pressure; abdominal bruit.

DIAGNOSTIC TEST RESULTS

Standard Laboratory Tests (Table 2–1)

- Serum chemistries: Blood urea nitrogen (BUN) and creatinine to determine the degree of any renal function impairment.

Invasive Vascular Imaging Procedures (Table 2–2)

- Angiography: Used to demonstrate only the blood flow in the lumen, which may be occupied by thrombus. Also used to evaluate the number and location of the renal arteries; determine the pressure of renal, inferior mesenteric, iliac, and distal artery disease or aneurysm; confirm thoracoabdominal aneurysm; and determine whether the aortic abdominal aneurysm is above the level of the renal arteries.

Noninvasive Diagnostic Tests (Table 2–3)

- Abdominal aorta ultrasonography: Provides a record of aortic dimensions in both the sagittal and the transverse planes. Elective resection should be a serious consideration for aneurysms that are 4 cm in diameter and it is firmly indicated for those exceeding 5 cm. Reveals aortic aneurysm with or without thrombus.
- Computerized scans: Computed Tomographic (CT) Scan: Superior for the diagnosis and measurement of suprarenal aneurysm, thoracoabdominal aneurysm, and those involving the iliac arteries. Can provide information about symptomatic aneurysms associated with contained rupture or proximal dissection.
- Doppler flow or plethysomography: Used to assess peripheral pulses should peripheral vascular occlusive disease occur.
- Magnetic Resonance Imaging (MRI): Used to study the aorta in the sagittal plane.
- Roentgenogram: Anteroposterior and lateral plain roentgenogram can show the presence of an aortic aneurysm based on calcifications outlining the aneurysm. Large aneurysms may appear as soft masses, displace other organs, or cause abdominal gas patterns.

ECG

- Useful in assessing old myocardial infarction or ischemic ST changes as a part of generalized arteriosclerosis.

MEDICAL AND SURGICAL MANAGEMENT

SURGICAL INTERVENTION

- Resection of abdominal aortic aneurysm in patients who are at risk for aneurysmal rupture. An aneurysm of 4 cm has ≤ 15% chance of rupture within 5 years, whereas

TABLE 2-1. STANDARD LABORATORY TESTS

Test	Purpose	Normal Value Formulas	Abnormal Findings
Blood Studies			
Myoglobin	Index of damage in myocardial infarction and to detect muscle injury	30–90 ng/mL	>90 ng/mL can indicate AMI, polymyositis, or other muscle injury
Urinalysis			
Myoglobin	Used to evaluate a variety of conditions, including some metabolic diseases	Does not appear in urine	>2 μg MB/mL Found in hereditary myoglobinuria, unknown metabolic defects, crush injuries, progressive muscle disease, metabolic myoglobinuria
Serum Chemistry			
BUN (end products of metabolism)	Used as a gross index of glomerular function and the production and excretion of urea Aid in the assessment of hydration	8–20 mg/dL	Increased BUN can indicate impaired renal function, shock, dehydration, gastrointestinal hemorrhage, infection, excessive protein uptake, urinary tract obstruction Decreased BUN can indicate liver failure, malnutrition, impaired absorption, overhydration
Creatinine	Used to diagnose impaired renal function or renal glomerular filtration	Men: 0.8–1.2 mg/dL Women: 0.6–0.9 mg/dL	Increased creatinine can indicate impaired renal function, chronic nephritis, muscle disease Decreased creatinine can indicate muscular dystrophy

AMI, acute myocardial infarction; BUN, blood urea nitrogen.

an aneurysm of 8 cm has a 75% chance of rupture. Surgery is recommended for aortic aneurysms greater than 5 cm.

NURSING MANAGEMENT: NURSING DIAGNOSES AND COLLABORATIVE PROBLEMS

Nursing Diagnoses

Common nursing goals for patients with abdominal aortic aneurysm (AAA) are to increase tissue perfusion and maintain adequate fluid volume.

Altered peripheral and renal tissue perfusion related to atherosclerosis and subsequent reduced blood flow.

Expected Patient Outcomes. Patient maintains adequate peripheral and renal tissue perfusion, as evidenced by peripheral pulses +2; systemic vascular resistance (SVR) 900 to 1200 dynes/s/cm^{-5}, systemic vascular resis-

TABLE 2-1

TABLE 2-2

TABLE 2-2. INVASIVE VASCULAR DIAGNOSTIC PROCEDURES

Test	Purpose	Normal Value Formulas	Abnormal Findings
Arteriography	Digital subtraction angiography provides visualization of the abdominal aorta and renal arteries.		
	Used as part of the lower-extremity arteriogram or as a screening examination or renovascular hypertension.	Visualization of the abdominal aorta in anterior and lateral veins and extending from the level of the celiac artery to the common femoral vessels	Occluded mesenteric artery, abdominal aneurysm, peripheral vascular disease
	Provides information about the status of mesenteric circulation, specifically the inferior mesenteric artery.		
Digital Subtraction Arteriography (DSA)	Intravenous DSA can be used to assess extracranial carotid artery disease, renal vascular hypertension, the vasculature proximal and distal to abdominal aortic aneurysms, iliac arteries in patients with peripheral vascular disease, and aortic arch anomilies.	Normal carotid and vertebral arteries, abdominal aorta and branches, renal arteries, and peripheral arteries	Reveals stenosis of arteries, large aneurysms, total occlusion of arteries, thoracic outlet syndrome, large jugular tumors, masses
Venography (Phlebography)	Studies deep leg veins as a definitive test for deep vein thrombosis.	Normal popliteal, femoral, and iliac venous system and superficial vasculature	Unfilled deep veins and diversion of blood indicate thrombotic formation in deep veins of the leg, incompetent veins, and obstruction or blockage of a vein
	Identifies a suitable vein for use in arterial bypass grafting.		If a red thrombus appears, thrombolytic therapy or thromboectomy can be done
		The media, with smooth muscle fibers, shows up as a dark ring	
Vascular Endoscopy	Allows imagery of intra-arterial disease in color and in three dimensions using fiberoptic technology.	The internal and external elastic lamina, with elastic fibers and some collagen, cast a brighter echo	
	Allows evaluation of the nature of the lesion prior to a procedure.		

TABLE 2-2

TABLE 2-2. CONTINUED

Test	Purpose	Normal Value Formulas	Abnormal Findings
Intravascular Ultrasound	Provides information about atherosclerotic intima beneath the luminal surface. Guides the complete and safe removal of atheroma without injuring the underlying media and adventitia. Allows evaluation of precision of stent inflation.		Distinguishes four components of atherosclerotic intima Lipid deposits are hyperechoic; fibromuscular tissue casts soft echoes; fibrous tissue elicits bright echoes; and calcification causes bright echoes with shadowing
Isotope Angiography	Visualizes flow in vessels as large as the aorta and as small as the digital arteries of the hand. Diagnosis and evaluation of vascular trauma, vascular occlusion and stenosis, bypass and shunt integrity, and false and true aneurysms.	The static image of the isotope arteriogram shows larger vessels of the arterial tree against a relatively homogenous background of activity The distribution of activity in the major veins of the trunk and limbs following equilibration of the tagged red blood cells in the circulation because most intravascular blood resides in the venous system	Decreased perfusion of portions of the hand because of obstruction at the level of the distal radial or ulnar artery Aortic and peripheral artery aneurysms Traumatic iliac artery disruption Bleeding into and clotting within aneurysms of peripheral vessels Thrombosis within the venous system
Aortography	A confirming test for abdominal or thoracic aortic aneurysm.		Opacification, dilation, and calcification of aorta, false channel along the aortic lumen
Duplex Scanning	Localizing the artery and recognizing the presence of anatomic variations.		Thrombosis in deep veins

tance index (SVRI) 1970 to 2390 dynes/s/cm^{-5}/m^2, bilateral equal systolic blood pressure (BP); mean arterial pressure (MAP) 70 to 100 mm Hg; absence of edema; skin color pink; capillary refill ≤3 seconds; urinary output (UO) ≥30 mL/h or ≥0.5 mL/kg/h; absence of neck vein distention; blood urea nitrogen (BUN) 8 to 10 mg/dL; creatinine clearance in men 90 mL/min/1·73 m^2 of body surface, in women 84 mL/min/1.73 m^2, central venous pressure (CVP) 2 to 6 mm Hg; serum electrolytes within normal range.

- Confer with the physician as to the size of the AAA (≤6 cm in diameter requires medical therapy, whereas ≥6 cm requires surgery).
- Confer with physician to validate the expected patient outcomes used to evaluate peripheral and renal tissue perfusion.
- Consult with physician about desired UO for patient with a AAA ≥ 6 cm in diameter.
- Review test results: Abdominal ultrasonography, arteriography, Doppler flow, computerized scans, serum electrolytes, UO, BUN, creatinine and creatinine clearance.

TABLE 2-3

TABLE 2–3. NONINVASIVE VASCULAR DIAGNOSTIC PROCEDURES

Test	Purpose	Normal Value Formulas	Abnormal Findings
Abdominal Aorta Ultrasonogram	Used to assess abdominal aortic aneurysms Used to evaluate presence of clots within the aorta	Pattern images of contour and diameter	Aortic aneurysm with or without thrombus
Doppler Ultrasonography	Used to diagnose chronic venous insufficiency and superficial and deep vein thrombosis (popliteal, femoral, iliac) Used to diagnose peripheral artery disease and arterial occlusion Used to evaluate arterial trauma		
Ankle Pressure Index (API)	The ratio between ankle systolic pressure and brachial systolic pressure is used to assess arterial circulation	≥ 1.0 Proximal thigh pressure is normally 20–30 mm Hg higher than arm pressure In arms, pressure readings should remain unchanged despite postural changes Segmented pressures in the limbs are equal	0.85–0.95: Mild ischemia including claudication 0.51–0.84: Moderate ischemia 0.26–0.50: Severe ischemia with foot becoming red when it hangs down 0.25 and below: Gangrene or ischemic ulcers are present
Segmental Pressure	Study of systolic pressure at various levels of the limb. Measurements are taken at high-thigh (HT), above the knee (AK), below the knee (BK), and at the ankle level	The indirect pressure measurement at the upper part of the thigh exceeds the brachial blood pressure by 30–40 mm Hg because of cuff artifact The pressures measured in the two thighs should be within 20 mm Hg of each other A thigh/brachial index greater than 1.20 indicates no significant aortoiliac occlusive disease The pressure gradient in the leg does not exceed 20–30 mm Hg between any two levels	A gradient >30 mm Hg indicates a significant degree of arterial obstruction A gradient >40 mm Hg indicates an occluded artery A thigh-brachial index between 0.8 and 1.2 indicates aortoiliac disease Indices less than 0.8 indicate complete occlusion

TABLE 2–3. CONTINUED

TABLE 2-3

Test	Purpose	Normal Value Formulas	Abnormal Findings
Toe Pressure	Used to identify obstructive decrease in the digital vessels and in the pedal arch	Systolic pressure in the toe is 80%–90% of the brachial artery pressure	A toe-brachial pressure index less than 0.6 is abnormal Values less than 0.5 can be found in patients with rest pain or toe pressure less than 20 mm Hg
Stress Testing			
Treadmill Exercise	Determines the degree of disability under controlled conditions Permits an assessment of some nonvascular factors that may affect performance, such as musculoskeletal or cardiopulmonary disease	Response to exercise is a slight increase or no change in ankle systolic pressure compared with resting value	If ankle pressure is decreased immediately after exercise, test result is positive and test is repeated 2 minutes for 10 minutes When patient is forced to stop walking by symptoms associated with arterial occlusive disease, ankle systolic pressure is less than 60 mm Hg When symptoms occur without a significant decreases in ankle pressure, a nonvascular cause of leg pain is considered
Reactive Hyperemia Testing	Used to assess peripheral circulation in patients unable to walk on the treadmill	Suprasystolic cuff inflation at the thigh level is maintained for 3 to 5 min Ischemic vasodilation occurs and resistant changes in ankle pressure are recorded and interpreted as in treadmill test	
Doppler Signal Velocity Wave-form Analysis			
Pulsatility Index (PI)	PI, calculated by dividing peak-to-peak frequency difference by mean forward frequency, is an approach to quantitate degree of wave form damping	In a femoral artery, PI is over 4 with a mean of 6.7. Distally, PI increases to 8 for the popliteal artery and 14.1 for the posterior tibial artery	With occlusion or stenosis, PI distal to site of disease decreases

TABLE 2-3

TABLE 2–3. CONTINUED

Test	Purpose	Normal Value Formulas	Abnormal Findings
Damping Factor	The ratio of pulsability indexes proximal and distal to a stenosis Used to assess severity of disease.		Increases according to the extent of obstruction in the intervening segment
Transit Time	Assesses the time taken by a pulse wave to travel from heart to an artery or thigh in an arterial segment		
Plethysmography	Records the dimensional changes of a finger, toe, arm, leg, eye, or other part of the body with each heartbeat or in response to temporary obstruction of venous return	Mean blood flow can be measured by recording the rate of increase in volume that occurs as a result of sudden interruption of venous outflow (venous occlusion plethysmography)	Shows peripheral artery disease from tests such as: digital plethysmography, segmental limb plethysmography, digital blood pressure, and limb blood flow Shows cerebrovascular disease through occular plethysmography Shows venous disease with test such as venous outflow with strain gauge (SIG) or impedance (IPG), venous volume changes using air (PRG), and venous reflux or photoelectric
Oculoplethysmography (OPG)	Used to study blood flow in the carotid arteries Helpful in identifying candidates for endarterectomy	Blood flow equal in both carotid arteries evidenced by no delay in wave tracings	A positive test is defined as a delay in pulse arrival when comparing right eye to left eye or eye to ear Pulse delay in eye signifies narrowing or blockage of the internal carotid artery on the affected side
Carotid Phono-angiography (CPA)	Used to evaluate cerebrovascular circulation; is the quantitative analysis of arterial bruits	First and second heart sounds are well defined with no cervical bruits present	Associated with areas of carotid stenosis

TABLE 2–3. CONTINUED

Test	Purpose	Normal Value/ Formulas	Abnormal Findings
Pulse Volume Recorder (PVR) testing of Peripheral Vasculature	Measurement of changes peripheral blood flow at various segments or locations in arms and legs Used to evaluate the severity of arterial occlusion before arteriography Used to determine the differential diagnosis of intermittent claudication of vascular origin versus neurogenic claudication and to monitor long-term treatment of peripheral occlusive disease	Maximum venous outflow (MVO) is normal; no significant pressure difference, no exercise symptoms, and open aortoiliac and distal system	A difference in pressure of 30 torr in segments of an arm or leg indicates increased arterial resistance and contributes to diagnosis of arterial occlusion Reduced maximum venous outflow is associated with deep venous thrombosis
Impedance Phlebograph (IPG)	Used to detect deep vein thrombosis Used as a screening test for patients considered at high risk for developing thrombophlebitis and for evaluating anticoagulant therapy	High degree of filling within a short period of time Electrical resistance falls quickly when cuff is released and indicates unobstructed blood flow Conductivity normally increases as the veins fill when a pneumatic cuff is inflated around the thigh	Little or no change in venous capacitance and venous outflow is indicative of deep vein thrombosis
Abdominal roentgenogram	Used to diagnose intra-abdominal diseases such as nephro-lithiasis, intestinal obstruction, soft tissue masses, or ruptured viscus	Normal abdominal structure	Calcium in blood vessels, tumors, or stones
Abdominal Aorta Ultrasonography	Used to detect and measure abdominal aortic aneurysm Used to measure expansion of known abdominal aortic aneurysm	The abdominal aorta tapers from 1" to ½" (2.5–1.5 cm) in diameter along its length from the diaphragm to the bifurcation Four of its major branches are usually well visualized: celiac trunk, renal arteries, superior mesenteric arteries, and common iliac arteries	Luminal diameter of the abdominal aorta greater than 1½" (4 cm) is aneurysmal; greater than 2¾" (7 cm), aneurysmal with high risk of rupture

TABLE 2-3

TABLE 2-3

TABLE 2–3. CONTINUED

Test	Purpose	Normal Value Formulas	Abnormal Findings
Scans			
Computed Tomographic Scan	Used to give a clear image of the chest, abdomen, and pelvis in identifying cysts and tumors	No tumor or pathological activity shown	Of significance to the vascular system is presence of an aneurysm of abdominal aorta
Magnetic Resonance Imaging	Used to quantitate blood flow and evaluate arterial system architecture	Image shows normal arterial and biochemical tissue details on any plane	Detection of plaque formation, tumors, blood clots, or hemorrhage
	Used to evaluate the vena cava and mesenteric veins		
Venous Reflex Plethysmography	Used to identify incompetent valves in either deep or superficial venous system	Calf volume decreases by at least 1% during exercise and returns to baseline in 10–30 s	Peripheral vascular disease or peripheral vascular occlusion
	Used to determine refilling time of calf veins after exercise or manual compressions	Skin blood content decreases during exercise and returns to baseline in ≤10 s	
	A photophlethysmography transducer (PPG) is used to record skin blood content response to leg exercise		

Baker, JD (1991), Loeb, S (1991), Ford, RD (1987)

- Limit physical activity to patient's comfort level when the AAA is ≤6 cm in diameter.
- Obtain and report hemodynamic parameters associated with altered peripheral tissue perfusion: SVR ≥1200 dynes/s/cm^{-5} and SVRI ≥2390 dynes/s/cm^{-5}/m^2.
- Monitor clinical indicators of peripheral perfusion: skin color, presence of edema, MAP, capillary refill, peripheral pulses, and UO.
- Obtain and report other clinical findings associated with altered tissue perfusion: pain, pulsatile abdominal mass, cyanotic and cool skin, capillary refill ≥3 seconds, peripheral pulses ≤+2, peripheral edema, thigh BP ≤ than arm BP, and MAP ≥90 mm Hg.
- Obtain and report clinical findings associated with decreased renal tissue perfusion: UO ≤30 mL/h or ≤0.5 mL/kg/h, specific gravity ≤1.010, peripheral edema, and neck vein distention.
- Monitor daily weight, intake, and output to assess renal function and presence of fluid gain.
- Administer prescribed IV fluid to maintain adequate hydration and UO ≥30 mL/h.
- Administer prescribed diuretics to maintain UO ≥30 mL/h (see Table 1–13, p. 76).
- Administer antihypertensive medication as ordered to maintain BP within patient's normal range and MAP 70–100 mm Hg (see Table 1–16, p. 146).
- Administer prescribed beta-blockers (see Table 1–5, p. 24).

- Teach patient with an AAA ≥ 6 cm in diameter to remain in bed until surgery.
- Teach patient to use alternative pain relief measures: progressive relaxation, repositioning, guided imagery, and meditation.
- Instruct patient regarding the need to modify risk factors: weight loss, exercise, ceasing smoking, and proper diet to reduce blood pressure and disease progression.
- Teach patient common side effects of diuretics.
- Teach patient to report any sudden changes in UO.

Fluid volume deficit related to hemorrhage from ruptured aneurysm or surgical trauma.

Expected Patient Outcomes. Patient maintains adequate fluid volume, as evidenced by capillary refill ≤3 seconds BP within patient's normal range, MAP 70 to 100 mm Hg, CVP 2 to 6 mm Hg, pulmonary capillary wedge pressure (PCWP) 6 to 12 mm Hg, cardiac output (CO) 4 to 8 L/min, skin color normal, and hemoglobin or hematocrit within normal limits.

- Review test results: hemoglobin, hematocrit, platelet count, and serum electrolytes.
- Obtain and report hemodynamic parameters associated with decreased fluid volume: CO ≤4.0 L/min, cardiac index (CI) ≤2.7 L/min/m², CVP ≤2 mm Hg, MAP ≤70 mm Hg, and PCWP ≤6 mm Hg.
- Obtain and report other clinical findings associated with decreased fluid volume: BP≤ 70 mm Hg, pallor, cool skin, UO ≤30 mL/h or ≤0.5 mL/kg/h, specific gravity ≤1.010, peripheral pulses ≤+2, and capillary refill ≥3 seconds.
- Should patient experience acute abdominal pain and BP≤ 70 mm Hg, prepare patient for emergency surgery.
- Prepare patient for surgery: aneurysm ≥6 cm in diameter or ruptured aneurysm.
- Administer oxygen by nasal cannula or mask.
- Administer oral and IV fluids, colloids, or blood products to maintain adequate circulating volume.

Collaborative Problems

A common collaborative goal for patients with AAA is to correct dysrhythmias.

Potential Complication: Dysrhythmias. Dysrhythmias related to coronary artery disease secondary to atherosclerosis.

Expected Patient Outcome. Patient maintains normal cardiac rhythm.

- Consult with physician about the underlying causes of dysrhythmias.
- Review test results of ECG, roentgenogram, serum electrolytes, and serum enzymes.
- Provide patient with prescribed low-salt, low-fat, and low-cholesterol diet.
- Limit physical activity to bed rest if the abdominal aneurysm is ≥6 cm in diameter and requires surgery.
- Monitor ECG continuously to assess heart rate and rhythm. Document ECG rhythm strips every 2 to 4 hours in patients with dysrhythmias.
- Monitor serum potassium levels that may contribute to dysrhythmias: hyperkalemia ≥5.5 mEq/L.
- Administer prescribed oxygen 2 to 4 L/min by means of a nasal cannula or mask.
- Administer prescribed IV fluids to maintain adequate hydration.
- Administer prescribed antidysrhythmias agents (see Table 1–11, p. 54).
- Prepare patient for surgery when the AAA is ≥ 6 cm in diameter.
- Teach patient to report an abnormal heart rate, chest pain, or syncope.
- Teach patient to avoid foods high in fat, cholesterol, and salt content.
- Teach patient to avoid behaviors that increase heart rate such as excessive physical activity, straining at stool, anger, or irritability.

DISCHARGE PLANNING. The critical care nurse will provide patient and significant other(s) with verbal or written discharge notes regarding the following subjects:

1. The signs and symptoms that warrant immediate medical attention when aortic abdominal aneurysm is 6 cm: abdominal or back pain or syncope.
2. The ways to reduce or modify risk factors: weight loss, exercise, ceasing smoking, and proper diet to reduce BP and disease progress.
3. A written list of side effects associated with patient's specific medication.

■ ACUTE AORTIC DISSECTION

(For related information see Cardiac Deviations, Part I: Acute myocardial infarction, p. 35; Shock, p. 174; Dysrhythmias, p. 184. Part III: Hemodynamic monitoring, p. 219. Part I: Hypertensive crisis, p. 141; Deep vein thrombosis, p. 304; Part II: Aneurysmectomy, p. 316).

Diagnostic Category and Length of Stay
DRG: 132 Atherosclerosis with complications
LOS: 4.00 days.
DRG: 133 Atherosclerosis without complications
LOS: 3.00 days

Definition
Acute aortic dissection results from hemorrhage that causes lengthwise splitting of the arterial wall. This causes a tear in the inner wall (intima) and the establishment of communication with the lumen of the vessel. Acute aortic dissection occurs in aortas with extensive medial disease or necrosis.

Pathophysiology
When hypertension is present, the aortic wall is exposed to additional hemodynamic stenosis that can cause medial degeneration. Dissection begins either in the proximal aorta above the aortic valve or just beyond the origin of the left subclavian artery. Proximal dissections occur more often in aortas involved with abnormalities of the smooth muscle, elastic tissue, or collagen. Dissections are characterized according to the originating tear and the extent of the dissection. DeBakey's classification model consists of three types. Type I dissections contain tear in the ascending aorta, with further dissection into the descending aorta. The intimal tear is found above the aortic valve and involves the valve leaflets, leading to aortic valve insufficiency. Type II dissections are limited to the ascending aorta. Finally, type III dissections are found distal to the left subclavian artery and can extend distally to the descending thoracic aorta.

Nursing Assessment

PRIMARY CAUSES
• Arteriosclerosis, cystic medial necrosis, third trimester pregnancy or labor, blunt chest trauma, rapid deceleration injuries in the aorta, injection of contrast material during angiography or during femoral artery cannulation for cardiopulmonary bypass, or hypertension from pheochromocytoma or Cushing's disease.

RISK FACTORS
• Family history of atherosclerosis, hyperlipidemia, hypertension, or diabetes.

PHYSICAL ASSESSMENT
• Inspection: Anterior chest pain (ripping, tearing, or stabbing sensation), epigastric pain, severe back pain, syncope, dyspnea, decreased level of consciousness, confusion, lethargy, anuria, peripheral cyanosis, pallor, hemiplegia, sternoclavicular pulsations, paralysis of the lower extremities, or clammy skin.
• Palpation: Peripheral pulses absent or unequal, pulse deficit in the upper extremities, cool skin, abrupt or abdominal tenderness.
• Auscultation: Blood pressure decreased or unequal, tachycardia, pericardial friction rub, murmurs over arteries, aortic diastolic murmur from dissection close to aortic valve, or aortic regurgitation murmur.

DIAGNOSTIC TEST RESULTS

Invasive Vascular Imaging Procedures (see Table 2–3)

- Arteriography: Visualization of the aortic phase.
- Aortography: Findings may include a false lumen, splitting of the contrast column, evidence of intraluminal thrombus, increased thickness of the aortic wall, narrowing or occlusion of aortic branches, and chances in flow patterns.

Noninvasive Vascular Diagnostic Procedure (see Table 2–3)

- Chest roentgenogram: An anteroposterior chest roentgenogram may show widened mediastinum, increase in the size of the aortic shadow, loss of the aortic knob, increased aortic diameter, deviation of the trachea to the right, and cardiac enlargement.
- Computerized Tomography (CT) scan: A CT scan can reveal the intimal tear and false channels within the aorta. It can also be used to visualize collection of fluid in the pericardial, pleural, and mediastinal spaces.
- Echocardiogram: Reveals the site of the dissection. Hemorrhage in the vessel is shown as an area of absent echoes.
- Magnetic Resonance Imaging (MRI): The MRI can be used to show the site and extent of the intimal flap and the false channel.

ECG

- Left ventricular hypertrophy, inferior wall abnormalities, since dissection compromises the right rather than the left coronary artery.

MEDICAL AND \SURGICAL MANAGEMENT

PHARMACOLOGY

- Vasodilators: Nitroprusside at an infused dose of 0.5 $\mu g/kg/min$ is titrated to lower blood pressure. Reserpine given at dose of 1 to 2 mg every 4 to 6 hours intramuscularly (IM) is used to decrease blood pressure and pulsatile force (see Table 1–4, p. 20).
- Beta-adrenergic blocker: Propranolol can be used to decrease myocardial contractility. It is administered in conjunction with nitroprusside, since the latter can increase ejection force. Propranolol is contraindicated if bradycardia, asthma, or congestive heart failure (CHF) occurs (see Table 1–5, p. 24).
- Diuretics: Diuretics such as furosemide can decrease cardiac workload, limit contractility, and limit progression of the dissection.
- Morphine: Can be used to control pain.

HEMODYNAMIC MONITORING

- Used to optimize fluid management by frequently measuring pulmonary artery pressure (PAP), pulmonary capillary wedge pressure (PCWP), cardiac output (CO), and continuous mixed venous oxygen saturation ($S\bar{v}O_2$).

SURGICAL INTERVENTION

- Proximal dissection: Indications for surgical intervention consist of aortic valve insufficiency, failure of drug therapy, cardiac tamponade, progression of the dissection, and symptoms of cerebral or coronary ischemia. Replacement of the excised segment is accomplished with prosthetic graft material.
- Descending dissection: Indications for surgical intervention include type III dissection, hypertension, pain, compromise of a major branch of the aorta, cardiac tamponade, and impending rupture. The segment is replaced with a graft. A femorofemoral, atriofemoral, or ventriculofemoral bypass or shunt can be used to facilitate blood supply.

NURSING MANAGEMENT: NURSING DIAGNOSES AND COLLABORATIVE PROBLEMS

Nursing Diagnoses

Common nursing goals for patients with acute aortic dissection are to increase tissue perfusion, reduce anxiety, and minimize pain.

Altered cardiopulmonary, cerebral, renal, and peripheral tissue perfusion related to reduced arterial blood flow secondary to decreased myocardial contractility or vasoconstriction causing impaired cellular function of vital organs.

Expected Patient Outcomes. Patient maintains adequate tissue perfusion, as evidenced by systolic blood pressure (SBP) 110 to 140 mm Hg or diastolic blood pressure (DBP) 70 to 90 mm Hg (or within patient's normal range); coronary artery perfusion pressure (CAPP) 60 to 80 mm Hg; CO 4 to 8 L/min; cardiac index (CI) 2.7 to 4.3 L/min/m^2; mean arterial pressure (MAP) 70 to 100 mm Hg; ($S\bar{v}o_2$) 60% to 80%; heart rate (HR) $\leq$ 100 bpm; absence of dysrhythmias; absence of chest pain; pulmonary vascular resistance (PVR) 155 to 255 dynes/s/cm^{-5}, pulmonary vascular resistance index (PVRI) 200 to 450 dynes/s/cm^{-5}/m^2, respiratory rate (RR) 12 to 20 BPM; partial pressure of arterial oxygen (Pao$_2$) 80 to 100 mm Hg; partial pressure arterial carbon dioxide (Paco$_2$) 35 to 45 mm Hg; arterial oxygen saturation Sao$_2$ $\geq$95%; absence of dyspnea; absence of rales; systemic vascular resistance (SVR) 900 to 1200 dynes/s/cm^{-5}/m^2, pupils equal and normoreactive; absence of confusion and irritability; oriented to person, place, and time; normal sensorimotor function; urinary output (UO) $\geq$30 mL/h or $\geq$0.5 mL/kg/h, specific gravity 1.010 to 1.030; blood urea nitrogen (BUN) $\leq$20 mg/dL, creatinine clearance, M: 95 to 135 mL/min or W: 85 to 125 mL/min; serum creatinine 0.6 to 1.2 mg/dL; capillary refill $\leq$3 seconds; peripheral pulses; and absence of peripheral edema.

- Consult with cardiologist to validate the expected patient's outcomes that indicate adequate tissue perfusion.
- Review results from arterial blood gas measurement, serum enzyme tests, and chest roentgenogram.
- Review results of 12-lead ECG to help evaluate the location, progression, resolution of infarction and ventricular function.
- Review results of serum electrolyte tests.
- Limit physical activity to bed rest to decrease myocardial work load and myocardial oxygen demand.
- Obtain, document, and report hemodynamic parameters that indicate decreased cardiopulmonary tissue perfusion: CO$\leq$4 L/min, CI $\leq$1.8 L/min/m^2, CAPP $\leq$60 mm Hg, MAP $\leq$ 70 mm Hg, PVR $\geq$255 dynes/s/cm^{-5} and PVRI $\geq$ 450 dynes/s/cm^{-5}/m^2.
- Obtain, document, and report other clinical findings suggestive of decreased cardiopulmonary tissue perfusion: HR $\geq$100 bpm, dysrhythmias, chest pain, RR 12 to 20 BPM, dyspnea, and rales.
- Initiate continuous monitoring of ECG to assess HR and rhythm. Document ECG rhythm strips every 2 to 4 hours in patients with dysrhythmias.
- Administer prescribed oxygen 2 to 4 L/min (24% to 36% O$_2$) by means of nasal cannula or function of inspired oxygen Fio$_2$ $\leq$50% by mask to maintain Pao$_2$ $\geq$ 80 mm Hg, Sao$_2$ $\geq$95%, or $S\bar{v}o_2$ $\geq$60%.
- Administer prescribed IV fluids to maintain adequate circulating volume.
- Administer prescribed morphine to relieve chest pain.
- Administer positive inotropes (dopamine or dobutamine) and phosphodiesterase inhibitor (amrinone) to maintain CO $\geq$4 L/min and CI $\geq$2.7 L/min/m^2 (see Table 1–10, p. 50).
- Should pharmacological therapy be ineffective in correcting dysrhythmias or heart block occur, prepare patient for a pacemaker (see Cardiac Durations, Pacemaker, p. 270).
- Monitor neurological status of patient: orientation to person, place and time; pupils equal and reactive; and normal sensorimotor function.

- Obtain, document, and report clinical findings suggestive of decreased cerebral tissue perfusion; confusion, irritability, unequal pupils, disorientation, and abnormal sensorimotor function.
- Evaluate distal pulses and carotid pulses during the initial phase of aortic dissection every hour, then every 4 hours.
- Obtain, document, and report clinical findings indicating decreased renal tissue perfusion: UO $\leq$30 mL/h or $\leq$0.5 mL/kg/h for 2 consecutive hours, specific gravity $\leq$1.010, and peripheral edema.
- Administer prescribed volume-reducing agents: thiazide (chlorothiazide, hydrochlorothiazide, chlorthalidine, metolazone), loop diuretics (furosemide or bumetanide) or potassium-sparing (spironolactone, amiloride, or triamterene) to maintain UO $\geq$30 mL/h or $\geq$0.5 mL/kg/h and specific gravity 1.010 to 1.030 (see Table 1–13, p. 76).
- Obtain, document, and report hemodynamic parameters that indicate decreased peripheral tissue perfusion: SVR $\geq$1200 dynes/s/cm^{-5} and SVRI $\geq$2390 dynes/s/cm$^{\geq 5}$/m^2.
- Obtain, document, and report other clinical findings suggestive of decreased peripheral tissue perfusion: capillary refill $\geq$ 3 seconds, peripheral pulses $\leq$+2, and peripheral edema.
- Administer prescribed vasodilator (nitroprusside) should SVR and SVRI be elevated as a result of vasoconstriction, thereby causing increased afterload (see Table 1–4, p. 20).
- Prepare patient for possible aneurysm resection should neurological status deteriorate.
- Teach patient common side effects of antidysrhythmia or diuretic medications.
- Instruct patient as to the potential need for surgery.

Anxiety related to the potential for aortic rupture, need for corrective surgery, or fear of potential complications.

Expected Patient Outcome. Patient experiences reduced verbalization of anxiety.

- Encourage patient to express feelings of anxiety regarding the disease, treatment, need for surgery, and prognosis.
- Assess patient and family's knowledge and understanding of disease process, therapeutic regimen, diagnostic procedures, and potential surgery.
- Provide opportunity for and encourage questions and verbalization of fears and anxieties.
- Provide a calm and quiet environment.
- Provide support for patient who is about to experience surgical correction of aortic dissection.
- Involve patient and family in planning of care.
- Instruct patient regarding ways to reduce risk factors.
- Instruct patient as to the use of progressive relaxation or meditation to reduce stress and subsequent BP.
- Explain nature of patient's circulatory problem and symptoms patient is experiencing.
- Teach patient the purpose and nature of possible surgery and expected outcomes.

Pain related to acute aortic dissection.

Expected Patient Outcome. Patient experiences absence or reduced verbalization of pain.

- Obtain and report clinical findings associated with acute aortic dissection: severe pain, diaphoresis, flushed or pale skin, tremors, restlessness, or grimacing.
- Monitor for increasing pain as an indicator of expansion of the aneurysm.
- Maintain proper positioning or alignment to reduce pain.
- Encourage patient to describe pain using a scale of 1 to 10.
- Monitor patient's response to procedure or treatment.
- Plan activities to provide rest periods after therapies.

- Administer prescribed analgesic or narcotic to reduce pain.
- Teach patient stress-reduction strategies: progression relaxation, meditation, or guided imagery.

Collaborative Problems

Common collaborative goals for patients with acute aortic dissection are to increase CO and maintain fluid balance.

Potential Complication: Decreased Cardiac Output.

Decreased CO related to increased afterload secondary to arteriosclerosis or hypertension.

Expected Patient Outcomes. Patient maintains adequate CO, as evidenced by SVR 900 to 1200 dynes/s/cm^{-5}, SVRI 1970 to 2390 dynes/s/cm^{-5}/m^2, PCWP 5 to 12 mm Hg, pulse pressure (PP) 30 to 40 mm Hg, BP within patient's normal range, MAP 70 to 100 mm Hg, peripheral pulses +2, capillary refill ≤3 seconds absence of peripheral edema, peripheral skin normal color, peripheral skin warm, and CVP 2 to 8 mm Hg.

- Consult with physician to validate expected patient outcomes used to evaluate CO.
- Confer with physician as to the desired level of arterial BP.
- Review test results: chest roentgenogram, CT scan, arteriography, and aortography.
- Limit physical activity when aneurysm is diagnosed to be ≥6 cm in diameter or hematoma in the arterial walls.
- Obtain and report hemodynamic parameters associated with increased afterload: PP ≤30 mm Hg, SVR ≥1200 dynes/s/cm^{-5} and SVRI ≥2390 dynes/s/cm^{-5}/m^2.
- Obtain and report other clinical findings associated with increased afterload: MAP ≥ 90 mm Hg, peripheral edema, SBP ≥ 100 mm Hg, peripheral cyanosis, cool skin, capillary refill ≥ 3 seconds and diastolic murmur.
- Monitor peripheral pulses every 2 to 4 hours, as diminished or unequal pulses can signify occlusion of the lumbar arteries.

- Assess patient's SBP while receiving nitroprusside 0.5 mL/min. Infusion can be increased by 0.5 mL every 5 min until SBP is ≤ 100 mm Hg.
- Monitor and report UO ≤ 30 mL/h or ≤ 0.5 mL/kg/h.
- Should patient experience severe chest pain radiating to the back and shock, prepare patient for surgery (see Aneurysectomy, p. 318).
- Administer prescribed oxygen at 2 to 4 L/min by nasal cannula or mask.
- Administer prescribed IV fluid to maintain adequate circulatory volume.
- Administer prescribed rapid-acting antihypertensive agent, nitroprusside (50 mg in 100 mL of 5% dextrose in water) to maintain PP ≤40 mm Hg, SBP ≤100 mm Hg, SVR ≤ 1200 dynes/s/cm^{-5}, and SVRI ≤ 2390 dynes/s/cm^{-5}/m^2 (see Table 1–16, p. 146).
- Administer prescribed rapid-acting antihypertensive agent, trimethaphan (1 to 2 mg/mL) infused while patient is in semi-Fowler's position to maintain SBP ≤ 100 mm Hg.
- Administer prescribed beta-blocker, IV propranolol (0.15 mg/kg over a 5-minute period), to maintain HR 60 bpm (see Table 1–5, p. 24).
- Should beta-blocker be ineffective, administer prescribed reserpine to maintain SBP ≤100 bpm.
- Should pharmacological therapy be ineffective in reducing SBP and chest pain not relieved, prepare patient for emergency surgery.
- Instruct patient to report any pain.

Potential Complication: Fluid Volume Deficit.

Fluid volume deficit related to hemorrhage secondary to acute aortic dissection.

Expected Patient Outcomes. Patient maintains adequate fluid balance, as evidenced by CO 4 to 8 L/min, CI 2.7 to 4.3 L/min/m^2, SBP ≤100 mm Hg, MAP 70 to 100 mm Hg, absence of syncope, capillary refill ≤3 seconds, peripheral pulses +2, and UO ≥30 mL/h.

- Consult with physician to validate expected patient outcomes used to evaluate fluid volume balance.
- Review results from chest roentgenogram, ECG, and cardiac enzymes.
- Limit activity to bed rest while patient is experiencing chest pain.
- Obtain and report hemodynamic parameters associated with fluid volume deficit: CO ≤4 L/min, CI ≤2.7 L/min/m², and MAP ≤70 mm Hg.
- Obtain and report other clinical findings associated with fluid volume deficit associated with acute aortic dissection: sudden hypotension, extension of pain area, UO ≤30 mL/h, peripheral pulses ≤ +2 or absent, altered level of consciousness, or aortic diastolic murmur.
- Provide a quiet and restful environment.
- Monitor ECG continuously to assess HR and rhythm. Document ECG rhythm strips every 2 to 4 hours in patients with dysrhythmias.
- Monitor BP continuously while patient is receiving antihypertensive agents.
- Administer prescribed IV fluids to maintain adequate hydration.
- Administer colloid or blood to maintain adequate circulating volume.

DISCHARGE PLANNING

The critical care nurse will provide patient and significant other(s) with verbal or written discharge notes regarding the following subjects:

1. The signs and symptoms that warrant immediate medical attention when aortic abdominal aneurysm is 6 cm: abdominal or back pain or syncope.
2. The ways to reduce or modify risk factors: weight loss, exercise, ceasing smoking, and proper diet to reduce BP and disease progress.
3. A written list of side effects associated with patient's specific medication.

■ PERIPHERAL VASCULAR OCCLUSIVE DISEASE

(For related information see Cardiac Deviations, Part I: Shock, p. 174; Part I: Deep vein thrombosis, p. 304; Peripheral vascular trauma, p. 308; Part II: Peripheral vascular bypass graft, p. 319. Part III: Laser-assisted balloon angioplasty, p. 321, Peripheral atherectomy, p. 323, Intravascular stent, p. 324.)

Diagnostic Category and Length of Stay

DRG: 130 Peripheral vascular disorder with complications
LOS: 6.10 days
DRG: 131 Peripheral vascular disorder without complications
LOS: 4.50 days

Definition

Peripheral vascular occlusive disease is defined as any pathophysiological process that disrupts blood flow through arteries or veins of the extracranium, thorax, abdomen, or extremities. The term is usually applied to lower-extremity arterial insufficiency. Atherosclerosis is the common cause of peripheral vascular disease.

Pathophysiology

Atherosclerosis is characterized by structural changes in the arterial wall and the development of intraluminal plaque, causing narrowing of blood flow through the artery. There is also an accumulation of lipids and connective tissue in the arterial wall, increased intimal permeability, platelet aggregation secondary to injury, and proliferation of smooth muscle cells. Peripheral vascular disease is classified in two ways. (1) Aortoiliac disease involves the occlusion of the common iliac vessel, which leads to severe vascular insufficiency of the lower limb. There is often adequate collateral circulation, so that symptoms may be minimized. (2) Femoropopliteal disease is a common form of occlusion, which affects the common femoral, superficial femoral, profunda femoris, or popliteal arteries.

Physical Assessment

PRIMARY CAUSES
- Causes include atherosclerosis, hypertension, and diabetes mellitus.

RISK FACTORS
- Risk factors include cigarette smoking, unfavorable family history, obesity, advanced age, male sex, and stress.

PHYSICAL ASSESSMENT
- Inspection: Atrophic skin and nail changes in the toes and foot. The nails are thickened and misshapen, while the skin of the foot is thin, shiny, and scaly. Blanching occurs because the capillary perfusion is unable to pump blood uphill to the distal portion of the limb. The dependent ischemic limb develops rubor or cyanosis. Arterial ulcer can develop on the toes and over bony prominences.
- Palpation: Weakness or absence of a pulse can indicate stenosis or occlusion of an artery proximal to the anatomic location; affected limb is cool and capillary refill prolonged.
- Auscultation: Bruit heard over the stenotic lesion in the carotid arteries, abdominal aorta, and femoral arteries.

DIAGNOSTIC TEST RESULTS

Invasive Vascular Diagnostic Procedures (see Table 2–2)

- Angioscopy: A fiberscope is used to provide direct intravascular visualization of peripheral arteries. Provides information about atherosclerotic plaque formation and composition and results of angioplasty or atherectomy.
- Aortography: Translumbar aortography is used in patient with aortoiliac disease.
- Arteriography: Used to delineate specific anatomic location of obstruction, depict the etiology, and determine the condition of the arteries proximal and distal to the obstructive lesion. Also helps to clarify the surgical treatment options. Oblique or lateral views are necessary to fully evaluate the presence of an ulcerated plaque. Lateral or ipsilateral posterior oblique view is used to evaluate the common iliac bifurcation and the internal iliac artery at its origin. Lesions greater than 50% are of hemodynamic significance. Enlarged collateral vessels indicate that a hemodynamically significant stenosis is present. Significant slowing in one branch of a trifurcated vessel is a useful sign of a stenosis.

Noninvasive Diagnostic Tests (see Table 2–3)

- Doppler ultrasound: Used to detect pulsatile flow through an artery in the absence of a palpable pulse.
- Plethysmography: The pulse volume recorder is used to detect blood volume changes in a limb through the placement of air-filled cuffs around the extremity. Vessels occluded by arteriosclerosis show less pulsatile wave forms.
- Pulse volume wave-form analysis: Normally, the pulse volume wave form is characterized by a rapid upstroke that peaks and declines rapidly. With progressive arterial occlusive disease, there is first an absence of the diastolic wave, then broadening of the wave form, and finally loss of amplitude.
- Treadmill testing: In occlusive disease, the individual experiences pain during exercise from decreased blood flow to the extremity.
- Segmental limb pressures: Segmental limb pressure (SLP) is used to assess the location and significance of arterial occlusions. Normal thigh pressure is usually no more than 20 mm Hg below the brachial systolic pressure, and a gradient of greater than 20 mm Hg between limb segments suggests a hemodynamically significant lesion in the intervening artery. With a major arterial occlusion, there is a pronounced decrease in the ankle–brachial pressure index (ABI). The ABI is determined by dividing the an-

kle pressure by the arm pressure. Patients with intermittent claudication may have an ABI in the symptomatic limb of 0.4 to 0.8, while for those with severe ischemic rest pain it is between 0.0 and 0.4.

- Velocity wave form analysis: The VWF tracing of an artery with occlusive disease shows a rounding of the systolic peak, no second or third deflection, and a widening of the entire wave form.

MEDICAL AND SURGICAL MANAGEMENT

PHARMACOLOGY

- Pentoxifylline (Trental): Used to reduce blood viscosity and thereby increase blood flow in the microcirculation by increasing red blood cell flexibility and decreasing platelet aggregates and fibrinogen (Table 2–4).
- Thrombolytic therapy: Used to treat acute thromboembolic events and occlusion of arterial bypass grafts. Thrombolytic agents of choice are streptokinase and recombinant tissue plasminogen activator (rt-PA). The goal is to convert plasminogen to plasmin, resulting in the degradation of fibrin clots, fibrinogen, and other plasma proteins (see Table 1–7, p. 30).

PHYSICAL ACTIVITY

- Walking to the point of discomfort, resting a short time, then continuing to walk can stimulate exercising leg muscles to develop collateral circulation. The collaterals can bypass a localized arterial obstruction, thereby increasing in diameter to improve blood flow and subsequently improve symptoms.

PERCUTANEOUS TRANSLUMINAL ANGIOPLASTY (PTA)

- Used to manage atheromatous lesions, especially in the focal narrowing of the iliac or common femoral arteries. The intimal plaque is cracked, leaving a rough intimal surface that results in platelet aggregation and potential for thrombus formation. Fol-

lowing PTA, patients are treated with anticoagulant or antiplatelet-aggregating agents (see Cardiac Deviations, Percutaneous transluminal coronary angioplasty, p. 226).

LASER-ASSISTED ANGIOPLASTY

- Used to open a totally occluded artery so that an angioplasty catheter can be passed through the occlusion to dilate the narrowed vessel (see Laser-assisted balloon angioplasty, p. 226).

ULTRASOUND ANGIOPLASTY

- Used to recanalize totally occluded peripheral arteries.

SURGICAL INTERVENTION

- Arterial revascularization is accomplished by use of bypass procedures. Bypass approaches for aortoiliac occlusion include aortofemoral, unilateral aortofemoral grafting, or extra-anatomic bypass. The procedures are done with synthetic graft material such as Dacron or polytetrafluoroethylene (PTFE) (see Peripheral vascular bypass graft, p. 319).

NURSING MANAGEMENT: NURSING DIAGNOSES AND COLLABORATIVE PROBLEMS

Nursing Diagnoses

Common nursing goals for patients with peripheral vascular occlusive disease (PVOD) are to maintain skin integrity, enhance tissue perfusion, promote activity tolerance, and prevent pain.

Impaired skin integrity of foot and leg related to ischemic ulceration, tissue necrosis, or gangrene secondary to reduced blood flow.

Expected Patient Outcomes. Patient's skin remains intact without mechanical, thermal, or chemical skin breakdown of the ischemic foot or leg.

- Monitor and report clinical findings associated with impaired skin integrity: pallor, ru-

TABLE 2-4

TABLE 2–4: VASCULAR-RELATED MEDICATIONS

Medications	Route/Dose	Uses and Effects	Side Effects
Alpha Blocking Agents			
Phenoxybenzamine hydrochloride (Dibenzyline)	PO: 10 mg once daily, increase by 10 mg/d at 4-d intervals Maintenance dose 20–40 mg/d, divided bid or tid	Long-acting alpha-adrenergic blocking agent used to improve circulation in peripheral vasospastic conditions, such as Raynaud's cyanosis and adjunct treatment of shock or hypertensive crisis	Dry mouth, drooping of eyelids, postural hypotension, tachycardia, palpitation, dizziness, drowsiness, tiredness, confusion, GI irritation, headache, shock
Antihypertensive			
Methyldopa (Aldomet)	PO: 250 mg bid or tid; can be increased up to 3/g d in divided doses IV: 250–500 mg q 6 h infused over 30–60 min up to 1 g in 6 h	Treatment of severe hypertension	Fever, drowsiness, headache, weakness, fatigue, paresthesia, depression, orthostatic hypotension, syncope, bradycardia, myocarditis, edema, jaundice, impotence, pancreatitis
Trimethaphan camsylate (Arfonad)	Emergency IV: 0.5–1.0 mg/min initially and can be increased to range of 1–5 mg/min Aortic dissection 1–2 mg/min and increased to maintain BP of 100–200 mm Hg	Management of hypertensive emergencies and acute aortic dissection	Weakness, restlessness, apnea, hypotension, angina, tachycardia, anorexia, nausea, vomiting, urticaria, itching, dry mouth
Antiplatelet Agent			
Sulfinpyrazone (Anturane)	PO: 100–200 mg bid for 1 wk, then increase to 200–400 mg bid, may be reduced to 200 mg/d Serum urate levels are controlled to maximum of 800 mg/d	Treatment of chronic gouty arthritis To decrease platelets after aggregation	Nausea, vomiting, epigastric pain, ataxia, dizziness, vertigo, edema, convulsions, skin rash, fever, precipitation of acute gout
Vasodilators			
Nylidrin hydrochloride (Adrin)	PO: 3–12 mg tid or qid	Used in vasospastic disorders, such as peripheral vascular disease as in Raynaud's syndrome, night leg cramps, thromboangiitis obliterans, diabetic vascular disease	Nervousness, weakness, dizziness, palpitation, nausea, vomiting, postural hypotension

TABLE 2-4

TABLE 2–4. CONTINUED

Medications	Route/Dose	Uses and Effects	Side Effects
		Acts on beta-adrenergic receptors to increase blood flow to skeletal muscle by vasodilation of arteries and arterioles	
		Increases cerebral blood flow and cardiac output	
Cycloandelate (Cyclospasmol)	Oral: 200–400 mg qid and bed time; usual range is 400–800 mg/d in 2–4 divided doses	Used to manage atherosclerosis obliterans, intermittent claudication, thrombophlebitis, nocturnal leg cramps, or Raynaud's phenomenon	Dizziness; facial flushing; sweating; tingling sensation in face, fingers, and toes; tachycardia; weakness; headache; GI disturbance; heartburn; stomach pain
Papaverine hydrochloride (Pavabid)	PO: 1000–300 mg 3–5 times/d, 150 mg sustained release q 8–12 h IM/IV: 30–120 mg q 3 h as needed	Relief of cerebral and peripheral ischemia associated with arterial spasm Relaxes smooth muscle of bronchi	Nausea, vomiting, dizziness, headache, hepatotoxicity, respiratory depression, arrhythmias, fatal apnea
Pentoxifylline (Trental)	PO: 400 mg tid	Used to manage intermittent claudication associated with peripheral vascular disease	Agitation, nervousness, dizziness, headache, tremor, confusion, angina, dyspnea, blurred vision, abdominal discomfort, flatus, bloating, dyspepsia, nausea, vomiting, pruritus, rash, weight change, unpleasant taste

BP, blood pressure; GI, gastrointestinal; IM, intramuscular; IV, intravenous; PO, by mouth.

Govmi LE, Hayes JE, Shannon MT, et al. (1995). Doglin JH, Vallerand AH, Russin MM (1995) Loeb S (1993).

bor or purplish discoloration, ulceration, and pain.

- Use lamb's wool between toes to prevent interdigital friction necrosis.
- Moisturize ischemic foot and leg with alcohol-free lubricant lotion to prevent cracking of skin.
- Monitor any open areas such as ulceration and initiate treatment protocol: wet-to-dry saline, bed rest, or topical or systemic antibiotics.

- Record the presence of arterial ulceration: location, size, and drainage.
- Inspect skin for pressure points or open areas that could become potential sites for infection.
- Instruct patient to inspect peripheral skin and report any openings.
- Teach patient about necessity of meticulous foot care, stressing the risk of skin breakdown resulting from compromised arterial circulation.

Altered peripheral tissue perfusion related to partial or complete occlusion of peripheral arterial vessels.

Expected Patient Outcomes. Patient maintains adequate tissue perfusion, as evidenced by systemic vascular resistance (SVR) 900–1200 dynes/s/cm^{-5}, systemic vascular resistance index (SVRI) 1970 to 2390 dynes/s/cm^{-5}/m^2, blood pressure (BP) within patient's normal range, mean arterial pressure (MAP) 70 to 100 mm Hg, peripheral pulses +2, capillary refill ≤3 seconds, improved ABI, normal sensorimotor function, extremity warm and pink, and absence of pain.

- Confer with physician to validate expected patient outcomes used to evaluate tissue perfusion.
- Confer with physician about surgical procedures used to correct the disease process or symptoms associated with PVOD: arterial resection to restore unimpeded flow and to redirect blood flow around the site of the occlusion or lumbar sympathectomy to decrease sympathetic tone and increase peripheral vasodilation.
- Confer with Rehabilitation to develop an activity or exercise program that incorporates reduction in peripheral tissue perfusion.
- Review results of Doppler ultrasound, plethysmography, treadmill testing, velocity wave-form analysis, pulse volume wave-form analysis or segmental limb pressure.
- Maintain the extremity in a flat or dependent position to increase arterial blood supply.
- Ambulate patient, when appropriate, to increase collateral blood flow.
- Monitor clinical indicators of peripheral perfusion: peripheral pulses, capillary refill, skin color and temperature, BP, and urinary output.
- Assess extremity for color. The extremity is pale in the supine position and, with less advanced disease, blanching occurs when the leg is elevated 30 to 40 degrees.

- Monitor the extremity for muscle asymmetry, which reflects atrophy from long-standing arterial insufficiency.
- Monitor the following leg pulses for strength and equality: common femoral, popliteal, dorsalis pedis, and posterior tibial branches. Pulses that are greater than expected may signify an aneurysm.
- Obtain and report other clinical findings associated with decreased peripheral tissue perfusion resulting from PVOD: extremity pallor on elevation, extremity redness when dependent, hair loss in lower leg, sensorimotor impairment, peripheral pulses ≤+2, capillary refill ≥3 seconds, and presence of a bruit or murmur over the abdomen in the groin.
- Auscultate the abdomen or groin for the presence of a bruit or murmur indicating stenosis in either the iliac or femoral system. High-pitched bruits that extend throughout systole and into diastole indicate severe plaques, which decrease distal blood flow. Low-pitched, short bruits signify less advanced disease.
- Provide adequate foot care to preserve tissue integrity.
- Administer pentoxifylline for intermittent claudication: increases blood flow by decreasing blood viscosity through an increase in red blood cell flexibility and decrease in platelet adhesiveness and blood fibrinogen (see Table 2–4).
- Administer prescribed vasodilator (nitroprusside) to maintain SVR ≤1200 dynes/s/cm^{-5}, SVRI ≤2390 dynes/s/cm^{-5}/m^2, peripheral pulses +2, and capillary refill ≤3 seconds (see Table 1–4, p. 20).
- Administer prescribed anticoagulants to maintain vessel patency.
- Administer prescribed analgesic to reduce peripheral pain.
- Should pharmacological therapy be ineffective, prepare patient for peripheral laser assisted angioplasty (see Laser-assisted balloon angioplasty, p. 321).
- Should pharmacology therapy be ineffective, prepare patient for peripheral

atherectomy or intravascular stent (see Peripheral atherectomy, p. 323; intravascular stent, p. 324).

- Should pharmacological therapy or supportive procedures be ineffective, prepare patient for peripheral vascular bypass graft (see Peripheral vascular bypass graft, p. 319).
- Teach patient to avoid sitting or standing for long periods of time, which reduces venous pooling.
- Teach patient to avoid crossing legs when sitting or lying flat.
- Teach patient to place extremity in position of comfort.
- Instruct patient to wear cotton or wool stockings.
- Instruct patient to cease smoking: Nicotine may cause further vasoconstriction of the blood vessels.
- Instruct patient as to the need to identify stressors and cope with them through meditation and progressive relaxation.

Activity intolerance related to intermittent claudication secondary to PVOD.

Expected Patient Outcomes. Patient tolerates activity, as evidenced by decreased calf pain on ambulation, diminished or absence of peripheral pain, absence of edema, BP within patient's normal range, heart rate (HR) ≤100 bpm, and respiratory rate (RR) 12 to 20 BPM.

- Consult with physical therapist about creating an incremental activity program.
- Monitor for the presence of calf pain during increased physical activity: type of activity, timing of pain, and intensity of pain.
- Monitor patient's tolerance of gradual but progressive increases in physical activity: reduced or absent leg pain; HR ≤120 bpm, which is within 20 bpm of resting HR; RR ≤24 BPM; and absence of peripheral edema.
- Obtain and report clinical findings associated with activity intolerance resulting from PVOD: severe pain, loss of peripheral pulses, collapse of superficial veins, cold-

ness and pallor, and impaired sensorimotor function.

- Assist patient during gradual increments in activity: walking to chair, in room, or in hallway.
- Assist patient to develop an exercise program that will increase blood flow to the tissues, which improves muscle tone and size.
- Instruct patient to note and report when claudication pain occurs.

Pain related to partial or complete obstruction of the arterial vessels.

Expected Patient Outcomes. Patient experiences absence of or controlled pain, as evidenced by verbalization of decrease in pain severity and increase in activities of daily living.

- Confer with Physical Therapy regarding a postdischarge exercise program.
- Provide arterial positioning (if not contraindicated) using 6-inch shock blocks at head of bed to achieve leg dependency.
- Limit physical activity to minimize tissue oxygen demands.
- Document the presence of intermittent claudication: location of pain, timing of pain to physical activity, and duration of pain.
- Avoid using restrictive clothing such as antiembolism stockings.
- Teach patient distraction methods, such as listening to music or guided imagery.
- Teach patient noninvasive pain relief measures such as relaxation techniques, massages, or warm or cold compresses.
- Instruct patient regarding the importance of life-style changes: cessation of smoking, dietary limitations, and exercise tolerance.

DISCHARGE PLANNING
The critical care nurse will provide patient and significant other(s) with verbal or written discharge notes regarding the following subjects:

1. The signs and symptoms that warrant immediate medical attention: severe pain, loss of pulses, collapse of superficial veins, coldness and pallor, and impaired motor and sensory function.
2. The ways to preserve tissue integrity such as carefully drying feet each day, wearing cotton or wool stockings, and avoiding restrictive footwear.
3. The ways to increase arterial blood supply by maintaining extremity in a flat or elevated position, ambulating, and active range of motion exercises.
4. The ways to decrease venous pooling by not sitting or standing for long periods of time.

■ DEEP VEIN THROMBOSIS

(For related information see Cardiac Deviations, Part I: Acute myocardial infarction, p. 38. Part III: Thrombolytic therapy, p. 265; Respiratory Deviations, Part I: Pulmonary embolism, p. 397.)

Diagnostic Category and Length of Stay
DRG: 128 Deep vein thrombophlebitis
LOS: 7.40 days

Definition
Thrombophlebitis is the inflammation of the vein associated with thrombus formation. It can be a recurrent condition that produces segmental lesions in the small and medium-sized veins. The thrombus may be recanalized and the lumen restored, but more frequently the vein becomes completely obliterated.

Pathophysiology
Deep vein thrombus (DVT) usually affects the veins of the lower extremities in the following order: deep calf, femoral, popiteal, and iliac veins. While venous thrombi are usually attached to the vessel at the point of origin, they may or may not be attached. Three factors (Virchow's triad) predispose

the patient to thrombosis, namely endothelial injury, impaired blood flow, and hypercoagulation. One or more of these factors produce a thrombus. A thrombus develops as a result of slowed flow in the venous bloodstream and is associated with platelet aggregation. A thrombus organizes from its outer margins toward the center. In a large thrombus, involution usually occurs by a process of partial fibrosis and partial lysis. Usually the center disappears and a portion of the periphery may organize in a fibrous ring. At other times, bands of fibrous tissue extend across the old lumen of the vein and divide it into many small lumina. Inflammatory cells, leukocytes, lymphocytes, and fibroblasts accumulate and cause congestion of capillaries in and around the venous wall.

Physical Assessment

PRIMARY CAUSES
• The causes of DVT are delineated according to Virchow's triad: hypercoagulability, venous stasis, and intimal damage. Hypercoagulability involves blood dyscrasias, trauma, malignant disease, estrogen therapy, systemic infection, and cigarette smoking. Venous stasis is due to heart failure, dehydration, immobility, and incompetent vein valves. Finally, intimal damage occurs from trauma, infection, and venipuncture.

RISK FACTORS
• History of varicose veins or decreased activity.

PHYSICAL ASSESSMENT
• Inspection: Tenderness, induration, and redness along a superficial vein; warmth in the affected extremity; edema in the extremity; chills and fever; or cyanotic skin if venous obstruction is marked and pale if a reflex arterial spasm exists; lower extremity pallor, cyanosis, or edema; asymmetry of leg circumference; and extremity hair loss.
• Palpation: Extremity coldness and edema.

DIAGNOSTIC TEST RESULTS

Standard Laboratory Tests (see Table 1–1, p. 3)

- Serum chemistry: Elevated cholesterol and lipids suggesting atherosclerosis.

Invasive Vascular Diagnostic Procedures (see Table 2–2)

- Peripheral arteriography: Demonstrates narrowed or calcified area in the vascular system, leading to ischemic or blocked areas.
- Radioisotope scanning: Fibrin thrombi can be detected by scanning the extremities for accumulation of radioisotopes. In venous thrombosis, isotope accumulates at the clot and is not cleared. The test can also detect intra-abdominal venous thrombi.
- Venography: Ascending contrast venography defines the location, extent, and degree of attachment of the thrombus. Roentgenograms are taken and positive findings include filling defects in the veins of the affected limb, sharp termination of a column of contrast, or nonfilling of the deep vein system.

Noninvasive Vascular Diagnostic Tests (see Table 2–3)

- Doppler ultrasonography: In DVT, the normal peak-and-valley pattern caused by the continuous surging and diminishing of venous blood flow is absent. In addition, when squeezing is caused, the calf muscle will cause an audible surge of blood through the common femoral vein in the normal patient, but not in the patient with DVT.
- Duplex scanning: The imaging technique consists of brightness (B mode), ultrasound, which gives high-resolution images, and pulsed Doppler, which shows blood flow characteristics within a vein or artery. The technique provides anatomic (B-mode ultrasound) and hemodynamic measurements (pulsed Doppler).

- Impedance plethysmography: If a DVT is present, venous volume won't increase nearly as much because blood will already be trapped in the calf.

MEDICAL OR SURGICAL MANAGEMENT

PHARMACOLOGY

- Anticoagulant therapy: Continuous intravenous heparin is used to prevent the propagation of the DVT and minimize the rest of embolization. Heparin acts directly in both the intrinsic and extrinsic coagulation pathways. Warfarin is used as a long-term oral anticoagulant.

PHYSICAL ACTIVITY

- Physical activity includes active or passive exercises for patient at bed rest until acute symptoms subside; early ambulation when appropriate; leg elevation; and application of warm, moist heat.
- Use of graduated compression stockings or treatment with pneumatic compression boot devices to reduce the element of Virchow's triad, such as venous stasis.

NURSING MANAGEMENT: NURSING DIAGNOSES AND COLLABORATIVE PROBLEMS

Nursing Diagnoses

Common nursing goals for patients with DVT are to increase tissue perfusion, promote activity tolerance, and provide knowledge.

Altered peripheral tissue perfusion related to arterial and venous thrombus formation secondary to venous stasis or hypercoagulability.

Expected Patient Outcomes. Patient maintains adequate peripheral tissue perfusion, as evidenced by absence of redness, tenderness, and edema in both extremities; peripheral pulses +2; capillary refill ≤3 seconds, heart rate (HR) ≤100 mm Hg; respiratory rate, (RR) 12 to 20 BPM, blood pressure (BP)

within patient's normal limits; mean arterial pressure (MAP) 70 to 100 mm Hg; and absence of cyanosis.

- Consult with physician to validate expected patient outcomes used to evaluate tissue perfusion.
- Review results of coagulation studies, Doppler ultrasonography, impedance plethysmorgraphy, venography, peripheral arteriography, ECG, and radioisotope scanning.
- Limit physical activity to bed rest when DVT is diagnosed.
- Encourage active and passive range of exercises to promote circulation and formation of collateral flow.
- Encourage movements of lower limbs to improve venous return and prevent DVT by muscle pumping action: leg exercises of ambulation.
- Encourage patient to turn and deep breathe every 2 hours.
- Monitor and report clinical findings associated with decreased peripheral tissue perfusion: peripheral pulses ≤+2, capillary refill ≥3 seconds, edema in the affected extremity, and tenderness and redness in affected extremity.
- Obtain and report clinical manifestations of altered coagulation: epistaxis, ecchymoses, hematuria, and black and tarry stools.
- Apply antiembolism stockings to minimize venous stasis and promote venous return.
- Place affected extremity in an elevated position to promote venous return.
- Apply warm and moist heat to the affected extremity to increase blood flow.
- Provide a restful, quiet environment to minimize stresses that stimulate a vasoconstrictive response.
- Administer analgesics to decrease discomfort.
- Administer anticoagulation therapy, heparin or warfarin to increase clotting time, decrease formation of clots within the vascular system, and decrease platelet aggregation. Intravenous heparin bolus 5,000 to 10,000 U to 1000 U/h; or oral warfarin 5 to 15 mg/d (see Table 1–8, p. 32).
- Administer intravenous low-molecular-weight dextran.
- Administer Embolex, which combines heparin and dehydroerogotamine mesylate to prevent fibrin clot formation and stimulation of venous constriction, which enhances overall venous blood flow.
- Administer thrombolytic therapy in patients with extremities swollen from acute iliofemoral thrombophlebitis or if ischemia of the foot appears imminent (see Cardiac Deviations, Thrombolytic therapy, p. 265).
- Prepare patient for possible surgery: Vena caval interruption through the transverse placement of an umbrella filter into the inferior vena cava or by partial ligation of the caval segment.
- Instruct patient to report any lower-extremity pain.
- Teach patient to avoid smoking and vasoconstricting drugs, which further impede circulation.

Activity intolerance related to pain.

Expected Patient Outcomes. Patient is able to increase physical activity upon resolution of DVT and absence of extremity pain, redness, or edema.

- Consult with Physical Therapy about the development of an incremental exercise program to avoid stasis of circulation and further DVT.
- When appropriate, encourage leg exercises, frequent positional changes, and ambulation.
- Obtain and report clinical findings associated with activity intolerance: pain in the affected extremity, HR ≥100 bpm, cyanosis of extremity, or edematous extremity.
- Evaluate the affected extremity after exercises for tenderness, redness, coldness, or swelling.
- Instruct patient to report any changes in calf pain.

- Instruct patient to report any difficulty in beginning incremental increases in physical activity.

Knowledge deficit related to the causes, risk factors, and treatments associated with DVT.

Expected Patient Outcomes. Patient is able to state the causes, risk factors, and reasons behind treatment of DVT.

- Encourage patient to rest the affected extremity. Rest will allow the vessel to heal, absorb clot, and reduce the risk of embolization.
- Encourage patient to walk instead of sitting or standing, which will decrease venous stasis.
- Provide patient with knowledge of DVT causes in relation to risk factors, using drawings.
- Prepare patient for the possibility of surgery and explain its purpose.
- Encourage patient and family to ask questions and share their concerns.
- Instruct patient as to the importance of taking oral anticoagulants as prescribed.
- Instruct patient to report any bleeding in association with anticoagulant therapy.

Collaborative Problems

A common collaborative goal for patients with DVT is to prevent pulmonary embolism.

Potential Complication: Pulmonary Embolism. Pulmonary embolism related to blood clot secondary to deep vein thrombosis.

Expected Patient Outcomes. Patient maintains adequate pulmonary perfusion, as evidenced by pulmonary vascular resistance (PVR) 155 to 255 dynes/s/cm^{-5}, peripheral vascular resistance index (PVRI) 200 to 450 dynes/s/cm^{-5}/m^2, partial pressure of arterial oxygen (Pao$_2$) 80 to 100 mm Hg, partial pressure of arterial carbon dioxide (Paco$_2$) 35 to 45 mm Hg, bicarbonate (HCO$_3$) 22 to 26 mm Hg, arterial oxygen saturation Sao$_2$ 95.5% to 97.5%, HR $\leq$24 BPM, absence of dyspnea, BP within patient's normal range, skin color normal, normal cardiac rhythm, and normal breath sounds.

- Consult with physician to validate expected patient outcomes used to evaluate pulmonary perfusion.
- Review results of arterial blood gas measurements, chest roentgenogram, and ventilation-perfusion scan.
- Monitor for signs and symptoms of embolization: dyspnea, chest pain, restlessness, cyanosis, neck vein distention, hypotension, dysrhythmias, tachypnea, or alterated level of consciousness.
- Monitor ECG continuously to assess HR and rhythm. Document ECG rhythm strips every 2 to 4 hours in patients with dysrhythmias.
- Auscultate chest for breath sounds such as crackles, rales, or wheezes.
- Apply antiembolic stockings to increase deep vein flow and decrease stasis or clot predisposition.
- Administer prescribed IV fluids to maintain adequate hydration.
- Administer prescribed oxygen at 2 to 4 L/min by means of nasal cannula or mask to maintain Pao$_2$ $\geq$80 mm Hg, Paco$_2$ $\geq$35 mm Hg, HCO$_3$ $\geq$22 mEq/L, and Sao$_2$ $\geq$95%.
- Administer prescribed thrombolytic therapy, streptokinase or t-PA, to enhance lysis of emboli and increase pulmonary capillary perfusion (see Table 1–8, p. 32).
- Administer prescribed narcotic (morphine) to reduce anxiety and decrease metabolic demands.
- Administer prescribed anticoagulant (heparin or warfarin) to increase clotting time, decrease formation of clots within the vascular system, and decrease platelet aggregation: intravenous heparin bolus 5000–10,000 U to 1000 U/h; or oral warfarin 5 to 15 mg/d (see Table 1–8, p. 32).
- Teach patient to report any chest pain.
- Teach patient common side effects of thrombolytic therapeutic agents.

DISCHARGE PLANNING

The critical care nurse will provide patient and significant other(s) with verbal or written discharge notes regarding the following subjects:

1. Signs and symptoms that warrant medical attention: pallor, cyanosis, coldness, redness, edema, loss of hair, atrophy, chest pain, or dyspnea.
2. Factors that affect the progression of atherosclerosis: hypertension, stress, obesity, hyperlipidemia, smoking, and sedentary living.
3. Importance of keeping up follow-up visits and laboratory studies.
4. Common side effects of anticoagulants.

■   PERIPHERAL VASCULAR TRAUMA

(For related information see Cardiac Part I: Shock, p. 174 and Part III: Hemodynamic monitoring, p. 219. Vascular Part II: Peripheral vascular bypass graft, p. 319.)

Diagnostic Category and Length of Stay

DRG: 130 Peripheral vascular disorders age over 69 with complications
LOS: 6.10 days.
DRG: 131 Peripheral vascular disorders, age less than 70 without complications
LOS: 4.50 days.

Definition

Peripheral vascular trauma includes arterial or venous trauma that can result from both penetrating and nonpenetrating injuries.

Pathophysiology

Penetrating injuries are caused by high-velocity weapons, which cause the artery to be severely contused proximal and distal to the penetration. High-velocity injuries have a cavitational effect and cause extensive soft tissue damage. Low-velocity gunshot wounds can push the blood vessels forward and stretch them, causing less extensive soft tissue injury. Penetrating trauma can cause laceration, perforation or transection of the involved artery or vein. Blunt injury, caused by motor vehicle accident, crush injuries, or athletic injuries, produce laceration, contusion, or penetration of the vessels by displaced bone or sharp edges of bone fragments. Iatragenic vascular injury can result from diagnostic and therapeutic procedures. Peripheral vascular injury consists of compression, spasm, contusion, laceration, or perforation, and false aneurysm. Injuries of the lower extremities involve arteries, veins, and nerves. The superficial femoral artery is the most frequently injured because it is near the distal femur and can be injured from a fracture.

Nursing Assessment

PRIMARY CAUSES

• Penetrating injuries include gunshot or stab wounds. Stab wounds can be caused by knives, metal strips, fragments of glass, or long bone fractures. Blunt injuries are due to motor vehicle accidents, crush injuries, or athletic injuries. Iatrogenic injuries may be due to procedures such as arteriography, arterial lines, repeated punctures of the radial or brachial artery for arterial blood gases, or insertion of an intra-aortic balloon pump.

PHYSICAL ASSESSMENT

• Inspection: Bright blood spurting from a wound at the time of injury, hematoma, pallor, poikilothermy, pain, paresthesia, paralysis, or nerve deficit distal to the injury.
• Palpation: Hard signs: absent distal pulse, expanding or pulsatile hematoma, bruit or thrill at injury site. Soft signs: diminished distal pulse or small, nonpulsatile hematoma.
• Auscultation: General hypotension, tachycardia, or bruit over a hematoma.

DIAGNOSTIC TEST RESULTS

Invasive Vascular Diagnostic Procedures (see Table 2–2)

- Arteriogram: Used to identify and confirm arterial injury, such as complete disruption, thrombosis, intimal defect, traumatic aneurysm, traumatic arteriovenous fistula, or spasm. The procedure also helps to determine the extent of injury.
- Intra-arterial digital subtraction angiography (DSA): used to further clarify vascular injuries or small area of injury.

Noninvasive Diagnostic Tests (see Table 2–3)

- Doppler ultrasound and Doppler ankle-brachial index (ABI): used to assess the extremity in patients with absent or diminished pulses. A decreased ABI and an abnormal arterial wave form can indicate significant arterial injury.
- Roentgenogram: A roentgenogram of the injured extremity can confirm a fracture.

MEDICAL AND SURGICAL MANAGEMENT

PHARMACOLOGY

- Antibiotic therapy: Given preoperatively for patients with penetrating wounds.
- Anticoagulant therapy: Heparin infusion may be necessary to prevent clot formation in vessels that may occlude collateral blood supply to an extremity.

SURGICAL INTERVENTIONS

- Surgical techniques include simple suturing of lacerations, end-to-end anastomosis, and interposition bypass grafts. Saphenous veins are used when appropriate, but should extensive injury occur, synthetic graft can be used.
- Venous ligation may be necessary when multiple injuries occur.
- Fasciotomy: Used on the extremity to prevent compartment syndrome or for the relief of increased compartment pressure.

NURSING MANAGEMENT: NURSING DIAGNOSES AND COLLABORATIVE PROBLEMS

Nursing Diagnoses

Common nursing goals for patients with vascular trauma are to increase tissue perfusion, maintain fluid volume, facilitate adequate breathing pattern, maintain skin integrity, and promote physical mobility.

Altered peripheral tissue perfusion related to interruption of arterial or venous blood flow secondary to trauma or compartment syndrome.

Expected Patient Outcomes. Patient maintains adequate peripheral tissue perfusion, as evidenced by absence of pain on passive motion of the ankle or great toe, ankle pressure equal to or greater than the brachial systolic pressure, blood pressure (BP) within patient's normal range, absence of edema, peripheral pulses +2, capillary refill ≤ 3 seconds, skin warm, and absence of pallor or cyanosis.

- Consult with physician to validate expected patient outcomes used to evaluate peripheral tissue perfusion.
- Review results of coagulation studies, Doppler ultrasound, and Doppler ABI, roentgenogram, arteriography, and intra-arterial digital subtraction angiography.
- Monitor affected extremity for the presence of the six Ps of vascular injury: pallor, poikilothermy, pain, pulselessness, paresthesia, or paralysis. The presence of the six Ps signifies an extremity ischemic from interruption of the arterial circulation.
- Monitor and report clinical findings associated with decreased peripheral tissue perfusion: diminished or absent peripheral pulses, capillary refill ≥ 3 seconds, ankle perfusion pressure ≤ 30 Hg, extremity coolness and cyanosis, and peripheral pain.
- Position the affected extremity to facilitate peripheral perfusion.

- Monitor and report a large, firm, pulsatile hematoma with ill-defined margins surrounding the wound. The hematoma may suggest arterial injury.
- Auscultate the peripheral vessel and report a thrill or bruit over a hematoma, which may indicate the development of an arteriovenous fistula.
- Administer prescribed IV fluids to maintain adequate hydration and adequate circulating volume.
- Administer prescribed anticoagulant, when appropriate, to prevent thrombus formation.

Fluid volume deficit related to hemorrhage from an arterial or venous tear.

Expected Patient Outcomes. Patient maintains adequate fluid volume, as evidenced by BP within patient's normal range, pulmonary capillary wedge pressure (PCWP) 4 to 12 mm Hg, mean arterial pressure (MAP) 70 to 100 mm Hg, capillary refill $\leq$3 seconds, peripheral pulses +2, urinary output (UO) $\geq$ 30 mL/h or 0.5 mL/Kg/h, cardiac output (CO) 4 to 8 L/min, cardiac index (CI) 2.7 to 4.3 L/min/m², central venous pressure (CVP) 2 to 6 mm Hg, pulmonary artery pressure (PAP) 20 to 30 and 8 to 15 mm Hg, or heart rate (HR) $\leq$100 bpm.

- Consult with physician to validate expected patient outcomes used to evaluate adequate fluid volume.
- Limit physical activity to bed rest until the patient's condition stabilizes.
- Keep the affected extremity immobilized until the vascular problem has been corrected.
- Apply direct digital pressure over the wound or on the artery proximal to the wound for 5 to 10 minutes to produce hematoma.
- Obtain and report hemodynamic parameters associated with fluid-volume deficit: CO$\leq$4 L/min, CI $\leq$2.7 L/min/m², CVP $\leq$2 mm Hg, and PCWP $\leq$4 mm Hg.
- Obtain and report other clinical findings associated with fluid-volume deficit: BP $\leq$70

mm Hg, MAP $\leq$70 mm Hg, HR $\geq$100 bpm, UO $\leq$30 mL/h or $\leq$0.5 mL/kg/h, peripheral pulses $\leq$+2 and capillary refill $\geq$3 seconds.
- Measure the amount of bleeding from the wound site.
- Measure intake, output, and specific gravity every 1 to 2 hours to evaluate fluid balance.
- Monitor BP: Systolic BP between 80 and 90 mm Hg is associated with bleeding at a rate of 60 to 200 mL/min.
- Administer IV fluids to provide volume lost during active bleeding.
- Administer prescribed oxygen 2 to 4 L by means of nasal cannula or mask.
- Prepare patient for autotransfusion: collect hemothorax or mediastinal blood and infuse it directly without processing; intraoperative blood may be collected, concentrated, washed, and reinfused using a variety of devices.
- Administer aspirin, dypyridamole, or nonsteroidal antinflammatory agents to maintain short-term patency in small graft $\leq$8 mm.
- Should pharmacological and fluid therapy be ineffective, prepare patient for surgery.

Impaired skin integrity related to penetrating injury.

Expected Patient Outcome. Patient regains and maintains skin integrity.

- Assess and record the characteristics of the wound: redness, tenderness, edemas, or drainage.
- Cleanse the wound and apply a clear occlusive dressing following unit protocol.
- Change dressings using aseptic technique and apply antimicrobial ointment as ordered.
- Administer antibiotics as prescribed.

Mobility, impaired physical related to nerve deficit, paresthesia, or paralysis.

Expected Patient Outcomes. Patient maintains physical mobility and absence of peripheral nerve dysfunction.

- Consult with physician regarding the origin of impaired physical mobility from injury to peripheral nerves that result in neuropraxia with eventual complete return of function, in partial disruptions, or in complete nerve dysfunction and the expected degree of impaired physical mobility.
- Immobilize patient until the amount of sensorimotor damage can be determined.
- Position patient to maintain optimal body alignment by supporting the affected extremity in a functional position.
- Assist with sensorimotor testing in the involved area.
- Monitor all peripheral pulses for equality and quality.
- Instruct patient to report any changes in sensorimotor function.
- Instruct patient as to the purpose behind the surgery.

Anxiety related to potential loss of an extremity or need for surgery.

Expected Patient Outcome. Patient experiences reduced anxiety as verbalized by patient.

- Listen to patient's concerns regarding the trauma, vascular injury, treatment outcomes, and possible need for surgery.
- Support family throughout the vascular trauma episode.
- Instruct patient about the injury and its relationship to physical changes or need for corrective surgery.
- Instruct patient to report any changes in sensorimotor sensations.

Collaborative Problems

Common collaborative goals for patients with peripheral vascular trauma are to prevent compartment syndrome and correct deep vein thrombosis.

Potential Complication: Compartment Syndrome. Compartment syndrome related to massive swelling of the soft tissue secondary to impairment of distal blood flow.

Expected Patient Outcomes. Patient maintains adequate distal perfusion, as evidenced by normal muscle tissue pressure, compartment pressure normal 9 to 15 mm Hg, capillary refill $\leq$ 3 seconds, and absence of fluid extravasation from capillaries.

- Consult with physician to validate expected patient outcomes used to evaluate compartment syndrome.
- Review results of intracompartmental pressure.
- Obtain and report clinical findings indicating compartment syndrome; pain with passive stretch, hyperesthesia, loss of motor function, cool skin, pallor or cyanosis, palpable compartment tension, decreased or absent pulse, tingling or numbness, and high compartment tension.
- Assist with the measurement of intracompartment pressures: A wick catheter is connected to a standard pressure transducer and inserted into the appropriate muscle compartment.
- Obtain and report clinical findings associated with the need for a fasciotomy when there is injury to both arteries and veins: hypotension, massive swelling, and soft tissue damage.
- Should intracompartment pressure $\geq$30 mm Hg, one of three types of faciotomies can be performed to decompress the compartment: blind incision of the fascia with limited skin incision, open incision of the fascia with extensive skin incision, or resection of a part of the fibula with fasciotomy.
- After fasciotomy, keep the exposed muscle moistened with normal saline or quarter-strength (isotonic) povidine-iodine–soaked gauze. This procedure is maintained until secondary closure occurs or the area receives a skin graft. Report any muscle necrosis, since bone and soft tissue infection can occur.
- Should massive swelling occur, prepare patient for a split-thickness graft. A secondary skin graft may be necessary when there is

excessive swelling and a wide fasciotomy has been done.

- Elevated the affected extremity and apply ice for the first 24 to 48 hours after opening to reduce edema, if not contraindicated.
- Prepare patient for fasciotomy, which is performed when intracompartment pressure is increased 30 to 40 mm Hg, or there are signs of distal ischemia or massive edema.
- Should necrotic muscle tissue occur, prepare patient for surgical debridement.
- Administer IV fluids to maintain adequate hydration.
- Administer prescribed analgesic to relieve pain.
- Teach patient to report any changes in sensation or appearance.
- Instruct patient to report indicators of compartment syndrome: pain, paresthesia, hyperesthesia, paralysis, or coolness.

Potential Complication: Deep Vein Thrombosis. Deep vein thrombosis related to puncture or tear in the intima secondary to vessel cannulation or trauma.

Expected Patient Outcomes. Patient maintains adequate peripheral vessel circulation, as evidenced by normal coagulation studies, peripheral pulses ≥2, capillary refill ≤3 seconds, skin warm, absence of redness or cyanosis, HR ≤100 bpm, and absence of pain.

- Consult with physician to validate expected patient outcomes used to evaluate peripheral vessel circulation.
- Review results of angiography, venography, or coagulation studies.
- Limit activity to bed rest and provide positional support for the affected extremity.
- Obtain and report clinical findings associated with venous thrombosis: peripheral pulse ≤+2 or absent, unusual warmth and redness or coolness and cyanosis, leg pain, and positive Homans' sign.
- Monitor intake, urine output, and specific gravity to evaluate fluid balance.

- Encourage patient to perform isotonic leg exercises to promote venous return.
- Monitor for abnormal bleeding in patients receiving anticoagulant therapy: hematuria, bleeding gums, ecchymoses, petechiae, or epistaxis.
- Evaluate the affected extremity to reduce interstitial swelling by enhancing venous return.
- Administer prescribed IV fluids to maintain adequate hydration.
- Administer prescribed anticoagulant therapy, if not contraindicated, to prevent extension of the thrombus by prolonging clotting time.
- Administer prescribed analgesics for leg pain.
- Instruct patient about the hazards of smoking and that nicotine can cause vasospasm.
- Teach patient the common side effects of anticoagulants.

DISCHARGE PLANNING

The critical care nurse will provide patient and significant other(s) with verbal or written discharge notes regarding the following subjects:

1. The signs and symptoms that warrant medical attention; sensorimotor changes, pain, pallor or cyanosis, and absent or decreased peripheral pulses.
2. Common side effects of diuretics
3. Importance of keeping up follow-up visits and laboratory studies.

■   REPERFUSION INJURY

(For related information see Part I: Deep vein thrombosis, p. 304; Peripheral vascular occlusive disease, p. 297. Part III: Laser-assisted balloon angioplasty, p. 321; Peripheral atherectomy, p. 323; intravascular stent, p. 324. See also Renal Deviations, Part I: Acute renal failure, p. 459.)

Diagnostic Category and Length of Stay

DRG: 130 Peripheral vascular disorder with complications

LOS: 6.10 days

DRG: 131 Peripheral vascular disorder without complications

LOS: 4.50 days

Definition

Reperfusion injury concerns events that occur causing injury during the early phases of reperfusion from acute arterial occlusion.

Pathophysiology

An extremity can be viewed as an organ system composed of different tissue types. The various tissues, such as nerve, muscle, skin, subcutaneous tissue, and bone, vary in their ability to tolerate ischemia, depending on their metabolic demands. During the early phases of reperfusion, there is progressive microcirculatory obstruction, called the no-reflow phenomenon. This process occurs with progressive ischemic intervals. In the extremity, the consequences of an arterial occlusion depends on the presence or absence of collateral circulation. With prolonged ischemia, thrombus formation in the venous effluent can occur as a secondary event caused by low flow and thrombogenicity of the system. The result is an aggravation of the ischemic process and complicated revascularization.

There are two major components responsible for the injury that occurs in tissues after ischemia. Cellular injury occurs with the introduction of oxygen without adequate preparation of the cell to handle it. The second component is the reflow phenomenon. The deposition of fibrin in the microcirculation may contribute to the inability to reperfuse tissues after prolonged ischemia. Following the initial event, the ischemia may be aggravated by proximal or distal thrombus development. Collateral circulation is impaired and ischemia worsens.

Nursing Assessment

PRIMARY CAUSES

- Embolic causes include atherosclerotic heart disease, valvular heart disease, aneurysm, or paradoxical embolus. Traumatic causes are penetrating trauma, blunt trauma, dissection, presence of medical device, external compression, or drug abuse. Thrombosis causes can be atherosclerosis; low-flow states such as congestive heart failure, hypovolemia, or hypotension; hypercoagulable states, or vascular grafts. Outflow venous occlusion can be caused by compartment syndrome and phlegmasia. Low-flow state involves cardiogenic shock, hypovolemic shock, or drug effect.

RISK FACTORS

- Risk factors are cigarette smoking or drug abuse.

PHYSICAL ASSESSMENT

- Inspection: Edema of the affected tissue, muscle weakness, difficulty in moving the extremity, and mild pain throughout the involved limb.
- Palpation: Decreased or absent peripheral pulses.

DIAGNOSTIC TEST RESULTS

Standard Laboratory Tests (see Table 2–1)

- Serum myoglobin: Increased in skeletal muscle injury and shock.
- Urine myoglobin: Increased in severe trauma to the skeletal muscles.

MEDICAL AND SURGICAL MANAGEMENT

PHARMACOLOGY

- Diuretics: Hyperosmotic diuretics such as mannitol exert an osmotic effect across the cell membrane, thereby pulling fluid from the cells and clearing this fluid via the kidneys. The osmotic effect can alleviate the complications of compartment syndrome.

- Calcium channel blockers: Used to prevent reperfusion injury because of increased cytosolic calcium, which is involved in oxygen-radical generation (see Table 1–6, p. 28).
- Glucose and insulin: Administered in the treatment of hyperkalemia should myeonephrotic-metabolic syndrome occur.
- Sodium bicarbonate: Should hyperkalemia occur, sodium bicarbonate will promote cellular uptake of potassium.
- Low-dose dopamine alone or in conjunction with prostaglandin E_1 (PGE): The PGE can serve to lower the blood pressure as does low-dose dopamine.

NURSING MANAGEMENT: NURSING DIAGNOSES AND COLLABORATIVE PROBLEMS

Nursing Diagnoses

Common nursing goals for patients with reperfusion injury are to increase tissue perfusion and maintain urinary elimination.

Altered peripheral tissue perfusion related to rethrombosis secondary to vessel trauma.

Expected Patient Outcomes. Patient maintains adequate peripheral tissue perfusion, as evidenced by normal coagulation studies, peripheral pulses ≥ 2, capillary refill ≤ 3 seconds, skin warm, skin color normal, absence of redness or cyanosis, normal sensorimotor function, and absence of pain.

- Consult with physician to validate expected patient outcomes used to evaluate peripheral tissue perfusion.
- Review results of coagulation studies.
- Limit activity to bed rest and provide positional support for the affected extremity.
- Limit activity to bed rest until peripheral tissue perfusion has been established.
- Obtain and report clinical findings associated with decreased peripheral tissue perfusion: peripheral pulse $\leq +2$ or absent,

capillary refill ≥ 3 seconds, peripheral pallor or cyanosis, and decreased sensorimotor function.

- Monitor intake, urine output, and specific gravity to evaluate fluid balance.
- Encourage patient to perform isotonic leg exercises to promote venous return.
- Monitor for abnormal bleeding in patients receiving anticoagulant therapy: hematuria, bleeding gums, ecchymoses, petechiae, or epistaxis.
- Evaluate the affected extremity to reduce interstitial swelling by enhancing venous return.
- Administer prescribed IV fluids to maintain adequate hydration.
- Administer prescribed analgesics for leg pain.

Urinary elimination decreased related to increased myoglobulin from the breakdown of ischemic muscle, which then precipitates in the renal tubule.

Expected Patient Outcomes. Patient maintains adequate urinary output, as evidenced by urinary output (UO) ≤ 0.5 mL/kg/h, normal specific gravity, normal color, and serum myoglobin within normal range.

- Review results of serum and urine myoglobin.
- Obtain and report clinical findings associated with altered UO resulting from myoglobin in urine: UO ≤ 30 mL/h or ≤ 0.5 mL/kg/h, specific gravity ≤ 1.010, brown pigmentation in urine, and myoglobinuria.
- Monitor UO for amount, color, and specific gravity.
- Monitor urine for the presence of myoglobin (urine will have a brown pigmentation).
- Monitor blood pressure to ensure adequate perfusion of the renal vasculature and patency of the affected vessel.
- Administer prescribed IV fluids to maintain adequate hydration.
- Administer mannitol and loop diuretics to help prevent acute renal failure by pulling

fluid from the cells and clearing the fluid through the kidneys.

- Administer sodium bicarbonate or acetazolamide to alkalinize the urine.
- Administer low-dose dopamine alone or in conjunction with PGE in continuous drip form to increase renal perfusion (see Table 1–10, p. 50).

Pain related to the ischemic limb.

Expected Patient Outcome. Patient experiences reduced or absence of extremity pain.

- Encourage patient to rate the severity of pain on a scale of 1 to 10.
- Encourage patient to report the presence of extremity pain.
- Assess the affected extremity for pain, which may indicate compartment syndrome.
- Administer analgesics or narcotics and document the degree of pain relief achieved.
- Instruct patient to report any extremity pain and identify its location (ischemic pain can be generalized in the large muscle or limited to metatarsal pain).

Collaborative Problems

Common collaborative goals for patients with reperfusion injury are to prevent compartment syndrome and correct electrolyte imbalance.

Potential Complication: Compartment Syndrome.
Compartment syndrome related to endothelial swelling in the affected extremity secondary to revascularization or reperfusion.

Expected Patient Outcomes. Patient maintains adequate peripheral tissue perfusion, as evidenced by absence of edema, normal sensorimotor function in the affected extremity, capillary refill ≤3 seconds, skin color and temperature normal, and peripheral pulses +2.

- Consult with physician regarding the possibility of reperfusion injury following an ischemic episode.

- Monitor for edema of the reperfused extremity after revascularization.
- Monitor for and report the signs of compartment syndrome: fullness or tenseness of the muscle, pain out of proportion to the physical findings, paresthesia, weakness, and motor dysfunction.
- Measure ankle-arm indices and compare the ratio for decreases signifying hypoperfusion.
- Monitor peripheral nerve function, since nerve function can be injured from ischemia and reperfusion.
- Measure compartment pressures to determine whether or not there is expansion of the muscle tissue inside the fascial compartment (cessation of microcirculation occurs when tissue pressure in the compartment increases to a level equal to the diastolic blood pressure).
- Monitor thromboectomized site for hematoma formation.
- Assist physician with a fasciotomy to prevent further ischemia, necrosis, and limb loss.
- Administer prescribed hyperosmotic diuretics (mannitol) which exerts an osmotic effect across the cell membrane to alleviate the complication of compartment syndrome.
- Administer calcium channel blockers to prevent reperfusion injury because increased cytosolic calcium is involved in oxygen-radical generation. (see Table 1–6, p. 28).
- Administer fibrinolytic agents during reperfusion to reduce problems associated with the no-flow phenomenon.

Potential Complication: Electrolyte Imbalance.
Electrolyte imbalance related to hyperkalemia secondary to the leakage of potassium during cell death and acute renal failure.

Expected Patient Outcomes. Patient maintains adequate electrolyte balance, as evidenced by potassium of 3.8 to 5.5mEq/L and UO

≥0.5mL/kg/h, absence of dysrhythmias, and normal sensorimotor function.

- Review results of potassium, blood urea nitrogen (BUN), and ECG.
- Monitor for the signs and symptoms of hyperkalemia: weakness, flaccid paralysis, abdominal distention, and diarrhea.
- Monitor patient's cardiac rhythm for changes associated with hyperkalemia: peaked T waves, atrial arrest, widening in the QRS and biphasic QRS-T complexes.
- Administer IV fluids to maintain adequate hydration.
- Administer glucose, insulin, or sodium bicarbonate to promote cellular uptake of potassium.
- Administer prescribed ion exchange resin (sodium polystyrene sulfonate [kayexalate]) to reduce potassium levels.
- Administer prescribed diuretics to eliminate excess potassium (see Table 1–13, p. 75).
- Administer prescribed sodium bicarbonate, which will promote cellular uptake of potassium.

DISCHARGE PLANNING

The critical care nurse will provide patient and significant other(s) with verbal or written discharge notes regarding the following subjects:

1. The signs and symptoms that warrant medical attention: sensorimotor changes, pain, pallor, or cyanosis and absent or decreased peripheral pulses.
2. Common side effects of diuretics
3. Importance of keeping up follow-up visits and laboratory studies.

PART II: SURGICAL CORRECTION AND NURSING MANAGEMENT

■   ANEURYSMECTOMY

(For related information see Cardiac Deviations, Part I: Shock, p. 174; Congestive heart failure, p. 87; Dysrhythmias, p. 184. Part III: Hemodynamic monitoring, p. 219. Part I: Deep vein thrombosis, p. 304; Peripheral vascular trauma, p. 308. Respiratory Deviations, Part I: Pulmonary embolism, p. 397. Part III: Mechanical ventilation, p. 428. Multisystem Deviations, Part I: Sepsis, p. 772.)

Diagnostic Category and Length of Stay
DRG: 108 Other cardiothoracic or vascular procedures with pump
LOS: 12.70 days.

Definition
Aneurysmectomy is the excision of an aneurysm and its replacement with a Dacron graft.

Patient Selection

INDICATIONS. Elective surgery is advised for all aortic aneurysms larger than 6 cm.

CONTRAINDICATIONS. Patients for whom the surgery would place them at risk for other problems.

Procedure

TECHNIQUE. Prosthesis, which is a fabric Dacron graft of approximate diameter, is preclotted, and heparin (1 mg/kg bodyweight) is given intravenously. In general, the proximal and distal aortic clamps are applied, and the aneurysm incised. All mural thrombi and arteriosclerotic plaques are evacuated to identify the lumbar arteries along the posterior wall. After removing debris from the proximal and distal ends of the aorta, the fabric graft is sutured in place. The walls of the aneurysm are approximated over the graft to isolate it from contact with the abdominal viscera.

Abdominal Aortic Aneurysm. The distal aorta and iliac vessels are exposed. If there is no aneurysmal involvement of the common iliac arteries and no significant distal occlusive disease, the distal graft anastomosis can be made proximal to the aortic bifurcation. If aneurysmal involvement of iliac arteries or distal occlusive disease is present, distal anastomoses to the external iliac arteries are preferred. Finally, if the external iliac or common femoral arteries are diseased, both femoral arteries should be exposed through a small groin incision.

Descending Aortic Aneurysm. Resection of descending aneurysm involves protecting the spinal cord and kidneys from ischemia during aortic interruption. The aorta is clamped proximal and distal to the aneurysm, and the wall of the aneurysm is incised. Thrombus within the aneurysm is removed and segmental intercostal, bronchial, and mediastinal vessels within the aorta are oversewn.

Dissecting Aneurysm. Cardiopulmonary bypass is used. If the aneurysm is confined to the thoracic aorta, the aorta distal to the aneurysm is dissected. If the dissection process extended below the diaphragm, the aorta is mobilized at a level above the diaphragm where the distal anastomoses will be made.

EQUIPMENT. Dacron fabric prosthesis.

Complications

Myocardial infarction, arrhythmias, congestive heart failure, renal failure, respiratory insufficiency, infection, pulmonary embolus, and stroke.

NURSING MANAGEMENT: NURSING DIAGNOSES AND COLLABORATIVE PROBLEMS

Nursing Diagnoses

Common nursing goals for patients undergoing aneurysmectomy are to maintain tissue perfusion and enhance gas exchange.

Altered cardiopulmonary, peripheral, renal, or cerebral tissue perfusion related to aorta leaking or occlusion secondary to aortic graft rupture.

Expected Patient Outcomes. Patient maintains adequate tissue perfusion, as evidenced by systolic blood pressure (SBP) 110 to 140 mm Hg or diastolic blood pressure (DBP) 70 to 90 mm Hg (or within patient's normal range); coronary artery perfusion pressure (CAPP) 60 to 80 mm Hg; cardiac output (CO) 4 to 8 L/min; cardiac index (CI) 2.7 to 4.3 L/min/m^2, mean arterial pressure (MAP) 70 to 100 mm Hg; continuous mixed venous oxygen saturation (S$\bar{v}$o$_2$) 60% to 80%; heart rate (HR) $\leq$100 bpm; absence of dysrhythmias; absence of chest pain; pulmonary vascular resistance (PVR) 155 to 255 dynes/s/cm^{-5}; pulmonary vascular resistance index (PVRI) 200 to 450 dynes/s/cm^{-5}/m^2; respiratory rate (RR) 12 to 20 BPM, partial pressure of arterial oxygen (Pao$_2$) 80 to 100 mm Hg; partial pressure of arterial carbon dioxide (Paco$_2$) 35 to 45 mm Hg; arterial oxygen saturation Sao$_2$ $\geq$95%; absence of dyspnea; absence of rales; systemic vascular resistance (SVR) 900 to 1200 dynes/s/cm^{-5}; systemic vascular resistance index (SVRI) 1970 to 2390 dynes/s/cm^{-5}/m^2; pupils equal and normoreactive; absence of confusion and irritability; oriented to person, place, and time; normal sensorimotor function; urinary output (UO) $\geq$30 mL/h or $\geq$0.5mL/kg/h, specific gravity 1.010 to 1.030; blood urea nitrogen (BUN) $\leq$20 mg/dL; creatinine clearance, M:95 to 135 mL/min or W: 85 to 125 mL/min; serum creatinine 0.6 to 1.2 mg/dL; capillary refill $\leq$3 seconds; peripheral pulses; and absence of peripheral edema.

- Consult with cardiologist to validate expected patient outcomes that indicate adequate tissue perfusion.
- Review results of ECG, chest roentgenogram, serum enzymes, serum electrolytes, complete blood count (CBC), coagulation profile, BUN, and creatinine.
- Elevate head of bed to no more than 45 degrees to avoid hip flexion and subsequently cause a kink in the abdominal aortic graft.
- Obtain, document, and report hemodynamic parameters that indicate decreased

cardiopulmonary tissue perfusion: CO≤4 L/min, CI ≤1.8 L/min/m^2, CAPP ≤60 mm Hg, MAP ≤ 70 mm Hg, PVR ≥255 dynes/s/cm^{-5}, and PVRI ≥450 dynes/s/cm^{-5}/m^2.

- Obtain, document, and report other clinical findings suggestive of decreased cardiopulmonary tissue perfusion: HR ≥100 bpm, dysrhythmias, chest pain, RR 12 to 20 BPM, dyspnea, and rales.
- Initiate continuous monitoring of ECG to assess HR and rhythm. Document ECG rhythm strips every 2 to 4 hours in patients with dysrhythmias.
- Administer prescribed oxygen 2 to 4 L/min (24% to 36% O$_2$) by means of nasal cannula or fraction of inspired oxygen (F$_1$O$_2$) ≤50% by mask to maintain Pao$_2$ ≥ 80 mm Hg, Sao$_2$ ≥95%, or S$\bar{\text{v}}$o$_2$ ≥60%.
- Administer the prescribed intravenous fluid to correct hypovolemia and potential graft collapse.
- Administer prescribed morphine to relieve chest pain.
- Administer prescribed antidysrhythmic agents appropriate for the particular dysrhythmia resulting from decreased myocardial tissue perfusion (see Table 1–11, p. 54).
- Administer positive inotropes (dopamine or dobutamine) and phosphodiesterase inhibitor (amrinone) to maintain CO ≥4 L/min and CI ≥2.7 L/min/m^2 (see Table 1–10, p. 50).
- Obtain, document, and report clinical findings suggestive of decreased cerebral tissue perfusion: confusion, irritability, unequal pupils, disorientation, and abnormal sensorimotor function.
- Obtain, document, and report clinical findings indicating decreased renal tissue perfusion: UO ≤30 mL/h or ≤ 0.5 mL/kg/h for 2 consecutive hours, specific gravity ≤1.010, and peripheral edema.
- Administer prescribed volume-reducing agents: thiazide (chlorothiazide, hydrochlorothiazide, chlorthalidine, metolazone), loop diuretics (furosemide or bumetanide) or potassium-sparing (spironolactone, amiloride, or triamterene) to maintain

UO ≥30 mL/h or ≥0.5 mL/kg/h and specific gravity 1.010 to 1.030 (see Table 1–13, p. 76).
- Obtain, document, and report hemodynamic parameters that indicate decreased peripheral tissue perfusion: SVR ≥1200 dynes/s/cm^{-5} and SVRI ≥2390 dynes/s/cm^{-5}/m^2.
- Obtain, document, and report other clinical findings suggestive of decreased peripheral tissue perfusion: capillary refill ≥3 seconds, peripheral pulses ≤+2, and peripheral edema.
- Monitor BP in all extremities: Unequal BP in extremities with a difference ≥10 mm Hg indicates possible graft defect.
- Avoid engaging the knee gatch so not to compress popliteal vessels, thereby restricting venous return.
- Apply antiembolic hose to lower extremities, thereby facilitating venous return.
- Administer antihypertensive and beta-blocker agents to reduce hemodynamic stressor that could affect graft anastamoses (see Table 1–16, p. 146, and Table 1–5, p. 24).
- Teach patient common side effects of antidysrhythmia or diuretic medications.
- Instruct patient to report any pain in the surgical site.
- Instruct patient about the surgery and need to comply with post surgical treatments.

Impaired gas exchange related to retained alveolar secretion or alveolar atelectasis secondary to cardiopulmonary bypass.

Expected Patient Outcome. Patient maintains adequate gas exchange, as evidenced by absence of adventitious breath sounds, RR 12 to 20 BPM, absence of cyanosis, arterial blood gases within normal range, Sao$_2$ 95.0% to 97.5%, S$\bar{\text{v}}$o$_2$ 60% to 80%, and BP within patient's normal range.

- Consult with physician and respiratory therapist regarding the type of ventilatory support required by patient.
- Review results of arterial blood gas measurement and chest roentgenogram.

- Monitor clinical indicators of respiratory status: lung sounds, RR and rhythm, skin color and warmth, symmetry of chest movement, level of consciousness, and use of accessory muscles.
- Obtain and report clinical findings associated with impaired gas exchange: RR ≥ 20 BPM, cyanosis, crackles or wheezes, asymmetry of chest movement, and use of accessory muscles.
- Obtain and report $Sao_2 \leq 90\%$ and $S\bar{v}o_2 \leq 60\%$.
- Encourage patient to cough and deep breathe to deter alveolar hypoventilation and retention of secretions.
- Encourage patient to use incentive spirometry to enhance lung expansion and prevent atelectasis.
- Administer prescribed IV fluids to maintain adequate fluid hydration.
- Administer prescribed oxygen at 2 to 4 L by means of nasal cannula or mask to maintain $Pao_2 \geq 80$ mm Hg and $Paco_2 \leq 45$ mm Hg.

Mobility, impaired physical related to spinal cord injury from surgical manipulation.

Expected Patient Outcomes. Patient is able to move all extremities and mobility remains unimpaired.

- Assist patient, when realistic, with gradual increase in physical activity.
- Assess peripheral sensorimotor function hourly to determine changes in sensation or mobility.
- Encourage the use of isometric leg exercises to maintain muscle tone.
- Monitor extremities for color, pulses, warmth, and presence of edema.
- Instruct patient to report any decreased sensation in the extremities.

DISCHARGE PLANNING
The critical care nurse will provide patient and significant other(s) with verbal or written discharge notes regarding the following subjects:

1. Importance of keeping up follow-up visits and laboratory studies.
2. Importance of reducing risk factors by limiting fats and salt in diet, ceasing smoking, and maintaining an exercise program.
3. Common side effects of medications.

■ PERIPHERAL VASCULAR BYPASS GRAFT

(For related information see Part I: Deep vein thrombosis, p. 304; Peripheral vascular trauma, p. 308. Part III: Laser-assisted balloon angioplasty, p. 321; Peripheral atherectomy, p. 323; Intravascular stent, p. 324)

Diagnostic Category and Length of Stay
DRG: 110 Major cardiovascular procedures with complications
LOS: 10.30 days
DRG: 111 Major cardiovascular procedures without complications
LOS: 7.50 days
DRG: 120 Other circulatory system OR procedures
LOS: 7.40 days

Definition
Peripheral vascular bypass graft involves the anastamosis of a synthetic graft proximal and distal to the lesion.

Patient Selection

INDICATIONS. Patients with a rapidly deteriorating ability to walk and those with impending ulceration or gangrene.

CONTRAINDICATIONS. Patients who are at risk for surgical procedure or at risk for developing other problems.

Procedure

TECHNIQUE. Femoropopliteal graft bypass: The technique consists of a parallel shunt with the occluded artery, using end-to-end anastomoses both proximally and distally. The approach permits the transporting of arterial blood around an occluded segment while avoiding operative trauma and interference with collateral veins or damage to concomitant veins. The procedure can be carried out above or below the knee.

EQUIPMENT

Autogenous Veins. Used for reconstructive occlusive arterial lesions. The autogenous saphenous vein is considered the optimal graft material.

Polytetrafluoroethylene (PTFE) graft. This is composed of expanded Teflon, arranged as nodules connected by thin fibrils. There is little perigraft inflammation, yet the inner surface of the graft has a strong electronegative potential. These two factors account for the graft's resistance to thrombosis.

Glutaraldehyde-stabilized Human Umbilical Cord Vein Graft. The graft is covered with a net like polyester mesh. The umbilical vein graft is a musculocollagenous tube, lined by a thromboresistant basement membrane. A high incidence of aneurysmal degeneration has been reported with the graft, which deters its widespread use.

Complications

Failure of the extremity to revascularize, infection, or bleeding.

NURSING MANAGEMENT: NURSING DIAGNOSIS AND COLLABORATIVE PROBLEMS

Nursing Diagnoses

Common nursing goals in patients with peripheral vascular bypass graft are to increase tissue perfusion, enhance activity tolerance, and prevent infection.

Altered peripheral tissue perfusion related to thrombosis or graft rupture, occlusion, or leakage.

Expected Patient Outcomes. Patient maintains adequate peripheral tissue perfusion, as evidenced by peripheral pulses +2, capillary refill ≤3 seconds, peripheral skin color normal, skin warm and dry, absence of edema, and absence of pain.

- Review results of coagulation studies.
- Limit activity to bed rest while there is thrombus in the affected vessel.
- Monitor clinical indicators of peripheral tissue perfusion: peripheral pulses, capillary refill, skin color, and skin temperature.
- Monitor and report clinical findings associated with decreased peripheral tissue perfusion: peripheral pulses ≤+2 or absent, capillary refill ≥3 seconds, pallor or cyanosis, cool extremity, edema, and pain.
- Position the affected extremity to ensure proper alignment and to avoid occlusion of graft.
- Evaluate the affected extremity to reduce interstitial swelling by enhancing venous return.
- Encourage patient to perform isotonic leg exercises, when appropriate, to promote venous return.
- Monitor for abnormal bleeding in patients receiving anticoagulant therapy: hematuria, bleeding gums, ecchymoses, petechiae, or epistaxis.
- Administer prescribed IV fluids to maintain adequate hydration.
- Administer prescribed anticoagulant therapy, if not contraindicated, to prevent extension of the thrombus by prolonging clotting time.
- Administer prescribed analgesics for leg pain.
- Instruct patient to report any pain in the affected extremity.

Activity intolerance related to graft dysfunction or incisional pain or peripheral vascular graft bypass.

Expected Patient Outcomes. Patient is able to move both extremities and ambulate without pain.

- Provide incremental increases in physical activity when ambulation is realistic.
- Evaluate peripheral pulses in the affected extremity before and after ambulation.
- Evaluate skin color, temperature, and sensation in the affected extremity.
- Instruct patient to report any pain during ambulation.

High risk for infection related to perigraft inflammation or incisional inflammation.

Expected Patient Outcome. Patient experiences no infection, as evidenced by absence of redness, edema, tenderness, or drainage from the incision; negative cultures; no fever; and white blood count (WBC) $\leq 11,000/\mu L$.

- Review test results: WBC and cultures.
- Provide prescribed nutritional support to ensure that negative nitrogen balance is achieved.
- Culture any drainage from incision site.
- Change all dressings per agency protocol, using aseptic technique.
- Monitor and report clinical findings associated with infection: hyperthermia, fatigue, swelling, tenderness, redness, or drainage from incisional site.
- Administer prophylactic IV antibiotics as prescribed.

DISCHARGE PLANNING

The critical care nurse will provide patient and significant other(s) with verbal or written discharge notes regarding the following subjects:

1. Importance of keeping up follow-up visits and laboratory studies.
2. Importance of reducing risk factors by limiting fats and salt in diet, ceasing smoking, and maintaining an exercise program.
3. Reporting any swelling, tenderness, or pain in the affected extremity.
4. Common side effects of medications.

PART III: SUPPORTIVE PROCEDURES AND NURSING MANAGEMENT

■ LASER-ASSISTED BALLOON ANGIOPLASTY

(For related information see Part III: Peripheral atherectomy, p. 323; Intravascular stent, p. 324)

Diagnostic Category and Length of Stay
DRG: 112 Percutaneous cardiovascular procedures
LOS: 4.80 days

Definition
Laser angioplasty converts electrical or chemical energy into a unidirectional beam of light to vaporize or thermally abolish atherosclerotic lesions.

Patient Selection

INDICATIONS. Symptomatic peripheral vascular disease, angiographic documentation of a 100% arterial obstruction, surgical candidate for repair if not possible to open the artery using percutaneous technique and renal function adequate to handle the insult of the contrast agent.

CONTRAINDICATIONS. Patients whose arteries have ≥ 2 cm concentricto stenosis with low flow, those with multilevel vascular disease, and diabetes on insulin agent.

Procedure

TECHNIQUE. The femoral artery is cannulated in an antegrade fashion. A guiding catheter is positioned at the site of the obstruction, and an injection of contrast material verifies its position. The laser's fiberoptic catheter is threaded through the guiding catheter until it bumps against the lesion. After crossing the area of blockage, using laser energy, the fiberoptic is replaced with a balloon catheter, which enlarges the primary laser channel.

EQUIPMENT. Laser Probe: A round-tipped, metal-capped laser probe indirectly uses the laser energy as an instantaneous heat source for the tip, providing a temperature of 400°C. Thermal ablation is produced rather than the vaporization that would result from an open beam. The result is a less-traumatized arterial lumen than would be created by the use of balloon angioplasty or laser fibers. Balloon angioplasty frequently follows the initial laser recanalization to widen the lumen. (For information about the types of lasers, see Coronary laser angioplasty, p. 228.)

Complications

Perforation, dissection, spasm, pain, and thrombosis.

NURSING MANAGEMENT: NURSING DIAGNOSES AND COLLABORATIVE PROBLEMS

Nursing Diagnoses

Common nursing goals for patients undergoing laser-assisted balloon angioplasty are to increase tissue perfusion and maintain fluid volume.

Altered peripheral tissue perfusion related to vasospasm, ruptured artery, or thrombus.

Expected Patient Outcome. Patient maintains adequate peripheral tissue perfusion, as evidenced by right and left side peripheral pulses equal and +2, blood pressure (BP) equal in both arms and within patient's normal range, peripheral skin color normal, skin warm, absence of edema, capillary refill ≤3 seconds, normal peripheral sensation, and absence of pain on walking.

- Consult with physician regarding the desired effect of laser angioplasty.
- Review test results: ankle-brachial index (ABI) which is a ratio of the systolic pressure at the ankle divided by the brachial systolic pressure; arteriogram, which indicates the obstructed vessel during the injection of a radiopaque contrast medium; and activated clotting time (ACT), prothrombin time (PT), and partial thromboplastin time (PTT).
- Limit physical activity to bed rest after the procedure: Keep head of bed no higher than 30 degrees and the affected leg straight for 8 hours.
- Monitor extremities for clinical indicators of perfusion: peripheral pulses, capillary refill, temperature, color, sensation, and mobility.
- Obtain and report clinical findings associated with decreased peripheral tissue perfusion: peripheral pulses ≤+2, capillary refill ≥3 seconds, pallor or cyanosis, coolness, and sensorimotor dysfunction.
- Palpate pulses bilaterally for comparison and baseline values: femoral, popiteal, dorsalis pedis, and posterior tibial arteries.
- Encourage patient to flex toes during immobile period.
- Inspect patient for hematoma: femoral and distal arterial procedures present with a palpable mass around or near the skin puncture site; or patients with iliac procedures may exhibit no palpable masses, but rather, a hematoma appears as a retroperitoneal hemorrhage.
- Measure abdominal girth every 4 hours in patients with an iliac procedure.
- Administer a heparin drip 12,500 U in 250 mL normal saline for 18 to 36 hours postoperatively or as needed (see Table 1–8, p. 32).

- Instruct patient to keep extremity straight.
- Instruct patient to report any changes in sensation or pain.

Fluid volume deficit related to hemorrhage secondary to ruptured vessel.

Expected Patient Outcomes. Patient maintains adequate fluid volume, as evidenced by absence of bleeding from insertion site, BP within patient's normal range, mean arterial pressure (MAP) 70 to 100 mm Hg, urinary output (UO) $\geq$30 mL/h or $\geq$0.5 mL/Kg/h, good skin turgor, skin warm and dry, and heart rate (HR) $\leq$100 bpm.

- Review test results: hemoglobin and hematocrit, blood urea nitrogen (BUN) and creatinine.
- Monitor and report clinical findings associated with fluid volume deficit: hypotension, MAP $\leq$70 mm Hg, tachycardia, poor skin turgor, and peripheral pulses $\leq +2$.
- Inspect groin for oozing and palpate site for swelling or hematoma formation.
- Monitor intake, UO, specific gravity, and weight to evaluate fluid balance.
- Measure abdominal girth every 4 hours in iliac procedure patient: 1 liter of fluid can be sequestered in the abdominal cavity.
- Administer IV fluids at the prescribed amount.
- Provide oxygen at the prescribed flow rate 2 to 4 L/min by nasal cannula or mask.

■ PERIPHERAL ATHERECTOMY

(For related information see Part III: Intravascular stents, p. 324).

Diagnostic Category and Length of Stay
DRG: 112 Percutaneous cardiovascular procedures
LOS: 4.80 days

Definition
Atherectomy is the selective removal of atheroma from atherosclerotic arteries. The procedure can be performed percutaneously or through a small arteriotomy remote from the disease site.

Patient Selection

INDICATIONS. For the Simpson Atherocath: A short, discrete, eccentric atheroma, ulcerated atherosclerotic intima, concentric stenosis, and intimal hyperplasia. For a Kensey Atherectomy: Occlusive lesions of the superficial femoral artery. For the Auth Rotablator: Hard, calcified atherosclerotic intima in diabetes; tibial, popliteal, superficial femoral, and iliac artery lesions; and eccentric atherosclerotic intima. For the transluminal extraction catheter: Same as for Simpson Athercath.

CONTRAINDICATIONS. Hard-calcified lesions at the adductor's canal that may be resistant to atherectomy.

Procedure

TECHNIQUE. The procedure can be performed percutaneously or through a small arteriotomy remote from the diseased site. There are several atherectomy devices with their own unique feature.

EQUIPMENT

Simpson Atherocath. This is a flexible catheter whose cutting equipment is a small circular cutter spinning at 2000 rpm inside a metal housing with a 15- to 20-mm window. The plaque is pulled into the housing unit via the window by a balloon inflated on the opposite side of the housing. The rotating cutter in the housing advances, thereby removing the plaque. The radial rotation of the catheter in the artery removes most of the lesion.

Kensey Atherectomy. This is also called the Trac-Wright system. It is a flexible catheter with a distal cam-tip attached to a central drive shaft. A high-pressure irrigating system dilates the artery, while the rotating cam pulverizes the atheromatous intima. Only the fibrous or firm athermatous tissue is pulverized.

Auth Rotablator. This is a flexible catheter with a deliverable atherectomy device with a variable-sized, football-shaped metal burr on the distal tip. The high-speed rotation allows the diamond microchips in the burr to attack hard-calcified atherma preferentially, while leaving the surrounding elastic soft tissue of the normal artery wall intact. The small pulverized particles circulate harmlessly through the body.

Transluminal Extraction Catheter. This is a semi-flexible torque-controlled hollow catheter that is passed via an introducer sheath over a guide wire and positioned proximal to the atherosclerotic lesion. The plaque is cut as it enters into a short, rotating, conical housing with internal cutting blades. The cut plaque is aspirated into vacuum bottles.

Complications

Intimal dissection, limb loss, peripheral emboli, wound hematoma, infection, re-stenosis, or intimal hyperplasia.

NURSING MANAGEMENT: NURSING DIAGNOSES AND COLLABORATIVE PROBLEMS

NURSING DIAGNOSIS

A common nursing goal in patients with peripheral atherectomy is to increase tissue perfusion.

Altered tissue perfusion related to perforated artery, arterial wall trauma, and re-stenosis.

Expected Patient Outcomes. Patient maintains adequate peripheral tissue perfusion, as evidenced by peripheral pulses +2, capillary refill ≤ 3 seconds, skin color and temperature normal, absence of edema, and absence of pain.

- Consult with the physician regarding the desired peripheral tissue response post-atherectomy.
- Review test results: hemoglobin, hematocrit, and PTT.
- Obtain and report clinical findings associated with decreased peripheral tissue perfusion: peripheral pulses ≤+2, capillary refill ≥3 seconds, pallor or cyanosis, cool extremity, edema, and sensorimotor dysfunction.
- Monitor the insertion site for bleeding.
- Administer prescribed aspirin and warfarin postoperative for pain and to prevent thrombus formation.

DISCHARGE PLANNING

The critical care nurse will provide patient and significant other(s) with verbal or written discharge notes regarding the following subjects:

1. Importance of keeping follow-up visits.
2. Importance of reducing risk factors by limiting fats in diet, ceasing smoking, and maintaining an exercise program.
3. Report any swelling, tenderness, or pain in the affected extremity.

■ INTRAVASCULAR STENT

(For related information see Part III: Laser-assisted balloon angioplasty, p. 321; Peripheral atherectomy, p. 323).

Definition

A stent is a device designed to provide a scaffold to maintain the intraluminal structure and patency of the artery.

Patient Selection

INDICATIONS. Patients who require treatment of residual stenosis or dissections following balloon angioplasty, infrarenal aortic aneurysms, proximal renal artery balloon angioplasty, aneurysmal disease, or recurrent stenosis of hemodialysis access graft.

CONTRAINDICATIONS. Patients not candidates for angioplasty or surgery.

Procedure

TECHNIQUE. Superficial femoral arteries are stented with 6 mm-diameter stents, whereas iliac arteries are stented with 8-10-mm stents.

Balloon Expandable Stent. The stent balloon is advanced to the level of the stenotic lesion. The balloon is inflated to expand the stent and the lesion simultaneously, leaving the stent mesh flush with the inner lumen. After the stent expands, the balloon is deflated and withdrawn.

Self-expanding Stent. The stent is delivered through an introducer catheter, with a rolling membrane or sheath covering the stent. Gradual retraction of the outer membrane or sheath deploys the stent.

EQUIPMENT. The stainless steel Patmaz-Schatz stent is rigid and balloon-expandable; the Gianturco-Wallace stent is rigid and self-expandable; the Strecker stent is flexible and balloon-expandable; and the stainless steel Wallstent is flexible and self-expandable.

Complications

Re-stenosis of the affected artery.

NURSING MANAGEMENT: NURSING DIAGNOSES AND COLLABORATIVE PROBLEMS

NURSING DIAGNOSES

Common nursing goals for patients with an intravascular stent are to increase tissue perfusion and maintain fluid balance.

Altered peripheral tissue perfusion related to re-stenosis of the iliac, superficial femoral, or popliteal artery.

Expected Patient Outcomes. Patient maintains adequate peripheral tissue perfusion, as evidenced by peripheral pulses +2, skin color and temperature normal, absence of edema, and absence of claudication.

- Consult with cardiologist as to the expected behaviors reflecting embolus or claudication: cool, mottled skin; peripheral pulses in affected limb ≤2+; numbness of limb; and decreased motility of toes.
- Consult with cardiologist as to the specific intracoronary stent used and potential complications.
- Review test results: platelets, hemoglobin, hematocrit, and PTT.
- Monitor clinical indicators of perfusion in the affected limb: Pulses, temperature, color, and sensation every 30 minutes for 2 hours, then every 2 hours.
- Monitor and report clinical findings associated with decreased peripheral tissue perfusion: peripheral pulses ≤+2, capillary refill ≥3 seconds, pallor or cyanosis, cool skin, edema, sensorimotor dysfunction.
- Administer anticoagulant as ordered or as needed.
- Instruct patient to report any numbness, tingling, or pain in the affected limb.

Fluid volume deficit related to abnormal volume loss secondary to bleeding at the catheter insertion site.

Expected Patient Outcomes. Patient maintains adequate fluid volume, as evidenced by absence of bleeding at the catheter insertion site, blood pressure (BP) within patient's normal range, heart rate (HR) ≤100 bpm, good skin turgor, mean arterial pressure (MAP) 70 to 100 mm Hg, and coagulation studies within normal range.

- Consult with physician to validate expected patient outcomes used to evaluate adequate fluid volume.
- Confer with cardiologist as to the potential for bleeding based on events occurring during intracoronary stenting.

- Review results of hemoglobin, hematocrit, coagulation profile, and quantitative coronary angiography.
- Monitor catheter site for signs of external bleeding: swelling, tenderness, or blood on dressing.
- Position sandbag on insertion site until discontinued by physician.
- Maintain immobilization of the involved limb until discontinued by physician.
- Obtain and report clinical findings associated with fluid-volume deficit related to bleeding: hypotension, MAP ≤70 mm Hg, poor skin turgor, and tachycardia.
- Administer prescribed IV fluids to maintain adequate circulating volume.
- Instruct patient to keep sandbag in place until otherwise discontinued.

DISCHARGE PLANNING

The critical care nurse will provide patient and significant other(s) with verbal or written discharge notes regarding the following subjects:

1. Importance of keeping follow-up visits.
2. Importance of reducing risk factors by limiting fats in diet, ceasing smoking, and maintaining an exercise program.
3. Report any swelling, tenderness, or pain at the procedural site.

SELECTED BIBLIOGRAPHY

Baker MB. Patients with vascular emergencies. In: Clochesy JM, Breu C, Cardin S, et al., eds. *Critical Care Nursing*. Philadelphia: WB Saunders Co; 1993;437–460.

Baker JD. Assessment of peripheral arterial occlusive disease. *Crit Care Nurs Clin North Am* 1991;3:325–355.

Bauer-Creamer C, Webber M. Patient teaching strategies for peripheral laser procedures. *Prog Cardiovasc Nurs*. 1990;5(2):50–58.

Bilodeau ML, Capasso VC. Peripheral arterial thrombolytic therapy. *Crit Care Nurs Clin North Am*. 1990;2:673–680.

Blank CA, Irwin GH. Peripheral vascular disorders. *Nurs Clin North Am*. 1990;25:777–793.

Bullock BL, Rosendahl PP. *Pathophysiology: Adaptations and Alterations in Function*, 3rd ed. Philadelphia, Pa: JB Lippincott Co; 1992.

Cardelli MB, Kleinsmith DM. Raynaud's phenomenon and disease. *Med Clin North Am*. 1989;73:1127–1141.

Delgin JH, Vallerand AH, Russin MM. *Davis's Drug Guide for Nurses*, 3rd ed. Philadelphia, Pa: FA Davis Co; 1995.

Dixon MB. Patients with vascular emergencies. In: Clochesy JM, Breu C, Cardin S, et al, eds. *Critical Care Nursing*. Philadelphia, Pa: WB Saunders Co; 1993: 437–430.

Dolan JT. *Critical Care Nursing: Clinical Management Through the Nursing Process*. Philadelphia, Pa: FA Davis Co; 1991; 173–204.

Dossey BM, Guzzette CE, Kenner CV. *Critical Care Nursing Body-Mind-Spirit*, 3rd ed. Philadelphia, Pa: JB Lippincott Co; 1992.

Doyle J, Johantgen M, Cicciu-Vitello J. Vascular disease. In: Kinney MR, Packa DR, Dunbar SB, eds. *AACN Critical Care Nursing*, 3rd ed. St. Louis, Mo: Mosby-Year Book; 1993;607–634.

Eton D, Ahn SS. Trends in endovascular surgery. *Crit Care Nurs Clin North Am*. 1991;3:535–549.

Grundfest WS, Litvack F. Angioplasty and laser angioplasty. In: Haimovici H, Callow AD, DePalma RG, et al, eds. *Vascular Surgery Principles and Techniques*, 3rd ed. Norwalk, Conn.: Appleton & Lange; 1989;324–329.

Loeb S. Nurse's Handbook of Drug Therapy. Springhouse, Pa: Springhouse Corp, 1993.

Loeb S. *Clinical Laboratory Tests*. Springhouse, Pa: Springhouse Corp; 1991.

Paul MC, Franey-Halfman M. Laser angioplasty in peripheral vascular disease. *Crit Care Nurse*. 1990;10(5):65–77.

Govoni LE, Hayes JE, Shannon MT, et al, eds. *Drugs and Nursing Implications*, 8th ed. Norwalk, Conn.: Appleton & Lange, 1995.

Swearingen PL, Keen JH. *Manual of Critical Care*, 2nd ed. St. Louis, Mo: Mosby-Year Book, 1992.

Ting M. Wound healing and peripheral vascular disease. *Crit Care Nurs Clin North Am* 1991; 3:515–523.

Webber M, Jenkins N. Laser treatment of peripheral vascular disease. *Prog Cardiovasc Nurs* 1988;(3): 81–88.

Respiratory Deviations

■ ADULT RESPIRATORY DISTRESS SYNDROME

(For related information see Cardiac Deviations, Part I: Shock, p. 174; Dysrhythmias, p. 184. Part III: Hemodynamic monitoring, p. 219; Part I: Acute pulmonary edema, p. 346; Pulmonary embolism, p. 397; Pulmonary hypertension, p. 404; Respiratory acidosis, p. 412. Part III: Pulse oximetry, p. 426; Mechanical ventilation, p. 428; Extracorporeal membrane oxygenation, p. 437; Capnography, p. 439; Transcutaneous Pao$_2$ and Paco$_2$, p. 441; Indirect calorimetry, p. 441; Implantable intravascular oxygenator, p. 442.)

Case Management Basis

DRG: 101 Other respiratory system diagnoses with complications
LOS: 5.10 days
DRG: 102 Other respiratory system diagnoses without complications
LOS: 3.20 days

Definition

Adult respiratory distress syndrome (ARDS) is pulmonary edema that is noncardiac in origin. ARDS occurs when there is injury to the alveolar-capillary membrane. The condition is characterized by severe hypoxemia and progressive loss of lung compliance.

Pathophysiology

After a direct or indirect pulmonary injury, changes occur in the alveolar-capillary membrane that permit fluid and protein to accumulate first in the interstitium and then in the alveoli. When the interstitial fluid overwhelms oncotic pressure, capillary hydrostatic pressure, and lymphatic drainage, the terminal bronchioles are compressed and eventually collapse. In time, fluid and protein enter the alveoli. Endothelial cell damage occurs as well as malfunction of type II pneumocytes. As the activity of type II pneumocytes decreases, there is decreased surfactant production. As fluid continues to move into the alveolar spaces, lung compliance and functional residual capacity decrease. At the same time, the work of breathing, oxygen consumption, and dead space area increase. Eventually the protein in the interstitium and alveoli form a hyaline membrane, further decreasing compliance and increasing hypoxemia, as measured by a widening alveolar-arteriolar oxygen gradient.

Nursing Assessment

PRIMARY CAUSES
- Direct injury to the lung resulting from aspiration of gastric contents, aspiration of fresh and salt water, aspiration of hydrocarbons, oxygen toxicity, inhaled toxic gases, pneumonitis, radiation, thromboembolism, pulmonary contusion, drugs, or embolism. Indirect injury to the lung is due to hypoperfusion of the lung, endotoxins and other bacterial products, humoral substances, cellular elements of the blood, hematological disorders, neurological mechanisms, multiple trauma, pancreatic disorder after cardiopulmonary bypass, and anaphylaxis.

PHYSICAL ASSESSMENT
- Inspection: Hyperventilation, dyspnea, tachypnea, grunting respirations, intercostal and suprasternal retractions, cyanosis or pallor, diaphoresis, restlessness, obtun, or fatigue.
- Palpation: Tactile fremitus or unequal or decreased chest excursion.
- Percussion: Dullness over consolidated areas.
- Auscultation: Fine rales and crackles, wheezes and bronchial breath sounds, tachycardia, S_2 with pulmonary hypertension or hypotension.

DIAGNOSTIC TEST RESULTS

Hemodynamic Parameters (Table 3–1)
- Pulmonary capillary wedge pressure (PCWP) is normal (≤ 12 mm Hg), cardiac output (CO) is increased initially then decreased in later stages, increased right-to-left shunt ($\dot{Q}s/\dot{Q}t$) $\geq 20\%$ of CO, and increased alveolar-arterial gradient (P_{AO_2}–Pa_{O_2}).

Standard Laboratory Tests (Table 3–2)
- Alveolar fluid: plasma protein ratio: ≥ 0.6.
- Arterial blood gases: Partial pressure of arterial carbon dioxide (Pa_{CO_2}) decreased initially then increased in later stages, partial pressure of oxygen (Pa_{O_2}) decreased ≤ 55 mm Hg, pH initially increased then decreased, and base excess initially increased ($+3$) then decreased (-13) in later stages.

Invasive Respiratory Diagnostic Procedures (Table 3–3)
- Ventilation-Perfusion Scan: May show reduced ventilation and eventually mismatching ventilation and perfusion.

Noninvasive Respiratory Diagnostic Procedures (Table 3–4; see Table 3–2)
- Chest roentgenogram: Reveals microatelectasis; elevated diaphragm consistent with decreased, functional residual capacity (FRC); and consolidation and coalescing infiltrates. Also can reveal diffuse bilateral pulmonary infiltrates ("alveolar pattern").
- Pulmonary functions tests: Decreased static and dynamic compliance, decreased FRC, decreased vital capacity, increased minute ventilation, increased deadspace/waster ventilation, and increased venous admixture.

MEDICAL AND SURGICAL MANAGEMENT

PHARMACOLOGY
- Morphine: Used to decrease respiratory rate so patient won't hyperventilate when receiving continuous positive-pressure ventilation (CPPV) and breathe out of phase with the ventilator.
- Neuromuscular blocking agents: Used in patients requiring mechanical ventilation to reduce or eliminate spontaneous breathing effort; to prevent motor activity that might dislodge vascular catheters, access tubes, and surgical dressings; and to reduce oxy-

TABLE 3–1. STANDARD RESPIRATORY LABORATORY TESTS

Test	Purpose	Normal Value	Abnormal Findings
Pleural fluid analysis (Thoracentesis)	To provide a fluid specimen to determine the cause and nature of pleural effusion	Pleural cavity maintains negative pressure and contains less than 20 mL of serous fluid	Transudate Appearance: Clear Specific gravity: <1.016 Clot (fibriniogen): Absent Protein: <3g/dL WBCs: Few lymphocytes RBCs: Few Glucose: Equal to serum level LDH: Low Transudate pleural fluid effusion can result from ascites, systemic or pulmonary venous hypertension, congestive heart failure, hepatic cirrhosis, nephritis Exudate Appearance: Cloudy, turbid Specific gravity: >1.016 Clot (fibrinogen): Present Protein: >3g/dL WBCs: Many; may be purulent RBCs: Variable Glucose: May be less than serum level LDH: High Exudative effusion can result from lymphatic drainage interference, infections, pulmonary infarctions, or neoplasms
Pleural biopsy	To differentiate between nonmalignant and malignant disease To diagnose viral, fungal, or parasitic disease To diagnose collagen vascular disease of the pleura	The pleura consists of mesothelial cells, flattened in a uniform layer	Examination of the tissue may detect malignant disease, tuberculosis, viral disease, fungal disease, parasitic disease, collagen vascular disease
Respiratory tract cultures Sputum	To diagnose infectious disease of respiratory tract: bacterial pneumonia, tuberculosis, chronic bronchitis, bronchiectasis, viral pneumonia		

TABLE 3-1

TABLE 3-1

TABLE 3–1. CONTINUED

Test	Purpose	Normal Value	Abnormal Findings
Throat culture (swab)	To diagnose streptococcal sore throat, diphtheria, thrush, tonsillar infection To determine the focus of infection: scarlet fever, rheumatic fever, acute hemorrhagic glomerulonephritis Helpful in determining the carrier state of organisms: beta-hemolytic streptococci or *Staphylococcus aureus*		
Nasal culture (swab)	Used in acute leukemia, transplant, intermittent dialysis patients		
Nasopharyngeal culture (swab)	When present in significant titer, the following organisms are revealed as pathogenic: *Candida albicans, Haemophilus influenzae, Meningococcus,* pneumococci, *Staphylococcus aureus,* streptococci		
Alveolar to arterial O_2 gradient ($AO_2 - Pao_2$, ratio)	To identify the cause of hypoxemia and intrapulmonary shunting (ventilated or unventilated alveolus)	9 torr or less in a patient breathing room air	Increased value can be attributed to mucus plugs, bronchospasm, or airway collapse Hypoxemia due to increased A-aO2 difference caused by pneumothorax, atelectasis, emboli or edema
Arterial:alveolar O_2 tension ratio $P(a/A)O_2$	To show the ratio between Pao_2 (arterial oxygen tension) and Pao_2 (alveolar oxygen tension) The ratio remains stable within the Fio_2 changes as long as the underlying lung condition is stable	Pao_2 Pao_2 ratio is 0.75–0.90 for any Fio_2	A ratio of <0.75–0.90 indicates ventilation-perfusion inequality, shunt, or diffusion limitation

TABLE 3-1

TABLE 3–1. CONTINUED

Test	Purpose	Normal Value	Abnormal Findings
Arterial-mixed Venous Oxygen Content Difference (a-VD)$_{O2}$	The (a-VD)$_{O2}$ is an assessment of CO in relation to metabolic needs Used to determine oxygen extraction and whether CO is sufficient to meet the body's metabolic needs	A-VD$_{O2}$ is 5.0 vol % with the normal range of 4.5–6.0 vol %	Critically ill patients with inadequate cardiovascular reserves have a A-VD$_{O2}$ >6.0 vol%
WBC Differential	To determine the stage and severity of an infection To identify the various types of leukemia		
Neutrophil	To evaluate the body's reaction to inflammation	Relative value: 47.6%–76.8% Absolute value: 1950–8400/μL	Increased neutrophils can indicate infection, ischemic necrosis, metabolic disorders, stress response, inflammatory disease Decreased neutrophils can indicate bone marrow depression, hepatic disease, collagen vascular disease, deficiency of folic acid or vitamin B$_{12}$
Eosinophils	To diagnose allergic infections, severity of infestations with worms and other large parasites	Relative value: 0.3%–7% Absolute value: 12–760/μL	Increased eosinophils can indicate allergic disorders, parasitic infections, skin diseases, neoplastic diseases, collagen vascular disease, ulcerative colitis, pernicious anemia, excessive exercise Decreased eosinophils can indicate stress resulting from trauma, shock, burns, surgery, Cushing's syndrome

TABLE 3-1

TABLE 3–1. CONTINUED

Test	Purpose	Normal Value	Abnormal Findings
Serum electrolytes Phosphate	To evaluate diaphragmatic contractility	2.5–4.5mg/dL	To determine if hypophosphatemia is contributing to poor ventilatory dynamics in acute respiratory failure
			Increased phosphate level can indicate healing fractures, hypoparathyroidism, diabetic acidosis, and renal failure
			Decreased phosphate level can indicate malnutrition, malabsorption syndrome Hyperparathyrodism, renal tubular necrousis, and treatment of diabetic acidosis
Physiological shunt (Qs/Qt)	To measure the efficiency of the oxygenation system	0%–8%	High value indicates lung dysfunction such as pulmonary edema
	Indicates the portion of venous blood that is not involved in the gas exchange		
Compliance Dynamic compliance	To measure maximum airway pressure required to deliver a given tidal volume	35–55 mL/cm H_2O	Low value reflects reduced compliance, as from secretions in the airway
	To reflect the lung's elasticity and airway resistance to the breathing cycle		
Static compliance	To measure airway pressure required to hold the lungs at end-inspiration after a tidal volume has been delivered and no air flow is present	50–100 mL/cm H_2O	Low value reflects lung stiffness
	To reflect lung elasticity not affected by gas flow		

CO, cardiac output; F_{IO_2}, fraction of inspired oxygen; LDA, low-density lipoprotein; RBC, red blood cells; WBC, white blood cells.

From Ford RD, 1987; Thelan LA, Davie JK, Urden LD, 1990; Stillwell SB, 1992; and Loeb S, 1991.

TABLE 3–2. RESPIRATORY FUNCTION TESTS

Test	Purpose	Normal Value	Abnormal Findings
Spirometry	To determine the effectiveness of the forces involved in the movement of the lungs and chest wall		
	To determine the degree of obstruction of air flow and the restrictive amount of air that can be inspired		
Functional Residual Capacity (FRC)	To evaluate both the restrictive and obstructive defects of the lung	Approximately 2400–3000 mL	A value less than 75% is indicative of restrictive disease
	Measures the volume of gas contained in the lungs at the end of a normal quiet expiration	The observed value is 75–125% of the predicted value	A value greater than 125% represents air trapping
Total Lung Capacity (TLC)	To evaluate obstructive defects of the lungs	Approximately 5500 mL	Increased TLC can indicate obstructive defect, bronchiolar obstruction, emphysema
	Measures the volume of gas contained in the lungs at the end of a maximal inspiration	Predicted values are based on age, height, and sex	Decreased TLC can indicate edema, atelectasis, neoplasms, pulmonary congestion
Vital Capacity (VC)	To identify defects that can be due to lung or chest wall restriction	Approximately 4000–4800 mL	Decreased VC is less than 80% of the predicted value in either a restrictive or obstructive disorder
	Measures the largest volume of gas that can be expelled from the lungs after the lungs are first filled to the maximum extent and then emptied to the maximum extent	Predicted values are based on age, height, and sex	
Residual Volume (RV)	To differentiate between a restrictive or obstructive ventilatory effort	Approximately 1200–1500 mL	Increased RV may be due to emphysema, chronic air trapping, chronic bronchial obstruction
	Measures the volume of gas remaining in the lungs after a maximal exhalation	Predicted values are based on age, height, and sex	
Expiratory Reserve Volume (ERV)	Measures the largest volume of gas that can be exhaled following normal resting expiration	Approximately 1200–1500 mL	Decreased ERV may be due to elevated diaphragm in massive obesity, ascites, pregnancy, pleural effusion, thoracoplasty
	To identify lung or chest wall restriction	Predicted values based on age and height	
Forced Vital Capacity (FVC)	To evaluate the severity of airway obstruction	FVC is approximately 4800 mL	Decreased values can be due to emphysema, pulmonary fibrosis, asthma
Forced Expiratory Volume (FEV1)	Measures the maximum amount of air that can rapidly be exhaled after a maximum deep inspiration is recorded	FEV1 is approximately 80% of this value	

TABLE 3-2

TABLE 3-2

TABLE 3–2. CONDITION

Test	Purpose	Normal Value	Abnormal Findings
Peak Inspiratory Flow Rate (PIFR)	To identify reduced breathing on inspiration and is totally dependent on the effort patient makes in inspiration Measures the maximum flow of air achieved during a forced maximal inspiration	An average value of 300 L/min	Decreased value in neuromuscular disorders, weakness, poor effect, extrathoracic airway obstruction
Peak Expiratory Flow Rate (PEFR)	Index of large-airway function Measures the maximum flow of expired air attained during a forced vital capacity (FVC) maneuver	An average of 450 L/min	Decreased value in emphysema
Maximum Voluntary Ventilation (MVV)	To measure several factors simultaneously: thoracic cage compliance, lung compliance, airway resistance, and muscle force available Measures the liters of air that a person can breathe per minute by a maximum voluntary effort	Approximately 170 L/min	Decreased MVV can be due to chronic obstructive pulmonary disease, abnormal neuromuscular control, poor patient effort
Closing Volume (CV)	An index of pathological changes in the small airways in the lower alveoli	Average is about 10% to 20% of vital capacity	Increased value in bronchitis, chronic smokers, and the elderly

From Ford RD, 1987; Thelan LA, Davie K, Urden DL, 1990; Loeb S, 1991.

gen consumption in patients with cardiopulmonary compromise (Table 3–5).
- Antibiotics: Used to treat infections associated with ARDS.

MECHANICAL VENTILATION

- Positive end-expiratory pressure (PEEP): PEEP augments the reduced lung volume in patients with ARDS by providing a continually positive distending pressure in the airways and alveoli, thereby reducing intrapulmonary shunting. Tidal volumes of 10 to 15 mg/kg are used to minimize atelectasis. The combination of PEEP therapy with continuous positive pressure (CPAP) or intermittent mandatory volume (IMV) can enhance the therapeutic potential of PEEP in ARDS. PEEP is initiated in 3 to 5 cm H_2O increments until a predetermined level of tissue oxygenation is altered. The range of PEEP is 1 to 20 cm H_2O (see Mechanical ventilation, p. 428).
- Inverse Ratio Ventilation: In inverse ratio ventilation the inspiratory positive pressure is prolonged to recruit collapsed alveoli, and the quick expiratory period may control expiration long enough to keep alveoli above their closing volume (see Mechanical ventilation, p. 428).

OXYGEN THERAPY

- Oxygen delivery is accomplished with fraction of inspired oxygen (F_iO_2)≤0.50 to prevent further hyperoxia and oxygen free radical production. Should Pao_2 remain at 60 mm Hg with a maximum F_{IO_2} of 0.45, intra-alveolar edema may be developing.

FLUID THERAPY

- Crystalloid solutions: Crystalloids restore intravascular volume and functional extra-

TABLE 3–3: INVASIVE RESPIRATORY DIAGNOSTIC PROCEDURES

Test	Purpose	Normal Value	Abnormal Findings
Pulmonary angiography (Pulmonary arteriography)	To detect thromboembolic disease of the lung and delineation of masses	Normal pulmonary circulatory system	Interrupted blood flow, which can suggest pulmonary emboli, vascular filling defect, or stenosis
Bronchoscopy	To diagnose tumors or granulomatous lesions, find the site of hemorrhage, improve drainage, and remove foreign bodies To take brushings for cytologic examination or biopsy	Normal trachea, bronchi, and alveoli	Bronchitis, tumors, alveolitis, carcinoma, tuberculosis, abscesses
Laryngoscopy (direct)	To detect lesions, strictures in the larynx; diagnose laryngeal cancer; or remove benign lesions or foreign bodies	The larynx shows no evidence of inflammation, lesions, strictures, or foreign bodies	Lesions, strictures, foreign bodies can distinguish laryngeal edema from radiation reaction or tumor
Mediastinoscopy	To biopsy nodes in the mediastinum	Lymph nodes appear as small, smooth, flat oval bodies of lymphoid tissue	Lung cancer, sarcoidosis, lymphomas
Lung perfusion scan (Lung scintiscan)	To determine arterial perfusion of the lungs Detect pulmonary emboli	Hot spots are areas with normal blood perfusion and show a high uptake of the radioactive substance	Vasculitis, pulmonary hypertension, tumors of hilum, diffuse interstitial fibrosis, pulmonary infarction
Ventilation scan	To discover areas of the lung capable of ventilation Evaluate regional respiratory function Locate regional hypoventilation	Normal lung shows a uniform uptake pattern	
Ventilation/perfusion scan	To measure the matching of ventilation and perfusion	Equal distribution of gas in both lungs	Chronic obstructive pulmonary disease, bronchiectasis, airway obstruction, pneumonia, pulmonary infarction, severe pulmonary edema
		$\dot{V}/\dot{Q}$ ratio is 1:0	Pulmonary embolism and $\dot{V}/\dot{Q}$ mismatch

From Ford RD, 1987; Thelan LA, Davie JK, Urden LD, 1990; Loeb S, 1991.

TABLE 3-3

TABLE 3-4

TABLE 3-4. NONINVASIVE RESPIRATORY DIAGNOSTIC PROCEDURES

Test	Purpose	Normal Value	Abnormal Findings
Chest fluoroscopy	To evaluate lung expansion and contraction during quiet breathing, deep breathing, and coughing To detect bronchiolar obstruction and pulmonary disease	Diaphragmatic movement is synchronous and symmetric Normal diaphragmatic excursion is 2–4 cm	Abnormal results can indicate pulmonary disease, bronchial obstruction, and diaphragmatic paralysis
Chest roentgenography	To detect pneumonia, atelectasis, pneumothorax, tumors, mediastinal abnormalities, and cardiac disease To determine the location and size of a lesion	Lung fields usually are not visible throughout except by the blood vessels Trachea: Midline in the anterior mediastinal cavity Ribs: Visable as thoracic cavity encasement or widening of intercostal spaces Hila: Visible above the heart and appear as small, white, bilateral densities Main-stem bronchus: Visible and part of the hili as a transluent tube Hemidiaphragm: Round, visible, and right higher than the left	Visible, irregular, patchy densities suggesting atelectasis, resolving pneumonia, or metastatic neoplasm Deviation from midline from pneumothorax, atelectasis, pleural effusion, or consolidation Break or misalignment from fractured ribs, sternum, or emphysema Shift to one side as a result of atelectasis Accentuated shadows from emphysema, pulmonary abscess, tumor, or enlarged lymph nodes Spherical or oval density a bronchogenic cyst Elevation of diaphragm caused by pneumonia, pleurisy, acute bronchitis, or atelectasis Flattening of diaphragm the result of asthma or emphysema
Scans Chest tomography	To demonstrate pulmonary densities, tumors, or lesions	Structures equivalent to a normal chest roentgenographic	Can differentiate blood vessels from nodes at the hilus; identify bronchial dilation, stenosis, or endobronchial lesions; detect tumor extension into the hilar lung area; and identify extension of a mediastinal lesion

TABLE 3–4. CONTINUED

TABLE 3-4

Test	Purpose	Normal Value	Abnormal Findings
Thoracic computed tomography (CT)	To locate neoplasms; differentiate calcified lesions from tumors; distinguish tumors next to the aorta from aortic aneurysms; evaluate primary malignancy; evaluate mediastinal lymph nodes	Lungs, great vessels, and mediastinal lymph nodes are normal density, size, shape and position	May suggest tumors, cysts, aortic aneurysm, enlarged mediastinal lymph nodes, pleural effusion, abscesses

cellular fluid volumes. They can be used early in ARDS when the increase in permeability is the greatest.

- Colloid solutions: Colloids can be used later, should the serum protein concentration be low.

HEMODYNAMIC MONITORING

- Used to measure CO, CI, PCWP, pulmonary vascular resistance (PVR) and index (PVRI), stroke volume (SV), left ventricular stroke work index (LVSWI), systemic vascular resistance (SVR) and index (SVRI), and mixed venous oxygen saturation ($S\bar{v}o_2$).

PHYSICAL ACTIVITY

- Rotorest bed: Can be used to position patient with unilateral lung disease so that the diseased lung is elevated and the unaffected lung is in the dependent position. In this position, ventilation and perfusion can be delivered to the unaffected lung, causing less perfusion to nonventilated areas of the diseased lung. This will also reduce intrapulmonary shunting and microvascular pressure in the diseased lung. Other benefits include mobilization of secretions, facilitation of selective suctioning, provision for continuous postural drainage, and elimination of negative aspects of prone positioning.

DIET

- Nutritional supplementation is controlled in conjunction with the dietitian and physician

so that a positive protein balance is achieved. The goal is to prevent protein-calorie malnutrition. Should carbohydrate load exceed energy need, lipogenesis and a greater production of carbon dioxide relative to oxygen consumption may occur. This can ultimately cause hypercapnia.

EXTRACORPOREAL MEMBRANE OXYGENATION (ECMO)

- Blood is taken from the inferior vena cava via the femoral vein, passed at high flow rates through a membrane oxygenator where it undergoes gas exchange, and then is returned to the circulation through the femoral artery. A modified form of extracorporeal gas exchange, termed extracorporeal carbon dioxide removal, still uses the lungs for oxygenation, which are supplied with low-frequency positive-pressure ventilation. Carbon dioxide is removed through the membrane (see ECMO, p. 437).

NURSING MANAGEMENT: NURSING DIAGNOSES AND COLLABORATIVE PROBLEMS

Nursing Diagnoses

Common nursing goals for patients with ARDS are to promote effective airway clearance, support activity tolerance, prevent infection, and maintain adequate nutrition.

Ineffective airway clearance related to increased secretion production secondary to

TABLE 3-5 *(vertical, left margin)*

TABLE 3–5: NEUROMUSCULAR BLOCKING AGENTS

Medication	Route/Dose	Uses and Effects	Side Effects	Nursing Implications
Depolarizing				
Succinylcholine chloride (Anectine)	IV push: 0.75–1.5 mg/kg over 10–30 s Intubation dose: 1.3–1.1 mg/kg Maintenance dose: 0.04–0.07 mg/kg	Facilitates tracheal intubation	Sinus bradycardia, junctional dysrhythmias, PVC, ventricular fibrillation	Monitor BP and HR Monitor ECG for dysrhythmias Apprise patient that drug may cause muscle soreness
Nondepolarizing				
Atracurium besylate (Tracrium)	IV push: 0.4–0.5 mg/kg Intubation dose: 0.4–0.5 mg/kg Maintenance dose: 0.08–0.10 mg/kg Continuous infusion: 5.0–9.0 µg/kg/min	Optimizes mechanical ventilation	Skin flushing on upper thorax, decreased BP, increased HR lasting 5–30 min, bronchospasm	Monitor BP and HR Monitor RR, rhythm, and pattern
Vecuronium bromide (Norcuron)	IV push dose: loading dose 0.04–1.0 mg/kg Intubation dose: 0.08–0.1 mg/kg Maintenance dose: 0.001–0.015 Continuous infusion: 1.0 µg/kg/min	Optimizes mechanical ventilation	Patient with renal failure may have prolonged effects of drug	Monitor ABGs since recovery is prolonged by acidosis
Pancuronium bromide (Pavulon)	IV push: 0.04–1.0 mg/kg loading dose Intubation dose: 0.06–0.1 mg/kg Maintenance dose: 0.01–0.015 mg/kg	Adjunct to sedatives and analgesics in patients requiring prolonged ventilation Used in patients with tetanus and asthma	Tachycardia and active metabolites that can accumulate in renal failure	Monitor HR, BP and CO, since drug can cause increase Monitor temperature, since hypothermia can reduce drug's effectiveness
New Agent				
Mivacurium (Mivacron)	Initial dose: 0.28 mg/kg	Alternative to succinylcholine in patients with burns, crush injuries, trauma, renal failure	Hypotension, asthma, or allergies where histamine release could cause bronchospasm	Monitor BP Monitor RR, since drug may cause asthma or bronchospasm

ABG, arterial blood gases; BP, blood pressure; CO, cardiac output; ECG, electrocardiogram; HR heart rate; IV, intravenous; PVC, premature ventricular contraction; RR, respiratory rate.

From Susla, 1993; Ford R, 1987; Deglin JH, Vallerand AH, 1995; Thelan LA, Davie JK, Urden LD, 1990; and Loeb S, 1991).

loss of compliance, increased hydrostatic pressure, and ineffective cough.

Expected Patient Outcomes: Patient maintains effective airway clearance, as evidenced by absence of crackles, respiratory rate (RR) 12 to 20 BPM, tidal volume ≥5 to 7 mL/kg, vital capacity ≥12 to 15 mg/kg, minute ventilation 6 to 10 L/min, absence of cyanosis, and ability to cough up secretions.

- Consult with Physical Therapy about developing an exercise program to mobilize secretions and increase muscle tone.
- Review results of arterial blood gas measurement and chest roentgenogram.
- Place patient in semi- to high Fowler's position with knees bent and a pillow over the abdomen to augment expiratory pressures and reduce pain.
- Turn patient every 2 hours if crackles or rhonchi are auscultated.
- Obtain and report clinical findings associated with ineffective airway clearance requiring ventilatory support: altered level of consciousness, crackles or wheezes, cyanosis, pH ≤ 7.24, $Paco_2 \geq 60$ mm Hg, and $Pao_2 \leq 60$ mm Hg.
- Encourage patient to cough and deep breathe every 2 hours.
- Remove excess pulmonary secretions by suctioning, using unit protocol for pre- and postoxygenation.
- Monitor continuous ECG to assess heart rate and rhythm for dysrhythmias during suctioning.
- Should positional changes or suctioning be ineffective in removing excess secretion and maintaining normal arterial blood gases, prepare patient for mechanical ventilatory support.
- Obtain and report respiratory function results that might reflect ineffective breathing pattern while patient is receiving ventilatory support: tidal volume ≤ 5 mk/kg, vital capacity ≤ 10 mL/kg, and minute ventilation ≤ 6 L/min.
- Monitor intake, output, drainage from tubes, and specific gravity.
- Implement chest physiotherapy to aid in the removal of excess secretions.
- Administer prescribed FIo_2 at ≤ 0.50 with humidification to maintain $Pao_2 \geq 60$ mm Hg and loosen secretions.
- Administer prescribed IV fluids to maintain adequate hydration.
- Administer prescribed bronchodilators such as isoetharine Bronkosol to enhance mucociliary drainage of secretions and smooth muscle relaxation.

- Administer prescribed diuretics to reduce interstitial edema.
- Administer prescribed mucolytic agents to improve ventilation and aid in the removal of secretions.
- Instruct patient to deep breathe and cough.

Activity intolerance related to dyspnea, weakness, or fatigue.

Expected Patient Outcomes. Patient is able to tolerate gradual increases in activity, RR ≤ 24 BPM, normal sinus rhythm, blood pressure (BP) within patient's normal range, and heart rate (HR) within 20 bpm of patient's resting HR.

- Consult with physician regarding the desired physiological responses to increased physical activity.
- Consult with Rehabilitation regarding the appropriate incremental activity program for the ARDS patient.
- Review results of arterial blood gases and pulmonary function tests.
- Position patient from the supine to the prone position, which can improve gas exchange by favoring blood distribution to the healthier lung region.
- Monitor patient's RR, HR, cardiac rhythm, and BP when beginning gradual increases in physical activity.
- Teach patient how to safely increase physical activity: Breathe deeply, change position frequently, assume an upright position, and when walking is realistic.

High risk for infection related to invasive monitoring devices.

Expected Patient Outcomes. Patient experiences absence of infection, as evidenced by normal temperature; negative cultures; white blood count (WBC) $\leq 11,000/\mu L$ and absence of redness, tenderness, edema, or drainage from cannulation sites.

- Review results of chest roentgenogram, cultures, and WBC.

- Monitor oral and skin temperatures, amount and consistency of sputum, and the presence of drainage from cannulation sites.
- Change dressings per unit protocol, using aseptic technique, and apply antimicrobial ointment.
- Change IV tubing per unit protocol and suction while using aseptic technique.
- Administer antibiotics as prescribed.

Nutritional alteration, less than body requirement related to increased metabolic activity, endotracheal intubation, or ventilatory support.

Expected Patient Outcomes. Patient maintains body weight within 5% of baseline weight, total serum protein 6.0 to 8.4 g/100 mL, and blood urea nitrogen (BUN), serum creatinine, electrolytes, fasting blood sugar, serum albumin, hemoglobin, and hematocrit within normal range.

- Consult with a nutritionist to obtain a nutritional assessment and dietary program for patient.
- Review results of total serum protein, BUN, serum creatinine, electrolytes, fasting blood sugar, serum albumin, hemoglobin, and hematocrit.
- Provide prescribed nutrition with the enteral or parenteral feedings: Mechanically ventilated patients require nutritional supplements to meet hypermetabolic needs.
- Monitor daily weight to determine whether patient's weight is being maintained within an acceptable range.
- Encourage patient to eat the prescribed diet.
- Monitor indirect calorimetry to measure caloric and substrate requirement by measuring oxygen consumption (Vo_2) and carbon dioxide production.
- Place patient in optimal position during feedings to reduce risk of aspiration.
- Confirm placement of nasogastric tube in stomach before initiating feedings.
- Monitor the ratio of carbon dioxide produced to oxygen consumed, which is called

the respiratory quotient. RQ = VCO_2 L/min: VO_2 L/min.
- Administer prescribed IV fluids to maintain adequate hydration.
- Administer prescribed total parenteral nutrition to supplement patient's nutritional needs.

Collaborative Problems

Common collaborative goals for patients with ARDS are to correct pulmonary edema, maintain ventilation-perfusion balance, increase functional residual capacity, prevent hypoxemia, maintain acid-base balance, increase CO, and enhance pulmonary muscle function.

Potential Complication: Pulmonary Edema. Pulmonary edema related to increased intraalveolar fluid volume secondary to altered alveolar-capillary membrane, increased oncotic pressure, capillary hydrostatic pressure and decreased lymphatic drainage.

Expected Patient Outcomes. Patient maintains normal intraalveolar fluid volume, as evidence by absence of crackles; absence of dyspnea; BP within patient's normal range; mean arterial pressure (MAP) 70 to 100 mm Hg; Pao_2 ≥80 mm Hg; $Paco_2$ 35 to 45 mm Hg; RR 12 to 20 BPM with normal depth; absence of dyspnea, crackles, and persistent cough; CO 4 to 8 L/min; CI 2.7 to 4.3 L/min/m²; arterial oxygen saturation (Sao_2) ≥95%; $S\bar{v}o_2$ 60% to 80%; and arterial-alveolar oxygen tension ratio (P[a/A]O_2) of 0.75 to 0.90.

- Consult with physician to validate expected patient outcomes used to determine the resolution of pulmonary edema.
- Consult with physician about criteria used to determine when ventilatory support is needed: oxygenation (Pao_2 ≤60 mm Hg on Fio_2 50%), ventilation ($Paco_2$ ≥50 to 60 mm Hg, which is ≥10 mm Hg above patient's normal $Paco_2$), and respiratory mechanisms (apnea, sustained RR ≥35 BPM, and vital capacity ≤10 to 15 mL/kg).

- Consult with respiratory therapist about patient's compatibility with mechanical ventilator and need for prescribed changes in tidal volume, oxygen, or PEEP.
- Review results from arterial blood gas measurement, chest roentgenogram, protein alveolus: protein plasma ratio (≥ 0.6 in ARDS), and pulmonary function tests.
- Limit physical activity to chair rest or bed rest. The position promotes diuresis by recumbency-induced increase of glomerular filtration and reduction of antidiuretic hormone production. Keeping legs dependent will decrease venous return, increase venous pooling, and decrease preload.
- During periods of breathlessness, physical activity is restricted to bed rest, with the head of bed elevated to allow for maximum lung expansion and legs placed in a dependent position to encourage venous pooling, which decreases venous return.
- Change patient's position every 2 hours. Limiting the time spent in a position that compromises oxygenation will improve Pao_2.
- Obtain and report the following signs and symptoms reflective of left ventricular failure and pulmonary edema: ineffective cough, dyspnea, bronchial wheezing, paroxysmal nocturnal dyspnea, orthopnea, cyanosis, pallor, confusion, pulsus alternans, S_3, S_4, and gallop rhythm.
- Obtain and report hemodynamic parameters associated with ARDS related to pulmonary edema: CO ≤ 4 L/min, CI ≤ 2.7 L/min/m^2, PCWP 12 mm Hg, and Svo_2 $\leq 60\%$.
- Obtain and report clinical findings associated with pulmonary edema: dyspnea, crackles, cyanosis, tachypnea, and tachycardia.
- Monitor the adequacy of fluid therapy through specific indexes: skin temperature and turgor, urine output (UO), daily body weight, central nervous system function, blood lactate levels, and presence or absence of metabolic acidosis.
- Initiate continuous monitoring of ECG readings to assess HR and rhythm. Document ECG rhythm strips every 2 to 4 hours.
- Continuously calculate arterial-alveolar oxygen tension ratio ($P[a/A]O_2$ as a measurement of the efficiency of gas exchange in the lungs. Report a value ≤ 0.75, which indicates diffusion problems.
- Monitor and report physiological shunt ($\dot{Q}s/\dot{Q}t$) $\geq 20\%$, static compliance (Cst) ≤ 50 mL/cm H_2O, and dynamic compliance (Cdyn) ≤ 35 mL/cm H_2O.
- Monitor intake, output, specific gravity, and daily weight. Report UO ≤ 30 mL/h or ≤ 0.5 mL/kg/h, specific gravity ≥ 1.010, and weight gain 0.5 kg (1.1 lb)/d or ≥ 2.5 kg (5 lb)/w, indicating fluid retention.
- Administer prescribed supplemental oxygen Fio_2 $\leq 50\%$ by mask or oxygen 2 to 4 L/min (24% to 36% O_2) by means of nasal cannula to maintain or improve oxygenation.
- Use criteria for determining when ventilatory support is necessary: RR ≥ 30 to 35 BPM, Pao_2 ≤ 55 mm Hg with Fio_2 21% and $Paco_2 \geq 45$ mm Hg.
- Assist with prescribed IMV or synchronized IMV (SIMV) at a tidal volume of 10 to 15 mL/kg by endotracheal intubation to maintain normal arterial blood gases.
- Monitor clinical indicators requiring IMV or SIMV rate adjustment: difficulty breathing, breathlessness, or increasing anxiety.
- Provide prescribed PEEP to recruit alveoli and decrease the loss of FRC by opening alveoli, decreasing pulmonary shunting, and decreasing hypoxemia.
- Suction patient by means of a closed suctioning system to avoid ventilation disconnection and loss of PEEP.
- Use intratracheal or intraendotracheal instillation of 2 mL to 5 mL of normal saline during suctioning to enhance the removal of secretions by stimulating a cough.
- Monitor and evaluate patient's oxygen (Sao_2, Svo_2) and hemodynamic status (MAP, CO) before, during, and after suctioning.
- Assist with weaning patient from ventilatory support using prescribed or unit crite-

ria: pH $\geq$7.35, $Paco_2$ $\leq$45 mm Hg, RR $\leq$30 BPM, $Pao_2$$\geq$55 mm Hg, Pio_2 21% on constant positive airway pressure of 5 cm H_2O without supplemental IMV or SIMV breaths.

- Administer crystalloid (Ringer's lactate or isotonic salt solution) IV solution to maintain PCWP $\leq$12 mm Hg, MAP $\geq$70 mm Hg, and $Svo_2$$\geq$70%.
- Administer prescribed volume-reducing agents (furosemide or bumetanide) to maintain UO $\geq$30 mL/h or $\geq$0.5 mL/kg/h, specific gravity $\leq$1.030, decrease neck vein distention, decrease venous return to the heart, and decrease preload (see Table 1–13, p. 76).
- Administer prescribed low-dose morphine sulfate to promote decreased venous and arterial vasoconstriction, which reduces preload and afterload, to reduce edema, lessen pain, and reduce adventitious breath sounds, such as crackles.
- Administer prescribed bronchodilators to improve ventilation and facilitate the removal of secretions.
- Administer prescribed antibiotics to minimize the growth of bacteria in the pooled secretions.
- Administer prescribed inotropic agents (dopamine or dobutamine) to increase peripheral perfusion and enhance myocardial contractility (see Table 1–10, p. 50).
- Administer peripheral vasodilator (nitroprusside) to decrease afterload (see Table 1–4, p. 20).
- Should mechanical ventilatory support be ineffective, prepare patient for ECMO (see ECMO, p. 437).
- Teach patient to cough, turn, and deep breathe every 1 to 2 hours if congested to clear airways and every 2 to 4 if not congested.

Potential Complication: Decreased Ventilation/Perfusion. Decreased ventilation/perfusion related to fluid accumulation in the pulmonary interstitial and alveolar space secondary to altered alveolar-capillary membrane.

Expected Patient Outcomes. Patient maintains adequate ventilation/perfusion balance, as evidenced by ventilation/perfusion ratio ($\dot{V}/\dot{Q}$) 1.0, Sao_2 97%, Svo_2 75%, alveolar-arterial oxygen gradient ($P[A-a]O_2$) $\leq$15 mm Hg on room air to 10 to 65 mm Hg on 100% O_2, arterial-alveolar oxygen tension ratio ($P[a/A]O_2$) 0.75 to 0.90, static compliance (Cst) $\geq$50 mL/cm H_2O, dynamic compliance (Cdyn) $\geq$45 mL/cm H_2O, RR 12 to 20 BPM, absence of adventitious breath sounds, absence of cyanosis, absence of dyspnea, CO 4 to 8 L/min, CI 2.7 to 4.3 L/min/m^2, PCWP 4 to 12 mm Hg, MAP 70 to 100 mm Hg, BP within patient's normal range, arterial blood gases within normal range, and HR $\leq$100 bpm.

- Consult with physician to validate expected patient outcomes used to evaluate ventilation-perfusion balance.
- Confer with Respiratory Therapy regarding the appropriate ventilatory support for ARDS patient.
- Review of results arterial blood gas measurement, static lung compliance, dynamic lung compliance, physiological shunting, alveolar-arterial oxygen gradient, arterial: alveolar oxygen tension ratio, or ventilation-perfusion scan.
- Limit physical activity to bed rest to decrease the work of breathing.
- Obtain and report hemodynamic parameters that could affect ventilation-perfusion balance: CO $\leq$4 L/min, CI$\leq$2.7 L/min/m^2, PCWP $\leq$12mm Hg, MAP $\leq$70 mm Hg, and Svo_2 $\leq$60%.
- Obtain and report other clinical findings associated with decreased $\dot{V}/\dot{Q}$: tachypnea, cyanosis, crackles, dyspnea, and tachycardia.
- Monitor $\dot{V}/\dot{Q}$ ratio and report value $\leq$1.0, which signifies reduced alveolar ventilation. A low $A\dot{Q}$ ratio is referred to as an intrapulmonary shunt (blood flow [$\dot{Q}s$]/ total flow [$\dot{Q}t$] $\geq$15% to 30%.
- Provide prescribed PEEP and inverse ratio ventilation for high $\dot{Q}s/\dot{Q}t$ levels.
- Obtain the following information in order to measure $\dot{Q}s/\dot{Q}t$: hemoglobin level, Fio_2

level, arterial and mixed venous blood gas results, and arterial and mixed venous oxyhemoglobin (oxygen saturation) values.

- Monitor alveolar partial pressure of oxygen (P_{AO_2}) and P_{AO_2}, which are approximately equal. Report discrepancy between P_{AO_2} and Pa_{CO_2}, which signifies the development of an intrapulmonary shunt.
- Estimate $\dot{Q}s/\dot{Q}t$ using the following methods: $P_{AO_2}:F_{IO_2}$ ratio ≥ 286, arterial:alveolar (a:A) ratio ≥ 0.60, alveolar-arterial (A−a) gradient ≤ 20 mm Hg with an F_{IO_2} of 0.21, respiratory index ≤ 1, and shunt equation $\leq 5\%$.
- Monitor and report $P_{AO_2}:F_{IO_2} \geq 200$, which is considered to be a large intrapulmonary shunt (20%). The lower the value, the more severe the $\dot{Q}s/\dot{Q}t$ disturbance.
- Obtain and report $Sa_{O_2} \leq 90\%$, which can signify intrapulmonary shunting.
- Evaluate the effectiveness of PEEP according to the following criteria: arterial blood gases, mixed venous oxygen tension, lung compliance, PCWP, and CO.
- Increase PEEP, as prescribed, in increments of 3 to 5 cm H_2O pressure until the desired PEEP is achieved to keep $Pa_{O_2} \geq 60$ mm Hg.
- Monitor and report complications associated with PEEP: reduced venous return, reduced CO, reduced cerebral perfusion, and barotrauma.
- Measure intake, output, specific gravity, and daily weight. Excessive fluid accumulation increases total lung water, contributing to an increase in ventilation-perfusion imbalance.
- Monitor skin color for the presence of cyanosis, which can reflect the desaturation of at least 5 g of hemoglobin and ventilation-perfusion mismatch.
- Evaluate the adequacy of oxygenation: oxygen delivery ≥ 600 mL/min/m^2, CI ≥ 2.7 L/min/m^2, and $V_{O_2} \geq 156$ mL/min/m^2.
- Administer prescribed humidified oxygen to keep $Pa_{O_2} \geq 60$ mm Hg.
- Administer IV fluids at the prescribed flow rate to maintain adequate hydration and to avoid excess fluid accumulation, which increases lung water, causing increased $\dot{V}/\dot{Q}$ mismatch.

Potential Complication: Decreased Functional Residual Capacity. Decreased FRC related to decreased surfactant production or decreased lung compliance secondary to intra-alveolar fluid and protein accumulation.

Expected Patient Outcomes. Patient maintains adequate FRC, as evidenced by RR 12 to 20 BPM, arterial blood gases within normal range, reduced work of breathing, absence of cyanosis, alveolar-arterial oxygen gradient ≤ 15 mm Hg, Sa_{O_2} 97%, and FRC 2400 to 300 mL of air, and $\dot{Q}s/\dot{Q}t$ within normal limits.

- Consult with physician to validate expected patient outcomes used to evaluate adequate FRC.
- Review results of lung volumes (vital capacity, residual volume, and total lung capacity), static lung compliance (Cst), dynamic compliance (Cdyn), tidal volume, and arterial blood gases.
- Position patient for comfort and to promote adequate gas exchange.
- Obtain and report parameters reflecting decreased FRC: $\dot{Q}s/\dot{Q}t \leq 0.8$ P(A−a)$_{O_2} \geq 15$ mm Hg, $Pa_{O_2} \leq 60$ mm Hg, $Pa_{CO_2} \geq 45$ mm Hg, and $Sa_{O_2} \leq 95\%$.
- Obtain and report clinical findings that might suggest decreased FRC: RR ≥ 24 BPM, increased work of breathing, and cyanosis.
- Monitor patient for complications of PEEP therapy: decreased venous return, barotrauma, reduced cerebral perfusion, oxygen toxicity, obstruction to tracheal tube, and hemodynamic complications.
- Auscultate patient's lungs for adventitious breath sounds.
- Monitor compliance: Static lung compliance (Cst) 50 mL/cm H_2O to 100 mL/cm H_2O and dynamic compliance (Cdyn) 50 mL/cm H_2O in relationship to mechanical support are considered optimal.

- Monitor static lung compliance in relation to weaning from mechanical ventilation: ideal static compliance for weaning is 35 mL/cm H_2O.
- Encourage the use of incentive spirometer to prevent the development of atelectasis and pneumonia.
- Provide PEEP therapy in conjunction with traditional ventilatory modes. PEEP therapy distends airway pressure, thereby increasing FRC.
- Provide PEEP in conjunction with non-traditional ventilatory modes that result in increased inspiratory time and decreased expiratory time, such as inverse ratio ventilation.

Potential Complication: Hypoxemia. Hypoxemia related to intrapulmonary shunting secondary to loss of compliance and atelectasis.

Expected Patient Outcomes. Patient maintains adequate oxygen gas exchange, as evidenced by intrapulmonary physiological shunt within normal limits, Pao_2 100 mm Hg, $Paco_2$ 40 mm Hg, oxygen consumption (resting) 250 mL/min, oxygen transport (resting) 1000 mL/min, and skin color normal.

- Review results of arterial blood gas measurement, hemoglobin, hematocrit, and intrapulmonary physiological shunt ($\dot{Q}s/\dot{Q}t$) fraction.
- Position patient with bilateral lung involvement in a prone Trendelenburg position, if not contraindicated, to promote blood flow to the areas of lung that receive the largest tidal volume during mechanical ventilation.
- Assess breath sounds and presence of adventitious breath sounds every 1 to 2 hours. Pulmonary congestion, documented as crackles and wheezes, can indicate increased hydrostatic force in the pulmonary vascular system, causing fluid to move across the alveolar-capillary membrane.
- Should mechanical ventilation and intubation not be necessary, pulse oximetry measurement of Sao_2 and incentive spirom-

etry measurement can be used to provide indirect data about lung compliance and hypoxemia.
- Monitor and report changes in the major factors of oxygen transport: CO $\leq$4 L/min hemoglobin (Hgb)$\leq$12 g/dL, Sao_2 $\leq$90%, and Pao_2 $\leq$80 mm Hg.
- Use chest physiotherapy, postural drainage, chest vibration, and cough enhancement to improve mucus and sputum clearance from the airways.
- Encourage the use of cascade (normal) cough by having patient take a deep breath, followed by three to four coughs until almost all of their air is out of the lungs. Cascade coughing moves secretions from the periphery of the lungs to the central airways.
- Monitor $\dot{Q}s/\dot{Q}t$ fraction at Fio_2 50% to 60%: Normal shunt fraction without a ventilator is 6% and with a ventilator is 10%.
- Suction patient using the principles of preoxygenation, short suctioning time, post-suctioning hyperinflation to reverse atelectasis and uninterrupted PEEP.
- Monitor alveolar-arterial gradient $P(A-a)o_2$ to $\leq$250 to 300 mm Hg with an Fio_2 of 100% is a classic hallmark of ARDS.
- Provide inverse ratio ventilation ventilatory support, if necessary and prescribed, to slowly improve $\dot{Q}s/\dot{Q}t$ and Static Compliance (Cst) over 24 hours.
- Administer prescribed sedation or muscle relaxant to mechanically ventilated patients to reduce prolonged coughing, breathing out of phase with the ventilator, agitation, and decerebrate or decorticate posturing, which may cause trauma to the tracheal mucosa.
- Monitor chest expansion, since patients receiving paniuromium bromide may have a predominance of tidal volume distributed to the apices of the lung.
- Administer prescribed bronchodilators to improve ventilation and facilitate removal of secretions.
- Administer prescribed IV fluids, such as crystalloids, to maintain adequate intra-

vascular volume and PCWP 10 to 12 mm Hg.

- Instruct patient to cough, turn, and deep breathe to enhance oxygen–carbon dioxide exchange.

Potential Complication: Respiratory Alkalosis. Respiratory alkalosis related to tachypnea or hyperventilation secondary to ventilatory support.

Expected Patient Outcomes. Patient maintains adequate acid-base balance, as evidenced by RR 12 to 20 BPM, arterial blood gases within normal limits, BP within the patient's normal range, MAP 70 to 100 mm Hg, absence of dysrhythmias, tidal volume $\geq$5 to 7 mL/kg, vital capacity $\geq$12 to 15 mL/kg, absence of adventitious breath sounds, absence of signs and symptoms associated with respiratory alkalosis.

- Consult with Respiratory Therapy regarding patient's tidal volume and vital capacity values.
- Review arterial blood gas and electrolyte values.
- Position patient to allow for best lung expansion, which may increase ventilation-perfusion matching.
- Monitor and report clinical findings associated with respiratory alkalosis: light-headedness, weakness, muscle cramps, twitching, paresthesia, seizures, tetany, or hyperactivity.
- Monitor ventilatory support in relation to patient's RR, tidal volume, and arterial blood gases to avoid respiratory alkalosis.
- Monitor continuous ECG to assess HR and rhythm. Document ECG rhythm every 2 to 4 hours in patients with dysrhythmias.
- Administer prescribed oxygen, FIO_2 at $\leq$50% to maintain PaO_2 $\geq$60 mm Hg.
- In mechanically ventilated patients, increase dead space ventilation and minute ventilation, as prescribed and necessary, to allow $PaCO_2$ and $PaCO_2$ to return to a normal range of 35 to 45 mm Hg.

- Instruct patient to control respirations through meditation, progressive relaxation, or guided imagery.

Potential Complication: Decreased Pulmonary Muscle Function. Decreased pulmonary muscle function related to nutritional deficit or dependency upon ventilatory support secondary to loss of compliance and endotracheal intubation.

Expected Patient Outcomes. Patient maintains adequate pulmonary muscle function, as evidenced by RR $\leq$24 BPM, tidal volume $\geq$5 to 7 mL/kg, vital capacity $\geq$12 to 15 mL/kg, alveolar-arterial oxygen gradient $P(A-a)O_2$ $\leq$15 mm Hg on room air, static compliance (Cst) $\geq$50 mL/cm H_2O, dynamic compliance (Cdyn) $\geq$45 mL/cm H_2O, absence of fatigue, and absence of adventitious breath sounds.

- Review results of alveolar ventilation, minute volume, lung volumes, and arterial blood gases.
- Place patient in semi- to high Fowler's position to allow more effective lung expansion.
- Evaluate respiratory muscle efficiency through measurements of tidal volume, minute ventilation, RR, vital capacity, and maximum inspiratory pressure.
- Monitor symmetry of chest wall, diaphragmatic excursion, and use of accessory muscles.
- For patient not requiring mechanical ventilation or intubation, use incentive spirometry to facilitate lung expansion and prevent atelectasis.
- Assess static compliance (Cst) and dynamic compliance (Cdyn) as a measure of lung compliance.
- Encourage use of deep-breathing therapy with chest physiotherapy to improve ventilation and increase muscle tone.
- Instruct patient to deep breathe, thereby stimulating respiratory muscles and enhancing gas exchange.

• Teach patient to report any shortness of breath, fatigue, or exhaustion.

DISCHARGE PLANNING

The critical care nurse will provide patient and significant other(s) with verbal or written discharge notes regarding the following subjects:

1. The signs and symptoms that warrant medical attention: shortness of breath, fatigue, activity intolerance, tachypnea, and tachycardia.
2. Need to cease any activity that increases HR and BP or causes fatigue, because these behaviors can increase tissue oxygen demand.
3. The names of community agencies that can provide support if the patient should require portable oxygen unit (American Lung Association).
4. A written list of side effects associated with patient's specific medications.
5. The need to use of a weekly schedule of exercise and rest.

■ ACUTE PULMONARY EDEMA

For related information see Cardiac Derivations, Part I: Shock, p. 174; Dysrhythmias, p. 184. Part III: Hemodynamic monitoring, p. 219. Part I: Adult respiratory distress syndrome, p. 327; Pulmonary embolism, p. 397; Pulmonary hypertension, p. 404; Respiratory acidosis, p. 412. Part III: Pulse oximetry, p. 426; Mechanical ventilation, p. 428; Extracorporeal membrane oxygenation, p. 437; Capnography, p. 439; Transcutaneous Pao$_2$ and Paco$_2$, p. 441; Indirect calorimetry, p. 441.

Case Management Basis
DRG: 87 Pulmonary edema and respiratory failure
LOS: 6.00 days

Definition
The pulmonary vascular system is able to accommodate three times its normal volume. When the normal volume is exceeded, however, and fluid moves across the alveolar-capillary membrane, pulmonary edema occurs in the interstitial and air spaces of the lungs.

Pathophysiology
Pulmonary edema occurs in two stages. The first stage is interstitial edema in which fluid accumulates in the peribronchial and perivascular spaces. Interstitial pulmonary edema increases the distance between the alveoli and pulmonary capillaries. The second stage occurs when interstitial hydrostatic pressure in the pulmonary capillaries increases ≥25 to 30 mm Hg and pushes fluid into the alveoli, causing alveolar edema. Plasma oncotic pressure also increases to ≥25 mm Hg. As the alveoli gradually fill, surfactant is diluted, eventually causing the alveoli to collapse. The alveoli that aren't collapsed may be compressed by edematous alveoli. Since the affected alveoli are void of oxygen, a right-to-left shunt occurs.

Acute pulmonary edema may show different patterns of distribution as a result of variations in the transmission of pleural pressures in the lungs. Normally, lymphatic drainage is sufficient to drain excess protein and fluid that does not reenter the capillary. A sustained increase in hydrostatic pressure can normally be compensated for by increased lymphatic drainage. Excess blood in the pulmonary vascular system increases pulmonary capillary hydrostatic pressure in the dependent areas of the lungs. When hypoxemia occurs, there is reflex vasoconstriction, which leads to increased pulmonary blood pressure. As the pulmonary pressure increases, transudation of fluid into the pulmonary interstitial space occurs.

Nursing Assessment

PRIMARY CAUSES

- Cardiogenic pulmonary edema: Occurs as a result of heart failure or cardiogenic shock, caused by an imbalance between the hydrostatic and osmotic pressures that control fluid movement within the lungs. The permeability of the microvascular membrane remains intact, limiting movement of protein out of the capillaries.
- Noncardiogenic pulmonary edema: Occurs in adult respiratory distress syndrome, where there is an increase in the permeability of the alveolar-capillary membrane in the presence of normal pulmonary capillary hydrostatic pressure. Fluid moves out of the intravascular space and into the pulmonary interstitium.

PHYSICAL ASSESSMENT

- Inspection: Dyspnea, cough, orothopnea, cyanosis, apprehension, restlessness, pallor, anxiety, diaphoresis, pink frothy sputum, tachypnea, or jugular venous distention.
- Palpation: Tactile fremitus or peripheral edema.
- Auscultation: Bilateral basilar or diffuse rales, wheezes, rhonchi, tachycardia, normal blood pressure (BP) to hypotension, or S_3 gallop rhythm.

DIAGNOSTIC TEST RESULTS

Hemodynamic Monitoring

- Left atrial pressure (LAP) 25 to 30 mm Hg and pulmonary capillary wedge pressure (PCWP) $\geq$ 15 mm Hg.

Standard Laboratory Tests (see Table 3–1)

- Alveolar fluid shows protein concentration.
- Arterial blood gases: Hypoxemia reflected as partial pressure of arterial oxygen (Pao_2) $\leq$ 60 mm Hg and partial pressure of arterial carbon dioxide ($Paco_2$) $\geq$ 40 mm Hg.

Noninvasive Respiratory Diagnostic Procedures (see Table 3–4)

Chest roentgenogram: Cardiomegaly, aortic valve calcification, mitral valve calcification, pleural effusion, redistribution of pulmonary blood flow to upper-lung zones, blurring of vascular markings, increased bronchial wall thickness, or periphilar distribution of infiltrates.

ECG

- New Q waves of infarction, ST-T wave changes of injury and ischemia, and P wave changes of mitral or left atrial disease.

MEDICAL AND SURGICAL MANAGEMENT

Pharmacology

- Dobutamine hydrochloride (Dobutrex): A synthetic catecholamine that acts on the beta-adrenergic receptors, which enhance contractility. It is used, at a dose of 0.5 mg/kg/min, in any stage of cardiogenic shock that can be a cause of pulmonary edema (see Table 1–10, p. 50).
- Dopamine hydrochloride (Intropin): It is used to increase contractility through its beta-adrenergic receptor activity at a dose of 1 to 2 μg/kg/min (see Table 1–10, p. 50).
- Amrinone lactate: It inhibits the enzyme phosphodiesterase. This enhances the availability of cyclic adenosine monophosphate (cAMP), which is a major factor in cardiac contractility. It is given as IV bolus 0.75 mg/kg over 2 to 3 minutes, then titrated at 5 to 10 μg/kg/min (see Table 1–10, p. 50).
- Antidysrhythmic agents: These are administered to treat dysrhythmias that can occur from injury to the myocardium, such as acute myocardial infarction, or in response to hypoxia or acidosis (see Table 1–11, p. 54).
- Diuretics: These are used to maintain patency of the renal tubules and reduce preload. The latter helps to decrease pulmonary congestion. The furosemide IV

push is infused at a rate of 10 mg/min and the 0.5 to 1.0 mg bumetanide IV push at rate of 0.5 mg/min.

- Vasodilators: Nitroprusside is used to reduce preload and afterload at a dose of 10 μg/kg/min when systolic blood pressure is $\geq$100 mm Hg. Morphine can be administered by IV push at a dose of 2 mg increments every 5 minutes (see Table 1–4, p. 20).

FLUID THERAPY

- Restrict fluid intake to avoid further pulmonary edema.

ROTATING TOURNIQUETS

- Apply tourniquets to three extremities. Set pressure midway between systolic BP (SBP) and diastolic BP (DBP). The tourniquets are rotated every 15 minutes and removed by rotating of one every 15 minutes.

MECHANICAL VENTILATION

- Assisted ventilation with positive endexpiratory pressure (PEEP) can improve gas exchange (see Mechanical ventilation, p. 428).

OXYGEN THERAPY

- Supplemental oxygen such as 2 to 4 L by nasal cannula or mask and/or $FIO_2 \leq$50% to maintain adequate tissue oxygenation.

NURSING MANAGEMENT: NURSING DIAGNOSES AND COLLABORATIVE PROBLEMS

Nursing Diagnoses

Common nursing goals for patients with pulmonary edema are to enhance gas exchange, maintain fluid balance, increase urinary elimination, support activity tolerance, and promote sense of powerfulness.

Impaired gas exchange related to alveolar-capillary membrane alteration secondary to increased hydrostatic pressure in the pulmonary bed contributing to pulmonary edema.

Expected Patient Outcomes. Patient maintains adequate gas exchange, as evidenced by arterial blood gases within the patient's normal range, respiratory rate (RR) 12 to 20 BPM, heart rate (HR) $\leq$100 bpm, arterial oxygen saturation (SaO_2) $\geq$95%, mixed venous oxygen saturation $S\bar{v}O_2$ 60% to 80%, $P(a/A)O_2$ ratio 0.75 to 0.95, absence of crackles or wheezes, absence of cyanosis, and normal skin color.

- Consult with physician to validate expected patient outcomes used to evaluate adequate gas exchange.
- Consult with physician about the criteria used to determine when ventilatory support is needed: oxygenation ($PaO_2 \leq$60 mm Hg on FIO_2 at 50%), ventilator ($PaCO_2 \geq$50 to 60 mm Hg, which is $\geq$10 mm Hg above patient's normal $PaCO_2$), and respiratory mechanics (apnea, sustained RR $\geq$35 BPM, and vital capacity $\leq$10 to 15 mL/kg).
- Review results of arterial blood gas measurement and chest roentgenogram.
- Maintain bed rest during the second stage of alveolar edema.
- Monitor clinical indicators of respiratory status: RR, lung sounds, skin color, symmetry of chest movement, skin warmth, and use of accessory muscles.
- Obtain and report clinical findings associated with impaired gas exchange: RR $\geq$24 BPM, crackles, cyanosis, diaphoresis, and use of accessory muscles.
- Monitor patient's tolerance of ventilatory support through the use of an individualized plan of care that includes data from chest, such as lung sounds, RR, chest expansion, and ventilator settings; hemodynamic parameters including HR, BP, temperature (T), cardiac output (CO), cardiac index (CI), pulmonary artery pressure (PAP), and PCWP; nutritional status, such as type of feedings, intake, and output; and level of anxiety.
- Assess ventilator function by verifying that the prescribed settings are being used and are effective. The settings include FIO_2 at

the lowest rate to maintain Pao_2 $\geq$60 mm Hg and 100% in acute situation to achieve adequate oxygenation; tidal volume 10 to 15 mL/kg; RR 10 to 14 BPM; and mode of ventilation.

- Evaluate the efficiency of deep-breathing ability by monitoring vital capacity and maximal inspiratory force (MIF).

- Administer Fio_2 through a mask at 35% to 65% when the oxygen flow rate is 6 to 12 L/min.

- Provide mechanical ventilation according to the required mode to keep Pao_2 $\geq$60 mm Hg: PEEP, intermittent mandatory ventilation (IMV), synchronized intermittent mandatory ventilation (SIMV), pressure support ventilation (PSV), or inverse ratio ventilation.

- Provide continuous positive airway pressure (CPAP) by mask, if necessary, to improve arterial oxygenation by increasing functional residual capacity and lung compliance.

Fluid volume excess related to abnormal intra-alveolar fluid gain secondary to increased permeability and fluid exudation into the alveoli and decreased CO.

Expected Patient Outcomes. Patient maintains adequate fluid volume, as evidenced by PCWP 6 to 12 mm Hg, PAP 20 to 30-8 to 15 mm Hg, central venous pressure (CVP) 2 to 6 mm Hg, right atrial pressure (RAP) 4 to 6 mm Hg, pulmonary vascular resistance (PVR) 155 to 255 dynes/sc/cm^{-5}, pulmonary vascular resistance index (PVRI) 200 to 450 dynes/sc/cm^{-5}/m^2, Svo_2 60 to 80 mm Hg, BP within patient's normal range, absence of cyanosis, absence of adventitious breath sounds, RR 12 to 20 BPM, and urinary output (UO) $\geq$30 mL/h.

- Consult with physician to validate expected patient outcomes used to evaluate adequate fluid volume.

- Review results of chest roentgenogram, 12-lead ECG, and arterial blood gas measurement.

- Restrict physical activity to bed rest and semi- to high-Fowler's position.

- Provide a low-salt diet.

- Obtain and report hemodynamic parameters indicating fluid volume excess: CVP $\geq$6 mm Hg, PAP systolic $\geq$30 mm Hg or PAP diastolic $\geq$15 mm Hg, PCWP $\geq$12 mm Hg, PVR $\geq$250 dynes/s/cm^{-5}, PVRI $\geq$450 dynes/s/cm^{-5}/m^2, and Svo_2 $\leq$60 mm Hg.

- Obtain and report other clinical findings that reflect increased intra-alveolar fluid excess: tachypnea, hypotension, tachycardia, crackles or rhonchi, peripheral edema, and cyanosis.

- Monitor daily weight, intake, specific gravity, and UO. Report UO $\leq$30 mL/h and weight gain $\geq$1 kg/d.

- Apply automatic rotating tourniquet, if necessary.

- Should fluid restriction, oxygenation, and diuretics be ineffective, prepare patient for mechanical ventilatory support and endotracheal intubation.

- Assess ventilator function by verifying that the prescribed settings are being used and are effective. The settings include Fio_2 at the lowest rate to maintain Pao_2 $\geq$60 mm Hg and 100% in acute situation to achieve adequate oxygenation; tidal volume 10 to 15 mL/kg; RR 10 to 14 BPM; and mode of ventilation.

- Move endotracheal tube to the other side of the mouth daily to prevent tissue necrosis.

- Use unit-prescribed method of endotracheal suctioning: preoxygenation, hyperinflation, hyperoxygenation, hyperventilation, maximal inflation, and oxygen insufflation.

- Use unit-prescribed suction devices that permit patient to remain on the ventilator during suctioning: oxygen insufflation devices (OID) or closed tracheal suction system (CTSS).

- Use intratracheal instillation of 2 mL to 5 mL of normal saline during suctioning to enhance the removal of secretions by stimulating a cough.

- Monitor and evaluate patient's oxygen (Sao_2, Svo_2) and hemodynamic status

(MAP, CO) before, during, and after suctioning.

- Evaluate patient's readiness to be weaned from full or partial ventilatory support to spontaneous unassisted breathing by using the following objective weaning criteria: oxygenation (Pao_2 ≥60 mm Hg on Fio_2 ≤0.4 to 0.5 and PEEP ≤5 cm H_2O); ventilation (minute ventilation ≤10 L/min, tidal volume ≥5 mL/kg, and $Paco_2$ within usual range for patient); and respiratory mechanics (spontaneous RR ≤30 to 35 BPM, maximal inspiratory force ≤ −20 cm H_2O).
- Administer prescribed Fio_2 at 50% and oxygen at 2 to 4 L/min by nasal cannula, mask, or ventilator to maintain Pao_2 ≥60 mm Hg and Sao_2 ≥95%.
- Administer prescribed IV fluids to maintain adequate hydration and UO ≥30 mL/h or ≥0.5 mL/kg/h.
- Administer volume-reducing agents. (For additional information see Table 1–13, p. 76).
- Administer prescribed sedative or muscle relaxant (or mechanically ventilated patient to reduce prolonged coughing, breathing out of phase with the ventilator, agitation, and decerebrate or decorticate posturing, which may cause trauma to the tracheal mucosa.

Urinary elimination, altered pattern related to decreased glomerular filtration and increased sympathoadrenergic stimulants secondary to decreased CO.

Expected Patient Outcomes. Patient maintains adequate urinary elimination, as evidenced by UO ≥30 mL/h or 0.5 mL/kg/h, specific gravity 1.010 to 1.030, stable body weight, blood urea nitrogen (BUN) ≤20 mg/dL, serum creatinine ≤1.5 mg/dL, serum potassium ≥3.5 mEq/L, absence of adventitious breath sounds, absence of peripheral edema, BP within patient's normal range, MAP ≥70 mm Hg, and absence of cyanosis.

- Review results of BUN, creatinine, serum electrolytes, and serum protein.

- Obtain and report clinical findings associated with altered urinary elimination: UO ≤30 mL/h or ≤0.5 mL/kg/h, crackles or wheezes, peripheral edema, and weight gain ≥0.5 to 1.0 kg/d.
- Administer prescribed IV fluids to maintain adequate hydration.
- Administer volume-reducing agents to maintain UO ≥30 mL/h (see Table 1–13, p. 76).
- Should pharmacological therapy be ineffective in increasing urinary volume, implement ultrafiltration to remove excess fluid and solutes (see Renal Deviations, Continuous renal replacement therapy, p. 505).

Activity intolerance related to generalized weakness and fatigue secondary to imbalance between oxygen supply and demand.

Expected Patient Outcomes. Patient tolerates increases in physical activity, peak HR ≤20 bpm over patient's resting HR, peak SBP ≤20 mm Hg over patient's resting SBP, Svo_2 ≥60%, RR ≤24 BPM, absence of angina, absence of shortness of breath, normal sinus rhythm, skin warm and dry, and absence of dyspnea.

- Confer with Rehabilitation as to the appropriate activity program for the patient.
- Consult with physical therapist about exercises patient can do to maintain muscle tone.
- Limit activity to bed rest while patient is experiencing alveolar edema.
- Monitor clinical indicators of activity intolerance: HR, BP, RR, cardiac rhythm, and skin color when patient is gradually increasing physical activity.
- Obtain and report clinical findings associated with activity intolerance: chest pain, HR ≥120 bpm, fatigue, shortness of breath, dysrhythmias, and BP ≥20 mm Hg from baseline or ≥160 mm Hg.
- Provide rest before and after physical activity.

- Administer oxygen at the prescribed amount before and after physical activity.
- Administer prescribed analgesics to relieve pain before and after gradual increases in physical activity.
- Teach patient to report any patient pain while ambulating.
- Teach patient to cease activity and rest should activity intolerance occur.
- Teach patient to perform passive range of motion (ROM) to prevent complications of immobility.
- Explain the need to exercise to tolerance while avoiding strenuous exercises.

Powerlessness related to the loss of control over heart failure, pulmonary alveolar edema, need for supportive therapies, or potential life-style changes.

Expected Patient Outcome. Patient demonstrates increase in ability to exercise control over own body, cognition, environment, and decision making.

- Encourage physiological control by helping patient reduce stress through clarification of the events leading to pulmonary edema and through active acceptance of the unavoidable physiological changes surrounding the current illness.
- Assist patient's cognitive control by providing educational information and thorough explanation of sensations to be expected during treatment.
- Provide environmental control by helping patient to establish positive interpersonal relations with members of the critical care health team and to place personal belongings in the environment.
- Assist patient to control decision making in so far as possible and to participate in own care by adhering to discharge treatments.

Collaborative Problem

Potential Complication: Decreased Cardiac Output.

Decreased CO related to increased left ventricular preload and afterload secondary to impaired myocardial contractility and impaired ventricular compliance as a result of ischemia or infarction.

Expected Patient Outcomes. Patient maintains adequate left ventricular preload and afterload, as evidenced by BP $\geq$90/60 mm Hg, CO 4 to 8 L/min, CI 2.7 to 4.3 L/min/m^2, mean atrial pressure (MAP) 70 to 100 mm Hg, PAP systolic $\leq$25 mm Hg and diastolic $\leq$15 mm Hg, PCWP 16 to 18 mm Hg, pulse pressure (PP) 30 to 40 mm Hg, PVR 155 to 250 dynes/s/cm^{-5}, PVRI 200 to 450 dynes/s/cm^{-5}$\neq$m^2, systemic vascular resistance (SVR) 900 to 1200 dynes/s/cm^{-5}, and systemic vascular resistance index (SVRI) 1970 to 2390 dynes/s/cm^{-5}$\neq$m^2.

- Consult with cardiologist to validate the expected patient outcomes that reflect adequate left ventricular preload and afterload.
- Limit physical activity to bed rest to decrease ventricular wall tension and myocardial oxygen demand.
- Place patient in a high Fowler's position to decrease myocardial work load, decrease venous return, and increase lung expansion.
- Obtain, document, and report hemodynamic values associated with decreased CO contributing to pulmonary edema: CO $\leq$4 L/min, CI $\leq$2.7 L/min/m^2, CVP $\geq$6 mm Hg, PAP systolic $\geq$30 mm Hg and diastolic $\geq$15 mm Hg, PCWP $\geq$18 mm Hg, PVRT cm^{-5}/m^2, PP $\leq$30 mm Hg, PVR $\geq$250 dynes/s/cm^{-5}, PVRI $\geq$450 dynes/sec/cm^{-5}/m^2, SVR $\geq$1200 dynes/s/cm^{-5} and SVRI $\geq$2390 dynes/s/cm^{-5}/m^2.
- Obtain and report other clinical findings associated with decreased CO contributing to pulmonary edema: RR $\geq$24 BPM, HR $\geq$100 bpm, hypotension, crackles, fatigue, cyanosis, and diaphoresis.
- Monitor continuous ECG to assess HR and rhythm. Document ECG strips every 2 to 4 hours in patients with dysrhythmias.
- Monitor UO in relation to volume reducing agents: $\geq$30 mL/h or 0.5 mL/Kg/h.

- Monitor daily weight: Each liter of fluid weighs 1 kg, and daily weight changes in excess of 0.25 kg are the result of loss or gain of water.
- Administered prescribed low-flow oxygen 2 to 4 L/min (24% to 36% O_2) by nasal cannula or $F_{IO_2} \leq 50\%$ by mask.
- Administer IV fluids as prescribed to maintain hydration, $CO \geq 4$ L/min, $CI \geq 2.7$ L/min/m^2, PCWP ≤ 18 mm Hg, and UO ≥ 30 mL/h or ≥ 0.5 mL/kg/h.
- Administer prescribed positive inotropes (dopamine or dobutamine) or phosphodiesterase inhibitor (amrinone) to maintain BP $\geq 90/60$ mm Hg, CO 4 to 8 L/min, CI ≥ 2.7 L/min/m^2, PAP systolic ≤ 25 mm Hg and diastolic ≤ 15 mm Hg, and PCWP ≤ 12 mm Hg. Be cautious, as drugs may increase ventricular ectopy, size of infarction, or be ineffective if beta blockers have been administered (see Table 1–10, p. 50).
- Administer vasodilators: to lower systemic afterload, peripheral vasodilators (nitroprusside); to lower preload, coronary vasodilators (nitroglycerin); or peripheral coronary vasodilators (verapamil, nifedipine, or diltiazem) to maintain BP$\geq 90/60$mmHg, PP 30 to 40 mm Hg, SVR 900 to 1200 dynes/s/cm^{-5}, and SVRI 1970 to 2390 dynes/s/cm^{-5}/m^2 (see Table 1–4, p. 20, and Table 1–6, p. 28).
- Administer volume-reducing agents to enhance renal excretion of sodium and water, decrease preload, reduce blood volume, reduce intracardiac filling pressures, and resolve interstitial peripheral and intraalveolar edema: furosemide or bumetanide. (For additional information see Table 1–13, p. 76).
- Administer morphine sulfate to dilate pulmonary vascular bed and decrease venous and arterial vasoconstriction.
- Should pharmacological therapy be ineffective in reducing preload and afterload, assist with the insertion of an intra-aortic balloon pump (see Intra-aortic balloon counter pulsation, p. 254).

- Teach patient the common side effects of diuretics and vasodilators.
- Instruct patient to report any chest pain.

DISCHARGE PLANNING

The critical care nurse will provide patient and significant other(s) with verbal or written discharge notes regarding the following subjects:

1. The importance of continuing follow-up care. If possible confirm the next appointment.
2. Reporting the signs and symptoms of weight gain, decrease UO, swollen feet and ankles, and persistent cough.
3. The name, dose, purpose, schedule, and side effects of all medications.

■ EMPHYSEMA

For related information see Cardiac Deviations, Part I: Shock, p. 174; Dysrhythmias, p. 184. Part III: Hemodynamic monitoring, p. 219. Part I: Adult respiratory distress syndrome, p. 327; Pulmonary embolism, p. 397; Pulmonary hypertension, p. 404; Respiratory acidosis, p. 412. Part III: Pulse oximetry, p. 426; Mechanical ventilation, p. 428; Capnography, p. 439; Transcutaneous PaO_2 and $PaCO_2$, p. 441; Indirect calorimetry, p. 441.)

Case Management Basis

DRG: 88 Chronic obstructive pulmonary disease
LOS: 5.90 days

Definition

Emphysema designates a lung disorder in which the terminal bronchioles become plugged with mucus. Emphysema is characterized by an abnormal enlargement of the distal terminal bronchioles with alveolar fragmentation and destruction of the alveolar septa.

Pathophysiology

Destruction of the alveolar structure leading to a loss of gas exchange surface area, loss of elastic recoil, and distention of remaining lung tissue are features of emphysema. The primary defect underlying emphysema involves the proteolysis of the complex structural protein, elastin, which is found in the walls of the alveoli. The breaking down of the elastin decreases elastic recoil of the lung. This leads to altered expiratory air flow and decreased respiratory epithelial surface area for gas exchange.

The alveoli enlarge, their walls are destroyed, and alveolar destruction leads to the formation of large air spaces. The latter reduces the alveolar diffusing surface. Alveolar destruction undermines the support structure for the airways, making them vulnerable to expiratory collapse. Ischemia may cause alveolar breakdown, thus leading to emphysema. When the alveolar walls are destroyed, fibrous and muscle tissues are lost, making the lungs more distensible.

Emphysema can be classified according to the site of pulmonary involvement. With centrilobular or centriacinar emphysema, the lesion is located in the center of the lobule. The disease involves the upper lung zones and is associated with chronic bronchitis. Panlobular or panacinar emphysema involves the entire acinus. The septa are lost, with enlargement of the air spaces causing loss of pulmonary parenchyma. Paulobular emphysema is found in the lower and anterior lungs and is also found in patients with alpha$_1$ proteinse inhibitor deficiency.

Nursing Assessment

PRIMARY CAUSES
• Air pollution and airway infection.

RISK FACTORS
• Cigarette smoking and familial factors.

PHYSICAL ASSESSMENT
• Inspection: Breathlessness, dyspnea, cyanosis, orthopnea, thin, underweight, increased anteroposterior diameter, hypertrophied accessory muscles, diminished di-aphragmatic excursion, productive cough, ankle edema, bird flapping tremor, distended neck veins, weight loss, weakness, or fatigue.
• Palpation: Right ventricular heave and unequal chest expansion.
• Percussion: Increased chest resonance.
• Auscultation: Distant breath sounds, distant heart sounds, full volume pulse of distended forearm veins, tachypnea, wheezing, or scattered crackles.

DIAGNOSTIC TEST RESULTS

Standard Laboratory Tests (see Table 3–1)

• Arterial blood gases: Show decreased partial pressure of arterial oxygen (Pao$_2$) and increased partial pressure of arterial carbon dioxide (Paco$_2$).
• Blood studies: Increased white blood count (WBC).
• Sputum cultures: May be positive for bacteria, pneumococci, or staphylococci.

Respiratory Function Tests (see Table 3–2)

• Lung volumes: Increased residual volume (RV) liters, functional residual capacity (FRC), total lung capacity (TLC), forced expiratory volume in 1 second (FEV$_1$) and maximal mid expiratory flow rate (MMFR). There is decreased vital capacity (VC) and diffusing capacity.
• Spirometry: Reduction in forced expiratory volume in the second (FEV$_1$) and in the ratio of forced expiratory volume to forced vital capacity (FEV$_1$:FVC).

Invasive Respiratory Diagnostic Procedures (see Table 3–3)

• Bronchoscopy: Shows mucopurulent secretions present in and around involved areas.
• Bronchogram: Shows areas of bronchial dilation.

Noninvasive Respiratory Diagnostic Procedures (see Table 3–4)

- Chest roentgenogram: In the latter stages of emphysema there is flattening of the diaphragm, hyperlucency, decreased vascular markings, widening of the rib spaces, and increased anteroposterior diameter.

ECG

- Sinus tachycardia, supraventricular arrhythmias (multifocal atrial tachycardia, atrial flutter, and atrial fibrillation), and ventricular irritability.

MEDICAL AND SURGICAL MANAGEMENT

PHARMACOLOGY

- Bronchodilator therapy: Bronchodilators such as theophylline relax the bronchial smooth muscle in the lung. The goal is to maintain blood levels of 10 to 20 μg/ml. (Table 3–6).
- Steroids: Can be used in patients with emphysema who have a strong component of asthma. Intravenous methylprednisolone can be given for 1 to 2 days, followed by oral prednisone.
- Antibiotics: Used to treat infections, which can be a precipitating factor causing respiratory failure in the emphysema patient.

OXYGEN THERAPY

- Supplemental oxygen is given at flow rates of 2 to 4 L/min to maintain Pao_2 between 55 and 65 mm Hg. An adequate Pao_2 improves tissue oxygen delivery. The fraction of inspired oxygen (Fio_2) varies, since it is determined by the tidal volume of room air the patient also inhales. Oxygen by Venturi-principle face mask allows more precise administration of oxygen when necessary.

MECHANICAL VENTILATION

- Endotracheal intubation and mechanical ventilation may be necessary should $Paco_2$ increase above normal levels for the patient, together with acidemia, hypoxemia, or loss of mental acuity.

HEMODYNAMIC MONITORING

- Used to measure pulmonary vascular pressure, pulmonary artery systolic and diastolic pressure, and mean pulmonary artery pressure, which are all elevated. Furthermore, the pulmonary artery diastolic pressure (PADP) may be 5 to 20 mm Hg higher than the pulmonary capillary wedge pressure (PCWP). When the gradient between PADP and PCWP is $\geq$2 mm Hg, the patient may have increased pulmonary vascular resistance (PVR).

DIET

- Treatment regimen may include an increase in calories; excess carbohydrates, when converted to fat, lead to increased production of carbon dioxide. It is recommended that less than one third of the calories provided be made up of carbohydrates.

NURSING MANAGEMENT: NURSING DIAGNOSES AND COLLABORATIVE PROBLEMS

Nursing Diagnoses

Common nursing goals for patients with emphysema are to improve gas exchange, maintain effective airway clearance, facilitate effective breathing patterns, prevent infection, support activity tolerance, and minimize anxiety.

Impaired gas exchange related to decreased lung compliance secondary to air trapping or hyperinflation.

Expected Patient Outcomes. Patient maintains adequate gas exchange, as evidenced by arterial blood gases within normal range; respiratory rate (RR) 12 to 20 BPM; heart rate (HR) $\geq$100 bpm; absence of cyanosis; normal sinus rhythm; absence of confusion, restlessness, or irritability; absence of lethargy; absence of crackles; (P[a:A]O_2) 0.075 to 0.90 (P[A−a]O_2) $\leq$15 mm Hg, and Pao_2 100 mm Hg.

TABLE 3-6. BRONCHIODILATORS

Medication	Route/Dose	Uses and Effects	Side Effects
Albuterol (Proventil)	PO: 2–4 mg 3–4 times/d, 4–8 mg sustained release bid Inhaled: 1–2 inhalations q4–6h	Relieves bronchospasm associated with chronic asthma, bronchitis, or COPD	Tremor, anxiety, nervousness, restlessness, palpitation, weakness, hypertension, bradycardia, nausea, vomiting, muscle cramps, hoarseness, hyperglycemia
Aminophylline (Corophyllin)	PO: Loading dose 500 mg, followed by 250–500 mg q6–8 h IV: Loading dose 5–6 mg/kg infused over 30 min, followed by 0.2–0.9 mg/kg/h continuous infusion Rectal: 500 mg retention enema every 6–8 h	Relieves symptoms of acute bronchial asthma and treatment bronchospasm associated with chronic bronchitis and emphysema	Nervousness, restlessness, depression, headache, tachycardia, chest pain, severe hyotension, nausea, vomiting, diarrhea
Ipratropium bromide (Atrovent)	Inhalation: 2 inhalations qid at no less than 4 h intervals; maximum 12 inhalations in 24 h	Maintenance therapy in chronic bronchitis and emphysema	Nervousness, dizziness, headache, blurred vision, tachycardia, hypotension, nausea, insomnia, GI distress, hoarseness, rash, drying of bronchial secretions
Isoetharine hydrochloride (Bronkosol)	Inhalation: 0.5–1 mL 0.5% or 0.5 mL 1% solution diluted 1:3 with normal saline, or 2–4 mL 0.125% solution undiluted, or 2–5 mL 0.2% solution diluted per nebulizer q 4 h up to 5 times/d 1–2 inhalations from a metered dose inhaler (MD) q 6 h up to 5 times/d	Bronchodilator in reversible air way obstruction produced by asthma or COPD	Nervousness, restlessness, tremor, nausea, vomiting, headache, tension, weakness, cough, bronchial irritation, edema
Isoproterenol hydrochloride (Aerolone)	Metered dose: 1–2 inhalations 4–6 times/d; no more than 6 inhalations in any hour during a 24-h period Compressed air or IPPB: 0.5 mL of 0.5% solution diluted to 2.0–2.5 mL with water or saline up to 5 times/d	Treatment of bronchial asthma and reversible bronchospasm, shock that persists after replacement of blood volume, or cardiac stimulant	Nervousness, headache, tremors, hypertension, arrhythmias, angina, nausea, vomiting, fatigue, flushing, hyperglycemia
Metaproterenol sulfate (Alupent)	PO: 20mg q 6–8 h Metered Dose Inhaler: 2–3 inhalations q3–4h; maximum 12 inhalations/day Nebulizer: 5–10 inhalations of undiluted 5% solution IPPB: 2.5 mL or 0.4%–6% solution q 4–6 h	Treatment of asthma, reversible bronchospasm associated with bronchitis, emphysema	Nervousness, restlessness, tremor, weakness, nausea, drowsiness, tachycardia, vomiting, muscle cramps, hyperglycemia

TABLE 3-6

TABLE 3-6

TABLE 3–6. CONTINUED

Medication	Route/Dose	Uses and Effects	Side Effects
Terbutaline sulfate (Bretnaire)	PO: 2.5–5.0 mg tid at 6 h intervals; maximum 15 mg/d. SC: 0.25 mg q 15–30 min up to 0.5 mg in 4 h Inhaled: 2 inhalations separated by 60 s q 4–6 h	Treatment of bronchial asthma, COPD	Nervousness, tremor, headache, light-headness, fatigue, tachycardia, angina, hypertension, anxiety, nausea, vomiting, hypokelemia
Theophylline (Acrolate)	PO: 5–6 mg/kg initially, followed by 4–16 mg/kg/d in divided doses q 6–12 h in range of 400–900 mg/d IV: Loading dose of 5mg/kg infused over 30 minutes, followed by 0.2–0.8 mg/kg/hr continuous infusion	Treatment of asthma and reversible bronchospasm that occurs with chronic bronchitis and emphysema Relaxes the respiratory smooth muscle, causing increased flow rates and vital capacity Dilates pulmonary arterioles, reduces pulmonary hypertension, reduces alveolar carbon dioxide tension, and increases pulmonary blood flow	Restlessness, dizziness, headache, tremor, muscle twitching, nausea, tachycardia, vomiting, abdominal pain, diarrhea, tachypnea, fever, activation of peptic ulcer

COPD, chronic obstructive pulmonary disease; GI, gastrointestinal; IPPB, intermittent positive-pressure breathing; IV, intravenous; PO, by mouth; SC, subcutaneous.

From Fischblach F, 1984; Ford RD, 1987; Deglin JH, Vallerand AH & Russin MM, 1991; Thelan LA, Davie JK, Urden LD, 1990; Loeb S, 1993.

- Consult with physician about the criteria used to determine when ventilatory support is needed: oxygenation ($Pao_2 \leq 60$ mm Hg on Fio_2 at 50%), ventilator ($Paco_2 \geq 50$ to 60 mm Hg, which is ≥ 10 mm Hg above patient's normal $Paco_2$), and respiratory mechanics (apnea, sustained RR ≥ 35 BPM, and VC ≤ 10 to 15 ml/kg).
- Consult with physician about alternative treatments to assist patient in removing excess or viscous secretions: bronchodilators and humidification.
- Review results of arterial blood gas measurement and chest roentgenogram.
- Elevate the head of bed 45–65° to facilitate lung expansion and reduce work of breathing.
- In patient with bilateral lung disease, position with right lung down, since this lung is larger than the left and provides a greater area for ventilation-perfusion.
- Obtain and report clinical findings that indicate impaired gas exchange: cyanosis, RR ≥ 20 BPM, HR ≥ 100 bpm, crackles,

confusion, restlessness, irritability, and lethargy.

- Obtain and report $P(a/A)O_2 \leq 0.75$, $P(A-a)O_2 \geq 15$ mm Hg, and $PAO_2 \leq 100$ mm Hg, which can indicate worsening gas exchange.
- Should mechanical ventilation be necessary, assess ventilator function by verifying that the prescribed settings are being used and are effective. The settings include FIO_2 at the lowest rate to maintain $PaO_2 \geq 60$ mm Hg and 100% in acute situation to achieve adequate oxygenation; tidal volume 10 to 15 mL/kg; RR 10 to 14 BPM; and mode of ventilation.
- Move endotracheal tube (ET) tube to the other side of the mouth daily to prevent tissue necrosis.
- Monitor patient's tolerance of ventilatory support through the use of an individualized plan of care, which includes data from chest such as lung sounds, RR, chest expansion and ventilator settings; hemodynamic parameters including HR, blood pressure (BP), (T), cardiac output (CO), cardiac index (CI), pulmonary artery pressure (PAP), and PCWP; nutritional status, as type of feedings, intake, and output; and level of anxiety.
- Use chest physiotherapy to augment the removal of mucus.
- Assist patient to turn, cough, and deep breathe, q 2–4 h.
- Administer prescribed IV fluids to maintain adequate hydration or circulating volume.
- Administer low-flow oxygen, 2 L/min with humidification, to maintain PaO_2 and $PaCO_2$ within patient's normal range.
- Administer prescribed bronchodilators to facilitate gas exchange.
- Utilize prescribed incentive spirometry for patient not on mechanical ventilation, to provide lung inflation, which helps reduce the risk of atelectasis.
- Teach patient to perform breathing exercises such as pursed-lip breathing and diaphragmatic breathing.

Ineffective airway clearance related to retained secretions secondary to impaired cough effort or thick secretions.

Expected Patient Outcomes. Patient maintains effective airway clearance, as evidenced by productive cough; absence of crackles, rhonchi, or wheezes; absence of dyspnea, restlessness, or anxiety; RR 12 to 20 BPM; skin color normal; sputum culture negative; and arterial blood gases within normal range.

- Review results of chest roentgenogram and bronchoscopy.
- Place patient in the prone position to improve ventilation and oxygenation.
- Elevate head of bed to facilitate ventilation.
- Provide opportunities for rest to decrease oxygen requirements.
- Provide 1.5 to 3.0 L of decaffeinated fluids, if not contraindicated, to prevent thick mucus and to facilitate cough.
- Monitor clinical indicators of respirations status: airway patency; rate, rhythm, depth of breathing; chest and diaphragmatic excursion.
- Obtain and report clinical findings that indicate ineffective airway clearance: crackles, wheezes, dyspnea, tachypnea, restlessness, cyanosis, and anxiety.
- Encourage use of cascade (normal) cough by having patient take a deep breath, followed by three to four coughs until almost all of the air is out of the lung. Cascade coughing moves secretions from the periphery of the lungs to the central airways.
- Should cascade cough be ineffective, encourage patient to use huff cough to move secretions from the smaller airways into the main-stem bronchi or trachea.
- Encourage patient to use a voluntary inhalation of 3 to 10 seconds after coughing to reinflate collapsed alveoli, avoid mucus pool, avoid decreased oxygenation, and avoid increased risk of infection.
- Chest physiotherapy (CPT) such as postural drainage, chest percussion, chest vibration, and cough enhancement is used to im-

prove mucus and sputum clearance from the airways.

- Should coughing be ineffective in removing excess secretions and Pao_2 ≤60 mm Hg, assist with endotracheal intubation and ventilatory support.
- Use unit-prescribed method of endotracheal suctioning: preoxygenation, hyperinflation, hyperoxygenation, hyperventilation, maximal inflation, and oxygen insufflation.
- Use unit-prescribed suction devices that permit the patient to remain on the ventilator during suctioning; oxygen insufflation devices (OID) or closed tracheal suction system (CTSS).
- Use intratracheal instillation of 2 mL to 5 mL of normal saline during suctioning to enhance the removal of secretions by stimulating a cough.
- Monitor and evaluate patient's oxygen (arterial oxygen saturation [Sao_2], mixed venous oxygen saturation [Svo_2]) and hemodynamic status mean arterial pressure ([MAP], CO) before, during, and after suctioning.
- Apply CPT techniques to mobilize secretions: postural drainage, percussion and vibration, coughing and deep breathing exercises, and incentive spirometry.
- Administer IV fluids to maintain adequate hydration, thereby decreasing mucus viscosity and enhancing mucociliary effectiveness and cough.
- Provide prescribed incentive spirometry to reduce the risk of atelectasis.
- Should patient be unable to remove excessive secretions and suctioning be ineffective, prepare patient for bronchoscopy.
- Administer prescribed bronchodilators to decrease mucosal edema and smooth muscle contraction.
- Provide prescribed humidification of inhaled gas by mechanical ventilation to keep secretions thin so they can be removed by suctioning.
- Administer prescribed antibiotics to correct infection.

- Teach patient to ambulate to tolerance, being careful to avoid overtiring and to maintain planned rest periods.
- Teach patient to cough to clear pulmonary secretions.
- Instruct patient as to the importance of deep breathing and coughing.
- Instruct patient in the use of incentive spirometry.

Ineffective breathing pattern related to decreased maximum expiratory air flow secondary to air trapping or respiratory muscle weakness.

Expected Patient Outcomes. Patient maintains effective breathing pattern, as evidenced by RR ≤35 BPM, tidal volume ≥5 to 7 mL/kg, vital capacity ≥12 to 15 mL/kg, absence of crackles, absence of diaphoresis, coordination of contraction of inspiratory and expiratory muscles and symmetry of chest wall and diaphragmatic breathing, absence of shortness of breath or orthopnea, and arterial blood gases within normal range.

- Consult with physician about the criteria used to determine when ventilatory support is needed: oxygenation (Pao_2 ≤60 mm Hg on Fio_2 at 5%), ventilator ($Paco_2$ ≥50 to 60 mm Hg, which is ≥10 mm Hg above patient's normal $Paco_2$), and respiratory mechanics (apnea, sustained RR ≥35 BPM, and VC ≤10 to 15 mL/kg).
- Consult with dietitian about providing dyspneic patient with small, frequent feedings.
- Review results of arterial blood gas measurement, pulmonary function tests, and serum electrolyte studies.
- Limit activity to bed rest to minimize tachypnea, work of breathing, and subsequent respiratory muscle weakness or fatigue.
- Provide prescribed protein-caloric diet to maintain respiratory muscle function and avoid excess carbohydrates, which increase $Paco_2$ beyond patient's ability to eliminate it.

- Obtain and report clinical findings that ineffective breathing pattern: tachypnea, crackles, diaphoresis, dyscoordination of contraction of inspiratory and expiratory muscles, asymmetry of chest wall, diaphragmatic breathing, shortness of breath or orthopnea.
- Obtain and report clinical findings that indicate respiratory muscle weakness or fatigue: $Paco_2 \geq 45$ mm Hg; rapid shallow ventilation; and paradoxical abdominal wall motion.
- Encourage use of pursed-lip and diaphragmatic breathing, if not contraindicated, to improve the control of ventilation and prolong pulmonary emptying time, thereby preventing premature airway collapse and retraining the diaphragm.
- Evaluate the efficiency of deep breathing ability by monitoring VC and maximal inspiratory force (MIF).
- Monitor FEV_1 and the ratio of FEV_1 to FVC to determine the patient's ability to generate high air flow and pressure needed for effective coughing.
- Position patient to facilitate diaphragmatic descent and avoid use of accessory muscles of breathing.
- Monitor fluid balance, since fluid retention may occur due to overhydration by airway humidification and urinary output (UO) ≤ 30 mL/h.
- Monitor for VC ≤ 12 mL/kg, weight gain, intake greater than output, and decreased compliance.
- Administer prescribed IV fluid to maintain adequate hydration.
- Administer prescribed oxygen 2 to 4 L/min to maintain $Pao_2 \geq 60$ mm Hg and $Sao_2 \geq 95\%$.
- Administer bronchodilators to stimulate beta receptors in the bronchial smooth muscle to relax bronchial smooth muscle and block cholinergic constricting influences in bronchial muscle.
- Administer corticosteroids to augment the effects of beta-agonist bronchodilators.

- Teach patient to avoid hyperventilation, which can predispose to metabolic alkalosis.
- Instruct patient to deep breathe hourly to minimize atelectasis, mobilize secretions, and improve ventilation.

High risk for infection related to bacterial pneumonias secondary to retained secretions.

Expected Patient Outcomes. Patient experiences absence of infection, as evidenced by normothermia; negative sputum culture; WBC $\leq 11,000/\mu l$; absence of redness, swelling, tenderness, or drainage from catheter insertion site.

- Review results of sputum culture, WBC, and chest roentgenogram.
- Monitor temperature and sputum for changes in color, quantity, consistency, and odor.
- Monitor and report clinical findings that indicate infection: temperature $\geq 101°F$, and redness, swelling, tenderness, or drainage from catheter insertion site.
- Initiate the use of CPT and bronchial hygiene to improve ventilation and decrease pooling of secretions that can serve as a medium for infection.
- Use aseptic technique when suctioning or changing invasive lines.
- Initiate CPT to remove excess secretions.
- Administer IV fluids to maintain hydration.
- Administer antibiotic therapy to treat bacterial infections.
- Teach patient to cough up excess secretions.

Activity intolerance related to reduced pulmonary capacity, fatigue, or muscle weakness.

Expected Patient Outcomes. Patient is able to tolerate gradual increases in activity, RR ≤ 24 BPM, normal sinus rhythm, BP within patient's normal range, HR within 20 bpm of patient's resting HR, and absence of cyanosis.

- Consult with physician as to the desired cardiopulmonary response to increased physical activity.
- Consult with rehabilitation regarding the appropriate incremental activity program for the chronic obstructive pulmonary disease (COPD) patient.
- Place the patient in a semi-Fowler's or high Fowler's position to enhance gas exchange and to decrease work of breathing.
- Monitor and report clinical findings that indicate activity intolerance: HR ≥20 bpm of patient's resting HR, RR ≥24 BPM, fatigue, chest pain, or diaphoresis.
- Monitor continuous ECG to assess HR and rhythm. Document ECG strips every 2 to 4 hours in patients with dysrhythmias.
- Organize nursing care activities to ensure planned rest periods.
- Assist patient with active or passive range of motion (ROM).
- Administer prescribed oxygen at 2 to 4 L/min.
- Teach patient how to safely increase physical activity and report any unusual increase in dyspnea.

Anxiety related to the progressive loss of pulmonary function or need for ventilatory support.

Expected Patient Outcome. Patient is able to express concerns without becoming anxious.

- Listen to patient's and family's concerns regarding the illness and treatment.
- Explain the purposes behind noninvasive or invasive procedures.
- Support patient when experiencing an invasive procedure such as pulmonary artery catherization or mechanical ventilation.
- Provide a quiet, unstressful environment.
- Encourage verbalization of fears and anxieties.
- Encourage communication with significant others.
- Teach patient about the disease process and risk factors.

- Teach patient how to become involved in self-care.
- Teach patient how to reduce anxiety through progressive relaxation, meditation, or guided imagery.

Collaborative Problems

Common collaborate goals for patients with emphysema are to increase maximal expiratory outflow, improve oxygenation, maintain ventilation-perfusion balance, increase pulmonary muscle function, increase CO, and maintain acid-base balance.

Potential Complication: Decreased Maximal Expiratory Outflow. Decreased maximal expiratory outflow related to changes in lung volume secondary to large air spaces.

Expected Patient Outcomes. Patient maintains maximal expiratory outflow, as evidenced by RR 12 to 20 BPM, tidal volume ≥7mL/kg, VC ≥15mL/kg, TLC 6.0 L, FRC 3 L, RV 1.5 L, absence of cyanosis, absence of adventitious breath sounds, and arterial blood gases within normal limits.

- Consult with physician about pulmonary function tests used to evaluate maximal expiratory outflow: tidal volume, VC, TLC, FRC, and RV.
- Consult with respiratory therapist about the types of ventilatory support needed in relation to pulmonary function tests.
- Review results of arterial blood gas measurement, pulmonary function tests, and chest roentgenogram.
- Monitor and report pulmonary function tests that indicate decreased maximal expiratory outflow: tidal volume ≤7 mL/kg, VC ≤15 mL/kg, TLC ≤6.0 L, FRC ≤3 L, and RV ≤1.5 L.
- Evaluate the efficiency of deep breathing ability by monitoring VC and MIF.
- Monitor chest excursion for symmetry, degree of expansion, and use of accessory muscles.

- Encourage patient to deep breathe in an attempt to improve ventilation and TLC. TLC is increased as a result of a loss of elastic recoil, which reduces the force opposing that generated by the inspiratory musculature.
- CPT such as postural drainage, chest percussion, chest vibration, and cough enhancement is used to improve mucus and sputum clearance from the airways.
- Encourage patient to increase physical activity as tolerated to maintain pulmonary muscular function and minimize immobility-related general weakness.
- Monitor patient's respirations for rate, depth, and relationship to inspiration and expiration: FRC increases if expiration is prolonged and the RR is rapid, thereby decreasing the time during expiration for patient to achieve the normal resting end-expiratory point.
- Monitor RV, which is the volume of gas left within the lungs when the stiff chest wall can be compressed no further by the expiratory muscles: increased because of early airway closure during a maximal expiration.
- Administer prescribed IV fluids to maintain adequate hydration.
- Administer prescribed oxygen via mask or nasal cannula to keep oxygen 2 to 4 L/min and FIO_2 ≤50 % to maintain PaO_2 ≥60 mm Hg.
- Administer prescribed ventilatory support to assist with ventilation and maintain PaO_2 80 to 100 mm Hg.
- Teach patient deep-breathing exercises, since ventilatory support may cause atrophy of the respiratory musculature, making the weaning process difficult.

Potential Complication: Hypoxemia. Hypoxemia related to intrapulmonary shunting secondary to destruction and compression of the capillary bed.

Expected Patient Outcomes. Patient maintains adequate oxygen gas exchange, as evidenced by intrapulmonary physiological shunt within normal limits, PaO_2 100 mm Hg, $PaCO_2$ 40 mm Hg, oxygen consumption (resting) 250 mL/min, oxygen transport (resting) 1000 mL/min, and skin color normal.

- Consult with physician about the criteria used to determine when ventilatory support is needed: oxygenation (PaO_2 ≤60 mm Hg on FIO_2 at 50%), ventilator $PaCO_2$ ≥50 to 60 mm Hg, which is ≥10 mm Hg above patient's normal $PaCO_2$), and respiratory mechanics (apnea, sustained RR ≥35 BPM, and VC ≤10 to 15 mL/kg).
- Review results of arterial blood gas measurement, hemoglobin, hematocrit, and intrapulmonary physiological shunt ($\dot{Q}s/\dot{Q}t$) fraction.
- Position the good lung down to improve oxygenation, since ventilation: perfusion ($\dot{V}/\dot{Q}$) matching is improved.
- Provide nutritional support with enteral alimentation and supplemental parenteral feedings.
- Assess breath sounds and presence of adventitious breath sounds every 1 to 2 hours. Pulmonary congestion, documented as crackles and wheezes, can indicate increased hydrostatic force in the pulmonary vascular system, causing fluid to move across the alveolar-capillary membrane.
- Use unit-prescribed method of endotracheal suctioning: preoxygenation, hyperinflation, hyperoxygenation, hyperventilation, maximal inflation, and oxygen insufflation.
- Use unit-prescribed suction devices that permit the patient to remain on the ventilator during suctioning: OID or CTSS.
- Use intratracheal instillation of 2 mL to 5 mL of normal saline during suctioning to enhance the removal of secretions by stimulating a cough.
- Use chest physiotherapy, postural drainage, chest vibration, and cough enhancement to improve mucus and sputum clearance from the airways.

- Monitor and report patient's oxygen (SaO_2, $S\dot{v}O_2$) and hemodynamic status (MAP, CO) before, during, and after suctioning.
- Evaluate patient's readiness to be weaned from full or partial ventilatory support to spontaneous unassisted breathing by using the following objective weaning criteria: oxygenation ($PaO_2 \geq 60$ mm Hg on $FIO_2 \leq 40\%$ to 50% and PEEP ≤ 5 cm H_2O); ventilation ≤ 10 L/min, tidal volume ≥ 5 mL/kg, and $PaCO_2$ when usual range for patient); and respiratory mechanics (spontaneous RR ≤ 30 to 35 BPM, MIF ≤ -20 cm H_2O).
- Should mechanical ventilation and intubation not be necessary, pulse oximetry measurement of SaO_2 and incentive spirometry measurement can be used to provide indirect data about lung compliance and hypoxemia.
- Monitor and report changes in the major factors of oxygen transport: CO ≤ 4 L/min, hemoglobin (Hgb) ≤ 12 g/dL, $SaO_2 \leq 90\%$, and $PaO_2 \leq 80$ mm Hg.
- Encourage the use of cascade (normal) cough by having patient take a deep breath, followed by three to four coughs until almost all of the air is out of the lungs. Cascade coughing moves secretions from the periphery of the lungs to the central airways.
- Monitor $\dot{Q}s/\dot{Q}t$ fraction at FIO_2 at .50 to .60: Normal shunt fraction without a ventilator is 6% and with a ventilator is 10%.
- Suction patient using the principles of preoxygenation, short suctioning time, postsuctioning hyperinflation to reverse atelectasis, and uninterrupted PEEP.
- Administer oxygen using FIO_2 of 24% to 28% by Venturi mask or 2 to 3 L by nasal cannula to achieve a $PaO_2 \geq 60$ mm Hg or $SaO_2 \geq 95\%$.
- Administer bronchodilator therapy (aminophyllin) to improve air flow and ventilation by decreasing bronchospasm.
- Administer prescribed IV fluids, such as crystalloids, to maintain adequate intravascular volume and PCWP 10 to 12 mm Hg.

- Instruct patient to cough, turn, and deep breathe to enhance oxygen–carbon dioxide exchange.
- Administer corticosteroids in combination with bronchodilators (see Table 1–15, p. 129).

Potential Complication: Decreased Pulmonary Muscle Function. Decreased pulmonary muscle function related to muscular weakness secondary to ventilatory dependence or nutritional deficit.

Expected Patient Outcomes. Patient maintains effective pulmonary muscle function, FRC 2400 to 3000 mL, TLC 5500 mL, VC 4000 to 4800 mL, RV 1200 to 1500 mL, expiratory reserve volume (ERV) 1200 to 1500 mL, FVC 4800 mL, maximum voluntary ventilation (MVV) 170 L/min, RR 12 to 20 BPM, absence of crackles, absence of dyspnea, absence of fatigue, and maintenance of normal body weight.

- Consult with physician to validate expected patient outcomes used to evaluate changes in pulmonary muscle function.
- Review results of pulmonary function tests and arterial blood gas measurement.
- Place patient in a position of low to semi-Fowler's or unaffected side down in side-lying position to improve oxygenation.
- Provide nutritional support with enteral alimentation and supplemental parenteral feedings.
- Monitor clinical indicators of respiratory muscle function: Rate, rhythm, depth, pattern of breathing, symmetry of chest wall, and diaphragmatic excursion.
- Monitor and report clinical findings that indicate decreased pulmonary muscle function: FRC ≤ 2400 mL, TLC ≤ 5500 mL, VC ≤ 4000 mL, FVC ≤ 4800 mL, RV ≤ 1200 mL, ERV ≤ 1200 mL, and MVV ≤ 170 L/min.
- Use CPT, postural drainage, chest vibration, and cough enhancement to improve mucus and sputum clearance from the airways.

- Evaluate the efficiency of deep breathing ability by monitoring VC and MIF.
- Monitor FEV_1 and the ratio of FEV_1 to FVC to determine patient's ability to generate high air flow and pressure needed for effective coughing.
- Administer bronchiodilator therapy to improve air flow and ventilation.
- Instruct patient how to use breathing techniques: Pursed-lip breathing and diaphragmatic breathing.
- Teach patient to avoid lying in a flat position which limits diaphragmatic excursion.

Potential Complication: Decreased Cardiac Output. Decreased CO related to altered preload and afterload secondary to related to positive-pressure mechanical ventilation or pulmonary hypertension.

Expected Patient Outcomes. Patient maintains adequate right ventricular preload, as evidenced by CO 4 to 8L/min, central venous paper (CVP) 2 to 6 mm Hg, RR 12 to 20 BPM, HR ≤100 bpm, PAP 20 to 30 8 to 15 mmHg, PCWP 6 to 12 mm Hg, PVR 155 to 255 dynes/s/cm^{-5}, PVRI 200 to 450 dynes/s/cm^{-5}/m^2, BP within patient's normal range, MAP 70 to 100 mm Hg, absence of neck vein distention, absence of weakness and peripheral edema, absence of dysrhythmias, UO ≥30 mL/h or ≥0.5 mL/kg/h, and absence of chest pain.

- Consult with physician to validate expected patient outcomes used to evaluate changes in CO.
- Obtain and report hemodynamic parameters that indicate altered preload: CO ≤4 L/min, CI ≤2.7 L/min/m^2, CVP ≤2 mm Hg, PAP systolic ≤20 mm Hg or diastolic ≤8 mm Hg, and PCWP ≤6 mm Hg.
- Obtain and report other clinical findings that indicate altered preload: distended neck veins, tachypnea, fatigue, weakness, UO 30 mL/h, peripheral pulse ≤+2, and capillary refill ≥3 seconds.

- Obtain and report hemodynamic parameters that indicate altered afterload: CO ≤4 L/min, PAP systolic ≥30 mm Hg or diastolic ≥15 mm Hg, PCWP ≥12 mm Hg, PVR ≥250 dynes/s/cm^{-5}, and PVRI ≥450 dynes/s/cm^{-5}/m^2.
- Obtain and report other clinical findings that indicate altered afterload secondary to pulmonary hypertension: tachypnea, dyspnea, fatigue, chest pain, syncope on exertion, distended neck veins, and S_1 split.
- Monitor ECG continuously to assess HR and rhythm. Document ECG rhythm strips every 2 to 4 hours in patients with dysrhythmias.
- Monitor hydration status: daily weight, specific gravity, intake, and output.
- Monitor patient's hemodynamic response to mechanical ventilation with PEEP. PEEP can impede venous return, thereby decreasing preload and CO.
- Provide oxygenation: FIO_2 of 25% to 28% by Venturi mask or 2 to 3 L by nasal cannula to achieve a PAO_2 ≥60 mm Hg.
- Administer IV fluids to maintain blood volume and keep pulmonary secretions moist.
- Administer prescribed bronchodilator to maintain PAP systolic ≤30 mm Hg or diastolic ≤15 mm Hg and PCWP ≤12 mm Hg (see Table 3–6).
- Administer prescribed vasodilators, calcium channel blockers, or ACE inhibitors to maintain PVR ≤250 dynes/s/cm^{-5} and PVRI ≤450 dynes/s/cm^{-5}/m^2 (see Table 1–4, p. 20; Table 1–6, p. 28; and Table 1–12, p. 60).

Potential Complication: Respiratory Alkalosis. Respiratory acidosis related to alveolar hypoventilation secondary to ventilatory support.

Expected Patient Outcomes. Patient maintains adequate acid-base balance, as evidenced by RR 12 to 20 BPM, arterial blood gases within normal limits, BP within the patient's normal range, MAP 70 to 100 mm Hg, absence of dysrhythmias, tidal volume ≥5 to 7 mL/kg, VC ≥12 to 15 mL/kg, absence of adventitious breath sounds, absence of signs and symptoms associated with respiratory alkalosis.

- Consult with Respiratory Therapy regarding the patient's tidal volume and VC values.
- Review arterial blood gas and electrolyte values.
- Position patient to allow for best lung expansion, which may increase ventilation-perfusion matching.
- Monitor and report clinical findings associated with respiratory alkalosis: light-headedness, weakness, muscle cramps, twitching, paresthesia, seizure activity, tetany, or hyperactivity.
- Monitor clinical indicators of respiratory function: rate, rhythm, depth, pattern of breathing, symmetry of chest wall, and diaphragmatic excursion.
- Monitor ventilatory support in relation to patient's RR, tidal volume, and arterial blood gases to avoid respiratory alkalosis.
- Monitor patient's tolerance of ventilatory support through the use of an individualized plan of care, which includes data from chest such as lung sounds, RR, chest expansion, and ventilator settings; hemodynamic parameters including HR, BP, T, CO, CI, PAP, and PCWP; nutritional status, such as type of feedings, intake, and output; and level of anxiety.
- Evaluate patient's readiness to be weaned from full or partial ventilatory support to spontaneous unassisted breathing by using the following objective weaning criteria: oxygenation ($Pao_2 \geq 60$ mm Hg on Fio_2 $\leq 40\%$ to 50% and PEEP ≤ 5 cm H_2O); ventilation (minute ventilation ≤ 10 L/min, tidal volume ≥ 5 mL/kg, and $Paco_2$ when usual range for patient); and respiratory mechanics (spontaneous RR ≤ 30 to 35 BPM, maximal inspiratory force ≤ -20 cm H_2O).
- Monitor ECG continuously to assess HR and rhythm. Document ECG rhythm every 2 to 4 hours in patients with dysrhythmias.
- Administer prescribed oxygen, Fio_2 at $\leq 50\%$ to maintain $Pao_2 \geq 60$ mm Hg.

- Instruct patient to control respirations through meditation, progressive relaxation, or guided imagery.
- Teach patient to avoid hyperventilation, which leads to respiratory alkalosis.

DISCHARGE PLANNING

The critical care nurse will provide patient and significant other(s) with verbal or written discharge notes regarding the following subjects:

1. The signs and symptoms that warrent medical attention: RR ≥ 30 BPM, HR ≥ 100 bpm, fatigue, dyspnea, dizziness, palpitation, diaphoresis, shortness of breath, or pain.
2. Need to cease any activity that increases HR and BP or causes fatigue because these behaviors can increase tissue oxygen demand.
3. The names of community agencies that can provide support should the patient require a portable oxygen unit (American Lung Association).
4. A written list of side effects associated with patient's specific medications.
5. Importance of maintaining the prescribed activity program.

■ ASTHMA

For related information see Cardiac Durations, Part I: Dysrhythmias, p. 184; Cardiac Part III: Hemodynamic monitoring, p. 219. Part I: Pneumonia, p. 375; Respiratory acidosis, p. 412; Respiratory alkalosis, p. 415. Part III: Pulse oximetry, p. 426; Mechanical ventilation, p. 428; Capnography, p. 439; Transcutaneous Pao_2 and $Paco_2$, p. 441; Indirect calorimetry, p. 441.

Case Management Basis

DRG: 96 Bronchitis and asthma age ≥ 17 with complications

LOS: 5.90 days

DRG: 97 Bronchitis and asthma age ≥17 without complications
LOS: 4.60 days

Definition

Asthma is a recurrent, reversible airway obstruction with prolonged expiratory length, air trapping during attacks, ventilation-perfusion mismatching, increased intrapulmonary shunting, cough, and tenacious sputum. Asthma is characterized by increased responsiveness of the trachea and bronchi to various stimuli, leading to widespread narrowing of the airways. Asthma causes recurrent attacks of dyspnea with wheezing as a result of spasmodic constriction of the bronchi.

Pathophysiology

In general, the pathological changes in asthma include bronchospasm, airway edema, and hypersecretion of mucus. The bronchoconstriction of the central and peripheral airways leads to edema, cellular infiltration, and hypersecretion. There is hypertrophy of the smooth muscle layer, thickening of the epithelial basement membrane, and infiltration of esosinophils within the bronchial wall.

During an asthma attack, chemical mediators in an IgE mast cell interaction are released. The chemical mediators cause constriction of the bronchial smooth muscle, increased bronchial secretion from the globlet cells, and mucosal swelling. These factors lead to narrowing of the airways. An allergen causes production of histamine and other chemicals by the lung. The acute respiratory obstruction and resistance to air flow are caused by bronchospasm, production of large amounts of thick mucus, inflammatory response, increased capillary permeability, and mucosal edema.

Nursing Assessment

PRIMARY CAUSES

- Allergies, infection, exercise, emotions, nasal polyps, and occupational irritants.

RISK FACTORS

- Genetic predisposition, such as the specific inheritable trait of a tendency of form IgE antibodies. Allergies, such as dust, molds; inhaled irritants, such as cigarette smoke or environmental dust; emotional factors; and exercise.

PHYSICAL ASSESSMENT

- Inspection: Tachypnea ≥18 to 50 BPM, dyspnea, use of accessory muscles, stridor, agitation, restlessness, productive cough, pulsus parodoxus, sternocleidomastoid retraction, diaphoresis, inability to speak, and fatigue.
- Palpation: Subcutaneous emphysema.
- Percussion: Hyperinflation of the lungs or hyperresonance.
- Auscultation: Wheezing (inspiration indicates constriction in larger proximal airway; expiration indicates constriction in smaller airways), tachycardia ≥130 bpm, prolongation of expiration, diminished breath sounds, and distant heart sounds.

DIAGNOSTIC TEST RESULTS

Standard Laboratory Tests (see Table 3–1)

- Arterial blood gases: Arterial partial pressure of oxygen (Pao_2) ≤60 mm Hg and partial pressure of arterial carbon dioxide ($Paco_2$) ≥40 mm Hg.
- Blood studies: white blood cells (WBC) 6.1 to 28.0 × 10/μL, hematocrit increased, esinophils ≥350/μL, sputum shows WBCs, and elevated serum immunoglobulin E (IgE).
- Skin testing: Test for allergens that trigger attacks; IgE increased in extrinsic asthma.
- Sputum: Reveals increased viscosity, mucus plugs, or microorganisms if infection is the causative event.
- Theophylline level: Acceptable range is 10 to 20 μg/mL.

Respiratory Function Tests. (see Table 3–2)

- Pulmonary function test: Decreased forced expiratory volume in 1, 2, and 3 seconds

(FEV$_{1-3}$), maximal mid-expiratory flow rate (MMF), peak expiratory flow rate (PEFR), and vital capacity (VC). Increased residual volume (RV), functional residual capacity (FRC), and total lung capacity (TLC).

Noninvasive Respiratory Diagnostic Procedures.
(see Table 3–4)

- Chest roentgenogram: Infiltrates can suggest a respiratory infection; atelectasis or collapse of a segment or lobe can indicate mucous plugging of a bronchus; and the presence of a pneumothorax or pneumomediastinum. Also can show hyperinflation during an asthmatic episode, identified by a low diaphragm. The heart may be long and narrow and the peripheral vessels poorly visualized.

ECG
- Right axis deviation, right bundle branch block, P in II≥III or I, or ST-T changes of ischemia.

MEDICAL AND SURGICAL MANAGEMENT

PHARMACOLOGY
- Sympathomimetics: These drugs, known as beta-adrenergics, have a direct bronchodilating effect in the airways and inhibit mast cell release of the mediators that can cause bronchonconstriction. Examples of sympathomimetics include epinephrine, isoproterenol, isoetharine, metaproterenol, terbutaline, albuterol, and bitolterol. They are administered by metered dose inhalers (MDI), jet nebulizers, and intermittent positive-pressure breathing (IPPB) (see Table 3–6).
- Xanthines: Theophylline and aminophylline are used to inhibit phosphodiesterase activity, thereby preventing breakdown of cyclic adenosine monophosphate (cAMP) and favoring bronchial relaxation. The desired therapeutic level of theophylline is 10 to 20 μg/ml. Amino-

phylline can be administered IV with a loading dose of 5 to 6 mg/kg, followed by 0.3 to 0.9 mg/kg via slow IV drip (see Table 3–6).
- Disodium cromoglycate (cromolyn sodium): This is used to block the release of chemical mediators of bronchospasm from the bronchial mucosa. It is administered as a propelled powder from a hand-held inhaler (Table 3–7).
- Corticosteroids: Can be used to potentiate the effect of bronchodilators and reduce inflammation. Prednisone and prednisolone can be administered 40 to 70 mg/d for 5 to 7 days, then titrated down to a maintenance dose of 5 to 20 mg/d. Intravenous hydrocortisone (Solu-Cortef) can be infused 250 to 500 mg initially, followed by 100 to 250 mg every 3 hours (see Table 1–15, p. 129).

MECHANICAL VENTILATION
- Endotracheal intubation and mechanical ventilation may be needed to relieve hypoxemia with resultant stabilization of the cardiovascular and central nervous system (see Mechanical ventilation, p. 428).

OXYGEN THERAPY
- High levels of supplemental oxygen may be necessary initially, with fraction inspired oxygen (F$_{IO_2}$) levels lowered following the asthmatic crises.

NURSING MANAGEMENT: NURSING DIAGNOSES AND COLLABORATIVE PROBLEMS

NURSING DIAGNOSES
Common nursing goals for patients with asthma are to promote effective airway clearance, maintain effective breathing pattern, facilitate acceptance, support activity tolerance, and minimize anxiety.

Ineffective airway clearance related to mucosal edema, excessive mucus production, and bronchospasm secondary to chemical mediators.

TABLE 3-7

TABLE 3–7. ANTIHISTAMINES

Medication	Route/Dose	Uses/Effects	Side Effects
Antiasthmatic (Mast Cell Stabilizer)			
Cromolyn sodium (Disodium Cromoglycate)	Inhalation: 20 mg qid Nasal: 1 spray (5.2 mg) each nostril 3–4 times daily up to 6 times/d	Treatment of bronchial asthma, or allergic rhinitis	Headache, rash, nasal irritation, sneezing, cough, irritation of throat, itchy and puffy eyes, rash, nausea, vomiting
Mucolytic			
Acetylcysteine (Airbron Mucosol)	Inhalation: 1–10 ml of 20% solution q 4–6 h or 2–20 mg of 10% solution q 4–6 h Direct instillation: 1–2 mL of 10%–20% solution q 1–4 h	Adjunctive therapy in patients with abnormal, viscid mucous secretions and atelectasis	Dizziness, drowsiness, nausea, vomiting, fever, chills, or urticaria
Iodinated Glycerol (Iophen Organidin)	60 mg qid	Adjunctive therapy in bronchial asthma, bronchitis, emphysema, and other respiratory disorders	Nausea, GI irritation, rash, headache, inflammation of salivary glands, skin eruptions, swelling of the eyelids, or parotitis
Sympathomimetic			
Epinephrine (Bronkaid Mist)	SC: 0.1–0.5 mL of 1:1000 q 20 min for 4 h Inhalation: 1 inhalation q 4 h prn	Treatment of acute asthma attack, mucosal congestion, hypersensitivity, and anaphylactic reactions	Dryness of nasal mucosa, rebound congestion, allergy, coroneal edema, nervousness, restlessness, fear, anxiety, severe headache, nausea, vomiting, pallor, dyspnea, tachyarrhythmias, or precordial pain

From Fischblach F, 1984; Ford R, 1987; Deglin JH, Vallerand AH, 1991; Thelan LA, Davie JK, Urden LD, 1990; Loeb S, 1993.

GI, gastrointestinal; SC, subcutaneous.

Expected Patient Outcomes. Patient maintains effective airway clearance, as evidenced by respiratory rate (RR) ≤30 BPM, absence of excessive cough, absence of abnormal or adventitious breath sounds, absence of cyanosis, or absence of fatigue.

- Review results of arterial blood gas measurement, chest roentgenogram, sputum, and pulmonary function tests.
- Elevate head of bed 60 to 90 degrees, support back with pillow and pad over bedtable so patient can lean forward.

- Monitor clinical indicators of respiratory status: rate, depth, regularity, chest expansion, skin color, use of excessory muscles, and respiratory effort.
- Obtain and report clinical findings associated with ineffective airway clearance: crackles, heart rate (HR) ≥100 bpm, RR ≥30 BPM, fatigue, cyanosis, diaphoresis, use of accessory muscles, intercostal and sternal retraction, prolonged expiratory wheeze, and nonproductive cough.
- Monitor ECG continuously to assess HR and rhythm. Document ECG rhythm strips

every 2 to 4 hours in patients with dysrhythmias.

- Evaluate the efficiency of deep-breathing ability by monitoring VC and maximal inspiratory force (MIF).
- Monitor FEV_1 and the ratio of FEV_1 to forced vital capacity (FVC) to determine the patient's ability to generate high air flow and pressure needed for effective coughing.
- Chest physiotherapy (CPT) such as postural drainage, chest percussion, chest vibration, and cough enhancement is used to improve mucus and sputum clearance from the airways.
- Encourage the use of cascade (normal) cough by having patient take a deep breath, followed by three or four coughs until almost all the air is out of the lungs. Cascade coughing moves secretions from the periphery of the lungs to the central airways.
- Encourage patient to use a voluntary inhalation of 3 to 10 seconds after coughing to reinflate collapsed alveoli, avoid mucus pool, avoid decreased oxygenation, and avoid increased risk of infection.
- Evaluate sputum for color, tenacity, and amount.
- Administer prescribed IV fluids to maintain adequate hydration.
- Administer oxygen by Venturi mask or nasal cannula.
- Administer prescribed bronchodilators such as epinephrine, terbutaline, or theophylline to dilate smooth vessels of airways (see Table 3–6).
- Administer corticosteroids to decrease the inflammatory response, stabilize membranes, decrease release of spasmogens, inhibit histamine release; inhibit chemotaxis; and inhibit type III immunologic actions (see Table 1–15, p. 129).

Ineffective breathing pattern related to overinflation from premature airway closure on expiration, fatigue, or anxiety.

Expected Patient Outcomes. Patient maintains effective breathing pattern, as evidenced by

arterial blood gases within normal range, absence of bronchial or adventitious breath sounds, RR $\leq$30 BPM, absence of cyanosis, HR $\leq$100 bpm, or productive cough.

- Consult with physician about the criteria used to determine when ventilatory support is needed: oxygenation ($Pao_2 \leq$60 mm Hg on Fio_2 at 50%), ventilator ($Paco_2 \geq$50 to 60 mm Hg, which is $\geq$10 mm Hg above patient's normal $Paco_2$), and respiratory mechanics (apnea, sustained RR $\geq$35 BPM, and VC $\leq$10 to 15 mL/kg).
- Review results of complete blood count (CBC), chest roentgenogram, or arterial blood gas measurements.
- Monitor clinical indicators of respiratory status: rate, depth, chest expansion, skin color, and presence of adventitious breath sounds.
- Evaluate clinical indicators for endotracheal intubation: increased $Paco_2$ not decreasing with optimal therapy; hypercarbia; hypoxemia causing altered level of consciousness; severe hypoxia unresponsive to supplemental oxygen; or cardiopulmonary arrest.
- Assess ventilator function by verifying that the prescribed settings are being used and are effective. The settings include Fio_2 at the lowest rate to maintain $Pao_2 \geq$60 mm Hg and 100% in acute situations to achieve adequate oxygenation; tidal volume 10 to 15 mL/kg; RR 10 to 14 BPM; and mode of ventilation.
- Evaluate patient's readiness to be weaned from full or partial ventilatory support to spontaneous unassisted breathing by using the following objective weaning criteria: oxygenation ($Pao_2 \geq$ 60 mm Hg on Fio_2 $\leq$40% to 50% and PEEP $\leq$5 cm H_2O); ventilation (minute ventilation $\leq$10 L/min, tidal volume $\geq$5 mL/kg, and $Paco_2$ within usual range for patient); and respiratory mechanics (spontaneous RR $\leq$30 to 35 BPM, MIF $\leq$ -20 cm H_2O).
- Monitor patient's tolerance of ventilatory support through the use of an individualized

plan of care, which includes data from chest such as lung sounds, RR, chest expansion, and ventilator settings; hemodynamic parameters including HR, blood pressure (BP), (T), cardiac output (CO), cardiac index (CI), pulmonary artery disease (PAP), and pulmonary capillary wedge pressure (PCWP); nutritional status as type of feedings, intake and output; and, level of anxiety.

- Monitor intake and urinary output (UO) ≥30mL/h.
- Encourage patient to breathe deeply and expectorate secretions.
- Provide CPT: postural drainage with percussion and vibration, deep breathing and coughing, and facilitation of removal of tracheobronchial secretion.
- Administer IV fluids at the prescribed amount to maintain hydration.
- Administer prescribed oxygen 2 to 4 L/min by nasal cannula or mask to improve oxygenation.
- Administer prescribed sympathomimetic bronchodilators to dilate smooth muscles of airways (see Table 3–6).

Denial related to the risk factors associated with asthmatic episode.

Expected Patient Outcomes. Patient complies and verbalizes acceptance of prescribed therapy.

- Instill a sense of hope by maintaining a positive attitude.
- Provide opportunity to perform activities such as administering medications and identifying clinical mediators to be avoided.
- Reinforce complaint behaviors indicating acceptance of asthma and its treatments.
- Encourage patient to verbalize concerns regarding risk factors causing asthmatic episode and its treatment.
- Teach patient the relationship between risk factors and asthmatic episode.

Activity intolerance related to reduced pulmonary capacity, fatigue, or muscle weakness.

Expected Patient Outcomes. Patient is able to tolerate gradual increases in activity, RR ≤24 BPM, normal sinus rhythm, BP within patient's normal range, HR within 20 bpm of patient's resting HR, and absence of cyanosis.

- Consult with physician as to the desired cardiopulmonary response to increased physical activity.
- Consult with Rehabilitation regarding the appropriate incremental activity program for the chronic obstructive pulmonary disease (COPD) patient.
- Place the patient in a semi-Fowler's or high Fowler's position to enhance gas exchange and to decrease work of breathing.
- Monitor and report clinical findings that indicate activity intolerance: HR ≥20 bpm of patient's resting HR, RR ≥24 BPM, fatigue, chest pain, or diaphoresis.
- Encourage patient to remain calm, which will decrease oxygen demand.
- Schedule rest time after meal to avoid increase oxygen demand.
- Assist patient with active or passive range of motion (ROM).
- Administer prescribed oxygen at 2 to 4 L/min.
- Teach patient how to safely increase physical activity and report any unusual increase in dyspnea.

Anxiety related to difficulty or breathing and fear of recurrent asthmatic episode.

Expected Patient Outcome. Patient is able to verbalize feelings of anxiety about asthmatic episodes.

- Place patient in semi-Fowler's position to facilitate ventilation.
- Support patient during the asthmatic episode with reassurance.
- Encourage patient to use diaphragmatic and pursed-lip breathing.
- Provide emotional support by remaining with patient when anxious, providing quiet reassurance, and anticipate patient's needs.

- Remain with patient during coughing episode.
- Perform active or passive ROM exercises q 4 hours if patient on bed rest.
- Teach patient to decrease anxiety through progressive relaxation, meditation, or guided imagery.

Collaborative Problems

Common collaborative goals for patients with asthma are to increase oxygenation and maintain ventilation-perfusion balance.

Potential Complication: Hypoxemia. Hypoxemia related to decreased alveolar ventilation secondary to narrowed airways.

Expected Patient Outcomes. Patient maintains adequate oxygen gas exchange, as evidenced by intrapulmonary physiological shunt within normal limits, Pao_2 100 mm Hg, $Paco_2$ 40 mm Hg, oxygen consumption (resting) 250 mL/min, oxygen transport (resting) 1000 mL/min, and skin color normal.

- Consult with physician about the criteria used to determine when ventilatory support is needed: oxygenation (Pao_2 ≤60 mm Hg on Fio_2 at 50%), ventilator ($Paco_2$ ≥50 to 60 mm Hg, which is ≥10 mm Hg above patient's normal $Paco_2$), and respiratory mechanics (apnea, sustained RR ≥35 BPM, and VC ≤10 to 15 mL/kg).
- Confer with physician regarding patient's desired lung volumes during bronchodilator therapy.
- Review results of pulmonary function tests, chest roentgenogram, and arterial blood gas measurement.
- Place patient in high Fowler's position with the patient leaning forward with elbows propped on the bedside table.
- Monitor FEV, in relation to the presence of pulsus paradoxus: FEV_1 ≤25% of predicted (≤1.0 L) is accompanied by pulsus paradoxus.
- Monitor asthma index score: pulse rate ≥120 bpm, RR ≥30 BPM, pulsus para-

doxus ≥18 mm Hg, PEFR ≤120 L/min, moderate to severe dyspnea, the use of accessory muscles, and wheezing.
- Monitor arterial blood gases: Pco_2 may initially be low; a normal $Paco_2$ may indicate impending respiratory muscle fatigue.
- Monitor ventilation ($\dot{V}$)/perfusion ($\dot{Q}$): Increasing $\dot{V}/\dot{Q}$ is the common early finding with low Pco_2; decreasing $\dot{V}/\dot{Q}$ is late with normal or increased $Paco_2$.
- Administer oxygen via Venturi mask or nasal cannula: Initially there is a fall in Pao_2 with the initiation of oxygen therapy because of a change in $\dot{V}/\dot{Q}$ matching; and sympathomimetics and aminophylline cause increased perfusion of poorly ventilated areas, thereby producing a decrease in Pao_2.
- Provide mechanical ventilation with humidification to asthmatic patient who shows signs of respiratory failure: tachycardia ≥130 bpm, sternocleidomastoid retractions, diaphoresis, inability to speak, central cyanosis, hypercarbia, PEFR ≤130 L/min, and FEV_1 ≤0.6 L.
- Administer sympathomimetic inhalant: isoproterenol 0.1 mg/puff; isoetharine 0.5 mL of a 1% solution diluted in normal saline; metaproterenol in nebulizer 0.2 to 0.3 mL of a 5% solution (see Table 3–6).
- Administer cromolyn sodium to act on the surface of mast cells to block the release of chemical mediators (see Table 3–7).
- Instruct patient to breathe slowly and deeply to increase lung expansion.

Potential Complication: Ventilation-Perfusion Imbalance. Ventilation-perfusion imbalance related to unequal ventilation secondary to airway narrowing, increased secretions, and edema.

Expected Patient Outcomes. Patient maintains adequate ventilation-perfusion balance, as evidenced by ventilation: perfusion ($\dot{V}/\dot{Q}$) ratio 1.0, saturation of arterial oxygen (Sao_2) 97%, mixed venous oxygen saturation ($S\bar{v}o_2$ 75%, alveolar-arterial oxygen gradient ($P[A-a]o_2$) ≤15 mm Hg on room air or 10 to 65 mm Hg on 100% O_2, arterial-alveolar oxygen tension ratio (P[a/A]O_2 0.75 to 0.90, static compliance (Cst) $\geq$ 50 mL/cm H_2O, dynamic compliance (Cdyn) $\geq$ 45 mL/cm H_2O, RR 12 to 20 BPM, absence of adventitious breath sounds, absence of cyanosis, absence of dyspnea, CO 4 to 8 L/min, CI 2.7 to 4.3 L/min/m^2, PCWP 4 to 12 mm Hg, mean arterial pressure (MAP) 70 to 100 mm Hg, BP within patient's normal range, arterial blood gases within normal range, and HR $\leq$ 100 bpm.

- Consult with physician to validate expected patient outcomes used to evaluate ventilation-perfusion balance.
- Confer with Respiratory Therapy regarding the appropriate ventilatory support for the asthma patient.
- Review of results arterial blood gas measurements, static lung compliance, dynamic lung compliance, physiological shunting, alveolar-arterial oxygen gradient, arterial-alveolar oxygen tension ratio, or ventilation-perfusion scan.
- Limit physical activity to bed rest to decrease the work of breathing.
- Obtain and report other clinical findings associated with decreased $\dot{V}$:$\dot{Q}$ ratio: tachypnea, cyanosis, crackles, dyspnea, and tachycardia.
- Monitor $\dot{V}$:$\dot{Q}$ ratio and report value $\leq$ 1.0, which signifies reduced alveolar ventilation. A low $\dot{V}/\dot{Q}$ ratio is referred to an intrapulmonary shunt (blood flow [$\dot{Q}s$] total flow [$\dot{Q}t$] $\geq$ 15% to 30%.
- Obtain the following information in order to measure $\dot{Q}s/\dot{Q}t$: hemoglobin level, FIO_2 level, arterial and mixed venous blood gas results, and arterial and mixed venous oxyhemoglobin (oxygen saturation) values.
- Monitor alveolar partial pressure of oxygen (PAO_2) and arterial pressure of oxygen (PaO_2), which are approximately equal. Report a diversion of PAO_2 from $PaCO_2$, which signifies the development of an intrapulmonary shunt.
- Estimate $\dot{Q}s/\dot{Q}t$ using the following methods: PaO_2/FIO_2 ratio $\geq$ 286, arterial/alveolar (a/A) ratio $\geq$ 0.60, alveolar-arterial (A$-$a) gradient $\leq$ 20 mm Hg with an FIO_2 of .21%, respiratory index $\leq$ 1, and shunt equation $\leq$ 5%.

- Monitor and report PAO_2/FIO_2 $\leq$ 200, which is considered to be a large intrapulmonary shunt (20%). The lower the value, the more severe the $\dot{Q}s/\dot{Q}t$ disturbance.
- Obtain and report SaO_2 $\leq$ 90%, which can signify intrapulmonary shunting.
- Measure intake, output, specific gravity, and daily weight. Excessive fluid accumulation increases total lung water, contributing to an increase in ventilation/perfusion imbalance.
- Monitor skin color for the presence of cyanosis, which can reflect the desaturation of at least 5 grams of hemoglobin and ventilation-perfusion mismatch.
- Evaluate the adequacy of oxygenation: oxygen delivery $\geq$ 600 mL/min/m$_2$, CI $\geq$ 2.7 L/min/m^2, and oxygen consumption (VO_2) $\geq$ 156 mL/min/m^2.
- Administer prescribed humidified oxygen to keep PaO_2 $\geq$ 60 mm Hg.
- Administer IV fluids at the prescribed flow rate to maintain adequate hydration and to avoid excess fluid accumulation, which increases lung water, causing increased $\dot{V}/\dot{Q}$ mismatch.

DISCHARGE PLANNING

The critical care nurse will provide patient and significant other(s) with verbal or written discharge notes regarding the following subjects:

1. Importance of preventing future attacks by avoiding chemical mediators, avoiding stressful situations, avoiding smoking, and providing adequate humidity.
2. Importance of breathing exercises and exercising to tolerance without becoming fatigued.
3. Importance of maintaining appropriate diet and fluids 2000 to 3000 mL/d unless contraindicated and avoiding gaining weight.

4. Importance of taking prescribed medications.

5. Signs and symptoms that require medical attention: respiratory distress, diaphoresis, cyanosis, tachycardia, shortness of breath, and RR 30 BPM.

6. Importance of keeping ongoing outpatient appointments.

7. A written list of purpose, dosage, schedule, and side effects associated with patient's specific medication.

■ CHRONIC BRONCHITIS

For related information see Cardiac Durations, Part I: Dysrhythmias, p. 184; Part III: Hemodynamic monitoring, p. 219. Part I: Pneumonia, p. 375; Respiratory acidosis, p. 412; Respiratory alkalosis, p. 415. Part III: Pulse oximetry, p. 426; Mechanical ventilation, p. 428; Capnography, p. 439; Transcutaneous Pao_2 and $Paco_2$, p. 441; Indirect calorimetry, p. 441.)

Case Management Basis
DRG: 96 Bronchitis & asthma age ≥17 with complications
LOS: 5.90 days
DRG: 97 Bronchitis & asthma age ≥17 without complications
LOS: 4.40 days

Definition
Bronchitis is a common condition caused by infection and inhalants, which results in inflammation of the mucosal lining to the tracheobronchial tree. Bronchitis causes cough and production of large amounts of purulent mucus.

Pathophysiology
With chronic bronchitis there is increased production of mucus resulting from the enlargement of the bronchial mucus glands and an increase in the number of goblet cells. Additional changes include inflammation of the bronchial and bronchiolar walls, loss of cilia, and the presence of mucus plugs. In chronic bronchitis, the degree of tapering is nonuniform, and airway wall surface and outpouchings are irregular. The changes account for the increased airway resistance that results in inspiratory and expiratory air-flow obstruction, overinflation of the alveoli, and abnormal distribution of ventilation. The expiratory air flow is decreased as a result of increased airway resistance.

Nursing Assessment

PRIMARY CAUSES
• Air pollutants, industrial irritants, or bacterial infections.

RISK FACTORS
• Cigarette smoking

PHYSICAL ASSESSMENT
• Inspection: Cough, purulent sputum, cyanosis, edema, dyspnea, jugular venous distention, diaphoresis, or headache.
• Palpation: Peripheral edema and hepatomegaly.
• Auscultation: Wheezing, coarse rales, loud S_2 in the pulmonic area or S_3 and S_4, or tachycardia.

DIAGNOSTIC TEST RESULTS

Standard Laboratory Tests (see Table 1–9, p. 40)

• Arterial blood gases: partial pressure of arterial oxygen (Pao_2) ≤60 mm Hg and partial pressure of arterial carbon dioxide ($Paco_2$) ≥45 mm Hg.
• Blood studies: Hematocrit elevated (polycythemia).
• Sputum cultures: Variable number of leukocytes and a mixed flora of organisms.

Noninvasive Respiratory Diagnostic Procedures (see Tables 3–2, 3–4)

• Chest roentgenogram: Normal if chronic bronchitis alone; progressive disease shows pulmonary hypertension or cor pulmonale and increased peribronchial markings at both bases.

- Pulmonary function tests: Increased total lung capacity (TLC), functional residual capacity (FRC), and residual volume (RV). Reduced vital capacity (VC) and flow rate, with indications of moderate increase in airway resistance.

ECG

- When hypoxemia and air-flow obstruction occur, ECG shows P waves smaller in lead I but larger in lead II, III, and avF; shift of the P wave axis to the right; reduced voltage as a result of the hyperinflation; signs of right ventricular hypertrophy; and atrial or ventricular dysrhythmias.

MEDICAL AND SURGICAL MANAGEMENT

Pharmacology

- Bronchodilators: Metaproterenol and albuterol are selective beta$_2$ agents and are useful in managing patients with bronchospasm who also have hypoxemia and tachycardia.
- Antibiotics: Antibiotics, such as ampicillin, are given as a prophylaxis against infections.

NURSING MANAGEMENT: NURSING DIAGNOSES AND COLLABORATIVE PROBLEMS

Nursing Diagnoses

Common nursing goals for patients with chronic bronchitis are to maintain airway clearance, promote effective breathing pattern, improve oxygenation, reduce fatigue, and provide knowledge.

Ineffective airway clearance related to increased airway resistance or retained tenacious secretions secondary to inflammation.

Expected Patient Outcomes. Patient maintains effective airway clearance, as evidenced by RR ≤30 BPM, able to remove own secretions, absence of adventitious breath sounds, residual volume 1.5 L, negative sputum cul-

ture, no fever, and arterial blood gases within normal range.

- Review results of sputum culture and arterial blood gas measurement.
- Place patient in a semi- to high Fowler's position to improve ventilation.
- Obtain and report clinical findings that indicate ineffective airway clearance: elevated temperature, chills, nonproductive cough, mucopurulent sputum, crackles, wheezing respirations, and dyspnea.
- Monitor temperature: Patient febrile for 2 to 3 days may require antibiotic therapy.
- Chest physiotherapy (CPT) such as postural drainage, chest percussion, chest vibration, and cough enhancement is used to improve mucus and sputum clearance from the airways.
- Encourage the use of cascade (normal) cough by having patient take a deep breath, followed by three to four coughs until almost all of the air is out of the lungs. Cascade coughing moves secretions from the periphery of the lungs to the central airways.
- Encourage patient to use a voluntary inhalation of 3 to 10 seconds after coughing to reinflate collapsed alveoli, avoid mucus pool, avoid decreased oxygenation, and avoid increased risk of infection.
- Assist patient to turn, cough, and deep breathe every 2 h.
- Provide prescribed humidified air to loosen tenacious secretions.
- Encourage incentive breathing via incentive spirometry.
- Administer IV fluids to maintain hydration and mobilize secretions.
- Administer oxygen at the prescribed amount via Venturi mask or nasal cannula.
- Administer prescribed bronchodilators to relieve bronchospasm and facilitate mucociliary clearance: beta-adrenergic agonists or methylxanthines.
- Administer adrenocortical hormones to relieve persistant airway obstruction: oral prednisone or inhaled beclomethasone dipropionate.

- Administer mucolytic agents in conjunction with bronchodilator therapy to decrease viscosity of pulmonary secretions.
- Administer prescribed antibiotics to treat infection caused by retained secretions.
- Instruct patient as to the purpose behind CPT.

Ineffective breathing pattern related to reduced maximal expiratory outflow.

Expected Patient Outcomes. Patient maintains effective breathing pattern, as evidenced by respiratory rate (RR) 12 to 20 BPM, TLC 6.0 L, FRC 3 L, RV 1.5 L, arterial blood gases within normal range, absence of diaphoresis, absence of dyspnea, and absence of cyanosis.

- Review results of arterial blood gas measurement, chest roentgenogram and lung volumes.
- Place patient in high Fowler's position to maximize chest expansion.
- Obtain and report clinical findings that indicate ineffective breathing pattern: dyspnea, heart rate (HR) ≥24 bpm, diaphoresis, and use of accessory muscles.
- Evaluate the efficiency of deep-breathing ability by monitoring VC and maximal inspiratory force (MIF).
- Monitor chest excursion for symmetry, degree of expansion, and use of accessory muscles.
- Monitor RV in relation to the administration of bronchodilators: RV is increased in bronchitis as a result of the air trapping that occurs during expiration, when small airways are narrowed or occluded.
- Encourage deep breathing by using incentive spirometry.
- Administer prescribed oxygen 2 to 4 L/min to facilitate oxygenation.
- Administer prescribed IV fluids to maintain adequate hydration.
- Administer the prescribed bronchodilators to reduce bronchospasm (see Table 3–6).
- Instruct patient how to use the incentive spirometer.

Fatigue related to chronic cough.

Expected Patient Outcome. Patient is able to ambulate and maintain activities of daily living (ADL) without feeling fatigued.

- Consult with Rehabilitation therapist about an activity program that increases patient's endurance.
- Limit activity to bed rest should patient experience severe fatigue secondary to chronic cough or increased oxygen consumption.
- Provide frequent rest periods to conserve energy.
- Organize care to avoid fatigue by providing rest periods between procedures, having patient rest before and after meals, and maintaining planned rest periods.
- Monitor patient's intolerance for gradual increases in physical activity: HR ≥100 bpm, RR ≥24 BPM, dyspnea, pale skin, or cyanosis.
- Support chest muscle while patient coughs.
- Administer oxygen before and after increased physical activity.
- Administer bronchodilators before patient begins ambulating.
- Teach patient to report when he or she feels unusual fatigue.
- Instruct patient to pace and prioritize activities: identify priorities and eliminate nonessential activity, distribute difficult tasks throughout the day, and rest before difficult activities.
- Teach patient the causes of fatigue.

Knowledge deficit related to the causes, risk factors, or treatments associated with bronchitis.

Expected Patient Outcome. Patient is able to verbalize the risk factors and treatments associated with bronchitis.

- Consult with physician about content to be covered in an individualized teaching plan.

- Explain the need to exercise to tolerance to avoid fatigue.
- Encourage patient to eat the prescribed diet.
- Provide fluid of 2000 to 3000 mL/d, if not contraindicated, to loosen secretions.
- Encourage patient to maintain weight within normal limits.
- Provide knowledge regarding the risk factors associated with bronchitis.
- Teach patient importance of not smoking and avoidance of exposure to air pollution.
- Teach patient the purposes of bronchodilators in relation to the bronchial airways.
- Teach patient diaphragmatic breathing and coughing techniques.
- Teach patient how to administer medications, noting any side effects.
- Instruct patient to report any increase in temperature or change in mucus production, which may reflect an impending infection.

DISCHARGE PLANNING

The critical care nurse will provide patient and significant other(s) with verbal or written discharge notes regarding the following subjects:

1. Importance of preventing future attacks by avoiding chemical mediators, avoiding stressful situations, avoiding smoking, and providing adequate humidity.
2. Importance of breathing exercises and exercising to tolerance without becoming fatigued.
3. Importance of maintaining appropriate diet and fluids 2000 to 3000 mL/d unless contraindicated and avoiding gaining weight.
4. Importance of taking prescribed medications.
5. Signs and symptoms that warrant medical attention: elevated temperature, HR ≥ 100 bpm, RR 24 BPM, cough, and fatigue.
6. Importance of keeping ongoing outpatient appointments.
7. Discussion of medications's purpose, dosage, route, schedule and side effects.

■ PNEUMONIA

For related information see Cardiac Deviations, Part I: Hemodynamic monitoring, p. 219. Part I: Pneumonia, p. 375; Respiratory acidosis, p. 412; and Respiratory alkalosis, p. 415. Part III: Pulse oximetry, p. 426; Mechanical ventilation, p. 428; Capnography, p. 439; Transcutaneous Pao_2 and $Paco_2$, p. 441; Indirect calorimetry, p. 441.

Case Management Basis

DRG: 89 Simple pneumonia and pleurisy
   age ≥ 17 with complications
LOS: 7.10 days
DRG: 90 Simple pneumonia and pleurisy
   age ≥ 17 without complications
LOS: 5.40 days

Definition

Acute pneumonia is an acute infection that leads to inflammation of the alveolar spaces and interstitial tissue. The inflammation eventually causes impaired gas exchange. Virulent organisms multiply in the lower respiratory system.

Pathophysiology

In acute viral pneumonia, the alveoli are filled with fibrin, fluid, red blood cells, and macrophages; patients with viral pneumonia have hypoxemia, which may fail to improve with oxygen administration. Aspiration of gastric contents causing aspiration pneumonia leads to chemical pneumonitis with diffuse alveolar filling. Chronic aspiration pneumonia is more localized as consolidation in dependent portions of the lungs or bilateral midzones as a result of repeated aspiration of small quantities of infected pharyngeal secretion. Radiation pneumonia, a result of radiation near the lungs, can cause loss of lung volume. Bacterial pneumonia is a consolidative inflammation caused by pathogenic microorganisms.

In general with pneumonia, there is disruption of the mechanical defense of cough and ciliary motility, which leads to colonization of the lungs and subsequent infection. Infection causes pulmonary inflammation with or without significant exudates. The overall result is ventilation/perfusion ($\dot{V}/\dot{Q}$) mismatch.

Nursing Assessment

PRIMARY MECHANISMS

- Bacterial pneumonia is caused by gram-positive cocci such as *Streptococcus pneumoniae, Staphylococcus aureus, Streptococcus pyogenes,* and anaerobes; gram-negative cocci such as *Neisseria meningitidis;* gram-positive rods from *Nocardia* or *Actinomyces* species or *Bacillus anthracis;* and gram-negative rods such as *Haemophilus influenzae, Klebsiella pneumoniae, Pseudomonas aeruginosa, Escherichia coli, Acinetobacter* species, *Legionella* species, or anaerobes. Viral pneumonia can be attributed to parainfluenza virus, influenza viruses A and B, varicella viruses, measles, and cytomegalovirus. Other pneumonias include aspiration, radiation, myoplasma, protoza and nosocomial.

RISK FACTORS

- History of diabetes mellitus, congestive heart failure (CHF), chronic obstructive pulmonary disease (COPD), alcohol abuse, or debilitating underlying disease; life-style factors such as smoking; being in middle-age or elderly population.

PHYSICAL ASSESSMENT

Bacterial Pneumonia

- Inspection: Shaking chills, fever, dry to productive cough with rusty or yellow green sputum, dyspnea, cyanosis, pleuritic chest pain, malaise, weakness, headache, or myalgia.
- Palpation: Tactile fremitus, dry skin, or poor turgor.
- Percussion: Dull over consolidated lung field.

- Auscultation: Tachycardia, tachypnea, hypotension, friction rub, or crackles (rales).

Atypical Pneumonia (Viral, Mycoplasmal)

- Inspection: Headache, rhinorrhea, dry cough, low-grade fever without chills, malaise, pharyngitis, muscle pain, and myalgias.

DIAGNOSTIC TEST RESULTS

Standard Laboratory Tests (see Table 1–9, p. 40)

- Arterial blood gases: partial pressure of arterial oxygen (Pao_2) $\leq$60 mm Hg, partial pressure of arterial carbon dioxide (Paco_2) $\leq$35 mm Hg, and pH $\geq$7.35.
- Blood cultures: Reveal the presence of bacteremia.
- Blood studies: Elevated white blood cells (WBC) $\geq$12,000 to 30000 μL and sedimentation rate.
- Serologic studies on serum or sputum: Cold agglutinins and specific complement-fixation antibody titers may identify myocoplasma infection in the acute phase.
- Serum chemistries: Reduced sodium and chloride; elevated bilirubin.
- Sputum of lower respiratory tract (LRT) secretions: Technique: sputum induction, nasotracheal suctioning, translaryngeal aspiration, fiberoptic bronchoscopy or transthoracic needle aspiration.

Invasive Respiratory Diagnostic Procedures (see Table 3–3)

- Bronchial washing and lung biopsy: Used to diagnose certain pneumonias (*Pneumocystis carinii,* millary tuberculosis or fungi).
- Thoracentesis: When pleural fluid is present, it is aspirated and analyzed for the presence of the pathogen and for early identification of emphysema.

Noninvasive Respiratory Diagnostic Procedures (see Table 3–4)

- Chest roentgenogram: With pneumococcal pneumonia there are dense infiltrates of one or more lobes or a patchy pattern with no consolidation. Gram-negative pneumonia shows interstitial infiltrates that may be unilateral or bilateral, progressing to consolidation. Chest roentgenogram of viral pneumonia reveals scattered and diffuse interstitial infiltrates involving one or more lower lobes. Finally, mycoplasmal pneumonia shows segmental areas of consolidation, which are isolated in the lower lobes.

ECG
- Reveals tachycardia.

MEDICAL AND SURGICAL MANAGEMENT

PHARMACOLOGY
- Antibiotics: The specific antibiotics used depend on the organisms causing pneumonia. Antibiotics commonly used include penicillin, erythromycin, cephalosporin, nafcillin, ampicillin, gentamicin, vancomycin, sulfamethoxazole (see Table 1–14, p. 122).
- Bronchodilators: Used for patients who may develop bronchospasm as a result of aspiration (see Table 3–6).

PHYSICAL ACTIVITY
- Position with head of bed elevated, which can decrease gastric reflux and facilitate swallowing.
- Coughing, turning, and deep-breathing exercises are facilitated.

AIRWAY MANAGEMENT
- Airway management includes chest percussion and drainage for improved sputum clearance and nasotracheal or endotracheal suctioning.
- A cuffed endotracheal intubator is used to restore adequate oxygenation and protect airway from aspiration.

OXYGEN THERAPY
- Supplemental humidified oxygen can help to liquify and mobilize secretions.

MECHANICAL VENTILATION
- Mechanical ventilation with positive end-expiratory pressure (PEEP) may be necessary to reverse arterial hypoxemia.

FLUID THERAPY
- IV fluid therapy may be necessary in patients who are unable to ingest an adequate amount of oral fluids. The fluids replace intravascular volume.
- Fruit juices can be used in febrile patients to replace electrolytes lost during diaphoresis.

NURSING MANAGEMENT: NURSING DIAGNOSES AND COLLABORATIVE PROBLEMS

Nursing Diagnoses
Common nursing goals in patient with pneumonia are to improve oxygenation, support airway clearance, maintain fluid balance, prevent infection, provide adequate nutritional intake, and correct complication of fatigue.

Impaired gas exchange related to tracheobronchial secretion in the alveolar space or alveolar hyperventilation secondary to pulmonary inflammation.

Expected Patient Outcomes. Patient maintains adequate gas exchange, as evidenced by Pao_2 80 to 100 mm Hg, $Paco_2$ 35 to 45 mm Hg, alveolar oxygen tension (Pao_2) 100 mm Hg, arterial-alveolar tension ratio ($P[a/A]o_2$) 0.75 to 0.90, alveolar-arterial oxygen gradient ($P[A-/a]o_2$) $\leq$15 mm Hg, arterial oxygen content (Cao_2) 18 to 20 mL/100mL, arterial oxygen saturation (Sao_2) 95 %, mixed venous oxygen saturation ($S\bar{v}o_2$) 60% to 80%, respiratory rate (RR) $\leq$30 BPM, heart rate (HR) $\leq$100 bpm, no fever, no shortness of breath, and absence of pleuritic pain.

- Consult with physician about the criteria used to determine when ventilatory support is needed: oxygenation (Pao_2 $\leq$60 mm Hg on fraction of inspired oxygen [Fio_2] at 50%), ventilator ($Paco_2$ $\geq$50–60 mm Hg, which is $\geq$10 mm Hg above patient's normal $Paco_2$), and respiratory mechanics (apnea, sustained RR ≥ 35 BPM, and VC ≤ 10 to 15 mL/kg).

- Review results of arterial blood gas measurement and chest roentgenogram.
- Elevate head of bed 45 to 60 degrees to facilitate ventilation.
- Limit activity to bed rest while patient febrile.
- Obtain and report clinical findings that indicate impaired gas exchange: cyanosis, shortness of breath, tachypnea, restlessness, tachycardia, crackles, and pleuritic pain.
- Obtain and report $Pao_2 \leq 60$ mm Hg, $Paco_2 \geq 45$ mm Hg, $PAO_2 \leq 100$ mm Hg, $P[a/A]O_2 \leq 0.75$, $P[A/a]O_2 \geq 15$ mm Hg, and $Cao_2 \leq 18$ mL/100mL.
- Should ventilatory support be required, assess ventilator function by verifying that the prescribed settings are being used and are effective. The settings include FIO_2 at the lowest rate to maintain $Pao_2 \geq 60$ mm Hg and 100% in acute situation to achieve adequate oxygenation; tidal volume 10 to 15 mL/kg; RR 10-14 BPM; and mode of ventilation.
- Use unit-prescribed method of endotracheal suctioning: preoxygenation, hyperinflation, hyperoxygenation, hyperventilation, manual inflation, and oxygen insufflation.
- Monitor patient's tolerance of ventilatory support through the use of an individualized plan of care, which includes data from chest such as lung sounds, RR, chest expansion and ventilator settings; hemodynamic parameters including HR, blood pressure (BP), (T), cardiac output (CO), cardiac index (CI), pulmonary artery pressure (PAP), and pulmonary capillary wedge pressure (PCWP); nutritional status as to type of feedings, intake, and output; and level of anxiety.
- Encourage patient to turn and deep breathe every 2 hours.
- Assist patient during coughing episodes by having sit upright and splinting the chest.
- Administer prescribed IV fluids to maintain adequate hydration.

- Administer prescribed humidified oxygen 2 to 4 L/min by means of nasal cannula or mask, $FIO_2 \leq 50\%$ to maintain $Pao_2 \geq 80$ mm Hg and $Sao_2 \geq 95\%$.
- Administer prescribed aminophylline to relieve bronchospasm and increase oxygenation of the lungs.
- Administer prescribed antibiotics, depending on the results of sputum or blood cultures.
- Administer prescribed antipyretics and analgesics to reduce temperature and pleuritic pain.
- Teach patient to cough, turn, and deep breathe every 2 to 4 hours.

Ineffective airway clearance related to increased or retained tracheobronchial secretions secondary to infection process of impaired cough.

Expected Patient Outcomes. Patient maintains effective airway clearance, as evidenced by arterial blood gases within normal range, RR ≤ 30 BPM, absence of adventitious breath sounds, absence of cyanosis, and productive cough.

- Review results of chest roentgenogram and arterial blood gases.
- Encourage patient to turn and deep breathe every 2 to 4 hours.
- Monitor clinical indicators of respiratory status: rate, depth, symmetry of chest excursion, skin color, presence of adventitious breath sounds, or presence of tactile fremitus.
- Maximize lung expansion: Deep breathing, incentive spirometry, chest physiotherapy, and frequent turning, and coughing.
- Encourage fluid intake, if not contraindicated, to maintain adequate hydration to help loosen secretions.
- Evaluate the efficiency of deep-breathing ability by monitoring vital capacity and maximal inspiratory force (MIF).
- Monitor forced expiratory volume in 1 second (FEV_1) and the ratio of FEV_1 to forced vital capacity (FVC) to determine patient's

ability to generate high air flow and pressure needed for effective coughing.

- Chest physiotherapy (CPT) such as postural drainage, chest percussion, chest vibration, and cough enhancement is used to improve mucus and sputum clearance from the airways.
- Encourage the use of cascade (normal) cough by having patient take a deep breath, followed by three to four coughs until almost all of the air is out of the lungs. Cascade coughing moves secretions from the periphery of the lungs to the central airways.
- Encourage patient to use a voluntary maximal inhalation of 3 to 10 seconds after coughing to reinflate collapsed alveoli, avoid mucus pool, avoid decreased oxygenation, and avoid increased risk of infection.
- Suction patient as necessary to stimulate cough and clear airway, using aseptic technique and following unit protocol.
- Monitor intake, output, and specific gravity to evaluate fluid balance.
- Administer prescribed IV fluids to maintain adequate hydration.
- Administer prescribed oxygen 2 to 4 L/min or $FIO_2 \leq 50\%$ to maintain PaO_2 80 to 100 mm Hg.
- Administer prescribed expectorant to assist patient in removing secretions.
- Teach patient to expectorate secretions.
- Teach patient postural drainage as tolerated.

Fluid volume deficit related to increased insensible loss secondary to hyperventilation, supplemental oxygen, and decreased fluid intake.

Expected Patient Outcome. Patient maintains adequate fluid volume, as evidenced by urinary output (UO) ≥ 30 mL/h or ≥ 0.5 mL/kg/h, specific gravity 1.010 to 1.030, stable weight, BP within patient's normal range, CO 4 to 8 L/min, CI 2.7 to 4.3 L/min/m², central venous pressure (CVP) 2 to 6 mm Hg, mean arterial pressure (MAP) 70 to 100 mm Hg, HR ≤ 100 bpm, RR 12 to 20 BPM, SaO_2 95%, peripheral pulses +2, absence of fatigue, normothermia, capillary refill ≤ 3 seconds, and skin turgor adequate.

- Review results of hemoglobin, hematocrit, and serum osmolality.
- Obtain and report hemodynamic parameters that may indicate fluid volume deficit: CO ≤ 4 L/min, CI ≤ 2.7 L/min/m², CVP ≤ 2 mm Hg, and MAP ≤ 70 mm Hg.
- Obtain and report clinical findings that indicate fluid volume deficit: hypotension, HR ≥ 100 bpm, dizziness, fatigue, dry mucus membrane, fever, poor skin turgor, peripheral pulses $\leq +2$, capillary refill ≥ 3 seconds.
- Monitor intake, output, specific gravity, and daily weight. Report UO ≤ 30 mL/h or ≤ 0.5 mL/kg/h, specific gravity ≤ 1.010, and weight loss ≥ 0.5 to 1.0 kg/d.
- Monitor ECG continuously to assess HR and rhythm. Document ECG every 2 to 4 hours in patients with dysrhythmias.
- Administer prescribed IV fluids to adequately maintain hydration and circulatory volume.
- Administer prescribed dopamine or dobutamine, if necessary, to improve CO and tissue perfusion (see Table 1–10, p. 50).

High risk of infection related to aspiration, immunosuppression, invasive respiratory procedures, or invasive cannulation.

Expected Patient Outcome. Patient is free of infection, as evidenced by WBC $\leq 11,000/\mu L$, negative sputum culture, no fever, and RR ≤ 30 BPM.

- Review results of WBC, sputum or LRT secretions, bronchial washings, or lung biopsy.
- Limit physical activity to bed rest until patient is no longer febrile.
- Insert nasogastric (NG) tube, if necessary, to provide desired calories or prevent aspiration.
- Monitor temperature every 2 hours or as needed while patient is febrile.

- Obtain and report clinical findings that may indicate infection: elevated temperature, RR $\geq$30 BPM, and drainage from wound of catheter insertion site.
- When cultures are positive and temperature $\geq$102°F, prepare for contact, respiratory, acid-fast bacilli, or body substance isolation.
- Utilize aseptic technique when suctioning, changing dressings, or changing tubings.
- Administer prescribed IV fluids to maintain adequate hydration and circulating volume.
- Administer prescribed antimicrobial therapy to treat infection (see Table 1–14, p. 122).
- Administer antipyretics and analgesics as prescribed.

Nutrition, alteration in: less than body requirements related to fatigue, weakness, dyspnea, or hypermetabolic state resulting from fever.

Expected Patient Outcome. Patient maintains adequate nutritional intake and body weight within normal range.

- Consult with dietitian as to the desired diet and schedule for patient.
- Provide adequate nutritional intake via nasogastric feedings, IV fluids, or hyperalimentation.
- Provide nutrition to offset high calorie expenditure secondary to infection: high-caloric and high-protein diet.
- Monitor patients respiratory quotient the ratio of carbon dioxide volume to oxygen volume ($RQ = Vco_2/Vo_2$).
- Monitor patency of NG tube to prevent aspiration.
- Provide foods, if necessary, taking into account patient's likes and dislikes.
- Teach patient the importance of maintaining an adequate nutritional intake.

Fatigue related to incessant cough.

Expected Patient Outcome. Patient is free of fatigue.

- Place on bed rest while patient febrile and fatigued.

- Provide frequent rest periods to conserve energy.
- Provide chest support while patient coughing.
- Organize care to avoid fatigue by maintaining rest periods between coughing, having patient rest before and after meals and maintaining planned rest periods.
- Administer prescribed expectorants to clear secretions.
- Administer prescribed analgesics to reduce discomfort caused by coughing.

Collaborative Problems

Common collaborative goals for patients with pneumonia are to maintain ventilation-perfusion balance and improve oxygenation.

Potential Complication: Ventilation-Perfusion Imbalance. Ventilation-perfusion imbalance related to alveolar infiltrates secondary to pulmonary inflammation.

Expected Patient Outcomes. Patient maintains adequate ventilation-perfusion balance, as evidenced by ventilation/perfusion ($\dot{V}/\dot{Q}$) ratio 1.0, Sao_2 97%, Svo_2 75%, alveolar-arterial oxygen gradient ($P[A-a]o_2$) $\leq$15 mm Hg on room air or 10 to 65 mm Hg on 100% O_2, arterial-alveolar oxygen tension ratio ($P[a/A)o_2$) 0.75 to 0.90, static compliance $\geq$50 mL/cm H_2O, dynamic compliance $\geq$45 mL/cm H_2O, RR 12 to 20 BPM, absence of adventitious breath sounds, absence of cyanosis, absence of dyspnea, CO 4 to 8 L/min, CO 2.7 to 4.3 L/min/m^2, PCWP 4 to 12 mm Hg, MAP 70 to 100 mm Hg, BP within patient's normal range, arterial blood gases within normal range, and HR $\leq$100 bpm.

- Consult with physician to validate expected patient outcomes used to evaluate ventilation-perfusion balance.
- Confer with Respiratory Therapy regarding the appropriate ventilatory support for the pneumonia patient.
- Review results of arterial blood gas measurement, static lung compliance, dynamic

lung compliance, physiological shunting, alveolar-arterial oxygen gradient, arterial-alveolar oxygen tension ratio, or ventilation-perfusion scan.

- Limit physical activity to bed rest to decrease the work of breathing.
- Obtain and report hemodynamic parameters that could affect ventilation-perfusion balance: CO $\leq$4 L/min, CI $\leq$2.7 L/min/m^2, PCWP $\leq$12 mm Hg, MAP $\geq$70 mm Hg, and S$\bar{v}$O$_2$ $\leq$60%.
- Obtain and report other clinical findings associated with decreased $\dot{V}/\dot{Q}$ ratio: tachypnea, cyanosis, crackles, dyspnea, restlessness, shortness of breath, and tachycardia.
- Monitor $\dot{V}/\dot{Q}$ ratio and report value 1.0 which signifies reduced alveolar ventilation. A low $\dot{V}/\dot{Q}$ ratio is referred to as an intrapulmonary shunt (blood flow [$\dot{Q}$s]/total flow [$\dot{Q}$t]) $\geq$15% to 30%.
- Obtain the following information in order to measure $\dot{Q}$s/$\dot{Q}$t: hemoglobin level, FIO$_2$ level, arterial and mixed venous blood gas results, and arterial and mixed venous oxyhemoglobin (oxygen saturation) values.
- Monitor alveolar partial pressure of oxygen (PAO$_2$) and arterial partial pressure of oxygen (PaO$_2$), which are approximately equal. Report a diversion of PAO$_2$ from PaOO$_2$, which signifies the development of an intrapulmonary shunt.
- Estimate $\dot{Q}$s:$\dot{Q}$t using the following methods: PaO$_2$/FIO$_2$ ratio $\geq$286. arterial/alveolar (a/A) ratio $\geq$0.60, alveolar-arterial (A$-$a) gradient $\leq$20 mm Hg with an FIO$_2$ of 0.21, respiratory index $\leq$1, and shunt equation $\leq$5%.
- Monitor and report PAO$_2$/FIO$_2$ $\leq$200, which is considered to be a large intrapulmonary shunt (20%). The lower the value, the more severe the $\dot{Q}$s/$\dot{Q}$t disturbance.
- Obtain and report SaO$_2$ $\leq$90%, which can signify intrapulmonary shunting.
- Measure intake, output, specific gravity, and daily weight. Excessive fluid accumulation increases total lung water, contributing to an increase in ventilation-perfusion imbalance.

- Monitor skin color for the presence of cyanosis, which can reflect the desaturation of at least 5 g of hemoglobin and ventilation/perfusion mismatch.
- Evaluate the adequacy of oxygenation: Oxygen delivery $\geq$600 mL/min/m^2, CI $\geq$2.7 L/min/m^2, and oxygen consumption (VO$_2$) $\geq$156 mL/min/m^2.
- Administer prescribed humidified oxygen to keep PaO$_2$ $\geq$60 mm Hg.
- Administer IV fluids at the prescribed flow rate to maintain adequate hydration and to avoid excess fluid accumulation, which increases lung water causing increased $\dot{V}$:$\dot{Q}$ mismatch.

Potential Complication: Hypoxemia. Hypoxemia related to lung consolidation and tracheobronchial secretion secondary to pulmonary inflammation.

Expected Patient Outcomes. Patient maintains adequate oxygen gas exchange, as evidenced by PaO$_2$ 100 mm Hg, PaCO$_2$ 40 mm Hg, oxygen consumption (resting) 250 mL/min, oxygen transport (resting) 1000 mL/min, and skin color normal.

- Review results of arterial blood gas measurement, hemoglobin, and hematocrit.
- Position patient with bilateral lung involvement in a prone Trendelenburg position, if not contraindicated, to promote blood flow to the areas of lung that receive the largest tidal volume, should mechanical ventilation be required.
- Assess breath sounds and presence of adventitious breath sounds every 1 to 2 hours. Pulmonary congestion, documented as crackles and wheezes, can indicate increased hydrostatic force in the pulmonary vascular system, causing fluid to move across the alveolar-capillary membrane.
- Should mechanical ventilation and intubation not be necessary, pulse oximetry measurement of SaO$_2$ and incentive spirometry measurement can be used to provide indirect data about lung compliance and hypoxemia.

- Monitor and report changes in the major factors of oxygen transport: $CO \leq 4$ L/min hemoglobin (Hgb) ≤ 12 g/dL, $Sao_2 \leq 90\%$, and $Pao_2 \leq 80$ mm Hg.
- Use CPT (postural drainage, chest vibration, and cough enhancement) to improve mucous and sputum clearance from the airways.
- Encourage the use of cascade (normal) cough by having patient take a deep breath, followed by three to four coughs until almost all of the air is out of the lungs. Cascade coughing moves secretions from the periphery of the lungs to the central airways.
- Monitor $\dot{Q}s/\dot{Q}t$ fraction at Fio_2 at 50% to 60%: Normal shunt fraction without a ventilator is 6% and with a ventilator is 10%.
- Suction patient using the principles of preoxygenation, short suctioning time, post-suctioning hyperinflation to reverse atelectasis and maintain uninterrupted PEEP.
- Monitor alveolar-arterial gradient $P(A-a)O_2$.
- Provide ventilatory support, if necessary and prescribed, to slowly improve $\dot{Q}s/\dot{Q}t$ and static lung compliance (Cst) over 24 hours.
- Monitor chest expansion, since patients receiving pancuronium bromide may have a predominance of tidal volume distributed to the apices of the lung.
- Administer prescribed antibiotics to treat infection.
- Administer prescribed IV fluids such as crystalloids, to maintain adequate intravascular volume and PCWP 10 to 12 mm Hg.
- Instruct patient to cough, turn and deep in order to enhance oxygen-carbon dioxide exchange.

DISCHARGE PLANNING

The critical care nurse will provide the patient and significant other(s) with verbal or written discharge notes regarding the following subjects:

1. Signs and symptoms that require medical attention, including elevated temperature, tachycardia, tachypnea, unproductive cough, diaphoresis, and shortness of breath.
2. Importance of gradual convalescence by limiting exercise and activity to tolerance.
3. Importance of postural drainage and deep-breathing exercises.
4. Using a humidifier at home.
5. Need to force fluids to 3000 mL/day, if not contraindicated.
6. A written list of drugs' purpose, dosage, schedule, and side effects.

◼ CHEST TRAUMA

For related information see Cardiac Deviations, Part I: Acute cardiac tamponade, p. 117; Shock, p. 174; Dysrhythmias, p. 184. Part III: Hemodynamic monitoring, p. 219. Part I: Acute pulmonary edema, p. 346; Pulmonary embolism, p. 397; Respiratory acidosis, p. 412; Respiratory alkalosis, p. 415. Part III: Pulse oximetry, p. 426; Mechanical ventilation, p. 428; Capnography, p. 439; Transcutaneous Pao_2 and $Paco_2$, p. 441; Indirect calorimetry, p. 441; Intravascular oxygenator, p.442.)

Case Management Basis

DRG: 83 Major chest trauma with complications
LOS: 6.20 days
DRG: 84 Major chest trauma without complications
LOS: 3.70 days
DRG: 94 Pneumothorax with complications
LOS: 7.10 days
DRG 95: Pneumothorax without complications
LOS: 4.40 days
DRG: 101 Other respiratory system diagnoses with complications
LOS: 5.10
DRG: 102 Other respiratory system diagnoses without complications
LOS: 3.30

Definition

Chest trauma is potentially life-threatening because of the sudden disturbance of the cardiopulmonary system. Chest trauma is divided into two categories: blunt or penetrating. Blunt injury results in diffuse pulmonary injury with the extent and distribution determined by the velocity and point of impact. The flail chest injury consists of multifocal anterior, lateral, or posterior fractures. The injured parts of the thorax no longer respond to the action of the respiratory muscles but now move according to changes in intrapleural pressures. Lung contusion occurs when the chest wall hits a steering wheel or is impacted by an outside force like an explosion. The force against the chest wall is transmitted to the lung, rupturing tissue, small airways, and alveoli. The contusion process is hemorrhagic and also involves interstitial and alveolar edema resulting from injury. Pleural space injury can occur from a blunt impact from a steering column or rib fragment. These injuries can produce laceration or perforation of an intrathoracic structure, such as lung or blood vessels. Tracheobronchial tears can be due to frontal crash injury, in which a vertical stretching of the trachea or bronchus and a sudden increased intra-airway pressure against a closed glottis occur.

Penetrating injury can be caused by gunshot, leading to crushed tissue, cavitation, and combustion, and by stab wounds from accidental impalement or intentional assaults. Penetrating wounds to the chest can lead to injuries of lung parenchyma and esophagus, to intrathoracic air, or to pneumothorax. In a pneumothorax or hemothorax, air or fluid can enter the pleural space, causing lung tissue to be displaced. Air or fluid may enter the pleural space from the lungs themselves or from an opening in the chest wall.

Pathophysiology

In general, chest trauma can cause hypovolemic shock, which leads to a cellular oxygen demand that may exceed the supply. The body responds through several compensatory mechanisms. The sympathetic nervous system releases epinephrine and norepinephrine to initiate arterial and venous vasoconstriction. This leads to increased systemic vascular resistance and subsequent increase in arterial blood pressure. Baroreceptors respond by increasing heart rate and myocardial contractility while enhancing vasoconstriction of the systemic vasculature. In hypovolemic shock resulting from chest trauma, fluid shifts from the interstitial space into the blood vessels. The fluid in the interstitial space acts as a buffer, allowing fluid to move into the intravascular space when blood volume is depleted. The renin-angiotensin-aldosterone mechanism maintains cardiac output by acting on cells of the distal tubules to increase the reabsorption of sodium and water. Finally, the antidiuretic hormone (ADH, vasopressin) acts on the epithelial cells of the distal tubules and collecting ducts to increase the reabsorption of water, thereby expanding the intravascular volume. In addition, ADH causes vasoconstriction of the systemic vasculature, which increases blood pressure and enhances tissue perfusion. In blunt injury, there is rupture of small blood vessels and alveoli, which leads to the extravasation of blood and edema fluid into the interstitium and air into the pleural space. In a penetrating injury, there is increased lung density representing focal hemorrhage after the passage of a sharp instrument or a relatively low-velocity bullet.

Chest trauma can lead to three types of pneumothorax. (1) Spontaneous (closed) pneumothorax can occur when a bleb in the surface of the lung ruptures and releases air into the pleural space. Partial or complete lung collapse occurs when air enters the pleural space from within the lung and causes increased pleural pressure. The lungs are unable to expand during normal inspirations. (2) Tension pneumothorax involves air in the pleural space that is under higher pressure than air in the adjacent lung and vascular structures. Sometimes air leaks into the pleural space on inspiration, but the tissues seals itself on expiration and outward leakage does not occur. Air builds up in the pleural space with mediastinal displacement, which ultimately affects the other lung and impedes venous return to the heart. (3) Traumatic (open or closed) pneumothorax occurs when atmospheric air flows directly into the pleural cavity through a chest wall opening. Air may be unable to escape because of a one-way valve effect and pressure accumulates. The result is a collapsed lung and eventual mediastinal shift.

Finally, pathologic changes found in lung contusion include alveolar capillary damage with disruption of alveolar membranes, interstitial and intra-alveolar extravasation of blood, and interstitial edema. As the lung edema increases, alveoli fill with edema fluid, and alveolar ventilation and blood flow decrease through the damaged lung, leading to impaired gas exchange.

Nursing Assessment

PRIMARY CAUSES

- Open pneumothorax is due to penetrating chest injury from gunshot or knife wound, motor vehicle accident, insertion of a central venous catheter, chest surgery, transbronchial biopsy, thoracentesis, or a closed pleural biopsy. Closed pneumothorax is caused by blunt chest trauma, air leakage from ruptures, congenital blebs adjacent to the visceral pleural surface, rupture of an emphysematous bulla, rupture from barotrauma caused by high intrathoracic pressures during mechanical ventilation, cancerous lesions that can erode into the pleural space, or interstitial lung disease. Tension pneumothorax is due to penetrating chest wound treatment with an airtight dressing, lung or airway puncture by a fractured rib associated with positive-pressure ventilation, aftermath of chest injury, high levels of positive end-expiratory pressure (PEEP) causing rupture of an alveolar bleb, or chest tube occlusion.
- Contusions occur with motor vehicle accident, fall, or crushing injuries.

PHYSICAL ASSESSMENT

Blunt Injury

- Inspection: Tenderness at site of impact; pale, mottled extremities; increased work of breathing; abnormal chest wall movement; hemoptysis; neck vein distention; dyspnea; shallow breathing; tachypnea; restlessness; nasal flaring; paradoxical chest wall motion; ineffective cough; or hoarseness.
- Palpation: Cool or cold, moist extremities; weak peripheral pulses; tenderness over affected chest area; subcutaneous emphysema; flail chest segment; or tracheal deviation.
- Percussion: Dullness over fluid-filled lung fields or hyperresonance over air-filled lung field.
- Auscultation: hypotension, decreased or absent breath sounds, pericardial friction rub, paradoxical pulse, respiratory stridor, muffled heart sounds, atrial tachycardia.

Penetrating Injury

- Inspection: Ecchymoses, abrasions, hematomas, restlessness, confusion, agitation, lethargy or coma, cyanosis of lips and nail beds, bloody sputum, entry and exit wounds, tachypnea, splinting, hyperpnea, use of accessory muscles, hemoptysis, or chest pain.
- Palpation: Subcutaneous emphysema, tracheal deviation, weak pulses, or cool extremities.
- Percussion: Dullness over fluid-filled lung fields or hyperresonance over air-filled lung fields.
- Auscultation: Decreased or absent breath sounds, muffled heart sounds, sucking sound over point of entry during inspiration, respiratory stridor, tachycardia, or bradycardia, or hypotension.

Spontaneous or Traumatic Pneumothorax

- Inspection: Pleuritic pain, shortness of breath, asymmetric chest wall movement, and dyspnea.

- Palpation: Tracheal shift toward unaffected side, subcutaneous emphysema (crepitus), tactile fremitus decreased, and egophony decreased.
- Percussion: Hyperresonance over air-filled area; dull over fluid-filled area.
- Auscultation: Absent or decreased breath sounds, tachypnea, and tachycardia.

Tension Pneumothorax
- Inspection: Apprehension, agitation, dyspnea, tachypnea, cyanosis, increased jugular venous pressure, decreased chest wall movement on affected side, and mediastinum shifted away from the affected side.
- Palpation: Tracheal shift toward unaffected side, subcutaneous emphysema in neck and chest.
- Percussion: Hyperresonance on affected side.
- Auscultation: Tachycardia, hypotension, and absent or decreased breath sounds, distant heart sounds.

Pulmonary Contusion
- Inspection: Chest pain, restlessness, apprehension, ineffective cough, or hemoptysis.
- Auscultation: Tachycardia and tachypnea.

DIAGNOSTIC TEST RESULTS

Chest Trauma

Standard Laboratory Tests (see Table 3–1)

- Arterial blood gases: partial pressure of arterial oxygen (Pao_2) ≤ 80 mm Hg, partial pressure of arterial carbon dioxide ($Paco_2$) ≤ 35 mm Hg, then ≥ 45 mm Hg, and pH ≤ 7.35.
- Blood studies: Reduced hematocrit 30% and elevated serum osmolality ≥ 300 to 310 mOsm/kg water.

Invasive Respiratory Diagnostic Procedure (see Table 3–3)

- Aortogram: Only done if patient is stable to confirm aortic disruption or tear.

Noninvasive Respiratory Diagnostic Procedures. (see Table 3–4)

- Chest roentgenogram: Widened mediastinum, fractures of first or second ribs; obliteration of aortic knob; pressure of pleural cap; obliteration of space between pulmonary artery and aorta; tracheal deviation to the right; depression of left mainstem bronchus; elevation and rightward shift of left bronchus.

ECG
- Peaked T waves, atrial tachycardia or bradycardia, or ventricular dysrhythmias.

Pneumothorax

Standard Laboratory Tests
- Arterial blood gases: Pao_2 ≤ 70 to 80 mm Hg, $Paco_2$ ≥ 45 mm Hg, and pH ≤ 7.35.

Noninvasive Respiratory Diagnostic Procedures (see Table 3–4)

- Chest roentgenogram: Air in the pleural space exceeding ambient pressure throughout the respiratory cycle, contralateral shift of mediastinal structures, and lowering of the diaphragm.

ECG
- Reveals decrease in QRS amplitude, precordial T wave inversion, and small precordial R voltage.

Pulmonary Contusion

Standard Laboratory Tests
- Arterial blood gases: Pao_2 ≤ 60 mm Hg and $Paco_2$ ≥ 45 mm Hg.

Noninvasive Respiratory Diagnostic Procedures (see Table 3–4)

- Chest roentgenogram: Shows a patchy, poorly outlined density that may be localized or diffuse. Also can show irregular, lineal densities with a peribronchial distribution. Contused lung may appear larger in size on chest roentgenogram and the ispsilateral diaphragm may appear lower than the opposite side.

MEDICAL AND SURGICAL MANAGEMENT

PHARMACOLOGY

- Paralytic agents: Succinylcholine at dose of 1.0 to 1.5 mg/kg and pancuronium bromide at dose of 0.5 to 2.0 mg/kg are used as muscle relaxants to cause complete flaccid paralysis in patients resisting intubation and mechanical ventilation (see Table 1–6, p. 28).
- Analgesics: Used to manage pain.
- Antibiotics: Used should a chest infection occur.

OXYGEN THERAPY

- Supplemental oxygen is given by mask or cannula to correct hypoxemia. Initially this may be achieved with 100% oxygen by a bag valve-mask (BVM) device in a hypoxic patient and it is initiated simultaneously with intubation.

INTUBATION AND MECHANICAL VENTILATION

- Intubation: Used to maintain a patent airway and improve oxygenation.
- Mechanical ventilation: Controlled mandatory ventilation or intermittent mandatory ventilation may be necessary with PEEP to enhance oxygenation. The flail chest can be stabilized by internal splinting through positive-pressure ventilation for approximately 3 weeks. Massive pulmonary contusions may require pharmacological paralysis and controlled mandatory ventilation or high-frequency ventilation to ventilate the poorly compliant and damaged lungs.

FLUID THERAPY

- Crystalloids: Rapid infusion of crystalloid solution can be administered at a ratio of 3 mL for every 1 mL of suspected blood loss associated with chest injury.
- Plasma expanders: Hetastarch may be used to augment crystalloids in patients who do not show improvement with crystalloids alone.
- Blood products: Blood products are administered using a formula of 1 mL for each 1 mL of blood loss to maintain a hemoglobin concentration $\geq$10 to 12 g/100 mL and a hematocrit of 30%.

CHEST TUBE

- A chest tube is used to remove the accumulation of fluid or air from the chest cavity. The catheter is connected to a one-way flutter valve or to a closed chest drainage system (see Chest drainage, p. 434).

CAPNOGRAPHY

- Allows for intermittent or continuous evaluation of carbon dioxide elimination. The capnogram is displayed as a wave form of carbon dioxide content in the exhaled gas (see Capnography, p. 439).

HEMODYNAMIC MONITORING

- A pulmonary artery (PA) catheter is used to measure cardiac output (CO), pulmonary capillary wedge pressure (PCWP) (preload), and systemic vascular resistance (SVR) (afterload). Mixed venous blood gases obtained via the distal port of the PA catheter permit the evaluation of the amount of oxygen utilized at the tissue level.

SURGICAL INTERVENTION

- Surgical internal stabilization of ribs and sternal fragments is recommended, especially if thoracotomy is necessary for another problem. Internal fixation can avoid the complications associated with prolonged ventilatory support.

NURSING MANAGEMENT: NURSING DIAGNOSES AND COLLABORATIVE PROBLEMS

Nursing Diagnoses

Common nursing goals for patients with chest trauma are to improve gas exchange, promote effective breathing, maintain airway clearance, balance fluid volume, prevent infection, and reduce pain.

Impaired gas exchange related to flail chest secondary to fractured ribs.

Expected Patient Outcomes. Patient maintains adequate gas exchange, as evidenced by blood pressure (BP) within the patient's normal range, absence of cyanosis, arterial blood gases within normal range, mean arterial pressure (MAP) 70 to 100 mm Hg, respiratory rate (RR) 12 to 20 BPM, absence of stridor, absence of chest pain, arterial oxygen saturation (Sao$_2$) 95%, symmetrical chest excursions, skin color normal, and absence of dyspnea.

- Consult with physician to validate expected patient outcomes used to evaluate adequate gas exchange.
- Consult with physician about criteria used to determine when ventilatory support is needed: oxygenation (Pao$_2$ ≤60 mm Hg on fraction of inspired oxygen [Fio$_2$] 50%), ventilation (Paco$_2$ ≥50-60 mm Hg, which is ≥10 mm Hg above patient's normal Paco$_2$), and respiratory mechanisms (apnea, sustained RR ≥35 BPM, and vital capacity ≤10 to 15 mL/kg).
- Review results of arterial blood measurement, chest roentgenogram, or lung volumes.
- Position patient to promote drainage, promote lung reexpansion, or facilitate alveolar perfusion.
- Monitor clinical indicators of respiratory status: rate, rhythm, symmetry of chest, depth of excursion, use of accessory muscles, and presence of adventitious breath sounds.
- Obtain and report clinical findings that indicate impaired gas exchange related to flail chest: paradoxical respirations (a collapse of the chest wall in inspiration and an expansion of the chest wall on expiration), dyspnea, stridor, cyanosis, chest pain, and shallow respirations.
- Encourage patient to take deep breaths to promote lung expansion.
- Observe patient for the presence of subcutaneous emphysema.
- Evaluate tissue oxygenation through use of oximetry.
- Monitor and report ventilatory mechanisms that indicate ineffective ventilation: tidal volume ≤7 mL/kg and vital capacity ≤15 mm Hg.
- Assist with initiation of mechanical ventilation with PEEP to maintain chest wall expansion and provide internal fixation of the fractured ribs.
- Assist with maximal stabilization of the flail segment by application of pressure during expiration or by sandbag. Be careful, as intervention may increase atelectasis.
- Monitor the type and amount of chest drainage.
- Should pneumothorax occur, assist with chest tube insertion using sterile technique: When pneumothorax is ≥25%, reexpansion of the involved lung and reestablishment of the physiological integrity of the interpleural space is required; assess, measure, and record chest drainage; promote ease of breathing and respiratory excursion; and facilitate more even matching of ventilation with perfusion.
- Administer prescribed IV fluids to maintain adequate hydration and circulatory volume.
- Administer prescribed high-flow oxygen 6 to 10 L/min by means of nasal cannula or mask or Fio$_2$ at 100% to maintain Pao$_2$ ≥80 mm Hg and Sao$_2$ ≥95%.
- Administer prescribed analgesic to reduce pain and splinting.
- Assist with prescribed thoracic epidural analgesic therapy for pain control.
- Assist with thoracentesis to remove fluid or air from the pleural space to relieve lung

compression and to obtain a fluid specimen for bacterial or cytological analysis.

- Should the flail segment require external fixation, prepare patient for surgery by wiring or attaching the segment to the intact body surface.

Ineffective breathing pattern related to unstable chest, muscular soreness, or inadequate chest expansion secondary to chest injury, chest tube dysfunction, increased pleural pressure, or pain.

Expected Patient Outcomes. Patient maintains effective breathing pattern, as evidenced by RR $\leq$30 BPM, heart rate (HR) $\leq$100 bpm, absence of tachypnea or dyspnea, symmetrical chest movements, absence of pleural pain, chest tube patent and draining, full lung expansion, and absence of adventitious breath sounds.

- Review arterial blood gas results and chest roentgenogram.
- Limit activity to bed rest with the head of bed elevated 60 to 90 degrees to maximize lung expansion and facilitate ventilation.
- Monitor progression of tension pneumothorax: apprehension, agitation, labored breathing, cyanosis, elevated jugular venous pressure, weak and thready pulse, and hypotension.
- Monitor cardiac rhythm for the presence of pulsus paradoxus, which may proceed hypotension and shock.
- Monitor clinical indicators of perfusion: BB, peripheral pulses, capillary refill, skin color and temperature, urinary output (UO), CO, and central venous pressure (CVP).
- Monitor respiratory excursion, depth, and rate in relation to the presence of tracheal deviation and displacement of point of maximal cardiac impulse (PMI), which could indicate a tension pneumothorax.
- Evaluate the efficiency of deep-breathing ability by monitoring vital capacity and maximal inspiratory force (MIF).
- Monitor forced expiratory volume in 1 second (FEV_1) and the ratio of FEV_1 to forced vital capacity (FVC) to determine patient's ability to generate high air flow and pressure needed for effective coughing.
- Chest physiotherapy (CPT) such as postural drainage, chest percussion, chest vibration, and cough enhancement is used to improve mucous and sputum clearance from the airways.
- Encourage the use of cascade (normal) cough by having patient take a deep breath, followed by three to four coughs until almost all of the air is out of the lungs. Cascade coughing moves secretions from the periphery of the lungs to the central airways.
- Encourage patient to use a voluntary maximal inhalation of 3 to 10 seconds after coughing to reinflate collapsed alveoli, avoid mucus pool, avoid decreased oxygenation, and avoid increased risk of infection.
- Monitor chest tube system for fluid level in seal chamber, pressure of air leaks, and drainage every 1 to 2 hours.
- Encourage patient to deep breathe, cough, and change position to reexpand atelectatic areas.
- Encourage the use of incentive spirometry to facilitate lung expansion.
- Administer oxygen at the prescribed amount and delivery system to maintain Pao_2 $\geq$80 mm Hg.
- Administer prescribed IV fluids to maintain adequate hydration.
- Place a sterile petrolatum gauze over an open wound to restore ventilation and respiration while having the patient inhales forcefully, then exhales forcefully against a closed glottis to expand the collapsed lung.
- Prepare patient for chest tube insertion to reestablish negative intrapleural pressure, which allows reexpansion of the lung and enhances healing of the parenchymal leak.
- Administer the prescribed analgesic to reduce pain and enhance ventilation by decreasing the work of breathing.
- Prepare patient with two or more spontaneous pneumothoraxes on one side for a thoracotomy.

- Teach patient to deep breathe every 2 to 4 hours.
- Teach patient to reduce anxiety through meditation, progressive relaxation, or guided imagery.

Ineffective airway clearance related to pain or inability to cough secondary to chest injury.

Expected Patient Outcomes. Patient maintains effective airway clearance, as evidenced by arterial blood gases within normal limits, RR ≤30 BPM, absence of adventitious breath sounds, BP within patient's normal range, HR ≤100 bpm, and productive cough.

- Review results of chest roentgenogram and arterial blood measurements.
- Insert nasogastric tube for feeding if necessary.
- Monitor clinical indicators of respiratory status: rate, depth, symmetry of chest excursion, skin color, and presence of adventitious breath sounds.
- Obtain and report clinical findings that indicate ineffective airway clearance: crackles, rhonchi, or wheezing; cyanosis; diaphoresis; RR ≥30 BPM; tachycardia; hypotension; and unproductive cough.
- Suction patient using the principles of preoxygenation, short suctioning time, postsuctioning hyperinflation to reverse atelectasis and maintain uninterrupted PEEP.
- Use intratracheal or intraendotracheal instillation of 2 mL to 5 mL of normal saline during suctioning to enhance the removal of secretions by stimulating a cough.
- CPT such as postural drainage, chest percussion, chest vibration, and cough enhancement is used to improve mucus and sputum clearance from the airways.
- Monitor and evaluate patient's oxygen (Sao_2, mixed venous oxygen saturation [$S\bar{v}o_2$]) and hemodynamic status (MAP, CO) before, during, and after suctioning.
- Assist with intubation to maintain patent airway and enables removal of airway secretion.

- Administer oxygen at the prescribed amount by Venturi mask or nasal cannula.
- Administer prescribed analgesics to reduce pain associated with coughing.
- Use prescribed capnography or transcutaneous oxygen monitoring to evaluate ventilation and gas exchange (see Capnography, p. 439, and Transcutaneous $Paco_2$ and Pao_2, p. 441).
- Provide ventilatory support with PEEP as ordered.

Fluid volume deficit related to bleeding secondary to a penetrating injury.

Expected Patient Outcomes. Patient maintains adequate fluid volume, as evidenced by hemoglobin and hematocrit within normal range, UO ≥30 mL/h or 0.5 mL/kg/h, HR ≤100 bpm, BP within patient's normal range, CO 4 to 8 L/min, cardiac index (CI) 2.7 to 4.3 L/min/m², CVP 2 to 6 mm Hg, pulse pressure ≥30 mm Hg, no internal or external signs of bleeding, alert, RR 12 to 20 BPM, chest drainage ≤100 mL/h, normal cardiac rhythm, capillary refill ≤3 seconds, peripheral pulses +2, and absence of bleeding from wound.

- Confer with physician regarding the expected blood volume loss in relation to patient's chest injury.
- Review arterial blood gas, blood urea nitrogen (BUN), creatinine, serum protein, hemoglobin or hematocrit, and chest roentgenogram results.
- Limit physical activity to bed rest until bleeding from a penetrating chest injury or pneumothorax has ceased.
- Obtain and report hemodynamic parameters that indicate fluid volume deficit: CO ≤4 L/min, CI ≤2.7 L/min/m², and CVP ≤2 mm Hg.
- Obtain and report clinical findings associated with decreased fluid volume: hypotension, tachypnea, tachycardia, dysrhythmias, capillary refill ≥3 seconds, peripheral pulses ≤+2, and cyanosis.
- Control external bleeding by applying direct pressure until other corrective measures can be taken.

- Monitor ECG continuously to assess HR and rhythm. Document ECG rhythm strips every 2 to 4 hours in patients with dysrhythmias.
- Monitor intake, output, specific gravity, chest tube drainage, daily weight to evaluate fluid balance. Report UO $\leq$30 mL/h or $\leq$0.5 mL/kg/h and weight loss $\geq$0.5 to 1.0 kg/d.
- Administer prescribed oxygen 2 to 4 L/min to maintain adequate tissue oxygenation.
- Administer IV fluids or blood as prescribed: crystalloids 3 mL/1mL of blood loss or blood 1 mL/1mL of blood loss.
- Administer IV colloids as prescribed: Dextran 40 reduces blood viscosity and improves microvascular blood flow; hetastarch, which rapidly expands blood volume, improves BP and enhances CO.
- Assist with autotransfusion if necessary.

High risk for infection related to invasive procedures or incisional drainage.

Expected Patient Outcomes. Patient is free of infection, as evidenced by normal temperature; white blood count (WBC) $\leq$11,000 μL; negative culture; or absence of redness, swelling, tenderness, or drainage from wound, incision, or cannulation site.

- Review results of WBC and cultures.
- Monitor temperature every 2 hours or as necessary if patient is febrile.
- Use aseptic technique when changing dressing or suctioning patient.
- Obtain culture or drainage from wound, incision, or cannulation site.
- Administer prescribed IV fluids to maintain adequate hydration.
- Administer antipyretics as prescribed.
- Instruct patient to report any discomfort at wound, incision, or cannulation site.

Pain related to altered pleural integrity.

Expected Patient Outcome. Patient experiences absence of or reduces verbalization of pain.

- Place patient on the unaffected side to decrease pain from the chest tube insertion site.
- Monitor the type, duration, and intensity of pain.
- Secure the chest tube to avoid its accidental removal.
- Administer analgesic as prescribed.
- Instruct patient to report pain on inspiration or expiration.
- Teach patient to splint the affected side while turning, coughing, or deep breathing.

Collaborative Problems

Common collaborative goals for patients with chest trauma are to prevent hypovolemic shock, increase CO, promote ventilation-perfusion balance, and correct hypoxemia.

Potential Complication: Hypovolemic Shock. Hypovolemic shock related to depleted intravascular volume secondary to hemorrhage.

Expected Patient Outcomes. Patient maintains adequate circulating volume, as evidenced by CO to 4 to 8 L/min, CI 2.7 to 4.3 L/min/m², CVP 2 to 6 mm Hg, pulmonary artery pressure (PAP) systolic 20 to 30 mm Hg or diastolic 8 to 15 mm Hg, PCWP 6 to 12 mm Hg, UO $\geq$30 mL/h or $\geq$0.5 mL/kg/h, specific gravity 1.010 to 1.030, peripheral pulses +2, capillary refill $\leq$3 seconds, BP within patient's normal range, MAP 70 to 100 mm Hg, absence of cyanosis, normal skin turgor, HR $\leq$100 bpm, RR 12 to 20 BPM, alertness, and absence of internal bleeding.

- Consult with physician to validate expected patient outcomes used to evaluate adequate circulating volume.
- Review results of hemoglobin, hematocrit, serum osmolality, serum electrolyte, and arterial blood gas measurements.
- Limit activity to bed rest while patient is hypotensive.
- Obtain and report hemodynamic parameters indicating hypovolemic shock: CO $\leq$4 L/min, CI $\leq$2.7 L/min/m², CVP $\leq$2 mm

Hg, and PAP systolic 20 to 30 mm Hg or diastolic 8 to 15 mm Hg.

- Obtain and report clinical findings associated with hypovolemic shock: hypotension, diaphoresis, tachycardia, tachypnea, capillary refill ≥3 seconds, peripheral pulses ≤+2, altered level of consciousness.
- Monitor intake, output, specific gravity, and daily weight. Report UO ≤30 mL/h or ≤0.5 mL/kg/h or weight loss ≥0.5 kg/d.
- Position patient in Trendelenburg, if not contraindicated, to enhance venous return, thereby augmenting arterial BP.
- Monitor for the presence of external bleeding and control with direct pressure to prevent further hemorrhaging.
- Monitor ECG continuously to assess HR and rhythm. Document ECG rhythm strips every 2 to 4 hours.
- Administer prescribed IV fluids to maintain adequate hydration and circulating volume: crystalloids 3 mL/1mL blood loss or 1 mL/1 mL blood loss.
- Administer prescribed oxygen 2 to 4 L/min or FIO_2 ≤50% to maintain PaO_2 ≥80 mm Hg or SaO_2 ≥95%.

Potential Complication: Decreased Cardiac Output. **Decreased CO** related to bleeding into the pleural space secondary to a hemothorax.

Expected Patient Outcomes. Patient maintains adequate CO, as evidenced by cardiac rhythm normal, CO 4 to 8 L/min, CI 2.7 to 4.3 L/min/m², CVP 2 to 6 mm Hg, PAP systolic 20 to 30 mm Hg or diastolic 8 to 15 mm Hg, PCWP 6 to 12 mm Hg, MAP 70 to 100 mm Hg, normal heart sounds, skin turgor normal, RR 12 to 20 BPM, normothermia, symmetric chest movement, normal breath sounds, absence of dysrhythmias, HR ≤100 bpm, and capillary refill ≤3 seconds.

- Consult with physician about the size of hemothorax and criteria needed for chest tube insertion and drainage: 200 mL blood loss/h for 3 to 4 h or when bleeding increases over

3 to 5 hours or more than 300 to 500 mL blood loss in 2 hours.
- Review results of blood studies, coagulation profile, and chest roentgenogram.
- Limit activity to bed rest to decrease bleeding into the pleural space.
- Elevate head of bed 45 to 60 degrees to enhance ventilation.
- Obtain and report hemodynamic parameters that indicate decreased CO: CO ≤4 L/min, CI ≤2.7 L/min/m², CVP ≤2 mm Hg, MAP ≤70 mm Hg, PAP systolic ≤20 mm Hg or diastolic ≤8 mm Hg, and PCWP ≤6 mm Hg.
- Monitor clinical indicators of perfusion; skin color, capillary refill, peripheral pulses, BP and pulse.
- Obtain and report clinical findings that indicate decreased CO secondary to hemothorax; difficulty breathing, distant or absent breath sounds on affected side, asymmetric chest movement, tachycardia, tachypnea, hypotension, narrow pulse pressure, restlessness, and elevated temperature.
- Assist with chest tube insertion to remove blood in the pleural space. Chest tube replacement is made after fluid resuscitation in order to prevent irreversible shock.
- Monitor the amount of chest tube drainage every hour. Report amount ≥100 mL/h.
- Secure chest tube to limit movement and subsequent irritation.
- Report any sudden increase in bright-red blood or excessive drainage from chest tube.
- Administer prescribed IV fluids or blood to maintain CO and tissue perfusion.
- Administer prescribed oxygen 2 to 4 L/min or FIO_2 ≤50% to maintain PaO_2 ≥80 mm Hg.
- Assist with autotransfusion to replace blood loss.
- Should an infected hemothorax exist, prepare patient for surgery.
- Administer prescribed analgesics to reduce pain.

- Teach patient to deep breathe and cough to expand lungs, prevent atelectasis, and remove secretions.
- Instruct patient to avoid stretching, reaching, or sudden movement, which could accidentally remove the chest tube.
- Instruct patient to report any chest pain.

Potential Complication: Ventilation-Perfusion Imbalance. Ventilation-perfusion imbalance related to parenchymal injury, altered alveolar-capillary membrane secondary to lung contusion, penetrating, or blunt chest injury.

Expected Patient Outcomes. Patient maintains adequate ventilation-perfusion balance, as evidenced by ventilation:perfusion ($\dot{V}/\dot{Q}$) ratio 1.0, physiological shunt ($\dot{Q}s/\dot{Q}t$) 0% to 8%, SaO_2 97%, $S\bar{v}O_2$ 75%, alveolar-arterial oxygen gradient ($P[A-a]O_2$) $\leq$15 mm Hg on room air or 10 to 65 mm Hg on 100% oxygen, arterial-alveolar oxygen tension ratio ($P[a:A]O_2$ 0.75 to 0.90, static compliance (Cst) $\geq$50 mL/cm H_2O, dynamic compliance (Cdyn) $\geq$45 mL/cm H_2O, RR 12 to 20 BPM, absence of adventitious breath sounds, absence of cyanosis, absence of dyspnea, CO 4 to 8 L/min, CI 2.7 to 4.3 L/min/m², PCWP 4 to 12 mm Hg, MAP 70 to 100 mm Hg, BP within patient's normal range, arterial blood gases within normal range, and HR $\leq$100 bpm.

- Consult with physician to validate expected patient outcomes used to evaluate ventilation-perfusion balance.
- Consult with physician about criteria used to determine when ventilatory support is needed: oxygenation (PaO_2 $\leq$60 mm Hg on FIO_2 50%), ventilation ($PaCO_2$ $\geq$50 to 60 mm Hg, which is $\geq$10 mm Hg above patient's normal $PaCO_2$), and respiratory mechanisms (apnea, sustained RR $\geq$35 BPM, and vital capacity $\leq$10 to 15 mL/kg).
- Confer with Respiratory Therapy regarding the appropriate ventilatory support for the chest trauma patient.
- Review results of arterial blood gas measurement, static lung compliance, dynamic lung compliance, physiological shunting, alveolar-arterial oxygen gradient, arterial-alveolar oxygen tension ratio, or ventilation-perfusion scan.
- Limit physical activity to bed rest in order to decrease the work of breathing.
- Obtain and report hemodynamic parameters that could affect ventilation-perfusion balance: CO $\leq$4 L/min, CI $\leq$2.7 L/min/m², PCWP $\leq$12 mm Hg, MAP $\leq$70 mm Hg, and $S\bar{v}O_2$ $\leq$60%.
- Obtain and report other clinical findings associated with decreased $\dot{V}/\dot{Q}$ ratio: tachypnea, cyanosis, crackles, dyspnea, and tachycardia.
- Monitor $\dot{V}/\dot{Q}$ ratio and report value $\leq$1.0, which signifies reduced alveolar ventilation. A low $\dot{V}/\dot{Q}$ ratio is referred to an intrapulmonary shunt (blood flow [$\dot{Q}s$]/total flow [$\dot{Q}t$] $\geq$15% to 30%.
- Obtain the following information in order to measure $\dot{Q}s/\dot{Q}t$: hemoglobin level, FIO_2 level, arterial and mixed venous blood gas results, and arterial and mixed venous oxyhemoglobin (oxygen saturation) values.
- Monitor alveolar partial pressure of oxygen (PAO_2) and arterial partial pressure of oxygen (PaO_2), which are approximately equal. Report a diversion of PAO_2 from $PaCO_2$ which signifies the development of an intrapulmonary shunt.
- Estimate $\dot{Q}s/\dot{Q}t$ using the following methods: PaO_2/FIO_2 ratio $\geq$286, arterial/alveolar (a/A) ratio $\geq$0.60, alveolar-arterial (A-a) gradient $\leq$20 mm Hg with an FIO_2 of 0.21, respiratory index $\leq$1, and shunt equation $\leq$5%.
- Monitor and report $PAO_2:FIO_2$ $\leq$200, which is considered to be a large intrapulmonary shunt (20%). The lower the value, the more severe the $\dot{Q}s/\dot{Q}t$ disturbance.
- Obtain and report SaO_2 $\leq$90%, which can signify intrapulmonary shunting.
- Assist with chest tube insertion.
- Monitor chest tube drainage for fluctuation and amount. Report $\geq$100 mL in first hour.
- Encourage patient to cough and deep breathe which increase ventilation and reinflate the lung.

- Encourage the use of the incentive spirometer to reexpand the lung and remove secretions.
- Measure intake, output, specific gravity, and daily weight. Excessive fluid accumulation increases total lung water, contributing to an increase in ventilation-perfusion imbalance.
- Monitor skin color for the presence of cyanosis, which can reflect the desaturation of at least 5 grams of hemoglobin and ventilation-perfusion mismatch.
- Evaluate the adequacy of oxygenation: oxygen delivery $\geq$600 mL/min/m^2, CI $\geq$2.7 L/min/m^2, and oxygen consumption (Vo_2) $\geq$156 mL/min/m^2.
- Administer prescribed humidified oxygen to keep Pao_2 $\geq$60 mm Hg.
- Administer IV fluids at the prescribed flow rate to maintain adequate hydration and to avoid excess fluid accumulation, which increases lung water causing increased $\dot{V}/\dot{Q}$ mismatch.
- Assist with intubation and initiation of mechanical ventilation in patients with Pao_2 $\leq$60 mm Hg on 40% Fio_2.
- Should fluid or air accumulate in the pleural space, removal is accomplished by means of thoracentesis before chest tubes are inserted.
- Administer analgesics to reduce voluntary splinting caused by pain and reduce gas exchange.
- Teach patient the importance of deep breathing and coughing.

Potential Complication: Hypoxemia. Hypoxemia related to decreased lung expansion, increased work of breathing, alveolar-capillary membrane damage secondary to blunt or penetrating injury and interstitial or interalveolar edema.

Expected Patient Outcomes. Patient maintains adequate oxygen gas exchange, as evidenced by intrapulmonary physiological shunt within normal limits, Pao_2 100 mm Hg, $Paco_2$ 40 mm Hg, oxygen consumption (resting) 250 mL/min, oxygen transport (resting) 1000 mL/min, $P(A-a)o_2$ $\leq$15 mm Hg, arterial oxygen concentration (Cao_2) 18 to 20 mL/100 mL, RR 12 to 20 BPM, HR $\leq$100 bpm, absence of crackles, and skin color normal.

- Review arterial blood gas, hemoglobin, and hematocrit values.
- Place in semi-Fowler's position to provide comfort and allow expansion of chest wall.
- Limit physical activity to bed rest to reduce oxygen demand.
- Assess breath sounds and presence of adventitious breath sounds every 1 to 2 hours. Pulmonary congestion, documented as crackles and wheezes, can indicate increased hydrostatic force in the pulmonary vascular system, causing fluid to move across the alveolar-capillary membrane.
- Should mechanical ventilation and intubation not be necessary, pulse oximetry measurement of Sao_2 and incentive spirometry measurement can be used to provide indirect data about lung compliance and hypoxemia.
- Monitor and report changes in the major factors of oxygen transport: CO $\leq$4 L/min, hemoglobin (Hgb) $\leq$12 g/dL, Sao_2 $\leq$90%, and Pao_2 $\leq$80 mm Hg.
- Monitor the amount and type of chest tube drainage.
- Change patient's position every 2 hours to enhance lung reexpansion, alveolar perfusion, and drainage.
- Monitor $\dot{Q}s/\dot{Q}t$ fraction at Fio_2 at 50% to 60%: Normal shunt fraction without a ventilator is 6% and with a ventilator is 10%.
- Suction patient using the principles of preoxygenation, short suctioning time, postsuctioning hyperinflation to reverse atelectasis and maintain uninterrupted PEEP.
- Administer prescribed IV fluids, such as crystalloids, to maintain adequate intravascular volume and PCWP 10 to 12 mm Hg.
- Administer prescribed analgesics to reduce pain during deep-breathing exercises.
- Instruct patient to cough, turn, and deep breathe to promote lung expansion

and to enhance oxygen–carbon dioxide exchange.

DISCHARGE PLANNING

The critical care nurse will provide patient and significant other(s) with verbal or written discharge notes regarding the following subjects:

1. Need to exercise to tolerance to avoid fatigue and need to plan rest periods.
2. Signs and symptoms that warrant medical attention: elevated temperature; cough; sudden, sharp chest pain; difficulty breathing; redness, pain, swelling, or tenderness of puncture wound.
3. Information about medications: name, dosage, schedule, or side effects.
4. Need to restrict activity that might stress the ribs or thoracic musculature.
5. How to use a pillow to decrease discomfort.

■ PLEURAL EFFUSION

For related information see Cardiac Deviations, Part I: Acute cardiac tamponade, p. 117; Dysrhythmias, p. 184; Part III: Hemodynamic monitoring, p. 219. Part I: Respiratory acidosis, p. 412; Respiratory alkalosis, p. 415. Part III: Pulse oximetry, p. 426; Mechanical ventilation, p. 425; Capnography, p. 439; Transcutaneous Pao_2 and $Paco_2$, p. 441; Indirect calorimetry, p. 441.

Case Management Basis
DRG: 85 Pleural effusion with complications
LOS: 6.80 days
DRG: 86 Pleural effusion without complications
LOS: 4.30 days

Definition
Normally pleural fluid, 25 mL, is produced to lubricate the surfaces of the visceral and parietal pleura. Pleural effusion is the accumulation of fluid in excess of fluid in the pleural space, which may reflect an increase in pleural fluid formation or decrease in fluid absorption from the intrapleural space.

Pathophysiology
Pleural effusions are frequently categorized as exudative and transudative. Exudative pleural effusion is associated with a disease of the pleural surface and is due either to increased permeability of capillaries with resultant leakage of proteins or to an obstruction in the lymphatic system inhibiting drainage of proteins. The pleural fluid protein: serum protein ratio is ≥ 0.5; the pleural fluid LDH:serum LDH ratio is ≥ 0.6; or pleural fluid LDH is more than two thirds the amount of the upper limit of normal serum LDH. Transudative pleural effusion leads to changes in pressure gradients between parietal and visceral pleura, involving an increase in hydrostatic pressure within pleural capillaries or decrease in colloidal osmotic pressure.

Fluid in the intrapleural space occupies space and displaces lung tissue by decreasing lung expansion, causing atelectasis. Pleural effusion may cause a mediastinal shift, leading to decreased compliance and altered ventilation-perfusion.

Nursing Assessment

PRIMARY CAUSES
- Exudative pleural fluid: Parapneumonic effusion, cancer, pulmonary embolism, emphysema, tuberculosis, connective tissue disease, viral infection, fungal infection, rickettsial infection, parasitic infection, asbestos pleural effusion, Meigs' syndrome, pancreatic disease, uremia, chronic atelectasis, chylothorax, sarcoidosis, drug reaction, or postmyocardial infarction syndrome.
- Transudative pleural fluid: Congestive heart failure, cirrhosis with ascites, nephrotic syndrome, peritoneal dialysis, myxedema, acute atelectasis, constrictive pericarditis, supe-

rior vena cava obstruction, or pulmonary embolism.

PHYSICAL ASSESSMENT

- Inspection: Pleurtic chest pain, fever, fatigue, shortness of breath, asymmetric chest expansion, dyspnea, or dry cough.
- Percussion: Dullness over effusion.
- Auscultation: Decreased or absent breath sounds over the affected area, egophony at upper level of the effusion, or friction rub.

DIAGNOSTIC TEST RESULTS

Standard Respiratory Laboratory Tests (see Table 3–1)

- Pleural fluid analysis: Transudates show white blood cells (WBC) ≤1000/μ, mononuclear cells in the differential, glucose level in pleural fluid equal to that of serum, and normal pH. Exudates show serum protein ratio ≥0.5 or pleural fluid LDH:serum LDH ratio ≥0.6.
- Laboratory tests of pleural fluid: Total and differential WBC, protein amylase, glucose, and LDH.

Invasive Respiratory Diagnostic Procedures (see Table 3–3)

- Computerized tomographic (CT) scanning: Detects small amount of free or loculated pleural fluid.
- Pleural biopsy: Used to evaluate tissues for causes of pleural effusion.

Noninvasive Respiratory Diagnostic Procedures (see Table 3–4)

- Chest roentgenogram: Free pleural fluid collects in the subpulmonic area, while larger amounts of fluid spill over into the costophrenic sulcus to form a meniscus; thickening of major and minor fissures; lateral displacement of the apex of the diaphragm and abrupt obliteration of lung markings at the level of the diaphragm are features of subpulmonic effusion; or round to oval collections of fluid in fissures resemble tumors. Less than 100 mL may be undetectable if the effusion is small.
- Ultrasound: Locates loculated or small effusions.

MEDICAL AND SURGICAL MANAGEMENT

THORACENTESIS

- A needle is inserted into the intercostal space along the upper surface of the lower rib. No more than 100 mL of fluid is drained and less if the patient experiences signs of respiratory distress.

NURSING MANAGEMENT: NURSING DIAGNOSES AND COLLABORATIVE PROBLEMS

Nursing Diagnoses

Common nursing goals for patients with pleural effusion are to restore normothermia, reduce fatigue, and support effective breathing pattern.

Hyperthermia related to pleural inflammation secondary to pleural effusion.

Expected Patient Outcomes. Patient's temperature is normal, pressure in pleural cavity is negative, and there is ≤20 mL of serous fluid in pleural cavity.

- Review results of pleural fluid (appearance, specific gravity, protein, WBC, red blood cells [RBC], glucose, and LDH), chest roentgenogram, ultrasound, or CT scan.
- Elevate the head to bed to facilitate breathing.
- Encourage patient to eat the prescribed amount of high protein or high carbohydrate.
- Monitor temperature every 2 hours or as necessary to evaluate the presence of infection.
- Administer prescribed IV fluids to maintain adequate hydration and circulating volume.

- Administer antibiotics as prescribed.
- Administer antipyretics as prescribed.

Fatigue related to dyspnea or pleural pain.

Expected Patient Outcome. Patient is able to maintain daily activities without fatigue.

- Monitor patient's activity tolerance; blood pressure (BP) within normal range, respiratory rate (RR) 12 to 20 BPM, and heart rate (HR) ≥20 bpm from patient's normal rate.
- Evaluate situations that contribute to patient's feeling fatigued.
- Provide rest periods before and after activity.
- Administer analgesics before increasing physical activity to lessen pleuritic pain.
- Instruct patient to report unusual feelings of fatigue.

Anxiety related to respiratory distress, fatigue, or pain.

Expected Patient Outcome. Patient verbalizes less anxiety and demonstrates relaxed position.

- Encourage patient to identify anxious feelings and when they occur.
- Evaluate the patient's and family's coping behaviors and their effectiveness in dealing with the current illness.
- Monitor patient's behavioral response to chest tube insertion.
- Teach patient strategies to reduce anxiety: meditation, progressive relaxation, or guided imagery.
- Teach patient the purposes behind invasive procedures and support patient through the procedure.

Ineffective breathing pattern related to decreased lung expansion secondary to increased fluid in the pleural space.

Expected Patient Outcomes. Patient maintains effective breathing pattern, as evidenced by RR ≤30 BPM, HR ≤100 bpm, absence of tachypnea or dyspnea, symmetrical chest movements, absence of pleural pain, chest tube patent and draining, full lung expansion, and absence of adventitious breath sounds.

- Review arterial blood gas results and chest roentgenogram.
- Limit physical activity to bed rest while patient is experiencing chest pain.
- Obtain and report clinical findings that indicate ineffective breathing pattern secondary to fluid accumulation in the pleural space: shortness of breath, dyspnea, cyanosis, jugular vein distention, diminished or absent breath sounds, pleural friction rub, elevated temperature, and cough.
- Encourage patient to use incentive spirometer to facilitate lung expansion and prevent atelectasis.
- Splint patient's chest when coughing to reduce pain.
- Administer prescribed IV fluids to maintain adequate hydration.
- Administer prescribed oxygen 2 to 4 L/min by means of nasal catheter or mask to maintain partial pressure of arterial oxygen (Pao_2) ≥70 mm Hg.
- Administer prescribed antibiotics should an infection occur.
- Administer prescribed antipyretics when patient is febrile.
- Administer prescribed analgesics to relieve pain.
- Teach patient to cough, turn, and deep breathe every 2 to 4 hours.
- Teach patient to perform active range of motion exercises to all extremities every 2 to 4 hours.

DISCHARGE PLANNING

The critical care nurse will provide patient and significant other(s) with verbal or written discharge notes regarding the following subjects:

1. Signs and symptoms that require medical attention: difficulty in breathing, chest pain, elevated temperature, or persistent cough.
2. Medication's dosage, schedule, route, and side effects.

3. Importance of keeping all postdischarge appointments.

■ PULMONARY EMBOLISM

For related information see Cardiac Deviations, Part I: Dysrhythmias, p. 184; Part III: Hemodynamic monitoring, p. 219. Part I: Pulmonary embolism, p. 397; Respiratory acidosis, p. 412; Respiratory alkalosis, p. 415. Part III: Pulse oximetry, p. 426; Mechanical ventilation, p. 428; Capnography, p. 439; Transcutaneous Pao_2 and $Paco_2$, p. 441; Indirect calorimetry, p. 441.

Case Management Basis

DRG: 78 Pulmonary embolism
LOS: 8.70 days

Definition

A pulmonary embolism is an occlusion of one or more pulmonary vessels by matter that has traveled from a source outside the lung. Most pulmonary embolisms are the result of thrombi that have dislodged from the deep veins of the leg and pelvis. Pulmonary embolism can be either acute or massive. Acute or submassive pulmonary embolism results from emboli that are small in size and several in number. Small emboli tend to lodge in the distal branches of the pulmonary artery at the periphery of the lung. Massive pulmonary embolism involves one or more of the lobar arteries.

Pathophysiology

Virchow's triad is used to describe three conditions that favor clot formation: venostasis, endothelial disruption of the vessel lining, and hypercoagulability. Local concentration of coagulation factors in conjunction with vessel wall injury can provide a place for clots to form. As the flow of blood slows, clot forms and extends up to the vein. The clot pulls away from the vessel wall and floats as an embolus. Once the clot lodges in the pulmonary capillary bed, it obstructs blood flow beyond the point of lodgment. There are three primary consequences associated with pulmonary embolism: increased alveolar dead space, meaning an alveolar area that is ventilated but receives no blood flow; pneumoconstriction, where ventilated nonperfused lung zone is reduced in functional size; and loss of surfactant, which normally stabilizes and prevents the collapse of alveoli. Secondary pulmonary consequences consists of dyspnea and arterial hypoxemia. The primary hemodynamic consequence of pulmonary embolism is pulmonary arterial hypertension, which occurs when more than 50% of the pulmonary vascular bed is occluded, thereby reducing the available cross-sectional area. The reduction leads to three physiologic responses: increased pulmonary artery resistance, increased pulmonary artery pressure, and increased right ventricular work.

Nursing Assessment

PRIMARY CAUSES

- Venous stasis can occur from bed rest, prolonged standing, prolonged sitting, congestive heart failure, atrial fibrillation, or decreased cardiac output. Injury of vascular endothelium can be attributable to local trauma, venous disease, incision, sepsis, or atherosclerosis. Another cause may be hypercoagulability.

RISK FACTORS

- Elderly age group; surgery such as cholecystectomy or colectomy; injury from hip fracture; cardiopulmonary causes such as chronic obstructive pulmonary disease (COPD) or cor pulmonale; cancer of the pancreas, stomach, or lung; and pregnancy.

PHYSICAL ASSESSMENT

- Inspection: Dyspnea, apprehension, cough, diaphoresis, syncope, restlessness, weakness, cyanosis, hemoptysis, pleuritic chest pain, fever, edema, or jugular vein distention.
- Percussion: Lungs may be dull.

- Palpation: Pulses may be normal, weak, thready, or strong; right ventricular heave; localized edema; or tense muscle tissue.
- Auscultation: Tachycardia; tachypnea; rales, wheezing, and decreased breath sounds; S_3, S_4 gallop, split P_2 sound; murmur; and pleural friction rub.

DIAGNOSTIC TEST RESULTS

Standard Laboratory Tests (see Table 2–6)

- Arterial blood gases: pH ≥ 7.44, partial pressure of arterial oxygen (Pao_2) ≤ 80 mm Hg, partial pressure of arterial carbon dioxide ($Paco_2$) ≤ 35 mm Hg, increased alveolar-arterial oxygen tension difference $P(A-a)o_2 \geq 25$.
- Blood chemistry: white blood cells (WBC) $\geq 15,000/mm^3$, increased lactate dehydrogenase (LDH) and increased bilirubin.
- Coagulation studies: Increased serum fibrinogen degradation products (FDP).

Invasive Respiratory Diagnostic Procedures (see Table 3–3)

- Contrast venography: Deep vein thrombosis.
- Impedance phlebography: Increased pressure in distal vein leading to distention or decrease in the maximum rate at which blood can flow out of the leg.
- Pulmonary arteriography: The presence of a filling defect or cutoff of an artery confirms the diagnosis.
- Radioactive fibrinogen test: Detects small thrombi in the muscular veins of the calf.
- Radionuclide venography: Detects occlusive venous disease proximal to the knee.
- Ventilation-perfusion lung scan: *Perfusion:* Embolus denies the radioisotopes access to a segment of the lung and appears as a perfusion deficit. Shows absence of perfusion to the region of the lung supplied by the occluded blood vessel. *Ventilation:* Lung ventilation is immediately altered, since pulmonary embolism is a vascular abnormality.

Noninvasive Respiratory Diagnostic Procedures (see Table 3–4)

- Chest roentgenogram: Can reveal difference in the diameter of normally equal-sized vessels, since one vessel is blocked and the other may have to accommodate pulmonary blood flow; abrupt cessation of a vessel resulting from obstruction; shadow of a clot with no blood flow distally; and diaphragmatic elevation.

ECG

- Sinus tachycardia, peaked P wave, S wave in lead I, Q wave in lead III, ST segment depression, and T wave inversion in lead III.

MEDICAL AND SURGICAL MANAGEMENT

PHARMACOLOGY

- Anticoagulants: Continuous intravenous heparin at a loading dose of 2000 to 3000 U to prevent thrombus formation.
- Thrombolytic agents: Streptokinase and tissue type plasminogen activator (tPA) are used in patients with massive pulmonary thromboembolism with severe hemodynamic consequences (see Table 1–8, p. 32).

NONPHARMACOLOGICAL THERAPY

- The methods used to prevent thrombus formation are early ambulation, use of elastic stockings, leg elevation, and exercise machine.

SURGICAL INTERVENTION

- Vena caval interruption: Since most thrombi originate in the lower extremities, vena caval interruption is effective in preventing embolization to the pulmonary bed. There are a variety of techniques for vena caval interruption (ligation, plication a clips, and filter). Of these various techniques, the Greenfield filter is preferred. These devices block the passage of a clot yet allow blood to continue flowing through the vena cava (see Vena caval interruption, p. 417).

- Embolectomy: Should the patient experience a massive pulmonary embolus with significant hemodynamic instability, a transcatheter embolectomy is performed through either the common femoral or jugular vein.

NURSING MANAGEMENT: NURSING DIAGNOSES AND COLLABORATIVE PROBLEMS

Nursing Diagnoses

Common nursing goals for patients with pulmonary embolism are to increase pulmonary tissue perfusion, enhance physical mobility, promote effective breathing pattern, maintain fluid balance, reduce pain, prevent injury, and encourage communication.

Altered pulmonary tissue perfusion related to clot formation secondary to a thromboembolic disorder.

Expected Patient Outcomes. Patient maintains adequate pulmonary tissue perfusion, as evidenced by respiratory rate (RR) 12 to 20 BPM, heart rate (HR) $\leq$100 bpm, arterial blood gases within normal range, absence of adventitious breath sounds, pulmonary artery pressure (PAP) 20 to 30/8 to 15 mm Hg, pulmonary capillary wedge pressure (PCWP) 6 to 12 mm Hg, central venous pressure (CVP) 2 to 6 mm Hg, right atrial pressure (RAP) 4 to 6 mm Hg, right ventricular pressure (RVP) 25/0 to 5 mm Hg, absence of cyanosis, skin warm and dry or urine output (UO) $\geq$30 mL/h or $\geq$0.5 mL/kg/h, pulmonary vascular resistance (PVR) 155 to 255 dynes/s/cm^{-5}, or pulmonary vascu-lar resistance index (PVRI) 200 to 450 dynes/s/cm^{-5}/m^2.

- Consult with physician to validate expected patient outcomes used to evaluate pulmonary tissue perfusion.
- Review results of chest roentgenogram, ventilation-perfusion scan, ECG, pulmonary arteriography, WBC, coagulation profile, and arterial blood gas measurement.

- Position patient in semi- or high Fowler's position with frequent change of position from side to side: Turning improves gas exchange in different lung segments.
- Obtain and report hemodynamic parameters that indicate altered pulmonary tissue perfusion: CO $\leq$4 L/min, CI $\leq$2.7 L/min/m^2, PAP systolic $\geq$30 mm Hg or diastolic $\geq$15 mm Hg, PCWP $\geq$12 mm Hg, PVR $\geq$255 dynes/s/cm^{-5}, and PVRI $\geq$450 dynes/sec/cm^{-5}/m^2.
- Monitor clinical indicators of respiratory status: respiratory depth, regularity, skin color, use of accessory muscles, chest expansion, and respiratory effort.
- Obtain and report clinical findings that indicate altered pulmonary tissue perfusion: dyspnea, tachypnea, tachycardia, shortness of breath, chest and shoulder pain, restlessness, confusion, hypotension, and cyanosis.
- Obtain and report clinical findings associated with venous thrombosis: tenderness, warmth, pain, peripheral pulses $\leq$+2, capillary refill $\geq$3 seconds, and peripheral edema.
- Measure the circumference of each extremity every day or as necessary to assess the presence of edema secondary to altered venous blood flow.
- Monitor ECG continuously to assess HR and rhythm. Document ECG every 2 to 4 hours in patients with dysrhythmias resulting from pulmonary embolisms.
- Apply antiembolic hose to both lower extremities and remove for 20 minutes each shift to allow for the filling of superficial capillaries.
- Observe patient for clinical indicators of hypercoagulopathy: bleeding, bruising, petechiae, ecchymosis, or hematuria.
- Encourage patient to deep breathe hourly to expand the lungs.
- Provide oxygenation at the prescribed fraction of inspired oxygen (FIO$_2$) rate to support tissue oxygenation.
- Administer low-molecular-weight dextran as the plasma expander, if appropriate, because of its antithrombotic effect, facilita-

tion of clot lysis, and effect in reducing platelet activity.

- Administer heparin therapy to prevent clot development and allow lysis and endotheliazation of existing clots: loading does 5000 to 10,000 U IV and continuous infusion 1000 U/h (see Table 1–8, p. 32).
- Administer antiplatelet substance (dipyridamole [Persantine]), a mild vasodilator to reduce platelet aggregation by inhibiting the enzyme phosphodiesterase (see Table 1–8, p. 32).
- Administer thrombolytic agents to cause clot dissolution by activating plasminogen to form plasmin, a nonspecific proteolytic enzyme (see Cardiac Deviations, Thrombolytic therapy, p. 265).
- Administer warfarin to inhibit hepatic production of factors VII, IX, and X and prothrombin.
- Should pharmacological therapy be ineffective, prepare patient for pulmonary embolectomy when there is greater than 50% obstruction of the pulmonary circulation.
- Instruct patient to report any pain on breathing.

Mobility impaired physical related to deep vein thrombosis or surgical interruption of venous clot.

Expected Patient Outcomes. Patient maintains normal mobility, as evidenced by peripheral pulses +2; capillary refill ≤3 seconds; peripheral skin pink and warm; absence of redness, tenderness, or swelling in extremity; and ability to gradually increase mobility without complications.

- Review results of impedance phlebography, contrast venography, radioactive fibrinogen test, or fibrinogen degradation products.
- Limit physical activity to bed rest, then progress to out of bed as prescribed.
- Apply antithromboembolic or elastic stockings to promote venous return and to maintain peripheral blood flow.
- Monitor the extremities for tenderness, swelling, or pain in the calf or popliteal areas.

- Reduce venous stasis through active or passive exercises: Muscular activity promotes venous flow by alternately compressing and releasing the veins.
- Monitor all peripheral pulses for their quality and equality.
- Apply prophylactic intermittent pneumatic compression before patient develops deep vein thrombosis: Increase venous flow and hemodynamically increase the stress in the vein wall and reduce blood pooling. A sleeve-like cuff that fits over the calf or the calf and thigh is inflated at regular intervals by an external pump, which milks the calf and thigh by simple pneumatic compression.
- Prepare patient for ligation: Bilateral femoral vein ligation is attempted if the thrombi are located proximal to the groin.
- Prepare patient for other surgical techniques if embolization occurs despite femoral vein ligation: ligation of the inferior vena cava, plication, clipping, or suturing with mattress sutures to form a grid in the venous system.
- Prepare patient for the placement of an intraluminal umbrella to obstruct the passage of the emboli or a Greenfield filter, which has slender legs with little hooks in their ends that anchor the device to the vena caval wall.
- Prepare patient for possible embolectomy if manifesting severe hemodynamic compromise, such as shock, that does not respond to more conservative measures.
- Instruct patient as to risk factors causing deep vein thrombosis and possible thromboembolism.

Ineffective breathing pattern related to tachypnea or dyspnea secondary to pleuritic pain.

Expected Patient Outcomes. Patient maintains effective breathing pattern, as evidenced by RR ≤30 BPM, adequate thoracic expansion, symmetrical diaphragmatic excursion, absence of adventitious breath sounds, and normal skin color.

- Consult with respiratory therapist regarding the patient's ventilatory mode and settings.
- Review results of arterial blood gas measurement, chest roentgenogram, pulmonary function tests, and lung scan.
- Place patient in a semi- to high Fowler's position to allow more effective lung expansion.
- Monitor for evidence of diminished thoracic expansion, asymmetrical diaphragmatic excursion, accentuated point of maximal impulse (PMI), tenderness, and decrease in vocal or tactile fremitus.
- Auscultate the chest for abnormal breath sounds, diminished breath sounds, friction rub, rales (crackles), rhonchi, or wheezing.
- Obtain and report clinical findings associated with ineffective breathing pattern: tachypnea, crackles, use of accessory muscles, and cyanosis.
- Encourage patient to use incentive spirometer to facilitate lung expansion.
- Administer prescribed oxygen 2 to 4 L/min to support tissue oxygenation.
- Administer narcotic or analgesic to relieve pain.
- Instruct patient to deep breathe, thereby stimulating respiratory muscles and enhancing gas exchange.
- Teach patient to report pain upon inspiration or expiration.

Fluid volume deficit related to bleeding secondary to anticoagulants or thrombolytic therapy.

Expected Patient Outcomes. Patient maintains adequate fluid volume, as evidenced by coagulation profile within normal limits, absence of bleeding, blood pressure (BP) within patient's normal range, mean arterial pressure (MAP) 70 to 100 mm Hg, HR ≤100 bpm, peripheral pulses ≤+2, capillary refill ≥3 seconds, normal skin turgor and color, hemoglobin and hematocrit within normal range, stable weight, and UO ≥ 30 mL/h.

- Review results of coagulation profile, hemoglobin, and hematocrit.

- Place in high Fowler's position to enhance breathing and decrease oxygen demand.
- Limit activity to bed rest until pulmonary embolus has stabilized or corrected.
- Monitor patient for the presence of bleeding from cannulation site or incision.
- Obtain and report clinical findings associated with fluid volume deficit: poor skin turgor, skin pale or cyanotic, peripheral pulses ≤+2, capillary refill ≥3 seconds, tachycardia, and hypotension.
- Measure intake, output, and daily weight. Report UO ≤30 mL/h or ≤0.5 mL/kg/h.
- Administer the prescribed IV fluids to replenish or maintain a stable blood volume.
- Administer prescribed oxygen 2 to 4 L/min to support tissue oxygenation.

Pain related to pleural effusion or deep calf pain.

Expected Patient Outcome. Patient experiences absence of pleural or deep calf pain.

- Monitor and report the presence of pleuritic pain or deep calf pain.
- Encourage patient to describe any pleural or deep calf pain on a scale of 1 to 10.
- Assess complaints of pain including severity, location, radiation, duration, and quality.
- Encourage deep breathing to minimize atelectasis and improve distribution of gases.
- Provide comfort measures such as position change or back care to alleviate pain.
- Administer analgesics to relieve pain as prescribed.
- Instruct patient to report any pain or changes in the severity or duration of pain.
- Teach patient to splint chest with pillow when coughing, deep breathing, or repositioning to decrease pain.
- Teach patient how to reduce pain through meditation, progressive relaxation, or guided imagery.

High risk for injury related to bleeding secondary to anticoagulant therapy or thrombolytic therapy.

Expected Patient Outcomes. Patient is free of injury, as evidenced by absence of bleeding in stool, sputum, or urine, absence of petechiae, and coagulation tests are within normal range.

- Review results of coagulation profile.
- Monitor and report blood in the urine, sputum, or stool.
- Observe all invasive catheter sites for evidence of bleeding.
- Apply pressure dressings to puncture sites to prevent local hematoma formation.
- Follow safety protocol following thrombolytic therapy: provide safe environment for restless patient, limit cuff blood pressure use, and avoid venipuncture and intramuscular injections.
- Administer prescribed IV fluids to maintain adequate hydration and circulatory volume.
- Administer prescribed oxygen 2 to 4 L/min to maintain tissue oxygenation.
- Should bleeding be attributed to anticoagulation therapy, administer prescribed protamine sulfate to neutralize heparin.
- Instruct patient to avoid use of aspirin and nonsteroidal inflammatory drugs because they can prolong episodes of bleeding.
- Instruct patient to use electric razor, gentle teeth brushing, and avoid scratching skin.

Communication, impaired verbal related to intubation or mechanical ventilation.

Expected Patient Outcomes. Patient is able to express needs verbally or by using nonverbal devices.

- Encourage intubated patient to express needs and concerns nonverbally via a magic slate board.
- Explain any treatment or diagnostic procedures to patient.
- Encourage family to include the patient in family discussions.
- Teach the patient to use alternative ways to communicate.

Collaborative Problems

Common collaborative problems in patients with pulmonary embolism are to correct ventilation-perfusion imbalance, increase functional residual capacity and increase cardiac output.

Potential Complication: Ventilation-Perfusion Imbalance. Ventilation-perfusion imbalance related to thromboembolism disorder secondary to abnormal blood flow or abnormal vascular integrity.

Expected Patient Outcomes. Arterial blood gases within normal range, absence of pleuritic pain, absence of adventitious breath sounds, RR 12 to 20 BPM, HR ≤ 100 bpm, BP within patient's normal range, arterial oxygen saturation (Sao_2) 97%, mixed venous oxygen saturation ($S\bar{v}o_2$) 75%, cardiac output (CO) 4 to 8 L/min, cardiac index (CI) 2.7 to 4.3 L/min/m², arterial-alveolar oxygen tension ratio ($P(a-A)o_2$) ≤ 0.75, ventilation/perfusion ($\dot{V}/\dot{Q}$) ratio 1.0, physiological shunt ($\dot{Q}s/\dot{Q}t$) 0% to 8%, absence of cyanosis, MAP 70 to 100 mm Hg, PAP 20 to 30/8 to 15 mm Hg, PCWP 6 to 12 mm Hg, hemoglobin within normal range.

- Confer with physician to validate expected patient outcomes used to evaluate the presence of ventilation-perfusion imbalance.
- Review results of ventilation-perfusion scan, chest roentgenogram, arterial blood gas measurement, pulmonary arteriography, contrast venography, coagulation profile, radioactive fibrinogen test, or FDP.
- Position in semi- to high Fowler's position to enhance lung expansion.
- Obtain and report clinical findings that indicate ventilation-perfusion imbalance: dyspnea, shortness of breath, restlessness, cyanosis, altered level of consciousness, and tachypnea.
- Monitor and report changes in adequacy of oxygenation: CO 4 L/min, hemoglobin ≤ 12 g/dL, Sao_2 $\leq 90\%$, and Pao_2 ≤ 80 mm Hg.

- Obtain and report $\dot{V}/\dot{Q}$ ratio ≥ 0.8, which signifies reduced blood flow relative to alveolar ventilation. An increase in the $\dot{V}/\dot{Q}$ ratio is referred to as physiological dead space.
- Encourage patient to cough, deep breathe, and use incentive spirometer to increase oxygen–carbon dioxide exchange and increase Pao_2 concentration.
- Administer prescribed humidified oxygen 2 to 4 L/min by means of nasal cannula or mask to maintain $Pao_2 \geq 70$ mm Hg, $Sao_2 \geq 95\%$, keep mucous membrane moist, and mobilize secretions to enhance airway clearance.
- Administer prescribed bronchodilators (aminophylline) to decrease bronchoconstriction and enhance alveolar ventilation.
- Administer prescribed analgesics to relieve pain and reduce work of breathing.
- Administer prescribed thrombolytic therapy to lyse clots (see Table 1–8, p. 32, and Cardiac Deviations, Thrombolytic Therapy, p. 265).
- Administer prescribed heparin to inhibit thrombus growth, resolve formed thrombus, and prevent additional embolus formation.
- Should pharmacological therapy be ineffective, prepare patient for inferior vena caval interruption or pulmonary embolectomy (see Venal caval interruption, p. 417).
- Administer prescribed low-molecular-weight dextran to increase pulmonary blood flow to underperfused segments and increase oxygen saturation.

Potential Complication: Decreased Functional Residual Capacity.
Decreased functional residual capacity related to increased physiological dead space secondary to decreased pulmonary capillary perfusion.

Expected Patient Outcomes.
Patient maintains adequate functional residual capacity FRC, as evidenced by RR 12 to 20 BPM, arterial blood gases within normal range, Sao_2 95%, $S\bar{v}o_2$ 60% to 80%, and FRC 3.0 L.

- Consult with respiratory therapist regarding the desired positive end-expiratory pressure (PEEP) level to FRC.
- Review results of chest roentgenogram, arterial blood gas measurement, ECG, pulmonary arteriography, and lung scan.
- Monitor patient's lung compliance in relation to weaning from the ventilator, if necessary, and report static compliance ≤ 50 mL/H_2O and dynamic compliance ≤ 35 mL/H_2O.
- Monitor clinical indicators of respiratory status: rate, rhythm, and regularity of respiration; symmetry of chest movement; skin color; and use of accessory muscles.
- Suction patient using the principles of preoxygenation, short suctioning time, post-suctioning hyperinflation to reverse atelectasis and maintain uninterrupted PEEP.
- Encourage patient to cough, deep breathe, and change position.
- Monitor $\dot{V}/\dot{Q}$: Tidal volume minus dead space times respiratory rate divided by stroke volume, which is expressed as the formula $V_I - V_{DS} \times RR/SV$.
- Administer prescribed oxygen with humidification by mask or endotracheal tube to prevent the complication of hypoxemia: cardiac dysrhythmia, myocardial ischemia, and cerebral ischemia.
- Provide patient with prescribed ventilatory support, if necessary, including PEEP to improve gas exchange.

Potential Complication: Decreased Cardiac Output.
Decreased CO related to altered right ventricular preload and afterload secondary to pulmonary hypertension.

Expected Patient Outcomes.
Patient maintains adequate CO, as evidenced by CVP 2 to 6 mm Hg, right ventricular stroke work index (RVSWI) 7 to 12 g/m^2/beat, pulmonary vascular resistance (PVR) 155 to 255 dynes/s/cm^{-5}, pulmonary vascular resistance index (PVRI) 200 to 450 dynes/s/cm^{-5}/m^2, PAP 20 to 30/8 to 15 mm Hg, RAP 4 to 6 mm Hg, RVP 25/0

to 5 mm Hg, RR 12 to 20 BPM, HR ≤100 bpm, SaO_2 95%, normal heart sounds, absence of peripheral edema, and absence of distended neck veins.

- Consult with physician to validate expected patient outcomes used to evaluate effective right ventricular preload and afterload.
- Obtain and report hemodynamic parameters that suggest altered right ventricular preload and afterload: CVP ≥6 mm Hg, RVSWI ≤7 g/beat/m^2, PVR ≥250 dynes/s/cm^{-5}, PVRI ≥450 dynes/s/cm^{-5}/m^2, PAP systolic ≥30 mm Hg or diastolic ≥15 mm Hg, and RAP ≥6 mm Hg.
- Obtain and report clinical findings that suggest altered right ventricular preload and afterload: neck vein distention, tachycardia, tachypnea, S_3 and S_4, and peripheral edema.
- Monitor intake, output, and daily weight. Report UO ≤30 mL/h or ≤0.5 mL/kg/h and weight gain ≥0.5 kg/d.
- Administer prescribed oxygen at 2 to 4 L/min via nasal cannula or mask to maintain tissue oxygenation as evidenced by SaO_2 95%.
- Administer prescribed diuretics to maintain UO ≥30 mL/h or ≥0.5 mL/kg/h.
- Administer prescribed narcotic (morphine sulfate) to increase systemic vascular dilation and reduce venous return, thereby decreasing the work load of the heart.

DISCHARGE PLANNING

The critical care nurse will provide patient and significant other(s) with verbal or written discharge notes regarding the following subjects:

1. Technique used to prevent deep vein thrombosis: avoiding sitting or standing for long periods of time, elevation of legs while sitting, use of antiembolic stockings and exercise such as walking.
2. Importance of keeping scheduled appointments.
3. Signs and symptoms that need to be reported to physician: sharp, sudden chest pain; bloody urine, sputum, or stool; and elevated temperature.
4. Medication's purpose, dosage, route, schedule, and side effects.

■ PULMONARY HYPERTENSION

(For related information see Cardiac Deviations, Part I: Dysrhythmias, p. 184; Part III: Hemodynamic monitoring, p. 219. Part I: Pulmonary embolism, p. 397; Respiratory acidosis, p. 412; Respiratory alkalosis, p. 415. Part III: Pulse oximetry, p. 426; Mechanical ventilation, p. 428; Capnography, p. 439; Transcutaneous PaO_2 and PaCO_2, p. 441; Indirect calorimetry, p. 441.)

Case Management Basis

DRG: 101 Other respiratory system diagnosis with complications
LOS: 5.10 days
DRG: 102 Other respiratory system diagnosis without complications
LOS: 3.30 days

Definition

Pulmonary hypertension is a disorder of the pulmonary vasculature that is diagnosed when the pulmonary artery systolic pressures ≥30 mm Hg.

Pathophysiology

With pulmonary hypertension, the medial layer of the pulmonary arteries usually hypertrophies. The system then loses its ability to adapt to increased blood flow or hypoxia. The hypoxia causes vasoconstriction that increases PAP ≥40/15 mm Hg and increases pulmonary vascular resistance. The end-diastolic pressure in the right ventricle also elevates. The right ventricle undergoes hypertrophy and further increases systolic pressure. As the disease progresses, jugular venous distention, hepatomegaly, and peripheral edema occur. Increased pulmonary artery pressure increases pulmonary vascular resistance. The pulmonary capillaries tend to dilate to accommodate for the increased blood flow.

Nursing Assessment

PRIMARY CAUSES
- Reduction in cross-sectional areas of the pulmonary arterial bed, such as vasoconstriction resulting from hypoxia of any cause or acidosis; loss of vessels as a result of lung resection, emphysema, vasculitis, pulmonary fibrosis, or connective tissue disease; obstruction of vessels from pulmonary embolism, in situ thrombosis, or schistosomiasis; or narrowing of vessels because of structural changes resulting from pulmonary hypertension.
- Increased pulmonary venous pressure resulting from constrictive pericarditis, left ventricular failure or reduced compliance, mitral stenosis, left atrial myxoma, pulmonary veno-occlusive disease, or mediastinal diseases compressing pulmonary veins.
- Increased pulmonary blood flow from congenital left-to-right intracardial shunts.
- Increased blood viscosity caused by polycythemia.

PHYSICAL ASSESSMENT
- Inspection: Dyspnea, fatigue, chest pain or syncope on exertion, orthopnea, tachypnea, hyperventilation, cyanosis, peripheral edema, or distended neck veins.
- Palpation: Precordial palpation reveals right ventricular heave or impulse over the main pulmonary artery.
- Auscultation: Split S_2 with loud pulmonic component and pulmonary ejection click, crackles, or right ventricular diastolic gallop.

DIAGNOSTIC TEST RESULTS

Hemodynamic Parameters (see Table 1–9, p. 40)
- Pulmonary artery pressure (PAP) $\geq 40/15$ mm Hg, pulmonary vascular resistance (PVR) ≥ 255 dynes/s/cm^{-5}, pulmonary vascular resistance index (PVRI) ≥ 450

dynes/s/cm^{-5}/m^2, and mean PAP (MPAP) ≥ 20 mm Hg.

Standard Laboratory Tests (see Table 1–1, p. 3)
- Arterial blood gases: partial pressure of arterial oxygen (Pao$_2$) ≤ 60 mm Hg and partial pressure of arterial carbon dioxide (Paco$_2$) ≥ 45 mm Hg.
- Blood studies: Elevated complete blood count (CBC) and hematocrit.

Invasive Respiratory Diagnostic Procedures (see Table 3–3)
- Pulmonary angiography: Shows presence of embolus as a cause of pulmonary hypertension.
- Open lung biopsy: Can establish the type of pulmonary vascular disease.
- Ventilation-perfusion lung scan: Used to identify patient with major vessel thrombotic pulmonary hypertension.

Noninvasive Diagnostic Procedures
- Echocardiography: Reveals right ventricular enlargement and paradoxic motion of the interventricular septum.
- Chest roentgenogram: Dilation of the right and left main and lobar pulmonary arteries, enlargement of the pulmonary outflow tract, right ventricular and right atrial enlargement.

ECG
- Right ventricular hypertrophy, right atrial enlargement, or right axis deviation.

MEDICAL AND SURGICAL MANAGEMENT

PHARMACOLOGY
- Bronchodilators: Bronchodilators such as aminophylline, isoproterenol, or terbutaline are used to decrease PVR, improve gas exchange, and decrease vasoconstriction of the pulmonary vascular bed (see Table 3–6).
- Vasodilators: Vasodilators such as nitrates, hydralazone, and calcium channel blockers are used to reverse pulmonary vasocon-

striction (see Table 1–4, p. 20, and Table 1–6, p. 28).

- Diuretics: Used to reduce circulating volume, which decreases pulmonary artery pressure.

OXYGEN THERAPY

- Supplemental oxygen is given to reduce hypoxia and subsequently reduce pulmonary vascular vasoconstriction.

NURSING MANAGEMENT: NURSING DIAGNOSES AND COLLABORATIVE PROBLEMS

Nursing Diagnoses

Common nursing goals for patients with pulmonary hypertension are to increase pulmonary tissue perfusion and improve gas exchange.

Altered pulmonary tissue perfusion related to thromboembolism secondary to vasoconstriction.

Expected Patient Outcomes. Patient maintains adequate pulmonary tissue perfusion, as evidenced by respiratory rate (RR) ≤ 30 BPM, absence of cyanosis, normal coagulation profile, pulmonary capillary wedge pressure (PCWP) 6 to 12 mm Hg, PAP 20 to 30/8 to 15 mm Hg, PVR 100 to 250 dynes/s/cm^{-5}, blood pressure (BP) within patient's normal range, absence of adventitious breath sounds, arterial oxygen saturation (SaO_2) 95%, and arterial blood gases within normal range.

- Review results of ventilation-perfusion scanning, arterial blood gas measurements, ventilation/perfusion $\dot{V}/\dot{Q}$ ratio and chest roentgenogram.
- Limit physical activity to bed rest to reduce the work of breathing and oxygen demand.
- Obtain and report hemodynamic parameters that may indicate altered pulmonary tissue perfusion: PAP systolic ≥ 30 mm Hg or diastolic ≥ 15 mm Hg, PCWP ≥ 12 mm Hg and PVR ≥ 255 dynes/s/cm^{-5}.
- Monitor clinical indicators of respiratory status: rate, depth, symmetry of chest excursion, skin color, use of accessory mus-

cles, and presence of adventitious breath sounds.
- Obtain and report clinical findings associated with altered pulmonary tissue perfusion: tachypnea, tachycardia, cyanosis, and adventitious breath sounds.
- Apply antiembolic stockings to enhance venous return.
- Administer prescribed IV fluids to maintain adequate circulatory volume.
- Administer prescribed oxygen 2 to 4 L/min to maintain PaO_2 ≥ 80 mm Hg and SaO_2 ≥ 95%.
- Administer prescribed heparin to correct thromboembolism.

Impaired gas exchange related to alveolar-capillary membrane changes secondary to intra-alveolar fluid accumulation.

Expected Patient Outcomes. Patient maintains adequate gas exchange, as evidenced by RR ≤ 30 BPM, SaO_2 95%, mixed venous-oxygen saturation (S$\bar{v}O_2$ 60% to 80%, alveolar-arterial oxygen gradient (P[A$-$a]O_2 ≤ 15 mm Hg on room air, arterial oxygen content (CaO_2) 18 to 20 mL/100 mL, alveolar air equation (PAO_2) 100 mm Hg, arterial blood gases within normal range, absence of cyanosis, absence of dyspnea, no shortness of breath, and absence of adventitious breath sounds.

- Review results of chest roentgenogram, hemoglobin, arterial blood gas measurement, tidal volume, and vital capacity.
- Limit physical activity to bed rest.
- Place patient in semi- or high Fowler's position to enhance gas exchange.
- Obtain and report clinical findings that indicate impaired gas exchange: cyanosis, dyspnea, shortness of breath, tachypnea, and tachycardia.
- Obtain and report changes in oxygenation that indicate impaired gas exchange: PAO_2 ≤ 100 mm Hg, P(a/A)O_2 ≤ 0.75, P(A$-$a)O_2 ≥ 15 mm Hg, and CaO_2 ≤ 18 mL/100 mL.
- Administer prescribed IV fluids to maintain adequate hydration.
- Administer prescribed inspired oxygen fraction (FIO_2) ≤ 50% or oxygen 2 to 4

L/min by means of nasal cannula or mask to maintain PaO_2 ≥70 mm Hg and SaO_2 ≥95%.

- Administer prescribed bronchodilators (aminophylline, isoproterenol, or terbutaline) to decrease PVR and increase right ventricular ejection fraction.
- Instruct patient to report any shortness of breath or chest pain.

Collaborative Problems

A common collaborative problem in patients with pulmonary hypertension is to increase cardiac outputs.

Potential Complication: Decreased Cardiac Output. **Decreased CO** related to increased right ventricular preload and afterload secondary to pulmonary vasoconstriction, thickening of the initimal lining of the vessels, or noncompliance of the pulmonary vascular bed.

Expected Patient Outcomes. Patient maintains adequate right ventricular preload and afterload, as evidenced by cardiac output (CO) 4 to 8 L/min, cardiac index (CI) 2.7 to 4.3 $L/min/m^2$, central venous pressure (CVP) 2 to 6 mm Hg, right atrial pressure (RAP) 4 to 6 mm Hg, right ventricular pressure (RVP) 25/0 to 5 mm Hg, PVR 155 to 255 $dynes/s/cm^{-5}$, PVRI 200 to 450 $dynes/s/cm^{-5}/m^2$, BP within patients normal range, heart rate (HR) ≤100 bpm, PCWP 6 to 12 mm Hg, mean arterial pressure (MAP) 70 to 100 mm Hg, and PAP 20 to 30/8 to 15 mm Hg, pulse pressure (PP) 30 to 40 mm Hg, absence of neck vein distention, absence of peripheral edema, absence of orthopnea, normal lung sounds, and SaO_2 ≥95%.

- Consult with physician to validate expected patient outcomes used to evaluate adequate right ventricular preload and afterload.
- Review results of chest roentgenogram, 12-lead ECG, echocardiography, or ventilation-perfusion scan.
- Obtain and document hemodynamic parameters that may suggest altered right ventricular preload: CVP ≥6 mm Hg, RAP ≥6 mm Hg, RVP systolic ≥25 mm Hg or dias-

tolic ≥5 mm Hg, PAP systolic ≥30 mm Hg or diastolic ≥15 mm Hg, and MPAP ≥20 mm Hg.

- Obtain and report hemodynamic parameters that indicate increased right ventricular afterload: PAP systolic ≥40 mm Hg or diastolic ≥15 mm Hg, MPAP ≥15 mm Hg, PP ≤30 mm Hg, PVR ≥255 $dynes/s/cm^{-5}$, and PVRI ≥450 $dynes/s/cm^{-5}/m^2$.
- Obtain and report other clinical findings that indicate increased right ventricular preload and afterload: tachypnea, tachycardia, dyspnea, orthopnea, adventitious breath sounds, and cyanosis.
- Monitor intake, output, and daily weight. Report urinary output (UO) ≤30 mL/h or ≤0.5 mL/kg/h.
- Provide prescribed FIO_2 ≤50% or oxygen at 2 to 4 L/min by means of nasal cannula or mask to maintain PaO_2 at 80 mm Hg and SaO_2 ≥95%.
- Administer prescribed IV fluids to maintain adequate hydration.
- Administer prescribed diuretics to maintain UO ≥30 mL/h.
- Administer vasodilators to maintain PP 30 to 40 mm Hg, PVR ≤155 $dynes/s/cm^{-5}$, and PVRI ≤450 $dynes/s/cm^{-5}/m^2$.

DISCHARGE PLANNING

The critical care nurse will provide patient and significant other(s) with verbal or written discharge notes regarding the following subjects:

1. Signs and symptoms that require immediate medical attention: shortness of breath, dyspnea, chest discomfort, tachycardia, tachypnea, and peripheral edema.
2. Importance of keeping all outpatient appointments.
3. Medications' purpose, dosage, route, schedule, and side effects.

■ INTERSTITIAL LUNG DISEASE

(For related information see Cardiac Deviations, Part I: Dysrhythmias, p. 184; Part III: Hemodynamic monitoring, p. 219. Part I: Pneumonia, p. 375; Pulmonary embolism,

p. 397; Respiratory acidosis, p. 412; Respiratory alkalosis, p. 415. Part III: Pulse oximetry, p. 426; Mechanical ventilation, p. 428; Capnography, p. 439; Transcutaneous Pao_2 and $Paco_2$, p. 441; Indirect calorimetry, p. 441.

Case Management Basis

DRG: 92 Interstitial lung disease with complications
LOS: 6.90 days
DRG: 93 Interstitial lung disease without complications
LOS: 5.20

Definition

Interstitial lung disease (ILD) comprises a heterogeneous group of disorders that have in common the features of inflammation and fibrosis of the interalveolar septum, which represent a nonspecific reaction of the lung to diverse causes.

Pathophysiology

ILD involves inflammatory injury to alveolar cells or to pulmonary capillary endothelial cells. There is an influx of polymorphonuclear leukocytes and lymphocytes into the alveolar septa, which leads to alveolitus. Eventually ILD results in restrictive pathophysiological conditions. Vital capacity, total lung capacity, and lung compliance decrease.

Nursing Assessment

PRIMARY CAUSES

- Known causes consist of: inorganic dusts; organic dusts; gases, fumes, vapors; drugs; poisons; radiation; infections such as disseminated mycobacterial or fungal infections, viral pneumonia, *Pneumocystis carinii* pneumonia or residue of active infection of any type; pulmonary edema; or lymphangitis carcinomatosa.
- Unknown causes include cryptogenic fibrosing alveolitis; sarcoidosis; histiocytosis X; rheumatic disease; Goodpasture's syndrome; idiopathic pulmonary hemosiderosis; Wegener's granulomatosis; lym-

phomatoid granulomatosis; Churg-Strauss syndrome; angioimmunoblastic lymphadenopathy; inherited diseases; pulmonary veno-occlusive disease; ankylosing spondylitis; amyloidisis; chronic eosinophilic pneumonia; pulmonary lymphangiomyomatosis; Whipple's disease; alveolar proteinosis; and inflammatory bowel disease.

PHYSICAL ASSESSMENT

- Inspection: Dyspnea, dry cough, fever, chills, cyanosis, or digital clubbing.
- Auscultation: Mid-to-late inspiratory crackles, S_2, and tachypnea.

DIAGNOSTIC TEST RESULTS

Invasive Respiratory Diagnostic Procedures (see Table 3–3)

- Bronchoalveolar lavage: Used in diagnosis of opportunistic infections such as *Pneumocystis carinii* pneumonia in the immunocompromised host. Its role in diagnosing ILD is uncertain.
- Fiberoptic bronchoscopy and transbronchial biopsy: Used to establish the diagnosis of sarcoidosis, hypersensitivity pneumonitis, histiocytosis X, and inorganic dust diseases.
- Open-lung biopsy: The procedure is performed should transbronchial biopsy fail to definitively establish the diagnosis.

Noninvasive Respiratory Diagnostic Procedure (see Table 3–4)

- Chest roentgenogram: There may be widespread coalescence that produces a diffuse haziness on the chest roentgenogram and is referred to as ground-glass appearance. Nodular shadows may range in size from a few millimeters to 10 cm. Reticular shadows appear, such as linear or curvilinear densities, which form a ringlike network that can be fine to coarse, with a honeycomb appearance. The mediastinal or hilar lymph nodes may appear enlarged. There may also be cysts and bullae late in the disease process.

There may be diffuse, ground-glass, nodular, reticular, or reticulonodular infiltrates that may progress to honeycombing.

MEDICAL AND SURGICAL MANAGEMENT

PHARMACOLOGY

- Corticosteroids: Prednisone can be used to manage ILD associated with collagen-vascular disease at a dose of 1 mg/kg, up to 80 mg. The dose is slowly tapered at a rate of 2.5 to 5.0 mg/wk down to a daily maintenance dose of 15 to 20 mg.
- Cytotoxic agents: Used to treat the pulmonary vasculitides.

NURSING MANAGEMENT: NURSING DIAGNOSES AND COLLABORATIVE PROBLEMS

Nursing Diagnoses

Common nursing goals for patients with ILD are to improve gas exchange and promote effective breathing pattern.

Impaired gas exchange related to decreased diffusion of oxygen and carbon dioxide secondary to destruction of alveolar-capillary wall and decreased surface area for gas exchange.

Expected Patient Outcomes. Patient maintains adequate oxygen gas exchange, as evidenced by arterial blood gases within normal range, absence of adventitious breath sounds, arterial oxygen saturation (SaO_2) 95%, mixed venous oxygen saturation ($S\bar{v}O_2$ 60% to 80%, alveolar-arterial oxygen gradient ($P[A-a]O_2$ $\leq$15 mm Hg on room air, arterial oxygen content (CaO_2) 18 to 20 mL/100 mL, alveolar air equation (PAO_2) 100 mm Hg, respiratory rate (RR) $\leq$30 BPM, heart rate (HR) $\leq$100 bpm, blood pressure (BP) within patient's normal range, mean arterial pressure (MAP) 70 to 100 mm Hg, and skin color normal.

- Consult with physician to validate expected patient outcomes used to evaluate adequate gas exchange.

- Consult with physician about criteria used to determine when ventilatory support is needed: oxygenation (PaO_2 $\leq$60 mm Hg on inspired oxygen fraction [FIO_2] 50%, ventilation ($PaCO_2$ $\geq$50 to 60 mm Hg, which is $\geq$10 mm Hg above patient's normal $PaCO_2$), and respiratory mechanisms (apnea, sustained RR $\geq$35 BPM, and vital capacity $\leq$10 to 15 mL/kg).
- Review results of arterial blood gas measurement, chest roentgenogram, hemoglobin, and bronchoalveolar lavage.
- Limit physical activity to bed rest to reduce oxygen demand.
- Monitor clinical indicators of respiratory status: rate, depth, symmetry of chest excursion, skin color, use of accessory muscles, and presence of adventitious breath sounds.
- Monitor and report clinical findings that indicate impaired gas exchange: cyanosis, diaphoresis, dyspnea, tachypnea, and tachycardia.
- Assess ventilator function by verifying that the prescribed settings are being used and are effective. The settings include FIO_2 at the lowest rate to maintain PaO_2 $\geq$60 mm Hg and 100% in acute situations to achieve adequate oxygenation; tidal volume 10 to 15 mL/kg; RR 10 to 14 BPM; and mode of ventilation.
- Evaluate patient's readiness to be weaned from full or partial ventilatory support to spontaneous unassisted breathing by using the following objective weaning criteria: oxygenation (PaO_2 $\geq$60 mm Hg on FIO_2 $\leq$40% to 50% and positive end-expiratory pressure [PEEP] $\leq$5 cm H_2O); ventilation (minute ventilation $\leq$10 L/min, tidal volume $\geq$5 mL/kg, and $PaCO_2$ within usual range for patient); and respiratory mechanics (spontaneous RR $\leq$30 to 35 BPM, maximal inspiratory force $\leq$ -20 cm H_2O).
- Move endotracheal tube to the other side of the mouth daily to prevent tissue necrosis.
- Administer prescribed IV fluids to maintain adequate hydration.
- Administer oxygen by nasal cannula or mask to maintain a PaO_2 $\geq$70 mm Hg.

Ineffective breathing pattern related to generalized decrease in lung volume secondary to reduced lung compliance.

Expected Patient Outcomes. Patient maintains effective breathing pattern, as evidenced by RR ≤ 30 BPM, HR ≤ 100 bpm, physiological shunt ($\dot{Q}s/\dot{Q}t$) 0% to 8%, dynamic compliance (Cdyn) 35 to 55 mL/cm H_2O, static compliance (Cst) 50 to 100 mL/cm H_2O, $P(A-a)O_2$ ≤ 25 mm Hg, arterial-alveolar oxygen tension ratio ($P[a/A]O_2$ 0.75 to 0.90, functional residual capacity 3 L, arterial blood gases within normal range, skin color normal, and no adventitious breath sounds.

- Review results of arterial blood gas measurement, chest roentgenogram, tidal volume, and lung volume.
- Monitor clinical indicators of respiratory status: rate, depth, symmetry of chest excursion, skin color, presence of adventitious breath sounds.
- Obtain and report clinical findings associated with ineffective breathing pattern: dyspnea, tachypnea, tachycardia, cyanosis, and crackles.
- Evaluate respiratory muscle efficiency by pulmonary function by obtaining tidal volume, minute ventilation, vital capacity, and maximum inspiratory pressure.
- Monitor and report static lung compliance (Cst) ≤ 50 mL/cm H_2O, dynamic characteristic (Cdyn) ≤ 35 mL/cm H_2O, and pulmonary shunting ($\dot{Q}s/\dot{Q}t$) $\geq 8\%$.
- Administer prescribed IV fluids to maintain adequate hydration.
- Provide prescribed oxygen by nasal cannula and mask at the prescribed flow rate to maintain PaO_2 ≥ 70 mm Hg.
- Provide ventilatory support and PEEP to maintain adequate oxygenation.
- Administer immunosuppressive agents (azathioprene [Imuran]).

Collaborative Problems
Common collaborative goals for patients with ILD are to maintain ventilation-perfusion balance and increase CO.

Potential Complication: Ventilation-Perfusion Imbalance. Ventilation-perfusion related to interstitial fibrosis secondary to alveolitis.

Expected Patient Outcomes. Patient maintains adequate ventilation/perfusion balance, as evidenced by ventilation/perfusion ($\dot{V}/\dot{Q}$) ratio 1.0, SaO_2 97%, $S\bar{v}O_2$ 75%, alveolar-arterial oxygen gradient ($P[A-a]O_2$) ≤ 15 mm Hg on room air or 10 to 65 mm Hg on 100% oxygen arterial-alveolar oxygen tension ratio ($P[a/A]O_2$) 0.75 to 0.90, static compliance (Cst) ≥ 50 mL/cm H_2O, dynamic compliance (Cdyn) ≥ 50 mL/cm H_2O, RR 12 to 20 BPM, absence of adventitious breath sounds, absence of cyanosis, absence of dyspnea, cardiac output (CO) 4 to 8 L/min, cardiac index (CI) 2.7 to 4.3 L/min/m^2, pulmonary capillary wedge pressure (PCWP) 4 to 12 mm Hg, MAP 70 to 100 mm Hg, BP within patient's normal range, arterial blood gases within normal range, and HR ≤ 100 bpm.

- Consult with physician to validate expected patient outcomes used to evaluate ventilation-perfusion balance.
- Confer with Respiratory Therapy regarding the appropriate ventilatory support for the ILD patient.
- Review results of arterial blood gas measurement, static lung compliance, dynamic lung compliance, physiological shunting, alveolar-arterial oxygen gradient, arterial-alveolar oxygen tension ratio, or ventilation-perfusion scan.
- Limit physical activity to bed rest to decrease the work of breathing.
- Obtain and report hemodynamic parameters that could affect ventilation-perfusion balance: CO ≤ 4 L/min, CI ≤ 2.7 L/min/m^2, PCWP ≤ 12 mm Hg, MAP ≤ 70 mm Hg, and $S\bar{v}O_2$ $\leq 60\%$.
- Obtain and report other clinical findings associated with decreased ventilation:perfusion ratio: tachypnea, cyanosis, crackles, dyspnea, and tachycardia.
- Obtain and report parameters of oxygenation and compliance that indicate ventilation-perfusion imbalance: $\dot{Q}s/\dot{Q}t$ $\geq 8\%$,

static compliance ≤ 50 mL/cm H_2O, dynamic compliance ≤ 35 mL/cm H_2O, and $P(a{:}A)O_2 \leq 0.75$.

- Monitor $\dot{V}/\dot{Q}$ ratio and report value ≤ 1.0, which signifies reduced alveolar ventilation. A low $\dot{V}/\dot{Q}$ ratio is referred to as an intrapulmonary shunt (blood flow[$\dot{Q}s$]/total flow [$\dot{Q}t$]) $\geq 15\%$ to 30%.

- Provide prescribed ventilatory support, if necessary, and PEEP for high $\dot{Q}s/\dot{Q}t$ levels.

- Obtain the following information in order to measure $\dot{Q}s/\dot{Q}t$: hemoglobin level, FIO_2 level, arterial and mixed venous blood gas results, and arterial and mixed venous oxyhemoglobin (oxygen saturation) values.

- Monitor alveolar partial pressure of oxygen (PAO_2) and arterial partial pressure of oxygen (PaO_2), which are approximately equal. Report a diversion of PAO_2 from PaO_2, which signifies the development of an intrapulmonary shunt.

- Estimate $\dot{Q}s/\dot{Q}t$ using the following methods: PaO_2/FIO_2 ratio ≥ 286, arterial/alveolar (a/A) ratio ≥ 0.60, alveolar-arterial (A−a) gradient ≤ 20 mm Hg with an FIO_2 of 0.21, respiratory index ≤ 1, and shunt equation $\leq 5\%$.

- Monitor and report $PaO_2/FIO_2 \leq 200$, which is considered to be a large intrapulmonary shunt (20%). The lower the value, the more severe the $\dot{Q}s/\dot{Q}t$ disturbance.

- Monitor and report respiratory quotient ≤ 0.7 as lipolysis or starvation or ≥ 1.0 lipogenesis or overfeed to determine the relationship between oxygen consumption and carbon dioxide production.

- Obtain and report $SaO_2 \leq 90\%$, which can signify intrapulmonary shunting.

- Evaluate the effectiveness of PEEP according to the following criteria: arterial blood gases, mixed venous oxygen tension, lung compliance, PCWP and CO.

- If ventilatory support and PEEP are required, it can be increased, as prescribed, in increments of 3 to 5 cm H_2O pressure until the desired PEEP is achieved to keep $PaO_2 \geq 60$ mm Hg.

- Monitor and report complications associated with PEEP: reduced venous return, re-

duced CO, reduced cerebral perfusion, and barotrauma.

- Assess ventilator function by verifying that the prescribed settings are being used and are effective. The settings include FIO_2 at the lowest rate to maintain $PaO_2 \geq 60$ mm Hg and 100% in acute situations to achieve adequate oxygenation; tidal volume 10 to 15 mL/kg; RR 10 to 14 BPM; and mode of ventilation.

- Evaluate patient's readiness to be weaned from full or partial ventilatory support to spontaneous unassisted breathing by using the following objective weaning criteria: oxygenation ($PaO_2 \geq 60$ mm Hg on FIO_2 $\leq 40\%$ to 50% and PEEP ≤ 5 cm H_2O); ventilation (minute ventilation ≤ 10 L/min, tidal volume ≥ 5 mL/kg, and $PaCO_2$ within usual range for patient); and respiratory mechanics (spontaneous RR ≤ 30 to 35 BPM, maximal inspiratory force ≤ -20 cm H_2O).

- Move endotracheal tube to the other side of the mouth daily to prevent tissue necrosis.

- Monitor patient's tolerance of ventilatory support through the use of an individualized plan of care, which includes data from chest such as lung sounds, RR, chest expansion and ventilator settings; hemodynamic parameters including HR, BP, (T), CO, CI, PAP, and PCWP; nutritional status such as type of feedings, intake, and output; and level of anxiety.

- Measure intake, output, specific gravity, and daily weight. Excessive fluid accumulation increases total lung water contributing to an increase in ventilation-perfusion imbalance.

- Monitor skin color for the presence of cyanosis, which can reflect the desaturation of at least 5 grams of hemoglobin and ventilation-perfusion mismatch.

- Evaluate the adequacy of oxygenation: oxygen delivery ≥ 600 mL/min/m^2, CI ≥ 2.7 L/min/m^2, and oxygen consumption (VO_2) ≥ 156 mL/min/m^2.

- Administer prescribed humidified oxygen to keep $PaO_2 \geq 60$ mm Hg.

- Administer IV fluids at the prescribed flow rate to maintain adequate hydration and to avoid excess fluid accumulation, which increases lung water, causing increased $\dot{V}/\dot{Q}$ mismatch.

- Administer corticosteroids to decrease inflammatory process.
- Teach patient to cough, turn, and deep breathe.

Potential Complication: Decreased Cardiac Output.

Decreased CO related to increased right ventricular afterload secondary to pulmonary hypertension for bronchoconstriction or destruction of small pulmonary vessels.

Expected Patient Outcomes. Patient maintains adequate right ventricular preload and afterload, as evidenced by CO 4 to 8 L/min, CI 2.7 to 4.3 L/min/m², CVP 2 to 6 mm Hg, pulse pressure (PP) 30 to 40 mm Hg, pulmonary vascular resistance (PVR) 155 to 255 dynes/s/cm⁻⁵, pulmonary vascular resistance index (PVRI) 200 to 450 dynes/s/cm⁻⁵/m², BP within patient's normal range, HR ≤100 bpm, PCWP 6 to 12 mm Hg, MAP 70 to 100 mm Hg, and pulmonary artery pressure (PAP) 20 to 30/8 to 15 mm Hg, absence of neck vein distention, absence of peripheral edema, absence of orthopnea, normal lung sounds, and SaO_2 ≥95%.

- Consult with physician to validate expected patient outcomes used to evaluate adequate right ventricular preload and afterload.
- Review results of chest roentgenogram, 12-lead ECG, echocardiography, or ventilation-perfusion scan.
- Obtain and report hemodynamic parameters that indicate increased right ventricular afterload: PAP systolic ≥40 mm Hg or diastolic ≥15 mm Hg, mean PAP ≥15 mm Hg, PP ≤30 mm Hg, PVR ≥255 dynes/s/cm⁻⁵, and PVRI ≥450 dynes/s/cm⁻⁵/m².
- Obtain and report other clinical findings that indicate increased right ventricular afterload: tachypnea, tachycardia, dyspnea, orthopnea, adventitious breath sounds, and cyanosis.

- Monitor intake, output, and daily weight. Report urinary output (UO) ≤30 mL/h or ≤0.5 mL/kg/h.
- Provide prescribed FIO_2 ≤50% or oxygen at 2 to 4 L/min by means of nasal cannula or mask to maintain PaO_2 at 80 mm Hg and SaO_2 ≥95%.
- Administer prescribed IV fluids to maintain adequate hydration.
- Administer prescribed diuretics to maintain UO ≥30 mL/h.
- Administer vasodilators to maintain PP 30 to 40 mm Hg, PVR ≤100 dynes/s/cm⁻⁵ and PVRI ≤450 dynes/s/cm⁻⁵·m². (see Table 1–4, p. 20).

DISCHARGE PLANNING

The critical care nurse will provide patient and significant other(s) with verbal or written discharge notes regarding the following subjects:

1. Signs and symptoms that require immediate medical attention: shortness of breath, dyspnea, chest discomfort, tachycardia, tachypnea, and peripheral edema.
2. Importance of keeping all outpatient appointments.
3. Medications' purpose, dosage, route, schedule, and side effects.

■ RESPIRATORY ACIDOSIS

(For related information see Cardiac Deviations, Part I: Dysrhythmias, p. 184; Part III: Hemodynamic monitoring, p. 219. Part III: Pulse oximetry, p. 426; Mechanical ventilation, p. 428; Capnography, p. 439; Transcutaneous PaO_2 and $PaCO_2$, p. 441; Indirect calorimetry, p. 441.)

Case Management Basis

DRG: 99 Respiratory signs and symptoms with complications
LOS: 4.10 days
DRG: 100 Respiratory signs and symptoms without complications
LOS: 2.60 days

Definition

Respiratory acidosis (hypercapnia) results from ventilatory impairment and subsequent retention of carbon dioxide. Beside carbon dioxide retention, the pH is ≤7.35.

Pathophysiology

The underlying mechanism contributing to respiratory acidosis is alveolar hypoventilation. When the lungs fail to eliminate metabolically produced carbon dioxide, the partial pressure of arterial carbon dioxide ($Paco_2$) is ≥45 mm Hg, resulting in an increase hydrogen-ion concentration and an overall decrease in pH ≤7.35. The $Paco_2$ changes become a direct reflection of the degree of ventilatory function or abnormalities.

Nursing Assessment

PRIMARY CAUSES

- Airway obstruction causes include aspiration, foreign bodies, pulmonary embolus, severe bronchospasms, and pulmonary edema. Depressants of the respiratory center can be: sedatives, chronic narcotic abuse, metabolic alkalosis, increased intracranial pressure, medullary tumors, or vertebral artery embolism or thrombosis. Defects in the nerves and muscles of respiration are caused by myasthenia gravis, Guillain-Barré syndrome, spinal cord injury, or paralysis associated with hypo- or hyperkalemia. Lung diseases associated with respiratory acidosis include chronic obstructive pulmonary disease, pneumonia, atelectasis, asthma, interstitial lung disease, or bronchitis. Finally, thoracic cage disorders causing acidosis include flail chest, pneumothorax, or ankylosing spondylitis.

PHYSICAL ASSESSMENT

- Inspection: Restlessness, apprehension, disorientation, irritability, headache, drowsiness, confusion, coma, fatigue, flapping tremors, decreased reflexes, dysrhythmia, weakness, tremors, tachypnea, dyspnea, diaphoresis.
- Auscultation: Tachycardia.

DIAGNOSTIC TEST RESULTS

Standard Laboratory Tests (see Table 1–1, p. 30)

- Arterial blood gases: $Paco_2$ ≥45 mm Hg, pH ≤7.35, and bicarbonate (HCO_3) ≥26 mEq/L.
- Serum electrolytes: Within normal limits.

Noninvasive Respiratory Diagnostic Procedure

- Chest roentgenogram: Reveals underlying respiratory disease.

MEDICAL AND SURGICAL MANAGEMENT

PHARMACOLOGY

- Bicarbonate: Administered to treat the cause of acidosis in an attempt to correct or lessen the immediate effects of the imbalance.

OXYGEN THERAPY

- Given to correct or reduce the immediate effect of oxygen deficit.

MECHANICAL VENTILATION

- Depending on the severity of respiratory acidosis, patient may require an artificial airway or mechanical ventilation.

NURSING MANAGEMENT: NURSING DIAGNOSES AND COLLABORATIVE PROBLEMS

Nursing Diagnoses

Common nursing goals for patients with respiratory acidosis are to improve gas exchange, improve airway clearance, promote activity tolerance, and prevent confusion.

Impaired gas exchange related to alveolar hypoventilation secondary to factors depressing ventilatory function.

Expected Patient Outcomes. Patient maintains adequate gas exchange, as evidenced by respiratory rate (RR) 12 to 20 BPM, heart rate (HR) ≤100 bpm, absence of adventitious breath sounds and dyspnea, absence of cyanosis, arterial oxygen saturation (SaO_2) 95%, mixed venous oxygen saturation ($S\bar{v}O_2$) 60% to 80%, and arterial blood gases within normal range.

- Review results of chest roentgenogram, serum electrolytes, and arterial blood gas measurement.
- Monitor clinical indicators of respiratory status: rate, depth, use of accessory muscles, symmetry of chest excursion, skin color, and presence of adventitious breath sounds.
- Obtain and report clinical findings that indicate impaired gas exchange: tachypnea, tachycardia, crackles, dyspnea, cyanosis, and confusion.
- Initiate preventive pulmonary maintenance therapies to increase the removal of carbon dioxide by the lungs, turning, coughing, deep breathing, suctioning, and resistance breathing.
- Administer oxygen by nasal cannula or mask at the prescribed flow rate to maintain $PaO_2 \geq 70$ to 80 mm Hg.
- Provide ventilatory support, if necessary, to correct factors causing hypercarbia.
- Administer sodium bicarbonate ($NaHCO_3$) as prescribed.

Ineffective airway clearance related to retained secretions secondary to muscular weakness or hypoventilation.

Expected Patient Outcomes. Patient maintains effective airway clearance, as evidenced by productive cough, RR 12 to 20 BPM, HR ≤ 100 bpm, absence of muscular weakness, absence of cyanosis, absence of adventitious breath sounds, and arterial blood gases within normal limit.

- Review serum electrolyte and arterial blood gas results.
- Limit physical activity to bed rest until feelings of illness or fatigue subside and blood gases return to normal.
- Obtain and report clinical indicators associated with ineffective airway clearance: un-

productive cough, cyanosis, crackles, and muscular weakness.

- Encourage patient to cough, turn and deep breathe.
- Support patient's chest so retained sputum can be expectorated.
- Encourage use of an incentive spirometer to enhance lung expansion.
- Administer IV fluid as ordered to keep patient hydrated.

Activity intolerance related to weakness, confusion, or fatigue.

Expected Patient Outcomes. Patient tolerates increased increments of activity without fatigue, weakness, and absence of confusion.

- Monitor patient's tolerance of incremental physical activity.
- Monitor blood pressure (BP), HR, and RR before and after physical activity.
- Monitor for the presence of fatigue, weakness, or confusion in relation to patient's arterial blood gases.
- Instruct patient to report feelings of weakness or fatigue.

Altered thought process related to confusion and irritability.

Expected Patient Outcome. Absence of confusion or irritability.

- Provide a safe physical environment.
- Maintain a decreased activity level consistent with the level of hypoxia.
- Assist patient with all activities of daily living.
- Provide a quiet environment with enough stimuli to maintain orientation.
- Provide emotional support and reassurance.
- Monitor patient's thought process for signs of confusion or irritability.
- Evaluate patient's arterial blood gases in relation to behavior changes.
- Administer oxygen by normal cannula or mask at the prescribed amount to maintain $PaO_2 \geq 70$ to 80 mm Hg.
- Administer IV fluids as prescribed.

Collaborative Problem

A common collaborative goal for patients with respiratory acidosis is to correct dysrhythmias.

Potential Complication: Dysrythmias. Dysrhythmias related to hypercarbia secondary to respiratory dysfunction.

Expected Patient Outcomes. Patient remains in normal sinus rhythm, serum electrolytes are within normal range, HR ≤ 100 bpm, and BP within patient's normal range.

- Review results of arterial blood gas measurement and 12-lead ECG.
- Monitor continuous ECG to assess HR and rhythm. Document ECG rhythm strips every 2 to 4 hours in patients with dysrhythmias.
- Measure ECG components should hypokalemia occur in conjunction with diuretic therapy: decreased amplitude and broadening of T waves, prominent U waves, and sagging ST segment.
- Measure ECG components should hyperkalemia occur in conjunction with decreased renal arterial perfusion: peaked T waves of increased amplitude and biphasic QRS-T complexes.
- Administer prescribed IV fluids to maintain adequate hydration.
- Administer prescribed oxygen therapy 2 to 4 L/min to maintain adequate tissue oxygenation.
- Administer prescribed antidysrhythmia agents for hyperkalemia.
- Provide respiratory support, if necessary, to correct underlying cause of hypercapnia.

■ RESPIRATORY ALKALOSIS

(For related information see Cardiac Deviations, Part I: Dysrhythmias, p. 184; Part III: Thrombolytic therapy, p. 265. Hemodynamic monitoring, p. 219; ST segment monitoring, p. 264; Part III: Pulse oximetry, p. 426; Mechanical ventilation, p. 428.)

Case Management Basis

DRG: 99 Respiratory signs and symptoms with complications
LOS: 4.10 days
DRG: 100 Respiratory signs and symptoms without complications
LOS: 2.60 days

Definition

There is a loss of carbon dioxide from the lungs at a faster rate than it is produced in the tissue. The result is a partial pressure of arterial carbon dioxide ($Paco_2$) of ≤ 35 mm Hg. Respiratory alkalosis is a deficit of carbonic acid in the extracellular fluid.

Pathophysiology

As hypercapnia occurs with base excess, hydrogen ions are released from tissue buffers. This in turn lowers plasma bicarbonate (HCO_3) concentration.

Nursing Assessment

PRIMARY CAUSES

- Causes include alcoholic intoxication, anemia, meningitis, encephalitis, head trauma, brain lesions, congestive heart failure, exercise, fever, cirrhosis, pulmonary fibrosis, hypoxia, thyrotoxicosis, mechanical ventilation, anxiety, and voluntary hyperpnea.

PHYSICAL ASSESSMENT

- Inspection: Light-headedness, giddiness, breathlessness, decreased mental function, anxiety, confusion, paresthesias, weakness, muscle cramps, seizures, tetany, hyperactivity, tetany, or carpopedal spasm.
- Auscultation: Tachycardia, hypotension and dysrhythmias.

DIAGNOSTIC TEST RESULTS

Standard Laboratory Tests (see Table 1–1, p. 3)

- Arterial blood gases: $Paco_2 \leq 35$ mm Hg, $HCO_3 \leq 22$ mEq/L, and pH ≥ 7.43.
- Serum electrolytes: Hypokalemia and hypocalcemia.

ECG

• Reveals dysrhythmias.

MEDICAL AND SURGICAL MANAGEMENT

PHARMACOLOGY

• Sedatives or tranquilizers are used to reduce anxiety-induced respiratory alkalosis.

OXYGEN THERAPY

• Oxygen is administered should hypoxia be the cause of respiratory alkalosis.

NURSING MANAGEMENT: NURSING DIAGNOSES AND COLLABORATIVE PROBLEMS

Nursing Diagnoses

Common nursing goals for patients with respiratory alkalosis are to improve gas exchange, prevent injury, correct sensory-perceptual alteration, and reduce anxiety.

Impaired gas exchange related to alveolar hyperventilation secondary to factors increasing ventilatory effort.

Expected Patient Outcomes. Patient maintains adequate gas exchange, as evidenced by respiratory rate (RR) 12 to 20 BPM, heart rate (HR) $\leq$100 bpm, absence of restlessness or confusion, minute ventilation 6 L/min, respiratory dead space 150 mL, arterial oxygen saturation (SaO_2) 95%, and mixed venous oxygen saturation ($S\bar{v}O_2$) 60% to 80%.

• Review serum electrolyte and arterial blood gas results.
• Monitor clinical indicators of respiratory status: rate, depth, use of accessory muscles, skin color, and symmetry of chest excursions.
• Obtain and report clinical indicators suggesting impaired gas exchange: tachypnea, tachycardia, dyspnea, restlessness, and confusion.
• Monitor patient receiving ventilatory support for the presence of twitching, irritabil-

ity, or seizure: Decrease minute ventilation and increase dead space ventilation.
• Adjust ventilatory settings, as prescribed, to reduce risk of hypokalemia.
• Administer oxygen by nasal cannula or Venturi mask at the prescribed flow rate to maintain PaO_2 $\geq$70 mm Hg.
• Teach patient how to decrease respirations through progressive relaxation, meditation, or guided imagery.

High risk for injury related to seizure activity or tetany.

Expected Patient Outcome. Patient experiences no seizure activity or tetany that might cause injury.

• Review serum electrolyte and arterial blood gas results.
• Protect patient from potential injury during seizure activity.
• Monitor the type and duration of seizure activity.
• Monitor vital signs after a seizure episode.
• Administer sedatives as prescribed.

Sensory-perceptual alteration related to paresthesia, weakness, or tetany.

Expected Patient Outcome. Patient's sensory-perceptual activity is normal.

• Evaluate patient for paresthesia, weakness, or tetany.
• Support patient during incremental increases in physical activity.
• Inform patient regarding the reasons for the paresthesia or weakness.
• Instruct patient to report any changes in paresthesia.

Anxiety related to the underlying illness causing alkalosis or invasive procedures.

Expected Patient Outcomes. Patient verbalizes decreased anxiety.

• Encourage patient to verbalize when he or she feels anxious.

- Prepare patient for invasive procedures in order to lessen anxiety.
- Instruct patient regarding the relationship between the illness and alkalosis.
- Teach patient how to reduce anxious feelings through progressive relaxation, meditation, or guided imagery.

PART II: SURGICAL CORRECTIONS AND NURSING MANAGEMENT

■ VENA CAVAL INTERRUPTION

(For related information see Cardiac Deviations, Part I: Shock, p. 174; Dysrhythmias, p. 184; Part III: Hemodynamic monitoring, p. 219. Part I: Pulmonary embolism, p. 397; Part III: Pulse oximetry, p. 426; Mechanical ventilation, p. 428; Capnography, p. 439; Transcutaneous Pao_2 and $Paco_2$, p. 441; Indirect calorimetry, p. 441.)

Case Management Basis
DRG: 76 Other respiratory system OR procedures with complications
LOS: 10.60 days
DRG: 77 Other respiratory system procedures without complications
LOS: 4.50 days

Definition
Vena caval interruption is done to protect a patient from initial or recurrent pulmonary embolism when conventional anticoagulation is contraindicated or has failed.

Patient Selection

INDICATIONS. General indications include failure of successful anticoagulant therapy; recurrent pulmonary embolism while receiving adequate anticoagulation; or after pulmonary embolectomy. It is indicated as prophylaxis for chronic pulmonary hypertension; deep vein thrombosis (DVT) with severe respiratory impairment; free-floating thrombus in the iliofemoral system or vena cava; significant hip or pelvic fractures; a poor history of DVT in patients undergoing surgical procedures at high risk of pulmonary embolism.

CONTRAINDICATIONS. Patient is a poor surgical risk.

Procedure

TECHNIQUE

Vena Cava Ligation
Provides acceptable protection against recurrent pulmonary embolism. Mortality rates are high and acute vena caval occlusion may contribute to cardiac decompensation in patients with other diseases.

Extraluminal Interruption
- Suture grid: Using Dacron continuous mattress sutures, a grid is constructed by positioning sutures 2 to 3 mm apart without narrowing the caval lumen.
- Suture plication: Vena cava is mobilized 2 to 3 cm and interrupted mattress sutures are placed 5 mm apart, constructing channels that divide the cava into compartments, each measuring 3 mm in diameter.
- Staple of the vena cava: Stapled vena cava is closed but a 5 mm gap is left between staples to ensure adequate flow and reduce distal inferior vena caval (IVC) thrombosis.
- Teflon clip: The clip is placed below a sizable lumbar vein to prevent the formation of a cul-de-sac. Clips are adjusted so the apertures range between 3.0 to 3.5 mm in diameter.

Intraluminal Interruption
- Morbin-Uddin umbrella: Umbrella insertion is via the internal jugular vein. The collapsed umbrella is positioned at the level of

the third lumbar vertebra and with the guide wire in position, the filter is ejected, with fixation provided by firm upward traction in the guide wire.

- Greenfield vena cava filter: A cone-shaped device to provide a maximal entrapment area while preserving blood flow. Spacing between the six stainless steel wires ensures trapping of all emboli greater than 3 mm. The filter is inserted primarily through the internal jugular vein and positioned at the level of the third lumbar vertebra.
- Bird's nest filter: Consists of four thin strands of stainless steel wire, each 25 cm long, attached to a pair of short angle hooks at each end for fixation to the wall of the IVC. With percutaneous insertion through the femoral, internal jugular, or subclavian vein, the sheath is placed proximal to the renal veins for a femoral vein approach or at the inferior border of the third lumbar vertebra if the jugular or subclavian vein route is used.

Equipment. Prosthetic devices.

Complications

Bleeding, infection, edema in the extremity, or hematoma.

NURSING MANAGEMENT: NURSING DIAGNOSES AND COLLABORATIVE PROBLEMS

Nursing Diagnoses

Common nursing goals for patients with venal caval interruption are to correct fluid volume deficit, maintain peripheral tissue perfusion, prevent infection, and provide knowledge.

Fluid volume deficit related to bleeding from the incision or perforation of the vena caval wall by the struts.

Expected Patient Outcomes. Patient maintains adequate fluid volume, as evidenced by blood pressure (BP) within patient's normal range, mean arterial pressure (MAP) 70 to 100 mm Hg, heart rate (HR) ≤100 bpm, normal skin turgor, peripheral pulses +2, capillary refill ≤3 seconds, hemoglobin within normal range, urinary output (UO) ≥30 mL/h or ≥0.5 mL/kg/min, respiratory rate (RR) 12-2 BPM, and absence of excessive bleeding.

- Review hemoglobin, hematocrit, and serum electrolyte results.
- Limit patient's physical activity to bed rest until the source of bleeding is determined.
- Obtain and report clinical findings associated with fluid volume deficit resulting from bleeding: hypotension, tachycardia, MAP ≤70 mm Hg, poor skin turgor, peripheral pulses ≤+2, and capillary refill ≥3 seconds.
- Monitor daily weight, intake, specific gravity, and UO to evaluate fluid balance. Report UO ≥30 mL/h or ≤0.5 mL/kg/h and weight loss ≥0.5 kg/d.
- Assess incision and dressing for bleeding.
- Administer prescribed oxygen 2 to 4 L/min to maintain tissue oxygenation.
- Administer prescribed IV fluids to maintain adequate hydration and circulatory volume.

Decreased peripheral tissue perfusion related to postthrombotic syndrome.

Expected Patient Outcomes. Patient maintains adequate peripheral tissue perfusion, as evidenced by BP within patient's normal range, HR ≤100 bpm, absence of peripheral edema, peripheral pulses +2, capillary refill ≤3 seconds, absence of pain, peripheral skin color normal, skin warm and dry.

- Review test results that confirm venous thrombosis: Visualization of thrombus with sharp margins in a healthy opacified vein; thrombus present within a vein in at least two radiographs; nonvisualization of a long segment of vein; and demonstration of enlarged collateral vessels.
- Monitor clinical indicators of peripheral hypoperfusion: peripheral pulses, skin color and temperature, UO, presence of edema, and capillary refill.

- Obtain and report clinical findings suggesting decreased peripheral tissue perfusion: peripheral edema, peripheral pulses $\leq +2$, capillary refill ≥ 3 seconds, extremity pain, and peripheral skin cool, pale, or cyanotic.
- Administer anticoagulants as prescribed.
- Instruct patient to report any lower extremity pain, edema, or skin color changes.
- Teach patient the purpose behind anticoagulation therapy.
- Instruct patient to report any bleeding while taking anticoagulants.

High risk for infection related to vena caval incision or percutaneous cannulation site.

Expected Patient Outcomes. Patient is free of infection, as evidenced by white blood cells (WBC) $\leq 11,000/\mu L$; no fever; and absence of redness, tenderness, swelling, or drainage from incision.

- Review results of hemoglobin, hematocrit, WBC, or negative cultures.
- Monitor temperature every 2 hours or as needed when patient is febrile.
- Evaluate incision for redness, tenderness, swelling, or drainage.
- Change dressing using strict aseptic technique.
- Culture any drainage from incision or cannulation site.
- Instruct patient to report any incisional pain or drainage.

Knowledge deficit related to the type of vena caval interruption.

Expected Patient Outcomes. Patient is able to verbalize the type of vena caval interruption and postoperative care.

- Provide patient with information regarding the specific types of vena caval interruption.
- Explain the principles of postoperative care and need to monitor peripheral perfusion.
- Instruct patient regarding the purpose behind the anticoagulant, if ordered, and its continual use until discontinued.

- Instruct patient regarding the causes of DVT and its relationship to thromboembolism.

Collaborative Problem
A common collaborative goal for patients with venal caval interruption is to prevent peripheral edema.

Potential Complication: Peripheral Edema. Peripheral edema related to lower extremity edema secondary to venous stasis.

Expected Patient Outcomes. Patient maintains adequate peripheral fluid volume, as evidenced by absence of peripheral edema, peripheral pulses $+2$, capillary refill ≤ 3 seconds, warm and dry peripheral skin, equal circumferences of both extremities, and absence of peripheral pallor or cyanosis.

- Monitor both extremities for peripheral pulses and skin for color, temperature, and edema.
- Obtain and report clinical findings suggestive of peripheral edema: increased circumference of the affected extremity, peripheral pulses $\leq +2$, capillary refill ≥ 3 seconds, and extremity is cool, pale, or cyanotic.
- Elevate the affected extremity to decrease venous stasis and edema.
- Administer prescribed anticoagulant therapy to reduce the risk of DVT.
- Instruct patient to report any swelling in the affected extremity.
- Teach patient that peripheral edema will subside over subsequent months.
- Instruct patient to change position and avoid using the knee gatch.

DISCHARGE PLANNING
The critical care nurse will provide patient and significant other(s) with verbal or written discharge notes regarding the following subjects:

1. Signs and symptoms that require immediate medical attention: leg pain, peripheral edema, shortness of breath, chest pain.

2 Importance of keeping all outpatient appointments.

3. Medications[1] purpose, dosage, route, schedule, and side effects.

LUNG TRANSPLANTATION

(For related information see Cardiac Deviations, Part I, Shock, p.174; Dysrhythmias, p. 184. Part III: Hemodynamic monitoring, p. 219. Part I: Acute pulmonary edema, p. 346; Pulmonary embolism, p. 397; Respiratory acidosis, p. 412; Respiratory alkalosis, p. 415. Part III: Pulse oximetry, p. 426; Mechanical ventilation, p. 428; Capnography, p. 439; Transcutaneous Pao_2 and $Paco_2$, p. 441; Indirect calorimetry, p. 441).

Case Management Basis

DRG: 75 Major chest procedures

LOS: 11.50 days

DRG: 76 other respiratory system O.R. procedures with complications

LOS: 10.60 days

DRG: 77 Other respiratory system O.R. procedures without complications

LOS: 4.50 days

Definition

Lung transplantation can be single or double. The lung transplant candidate has a severe alteration in gas exchange, leading to hypoxemia, hypercarbia, or acidosis. Single lung transplantation can be used in patients with emphysema and pulmonary hypertension. Segmental bilateral lung replacement can take the place of en bloc double lung procedures.

Patient Selection

INDICATIONS. Single-lung transplantation indications are chronic obstructive pulmonary disease, pulmonary fibrosis, primary pulmonary hypertension, secondary pulmonary hypertension, and eosinophilic granuloma. Double-lung transplantation indications consist of emphysema, bronchiectasis, cystic fibrosis, and alpha$_1$-antitrypsin deficiency.

CONTRAINDICATIONS. Relative contraindications include atherosclerotic heart disease, renal failure, any systemic infection, malignancy, or history of alcoholism or drug abuse.

Procedure

TECHNIQUE. The surgical approach to a unilateral lung transplantation is made through either a right or left posterolateral throacotomy. The main pulmonary artery is temporarily clamped or the femoral artery and vein are cannulated for initiation of venoarterial bypass. After pneumonectomy, implantation of the single lung graft is accomplished by completing a left atrial anastomosis, a pulmonary artery anastomosis, and an end-to-end bronchial anastomosis. The bilateral approach uses an anterior transverse thoracosternotomy. The right lung is excised and replaced in a fashion similar to that used for single lung transplantation, while the patient is maintained with contralateral lung ventilation. Next, the recipient's left lung is excised and replaced with the donor left lung. Each bronchial anastomosis is wrapped with an omental pedicle.

Complications

Shock, intrathoracic tamponade, hemorrhage, dysrhythmias, and renal dysfunction. Rejection is classified as classic, atypical or alveolar, and vascular. Classic rejection occurs when there is a decrease in ventilation in the transplanted lung and perfusion with the alveolar exudate containing desquamated pneumocytes and a mixture of inflammatory cells. Atypical, or alveolar, rejection involves a decrease in ventilation without a concurrent reduction in blood flow. This leads to ventilation-perfusion imbalance. With vascular rejection, there is increased vascular resistance with decreased blood flow in the grafted tissue.

NURSING MANAGEMENT: NURSING DIAGNOSES AND COLLABORATIVE PROBLEMS

Nursing Diagnoses

Common nursing goals for patients with lung transplantation are to increase pulmonary tissue perfusion, maintain fluid balance, support airway clearance, prevent infection, and minimize pain.

Decreased pulmonary tissue perfusion related to embolism, bleeding at anastomosis site, or rejection secondary to coagulation abnormalities or surgical procedure.

Expected Patient Outcomes. Patient maintains adequate pulmonary tissue perfusion, as evidenced by arterial blood gases and coagulation studies within normal range, arterial oxygen saturation (SaO_2) 95%, absence of cyanosis, absence of adventitious breath sounds, respiratory rate (RR) 12 to 20 BPM, normothermia, heart rate (HR) $\leq$100 bpm, pulmonary artery pressure (PAP) 20 to 30 8-15 mm Hg, central venous pressure (CVP) 2 to 6 mm Hg, pulmonary capillary wedge pressure (PCWP) 6 to 12 mm Hg, pulmonary vascular resistance (PVR) 155 to 255 dynes/ s/cm^{-5}, pulmonary vascular resistance index (PVRI) 200 to 450 dynes/sc/cm$^{-5}\neq$m^2, and absence of bleeding.

- Consult with physician to validate expected patient outcomes used to evaluate effective pulmonary tissue perfusion.
- Review results of arterial blood gas measurement, coagulation studies, and chest roentgenogram.
- Obtain and report hemodynamic parameters that indicate altered pulmonary tissue perfusion: CVP $\leq$2 mm Hg, PAP $\leq$20/8 (if bleeding) and $\geq$30/15 (if embolic), PCWP $\leq$6 mm Hg (if bleeding) and $\geq$12 mm Hg (if embolic), PVR $\geq$255 dynes/sc/cm^{-5} or PVRI $\geq$450 dynes/s/cm^{-5}/m^2.
- Monitor clinical indicators of respiratory status: rate, depth, symmetry of chest excursions, skin color, use of accessory muscles, and presence of adventitious breath sounds.
- Obtain and report other clinical findings associated with decreased pulmonary tissue perfusion: elevated temperature, malaise, dyspnea, shortness of breath, cyanosis, tachypnea, tachycardia, and hypotension.
- Monitor ECG continuously to assess HR and rhythm. Document ECG strips every 2 to 4 hours in patients with dysrhythmias.
- Administer prescribed IV fluids or blood to maintain adequate hydration and circulating volume.
- Provide prescribed oxygen by Venturi mask or nasal cannula to maintain SaO$_2$ 95% and arterial partial pressure of oxygen (PaO$_2$) $\geq$70 mm Hg.
- Provide mechanical ventilation as needed.
- Administer prescribed anticoagulation therapy.

Fluid volume deficit related to bleeding or excess chest tube drainage secondary to coagulation abnormalities or surgical procedures.

Expected Patient Outcomes. Patient maintains adequate fluid volume, as evidenced by blood pressure (BP) within patient's normal range, mean arterial pressure (MAP) 70 to 100 mm Hg, HR $\leq$100 bpm, normal weight, normal skin turgor, peripheral pulses +2, capillary refill $\leq$3 seconds, chest tube drainage $\leq$100 mL/h, cardiac output (CO) 4 to 8 L/min, PAP 20 to 30 8 to 15 mm Hg, CVP 2 to 6 mm Hg, PCWP, 6 to 12 mm Hg, hemoglobin and hematocrit within normal range, and urinary (UO) $\geq$30 mL/h.

- Review hemoglobin, hematocrit, coagulation profile, and electrolyte results.
- Place patient in a comfortable position that will aid in ventilation and chest tube drainage.
- Limit activity to bed rest.
- Obtain and report hemodynamic parameters suggesting fluid volume deficit: CO $\leq$ L/min, CVP $\leq$2 mm Hg, PCWP $\leq$6 mm Hg, and MAP $\leq$70 mm Hg.

- Obtain and report other clinical findings associated with fluid volume deficit: tachycardia, hypotension, peripheral pulses ≤+2, capillary refill ≥3 seconds, and poor skin turgor.
- Monitor sites for potential bleeding: thoracotomy, bypass cannulation, chest tube, and incision.
- Monitor chest tube drainage hourly for the first 8 hours, then every 8 hours: ≤100 mL/h.
- Monitor daily weight, intake, specific gravity, and UO to determine fluid balance. Report UO ≤30 mL/h or ≤0.5 mL/kg/h.
- Monitor ECG continuously to assess HR and rhythm. Document ECG rhythm strips every 2 to 4 hours in patient with dysrhythmias.
- Monitor adequacy of fluid therapy through specific indexes: skin temperature, UO, daily body weight, central venous system function, and presence or absence of metabolic acidosis.
- Administer IV fluids or blood as needed according to patient's coagulation profile: cryoprecipitate, platelets, fresh-frozen or stored plasma.

High risk for ineffective airway clearance related to incisional pain, anesthesia, impaired cough, tracheal intubation, or decreased mobility.

Expected Patient Outcomes. Patient is able to maintain effective airway clearance, as evidenced by productive cough, RR 12 to 20 BPM, and absence of adventitious breath sounds.

- Review arterial blood gas, sputum, and chest roentgenogram results.
- Consult with physician about the inherent characteristics of transplanted lung that contribute to airway clearance, such as denervation, loss of cough reflex, and slowing of mucociliary clearance.
- Place patient with a single-lung transplant in the lateral decubitus position with the nonoperative side down to reduce postsurgical edema, facilitate gravitational drainage of the airway, and decrease mediastinal shift toward the operative side.
- Maintain a supine position for 6 to 8 hours in patients with bilateral lung transplantation. Then turn patient side to side every 1 to 2 hours.
- Evaluate mucociliary clearance by removal of inhaled radiolabeled aerosol, which is decreased in the graft but not in the native lung.
- Use chest physiotherapy (CPT) every 2 to 4 hours while the patient is awake: postural drainage of all lobes of the lung, vibration, deep breathing, and coughing.
- Administer prescribed inhalation of aerosolized albuterol before CPT.
- Use sterile suctioning with saline lavage after each drainage position and as needed.
- Use incentive spirometer after extubation to encourage deep breathing and coughing.
- Couch patient to cough and expectorate mucus. This is important because of loss of cough reflexes in the denervated lung.
- Provide frequent rest periods and uninterrupted sleep at night.
- Administer prescribed inspired oxygen fraction (FIO_2) and increase amount before and during repositioning, suctioning, and when patient sitting and getting out of bed.
- Administer prescribed intravenous or epidural morphine for the first few days and then oral analgesics to control pain during physiotherapy session.
- Administer prescribed sedation and avoid chest percussion in patients with a history of pulmonary hypertension or who develop pulmonary hypertension as a result of stimulation postoperatively.

Infection, high risk for related to impaired wound healing secondary to malnutrition or immunosuppressive agents.

Expected Patient Outcomes Patient experiences absence of infection, as evidenced by normal temperature; white blood cells (WBC) ≤11,000/μL; absence of adventitious lung sounds; negative cultures; and absence of redness, swelling, tenderness, or drainage from wound or catheter site.

- Consult with dietitian to individualize a dietary program that includes patient's prescribed diet while incorporating personal preferences.
- Review results of CBC, hemoglobin, hematocrit, and cultures.
- Limit physical activity to bed rest while patient is febrile.
- Restrict fresh unpeeled fruits and vegetables for 6 to 8 weeks after transplantation because of the presence of gram-negative bacteria.
- Change all intravenous solutions, tubings, stopcocks, and any heparin-locked lines using unit protocol (24 to 48 hours).
- Provide pulmonary care such as inspirometers, deep breathing, coughing, and early mobility to reduce risk of atelectasis and risk of pulmonary infection.
- Monitor and report findings indicating infection: temperature ≥37.5°C; WBC ≥11,000/µL; positive blood, urine, or wound cultures; presence of redness, swelling, tenderness, or drainage from wound or the IV site; discharge from chest tube site or Foley catheter; HR ≤100 bpm; and cloudy urine.
- Maintain isolation protocols and isolation technique for all visitors and staff entering patient's room to reduce the risk of infection.
- Monitor continuous ECG to assess HR and rhythm. Document ECG rhythm strips every 4 hours in patients with voltage alterations or dysrhythmias.
- Use strict sterile technique when changing dressing, lines, tubes, or pacemaker wire exit site.
- Monitor all wounds, IVs, and pacemaker wire sites daily for drainage, redness, swelling, or heat.
- Obtain culture of any suspicious drainage.
- Obtain temperature every 2 to 4 hours in febrile patient. Corticosteroid therapy reduces normal basal and maximal body temperature. A temperature ≥37°C can indicate presence of a systemic infection.
- Maintain isolation to protect patient receiving immunosuppressive agents.

- Monitor UO for color, clearance, odor, and specific gravity.
- Prepare patient for possible surgical debridement if mediastinitis or sternal wound infection occur.
- Administer prescribed IV fluids to maintain adequate hydration, UO ≥30 mL/h or ≥0.5 mL/kg/h, specific gravity, 1.010 to 1.030, peripheral pulses +2, and capillary refill ≤3 seconds.
- Administer prescribed nystatin oral suspension when patient is able to tolerate oral fluids.
- Administer prescribed acyclovir 1 week postoperatively and trimethoprim-sulfamethoxazole (Septra) 21 days posttransplant.
- Instruct patient to report any drainage or discomfort around incision or catheter sites.

Pain related to incision and fatigue.

Expected Patient Outcomes. Patient verbalizes a reduction in pain and fatigue.

- Encourage patient to describe pain on a scale of 1 to 10.
- Place in position of comfort that is appropriate for patient with a single or bilateral lung transplantation.
- Administer prescribed epidural analgesic, which is used for 5 to 7 days to control thoracotomy pain without reducing respiratory drive.
- Patient-controlled analgesics, if not contraindicated, can be used in place of an epidural or after the epidural is discontinued.
- Teach patient the rationale behind physiotherapy and exercise regimens.

Collaborative Problems

Common collaborative goals for patients experiencing lung transplantation are to prevent pulmonary edema, prevent airway dehiscence, correct rejection, and correct ventilation-perfusion imbalance.

Potential Complication: Pulmonary Edema. Pulmonary edema related to inadequate preservation of the lung, interruption of pulmonary branches of the vagal nerves secondary to unrecognized pulmonary injury occurring in the donor prior to transplantation.

Expected Patient Outcomes. Patient is free from pulmonary edema, as evidenced by arterial blood gases within normal range, absence of cyanosis, absence of adventitious breath sounds, RR 12 to 20 BPM, HR $\leq$100 bpm, PAP 20 to 30/8 to 15 mm Hg, CVP 2 to 6 mm Hg, PCWP 6 to 15 mm Hg, PVR 155 to 255 dynes/s/cm^{-5}, PVRI 200 to 450 dynes/s/cm$^{-5}\cdot$m^2, UO $\leq$30 mL/h, stable weight, absence of dyspnea or shortness of breath, and flat jugular neck veins.

- Review arterial blood gas, chest roentgenogram, serum electrolyte, and complete blood count (CBC) results.
- Elevate head of bed to enhance lung expansion.
- Place patient in comfortable position to enhance ventilation and oxygenation.
- Obtain and report hemodynamic parameters suggesting pulmonary edema: CVP $\geq$6 mm Hg, PAP systolic $\geq$30 mm Hg or diastolic $\geq$15 mm Hg$\leq$, PCWP $\geq$12 mm Hg$\leq$, PVR $\geq$255 dynes/s/cm^{-5}, and PVRI $\geq$450 dynes/s/cm^{-5}/m^2.
- Monitor clinical indicators of respiratory status: rate, depth, symmetry of chest excursions, skin color, use of accessory muscles, and presence of adventitious breath sounds.
- Obtain and report clinical findings that suggest pulmonary edema: shortness of breath, dyspnea, tachypnea, tachycardia, crackles or rales, distended neck veins, and cyanosis.
- Monitor daily weight, intake, specific gravity, UO, and chest tube drainage to evaluate fluid balance. Report UO $\leq$30 mL/h or $\leq$0.5 mL/kg/h and weight gain $\geq$0.5 kg/d.
- Should ventilatory support be necessary, use unit-prescribed method of endotracheal suctioning; preoxygenation, hyperinflation, hyperoxygenation, hyperventilation, manual inflation, and oxygen insufflation.
- Use unit-prescribed suction devices that permit patient to remain on the ventilator during suctioning: oxygen insufflation device (OID) or closed tracheal suction system (CTSS).
- Use intratracheal instillation of 2 mL to 5 mL of normal saline during suctioning to enhance the removal of secretions by stimulating a cough.
- Administer IV fluids at the prescribed amount and flow rate.
- Provide oxygen by Venturi mask or nasal cannula at the prescribed flow rate to maintain Pao$_2$ $\geq$80 mm Hg.
- Administer volume-reducing agents.

Potential Complication: Airway Dehiscence. Airway dehiscence related to ischemia secondary to donor airway's dependence on collateral pulmonary arterial circulation until revascularization occurs.

Expected Patient Outcomes. Patient maintains normal airway, as evidenced by normothermia, absence of hemoptysis, absence of secretion retention, and arterial blood gases within normal range.

- Consult with physician about technique used to prevent airway dehiscence: wrapping the airway anastomosis with omentum or pericardial fat or telescoping of the donor and recipient bronchi.
- Review results of bronchoscopy, will show airway necrosis or dehiscence.
- Monitor and report clinical findings associated with airway dehiscence: hemoptysis, fever, secretion retention, cyanosis, and signs of lung collapse.
- Monitor patient during airway dehiscence since most patients will heal spontaneously.
- Should healing leave a fibrous airway stricture and patient still be hospitalized, prepare for bronchoscopic placement of a silastic stent.

Potential Complication: Rejection. Rejection related to transplanted lung.

Expected Patient Outcomes. Patient is free from rejection or experiences recovery from rejection episode.

- Review results of chest roentgenogram, which may show the appearance of a fluffy hilar infiltrate, and radionuclide perfusion scan of patient with single lung transplant, which may show reduced perfusion to the transplanted lung.
- Obtain and report clinical findings associated with rejection: temperature elevation 0.5°C, decreased exercise tolerance, impaired oxygenation.
- Administer prescribed immunosuppressive agents such as cyclosporine (CSA) 4 mg/h IV, azathioprine 2 mg/kg/d IV, and antilymphocyte globulin (ALG) 15 mg/kg/d IV (see Table 1–15, p. 129).
- Monitor CSA blood levels until they are within the range of 350 to 450 mg/mL. Once the gastrointestinal tract is functioning, oral CSA is substituted for the IV infusion.
- Administer suspected rejection with prescribed bolus doses of steroids.
- Teach patient to report elevated temperature, activity, intolerance, and fatigue.

Potential Complication: Ventilation-Perfusion Imbalance. Ventilation-perfusion imbalance related to alveolar-capillary membrane changes secondary to intra-alveolar fluid accumulation or atelectasis.

Expected Patient Outcomes. Patient maintains adequate ventilation-perfusion balance, as evidenced by ventilation/perfusion ($\dot{V}/\dot{Q}$) ratio 1.0, SaO_2 97%), mixed venus oxygen saturation ($S\bar{v}O_2$) 75%, alveolar-arterial oxygen gradient ($P[A-a]O_2$) ≤ 15 mm Hg on room air or 10 to 65 mm Hg on 100% oxygen, arterial-alveolar oxygen tension ratio ($P[a/A]O_2$) 0.75 to 0.90, arterial oxygen content (CaO_2) 18 to 20 mL/100mL, alveolar air equation (PAO_2) 100 mm Hg, static compliance (Cst) ≥ 50 mL/cm H_2O, dynamic compliance (Cdyn) ≥ 35 mL/cm H_2O, RR 12 to 20 BPM, chest tube drainage ≤ 100 mL/h, absence of adventitious breath sounds, absence of cyanosis, absence of dyspnea, CO 4 to 8 L/min, cardiac index (CI) 2.7 to 4.3 L/min/m², PCWP 4 to 12 mm Hg, MAP 70 to 100 mm Hg, BP within patient's nor-

mal range, arterial blood gases within normal range, and HR ≤ 100 bpm.

- Consult with physician to validate expected patient outcomes used to evaluate ventilation-perfusion balance.
- Confer with Respiratory Therapy regarding the appropriate ventilatory support for patient.
- Review of results arterial blood gas measurement, static lung compliance, dynamic lung compliance, physiological shunting, alveolar-arterial oxygen gradient, arterial-alveolar oxygen tension ratio, or ventilation-perfusion scan.
- Limit physical activity to bed rest to decrease the work of breathing.
- Monitor clinical indicators of respiratory status: rate, rhythm, symmetry of chest excursions, skin color, use of accessory muscles, and presence of adventitious breath sounds.
- Report other clinical findings associated with decreased $\dot{V}:\dot{Q}$ ratio: tachypnea, cyanosis, crackles, dyspnea, and tachycardia.
- Monitor clinical indicators of adequate gas exchange: SaO_2 $\leq 90\%$, PaO_2 60 to 100 mm Hg, $PaCO_2$ 35 to 45 mm Hg, absence of cyanosis, $S\bar{v}O_2$ 60% to 80%, normal skin color, and MAP ≥ 70 mm Hg.
- Obtain and report changes in measures of oxygenation and compliance: CaO_2 ≤ 18 mL/100 mL, static compliance (Cst) ≤ 50 mL/cm H_2O, dynamic compliance (Cdyn) ≤ 35 mL/cm H_2O, $P[a/A]O_2$ ≤ 0.75, $P(A-a)O_2$ ≥ 15 mm Hg, PaO_2 ≤ 100 mm Hg, and $\dot{Q}s/\dot{Q}t$ $\geq 8\%$.
- Monitor $\dot{V}:\dot{Q}$ ratio and report value ≤ 1.0, which signifies reduced alveolar ventilation. A low A:Q ratio is referred to as an intrapulmonary shunt (blood flow [$\dot{Q}s$]: total flow [$\dot{Q}t$]) $\geq 15\%$ to 30%.
- Obtain the following information in order to measure $\dot{Q}s:\dot{Q}t$: hemoglobin level, FIO_2 level, arterial and mixed venous blood gas results, and arterial and mixed venous oxyhemoglobin (oxygen saturation) values.
- Monitor alveolar partial pressure of oxygen (PAO_2) and arterial partial pres-

sure of oxygen (Pa_{O_2}) which are approximately equal. Report a diversion of Pa_{O_2} from Pa_{CO_2}, which signifies the development of an intrapulmonary shunt.

- Estimate $\dot{Q}s/\dot{Q}t$ using the following methods: $Pa_{O_2}:F_{IO_2}$ ratio ≥ 286; arterial:alveolar (a:A) ratio ≥ 0.60, alveolar-arterial (A$-$a) gradient ≤ 20 mm Hg with an F_{IO_2} of 21%, respiratory index ≤ 1, and shunt equation $\leq 5\%$.
- Monitor and report $Pa_{O_2}:F_{IO_2} \leq 200$, which is considered to be a large intrapulmonary shunt (20%). The lower the value, the more severe the $\dot{Q}s/\dot{Q}t$ disturbance.
- Obtain and report $Sa_{O_2} \leq 90\%$, which can signify intrapulmonary shunting.
- Measure intake, output, specific gravity, and daily weight. Excessive fluid accumulation increases total lung water contributing to an increase in ventilation-perfusion imbalance.
- Monitor skin color for the presence of cyanosis, which can reflect the desaturation of at least 5 g of hemoglobin and ventilation-perfusion mismatch.
- Evaluate the adequacy of oxygenation: oxygen delivery ≥ 600 mL/min/m^2, CI ≥ 2.7 L/min/m^2, and oxygen consumption (V_{O_2}) ≥ 156 mL/min/m^2.
- Suction patient using the principles of preoxygenation, short suctioning time, postsuctioning hyperinflation to reverse atelectasis and maintain positive end-expiratory pressure uninterrupted (PEEP).
- Measure respiratory quotient (RQ) to determine the relationship of oxygen consumption and carbon dioxide production as they reflect the oxidase state of the cell. Report RQ ≥ 1.0.
- Administer prescribed humidified oxygen to keep $Pa_{O_2} \geq 60$ mm Hg.
- Administer IV fluids at the prescribed flow rate to maintain adequate hydration and to avoid excess fluid accumulation, which increases lung water causing increased $\dot{V}/\dot{Q}$ mismatch.
- Teach patient to deep breathe and cough.

DISCHARGE PLANNING

The critical care nurse will provide patient and significant other(s) with verbal or written discharge notes regarding the following subjects:

1. Signs and symptoms of rejection: elevated temperature, fatigue, and activity intolerance.
2. Importance of keeping all postdischarge appointments.
3. Importance of assuming self-care, including medication, exercise, and recording of relevant clinical data in a journal.
4. Use of a hand-held respiratory monitor daily. Need to report a decrease of 10% or more.
5. Medications: purpose, schedule, route, and side effects.

PART III: SUPPORTIVE PROCEDURES AND NURSING MANAGEMENT

■ PULSE OXIMETRY

(For related information see Cardiac Deviations, Part I: Dysrhythmias, p. 184. Part III: Hemodynamic monitoring, p. 219. Part III: Mechanical ventilation, p. 428; Capnography, p. 439; Transcutaneous Pa_{O_2} and Pa_{CO_2}, p. 441; Indirect calorimetry, p. 441, and Intravascular oxygenator, p. 442).

Case Management Basis
DRG: None

Definition
Pulse oximetry (Sp_{O_2}) allows for in noninvasive estimation of oxyhemoglobin saturation in the arteries (Sa_{O_2}). The Sp_{O_2} value usually overestimates Sa_{O_2} values by about 2% and 5%, depending on the degree of skin pigmentation and abnormal hemoglobin.

Patient Selection

INDICATIONS. Pulse oximetry is indicated in patients recovering from anesthesia, using oxygen therapy or ventilatory management, and experiencing hypoventilation. Pulse oximetry is used routinely for the patient requiring a high fraction of inspired oxygen (FIO_2) because of ventilation/perfusion ($\dot{V}/\dot{Q}$) mismatch, shunt, alveolar hypoventilation or, less commonly, impaired diffusion. In diagnostic and interventional procedures it is used to ensure oxygenation during suctioning and other routine nursing procedures; for patients with symmetric lung disease, refractory hypoxemia, significant ascites, or hemodynamic instability; for patient undergoing invasive procedures such as central venous pressure (CVP) monitoring; for patients using complex ventilatory modes; for patients with a low mixed venous oxygenations ($S\bar{v}O_2$) and patients receiving inotropic agents, vasopressors, and vasodilators; for patients undergoing hemodialysis; and for patients being transported to and from intensive care. Pulse oximetry can be also used in patients with specific disorders such as congestive heart failure, chronic obstructive pulmonary disease, adult respiratory distress syndrome, head trauma, stroke, and open heart surgery.

CONTRAINDICATIONS. None.

Procedure

TECHNIQUE. A pulse oximeter measures the absorption, or amplitude, of two wavelengths of light passing through body parts with a high perfusion of arterial blood. A lightweight probe is clipped onto the patient's earlobe or finger. The probe is connected by a cable to the oximeter unit. The probe consists of two light-emitting diodes and a light-sensitive photodetector. The photodetector measures the amplitude of the transmitted light as it passes through the pulsating vascular bed. Other fluids absorb the light, but because they do not pulsate, they do not modulate the light.

The pulsatile signal from the arterial blood flow is isolated for SaO_2 calculations.

EQUIPMENT. Pulse oximeter.

NURSING MANAGEMENT: NURSING DIAGNOSES AND COLLABORATIVE PROBLEMS

Nursing Diagnoses
Common nursing goals for patients with pulse oximetry are to improve tissue perfusion, maintain skin integrity, provide knowledge, and reduce fear.

Altered peripheral tissue perfusion related to vasoconstriction secondary to low perfusion.

Expected Patient Outcomes. Adequate perfusion in earlobe and digit with oximeter, SaO_2 95%, and capillary refill ≤3 seconds.

- Review arterial blood gases and hemoglobin results.
- Monitor clinical indicators of peripheral perfusion: peripheral pulses +2, capillary refill ≤3 seconds, skin color normal and warm, and blood pressure (BP) within normal range.
- Report clinical findings associated with altered peripheral perfusion: capillary refill ≥3 seconds, peripheral pulses ≤+2, cool earlobe or digit, and peripheral pallor or cyanosis.
- Obtain SaO_2 and correlate finding to clinical indicators of peripheral perfusion.
- Monitor placement of the probe to ensure correct reading: lower profusion alarm indicates too little or too much light entering the probe's photodetector.

High risk for skin integrity impaired related to earlobe or finger placement of oximeter.

Expected Patient Outcome. Patient's skin integrity remains intact.

- Monitor earlobe or digit for color, warmth, and capillary refill.

- Monitor skin turgor at the probe site.
- Evaluate probe site for adequate tissue perfusion every 4 hours and as necessary.
- Rotate probe site every 4 hours and as necessary.
- Apply hand lotion or vaseline to probe site if dryness persists from use of isopropyl alcohol.

Knowledge deficit related to the purpose of pulse oximetry.

Expected Patient Outcome. Patient verbalizes an understanding of ear or finger oximetry.

- Encourage patient to ask questions about the oximeter and its relationship to his or her disease.
- Provide clear information regarding the purpose of oximetry.
- Instruct patient not to remove the probe or to notify the nurse should the probe become disconnected.
- Instruct patient that changes in oximetry readings may require changes in patient care.

Fear related to the accidental removal of the pulse oximeter.

Expected Patient Outcome. Patient experiences lack of fear regarding the removal of the probe.

- Explain that the probe may become accidentally disconnected without any negative effect.
- Instruct patient to be careful not to accidentally remove the probe while changing positions.
- Inform patient that the probe off alarm will alert the staff that the probe is not functioning properly.

■ MECHANICAL VENTILATION

(For related information see Cardiac Deviations, Part I: Dysrhythmias, p. 184. Part III:
Hemodynamic monitoring, p. 219; Part III: Pulse oximetry, p. 426; Capnography, p. 439; Transcutaneous Pao_2 and $Paco_2$, p. 441; Indirect calorimetry, p. 441; Intravascular oxygenator, p. 442).

Case Management Basis
- DRG: None

Definition
Mechanical ventilation is used to treat hypoxemia and tissue hypoxia, to maintain positive pressure in the airways throughout the respiratory cycle, to improve oxygenation and ventilation, to decrease the work of breathing, and to promote rest and reconditioning of the respiratory muscle.

Patient Selection

INDICATIONS. Hypoxemia, tissue hypoxia, acute respiratory failure, chronic obstructive pulmonary disease, adult respiratory distress syndrome, hypoventilation resulting from chest wall or neuromuscular abnormalities, or patients who cannot affectively ventilate themselves.

Procedure

TECHNIQUE

Types of Mechanical Ventilators

- Volume-cycled ventilator: This delivers a preset volume despite a change in patient's lung compliance. The safety release pressure is set manually at about 10 cm H_2O above the peak-inspiratory pressure. The inspiratory time is determined by adjusting the flow rate of the gas to be delivered, while expiratory time is determined by setting a respiratory rate.
- Pressure-cycled ventilator: This delivers gas flows to patient until the preset pressure is reached throughout the system. When the pressure is reached, the gas flow is terminated and the patient exhales.

EQUIPMENT. Ventilator appropriate for patient's particular problem and availability.

Modes of Ventilators

- Continuous mandatory mode ventilation (CMV): CMV provides a preset number of breaths per minute or respiratory frequency (f) and tidal volume (V_T). The ventilator is sensitive to patient's inspiratory effort and subsequently delivers the preset V_T for patient-initiated breaths.
- Assisted mandatory control ventilation (AMV): AMV guarantees a preset minute ventilation and allows the patient to trigger the ventilator for additional breaths.
- Intermittent mandatory ventilation (IMV): IMV delivers a preset number of breaths at a given V_T while patient is allowed to breathe spontaneously through the ventilator circuit between the mandatory breaths. IMV breaths are independent of patient's breathing pattern.
- Synchronized intermittent mandatory ventilation (SIMV): SIMV delivers a preset V_T and f. Patient is able to breathe spontaneously while the ventilator provides a breath intermittently. SIMV is synchronized with patient's spontaneous breathing, which reduces competition between ventilator and spontaneous breathing patterns.
- High-frequency jet ventilation (HFJV): HFJV delivers low V_T (100 to 300 mL) at a rapid rate (60 to 100 BPM). The patient is connected to a volume ventilator set for continuous positive airway pressure. When the jet stream is propelled into the endotracheal tube, surrounding gases are propelled down the trachea.
- Continuous positive airway pressure (CPAP): CPAP is positive end-expiratory pressure applied to a spontaneously breathing patient and has the same effect as increasing functional residual capacity. It can be used in patients who require positive distending pressure to maintain adequate oxygenation but do not require mechanical ventilation.

- Positive end-expiratory pressure (PEEP): PEEP is applied to exhalation. The distending pressure in the airways and alveoli keeps small airways open throughout the entire ventilatory cycle. PEEP serves the purpose of increasing functional residual capacity.

Nontraditional Mechanical Ventilation

- Pressure support ventilation (PSV): PSV is a pressure-assist form of mechanical ventilatory support that augments the patient's inspiratory effort. Pressure support is sustained throughout the entire inspiratory cycle as the patient sets V_T, f, and timing. It is useful for the patient who is on IMV using a low flow rate and who is having difficulty being weaned from the ventilator. PSV can assist spontaneous effort and allow patient to exercise his or her own respiratory muscles, thereby reducing muscle atrophy.
- Differential lung compliance: This involves PEEP administered to a single lung, using a double-lumen endotracheal tube, which allows each lung to be ventilated independently. The V_T, fraction of inspired oxygen (F_{IO_2}), and airway pressure in each lung can be regulated independently to prevent exposing the unaffected lung to high pressures and toxic levels of oxygen.
- Inverse ratio ventilation (IRV): IRV provides an inspiratory time longer than expiratory time. The advantage of IRV is an improvement in arterial partial pressure of oxygen (Pa_{O_2}). Increased inspiratory time allows better stabilization of the alveoli and alveoli recruitment, thereby improving gas diffusion. With IRV, the increased Pa_{O_2} is related to an increase in mean airway pressure, which causes an increase in functional residual capacity.
- Extended mandatory minute ventilation: This provides patient with a constant level of minute ventilation, despite changes in his or her ability to breath. The patient can breathe more than the preset minute volume. The approach enhances the wean-

ing process by encouraging spontaneous breathing and by enabling patient to adjust to short-term changes in oxygen demand.

WEANING TECHNIQUES. Techniques include alternating assist control (A/C) or CMV, with periods of T-piece trials with and without CPAP; gradual reduction of the SIMV rate; or pressure support ventilation.

- Weaning parameters: Patient is awake and alert, oxygenation is $Pao_2 \geq 60$ mm Hg on $Fio_2 \leq 40\%$ to 50% and PEEP ≤ 5 cm H_2O. Ventilation is evaluated as minute ventilation ($\dot{V}E$) ≤ 10 L/min, $VT \geq 5$ mL/kg, and partial pressure of external carbon dioxide ($Paco_2$) within normal range for patient. Respiratory mechanisms reveal spontaneous respiratory rate (RR) ≤ 25 to 35 BPM, and maximal inspiratory force ≤ -20 cm H_2O.
- Criteria for termination of weaning: diastolic blood pressure (DBP) ≥ 100 mm Hg, decrease in level of consciousness, reduced systolic blood pressure (SBP), HR ≥ 110 bpm or ≥ 20 bpm increase over baseline, RR or f ≥ 30 BPM or ≥ 10 BPM increase over baseline, $VT \leq 250$ to 300 mL, pH ≤ 7.35, $Paco_2 \geq 45$ to 50 mm Hg, premature ventricular contractions ≥ 6/min, or changes in ST segment, such as elevation.

Complications

Complications include decreased venous return to the heart, barotrauma, oxygen toxicity, positive fluid balance, gastric distention and ileus, gastrointestinal bleeding, jaundice, pulmonary infection, malnutrition, respiratory muscle fatigue, acid-base disturbance, airway obstruction, dysrhythmias, and atelectasis.

NURSING MANAGEMENT: NURSING DIAGNOSES AND COLLABORATIVE PROBLEMS

Nursing Diagnoses

Common nursing goals for patients on mechanical ventilators are to improve gas ex-

change, promote airway clearance, maintain effective breathing pattern, prevent infection, provide nutritional intake, prevent injury, and promote alternative communication.

Impaired gas exchange related to increased ventilatory demand or inadequate PEEP ventilation secondary to increased work of breathing or improper ventilatory settings or asynchrony of patient and ventilation.

Expected Patient Outcomes. Patient maintains adequate gas exchange, as evidenced by arterial blood gases within normal range, RR 12 to 20 BPM, alveolar-arterial oxygen gradient ($P[A-a]O_2$) ≤ 15 mm Hg on room air or 10 to 65 mm Hg on 100% oxygen, arterial-alveolar oxygen tension ratio ($P[a/A]O_2$ 0.75 to 0.90, arterial oxygen content (Cao_2) 18 to 20 mL/100 mL, alveolar air equation (PAO_2) 100 mm Hg, static compliance (Cst) ≥ 50 mL/cm H_2O, dynamic compliance (Cdyn) ≥ 35 mL/cm H_2O, absence of dyspnea, no fever, respiratory function studies within normal range, proper ventilatory setting, adequate PEEP, Sao_2 95%, and synchrony between patient an ventilator.

- Consult with physician about the criteria used to determine when ventilatory support is needed: oxygenation ($Pao_2 \leq 60$ mm Hg on Fio_2 at 50%), ventilator ($Paco_2 \geq 50$ to 60 mm Hg, which is ≥ 10 mm Hg above patient's normal $Paco_2$), and respiratory mechanics (apnea, sustained RR ≥ 35 BPM, and vital capacity ≤ 10 to 15 mL/kg).
- Consult with physician about the criteria used to determine when weaning from a ventilator would be most effective for the patient: mechanical efficiency tests such as vital capacity ≥ 10 mL/kg, $V_T \geq 2$ mL/kg, RR ≤ 35 BPM, peak negative pressure ≤ -20 cm H_2O and minute ventilation 5 to 10 L/min; tests of oxygenation include $Pao_2 \geq 60$ torr on $\leq 40\%$ Fio_2, pulse oximetry ($SpO_2 \geq 92\%$ on ≥ 0.4 Fio_2, ($\dot{Q}s/\dot{Q}t$) $\leq 15\%$, PaO_2/Fio_2 ratio ≥ 200, and a:A ratio $\geq 25\%$; and tests of ventilation, which include ratio of volume of dead space

(V_{DS}) V_D/V_T ≤60%, pH ≤7.35, and $PaCo_2$ ≤45 mm Hg.

- Confer with Respiratory Therapy and physician regarding the desired type of ventilator and mode of ventilation.
- Review results of chest roentgenogram, arterial blood gas measurement, static compliance, dynamic compliance, and pulmonary function studies.
- Position patient in semi- to high Fowler's position to facilitate ventilation and oxygenation.
- Turn patient every 1 to 2 hours to enhance ventilation and perfusion delivered to lungs and promote drainage of some lung segments.
- Insert nasogastric tube to provide adequate nutritional intake.
- Monitor patient's diet to avoid increased carbon dioxide production: Decrease carbohydrate caloric intake.
- Monitor patient for clinical situations causing increased carbon dioxide production: fever, shivering, seizures, tissue injury, sepsis, stress, or trauma.
- Monitor respirations: rate, depth, symmetry of chest excursions, synchronization with ventilator, and presence of adventitious breath sounds.
- Obtain and report clinical findings associated with impaired gas exchange secondary to increased work of breathing: dyspnea, cyanosis, tachypnea, tachycardia, restlessness, and fatigue.
- Obtain and report changes in oxygenation and compliance indicating patient is not ready to be weaned from the ventilator: static compliance (Cst) ≤50 mL/cm H_2O, dynamic compliance (Cdyn) ≤35 mL/cm H_2O, and $\dot{Q}s/\dot{Q}t$ ≥8%.
- Monitor the efficiency of the patient ventilatory rate: A decrease in ventilatory efficiency leads to increased ventilatory demand.
- Monitor for factors increasing physiological dead space, which increases work load: rapid, shallow breathing pattern (high rate/low V_T ventilation); the length of the

ventilator connections and tubing; and positive-pressure ventilator.
- Assess ventilator function by verifying that the prescribed settings are being used and are effective. The settings include FIO_2 at the lowest rate to maintain Pao_2 ≥60 mm Hg and 100% in acute situations to achieve adequate oxygenation; V_T 10 to 15 mL/kg; RR 10 to 14 BPM; and mode of ventilation.
- Move endotracheal tube to the other side of the mouth daily to prevent tissue necrosis.
- Continuously monitor ECG during suctioning to assess HR and rhythm.
- Auscultate over artificial airway to assess for the presence of leaks.
- Use unit-prescribed method of endotracheal suctioning: preoxygenation, hyperinflation, hyperoxygenation, hyperventilation, maximal inflation, and oxygen insufflation.
- Evaluate patient's Sao_2 levels, as increased work of breathing causes increased ventilatory demand by increasing the metabolic need for oxygen.
- Teach patient use of techniques for inspiratory muscle training to increase muscle strength: Isocapnic hyperventilation requires many repetitions with a low load and increases the endurance of the respiratory muscle. Resistive breathing exercises are performed for one to three daily periods of 15 to 30 minutes.
- Monitor insensible and sensible fluid loss: daily weight, intake, specific gravity, and urine output.
- Administer IV fluids to maintain adequate hydration.
- Administer prescribed humidified oxygen FIO_2 50% to maintain normal secretion viscosity and Pao_2 80 to 100 mm Hg.
- Administer prescribed panaironium bromide to reduce patient's fighting the ventilator.
- Administer prescribed sedatives to relax patient while on the ventilator.

Ineffective airway clearance related to inability to remove excess secretion secondary to the presence of an artificial airway.

Expected Patient Outcomes. Patient maintains effective airway clearance, as evidenced by a patent airway, absence of adventitious breath sounds, RR 12 to 20 BPM, HR ≤100 bpm, skin color normal, or absence of restlessness.

- Review results of arterial blood gas measurement and chest roentgenogram.
- Obtain and report clinical findings indicating ineffective airway clearance: altered level of consciousness, crackles or wheezes, cyanosis, tachypnea, or tachycardia.
- Monitor clinical indicators of respiratory status: rate, rhythm, depth, symmetry of chest movement, skin color, use of accessory muscles, and lung sounds.
- Monitor for symptoms of excess secretions requiring suctioning: dyspnea, coughing, alarm system on ventilator, and increased secretions.
- In initiating endotracheal (ET) suctioning, preoxygenate with 100% oxygen or hyperinflation with a manual resuscitation bag and apply intermittent suction pressure according to unit protocol.
- Use unit-prescribed suction devices that permit patient to remain on the ventilator during suctioning: oxygen insufflation devices (OID) or closed tracheal suction system (CTSS). A closed-system, in-line suction catheter does not cause a clearly significant drop in SaO_2 or FIO_2 levels, thus eliminating suction-indiced hypoxemia. Change closed-system, in-line catheter every 24 hours or as indicated.
- Use intratracheal instillation of 2 mL or 5 mL of normal saline during suctioning to enhance the removal of secretion by stimulating a cough.
- Utilize chest physiotherapy (CPT) such as postural drainage, chest percussion, chest vibration, and cough enhancement to improve mucus and sputum clearance from the airways.
- Administer prescribed IV fluids to maintain adequate hydration.
- Maintain prescribed humidification of inspired gas to minimize drying of the tracheal mucosa.

- Administer prescribed bronchiodilators (aminophylline, metaproterenal or isoethasine) to relax bronchial smooth muscle and enhance removal of secretions (see Table 3–6).

Ineffective breathing pattern related to respiratory muscle weakness or increased dead space secondary to increased work of breathing or inability to inflate the lung.

Expected Patient Outcomes. Patient is able to maintain effective breathing pattern, as evidenced by arterial blood gases within normal range, RR 12 to 20 BPM, HR ≤100 bpm, synchrony with ventilator, absence of adventitious breath sounds, or absence of restlessness.

- Consult with physical therapist to assist patient with transfer, ambulation, and coordination of breathing with activity.
- Review results of arterial blood gas measurement and chest roentgenogram.
- Obtain and report clinical findings associated with ineffective breathing pattern: tachypnea, tachycardia, crackles, wheezes, restlessness, hyperventilation, and asynchrony with ventilation.
- Assess ventilator function by verifying that the prescribed settings are being used and are effective. The settings include FIO_2 at the lowest rate to maintain PaO_2 ≥60 mm Hg and 100% in acute situations to achieve adequate oxygenation; V_T 10 to 15 mL/kg; RR 10 to 14 BPM; and mode of ventilation.
- Monitor ventilator flow rate and note inspiratory:expiratory ratio. Both are adjusted so that inspiratory volume is completed in the time allowed. This is based upon the desired respiratory rate and inspiration:expiration ratio.
- Provide physical therapy to promote respiratory muscle strength, chest mobility, and general muscle tone.
- Ambulation promotes overall muscle conditioning and respiratory muscle functioning.
- Administer prescribed IV fluids to maintain adequate hydration.

- Administer prescribed analgesics or narcotics to relieve pain.
- Teach patient relaxation techniques such as progressive relaxation, meditation, biofeedback, or guided imagery.

High risk for infection related to intubation, immunosuppression, or malnutrition.

Expected Patient Outcomes. Patient is free of infection, as evidenced by negative sputum cultures, white blood cells (WBC) ≤11,000/μL, afebrile, heart rate (HR) ≤100 bpm, and RR 12 to 20 BPM.

- Consult with Respiratory Therapy regarding the schedule for changing ventilator tubing.
- Review results of WBC and sputum culture.
- Maintain adequate nutrition by nasogastric feedings: Protein malnutrition causes visceral protein (albumin) depletion.
- Obtain and report signs and symptoms of infection: elevated temperature ≥38°C (100°F), tachycardia, purulent sputum, drainage from endotracheal tube or tracheostomy stoma, and elevated WBC.
- Maintain aseptic technique when suctioning and caring for the endotracheal tube or tracheostomy.
- Monitor temperature every 2 hours while patient is febrile.
- Encourage patient to deep breathe, cough, and turn to promote mobilization and clearance of secretions.
- Measure respiratory quotient (RQ) to determine patient's nutritional status.
- Administer prescribed IV fluids to maintain adequate hydration.
- Administer prescribed hyperalimentation to provide nutrition.
- Administer prescribed antibiotics to treat ventilator-related infections.

Altered nutrition, less than body requirements related to increased energy expenditures from ventilatory support.

Expected Patient Outcomes. Patient's nutritional intake is adequate to meet metabolic needs, as evidenced by positive nitrogen balance and stable weight.

- Confer with dietitian as to the desired nutritional intake to meet caloric expenditures while patient on a ventilator.
- Consult with dietitian about the desired RQ.
- Review results of blood urea nitrogen (BUN) and serum electrolytes.
- Provide daily supplement of 200 to 300 mg nitrogen/kg body weight (1.2 to 1.9 g of protein/kg) for maintenance of ventilator-dependent patient.
- Provide enteral alimentation when patient has a functional gastrointestinal tract or parenteral nutrition as prescribed.
- Provide a positive caloric intake of 1.4 to 1.6 times the energy expenditure, a positive nitrogen balance with an intake of nitrogen 250 to 400 mg/kg of body weight, and half of the nonprotein calories as lipids.
- Assess gastrointestinal (GI) function such as presence and quality of bowel sounds, changes in abdominal girth, presence of anorexia, nausea, vomiting, constipation, or gastric bleeding.
- Monitor daily weight to ensure patient is receiving adequate nutritional intake.
- Monitor ventilatory mechanics in patients who are unable to maintain adequate nutrition intake: The malnourished patient may demonstrate decreased sighing, which can lead to decreased functional residual capacity and subsequent atelectasis or infection.
- Monitor serum albumin: ≤3.9 g/DL can contribute to decreased immune function and reduced oncotic pressure, which can lead to pulmonary edema.
- Monitor serum phosphorus levels: Low phosphorus can cause a decrease in the level of 2,3-diphosphoglycerate, which is a regulator of oxygen affinity at the cellular level, in red blood cells; and cause respiratory muscle weakness, since body is unable to produce sufficient adenosine triphosphate.
- Monitor clinical indicators of respiratory status: rate, depth, symmetry of chest ex-

cursions, use of accessory muscles, respiratory muscle fatigue, presence of inspiratory fatigue, or presence of adventitious breath sounds.

- Monitor daily weight, intake, specific gravity, and urine output to evaluate fluid balance.
- Utilize indirect calorimetry to reduce the incidence of overfeeding or underfeeding.
- Obtain the RQ by indirect calorimetry: Each substrate has its own RQ (carbohydrates 1.0, fat 0.7, protein 0.82, and lipogenesis 8.0). Carbohydrates provided in excess of energy needs cause lipogenesis, which increases carbon dioxide and an increase in RQ.
- Administer prescribed dextrose IV and multivitamins. Carbohydrate content is considered so as not to increase carbon dioxide production.

High risk of injury related to increased intrathoracic pressure, decreased cardiac output, and barotrauma secondary to PEEP and mechanical ventilation.

Expected Patient Outcomes. Patient is free of injury associated with mechanical ventilation, as evidenced by symmetry of chest movement, absence of adventitious breath sounds, intact skin, normal skin color, HR ≤ 100 bpm, BP within patient's normal range, cardiac output (CO) 4 to 8 L/min, central venous pressure (CVP) 2 to 6 mm Hg, and pulmonary capillary wedge pressure (PCWP) 6 to 12 mm Hg.

- Obtain and report clinical findings that indicate barotrauma: asymmetry of chest movement, diminished breath sounds on affected side, displacement of trachea to unaffected side, tachycardia, cyanosis, hypotension, or crepitus.
- Obtain and report hemodynamic parameters that indicated increased CO resulting from mechanical ventilation: CO ≤ 4 L/min, CVP ≤ 2 mm Hg, and PCWP ≤ 6 mm Hg.
- Assist with passive and active range of motion exercises to preserve muscle tone, enhance circulation, and improve ventilation.

- Provide lowest prescribed ventilatory pressure and level of PEEP to minimize risk of barotrauma.
- Assist with endotracheal or tracheostomy tube change.
- Administer prescribed IV fluids to maintain circulating volume and mean arterial pressure (MAP) ≥ 70 mm Hg caused by marginal or low flow states.
- Administer prescribed positive inotropes (dopamine) to maintain CO ≥ 4 L/min, BP within patient's normal range, MAP ≥ 70 mm Hg, and CVP ≤ 2 mm Hg.

Impaired verbal communication related to intubation or mechanical ventilation.

Expected Patient Outcomes. Patient is able to use alternative communication of needs.

- Establish an alternative means of communication, such as a Magic Slate or pencil and paper, so patient is able to share specific needs and concerns.
- Encourage family and friends to talk with patient about family events so patient feels included.
- Provide patient with simple information until he or she is able to confirm understanding verbally.
- Inform patient of the suctioning procedure.

■ CHEST DRAINAGE

For related information see Cardiac Deviations, Part I: Dysrhythmias, p. 184. Part III: Hemodynamic monitoring, p. 219. Part I: Pleural effusion, p. 394; Chest trauma, p. 382. Part III: Mechanical ventilation, p. 428; Capnography, p. 439; Transcutaneous Pao_2 and $Paco_2$, p. 441; Indirect calorimetry, p. 441.)

Case Management Basis
DRG: None

Definition
Chest tubes (CT) drain blood, fluid, or air that has accumulated in the thorax to restore

negative intrapleural pressure. Intermittent drainage can be accomplished via thoracentesis. Drainage by CTs reexpands the involved lung; reestablishes the integrity of the intrapleural sac; allows measurement and recording of chest drainage; promotes ventilation and decreases work of breathing; and facilitates ventilation-perfusion match.

Patient Selection

INDICATIONS. Traumatic pneumothorax, hemopneumothorax, spontaneous pneumothorax, iatrogenic pneumothorax, pyothorax, bronchopleural fistula, emphysema, and malignant hydrothorax.

Procedure

TECHNIQUE. The intraperative insertion of drainage tubes can be placed in the mediastinal or violated pleural cavities of the cardiothoracic patient. The mediastinal tube provides drainage of retrosternal fluid and reduction of mediastinal clot accumulation. Two transverse subdiaphragmatic incisions are made; then a right-angle catheter is used in the subdiaphragmatic position for retropericardial drainage. A second chest tube is positioned in the anterior mediastinum to the level of the fourth intercostal space. Closed-tube thoracotomy, the anatomic tube placement for treatment of pneumothorax, is at the anterior axillary line in the fourth interspace. The insertion site for drainage of a hemothorax or effusion is proximal to the fifth or sixth interspace in the midaxillary line.

- Suction: The amount and type of suction applied is determined by the type of medium to be drained, the amount of air leak from the lung, and the pressure or potential pressure of any factors that would influence suction (size of tubing, mode of connection of the bottles, or chamber to the chest tube, etc).
- Amount of suction: Apply 20 cm H_2O suction; if needed, increase suction to 40 to 60 cm H_2O, with an air-flow volume of 15 to 20 L/min.

EQUIPMENT
- Two-bottle: One serves as a one-way valve, allowing flow of the medium only from the pleural space into the chest bottles and not in the reverse direction, and as a collecting chamber; the second bottle controls the amount of suction applied to the pleural space.
- Three-bottle: The first bottle, connected to the tube, is the collecting chamber for fluid drainage from the pleural space; the second bottle functions as a one-way valve, allowing the flow of the drained medium only toward the chest bottle; and the third bottle controls the amount of suction used in the system.
- Pleur-evac: Disposable chest drainage system that functions on the same principle as the three chest bottles. The unit has a positive-pressure release valve, which prevent pressure buildup in the intrapleural space.

Complications
Ectopic insertion of chest tube into the lung, stomach, spleen, liver, or heart; infection in the pleural space; obstruction of chest tube from clotting or kinking and insufficient suction; or improper insertion of the chest tube.

NURSING MANAGEMENT: NURSING DIAGNOSES AND COLLABORATIVE PROBLEMS

Nursing Diagnoses
Common nursing goals for patients with chest tube drainage are to maintain fluid balance, prevent infection, and minimize pain.

Fluid volume deficit related to increased chest tube drainage or bleeding at insertion site.

Expected Patient Outcomes. Patient maintains adequate fluid volume, as evidenced by chest tube drainage within normal range and appropriate suction applied.

- Confer with physician regarding the amount of chest tube drainage expected for patient's problem and correct amount of suction.
- Review results of coagulation profile and chest roentgenogram.
- Place patient in a semi-Fowler's position, unless contraindicated, to facilitate air and fluid drainage.
- Splint chest tube insertion site during coughing or turning.
- Monitor and report bleeding ≥250 to 300 mL within first 2 hours. This can indicate the need for surgical reexploration.
- Measure chest tube drainage hourly until patient's condition stabilizes.
- Monitor and report chest tube output ≤50 mL or cessation of output; cessation with increased pulmonary capillary wedge pressure (PCWP) and cardiac output (CO) can indicate hemopericardium.
- Obtain and report the presence of clotted blood in the chest tubes, which can indicate active bleeding. Fresh blood pools and then clots when exposed to substernal air.
- Ensure that the water seal is at an appropriate level for the system being used and that all connections are tight.
- Monitor for the development of bubbling in the water-seal chamber, which can indicate a leak at a connector or the tracheobronchial tree. With mediastinal chest tubes there is no bubbling or fluctuation in the water seal chamber.
- Obtain and report respiratory rate (RR) ≥28 BPM, partial pressure of arterial oxygen (PaO_2) ≤60 mm Hg, restlessness, tachycardia, dyspnea, new bubbling in underwater seal chamber not caused by loose connection and deviated trachea.
- Apply occlusive dressing using petroleum jelly gauze and dry sterile gauze pads to reduce risks of air leak and infection.
- Secure excess chest drainage tubing loosely to bottom sheet so patient has sufficient tubing to move in bed: Securing tubing prevents accumulation of blood in the dependent tubing, which might interfere with drainage or serve as a milieu for bacterial growth.
- Administer prescribed IV fluids or blood products to maintain adequate circulating volume.
- Instruct patient as to the reasons for increased chest tube drainage.

High risk for infection related to incomplete drainage of the pleural space and lack of complete filling of the pleural space by the lung.

Expected Patient Outcomes. Patient is free from infection, as evidenced by white blood cells (WBC) ≤11,000/μL, absence or redness, tenderness, drainage, from incision site or chest tube, no fever; and negative cultures.

- Review results of CBC cultures.
- Monitor temperature every 1 to 2 hours or as needed.
- Encourage patient to turn, cough, and deep breathe to avoid stasis of secretions and atelectasis.
- Suction patient using unit protocol to aid in preventing pneumonia and maintain pulmonary integrity.
- Monitor chest tube site for redness, tenderness, swelling, or drainage.
- Change dressing using strict aseptic technique.
- Administer IV fluids as prescribed to maintain adequate hydration.
- Administer antipyretics as prescribed.

Pain related to the insertion of chest tube and removal of mediastinal or pleural tubes.

Expected Patient Outcomes. Patient evinces less nonverbal and verbal expression of pain.

- Secure excess chest drainage tubing to avoid pulling on sutures while patient turns.
- Evaluate when patient experiences pain.
- Splint chest tube insertion site during coughing or turning to reduce pain.
- Prepare patient for chest tube removal, which occurs when there is drainage ≤50 mL for 4 hours and ≤100 mL for 24 hours.

- Encourage patient to take a deep breath and hold while performing a gentle Valsalva's maneuver. A rapid motion is then used to extract the tube.
- Assist with removal of mediastinal tube, which involves a smooth, gentle technique to minimize tension or grafts.
- Teach patient that there may be sensation of burning, pain, pulling, or pressure when the chest tube is removed.
- Administer prescribed narcotic before chest tube is removed.
- Instruct patient to report any unusual pain.

■ EXTRACORPOREAL MEMBRANE OXYGENATION

(For related information see Cardiac Deviations, Part I: Dysrhythmias, p. 154. Part III: Hemodynamic monitoring, p. 219. Part I: Adult respiratory distress syndrome, p. 327; Pulmonary embolism, p. 397. Part III: Chest drainage, p. 434; Mechanical ventilation, p. 428; Capnography, p. 439; Transcutaneous Pao_2 and $Paco_2$, p. 441; Indirect calorimetry, p. 441.)

Case Management Basis
DRG: None

Definition
Extracorporeal membrane oxygenation (ECMO) is the use of a circuit and membrane lung to remove the majority of a patient's circulating blood volume for oxygenation and ventilation. It involves the partial removal of the patient's blood, infusion of oxygen, removal of carbon dioxide through an extracorporeal membrane, and return of the blood to the patient.

Patient Selection

INDICATIONS. Patients with reversible respiratory failure.

CONTRAINDICATIONS. Individual based.

Procedure

TECHNIQUE. Components of the ECMO circuit consist of a reservoir, a roller pump, a membrane oxygenator, and a heat exchanger. Venous blood is drained by gravity from the patient through a large-bore cannula placed in the saphenous, common iliac, or femoral vein. The blood is collected in a reservoir and circulated by a roller pump or Biopump through the membrane oxygenator. The membrane lung is connected to gas sources (oxygen and carbon dioxide) through a gas mixer. The blood is warmed with a heat exchanger, thereby maintaining normothermia, and returned to the patient through a second catheter.

EQUIPMENT
Venoarterial ECMO: This involves removing the patient's blood through a venous access catheter, exposing the blood to the membrane oxygenation, and returning the blood through a cannula in an artery. Venoarterial ECMO is less successful in adults than in children.

Venovenous ECMO: Venovenous ECMO drains venous blood by gravity into the extracorporeal circuit, infuses oxygen, removes carbon dioxide, and restores blood through a catheter into a large vein rather than an artery. Venovenous ECMO is used with less intensive pulmonary support, with low-frequency ventilation ≤5 breaths/min. It is used in patients with adult respiratory distress syndrome.

Complications
Technical difficulties of the circuit, cannula malposition, hemorrhage, or sepsis.

NURSING MANAGEMENT: NURSING DIAGNOSES AND COLLABORATIVE PROBLEMS

Nursing Diagnoses
Common nursing goals for patients undergoing ECMO are to maintain fluid balance,

improve oxygenation, prevent infection, and prevent injury.

Fluid volume deficit related to bleeding.

Expected Patient Outcomes. Patient maintains adequate fluid volume, as evidenced by blood pressure (BP) within patient's normal range, urinary output (UO) ≥30 mL/h, heart rate (HR) ≤100 bpm, central venous pressure (CVP) 2 to 6 mm Hg, patient maintains normal body weight, coagulation studies within normal range, and absence of bleeding.

- Review results of coagulation studies, hemoglobin, hematocrit, blood urea nitrogen (BUN) creatinine, electrolyte values, and total protein.
- Monitor all cannulation sites for bleeding.
- Measure daily weight, intake, specific gravity, gastric drainage, and UO to evaluate fluid balance. Report UO ≤30 mL/h.
- Obtain and report clinical findings associated with decreased fluid volume: hypotension, tachycardia, poor skin turgor, capillary refill ≥3 seconds, and peripheral pulse ≤+2.
- Monitor cannula site, incision, and invasive line sites for bleeding.
- Test nasogastric (NG) aspirate, urine, and stool for guiac.
- Administer prescribed IV fluids to maintain adequate hydration.
- Administer prescribed anticoagulants to maintain activated clotting time (ACT) 200 to 240 cc: 92-128 seconds. Initial dose of 100 to 200 U/kg is followed by a maintenance dose between 20 to 50 U/kg.
- Instruct patient to report any bleeding from invasive line sites, stool, or gums.

Impaired gas exchange related to respiratory failure.

Expected Patient Outcome. Patient maintains adequate gas exchange, as evidenced by RR 12 to 20 BPM, arterial blood gases within normal range, arterial oxygen saturation (SaO2) 95.0% to 97.5%, mixed venous oxygen saturation

(SvO2) 60% to 80%, absence of cyanosis, and absence of adventitious breath sounds.

- Review results of chest roentgenogram, arterial blood gas measurement, hemoglobin, and hematocrit.
- Change patient's position every 2 hours.
- Monitor for determinants in lung function: increased need for mechanical ventilation, declining arterial blood gas values, adventitious breath sounds, increased secretions, and increased pulmonary vascular resistance (PVR).
- Monitor clinical indicators of respiratory status: rate, depth, skin color, symmetry of chest wall movement, use of accessory muscles, presence of dyspnea, and presence of adventitious breath sounds.
- Obtain and report clinical findings associated with impaired gas exchange: tachycardia, hypotension, tachypnea, cyanosis, and crackles.
- Provide pulmonary hygiene with gentle suctioning, chest physiotherapy, and turning every 2 hours.
- Provide fraction of inspired oxygen (FIO2) at the prescribed amount to maintain SaO2 95%.
- Administer IV fluids as prescribed to maintain adequate hydration.
- Administer sedatives or paralytic agents as prescribed.

Infection related to cannulation sites.

Expected Patient Outcomes. Patient is free of infection, as evidenced by normal temperature; white blood cells (WBC) ≤11,000/μL; negative cultures; and absence of swelling, tenderness, redness, or drainage from cannulation site.

- Review results of WBC and cultures.
- Evaluate invasive line sites and cannulation sites for redness, tenderness, swelling or drainage.
- Monitor temperature every 2 to 4 hours while patient is febrile.

- Use strict aseptic technique when manipulating invasive lines or changing cannula.
- Clean cannula sites with povidone-idine solution and apply sterile dressing daily, using aseptic technique.
- Culture any suspicious drainage.
- Administer antibiotics as prescribed.

High risk for injury related to venovenous trauma from cannulation.

Expected Patient Outcome. Patient experiences no venovenous trauma from cannulation.

- Monitor clinical indicators of perfusion beyond the cannulation sites: skin color and warmth, peripheral pulses, and capillary refill.
- Report altered perfusion beyond the cannulation site: skin cool and pale or cyanotic, edema, peripheral pluses $\leq +2$, and capillary refill ≥ 3 seconds.
- Evaluate cannulation sites for bleeding or hematoma.
- Instruct patient to report any pain at the cannulation site.

Collaborative Problem

A common collaborative goal for patients undergoing ECMO is to increase cardiac output.

Potential Complication: Decreased Cardiac Output.

Decreased cardiac output related to decreased afterload related to blood flow through the ECMO circuit.

Expected Patient Outcomes. Patient maintains adequate cardiac output (CO), as evidenced by CO 4 to 8 L/min, cardiac index (CI) 2.7 to 4.3 L/min/m^2, CVP 2 to 6 mm Hg, systemic vascular resistance (SVR) 900 to 1200 dynes/s/cm^{-5}, systemic vascular resistance index (SVRI) 1970 to 2390 dynes/s/cm^{-5}/m^2, pulmonary artery pressure (PAP) 20 to 30 8 to 15 mm Hg, pulmonary capillary wedge pressure (PCWP) 6 to 12 mm Hg, HR ≤ 100 bpm, mean arterial pressure (MAP) 70 to 100 mm Hg, UO ≥ 30 mL/h, skin warm, dry and normal color, BP within patient's normal range, capillary refill ≤ 3 seconds and peripheral pulses $+2$.

- Consult with physician to validate expected patient outcomes used to evaluate adequate afterload.
- Obtain and report hemodynamic parameters that indicate altered afterload: CO ≤ 4 L/min, CI ≤ 2.7 L/min/m^2, CVP ≤ 2 mm Hg, SVR ≤ 900 dynes/s/cm^{-5}, SVRI ≤ 1970 dynes/s/cm^{-5}/m^2, PAP systolic ≤ 20mm Hg or diastolic ≤ 8 mm Hg, and PCWP ≤ 6 mm Hg.
- Monitor clinical indicators of perfusion: BP, HR, UO, cardiac rhythm, capillary refill, skin color and warmth, presence of edema, and peripheral pulses.
- Report other clinical findings that indicate decreased afterload: tachycardia, tachypnea, cyanosis, skin cool, hypotension, capillary refill ≥ 3 seconds, and peripheral pulses $\leq +2$.
- Monitor ECG continuously to assess HR and rhythm. Document ECG rhythm strips every 2 to 4 hours in patients with dysrhythmias.
- Measure daily weight, intake, specific gravity, and UO to evaluate fluid balance. Report UO ≤ 30 mL/h.
- Administer IV fluid replacement as prescribed to keep MAP 80 to 90 mm Hg, diastolic PAP 15 to 20 mm Hg, and left atrial pressure (LAP) 12 to 17 mm Hg.
- Administer vasoactive medications as prescribed to maintain CI ≥ 2.7 L/min/m^2 and MAP ≥ 70 to 100 mm Hg.

■ CAPNOGRAPHY

(For related information see Cardiac Deviations, Part I: Dysrhythmias, p. 184. Part III: Hemodynamic monitoring, p. 219. Part I: Respiratory acidosis, p. 412; Respiratory alkalosis, p. 415. Part III: Chest drainage, p. 434; Mechanical ventilation, p. 428 ; Tran-

scutaneous P_{O_2} and P_{CO_2}, p. 441; Indirect calorimetry, p. 441.)

Case Management Basis
DRG: None

Definition
Capnography is the continuous measurement of carbon dioxide exchange in the lungs. It is displayed as a wave form called the capnogram.

Patient Selection

INDICATIONS. During anesthesia and mechanical ventilation; for detection of esophageal intubation; induced hypocapnia in head-impaired patients; and to evaluate blood flow during resuscitation.

CONTRAINDICATIONS. None.

Procedure

TECHNIQUE. The normal capnogram is broken down into three phases. Phase I: The partial pressure of arterial carbon dioxide (P_{CO_2}) is zero during inspiration. At the beginning of exhalation, P_{CO_2} remains zero as gas from anatomic dead space leaves the airway. Phase II: The P_{CO_2} increases as alveolar gas mixes with dead-space gas. Phase III: During exhalation the curve levels from a plateau, called alveolar plateau. This represents the gas flow from alveoli. Finally, P_{CO_2} at the end of the alveolar plateau is called end-tidal P_{CO_2} ($P_{et}CO_2$). The $P_{et}CO_2$ represents alveolar P_{CO_2} ($P_{A}CO_2$). The $P_{A}CO_2$ is determined by how well carbon dioxide is added to the alveolus and the carbon dioxide is removed from the alveolus. Clinically, an increase or decrease in $P_{et}CO_2$ can result from changes in carbon dioxide production in metabolism, oxygen circulating to the lungs, or changes in alveolar ventilation. The gradient between $P_{a}CO_2$ and $P_{et}CO_2$ ($P(a-_{et}CO_2)$) is ≤ 5 mm Hg. In critically ill patients with dead space disease

causing high ventilation:perfusion, the $P_{et}CO_2$ may be less than $P_{a}CO_2$.

EQUIPMENT. The carbon dioxide is measured at the airway using mass spectrometry or infrared capnography. Bedside capnography uses either a mainstream capnograph or a sidestream capnograph.

- Mainstream capnograph: The measurement chamber is placed at the airway.
- Sidestream capnograph: Gas is aspirated through fine-bore tubing to the measurement chamber inside the capnograph.

NURSING MANAGEMENT: NURSING DIAGNOSES AND COLLABORATIVE PROBLEMS

Collaborative Problem
A common collaborative goal for patients using capnography is to maintain acid-base balance.

Potential Complication: Respiratory Acidosis. Respiratory acidosis related to inadequate weaning from mechanical ventilation secondary to weakness of respiratory muscles or inadequate compliance.

Expected Patient Outcomes. Patient maintains normal acid-base balance and $P_{et}CO_2$ 1 to 4 mm Hg below $P_{a}CO_2$.

- Consult with physician as to the desired value of $P_{et}CO_2$: $P_{et}CO_2$ can be as low as the inspired P_{CO_2} (zero) or as high as the mixed venous P_{CO_2} ($P_{\bar{v}}CO_2$).
- Consult with physician as to the patient's desired $P_{et}CO_2$ level during weaning from mechanical ventilation.
- Review arterial blood gas and serum electrolyte results.
- Monitor the gradient between $P_{a}CO_2$ and $P_{et}CO_2$.
- Report a decrease in $P_{et}CO_2$, which can be the result of changes in carbon dioxide production (metabolism), carbon dioxide de-

livery to the lungs (circulation), or change in alveolar ventilation.

- Report increased $P_{et}CO_2$, which can indicate increase in $PaCO_2$ caused by hypoventilation.
- Monitor $PaCO_2$, which is determined by the rate at which carbon dioxide is added to the alveolus and the rate at which carbon dioxide is cleared from the alveolus. The $PaCO_2$ is the result of ventilation:perfusion ($\dot{V}:\dot{Q}$) ratio.
- Monitor the shape of the capnogram as an indication of abnormal lung function.
- Instruct patient as to the purpose of capnography during surgery or mechanical ventilatory support.

■ TRANSCUTANEOUS Pa_{O2} AND Pa_{CO2}

(For related information see Cardiac Deviations, Part I: Dysrhythmias, p. 184. Part III: Hemodynamic monitoring, p. 219. Part III: Chest drainage, p. 434; Mechanical ventilation, p. 428; Capnography, p. 439; Indirect calorimetry, p. 441.)

Case Management Basis
DRG: None

Definition
Transcutaneous oxygen monitoring (TcP_{O2}) monitoring allows for continuous noninvasive measurement of oxygen level.

Patient Selection

INDICATIONS. Used to monitor ventilation: perfusion balance and in postoperative vascular surgery patients.

Procedure

TECHNIQUE. The $PtcO_2$ electrode is heated to approximately 44°C. The increase in oxygen pressure (PO_2) caused by heating roughly balances the decrease in PO_2 caused by skin oxygen consumption and the difference of oxygen across the skin. The $PtcO_2$ is less than the partial pressure of arterial oxygen (PaO_2). The $PtcO_2$ is affected by perfusion and can reflect the product of cardiac output and arterial oxygen content to the skin under the electrode.

EQUIPMENT. Severinghaus Electrode: Similar to ones used in blood gas analyzer. The $PtcO_2$ is greater than $PaCO_2$ and a correction factor is incorporated into the electrode so that Ptc_{CO2} approximates $PaCO_2$.

NURSING MANAGEMENT: NURSING DIAGNOSES AND COLLABORATIVE PROBLEMS

Nursing Diagnosis
A common nursing goal for patients with transcutaneous oxygen monitoring is to maintain skin integrity.

Skin integrity impaired related to electrode burn.

Expected Patient Outcome. Patient maintains skin integrity.

- Monitor patient's skin for evidence of redness or blistering.
- Change the location of the electrode as needed to maintain skin tissue integrity.
- Monitor the precise temperature of the skin electrode.
- Change membrane or electrode as needed.
- Instruct patient as to the relationship between heating the electrode and clinical data obtained about $PtCO_2$.

■ INDIRECT CALORIMETRY

(For related information see Part I: Adult respiratory distress syndrome, p. 327; Respiratory alkalosis, p. 412; Respiratory acidosis, p. 415. Part III: Mechanical ventilation, p. 428; Capnography, p. 439.)

Case Management Basis
DRG: None

Definition

Indirect calorimetry is the calculation of energy expenditure (EE) from measurements of oxygen consumption (Vo_2) and carbon dioxide production (Vco_2).

Patient Selection

INDICATIONS. Used to determine appropriate nutritional support in patients who are malnourished and patients with chronic obstructive pulmonary disease.

CONTRAINDICATIONS. None.

Procedure

TECHNIQUE. Indirect calorimetry is used to determine the respiratory quotient (RQ). RQ is used to evaluate substrate metabolism, with RQ = 0.7 for fat metabolism, RQ = 0.8 for protein metabolism, RQ = 1.0 for carbohydrate metabolism, and RQ $\geq$ 1.0 for lipogenesis.

EQUIPMENT. Indirect calorimeters use either open-circuit or closed-circuit techniques.

NURSING MANAGEMENT: NURSING DIAGNOSES AND COLLABORATIVE PROBLEMS

Nursing Diagnoses

A common nursing goal for patients with indirect calorimetry is to provide adequate nutrition.

Altered nutrition: more than body requirements related to increased metabolism, malnutrition, or prolonged dependency on mechanical ventilation.

Expected Patient Outcome. Patient maintains normal body weight.

- Consult with physician regarding the desired RQ.
- Consult with dietitian regarding patient's EE in relation to patient's diet.

- Provide patient with the appropriate diet to meet metabolic needs.
- Measure EE: EE = ($[Vo_2][3.94]$ + $[Vco_2][1.11]$) $\times$ 1440.
- Monitor the patient's RQ using either the open or closed circuit. RQ = Vco_2/Vo_2.
- Teach patient the purpose behind indirect calorimetry.

■ IMPLANTABLE INTRAVASCULAR OXYGENATOR

(For related information see Part I: Chest trauma, p. 382; Pneumonia, p. 375; Pulmonary embolism, p. 397; Adult respiratory distress syndrome, p. 327. Multisystem Deviations; Part I: Sepsis, p. 772.)

Case Management Basis
DRG: None

Definition

The implantable intravascular oxygenator still under phase II clinical evaluation, is a device for extrapulmonary gas exchange that provides oxygenation and carbon dioxide removal outside the lungs. The device provides supplemental gas exchange for dysfunctional lungs and provides temporary ventilatory support when reversible respiratory insufficiency occurs. The device is capable of delivery up to 170 mL O_2/min while removing up to 140 mL CO_2/min in an individual weighing 80 kg.

Patient Selection

INDICATIONS. The implantable intravascular oxygenator can be used in patients with respiratory insufficiency who have evidence of diffuse parenchymal or interstitial infiltrates in lungs, pulmonary capillary wedge pressure (PCWP) $\leq$ 16 mm Hg, and partial pressure arterial oxygen (Pao_2) $\leq$ 60 mm Hg when oxygen is given at $\geq$ 50 % or Pao_2 $\geq$ 40 mm Hg when minute volume of gas delivered is 150 mL/min/kg. Other indications consist of bronchopleural fistula, lung transplant, pneumonia, postshock lung injury, sepsis, surgery, trauma, postpartum, pulmonary resection, trauma with disrupted pulmonary tissue, and pulmonary embolisms.

CONTRAINDICATIONS. Contraindications include multiple organ failure, major sepsis unresponsive to treatment, recent major surgery or trauma in which systemic anticoagulation is contraindicated, venous or venal caval thrombosis at risk for embolization, invisible right femoral or right internal jugular access vein, irreversible pulmonary disease, low cardiac output unresponsive to therapy, intracranial bleeding, recent neurological dysfunction, or hepatic failure.

Procedure

TECHNIQUE. The intravascular oxygenator is placed within the vena cava and provides part of the body's total gas exchange requirements. The device is positioned between the mid-superior vena cava and the renal veins. Its goal is to assist the lungs by adding oxygen to and removing carbon dioxide from venous blood. Oxygen enters the venous blood and carbon dioxide is removed through an outer gas conduit of the double-lumen gas transport tube. The tube is attached to a gas controller unit so that adjustments can be made in either the rate of oxygen flow or amount of vacuum. The oxygen flow rate (inlet pressure) is between 1500 and 2500 mL/min and vacuum (outlet pressure) is between 200 and 400 mm Hg.

EQUIPMENT. The device consists of numerous hollow fibers that are permeable to gas, but not liquid. The crimped hollow fibers cause disordered blood flow through the vena cava while allowing maximum flow past each fiber.

Complications

Complications include impaired venous return, thrombosis, or bleeding.

NURSING MANAGEMENT: NURSING DIAGNOSES AND COLLABORATIVE PROBLEMS

Common nursing goals for patients with an implantable intravascular oxygenator are to maintain fluid balance, support tissue perfusion, or prevent infection.

Nursing Diagnoses

High risk for fluid volume deficit related to bleeding secondary to anticoagulation therapy.

Expected Patient Outcomes. Patient maintains adequate fluid volume, as evidenced by absence of bleeding, normal coagulation studies, blood pressure (BP) within patient's normal range, heart rate (HR) ≤100 bpm, absence of pallor or cyanosis, mean arterial pressure (MAP) 70 to 100 mm Hg, peripheral pulses +2, capillary refill ≤3 seconds, and urinary output (UO) ≥30 mL/h.

- Consult with physician about patient's risk for bleeding during use of intravascular oxygenator.
- Review results of coagulation studies.
- Assess the catheter insertion site for bleeding every hour and report the presence of subcutaneous collection of blood around the incision or pooling of blood under patient.
- Obtain data and report hypotension, tachycardia, MAP ≤70 mm Hg, peripheral pulses ≤+2, pallor or cyanosis, and capillary refill ≥3 seconds.
- Monitor and report presence of blood in the urine, stool, or nasogastric drainage; increase in chest tube drainage; or output from other drains.
- When the catheter is removed and heparin is discontinued, assess the surgical site for bleeding until coagulation studies are within normal limits.
- Administer prescribed packed red blood cells to replace volume loss and maintain hematocrit 30% to 35%.

• Teach patient to report any oozing or bleeding from catheter site.

Decreased tissue perfusion related to intravascular oxygenator device.

Expected Patient Outcomes. Patient maintains adequate tissue perfusion, as evidenced by peripheral pulses +2 in the catheterized extremity, pink and warm skin, and absence of edema in the cannulated extremity.

• Should the intravascular oxygenator be inserted through the right femoral vein, keep the right leg straight and restrained.
• Assess the cannulated extremity for quality of pulses, color, and temperature.
• Report changes in the quality of distal pulses, cool skin, pallor or cyanosis, or edema in the cannulated extremity.
• Encourage patient to described pain in the cannulated extremity on a scale of 1 to 10.
• Provide pneumatic compression stockings for patients immediately after the device is inserted to reduce edema formation.
• Teach patient to report pain in the catheter site.

High risk of infection related to invasive lines.

Expected Patient Outcomes. Patient is free of infection, as evidenced by white blood cells (WBC) $\leq 11,000/\mu L$; normothermia; absence of swelling; tenderness, redness, or drainage from catheter site and negative cultures.

• Review results of WBC and cultures.
• Provide sterile dressing to the insertion site daily or more frequently should there be drainage or bleeding.
• Assess and report tenderness, redness, swelling or drainage from the insertion site.
• Should a localized infection occur, obtain culture when temperature $\geq 38.3°C$.
• Monitor continuously temperature.
• Cleanse the insertion site with normal saline. This is followed by betadine spray and apply a dry, occlusive dressing.

• Administer prescribed prophylactic antibiotics, such as cephalosporins to prevent infection.

SELECTED BIBLIOGRAPHY

Adams SJ, Martin TG. The emergent approach to asthma. Chest. 1992;101:422S–425S.

Ahrens T. The cutting edge in pulmonary critical care. *Crit Care Nurse.* 1993; (suppl):4–5.

Ahrens T. Pulmonary data acquisition. In: Kinney MR, Packa DR, Dunbar SB, eds. *AACN's Clinical Reference for Critical Care Nursing,* 3rd ed. St. Louis, Mo: Mosby Year Book, 1993:689–700.

Ahrens T. Respiratory disorders. In: Kinney MR, Packa DR, Dunbar SB, eds. *AACN's Clinical Reference for Critical Care Nursing,* 3rd ed. St. Louis, Mo: Mosby Year Book, 1993:701–740.

Ahrens T. Pulmonary data acquisition. In: Kinney MR, Packa DR, Dunbar SB, eds. *AACN's Clinical Reference for Critical Care Nursing,* 3rd ed. St. Louis, Mo: Mosby Year Book; 1993:741–753.

Asskanaz J, Weissman C, Rosenbaum SH, et at. Nutrition and the respiratory system. *Crit Care Med.* 1982; 10:163–172.

Benz JJ. Adult respiratory distress syndrome. In: Hudak CM, Gallo BM, Benz JJ. *Critical Care Nursing,* 6th ed. Philadelphia, Pa: JB Lippincott, Co; 1994:502–514.

Booker KJ, Arnold JS. Respiratory-induced changes in the pulmonary capillary wedge pressure tracing. *Crit Care Nurse.* 1993; 13(3): 80–88.

Briones TL. Pressure support ventilation: new ventilatory techniques. *Crit Care Nurse.* 1992; 12(4):51–58.

Brown RB. Acute and chronic bronchitis. *Postgrad Med.* 1989; 85:249–254.

Bullock BL, Rosendahl PP. *Pathophysiology Adaptation and Alteration in Function,* 3rd ed. Philadelphia, Pa: JB Lippincott Co; 1992.

Carrougher GJ. Inhalation injury. *AACN Clin Issues Crit Care Nurs.* 1993; 4:367–377.

Caswell DR. Thromboembolic phenomena. *Crit Care Nurs Clin North Am.* 1993; 5:489–497.

Clochesy JM. *Advanced Technology in Critical Care Nursing.* Rockville, Md: Aspen Publishers Inc., 1989.

Cooper D. Patients with chronic obstructive pulmonary disease. In: Clochesy JM, Breu C, Cardin S, et al, eds. *Critical Care Nursing.*

Philadelphia, Pa: WB Saunders Co, 1993: 569–588.

Davidson JE. Neuromuscular blockade. *Focus Crit Care AACN*. 1991, 18:512–520.

Deglin JH, Vallerand AH. Davis's Drug Guide for Nurses, 3rd ed. Philadelphia, Pa: FA Davis Co; 1995.

Dettermeier PA, Johnson TM. The art and science of mechanical ventilation adjustment. *Crit Care Nurs Clin North Am*. 1990; 3:575–583.

Dirkes S, Dickinson S, Valentine J. Acute respiratory failure and ECMO. *Crit Care Nurse*. 1992; 12(7):39–47.

Doering LV. The effect of positioning on hemodynamics and gas exchange in the critically ill: a review. Am J Crit Care. 1993; 2:208–216.

Dolan JT. Nursing management of the adult respiratory distress syndrome in hypoxemic acute respiratory failure. *Critical Care Nursing: Clinical Management Through the Nursing Process.* Philadelphia, Pa: FA Davis Co; 1991:660–679.

Enger EL. Patients with adult respiratory distress syndrome. In: Clochesy JM, Breu C, Cardin S, et al, eds. *Critical Care Nursing*. Philadelphia, Pa: WB Saunders Co; 1993:546–565.

Geisman LK, Ahrens T. Auto-PEEP: An impediment to weaning in the chronically ventilated patient. *AACN Clin Issues Crit Care Nurs*. 1991; 2:391–397.

Goldhaber SZ. Tissue plasminogen activator in acute pulmonary embolism. *Chest*. 1989; 95:282S–289S.

Govon LE, Hayes JE, Shannon MT, et al. *Drugs and Nursing Implications,* 8th ed. Norwalk, Conn: Appleton & Lange, 1995.

Greenfield LJ, Michna BA. Venous interruption. In: Haimovici H, Callow AD, DePalma RG, et al. *Vascular Surgery: Principles and Techniques.* Norwalk, Conn: Appleton & Lang; 1989:929–940.

Gross SB. Current challenges, concepts and controversies in chest tube management. *AACN Clin Issues Crit Care Nurs*. 1993; 4:260–275.

Grossbach I. Pressure support ventilation. *Crit Care Nurse*. 1992; 12:50–52.

Groth ML, Hurewitz AM. Pharmacologic management of acute asthma. *Emer Med* 1989; 23–30.

Hammond SG. Chest injuries in the trauma patient. *Nurs Clin North Am*. 1990; 25:35–43.

Henneman EA. The art and science of weaning from mechanical ventilation. *Focus Crit Care.* 1991; 18:490–501.

Hess D. Noninvasive respiratory monitoring during ventilatory support. *Crit Care Nurs Clin North Am.* 1991;3:565–574.

Hinson JR, Marini JL. Principles of mechanical ventilation use is respiratory failure. *Ann Rev Med.* 1992; 43:341–361.

Hull RD, Moser KM, Salzman EW. Preventing pulmonary embolism. *Patient Care.* 1989; 23(4): 63–81.

Hurn PD, Hartsock RL. Blunt thoracic injuries. *Crit Care Nurs Clin North Am.* 1993;5:673–686.

Jarpe MB. Nursing care of patients receiving long-term infusion of neuromuscular blocking agents. *Crit Care Nurse.* 1992;12(7):58–63.

Juarez P. Mechanical ventilation for the patient with severe ARDS: pressure support and inverse ratio ventilation. *Crit Care Nurse.* 1992; 12(4):34–39.

Kearney ML. Adult respiratory distress syndrome following thoracic trauma. *Crit Care Nurs Clin North Am.* 1993; 5:723–734.

Kennedy JI, Fulmer JD. Diagnosis: interstitial lung disease. *Hosp Med* 1989; 25(2):82–103.

Knezevich BA. *Trauma Nursing Principles and Practice.* Norwalk, Conn: Appleton-Century-Crofts; 1986.

Loeb S. *Clinical Laboratory Tests.* Springhouse, Pa: Springhouse Publishing; 1991.

Luchtefeld WB. Pulmonary contusion. *Focus Crit Care.* 1990; 17:482–488.

Malen JF, Ochea LL, Sander MC. Lung transplantation. *Crit Care Nurs Clin North Am.* 1992; 4:111–130.

McIntosh D, Baun MM, Rogge J. Effects of lung hyperinflation and presence of positive end-expiratory pressure on arterial and tissue oxygenation during endotracheal suctioning. *Am J Crit Care Nurs.* 1993;2:317–325.

Mulla AD. One-lung ventilation. *Cur Rev Nurse Anesth.* 1989;9(6):66–72.

Peterson KJ, Brown MM. Extracorporeal membrane oxygenator in adults: a nursing challenge. *Focus Crit Care Nurs.* 1990; 17(1):40–49.

Prewill RM. Hemodynamic management in pulmonary embolism and acute hypoxemic respiratory failure. *Crit Care Med.* 1990; 18:561–569.

Reading PM, St. John RE. Aerosolized therapy for ventilator assisted patients. *Crit Care Nurs Clin North Am.* 1993; 5:271–280.

Roberts SL. Common nursing diagnoses for pulmonary adveolar edema patients. *Dimensions Crit Care Nurs.* 1992: 11(1):13–27.

Roberts SL. High-permeability pulmonary edema: nursing assessment, diagnosis and interventions. *Heart Lung.* 1990: 19:287–299.

Roberts SL. Pulmonary tissue perfusion altered: emboli. *Heart Lung.* 1987; 16:128–138.

Roberts SL. Pulmonary edema. In: Physiological Concepts and The Critically Ill Patient. Englewood Cliffs, NJ: Prentice-Hall; 1985: 134–176. [out of print]

Roberts SL. Pulmonary embolism. In: Physiological Concepts and The Critically Ill Patient. Englewood Cliffs, NJ: Prentice-Hall; 1985: 177–210. [out of print]

Roberts SL. Adult respiratory distress syndrome. In: Physiological Concepts and The Critically Ill Patient. Englewood Cliffs, NJ: Prentice-Hall; 1985:211–244. [out of print]

Ryan CJ. Patients with pulmonary infections. In: Clochesy JM, Breu C, Cardin S, et al, eds. *Critical Care Nursing.* Philadelphia, Pa: WB Saunders Co; 1993: 589–601.

Ryan B, Luer J. Respiratory pharmacology and the weaning patient: implications for critical care nursing. *AACN Clin Issues Crit Care Nurs.* 1991; 2:361–371.

Sachs FL. Bronchitis: a practical guide. *Hosp Med.* 1990; 26(4):95–106.

Sahd RL. Pulmonary contusion: the hidden danger in blunt chest trauma. *Crit Care Nurse.* 1991; 11(6):46–57.

Schactman M, Greene J. Rhythm disturbance in the patient with pulmonary disease. *Crit Care Nurse.* 1993; 13(2):41–46.

Schaffer SD. Current approaches in adult asthma: assessment, education and emergency management. *Nurse Practitioner.* 1991; 16(1):18–34.

Schrader KA. Penetrating chest trauma. *Crit Care Nurs Clin North Am.* 1993; 5:687–696.

Shekleton ME. Respiratory muscle conditioning and the work of breathing: a critical balance in the weaning patient. *AACN Clin Issues Crit Care Nurs.* 1991; 2:405–414.

Spector N. Nutritional support of the ventilator-dependent patient. *Nurs Clin North Am.* 1989; 24:407–415.

Somerson SJ, Sicilia MR. Emergency oxygen administration and airway management. *Crit Care Nurse.* 1992; 12(4):23–29.

Stamatos CA, Reed S. Nutritional needs of trauma patients: challenges, barriers and solutions. *Crit Care Nurs Clin North Am* 1994; 6:501–514.

Stauffer JL. Pulmonary diseases. In: Krupp MA, McPhee SJ, Papadakin MA, eds. *Current Medical Diagnosis and Treatment,* 33rd ed. Norwalk, Conn: Appleton & Lange; 1994:207–279.

Stillwell SB. *Mosby's Critical Care Nursing Reference.* St. Louis, Mo: Mosby Year Book; 1992.

Stone AV, Bone RC. Successful weaning from mechanical ventilation. *Postgrad Med.* 1989; 86:315–319.

Stratton MB. Ventilation-perfusion scintigraphy in diagnosis of pulmonary thromboembolism. *Focus on Crit Care.* 1990; 17:287–293.

Susla GM. Neuromuscular blocking agents in critical care. *Crit Care Nurs Clin North Am.* 1993; 5:297–311.

Swearingen PL, Keen JH. Mannual of Critical Care, 2nd ed. St. Louis, Mo: Mosby Year-Book; 1992.

Thelan LA, Davie JK, Urden LD. *Textbook of Critical Care Nursing,* 2nd ed. St. Louis, Mo; Mosby Year-Book; 1994.

Von Rueden KT, Dunham CM. Sequelae of massive fluid resuscitation in trauma patients. *Crit Care Nurs Clin North Am.* 1994; 6:463–472.

Weilitz PB. Weaning from mechanical ventilation: old and new strategies. *Crit Care Nurs Clin North Am.* 1991; 3:585–590.

White BS, Roberts SL. High permeability pulmonary edema: pathophysiology and mechanisms of injury. *Intensive Care Nurs.* 1990; 6:79–91.

White BS, Roberts SL. Nursing management of high permeability pulmonary edema. *Intensive Care Nurs.* 1991; 7:11–22.

White BS, Roberts SL. Powerlessness and the pulmonary edema patient. *Dimensions Crit Care Nurs.* 1993; 12(3):127–137.

White BS, Roberts SL. Pulmonary alveolar edema: preventing complications. *Dimensions Crit Care Nurs.* 1992; 11(2):90–103.

Wilson, RF. Trauma. In: Shoemaker WC, Ayres S, Grenvik A, et al, eds. *Textbook of Critical Care,* 2nd ed. Philadelphia, Pa: WB Saunders Co; 1989:929–940.

Wright J, Doylke PR, Yoshihara G. Advances in mechanical ventilation. In: Clochesy JM, Breu C, Cardin S, et al, eds. *Critical Care Nursing.* Philadelphia, Pa: WB Saunders Co; 1993: 602–622.

Renal Deviations

■ RENAL TRAUMA

(For related information see Cardiac Deviations, Part I: Shock, p. 174. Part I: Acute tubular necrosis, p. 455; Acute renal failure, p. 459; Metabolic acidosis, p. 474. Part II: Renal transplantations, p. 491. Part III: Hemodialysis, p. 496; Peritoneal dialysis, p. 502; Continuous renal replacement therapy, p. 505.)

Case Management Basis
DRG: 331 Other kidney and urinary tract diagnoses, age greater than 17 with complication
LOS: 5.30 days
DRG: 332 Other kidney and urinary tract diagnoses, age greater than 17 without complications
LOS: 3.00 days

Definition
Renal trauma resulting from penetrating or blunt injuries can cause hemorrhage, shock, infection, or organ dysfunction.

Pathophysiology
Renal trauma is classified as minor, major, or critical. Minor trauma involves kidney contusion, which causes some damage to the renal parenchyma but no rupture of the renal capsule or tear in the collecting system. Subcapsular hematoma and minor cortical lacerations are present in kidney contusion. Major trauma consists of a complete or incomplete laceration extending from the collecting system through the parenchyma and the renal capsule, allowing the mixture of blood and urine within collecting space. Critical trauma involves a fracture or fragmentation of the kidney or an extension of the injury into the renal pedicle. There may also be destruction of the renal parenchyma and extension of the injury into the renal pedicle.

Nursing Assessment

PRIMARY CAUSES
• Blunt, or nonpenetrating, renal injuries are caused by athletic accident; fall; blow to back, flank, or abdominal area; and motor vehicle accident involving an indirect deceleration injury in which the body stops but the kidney keeps going. This can cause tearing or rupture of the vascular pedicle.

- Penetrating renal injuries are caused by gunshot wounds and knife wounds. Approximately 8% of patients with a penetrating injury will have a renal injury.

RISK FACTORS
- Previously enlarged or diseased kidney or recent traumatic injury.

PHYSICAL ASSESSMENT
- Inspection: Weakness, fatigability, and lethargy; itching, scratching, purpura, and ecchymosis; nail beds thin, brittle, with white proximal section with darker brown distal edge and ridges; thirst; weight loss; myoclonic jerking, seizures; peripheral edema; Grey Turner's sign (bruising over the lower portion of the back and flank because of retroperitoneal hematoma over the 11th or 12th ribs); or vomiting.
- Palpation: Pulses are full, bounding, regular or irregular; abdominal pain or back tenderness.
- Auscultation: Hypotension, crackles or rhonchi, or dysrhythmias.

DIAGNOSTIC TEST RESULTS

Standard Laboratory Tests. (Table 4–1)

- Blood studies: Decreased hemoglobin and hematocrit. Elevated white blood cells (WBC) and polymorphonuclear leukocytes.
- Serum chemistry: Increased blood urea nitrogen (BUN) without an elevation in creatinine.
- Urinalysis: May show occult blood.

Invasive Renal Diagnostic Procedures. (Table 4–2)

- Renal angiography: Reveals thrombosis of the renal circulation.

Noninvasive Renal Diagnostic Procedures. (Table 4–3)

- Computerized tomography (CT): Can provide diagnosis of deep renal lacerations extending into subcapsular cortex, ruptured kidney, and hematoma.

- Excretory urogram (EU): Also referred to as intravenous pyelogram (IVP). The EU can reveal the stages of renal injury. Class I (renal contusion), the EU reveals enlarged renal outline. Class II (cortical laceration), the EU reveals intravasation of dye through cortical lacerations. The renal capsule is usually not torn but perinephric hematoma can occur. Class III (caliceal laceration), the EU will show intravasation of dye and disruption of pericaliceal system. The renal capsule is torn and the extravasation of urine can occur. Class IV (complete renal tear or fracture), there is expanding flank mass. The EU shows complete dye extravasation. Class V (vascular pedicle injury), the EU does not visualize the kidney.
- Kidney-ureter-bladder (KUB) radiography: Reveals retroperitoneal hematoma, fracture of lower ribs or pelvis, organ displacement, presence of foreign bodies, or fluid accumulation.

MEDICAL AND SURGICAL MANAGEMENT

PHARMACOLOGY
- Antibiotics: Used to treat infection from a penetrating renal injury.
- Analgesics: Used to relieve pain.

FLUID THERAPY
- Intravenous therapy: Provides rapid volume replacement.
- Blood or blood products: Used to restore normal blood volume in patient with critical renal trauma secondary to penetrating injury.

DIET
- Dietary restriction of protein, sodium, or potassium may be ordered should there be renal dysfunction.

HEMODIALYSIS
- Hemodialysis is the extracorporeal circulation of blood against dialysate separated by a semipermeable membrane. Used to remove excess water, electrolytes, and nitrogenous

TABLE 4–1. STANDARD LABORATORY TESTS

Test	Purpose	Normal Value	Abnormal Findings
Urinalysis			
General Characteristics of Urine			
Specific gravity	Measure of the kidney's ability to concentrate urine	1.003–1.035	Low specific gravity (1.001–1.0010): diabetes insipidus, glomerulonephritis, pyelonephritis, and severe renal damage
			Elevated specific gravity (1.025–1.035): diabetes mellitus, nephrosis, or excessive water loss
Concentration	Measures the kidney's ability to concentrate urine in patients at risk for renal disease	1.020	<1.020: renal disease; with severe involvement the specific gravity is 1.010 or less
	Measures kidney's ability to produce urine with a specific gravity ≥1.020		≥1.020: potassium deficiency, hypercalcemia, renal parenchymal disease such as pylenophritis, or acute renal failure
Color	The intensity of the normal amber color may be directly related to the concentration or specific gravity of the urine	Yellow (specific gravity 1.011–1.019), Straw color (specific gravity <1.010) Amber color (specific gravity ≥1.020)	Orange-colored urine may be due to restricted fluid intake, excess sweating, fever, or small amount of bile pigment
			Brownish yellow or greenish yellow color may indicate bilirubin in the urine
			Red or reddish dark brown color: hemoglobinuria, blood, hemoglobin, and myoglobin
			Port wine color: porphyrins or oxyhemoglobin
			Dark brown urine: porrphyrins or melanin
			Brownish-black urine: hemoglobin or melanin
			Black urine: alkaptonuria
Odor		Fresh urine in a healthy individual has an aromatic odor	Sweet smell of acetone in patients with diabetes ketosis
			Unpleasant smell in patients with infection
pH	Indicates the renal tubule's ability to maintain normal hydrogen ion concentration in the plasma and extracellular fluid	pH 4.6–8.0	pH ≤7.0: acidosis, uncontrolled diabetes, diarrhea, dehydration, or respiratory disease
			pH ≥7.0: urinary tract infection, renal tubular acidosis, or chronic renal failure
Turbidity	Cloudy urine provides a warning of possible problems such as pus, red blood cells, or bacteria	Fresh urine is clear	Turbid or cloudy urine: presence of red blood cells, white blood cells, or bacteria

TABLE 4-1

TABLE 4-1

TABLE 4–1. CONTINUED

Test	Purpose	Normal Value	Abnormal Findings
Osmolality	Measures urine concentration Assists in the diagnosis of polyuria, oliguria, or syndrome of inappropriate antidiuretic hormone	50–1400 mOsm/kg with a range of 300–800 mOsm/kg	Elevated osmolality: dehydration, hypovolemia, emotional stress, SIADH, trauma, hyperglycemia, Addison's disease, hypertonic saline Reduced osmolality: water diuresis, diabetes insipidus, hypertension, decreased sympathetic stimulation, thyroid hormone release, hyponatremia
Hemoglobin	Measures occult blood in the urine that has been hemolyzed or dissolved Determines whether or not there is bleeding in the urinary tract	Negative	Hemoglobinuria: burns, crushing injuries, transfusion reactions, malaria, or hemolytic anemias
Bacteria	Detects bacteria in the urine during routine urinalysis	Negative for bacteria	≥20 bacteria: urinary tract infection
Microscopic Elements			
Red cells/red cell casts	Evaluates presence of serious renal disease	1 or 2 in low-powered field Red blood cells: 0–3 in high-powered field Red cell casts: 0 in low-powered field	Red cell casts: acute glomerulonephritis, renal infarction, or collagen disease Red cells: pyelonephritis, lupus erythematosus, renal stones, cystitis, trauma to the kidney, malignancies of the genitourinary tract, or hemophilia
White cells (WBC)/white cell casts	Evaluates the presence of genitourinary tract or kidney tubule problems	WBC: 0 to 4 in high-powered field WBC casts: none–negative in low-powered field	Elevated WBC: bacterial infection in the urinary tract White cell casts: renal parenchymal infection
Hyaline casts	Casts' presence in urine depends on the rate of urine flow, urine pH, and degree of proteinuria	Occasional hyaline casts are found under low power	Associated with renal parenchymal disease, inflammation, and trauma to the glomerular capillary membrane
Crystals	The type and number of crystals vary with the pH of the urine	Some appear	Appearance of crystals may indicate urinary tract infection
Urine Chemistry **Electrolytes**			
Chlorides quantitative (24 h)	A means of evaluating dehydration A measurement to evaluate fluid and electrolyte balance	110–250 mEq/24 h 10–20 g NaCl/24 h 9 g/L (0.9 g/mL)	Reduced levels: malabsorption syndrome, pyloric obstruction, diaphoresis, CHF, diarrhea, prolonged gastric suction, or emphysema Elevated levels: dehydration, starvation, or salicylate toxicity

TABLE 4-1

TABLE 4–1. CONTINUED

Test	Purpose	Normal Value	Abnormal Findings
Sodium quantitative (24 h)	Measurement to evaluate renal problems including acid-base imbalance	130–200 mEq/ 24 h	Elevated levels: dehydration, starvation, chronic renal failure, diabetic acidosis, or adrenal cortical insufficiency
			Reduced levels can be associated with loss of chloride
Potassium quantitative (24 h)	Evaluation of renal disorders	40–80 mEq/24 h	Elevated levels: chronic renal failure, starvation, diabetes, renal tubular acidosis, dehydration, primary aldosteronism, Cushing's disease, or salicylate toxicity
			Reduced levels are due to diarrhea, acute renal failure, adrenal cortical insufficiency, or malabsorption syndrome
Calcium quantitative (24 h)	Evaluates the function of the parathyroid gland	100–250 mg/ average diet 150 mg/low-calcium diet	Elevated levels: hyperparathyroidism, breast or lung cancer, metastatic malignancies, myeloma with bone metastasis, renal tubular disease, or glucocorticoid excess
			Reduced levels: hypoparathyroidism, vitamin D deficiency, and malabsorption syndrome
Protein (albumin)	Differentiates diagnoses of renal disease Evaluates presence of proteinuria, which indicates renal disease	Negative 2–8 mg/dL	Proteinuria: nephritis, nephrosis, kidney stones, ascites, polycystic kidney, or cancer of the kidney
Glucose	Detects and confirms the diagnosis of diabetes	Random specimen is negative 24-h specimen is 100 mg/24 h	Elevated glucose: diabetes mellitus, lowered renal threshold exists
Acetone	Assesses the presence of diabetic ketoacidosis and diabetic coma	Negative	Ketonuria: fever, anorexia, fasting, starvation, vomiting, or GI disturbance

CHF, congestive heart failure; GI, gastrointestinal; SIADH, syndrome of inappropriate antidiuretic hormone.
From Loeb S, 1991; Baer CL, 1993; Stillwell SB, 1992.

waste products when renal dysfunction occurs (see Hemodialysis, p. 496).

SURGICAL INTERVENTION

- Surgery in renal trauma may be necessary for the following conditions: expanding hematoma, pulsatile hematoma, penetrating trauma with urinary extravasation, vascular injury and evidence of continued hemorrhage after patient has received three units of blood.

- Used to divert urine depending upon the location of renal injury.

NURSING MANAGEMENT: NURSING DIAGNOSES AND COLLABORATIVE PROBLEMS

Nursing Diagnoses

Common nursing goals for patients with renal trauma are to restore fluid volume, maintain urinary elimination, and maintain tissue integrity.

TABLE 4-2

TABLE 4–2. INVASIVE RENAL DIAGNOSTIC PROCEDURES

Test	Purpose	Normal Value	Abnormal Findings
Angiography	Evaluates configuration of renal vasculature prior to surgery Determines the cause of renovascular hypertension, chorionic renal failure, renal masses, or renal trauma Evaluates donors and recipients before renal transplantation and complications after renal transplantation	Normal appearance of renal vasculature and normal structure of the renal parenchyma	Renal artery stenosis, hypervascularity from renal tumors, renal infarction, renal artery aneurysms, renal abscesses, renal cysts, intrarenal hematoma, parenchymal laceration, shattered kidney, infarction from trauma
Antegrade pyelography	Evaluates the upper collecting system for obstruction by stricture, stone, clot, or tumor Enables placement of a percutaneous nephrostomy tube	The upper collecting system fills uniformly Normal structures clearly visualized	Enlargement of upper collecting system from obstruction Distention of the ureteropelvic junction resulting from hydronephrosis
Biopsy (percutaneous)	Diagnoses renal parenchymal disease Evaluates progression of renal disease	Normal configuration of tissue and structures	Renal cell carcinoma, amyloid infiltration, acute and chronic glomerulonephritis, renal vein thrombosis, pyelonephritis
Cystoscopy (cystourethroscopy)	Diagnoses urinary tract disorders	Normal appearance of urinary tract, mucosa lining the lower urinary tract, and bladder	Urethral stricture, bladder calculi, bladder tumors, bladder polyps, vesical neck obstruction
Digital subtraction angiography	Examines arteries of the body including renal arteries	Normal renal arteries	Large aneurysms, stenosis of arteries, large jugular masses, total occlusion of arteries, pulmonary emboli, thoracic outlet syndrome, or pheochromocytoma
Intravenous pyelography (IVP)	Diagnoses suspected renal disease or urinary tract infection Evaluates kidney function based on the length of time it takes the contrast material to appear and be excreted in each kidney	Normal size, shape, and position of the kidneys, ureters, and bladder	Presence of one kidney, hydronephrosis, renal or ureteral calculi (stones), tumors, and extent of renal injury following trauma

TABLE 4–2. CONTINUED

TABLE 4-2

Test	Purpose	Normal Value	Abnormal Findings
Retrograde cystography	Evaluates structure and integrity of the bladder	Normal bladder integrity	Vesical diverticula, ruptured bladder, bladder tumors, bladder calculi, hypo/ hypertonic bladder
Retrograde pyelography (Ureteropyelography)	Evaluates structure and integrity of the renal collecting system	Normal size and contour of ureters and kidneys	Intrinsic diseases of ureters and pelvis of the kidney
	Confirms findings suspected on the IVP		Extrinsic disease of ureters, such as obstructive tumor or stones
Retrograde urethrography	Diagnoses urethral strictures and lacerations	Normal urethra size, shape, and course	Urethral diverticula, fistulas, strictures, calculi, lacerations, or congenital anomalies
Renal scan	Evaluates patency of urinary system and rule out masses	Kidneys normal in shape, size, position and function	Decreased kidney function, masses within the kidney, obstruction, organ rejection posttransplant
	Evaluates kidney function and blood flow		
Renal venography	Detects and evaluate renal vein thrombosis, renal vein compression, renal tumors, and venous anomalies	Normal renal venous system	Renal vein thrombosis, renal tumor, venous anomalies, obstruction or compression of renal vein from extrinsic tumor or retroperitoneal fibrosis
	Collects renal venous blood samples for evaluation of renovascular hypertension	Renin content of venous blood 1.5–1.6 mg/mL/h	Elevated renin content in renal venous blood from both kidneys can indicate renovascular hypertension
			Elevated renin content in venous blood from one kidney can indicate unilateral lesions

Fluid volume deficit related to bleeding secondary to damaged renal artery.

Expected Patient Outcomes. Patient maintains adequate fluid volume, as evidenced by blood pressure (BP) within patient's normal range, heart rate (HR) ≤100 bpm, mean arterial pressure (MAP) 70 to 100 mm Hg, respiratory rate (RR) 12 to 20 BPM, urinary output (UO) ≥30 mL/h or ≥0.5 mL/kg/h, specific gravity ≥1.010, stable weight, central venous pressure (CVP) 2 to 6 mm Hg, pulmonary capillary wedge pressure (PCWP) 6 to 12 mm Hg, peripheral pulses +2, capillary refill ≤3 seconds, good skin turgor, and absence of bleeding and hematoma.

- Review results of hemoglobin, hematocrit, urinalysis, KUB radiography, renal angiography, and CT scan.
- Limit physical activity to bed rest until bleeding subsides.
- Place in position of comfort to reduce pain.

TABLE 4-3

TABLE 4–3. NONINVASIVE RENAL DIAGNOSTIC PROCEDURES

Test	Purpose	Normal Value	Abnormal Findings
Abdominal plain film kidney, ureters, bladder (KUB)	Assesses urinary tract Evaluates the size, structure and position of the kidneys	Normal abdominal structures	Renal enlargement, renal displacement, absence of a kidney, abnormal renal location or shape, urinary calculi, vascular calcifications, cystic tumor, ascites
Kidney sonogram	Differentiates renal masses and localizes urinary obstruction Monitors status of transplanted kidney Locates kidney and in planning radiation therapy for a renal tumor	Normal pattern image showing normal size and position of the kidney	Cysts, tumors, or abscesses of kidney or adrenal gland; advanced pyelonephritis or glomerulonephritis; obstruction of the ureters; renal hypertrophy; rejection of renal transplant
Renal computed tomography (CT)	Evaluates renal pathology, retroperitoneum, tumors Guides needle placement for percutaneous renal biopsy	Normal size, shape and position of kidneys	Renal cysts, renal tumors, adrenal tumors, renal calculi, polycystic kidney disease, perirenal hematomas

From Loeb S, 1991; Baer CL, 1993; Stillwell SB, 1992.

- Obtain and report hemodynamic parameters suggesting fluid volume deficit: CVP ≤2 mm Hg, MAP ≤700 mm Hg, and PCWP ≤6 mm Hg.
- Obtain and report clinical findings that indicate fluid volume deficit related to bleeding: hypotension, tachycardia, peripheral pulses ≤+2, capillary refill ≥3 seconds, skin cool and pale, and poor skin turgor.
- Observe for clinical indicators of renal trauma: anuria, hematuria, and difficult or unsuccessful catheterization.
- Measure intake, output, specific gravity, and daily weight to evaluate fluid balance. Report UO ≤30 mL/h or ≤0.5 mL/kg/h, specific gravity ≤0.010, and weight loss ≥0.5 kg/d.
- Monitor ECG continuously to assess HR and rhythm. Document ECG rhythm strips every 2 to 4 hours in patients with dysrhythmias.
- Assist with insertion of nephrostomy tube, if necessary, to divert urine.

- Administer prescribed IV fluids or blood to provide volume replacement.
- Administer prescribed fraction of inspired oxygen (FIO_2) by means of mask to provide tissue oxygenation.
- Should major renal injury exist and hemodynamic instability persist even after volume replacement, prepare patient for surgery.

Altered pattern of urinary elimination related to structural or functional injury secondary to renal injury.

Expected Patient Outcomes. Patient maintains adequate urinary elimination, as evidenced by UO ≥30 mL/h or ≥0.5 mL/kg/h; stable body weight; specific gravity 1.010 to 1.030; absence of hematuria; serum electrolytes, BUN, and creatinine within normal range.

- Review results of BUN, creatinine, or serum electrolyte tests.
- Test urine for occult blood.

- Obtain and report clinical findings that indicates altered pattern of urinary elimination: UO ≤30 mL/h or ≤0.5 mL/kg/h, specific gravity ≤1.010, and weight gain.
- Encourage patient to void to promote urinary outflow.
- Monitor daily weight, intake, specific gravity, and UO to evaluate fluid balance.
- Monitor nephrostomy tube, if present, to prevent occlusion from external pressure. Irrigate tube, as prescribed, with ≤5 mL of fluid.
- Monitor nephrostomy site for bleeding or leaking of urine. A catheter obstruction can decrease UO.
- Administer prescribed IV fluids to maintain adequate hydration and circulatory volume.

Impaired tissue integrity related to penetrating injury.

Expected Patient Outcome. Skin intact or reflects healing.

- Change patient's position to maintain skin integrity.
- Evaluate patient's skin for evidence of injury.
- Apply sterile dressing to lacerated skin over penetrating injury.
- Monitor skin laceration for swelling, tenderness, redness, or drainage.
- Change dressing using aseptic technique.

DISCHARGE PLANNING

The critical care nurse will provide patient and significant other(s) with verbal or written discharge notes regarding the following subjects:

1. Signs and symptoms that require immediate medical attention: edema, hypertension, weakness, pruritus, oliguria, or lethargy.
2. Importance of keeping all outpatient appointments.
3. Care of postoperative or postprocedure incisions and urinary drainage systems.
4. Medication purpose, dosage, route, schedule, and side effects.

■ ACUTE TUBULAR NECROSIS

(*For related information, see Part I: Acute renal failure, p. 459; Metabolic acidosis, p. 474. Part II: Renal transplantations, p. 491. Part III: Hemodialysis, p. 496; Peritoneal dialysis, p. 502; Continuous arteriovenous hemofiltration, p. 505. See also Behavioral Deviations, p. 725.*)

Case Management Basis
DRG: 331 Other kidney and urinary tract age ≥17 with complications
LOS: 5.30 days
DRG: 332 Other kidney and urinary tract diseases diagnoses age ≥17 without complications
LOS: 3.00 days

Definition
Acute tubular necrosis (ATN) is the sudden cessation of renal function, exemplified by the kidney's inability to concentrate urine, leading to the accumulation of nitrogenous waste products. Damage to the cellular structure in the tubules may prevent normal concentration of urine, filtration of waste, and regulation of acid-base, electrolytes, and water balance.

Pathophysiology
There are two types of ATN. In the first, ischemic, type patchy necrosis occurs in the straight portion of the proximal tubule. Lesions may also occur in the distal tubules. Should ischemia be prolonged, the basement membrane is injured and the tubular lumen is exposed to the interstitial space. Eventually the tubule lumina become blocked by casts. There may also be leukocyte in the vasa recta, dilatation of Bowman's spaces of the glomeruli, interstitial edema, and inflammation cells in the interstitium.

In the second, nephrotoxic, type lesions are located in the proximal tubules, basement membrane, and distal tubules. Nephrotoxic agents destroy tubular cells by direct cellular toxic injury, lysis of red blood cells (RBC), intravascular coagulation, and tissue hypoxia. These factors lead to blocking of the distal tubules, by casts, interstitial edema, leukocytes in the vasa recta, and inflammatory cells in the interstitium.

Nursing Assessment

PRIMARY CAUSES

- Postischemic causes include surgery such as abdominal aortic aneurysm repair, open heart surgery, major abdominal surgery, or transurethral prostatectomy; obstetric complaints such as postpartum hemorrhage, placenta previa, abrupto placentae, uterine rupture, or severe toxemia; septic infection by gram-negative bacteria; trauma such as crush injuries or burns; or transfusion reactions.
- Nephrotoxic causes include medications such as aminoglycosides, antimicrobials, cephalosporins, or antineoplastics; heme pigments from hemoglobinuria; traumatic rhabdomyolysis or nontraumatic rhabdomyolysis; radiocontrast hydrocarbon; or anesthetic agents.

RISK FACTORS

- History of kidney disease or recent kidney trauma.

PHYSICAL ASSESSMENT

- Inspection: Anorexia, nausea, lethargy, oliguria versus diuresis.
- Palpation: Pitting edema.
- Auscultation: Hypertension.

DIAGNOSTIC TEST RESULTS

Standard Laboratory Tests (Table 1–1, p.3, and Table 4–1)

- Serum chemistry: Blood urea nitrogen (BUN): creatinine ratio $\leq 10:1$. Elevated potassium, phosphate, or sulfate; decreased sodium, calcium, and bicarbonate.

- Urinalysis: Urinary sodium ≥ 40 mmol/dL, urine plasma creatinine ratio $\leq 20:1$, fractional excretion of sodium (FE_{Na}) $\geq 3\%$, osmolality ≤ 45 mOsm, specific gravity ≤ 1.015, and urinary sediment shows granular casts or epithelial cells.

MEDICAL AND SURGICAL MANAGEMENT

PHARMACOLOGY

- Diuretics: Mannitol, an osmotic diuretic, enhances the urine output by reducing sodium and water reabsorption in the proximal tubule and loop of Henle. It is used in conditions that cause postischemic ATN. The local results are prevention of tubular cellular swelling; clearance of cellular debris, which reduces the chance for tubular obstruction; and augmentation of renal blood flow. Furosemide augments renal blood flow and is enhanced when administered in conjunction with dopamine. The recommended dose of furosemide is 100 to 200 mg every 6 to 8 hours.
- Dopamine: Used to maintain renal blood flow, dopamine increases the glomerular filtration rate and preserves urine output in the face of impending acute renal failure. Low dose varying from 1–3 μg/kg/min may have either a preventive or augmenting effect (see Table 1–10, p. 50).
- Antibiotics: Used to treat gram-negative bacteria and staphylococci. The doses are closely monitored to avoid nephrotoxic changes.

FLUID THERAPY

- Crystalloid or colloid fluid therapy is used to reestablish renal blood flow before actual damage to the tubules occurs.

DIET

- Diet consist of low protein and high essential amino acid to minimize protein catabolism and increase BUN level. Sodium and potassium may need to be restricted because of the inability of the tubules to secrete these. The diet may be high in calories

(≥2200 calories/d) if the patient is healing from burns or trauma.

DIALYSIS

- Hemodialysis is used to remove water and solutes from the body. Hemodialysis is beneficial for patients with fluid volume overload and rapidly rising BUN and potassium level (see Hemodialysis, p. 496).
- Peritoneal dialysis is a renal replacement therapy that utilizes the peritoneum as the dialyzing semipermeable membrane. As a slow, continuous therapy, hourly exchanges may be required to control fluid and electrolyte abnormalities (see Peritoneal dialysis, p. 502).
- Continuous renal replacement therapy is an extracorporeal blood treatment used to control both fluid and solute balance (see Continuous renal replacement therapy, p. 505).

NURSING MANAGEMENT: NURSING DIAGNOSES AND COLLABORATIVE PROBLEMS

Nursing Diagnoses

Common nursing goals for patients with ATN are to maintain fluid volume, prevent infection, and promote positive body image.

Fluid volume excess related to interstitial edema secondary to hypoproteinemia in ischemic tubular injury.

Expected Patient Outcomes. Patient maintains adequate fluid volume, as evidenced by central venous pressure (CVP) 2 to 6 mm Hg, blood pressure (BP) within patient's normal range, heart rate (HR) ≤100 bpm, pulmonary capillary wedge pressure (PCWP) 6 to 12 mm Hg, serum osmolality 285 to 295 mOsm/kg, serum electrolytes within normal range, urinary output (UO) ≥30 mL/h or ≥0.5 mL/kg/h, absence of adventitious breath sounds, absence of edema, stable weight and specific gravity ≥1.030.

- Consult with physician about indicators that suggest the need for dialysis: glomerular filtration rate (GFR) falls ≤5 mL/min, BUN ≥99 mg/100 mL, creatinine ≥10 mg/100mL, and symptoms of nausea, vomiting, anorexia, lethargy, pruritus, and fatigue.
- Obtain and report clinical findings that indicate excess fluid volume: tachycardia, crackles or wheezes, hypertension, engorged neck veins, and peripheral edema.
- Monitor intake, output, specific gravity, and daily weight to evaluate fluid balance. Report UO ≤30 mL/h or ≤0.5 mL/kg/h, specific gravity ≥1.030, and weight gain ≥0.5 kg/d.
- Promote skin integrity of edematous areas by frequent repositioning and elevation of areas where possible.
- Organize patient care to provide rest periods to minimize exertional dyspnea.
- Obtain and report clinical findings that indicate complications associated with hemodialysis, if used: hypotension, hypertension, edema, muscle cramps, chest pain, and dysrhythmias.
- Obtain and report clinical findings that indicate dialysis disequilibrium syndrome if dialysis is rapid over an extended period: headache, rising BP, nausea, blurred vision, or seizures.
- Obtain and report complications associated with peritoneal dialysis, if used: abdominal hernia, hiatal hernia, dysrhythmias, acute myocardial infarction, stroke, peritonitis, or partial occlusion of the ileal femoral vessels.
- Monitor the peritoneal catheter sites for infection with localized cellulitis or a subcutaneous tunnel abscess extending into the deep cuff area.
- Maintain patency of subclavian, femoral vein, or arterioventricular (A-V) shunt by instilling 1000 units of heparin in 1 mL of normal saline solution in the catheter (heparin lock) between treatments.
- Administer prescribed hypertonic fluid therapy to avoid rapid fluid shifts or alteration in electrolyte balance. The goal is to reduce fluid volume approximately 0.5 kg of body weight/d.

- Administer prescribed peritoneal dialysate solution to the abdominal cavity via the catheter in intervals of 1 to 2 hours for intermittent peritoneal dialysis or every 4 to 6 hours for continuous therapy.
- Administer prescribed hypertonic dialysate containing a 4.12 g/dL of dextrose, which also increases peritoneal clearance. The addition of a vasodilator, such as nitroprusside, to dialysate can enhance the clearance by as much as 20%.
- Administer prescribed volume-reducing agents (furosemide or bumetanide) to maintain UO $\geq$30 mL/h or $\geq$0.5 mL/kg/h.
- Should pharmacological therapy and fluid restriction be ineffective, prepare patient for continuous arteriovenous hemofiltration, peritoneal dialysis, or hemodialysis (see Hemodialysis, p. 496; Peritoneal dialysis, p. 502; and Continuous renal replacement therapy, p. 505).
- Teach patient undergoing peritoneal dialysis to report abdominal pain from the use to dialysate with a high dextrose concentration and overfilling of the abdomen with dialysate.
- Teach patient the reasons behind fluid restriction.

High risk for infection related to bacterial sepsis secondary to malnutrition or invasive monitoring devices.

Expected Patient Outcomes. Patient is free of infection, as evidenced by white blood cells (WBC) $\leq$11,000/μL, normothermia, and negative cultures.

- Review results of lymphocyte count, differential, and cultures.
- Obtain temperature every 2 to 4 hours when patient is febrile.
- Obtain and report clinical findings that indicate infection: elevated temperature, drainage, swelling, tenderness and redness around catheter sites.
- Monitor urine for volume, color, and presence of precipitate.
- Use strict aseptic technique when changing dressings or catheters.

- Administer prescribed IV fluids to maintain adequate hydration.
- Administer prescribed antibiotics to treat bacterial sepsis.

Body image disturbance related to dependence on life-saving technology.

Expected Patient Outcomes. Patient shares feelings about view of self, achieves or maintains self-control, and assumes role-related responsibilities.

- Encourage patient to express feelings about how he or she feels or views himself or herself.
- Encourage patient to ask questions about health problem, treatment, progress, or prognosis.
- Support patient and family as they adapt to hemo- or peritoneal dialysis.
- Assess the meaning of renal functional loss for the individual and significant others.
- Explore realistic alternatives and provide encouragement.
- Provide information needed for patient and family.
- Assist patient to recognize his or her own functioning and performance when using hemodialysis or peritoneal dialysis.
- Encourage patient to establish body boundaries, separate from self and dialysis machine.
- Assist with the resolution of a surgically created alteration of body image such as A-V shunt.
- Explore strengths and resources with patient.

Collaborative Problems

Common collaborative goals in patients with ATN are to maintain electrolyte balance and correct dysrhythmias.

Potential Complication: Electrolyte Imbalance. Electrolyte imbalance related to hyperkalemia secondary to ACN during the diuretic phase.

Expected Patient Outcomes. Patient maintains electrolyte balance, as evidenced by serum electrolytes within normal range, UO ≥30 mL/h or 0 ≥.5 mL/kg/h, absence of dysrhythmias, specific gravity 1.010 to 1.030, and stable daily weight.

- Review serum electrolyte, serum osmolality, and urine osmolality results.
- Provide prescribed low-protein or low-potassium diet.
- Obtain and report clinical findings that indicate hypokalemia: irritability; restlessness; anxiety; nausea; vomiting; abdominal cramps; weakness; numbness and tingling; and tachycardia, then bradycardia.
- Continuously monitor ECG to assess heart rate and rhythm. Document ECG every 2 to 4 hours in patients with dysrhythmias.
- Obtain and report ECG findings associated with hyperkalemia (7.0 to 8.0 mmol/L(mEq/L): tall, peaked T waves, a lengthening PR interval, widening QRS complexes, and flattening P waves.
- Administer prescribed IV fluids, dextrose, and insulin, to force potassium (≥6.0 mEq/L) back into the cells.
- Administer prescribed calcium parenterally to block the effects of hyperkalemia in the heart muscle by stabilizing the cardiac membrane and moving potassium into the cells.
- Administer prescribed sodium bicarbonate to counteract effects of hyperkalemia and correct acidosis.
- Administer prescribed sodium polystyrene sulfonate (Kayexalate) to promote excretion of potassium. Potassium is exchanged across the gastrointestinal mucosa and is removed from the body in the feces. The Kayexalate is mixed in a 50:50 solution with sorbital to stimulate a diarrhea stool.
- Administer phosphate bonder or aluminum hydroxide gels to prevent or treat bone disease.

Potential Complication: Dysrhythmias. Dysrhythmias related to electrolyte imbalance secondary to diuretic therapy.

Expected Patient Outcomes. Patient remains in sinus rhythm, serum electrolytes within nor-

mal range, heart rate (HR) ≤100 bpm, and BP within patient's normal range.

- Review results of serum potassium levels that may contribute to dysrhythmias: hyperkalemia ≥5.5 mEq/L and hypokalemia ≤3.8 mEq/L.
- Monitor continuous ECG to assess HR and rhythm. Document ECG rhythm strips every 2 to 4 hours in patients with dysrhythmias.
- Assess for physical signs and symptoms of dysrhythmias: abnormal HR and rhythm, palpitations, chest pain, syncope, ECG change, and hypotension.
- Measure ECG components, should hyperkalemia occur in conjunction with decreased renal arterial perfusion: peaked T waves of increased amplitude and biphasic QRS-T complexes.
- Administer prescribed IV fluids to maintain adequate hydration.
- Withhold potassium and if potassium exceeds 6.0 mEq/L, administer prescribed Kayexalate, a sodium cycle sulfonic polystyrene exchange resin.
- Teach patient to report an abnormal HR, chest pain, or syncope.

DISCHARGE PLANNING

The critical care nurse will provide patient and significant other(s) with verbal or written discharge notes regarding the following subjects:

1. Signs and symptoms that require immediate medical attention: edema, hypertension, weakness, pruritus, oliguria, or lethargy.
2. Importance of keeping all outpatient appointments.
3. Purpose, dosage, route, schedule, and side effects of medication.

■ ACUTE RENAL FAILURE

(For related information see Part I: Renal trauma, p. 447; Acute tubular necrosis, p. 455; Metabolic acidosis, p. 474. Part II: Renal transplantations, p. 491. Part III: Hemodialysis, p. 496; Peritoneal dialysis, p. 502; Continuous renal replacement therapy, p. 505.)

Case Management Basis
DRG: 316 Renal failure
LOS: 6.30 days

Definition
Acute renal failure (ARF) is the sudden decrease in renal function manifested by rapid accumulation of waste metabolites in the patient's body. The onset of ARF is characterized by either anuria, oliguria, or polyuria.

Pathophysiology
Acute renal failure can be initiated by hypoperfusion or an ischemic episode. Hypoperfusion or ischemia alters cellular metabolism by converting the aerobic metabolism to anaerobic metabolism, in which less adenosine tryphosphate (ATP) is produced and acidosis occurs. Hypoperfusion leads to decreased renal blood flow and ischemia, thereby activating the renin-angiotensin system, which induces increased intrarenal vasoconstriction. Vasoconstriction further reduces renal blood flow and glomerular blood flow. Glomerular capillary pressure and permeability are also decreased, lowering the glomerular filtration rate and causing tubular dysfunction and oliguria. Nephrotoxic insult such as heavy metals, contrast media, pharmacological agents, microbial by-products, and circulating inflammatory mediators damage the tubular cells directly. The nephrotoxic agent destroys part of the tubule, causing intratubular obstruction and the back leak of glomerular filtrate. The overall result is tubular dysfunction and oliguria. In summary, hypoperfusion and nephrotoxic insult involve five specific mechanisms: increased intrarenal vasoconstriction, cellular edema, decreased glomerular capillary permeability, intratubular obstruction, and back leak of glomerular filtrate.

Nursing Assessment

PRIMARY CAUSES
- Prenal causes include primary cardiac failure from acute myocardial infarction, arrhythmias, pericardial tamponade, cardiomyopathy, hypovolemia from hemorrhage, plasma loss such as osmotic diuresis, diabetes insipidus, or third spacing, decreased systemic vascular resistance resulting from sepsis, or antihypertensive medication. Intrarenal causes consist of vascular disease resulting from renal artery embolism, bilateral renal artery stenosis or thrombosis, renal vein thrombosis, glomerular disease, tubular disease such as acute tubular necrosis, or tubular obstruction by myeloma proteins; and interstitial disease caused by allergic reaction to drugs. Postrenal causes include urinary stones, benign prostatic hypertrophy, tumors, retroperitoneal fibrosis, or neurogenic bladder dysfunction.

RISK FACTORS
- Chronic illness such as hypertension, diabetes mellitus, or infection; exposure to nephrotoxic drugs; recent blood transfusion; urinary tract disorder; recent severe muscular damage; or burn trauma.

PHYSICAL ASSESSMENT
- Inspection: Pallor, periorbital and peripheral edema, decreased attention span, confusion, drowsiness, weakness, decreasing level of consciousness, muscle irritability, twitching, abdominal cramps, jugular vein distention, tachypnea, or dyspnea.
- Palpation: Pulses weak, thready, full, bounding, or irregular; abdominal renal tenderness.
- Percussion: Renal tenderness.
- Auscultation: Soft, low-pitched murmur with renal artery stenosis, hum with inferior vena cava stenosis; crackles; S_3 or S_4 gallop, hypertension, or arrhythmias.

DIAGNOSTIC TEST RESULTS

Standard Laboratory Tests (See Table 4–1)

- Arterial blood gases: Decreased pH, partial pressure of arterial carbon dioxide bicarbonate ($Paco_2$), and bicarbonate (HCO_3).
- Blood studies: Decreased hematocrit and hemoglobin.

- Serum chemistry: Blood urea nitrogen (BUN): creatinine ratio increased 10:1; serum osmolality ≥285 mOsm/Kg; and increased uric acid, phosphorus, magnesium, and protein.
- Urinalysis: Casts with tubular epithelial cells, tubular casts and red blood cell (RBC) casts; protein 3+ or 4+; specific gravity 1.020; osmolality ≤350 mOsm/kg; urine: serum ratio 1.1; urine volume ≤400 mL/24h; creatinine clearance ≤50 mL/min; and urine sodium ≤10 mEq/L.

Invasive Renal Diagnostic Procedures. (see Table 4–2)

- Kidney-ureter-bladder (KUB): Demonstrates the size of kidneys and presence of stones.
- Intravenous pylography (IVP): Determines partial or complete obstruction in renal pelvis and ureters.
- Renal angiography: Allows visualization of renal blood flow. Visualizes stenosis, cysts, clots, tumors, infarcts, areas of trauma, or torn kidney.

Noninvasive Renal Diagnostic Procedures. (see Table 4–3)

- Renal computed tomography (CT) scan: Helps determine tumors, cysts, hemorrhage, calcification, adrenal tumors, or necrosis.
- Renal ultrasonography: It can detect hydronephrosis and help identify urethral obstruction or bladder outlet obstruction.

MEDICAL AND SURGICAL MANAGEMENT

PHARMACOLOGY
- Diuretics: Mannitol can be used to decrease endothelial cell swelling, which reduces renal vasoconstriction. A trial dose of 13.5 to 25.0 g IV is recommended for patient who is hypovolemic or normovolemic. Loop diuretics such as furosemide or bumetanide increase blood flow to the kidney's midcortical zone and cause vasodilation by aug-

menting synthesis of prostaglandins in the kidney. Furosemide 40 mg is considered equivalent to bumetanide 1 mg and ethacrynic acid 50 mg (see Table 1–13, p. 75).
- Vasopressors: Dopamine has sympathomimetic activity and acts at the dopaminergic receptors of the renal vasculature to cause vasodilation, which increases renal perfusion. A low dosage of 0.5 to 3.0 μg/kg/min is most effective (see Table 1–4, p. 20).
- Calcium channel blockers: Can be used to offer protection against renal ischemia and prevent the intracellular calcium overload (see Cardiac Table 1–6, p. 28).
- Sodium polystyrene sulfonate (Kayexalate): Ion exchange resin can be used to control serum potassium. Potassium is exchanged across the gastrointestinal mucosa and is removed from the body in the feces. The resin is mixed in a 50:50 solution with sorbital to stimulate a diarrheic stool. Each gram of Kayexalate removes 1 mEq of potassium (Table 4–4).
- Calcium gluconate: Used to stabilize cardiac membranes. It increases cellular threshold potential and acts as an antidysrhythmia agent (see Table 4–4).

HEMODYNAMIC MONITORING
- Used to monitor central venous pressure (CUP) or pulmonary capillary wedge pressure (PCWP) when determining appropriate fluid administration.

FLUID THERAPY
- Fluid restriction takes into account the patient's daily urine output (UO) and insensible fluid loss (500 mL). If the patient produces 300 mL of urine/d, the daily fluid restriction is 800 mL. Electrolyte intake is adjusted to maintain plasma electrolyte values within normal range. Intake of sodium and potassium should be in the range of 1 mEq/kg/d.

DIET
- Caloric requirements are in the range of 30 to 35 kcal/kg and protein requirements are

TABLE 4-4

TABLE 4-4. RENAL-RELATED MEDICATIONS

Medication	Route/Dose	Uses and Effects	Side Effects
Antacid			
Aluminum hydroxide	PO: 600 mg tid or qid	Decreases rate of gastric emptying Reduces acid concentration and pepsin activity by raising pH of gastric secretions	Constipation, fecal impaction, intestinal obstruction, hypomagnesemia
Antibiotics			
Amphotericin B (Fungizone)	IV: Test dose in 10–100 mL of D_5W over 1 h. Then increased up to 0.5–0.7 mg/kg/d	Used to treat fungal and protozoan infections	Shaking, fever, chills, headache, nausea, pain at injection site during IV infusion, nephrotoxicity
Clotrimazole (Lotrimin)	Topical: Apply small amount onto affected areas bid PO: 1 lozenge 5 times/d q 3 h for 14 d	Dermal infections and oropharyngeal candidiasis	Stinging, erythema, edema, pruritus, urticaria, nausea, vomiting, lower abdominal cramps, bloating, cystitis
Nystatin (Mycostatin)	PO: 500,000–1,000,000 U tid; 1–4 troches 4–5 times/d 400,000–600,000 U qid	Local infections of skin and mucous membrane caused by *Candida*	Nausea, vomiting, epigastric distress, diarrhea, hypersensitivity reactions
Pentamidine isethionate	IV: 4 mg/kg/d once daily Inhalation: 300 mg once every 4 wk for prophylaxis for *pneumocystis carinii*	*Pneumocystis carinii* pneumonia	Nephrotoxicity, fever, rash, abscess at the injection site
Sulfamethoxazole-trimethoprim (SMX-TMP) (Bactrim, Septra)	PO: 20 mg/kg/d SMX and 4 mg/kg/d TMP in 2 equally divided doses IV: 40–50 mg/kg/d SMX and 8–10 mg/kg/d TMP in 2 to 4 equally divided doses for gram-negative infection	Urinary tract infection, respiratory tract infection, soft tissue infections	Nausea, vomiting, anorexia, rash, urticaria, headache, phlebitis, muscle weakness, fever, dermatitis
Antidote			
Protamine sulfate	IV: 25–50 mg by slow IV push followed by the rest by continuous infusion over 8–16 h, depending on amount of heparin given	Antidote for heparin calcium or heparin sodium overdose	Hypotension, bradycardia, dyspnea, nausea, vomiting, lassitude, flushing, heparin rebound, urticaria, pulmonary edema, anaphyylaxis
Antispasmodic			
Propantheline bromide (Pro-Banthime)	PO: 15 mg 30 min a.c. and 30 mg h.s for a maximum of 120 mg/d	Adjunct treatment for peptic ulcer, pancreatitis, ureteral and urinary bladder spasm	Constipation, dry mouth, difficult urination, blurred vision, drowsiness, increased intraocular pressure, decreased sexual activity

TABLE 4–4. CONTINUED

Medication	Route/Dose	Uses and Effects	Side Effects
Oxybutynin chloride (Ditropan)	PO: 5 mg bid or tid for a maximum of 20 mg/d	Relieves symptoms associated with bladder spasm following transurethral surgical procedure	Drowsiness, dizziness, weakness, restlessness, palpitations, tachycardia, blurred vision, dry mouth, constipation, nausea, skin rashes, urticaria
Bone Metabolism Regulator			
Calcitonin (salmon) (Calcimar)	SC/IM: 4 IU/kg q 12 h and may increase to 8 IU/kg q 6 h if needed to treat hypercalcemia	Treatment of severe hypercalcemic emergencies	Nausea, vomiting, anorexia, abdominal pain, diarrhea, flushing of face or hands, edema of feet, headache, nocturia, analylaxis, hypersensitivity, feverish sensation
Carbonic Anhydrase Inhibitor			
Acetazolamide (Diamox)	PO: 250–375 mg every AM (5 mg/kg) for treatment of edema	Adjunct treatment of edema of CHF Also for glaucoma and seizures	Malaise, depression, fatigue, flaccid paralysis, anorexia, nausea, vomiting, weight loss, dry mouth, thirst, diarrhea, aplastic anemia
Electrolyte Balance Agents			
Ammonium chloride	PO: 4–12 g/d divided q 4–6 h as an urine acidifier IM/IV: Dose is calculated based on CO_2- combining power or serum chloride deficit for treatment of metabolic acidosis	As an acidifier for metabolic alkalosis	Headache, depression, drowsiness, twitching, excitability, bradycardia, gastric irritation, nausea, vomiting, anorexia, skin rash, metabolic acidosis, hyperventilation, glycosuria
Calcium chloride	IV: 0.5–1 g (7–14 mEq) at 1–3 day interval for hypocalcemia; 2.7–3.7 mEq × 1 CPR	Treatment during CPR when epinephrine fails to improve myocardial contractions and acute hypocalcemia occurs	Tingling, fainting, hypotension, bradycardia, dysrhythmias, cardiac arrest, venous thrombosis pain at the infusion site
Calcium gluconate	IV: 1.1–4.4 g/d for hypocalcemia IV: 0.5–1.1 g/d for hypocalcemia	Corrects hypocalcemia	Weakness, dizziness, irregular heartbeat, weak pulse, orthostatic hypotension, dry mouth, thirst, anorexia, diarrhea, aplastic anemia, blurred vision

TABLE 4-4

TABLE 4-4

TABLE 4-4. CONTINUED

Medication	Route/Dose	Uses and Effects	Side Effects
Sodium bicarbonate	PO: Antacid 0.3–2.0 g 1–4 times/d or 1/2 tsp of powder in a glass of water IV: Metabolic acidosis 2–5 mEq/kg by IV infusion over a 4–8 h time period	Used as a systemic alkalinizer to correct metabolic acidosis	Belching, gastric distention, flatulence, metabolic alkalosis, electrolyte imbalance
Renin Exchange Agent			
Sodium polystyrene sulfonate (Kayexalate)	PO: 15 g suspended in 70% sorbitol or 20–100 mL of other fluid 1–4 times/d PR: 30–50 g/100 mL 70% sorbitol q 6 h as warm emulsion high into sigmoid colon	Corrects hyperkalcemia	Constipation, fecal impaction, anorexia, gastric irritation, nausea, vomiting, diarrhea

CHF, congestive heart failure; CPR, ; D₅W, 5% dextrose in water; IM, intramuscular; IV, intravenous; PO, by mouth; PR, by the rectum; SC, subcutaneously.

From Deglin, Vallerand, MM 1993; Govoni LE, Hayes JE, 1992; Loeb S, 1993.

around 0.5 to 0.8 g/kg. The protein intake must be high biologic value (HBV), because these foods contain all the essential amino acids and less urea nitrogen is produced during metabolism than with low biologic value (LBV) proteins. The daily HBV protein intake for an individual with ARF who is being dialyzed is 1 g/kg of body weight; for the nondialyzed individual the intake is 40 g/d. Restrict diet to 0.5 to 1.0 g sodium and 20 to 50 mEq potassium.

- Total parenteral nutrition (TPN) is recommended for ARF patients who cannot eat. A TPN calorie:nitrogen ratio ≥450:1 is recommended to prevent body protein catabolism and BUN level elevation. Insulin may be necessary to maintain normal blood glucose level.

DIALYSIS THERAPY
- Hemodialysis, peritoneal dialysis (PD), or continuous renal replacement therapy is initiated early in the course of the renal failure to maintain the serum creatinine below 10 mg/dL and BUN ≤100 mg/dL.

NURSING MANAGEMENT: NURSING DIAGNOSES AND COLLABORATIVE PROBLEMS

Nursing Diagnoses
Common nursing goals for patients with ARF are to maintain fluid volume balance, enhance tissue perfusion, prevent infection, provide adequate nutrition, prevent injury, and provide information.

Fluid volume excess related to extracellular overhydration gain secondary to decreased intravascular colloidal osmotic pressure leading to fluid in the interstitial tissue and fluid overload.

Expected Patient Outcomes. Patient maintain adequate fluid balance, as evidenced by CVP 2 to 6 mm Hg, blood pressure (BP) within patient's normal range, heart rate (HR) ≤100 bpm, pulmonary artery pressure (PAP) 20 to 30 8 to 15 mm Hg, PCWP 6 to 12 mm Hg, cardiac output (CO) 4 to 8 L/min, absence of edema, absence of crackles, serum osmolality 285 to 295 mOsm/kg, serum sodium ≥135 to

148 mEq/L, UO $\geq$30 mL/h or 0.5 mL/kg/h, stable weight, and absence of edema.

- Consult with physician about indicators that suggest the need for dialysis: glomerular filtration rate (GFR) falls $\leq$5 mL/min; BUN $\geq$99 mg/100 mL; creatinine $\geq$10 mg/100 mL; and symptoms of nausea, vomiting, anorexia, lethargy, pruritis, and fatigue.
- Review results of urinalysis; measurements of serum osmolality, serum electrolytes, arterial blood gases; IVP; renal angiography; renal CT scan; or renal ultrasonography.
- Limit physical activity to bed rest until renal function stabilizes.
- Maintain adequate dietary intake through oral feeding, nasogastric tube feeding, or parenteral nutrition.
- Restrict total fluid intake, as ordered, to 1000 mL/d.
- Provide periodic sips of water, ice chips, or a cold wet gauze sponge to minimize thirst.
- Monitor daily weight, intake, specific gravity, and output such as urine, vomiting, diarrhea, or gastric drainage. An increase in weight of 1 kg is approximately equal to a fluid volume increase of 1 L. Report UO $\leq$30 mL/h or $\leq$0.5 mL/kg/h.
- Obtain and report clinical indicators of volume overload: peripheral edema, crackles, tachycardia, hypertension, shortness of breath, and increased jugular venous distention.
- Monitor and report hemodynamic parameters that suggest volume overload: CVP $\geq$6 mm Hg, PAP systolic $\geq$30 mm Hg or diastolic $\geq$15 mm Hg, and PCWP $\geq$12 mm Hg.
- Provide mouth care to control thirst and maintain the integrity of the oral mucosa.
- Administer hypertonic fluid therapy as prescribed to avoid rapid fluid shifts or alteration in electrolyte balance: Goal of fluid restriction is the loss of approximately 0.5 kg of body weight/d.
- Administer prescribed TPN to patients who are unable to eat. TPN may provide the largest volume of fluid given.

- Administer prescribed diuretics to increase removal of excess fluid.
- Administer prescribed dopamine to enhance the effect of diuretic therapy by increasing renal perfusion.
- Should pharmacological therapy and fluid restriction be ineffective, prepare patient for dialysis.
- Instruct patient as to the reasons behind fluid restriction.
- Inform patient about the types of invasive procedures to reduce fluid overload.

Fluid volume deficit related to fluid loss secondary to diuresis or clotting abnormalities.

Expected Patient Outcomes. Patient maintains adequate fluid volume, as evidenced by UO $\geq$30 mL/h or $\geq$0.5 mL/kg/h, stable weight, specific gravity 1.010 to 1.020, normal skin turgor, CVP 2 to 6 mm Hg, BP within patient's normal range, HR $\leq$100 bpm, and absence of thirst.

- Review results of coagulation profile, hemoglobin, hematocrit, and serum electrolytes.
- Obtain and report clinical findings associated with fluid volume deficit: poor skin turgor, hypotension, tachycardia, and thirst.
- Measure intake, output, specific gravity, and daily weight to evaluate fluid balance. Report UO $\leq$30 mL/h and weight loss 1.0 to 1.5 kg/d.
- Observe skin for bruising, petechiae, and hematoma formation.
- Test urine, stool, and nasogastric drainage for occult blood.
- Reduce blood loss by minimizing the number of times blood samples are drawn and drawing only the minimal amounts of blood for each specimen collection.
- Encourage the intake of oral fluids if not contraindicated.
- Administer prescribed IV fluids to maintain adequate circulatory volume.

Altered renal tissue perfusion related to hypoperfusion or ischemic episodes causing intrarenal vasoconstriction secondary to prerenal failure.

Expected Patient Outcomes. Patient maintains adequate renal tissue perfusion, as evidenced by UO ≥30 mL/h or ≥0.5 mL/kg/h, absence of peripheral edema, fractional excretion of sodium (FE_{Na}) no less than 1%, renal failure index (RFI) no less than 1%, BUN and creatinine within normal range, BP within patient's normal range, and urine:serum creatinine ratio ≤20.

- Review results of laboratory parameters suggesting prerenal oliguria: creatinine clearance 15 to 80 mL/min, urine sodium ≤20 mEq/L, urine osmolality ≥500 mOsm/kg H_2O, urine sediment normal with minimal casts, serum BUN:creatinine ratio ≥10, urine:serum creatinine ratio ≥20, and urine:serum osmolality ratio ≥1.2.
- Limit physical activity to bed rest until patient's hemodynamic status stabilizes.
- Restrict fluid intake to 1 L fluid if urinary output is 500 mL or less and insensible losses range from 500 to 700 mL/d.
- Measure and report a FE_{Na} ≤1% indicating a hypoperfusion state.
- Measure and report a RFI ≤1%, which expresses the urinary sodium concentration as a function of the ratio of the urine:plasma creatinine concentration.
- Monitor intake, output, and specific gravity hourly. Report UO ≤30 mL/h or ≤0.5 mL/kg/h and specific gravity ≥1.015.
- Monitor and report BP ≤70 mm Hg, mean arterial pressure (MAP) ≤70 mm Hg, and HR ≥100 bpm. A reduction in BP and increase in HR can further contribute to reduced renal tissue perfusion.
- Administer prescribed 500 to 1000 mL of 0.9% sodium chloride (NaCl) and diuretics to rule out decreased circulating blood volume as a cause of decreased renal perfusion.
- Administer IV fluids to maintain adequate circulatory volume.
- Administer prescribed vasoactive agents that increase renal blood flow (acetycholine, low doses of dopamine and isoproterenol).

High risk for infection related to altered immune system, invasive procedures, or poor nutritional status.

Expected Patient Outcomes. Patient is free of infection, as evidenced by normothermia; white blood cells (WBC) ≤11,000 μL; absence of redness, swelling, tenderness, or drainage from invasive lines; negative cultures; and normal breath sounds.

- Review results of WBC including neutrophils, lymphocytes, and cultures.
- Provide the prescribed diet: caloric intake 2000 to 3000 calories/24 h and low protein 1 g/kg of body weight/24 h.
- Monitor temperature every 1 to 2 hours or as needed while patient febrile.
- Observe all invasive lines and wound dressings and report redness, tenderness, swelling, and drainage from catheter site.
- Implement positive preventive pulmonary maintenance therapies such as turning, coughing, deep breathing, and suctioning at least every 2 hours or as necessary.
- Provide postural drainage, percussion, incentive spirometry, or ventilatory support to mobilize secretions and prevent atelectasis.
- Should the use of Foley catheter be necessary, provide perineal care and cleansing around catheter as per unit protocol. Maintain integrity of the closed drainage system.
- Examine urine for cloudiness of unusual odor.
- Use aseptic technique when suctioning or changing dressings or tubing.
- Administer prescribed nutritional supplements such as vitamins.
- Administer prescribed IV fluids to maintain adequate circulatory volume.

High risk of injury related to integumentary manifestations of acute renal failure or poor wound healing.

Expected Patient Outcomes. Patient has no injury or integrity shows improvement, as evidenced by intact integument.

- Review results of WBC and cultures.
- Inspect skin for breaks in integrity.
- Apply nonlanolin, light oil-based lubricating lotion every 4 hours to decrease pruritus.
- Provide skin care measures to prevent breakdown: antiembolic stockings to facil-

itate fluid mobilization; frequent position changes to increase circulation to the area; extra mattress padding or egg-crate mattress to prevent concentration of pressure over bony prominences; skin massage to increase circulation; and careful manipulation of the body to prevent trauma.
- Measure intake and output to evaluate fluid balance.
- Administer prescribed pharmacological agent to assist in controlling pruritus.
- Administer prescribed IV fluids to maintain adequate hydration and circulatory volume.
- Administer prescribed antibiotic therapy.

Altered nutrition: less than body requirements related to gastrointestinal manifestations of acute renal failure.

Expected Patient Outcomes. Patient's nutritional intake meets metabolic requirements, as evidenced by stable weight, caloric intake in excess of 2500 calories to prevent additional catabolism, energy level that is consistent with individual disease process, and positive nitrogen balance.

- Consult with physician as to the daily dietary requirements and restrictions: Water 400 to 600 mL plus the UO, calories 35 to 50 kcal/kg, protein 0.5 to 1.5 g/kg, sodium 500 to 1000 mg, potassium 20 to 50 mEq, phosphate 700 mg or less, calcium 800 to 1200 mg, carbohydrate unrestricted, and fats variable.
- Review results of laboratory tests for consistency with patient's pathophysiological process or within following range: total protein 6 to 8 g/dL, albumin 3.5 to 5.5 g/dL, transferrin 205 to 375 mg/dL, triglycerides 40 to 150 mg/dL, cholesterol 150 to 250 mg/dL, iron 75 to 175 mg/dL, vitamin B_{12} 180 to 1000 mg/dL, and folic acid 1.8 to 9.0 mg/dL.
- Provide high-caloric, low-protein, low-sodium, and low-potassium diet.
- Provide small frequent feedings at times patient has selected for eating.
- Monitor intake and output to prevent fluid excess during oliguric phase and fluid deficit during diuretic therapy.

- Maintain accurate record of body weight and dietary intake. Report weight loss 0.5 to 1.0 kg/d.
- Evaluate activity and energy levels daily.
- Encourage rest periods before and after meals.
- Provide frequent oral care to prevent stomatitis and stimulate appetite.
- Encourage family member to eat with patient.
- Should patient be unable to take oral diet, provide prescribed enteral or hyperalimentation.

Knowledge deficit related to causes, treatments, or prognosis.

Expected Patient Outcomes. Patient is able to verbalize risk factors, treatments, and prognosis of acute renal failure.

- Encourage patient to ask questions regarding his or her care.
- Inform patient about risk factors associated with ARF.
- Listen to the content of patient's questions.
- Provide specific information about the disease process, therapeutic regimen, and prognosis.
- Reinforce verbally the information that is provided by physician or other members of the health team.
- Include family members or significant others in the education process so they can reinforce important information with patient.
- Instruct patient regarding the use of renal supportive devices: hemodialysis, peritoneal dialysis, or continuous renal replacement therapy.
- Teach patient the relationship between the current illness and exercise or diet.

Collaborative Problems
Common collaborative goals for patients with ARF are to correct electrolyte imbalance, maintain acid-base balance, and correct dysrhythmias.

Potential Complication: Electrolyte Imbalance. Electrolyte imbalance related to hyperkalemia secondary to renal dysfunction.

Expected Patient Outcomes. Patient maintains electrolyte balance, as evidenced by potassium 3.5 to 4.5 mEq/L, absence of dysrhythmias, arterial blood gases within normal range, HR ≤100 bpm, and UO ≥30 mL/h.

- Consult with physician about indicators that suggest the need for dialysis: GFR falls ≤5 mL/min; BUN ≥99 mg/100 mL, creatinine ≥10 mg/100 mL; and symptoms of nausea, vomiting, anorexia, lethargy, pruritis, and fatigue.
- Review serum electrolyte, albumin:protein ratio, BUN, creatinine, hematocrit, serum osmolality, and urine osmolality results.
- Provide a low-protein and potassium diet.
- Monitor ECG continuously to assess HR and rhythm. Document ECG rhythm strips every 2 to 4 hours in patients with dysrhythmias.
- Obtain and report clinical findings indicative of hyperkalemia: weakness, cramps, paresthesia of face, tingle in extremities, hypotension, dysrhythmias, anorexia, and abdominal distention.
- Obtain and report ECG changes associated with potassium 5.5 to 6.0 mmol/L: tall, peaked, symmetric T wave in the precordia leads; QT interval is normal or decreased with occasional ST depression.
- Monitor and report ECG changes associated with potassium 6.0 to 7.0 mmol/L: prolonged PR interval and QRS duration.
- Obtain and report ECG changes associated with potassium 7.0 to 8.0 mmol/L: flattened P wave, QRS complex continues to widen with increased delays in atrioventricular conduction.
- Obtain and report ECG changes associated with potassium 8.0 to 10.0 mmol/L: irregular ventricular rhythm, absent P waves, and markedly increased QRS complexes with the eventual merging of the complexes with the T wave.
- Obtain and report ECG changes associated with potassium 10.0 to 12.0 mmol/L: ventricular fibrillation or asystole.

- Monitor for weight gain, specific gravity ≥1.030, or UO ≤400 mL/24 h, which indicate acute renal failure.
- Limit potassium intake in diet to reduce plasma and total body potassium content.
- Administer sodium polystyrene sulfonate, mixed in water and sorbitol and given orally, rectally, or through nasogastric (NG) tube: Renin captures potassium in the bowel and eliminates it in the feces.
- Administer prescribed diuretic (furosemide) to increase renal excretion of potassium.
- In patients with serum potassium ≥6.5 mEq/L, administer prescribed 10% calcium gluconate, 500 mL 10% glucose with 10 units regular insulin IV over 30 minutes and sodium bicarbonate 2 to 3 ampules in 500 mL glucose IV over 1 to 2 hours. This will shift the potassium intracellularly.
- Administer prescribed IV fluids to maintain adequate hydration. Replace serum electrolytes as prescribed: 5% normal saline solution.
- Administer phosphate binder or aluminum hydroxide gels to prevent or treat bone disease.
- Provide TPN to maintain adequate nutrition.
- Should pharmacological therapy be ineffective in reducing serum potassium, prepare patient for dialysis.

Potential Complication: Acid-Base Imbalance. Acid-base imbalance related to metabolic acidosis secondary to diarrhea, renal tubular acidosis, or dilutional acidosis.

Expected Patient Outcomes. Patient maintains acid-base balance, as evidenced by arterial blood gases within normal range; HCO_3 22 to 26 mEq/L, chloride 100 to 106 mEq/L; patient alert and oriented to person, time, and place; potassium 3.5 to 5.5 mEq/L; HR ≤100 bpm; and respiratory rate (RR) 12 to 18 BPM.

- Review result of serum electrolyte measurement.

- Review and report pH ≤7.35, PaCO₂ normal or decreased with compensation, and HCO₃ ≤20 mEq.
- Obtain and report clinical findings associated with metabolic acidosis: headache, drowsiness, confusion, coma, hypotension, tachycardia, Kussmaul's breathing, nausea, vomiting, and anorexia.
- Continuously monitor ECG to assess HR and rhythm. Document ECG rhythm strips every 2 to 4 hours in patients with dysrhythmias.
- Monitor potassium levels, since metabolic acidosis can predispose to hyperkalemia because excess hydrogen ions are moved into cells in exchange for potassium ions, which enter intravascular space.
- Administer prescribed IV sodium bicarbonate to raise pH to 7.20 and bicarbonate level to ≥15 mm/L in patients with pH ≤7.0.
- Monitor patient receiving continuous infusion with sodium bicarbonate since cerebrospinal fluid acidosis may worsen initially, causing changes in level of consciousness and retarded hemoglobin delivery to the tissues.
- Administer prescribed IV fluids to maintain adequate hydration.
- Prepare patient for hemodialysis, peritoneal dialysis, continuous ambulating peritoneal dialysis (CAPD), or continuous renal replacement therapy (see Hemodialysis, p. 496; Peritoneal dialysis, p. 502; Continuous renal replacement therapy, p. 505).

Potential Complication: Dysrhythmias. Dysrhythmias related to potassium imbalance.

Expected Patient Outcomes. Patient maintains a regular sinus rhythm and potassium is 3.5 to 5.5 mEq/L.

- Review results of serum electrolyte measurement and 12 lead-ECG.
- Continuously monitor ECG to assess HR and rhythm. Document ECG rhythm strips every 2 to 4 hours in patients with dysrhythmias.

- Administer sodium polystyrene sulfonate orally, rectally, or by NG tube to reduce potassium level.
- Administer antidysrhythmia agents should the rhythm not convert to normal sinus rhythm after potassium returns to normal range.
- Instruct patient as to the reasons for the cardiac dysrhythmia and possible treatment.

DISCHARGE PLANNING

The critical care nurse will provide patient and significant other(s) with verbal or written discharge notes regarding the following subjects:

1. Signs and symptoms that require immediate medical attention: bleeding, infection, and weight gain or loss.
2. Importance of keeping all outpatient appointments.
3. Importance of continuing with hemodialysis or ambulatory peritoneal dialysis, if necessary.
4. Care of hemodialysis or peritoneal dialysis access sites.
5. Patient's specific dietary needs and food that should be avoided.
6. Medication's purpose, dosage, route, schedule, and side effects.

■ RHABDOMYOLYSIS

(For related information see Part I: Renal trauma, p. 447; Acute tubular necrosis, p. 455; Acute renal failure, p. 459; Part II: Renal transplantations, p. 491. Part III: Hemodialysis, p. 496; Peritoneal dialysis, p. 502; Continuous renal replacement therapy, p. 505.)

Case Management Basis
DRG: 331 Other kidney and urinary tract diagnoses, age greater than 17 with complication
LOS: 5.30 days

DRG: 332 Other kidney and urinary tract diagnoses, age greater than 17 without complications
LOS: 3.00 days

Definition

Rhabdomyolysis is a nonspecific clinical syndrome resulting from the release of skeletal muscle cell contents into the plasma and leads to acute renal failure.

Pathophysiology

With rhabdomyolysis, cellular injury may increase the permeability of the cell membrane to sodium. This requires that the sodium-potassium pump increase its rate of sodium transport across the cell membrane, thus causing increased cellular oxygen consumption. In rhabdomyolysis, the contents of the sarcomere are released into the interstitium and the vasculature. Among these cellular contents is myoglobin. When myoglobulin is released into the vascular compartment, approximately 15 mg/L can be bound to protein and when 200 g of muscle is destroyed, enough myoglobin has been released to be seen in the urine as brown pigment. Myoglobin may accumulate within the proximal tubular cell and heme pigments may produce intratubular obstruction by local precipitation.

Nursing Assessment

PRIMARY CAUSES

- Abnormal energy production, including increased physical exertion, seizures, McArdle's syndrome, status asthmaticus, heat cramps, or malignant hyperthermia. Hypoxia due to arterial embolization, carbon monoxide poisoning, or prolonged immobility. Primary muscle injury from trauma, burns, and polymyositis. Infectious disease such as typhoid fever, legionnaire's disease, influenza, adenovirus infections, infectious mononucleosis, trichinosis, or streptococcal infection. Other causes include toxins, venoms, and lovastatin therapy.

RISK FACTORS

- Life-style factors such as alcohol or drugs.

PHYSICAL ASSESSMENT

- Inspection: Fever, weakness, malaise, pain, and swelling or tenderness of the involved extremities.

DIAGNOSTIC TEST RESULTS

Standard Laboratory Tests

- Serum chemistry: Serum color is clear straw, creatinine kinase ≥200,000 U/L, hypocalcemia (oliguric phase), hypercalcemia (diuretic phase), hyperphosphatemia, hyperkalemia, hyperuricemia, and normal haptoglobin.
- Urinalysis: Urine myoglobin and urine color brown.

MEDICAL AND SURGICAL MANAGEMENT

PHARMACOLOGY

- Antidysrhythmia agents: Used to correct dysrhythmias.

NURSING MANAGEMENT: NURSING DIAGNOSES AND COLLABORATIVE PROBLEMS

Nursing Diagnoses

Common nursing goals for patients with rhabdomylosis are to maintain fluid balance, increase urinary elimination, and support physical mobility.

Fluid volume excess related to oliguria.

Expected Patient Outcomes. Patient maintains adequate fluid balance, as evidenced by urinary output (UO) ≥30 mL/h or 0.5 mL/kg/h, stable weight, central venous pressure (CVP) 2 to 6 mm Hg, absence of neck vein distention, normal breath sounds, and absence of edema.

- Review results of serum hemoglobin and hematocrit.

- Provide nutrition up to 40 to 45 kcal/kg/d, including 1.5 to 2.0 g/kg/d of high biologic value protein.
- Obtain and report clinical findings associated with fluid volume excess: neck vein distention, peripheral edema, and crackles.
- Measure daily weight, intake, specific gravity, and UO to evaluate fluid balance. Report UO $\leq$30 mL/h or $\leq$0.5 mL/kg/h and weight gain $\geq$0.5 kg/d.
- Administer IV fluids as prescribed to prevent acute renal failure and oliguric phase: first 24 hours up to 11 L of 0.9% of saline to achieve a UO of up to 300 mL/h.
- Administer prescribed diuretics, if necessary, to increase UO.

Altered pattern of urinary elimination related to acute tubular necrosis.

Expected Patient Outcomes. Patient maintains normal pattern of urinary elimination, as evidenced by UO $\geq$30 mL/h or 0.5 mL/kg/h, specific gravity 1.010 to 1.020, absence of edema, CVP 2 to 6 mm Hg, and neck veins flat.

- Review results of evaluations of serum electrolytes, blood urea nitrogen (BUN), protein, creatinine, serum osmolality, urine osmolality, and sodium.
- Measure daily weight, intake, specific gravity, and UO to evaluate fluid balance. Report UO $\leq$30 mL/h or $\leq$0.5 mL/kg/h, specific gravity, 1.010, and weight loss.
- Administer prescribed mannitol, 100 mL of 25% solution administered over a period of 15 minutes.
- Teach patient the reasons for decreased UO.

Mobility, impaired physical related to musculoskeletal injury.

Expected Patient Outcome. Patient's physical mobility is maintained or restored.

- Evaluate patient's sensorimotor function.
- Monitor patient's ability to gradually increase physical activity after rhabdomyolysis is treated.

- Provide range of motion exercises to maintain muscle tone.
- Teach patient to report any increasing discomfort in the extremities.

Collaborative Problems

A common collaborative goal in patients with rhabdomyolysis is to prevent dysrhythmias.

Potential Complication: Dysrhythmias. Dysrhythmias related to electrolyte imbalance.

Expected Patient Outcomes. Patient maintains regular sinus rhythm and serum electrolyte within normal range.

- Review results of 12-lead ECG and serum electrolytes.
- Monitor cardiac rhythm for changes in configuration or presence of dysrhythmias associated with hyperkalemia: peaked T wave, widening of QRS, and biphasic QRS-T complexes.
- Obtain and report clinical findings associated with hyperkalemia: weakness, flaccid paralysis, abdominal distention, and diarrhea.
- Measure intake and output to determine fluid balance.
- Administer prescribed IV fluids to maintain adequate hydration and circulatory volume.
- Administer 44 mEq of sodium bicarbonate added to every other liter of 5% dextrose at 0.9% saline until urine pH exceeds 6.5, with acetazolamide given if plasma pH $\geq$7.45.

DISCHARGE PLANNING

The critical care nurse will provide patient and significant other(s) with verbal or written discharge notes regarding the following subjects:

1. Importance of keeping all outpatient appointments.
2. Importance of continuing with hemodialysis or ambulatory peritoneal dialysis, if necessary.
3. Care of hemodialysis or peritoneal dialysis access sites.

4. Patient's specific dietary needs and food that should be avoided.
5. Medication's purpose, dosage, route, schedule, and side effects.

■ RENAL ARTERY OCCLUSIVE DISEASE

(For related information see Part I: Acute tubular necrosis, p. 455; Acute renal failure, p. 459. Part II: Renal transplantations, p. 491. Part III: Hemodialysis, p. 496; Peritoneal dialysis, p. 502; Continuous renal replacement therapy, p. 505.)

Case Management Basis
DRG: 331 Other kidney and urinary tract diagnoses, age greater than 17 with complication
LOS: 5.30 days
DRG: 332 Other kidney and urinary tract diagnoses, age greater than 17 without complications
LOS: 3.00 days

Definition
Renal artery occlusive disease is unique in that critical stenosis of the renal artery occurs, causing hypertension and renal insufficiency.

Pathophysiology
Stenosis of the renal artery causes reduced kidney perfusion pressure. The juxtoglomerular apparatus causes increased renin production and activation of renin-angiotensin-aldosterone. The result is vasoconstriction, sodium resorption, increased vascular resistance, and increased blood pressure.

Nursing Assessment

PRIMARY CAUSES
• Atherosclerosis and fibrous dysplasia such as medial fibroplasia, intimal fibroplasia, perimedial fibroplasia, and fibromuscular hyperplasia.

RISK FACTORS
• Obesity, smoking, high sodium diet, and stress.

PHYSICAL ASSESSMENT
• Inspection: Retinopathy.
• Auscultation: Abdominal bruit and hypertension.

DIAGNOSTIC TEST RESULTS

Standard Laboratory Tests. (See Table 4–1)

• Serum chemistry: Decreased potassium and increased plasma renin activity (PRA).
• Urinalysis: A 24-hour urine sodium collection is compared against PRA.

Invasive Renal Diagnostic Procedures. (see Table 4–2)

• Intravenous pyelogram (IVP): In patients with unilateral renal artery stenosis, the poorly perfused kidney is 1.5 cm or smaller in length and slower by 1 minute or more to excrete contrast and hyperconcentrated contrast material.
• Renal arteriogram: Used to define the lesion and diagnosis of renovascular hypertension.

MEDICAL AND SURGICAL MANAGEMENT

PHARMACOLOGY
• Beta-adrenergic blockers: Propranolol and metaprolol are used to treat hypertension (see Table 1–5, p. 24).
• Vasodilators: Hydralazine and minoxidil are used to treat hypertension (see Table 1–4, p. 20).
• Alpha blockers. Methyldopa and clonidine are used to treat hypertension (see Table 1–16, p. 146).
• Diuretics: Furosemide or bumetanide are used to treat hypertension (see Table 1–13, p. 76).
• Angiotension converting enzyme (ACE) inhibitors: Enalapril and captopril are used to treat hypertension. The ACE inhibitors

are effective as single agents or in combination with diuretic therapy in patients with renovascular hypertension. Diastolic blood pressure can be maintained ≤ 90 mm Hg (see Table 1–12, p. 60).

DIET
- Dietary restrictions include reduced caloric and sodium intake.

PERCUTANEOUS TRANSLUMINAL ANGIOPLASTY (PCTA)
- The PCTA can be used in patients with atherosclerotic renal artery disease for nonostial plaques located within the main renal artery and in patients with fibrous dysplasias of the main renal artery including medial fibroplasia.

SURGICAL INTERVENTION
- Indications: Revascularization is indicated for aneurysm greater than 1 to 2 cm in size or fibrous dysplasia involving vessels branching from the main renal artery.
- Technique: Saphenous vein bypass grafting, end to end from the aorta and end to end beyond the lesion to normal renal artery. When the aorta is inadequate, bypass in the left splenorenal artery or in the right hepatorenal artery can be used. Should different lesions be present in the renal branch vessels, extracorporeal reconstruction with a bifurcated segment of hypogastric artery and renal autotransplantation can be used.

NURSING MANAGEMENT: NURSING DIAGNOSES AND COLLABORATIVE PROBLEMS

Nursing Diagnoses
Common nursing goals in patients with renal artery occlusive disease are to increase renal tissue perfusion, enhance urinary elimination, prevent injury, and maintain fluid balance.

Altered renal tissue perfusion related to renal artery stenosis secondary to atherosclerosis.

Expected Patient Outcomes. Patient maintains adequate renal tissue perfusion, as evidenced by blood pressure (BP) within patient's normal range, heart rate (HR) ≤ 100 bpm, stable weight, urinary output (UO) ≥ 30 mL/h or ≥ 0.5 mL/kg/h, specific gravity 1.010 to 1.025, renin plasmin activity, blood urea nitrogen (BUN), and creatinine within normal range.

- Review results of renin plasmin activity, BUN, and creatinine.
- Obtain and report clinical findings associated with reduced renal tissue perfusion: hypertension and tachycardia.
- Measure intake and output hourly for amount and color. Report persistent hematuria, which is indicative of bleeding. Urine volume may be affected by intraoperative administration of mannitol, which decreases intracellular swelling and increases renal perfusion.
- Continuously monitor arterial BP every 5 to 10 minutes while patient is receiving enalapril.
- Should hypotension occur, monitor UO. A UO ≤ 30 mL/h or ≤ 0.5 mL/kg/h may indicate reduced glomerular filtration rate secondary to decreased renal perfusion.
- Monitor arterial BP and report hypotension, since hypotension can cause inadequate flow and graft thrombosis.
- Calculate systemic vascular resistance (SVR) and systemic vascular resistance index (SVRI) values to determine the optimal titration of vasoactive drugs.
- Provide restful environment to reduce stress.
- Administer prescribed IV fluids to maintain adequate circulatory volume.
- Administer prescribed low-dose dopamine to enhance renal blood flow in conjunction with prostaglandin E_1.
- Prepare patient for PCTA to increase renal perfusion.
- Should PCTA be ineffective in restoring renal perfusion, prepare patient for revascularization surgery.

- Teach patient stress reduction strategies: progressive relaxation, guided imagery, and meditation.
- Teach patient to report common side effects of antihypertensive medications: dizziness, light-headedness, dry mouth, flushing, impotence, constipation, fatigue, and depression.

High risk for injury related to threatened graft integrity secondary to hypertension.

Expected Patient Outcomes. Patient is free of injury, as evidenced by graft remaining intact, BP $\leq$150/100 mm Hg, SVR 900 to 1200 dynes/s/cm^{-5}, SVRI 1970 to 2390 dynes/s/cm^{-5}/m^2, cardiac output (CO) 4 to 8 L/min, absence of pain, and normothermia.

- Consult with physician about causes of postoperative hypertension: elevated renin-aldosterone activity, hypothermia, surgical stress, environmental stress, altered fluid status, and pain.
- Monitor and report leakage at the anastomotic site, which threatens the viability of the kidney, as evidenced by hematoma in flank area, hypotension, and CO $\leq$4 L/min.
- Monitor BP by arterial line continuously in patient who requires vasoactive drip.
- Administer prescribed vasodilators (nitroprusside or nitroglycerin) to reduce BP, afterload, and myocardial oxygen demand by relaxing arterial and venous smooth muscle.
- Administer calcium channel blockers (nifedipine) to lower BP.
- Administer prescribed IV ACE inhibitor (enalapril) to reduce BP.

Fluid volume deficit related to postoperative bleeding.

Expected Patient Outcomes. Patient maintains adequate fluid volume, as evidenced by CO 4 to 8 L/min, cardiac index (CI) 2.7 to 4.3 L/min/m^2, central venous pressure (CVP) 2 to 6 mm Hg, pulmonary capillary wedge pressure (PCWP) 6 to 12 mm Hg, BP within patient's normal range, mean arterial pressure (MAP) 70 to 100 mm Hg, HR $\leq$100 bpm, peripheral pulses +2, capillary refill $\leq$3 seconds, normal skin turgor, UO $\geq$30 mL/h, hemoglobin and hematocrit within normal range, and absence of bruising or bleeding.

- Review results of hemoglobin and hematocrit.
- Obtain and report hemodynamic parameters that indicate fluid volume deficit: CO $\leq$4 L/min, CI $\leq$2.7 L/min/m^2, CVP $\leq$2 mm Hg, and PCWP $\leq$6 mm Hg.
- Obtain and report other clinical findings associated with fluid volume deficit: hypotension, tachycardia, peripheral pulses $\leq$2, capillary refill $\geq$3 seconds, and poor skin turgor.
- Measure intake, output, specific gravity, and daily weight. Report UO $\leq$30 mL/h or $\leq$0.5 mL/kg/h, specific gravity $\leq$1.010, and weight loss.
- Administer IV fluids to maintain adequate circulatory volume.
- Should bleeding occur at the anastomotic site, prepare patient for surgery.

DISCHARGE PLANNING

The critical care nurse will provide patient and significant other(s) with verbal or written discharge notes regarding the following subjects:

1. Inform patient of importance of taking antihypertensive medications, as prescribed.
2. Need to continue with low-calorie and low-salt diet.
3. Purpose, dose, schedule, and side effects of medications..
4. Importance of informing physician should side effects occur.
5. Need to keep appointments for regular medical visits to evaluate blood pressure and laboratory values.

■ METABOLIC ACIDOSIS

(For related information see Part I: Renal trauma, p. 447; Acute renal necrosis, p. 455; Acute tubular failure, p. 459; Hyperkalemia, p. 483. Part II: Renal transplantations, p.

491. Part III: Hemodialysis, p. 496; Peritoneal dialysis, p. 502; Continuous renal replacement therapy, p. 505.)

Definition

Metabolic acidosis is a deficit of bicarbonate in the extracellular fluid. It is related to a loss of bicarbonate from the body or increased amount of nonvolatile acids in the body.

Pathophysiology

The bicarbonate ion (HCO_3) concentration can be decreased by buffering activity of a strong acid with HCO_3; by loss of HCO_3 from gastrointestinal tract and kidneys; and by rapid hemodilution of fluid in extracellular spaces with isotonic saline.

Nursing Assessment

PRIMARY CAUSES

- Factors causing loss of bicarbonate include renal tubular acidosis, use of carbonic anhydrase inhibitors, extracellular fluid volume expansion, hyperalimentation, administration of chloride-containing acids, diarrhea, draining fistula of the pancreas or small bowel, ileal conduit or anion exchange resins such as cholestyramine.
- Increase in the amount of acid in the body as a result of renal failure, diabetic keto-acidosis, lactic acidosis, starvation, ethanol intoxication, tissue hypoxia, salicylate intoxication, and high-fat diets.

PHYSICAL ASSESSMENT

- Inspection: Thirst, shortness of breath, weakness, tachypnea, restlessness, impaired consciousness, headache, drowsiness, confusion, nausea, vomiting, anorexia, or Kussmaul's breathing.
- Auscultation: Dysrhythmia or hypotension.

DIAGNOSTIC TEST RESULTS

Standard Laboratory Tests. (see Table 4–1)

- Arterial blood gases: A pH of ≤ 7.35 arterial partial pressure of carbon dioxide ($PaCO_2$) normal or decreased, and $HCO_3 \leq 22 mEq/L$ to 15 mEq/L or base excess ≤ -2.
- Serum chemistry: Elevated urea nitrogen, creatinine, and potassium, positive test for ketone bodies if diabetic alcoholic keto-acidosis.
- Urinalysis: Reduced urine pH.

MEDICAL AND SURGICAL MANAGEMENT

PHARMACOLOGY

- Sodium bicarbonate ($NaHCO_3$): Used to raise pH ≥ 7.20 and bicarbonate levels ≥ 15 mM/L. Administered as IV drip 2 to 3 ampules in 1000 mL D_5W.
- Potassium replacement: Used if potassium deficit (K ≤ 3.5) occurs.
- Oral phosphate: Used if hypophosphatemia is present.

DIALYSIS

- Hemodialysis or peritoneal dialysis: Indicated in patients with underlying renal failure (see Hemodialysis, p. 496, and Peritoneal dialysis, p. 502).

NURSING MANAGEMENT: NURSING DIAGNOSES AND COLLABORATIVE PROBLEMS

Nursing Diagnoses

Common nursing goals for patients with metabolic acidosis are to improve thought process and support sensory-perceptual function.

Altered thought processes related to confusion, irritability, or drowsiness.

Expected Patient Outcome. Patient is alert and oriented.

- Monitor and report changes in neurological function: headache, drowsiness, confusion, and coma.
- Evaluate patient neurological function as metabolic acidosis is being corrected with sodium bicarbonate. Cerebrospinal fluid acidosis may worsen initially, causing changes in level of consciousness.
- Initiate seizure precautions.

- Provide stimuli appropriate to maintaining orientation.
- Clarify patient's questions and provide simple answers.
- Administer prescribed oxygen 2 to 4 L/min by mask or nasal cannula.
- Teach patient the reasons for temporary drowsiness, confusion, and restlessness.

Altered sensory-perceptual function related to weakness or fatigue.

Expected Patient Outcome. Absence of weakness or fatigue.

- Evaluate patient's overall muscle strength.
- Provide bed rest and institute active and passive range of motion exercises.
- Assist patient to assume a position of comfort.
- Establish a safe physical environment for patient.
- Monitor and report changes in sensorimotor function such as muscle weakness or inability to stand.
- Monitor patient's tolerance to gradually increased physical activity.
- Provide rest periods before and after patient gets out of bed.
- Encourage patient to sit at bedside before standing or walking.
- Administer $NaHCO_3$ to correct metabolic acidosis and weakness.

Collaborative Problem

A common collaborative goal for patients with metabolic acidosis is to correct electrolyte imbalance.

Potential Complication: Electrolyte Imbalance. Electrolyte imbalance related to hyperkalemia secondary to reduced bicarbonate level.

Expected Patient Outcomes. Patient maintains electrolyte balance, as evidenced by potassium 3.5 to 4.5 mEq/L, absence of dysrhythmias, arterial blood gases within normal range, heart rate (HR) $\leq$100 bpm, and urinary output (UO) $\geq$30 mL/h.

- Consult with physician about indicators that suggest the need for dialysis: glomerular filtration rate (GFR) falls $\leq$5 mL/min; blood urea nitrogen (BUN) $\geq$99 mg/100 mL; creatinine $\geq$10 mg/100 mL; and symptoms of nausea, vomiting, anorexia, lethargy, pruritus, and fatigue.
- Review of serum electrolyte, albumin: protein ratio, BUN, creatinine, hematocrit, serum osmolality, and urine osmolality results.
- Provide a low-protein low-potassium diet.
- Monitor ECG continuously to assess HR and rhythm. Document ECG rhythm strips every 2 to 4 hours in patients with dysrhythmias.
- Obtain and report clinical findings indicative of hyperkalemia: weakness, cramps, paresthesia of face, tingle in extremities, hypotension, dysrhythmias, anorexia, and abdominal distention.
- Obtain and report ECG changes associated with potassium 5.5 to 6.0 mmol/L: tall, peaked, symmetric T wave in the precordia leads; QT interval is normal or decreased with occasional ST depression.
- Monitor and report ECG changes associated with potassium 6.0 to 7.0 mmol/L: prolonged PR interval and QRS duration.
- Obtain and report ECG changes associated with potassium 7.0 to 8.0 mmol/L: flattened P wave, QRS complex continues to widen with increased delays in atrioventricular conduction.
- Obtain and report ECG changes associated with potassium 8.0 to 10.0 mmol/L: irregular ventricular rhythm, absent P waves, and markedly increased QRS complexes with the eventual merging of the complexes with the T wave.
- Obtain and report ECG changes associated with potassium 10.0 to 12.0 mmol/L: ventricular fibrillation or asystole.
- Limit potassium intake in diet to reduce plasma and total body potassium content.
- Administer sodium polystyrene sulfonate (Kayexalate), mixed in water and sorbitol

and given orally, rectally, or through naso-gastric tube: Renin captures potassium in the bowel and eliminates it in the feces.

- In patients with serum potassium ≥ 6.5 mEq/L, administer prescribed 10% calcium gluconate, 500 mL 10% glucose with 10 units regular insulin IV over 30 minutes and sodium bicarbonate 2 to 3 ampules in 500 mL glucose IV over 1 to 2 hours. This will shift the potassium intracellularly.
- Administer prescribed IV fluids to maintain adequate hydration. Replace serum electrolytes as prescribed: 5% normal saline solution.
- Administer small doses of IV sodium bicarbonate ($NaHCO_3$) 50 to 100 mmol to increase pH ≥ 7.2 and $HCO_3 \geq 15$ mM/L.
- Should pharmacological therapy be ineffective in reducing serum potassium, prepare patient for dialysis.

■ METABOLIC ALKALOSIS

(For related information see Part I: Renal trauma, p. 447; Acute tubular necrosis, p. 455; Acute renal failure, p. 459; Hypokalemia, p. 485. Part II: Renal transplantations, p. 491. Part III: Hemodialysis, p. 496; Peritoneal dialysis, p. 502; Continuous renal replacement therapy, p. 505.)

Definition
Metabolic alkalosis is an excess of bicarbonate in the extracellular fluid.

Pathophysiology
Bicarbonate gain can be attributed to a loss of hydrogen ion from extracellular fluid, an increase of bicarbonate HCO_3 to the extracellular fluid, or chloride loss from extracellular fluid in excess of HCO_3.

Nursing Assessment

PRIMARY CAUSES
- Causes include vomiting, gastrointestinal suctioning, diarrhea, diuretic therapy, laxative abuse, cystic fibrosis, primary and secondary hyperaldosteronism, Cushing's syndrome, excessive ingestion of bicarbonate, hypokalemia and hypercalcemia.

PHYSICAL ASSESSMENT
- Inspection: Hyperactive deep tendon reflexes, muscle weakness, confusion, seizures, stupor, nausea, vomiting, and diarrhea.
- Auscultation: Hypoventilation

DIAGNOSTIC TEST RESULTS

Standard Laboratory Tests
- Arterial blood gases: The pH is ≥ 7.43, $HCO_3 \geq 26$ mEq/L, base excess $\geq +2$, arterial partial pressure of carbon dioxide ($PaCO_2$) ≥ 45 mm Hg.
- Serum chemistry: Reduced potassium, chloride, and calcium.
- Urinalysis: Reduced urine chloride ≤ 10 mEq/L associated with extracellular fluid volume depletion.

MEDICAL AND SURGICAL MANAGEMENT

PHARMACOLOGY
- Arginine hydrochloride: Used if the sodium chloride in the saline solution is not sufficient to replace the lost anion.
- Potassium chloride: Used to correct potassium depletion.
- Acetazolamide: Acetazolamide, a sulfonamide derivative, is a potent, reversible inhibitor of carbonic anhydrase. Carbonic anhydrase (CA) is the enzyme that catalyzes the hydration of carbon dioxide and the hydration of carbonic acid in the renal tubular cells. The effects of acetazolamide in the kidneys are to increase urinary bicarbonate concentration and increase urine volume, thereby causing a fall in the extracellular pH (see Table 1–13, p. 76).
- Ammonium chloride (NH_4Cl): Used in compromised renal function problems (see Table 1–13, p. 76).

FLUID THERAPY

- Replace extracellular fluid volume deficit with saline.

NURSING MANAGEMENT: NURSING DIAGNOSES AND COLLABORATIVE PROBLEMS

Nursing Diagnoses

Common nursing goals for patients with metabolic alkalosis are to prevent injury and prevent fatigue.

High risk of injury related to altered neuromuscular function, seizure activity, or dysrhythmias.

Expected Patient Outcome. Absence of neuromuscular dysfunction, seizure activity, or dysrhythmias.

- Establish a safe physical environment.
- Initiate seizure precautions.
- Provide stimuli appropriate to maintaining orientation.
- Assist patient with activities of daily living.
- Monitor patient for the presence of weakness or muscle cramps.
- Prepare the patient for gradual increases in physical activity while he or she feels weak.
- Provide rest periods before incremental increase in activity.
- Instruct patient that once the metabolic dysfunction is corrected, neuromuscular alteration will be corrected.

Fatigue related to muscle weakness or muscle cramps.

Expected Patient Outcome. Absence of fatigue.

- Assist patient to identify when he or she experiences fatigue.
- Provide rest periods for patient before increasing activity.
- Provide passive and active range of motion exercises to maintain muscle tone.
- Administer oxygen by nasal cannula or Venturi mask at the prescribed amount.

Collaborative Problems

A common collaborative goal in patients with metabolic alkalosis is to prevent electrolyte imbalance.

Potential Complications: Electrolyte Imbalance. Electrolyte imbalance related to hypochloremia, hypokalemia, and hypocalcemia secondary to concentration of bicarbonate ions.

Expected Patient Outcomes. Patient maintains adequate electrolyte balance, as evidenced by potassium, chloride, and calcium within normal range; arterial blood gases within normal range; blood pressure (BP) within patient's normal range, urinary output (UO) $\geq$30 mL/h, central venous pressure (CVP) 2 to 6 mm Hg, and mean arterial pressure (MAP) 70 to 100 mm Hg.

- Review results of serum electrolyte measurement.
- Obtain and report clinical findings associated with hypokalemia: drowsiness, confusion, apathy, irritability, muscle weakness, paresthesia, muscle pain, muscle cramps, hyporeflexia, paralysis, hypoventilation, nausea, vomiting, abdominal distention, abdominal cramps, polyurea or nocturia.
- Monitor continuous ECG and report changes associated with hypokalemia ($\leq$3.5 mEq/L), which include a depressed ST segment; flattened, inverted T wave and U wave.
- Provide high-potassium foods or potassium supplement liquid should be potassium diluted to decrease gastrointestinal irritation.
- Administer prescribed IV potassium chloride in severe hypokalemia. Administer in a peripheral vein at 10 to 20 mEq/h using a concentration of 40 mEq/L.
- Obtain and report clinical findings associated with hypocalcemia: numbness and tingling of the extremities, muscle cramps, tetany, positive Chvostek's and Trousseau's signs, seizures, carpopedal spasm, laryngeal stridor, abdominal cramps, nausea, vomiting, diarrhea, and dry skin.

- Monitor continuous ECG and report changes associated calcium level ≤8.5 mg/100 mL: a lengthened ST segment and prolonged QT interval.
- Check Chvostek's sign periodically by percussing the facial nerve in the face anterior to the auricle of the ear. Hypocalcemia response is unilateral twitching of the facial muscles, eyelid, and lips.
- Test for Trousseau's sign periodically by inflating a BP cuff around the upper extremity for 3 to 4 minutes, which occludes blood supply to the extremity, thereby producing ischemia. Hypocalcemia is confirmed when the induced ischemia produces carpopedal spasm.
- Provide foods that are high in calcium and low in phosphorus.
- Administer prescribed IV infusion of calcium chloride or calcium gluconate.
- Obtain and report clinical findings associated with hypochloremia (≤96 mEq/L): muscle weakness; tetany; agitation; irritability; and slow, shallow respirations.
- Replace lost chloride with three fourths of the amount of the imbalance as sodium chloride and one fourth as potassium chloride. Sodium chloride or ammonium chloride is used in place of potassium chloride if serum potassium is ≥5.5 mEq/L.

■ HYPERNATREMIA

(For related information see Part I: Renal trauma, p. 447; Acute tubular necrosis, p. 455; Acute renal failure, p. 459; Hypokalemia, p. 485. Part II: Renal transplantations, p. 491. Part III: Hemodialysis, p. 496; Peritoneal dialysis, p. 502; Continuous renal replacement therapy, p. 505.)

Definition
Hypernatremia is an excess of sodium in the extracellular fluid.

Pathophysiology
Hypernatremia is found in conditions in which both water and sodium losses occur, but the water loss is greater than the sodium loss. Reduction of water in the extracellular fluid causes a rise in serum osmolality. Water is then drawn from the intracellular space, which stimulates the antidiuretic hormone (ADH) mechanism, with conservation of body water by a reduction in urine volume. When sodium concentration in extracellular fluid rises, water is drawn out of cells. The overall result is a combination of extracellular fluid (ECF) volume excess and intracellular fluid (ICF) volume deficit.

Nursing Assessment

PRIMARY CAUSES
- Water loss in excess of sodium loss: results from osmotic diuresis in conjunction with uncorrected hyperglycemia or glucosuria and extrarenal losses from sweating, fever, burns, and gastrointestinal losses.
- Water losses: result from renal losses from nephrogenic and central diabetes insipidus and extrarenal losses from excess respiratory loss.
- Pure sodium gain or sodium gain greater than water gain is due to administration of hypertonic dialysis, sodium bicarbonate ($NaCHO_3$) or sodium chloride ($NaCl$). Sodium gain greater than water gain is due to primary aldosteronism or Cushing's syndrome.

PHYSICAL ASSESSMENT
- Inspection: Thirst, dry and sticky mucous membranes, restlessness, irritability, muscular rigidity, weakness, agitation, lethargy, coma, confusion, tremors or seizures, fever, oliguria, or hyperpnea.
- Palpation: Flushed and loose skin.
- Auscultation: Tachycardia and hypotension.

DIAGNOSTIC TEST RESULTS

Standard Laboratory Tests. (see Table 4–1)

- Blood studies: Elevated hematocrit and hemoglobin.

- Serum chemistry: Elevated sodium ≥148 mEq/L, chloride ≥106 mEq/L, serum osmolality ≥29 mOsm/kg, and blood urea nitrogen (BUN).
- Urinalysis: Urine sodium ≤50 mEq/L, urine osmolality ≥800 mOsm/kg, urine chloride ≥50 mEq/L, and urine specific gravity ≥1.030.

MEDICAL AND SURGICAL MANAGEMENT

FLUID THERAPY

- Intravenous isotonic saline: Used when imbalance is due to a loss of ECF; urine osmolality is hypertonic, and urine sodium is ≤10 mEq/L.
- 5% dextrose and water (D_5W): Used to replace the ECF deficit created by the hypernatremia; urine osmolality is isotonic, hypertonic, or hypotonic and urine sodium ≥20 mEq/L.

DIET

- Daily sodium intake is restricted to 0.5 g to 2 g if the imbalance is due to a sodium excess.

NURSING MANAGEMENT: NURSING DIAGNOSES AND COLLABORATIVE PROBLEMS

Nursing Diagnoses

Common nursing goals for patients with hypernatremia are to prevent injury and correct fluid imbalance.

High risk of injury related to central nervous system alteration secondary to excess plasma sodium or cerebral edema.

Expected Patient Outcome. Patient is free of injury.

- Review results of urine osmolality and serum sodium tests.
- Provide prescribed low-sodium diet, which may provide a range from 0.5 g to 2 g/d.
- Obtain and report changes in neurological function resulting from hypernatremia: changes in mental status, restlessness, irritability, agitation, lethargy, confusion, tremors, or seizures.
- Institute seizure precautions.
- Provide a quiet, calm environment to decrease further stimulation.
- Provide protective measures such as placement of bed-rail padding when patient is restless and thrashing in bed.
- Administer prescribed IV isotonic or hypotonic solutions to maintain adequate hydration.
- Monitor patient's plasma sodium and infusion rate to avoid overhydration and too rapid a reduction in sodium.
- Promote comfort by using hard candy, gum, or sips of water to decrease thirst.
- Maintain skin integrity through the use of meticulous hygienic measures, moisturizing agents, and frequent repositioning.
- Obtain and record daily weight.
- Monitor intake, output, and specific gravity to evaluate fluid balance.

Fluid volume deficit related to excess water loss.

Expected Patient Outcomes. Patient maintains adequate fluid balance, as evidenced by urinary output (UO) ≥30 mL/h or 0.5 mL/kg/h, central venous pressure (CVP) 2 to 6 mm Hg, blood pressure (BP) within patient's normal range, cardiac output (CO) 4 to 8 L/min, mean arterial pressure (MAP) 70 to 100 mm Hg, pulmonary capillary wedge pressure (PCWP) 6 to 12 mm Hg, pulmonary artery pressure (PAP) systolic ≤25 mm Hg, normothermia, normal skin turgor, peripheral pulses +2, capillary refill ≤3 seconds, body weight stabilized within 5% of patient's baseline, heart rate (HR) ≤100 bpm, serum sodium 135 to 148 mEq/L, serum osmolality 285 to 295 mOsm/kg, and urine osmolality 500 to 800 mOsm/kg.

- Consult with physician about the causes of fluid volume deficit resulting from intracellular dehydration.
- Review results of BUN, creatinine, serum osmolality, serum electrolytes, serum

protein:albumin, hematocrit, hemoglobin, and urine osmolality tests.

- Obtain and report other clinical findings associated with intracellular dehydration: irritability; restlessness; listlessness; lethargy; thready, weak pulse; tachypnea; hypotension; tachycardia; fever; dry mucous membranes; constipation; and weight loss.
- Provide oral fluids as tolerated, using salt-free fluids.
- Measure all fluid output including urine, vomiting, diarrhea, gastric suctioning, wound or ostomy drainage, insensible loss by lungs, skin, and third spacing.
- Measure and document all fluid intake including oral and IV fluids, IV piggyback medications, irrigation of gastric tube, saline used for endotracheal suctioning, or humidified oxygen therapy.
- Report UO $\leq$400 mL/24 h; specific gravity $\geq$1.030, and weight loss.
- Administer prescribed IV D_5W to provide rehydration when fluid volume deficit is due to ECF imbalance.
- Administer prescribed antipyretics for fever.
- Teach patient the reasons behind increases in sodium and treatment.

■ HYPONATREMIA

(For related information see Part I: Renal trauma, p. 447; Acute tubular necrosis, p. 455; Acute renal failure, p. 459; Hyperkalemia, p. 485. Part II: Renal transplantations, p. 491. Part III: Hemodialysis, p. 496; Peritoneal dialysis, p. 502; Continuous arteriovenous hemofiltration, p. 505.)

Definition

Hyponatremia is a deficit of sodium in the extracellular fluid. The serum sodium can reach $\leq$134 mEq/L.

Pathophysiology

The predominant change in hyponatremia or hyposmolality occurs in water content, not solute concentration. Thirst is inactivated and inhibition of antidiuretic hormone (ADH) occurs. The response is excretion of a large volume of dilute urine.

Nursing Assessment

PRIMARY CAUSES

- Dilutional extracellular fluid (ECF) expansion: Causes of dilutional hyponatremia are excessive ingestion or infusion of electrolyte-free solutions, excessive use of tap water enema, irrigation of gastrointestinal tubes with electrolyte-free solutions, renal dysfunction, inappropriate secretion of ADH, cirrhosis, congestive heart failure, and hyperglycemia.
- Deficit of sodium: Occurs from inadequate ingestion of dietary sodium, infusion of solutions that are sodium-deficient, salt-wasting renal dysfunction, potent diuretic, adrenal insufficiency, severe vomiting, severe diarrhea, gastrointestinal suction, potassium depletion, burns, third-spacing, and severe malnutrition.

PHYSICAL ASSESSMENT

- Inspection: Headache, apprehension, lethargy, confusion, convulsions, coma, reduced jugular venous pressure, faintness, abdominal cramps, hyperreflexia, nausea, vomiting, fatigue, weakness, or coma.
- Auscultation: Tachycardia, postural hypotension, or orthostatic hypotension.

DIAGNOSTIC TEST RESULTS

Standard Laboratory Tests

- Serum chemistry: Serum sodium $\leq$136 mEq/L, serum chloride $\leq$96 mEq/L, and serum osmolality $\leq$285 mOsm/kg. Elevated urea and creatinine, and potassium may be low or high.
- Urinalysis: Variable urine sodium $\leq$20 mEq/L, osmolality $\leq$300 mOsm/L, and specific gravity $\leq$1.030.

MEDICAL AND SURGICAL MANAGEMENT

PHARMACOLOGY
- Diuretics: Furosemide is used to treat imbalance as the result of dilutional expansion of the ECF.

FLUID THERAPY
- Normal saline intravenous therapy: Used if the imbalance is due to sodium loss; urine osmolality is hypertonic and urine sodium is ≤10 mEq/L.

DIET
- Diet high in sodium content to replace sodium.

NURSING MANAGEMENT: NURSING DIAGNOSES AND COLLABORATIVE PROBLEMS

Nursing Diagnoses
Common nursing goals for patients with hyponatremia are to prevent injury and correct fluid imbalance.

High risk for injury related to central nervous system dysfunction secondary to decreased sodium plasma.

Expected Patient Outcomes. Patient is free from injury, as evidenced by absence of disorientation, confusion, or lethargy.

- Review results of serum sodium, serum osmolality, urine sodium, and urine osmolality.
- Obtain and report mental changes associated with sodium level ≤120 to 125 mEq/L: headache, lethargy, confusion, seizures, coma, malaise, nausea, and vomiting.
- Provide a bedside environment that prevents injury to the lethargic patient.
- Provide rest periods for the lethargic patient.
- Institute seizure precautions.
- Promote the conservation of energy by limiting activity.
- Maintain upper airway patency in the vomiting patient by suctioning or changing position.

- Administer prescribed diuretic (furosemide) to correct dilutional expansion of the ECF.

Fluid volume excess related to intracellular overhydration causing hyponatremia.

Expected Patient Outcomes. Patient maintains adequate fluid balance, as evidenced by heart rate (HR) ≤100 bpm, central venous pressure (CVP) 2 to 6 mm Hg, body weight stabilizes within 5% of patient's baseline, blood pressure (BP) within normal range, cardiac output (CO) 4 to 8 L/min, pulmonary artery pressure (PAP) systolic 15 to 25 mm Hg, pulmonary capillary wedge pressure (PCWP) 6 to 12 mm Hg, mean arterial pressure (MAP) 70 to 100 mm Hg, normal heart sounds, urinary output (UO) ≥30 mL/h, serum electrolytes within normal range, absence of crackles, absence of edema, and absence of neck vein distention.

- Consult with physician as to the causes of hyponatremia.
- Review results of tests for serum electrolytes, serum osmolality, urine sodium, and urine osmolality.
- Provide dietary provision of sodium if the fluid imbalance is due to sodium loss.
- Obtain and report hemodynamic parameters associated with fluid volume excess: elevated CO, CVP ≤8 mm Hg, PCWP ≥15 mm Hg, and PAP systolic ≥25 mm Hg.
- Obtain and report clinical findings associated with hyponatremia: altered mental status; seizure; dependent edema; skin pale, moist, or cool; tachycardia, tachypnea, elevated systolic BP, dyspnea, and crackles.
- Document fluid output such as urine, gastrointestinal losses from vomiting, gastric suctioning, insensible losses, and iatrogenic loss.
- Monitor daily weight and UO. Report UO ≤30 mL/h or ≤0.5 mL/kg/h and weight gain ≥0.5 kg/d.
- Provide progressive increase in activity as tolerated to reduce risk of fatigue, edematous tissue, and immobility.

- Administer prescribed hypertonic or isotonic saline IV if the fluid imbalance is due to sodium loss.
- Administer prescribed diuretic if fluid imbalance is due to expansion of the ECF. The goal is to increase excretion of excess fluid.
- Instruct patient about the significance of fluid restriction.

■ HYPERKALEMIA

(For related information see Part I: Renal trauma, p. 447; Acute tubular necrosis, p. 455; Acute renal failure, p. 459; Hyponatremia, p. 481. Part II: Renal transplantations, p. 491. Part III: Hemodialysis, p. 496; Peritoneal dialysis, p. 502; Continuous renal replacement therapy, p. 505.)

Definition

Hyperkalemia is an excess of potassium in the extracellular fluid. In hyperkalemia, serum potassium reaches a level of ≥5.5 mEq/L.

Pathophysiology

Potassium is primarily an intracellular ion and any disruption of cellular integrity will cause a loss of potassium into the extracellular fluid compartment.

Nursing Assessment

PRIMARY CAUSES

- Decreased renal excretion: Caused by renal dysfunction; adrenocortical insufficiencies such as Addison's disease and hyporeninemic hypoaldosteronism; and the use of potassium-sparing diuretics such as spironolactone or triamterene.
- Translocation from the cells: Translocations of potassium from the intracellular to extracellular fluid space include severe catabolism, burns, rhabdomyolysis, acute acidosis, and intravascular hemolysis.
- Excessive intake of potassium: Excessive intake of potassium is due to excess intravenous infusion or oral ingestion of medications or food substances high in potassium.

PHYSICAL ASSESSMENT

- Inspection: Irritability, confusion, weakness, cramps; paresthesia of face, tongue, extremities; flaccid paralysis, abdominal distention; neuromuscular hyperexcitability and, diarrhea.
- Auscultation: Hypotension and dysrhythmias.

DIAGNOSTIC TEST RESULTS

Standard Laboratory Tests

- Serum chemistry: Elevated potassium, urea nitrogen, creatinine, urate, and phosphate; decreased bicarbonate (HCO_3).

ECG

- Findings include peaked T waves of increased amplitude, widening of the QRS, reduced R wave amplitude, depressed ST segment, prolonged PR interval, and biphasic QRS-T complexes.

MEDICAL AND SURGICAL MANAGEMENT

PHARMACOLOGY

- Calcium chloride: Used to increase sodium flux through the sodium channels in muscle tissue, which also enhances conduction of the impulse (see Table 4–4).
- Sodium polystyrene sulfonate (Kayexalate): Used to remove potassium from the body. It can be administered as an oral preparation or by retentive enema. Kayexalate is administered with sorbital to enhance potassium loss via the bowel. Usually 50 g of Kayexalate can reduce serum potassium by 0.5 to 1.0 mEq/L (see Table 4–4).
- Sodium bicarbonate: Used to rapidly reduce potassium even in the absence of acidemia. It can be infused as a 50 mEq bolus over 5 to 10 minutes.
- Diuretics: Furosemide is used to remove potassium.

FLUID THERAPY

- 500 mL 10% glucose and regular insulin: Regular insulin (10%) with a glucose infusion is used for a rapid redistribution of potassium from the extracellular to the intracellular compartment. Insulin moves potassium intracellularly and glucose prevents hypoglycemia. When 1 g of glucose is converted to glycogen, approximately 3.6 mEq/L of potassium are retained intracellularly, it is effective in about 10 to 15 minutes after infusion.
- Hypertonic sodium chloride infusion: The infusion reduces the serum potassium level in hyponatremia patients but is most effective within 1 hour and has little effect on total body potassium.

DIALYSIS

- Hemodialysis is used to decrease both the serum level and total body level of potassium. Approximately 40 mEq/L of potassium can be removed during the first hour of dialysis.
- Peritoneal dialysis can be used to reduce serum potassium even though the process is slower than with hemodialysis.

DIET

- Low-potassium diet.

NURSING MANAGEMENT: NURSING DIAGNOSES AND COLLABORATIVE PROBLEMS

Nursing Diagnosis

A common nursing goal for patients with hyperkalemia is to maintain sensory-perceptual function.

High risk of sensory-perceptual alteration related to neuromuscular changes.

Expected Patient Outcomes. Patient maintains sensory-perceptual function, as evidenced by absence of paresthesia, normal deep tendon reflexes, and absence of weakness or neuromuscular hyperexcitability.

- Review results of serum potassium tests.
- Evaluate neuromuscular status at same time vital signs are assessed.
- Monitor for the presence of neuromuscular alteration, such as tremors.
- Obtain and report neuromuscular changes associated with hyperkalemia: paresthesia, twitching, seizure activity, muscle weakness, and hyperactive deep tendon reflexes.
- Protect patient from injury when increasing physical activity.
- Assist patient with eating while he or she is experiencing sensory-perceptual changes.
- Instruct patient as to the causes of neuromuscular changes associated with hyperkalemia.

Collaborative Problem

Potential Complication: Dysrhythmias. Dysrhythmias related to abnormalities in rhythm and conduction secondary to hyperkalemia.

Expected Patient Outcome. Patient maintains regular sinus rhythm.

- Review results of 12-lead ECG and serum potassium test.
- Provide low-potassium diet.
- Monitor continuous ECG rhythm and report tall, peaked, tented T wave and a depressed ST segment. As potassium imbalance progresses, the P wave decreases in amplitude and the PR interval is prolonged. Atrial systole can occur with a widened QRS complex that can merge with the T wave forming the sine wave characteristic of hyperkalemia.
- Monitor continuous ECG during calcium infusion.
- Should patient be receiving digitalis, calcium may potentate its effects. Calcium, in this situation, is diluted in 5% dextrose and water (D_5W) and the infusion rate is reduced to avoid toxic effects.
- Administer prescribed agents to antagonize the effect of potassium in the cell membrane. These include calcium salts, such as

calcium chloride, or hypertonic sodium salts, such as sodium chloride or sodium bicarbonate. A bolus (44 mEq) is followed by an infusion of 88 to 132 mEq $NaHCO_3$/L in D_5W.

- Administer prescribed diuretic (furosemide) to reduce potassium.
- Administer prescribed sodium polystyrene sulfonate (Kayexalate) with sorbital 15 to 30 g orally or by enema 2 to 3 times daily. This acts as an exchange resin that absorbs potassium in the gastrointestinal tract and eliminates it in the feces.
- Should pharmacological therapy be ineffective or slow in reducing potassium, prepare patient for peritoneal dialysis or hemodialysis (see Hemodialysis, p. 496, and Peritoneal dialysis, p. 502).

■ HYPOKALEMIA

(For related information see Part I: Renal trauma, p. 447; Acute tubular necrosis, p. 455; Acute renal failure, p. 459; Hypernatremia, p. 479. Part II: Renal transplantations, p. 491. Part III: Hemodialysis, p. 496; Peritoneal dialysis, p. 502; Continuous renal replacement therapy, p. 505.)

Definition

Hypokalemia is a deficit of potassium in the extracellular fluid. The serum potassium level can be ≤ 3.5 mEq/L.

Pathophysiology

Hypokalemia affects cardiac cell excitability by causing hyperpolarization of the resting membrane potential (RMP). The result is an irritable ventricular response with potential dysrhythmias.

Nursing Assessment

PRIMARY CAUSES

- Increased intracellular shifts of potassium: Results from alkalosis, intravenous infusion of glucose and insulin, and familial hypokalemic periodic paralysis.
- Decreased potassium intake: Results from the inability to ingest fluids or floods, infusion of large quantities of potassium-free intravenous solutions, and prolonged ingestion of diets low in potassium.
- Increased gastrointestinal potassium loss: Caused by vomiting, fistulas, diarrhea, inflammatory bowel disease, laxative abuse, or ureterosigmoidostomies.
- Excess renal potassium loss: Caused by diuretic therapy, renal tubular acidosis, chronic interstitial nephritis, primary and secondary hyperaldosteronism, Cushing's syndrome, adrenal steroid therapy, and diabetic ketoacidosis.
- Excess integumentary potassium loss: Results from excessive perspiration.

PHYSICAL ASSESSMENT

- Inspection: Fatigue, weakness, respiratory muscle weakness, hyporeflexia, muscle cramps, flaccid paralysis, anorexia, nausea, vomiting, constipation, abdominal distention, abdominal cramps, paralytic ileus, apathy, depression, irritability, drowsiness, lethargy, or paresthesia.
- Auscultation: Hypotension and dysrhythmias.

DIAGNOSTIC TEST RESULTS

Standard Laboratory Tests

- Serum chemistry: Potassium ≤ 3.5 mEq/L; elevated bicarbonate, pH, and phosphate; and reduced sodium, calcium, and magnesium.
- Urinalysis: Reduced osmolality and pH.

ECG

- Reveals peaked P wave, prolonged PR interval, flattened T wave, depressed ST segment, and elevated U wave.

MEDICAL AND SURGICAL MANAGEMENT

PHARMACOLOGY

- Oral potassium: Used when potassium levels are 2.5 to 3.5 mEq/L. Oral potassium therapy avoids potassium rebound because there is time for renal regulation to contribute to restoration of potassium balance.

- Intravenous potassium supplement: Given when potassium level is ≤2.5 mEq/L, at an infusion rate of 10 to 20 mEq/L up to 80 to 100 mEq/L in severe hypokalemia.

NURSING MANAGEMENT: NURSING DIAGNOSES AND COLLABORATIVE PROBLEMS

Nursing Diagnosis

A common nursing goal for patients with hypokalemia is to maintain effective breathing.

High risk for ineffective breathing pattern related to respiratory muscle weakness secondary to potassium ≤2.0 to 2.5 mEq/L.

Expected Patient Outcomes. Patient maintains effective breathing pattern as evidenced by respiratory rate (RR) 12 to 20 BPM; normal respiratory depth and pattern; deep, symmetrical chest expansion; and unlabored respirations.

- Review results of serum potassium and arterial blood gas measurements.
- Obtain and report clinical findings associated with ineffective breathing pattern resulting from potassium ≤2.0 to 2.5 mEq/L: tachypnea, dyspnea, shallow respirations, and labored breathing.
- Restrict physical activity to bed rest when patient's breathing is labored.
- Reposition patient every 2 hours to prevent stasis of secretions.
- Maintain muscle strength and monitor deep tendon reflex activity, since hypokalemia is associated with muscle weakness.
- Suction patient should compromised respiratory exercises and retention of secretions occur.
- Encourage deep breathing, coughing, and use of incentive spirometer.
- Provide prescribed oxygen 2 to 4 L/min by mask or nasal cannula to maintain adequate oxygenation.

Collaborative Problem

Common collaborative goals for patients with hypokalemia are to correct dysrhythmias and increase cardiac output.

Potential Complication: Dysrhythmias. Dysrhythmias related to altered conduction secondary to hypokalemia.

Expected Patient Outcome. Patient maintains regular sinus rhythm.

- Review results of 12-lead ECG and serum electrolyte and arterial blood gas measurements.
- Monitor cardiac rhythm for changes in configuration reflecting hypokalemia: peaked P wave, prolonged PR interval, flattened or inverted T wave, depressed ST segment, and elevated U wave.
- Encourage patient to eat foods high in potassium. These include apricots, bananas, dates, raisins, avocados, beans, potatoes, and orange juice.
- Monitor intake and urinary output (UO). Report UO ≤30 mL/h.
- Administer prescribed oral potassium supplements. Dilute liquid potassium to decrease gastrointestinal irritation.
- Administer prescribed potassium chloride in a central line at a rate not to exceed 20 mEq/100 mL/h.
- Teach patient to report any palpitations.

Potential Complication: Decreased Cardiac Output. Decreased cardiac output related to impaired contractility secondary to hypokalemia.

Expected Patient Outcomes. Patient maintains adequate cardiac output, as evidenced by cardiac output (CO) 4 to 8 L/min, cardiac index (CI) 2.7 to 4.3 L/min/m², central venous pressure (CVP) 2 to 6 mm Hg, pulmonary capillary wedge pressure (PCWP) 6 to 12 mm Hg, blood pressure (BP) within patient's normal range, heart rate (HR) ≤100 bpm, mean arterial pressure (MAP) 70 to 100 mm Hg, peripheral pulses +2, capillary refill ≤3 seconds, and UO ≥30 mL/h.

- Consult with physician when patient is receiving digitalis as to when the drug is to be withheld or reduced.
- Review results of ECG, serum potassium, serum enzymes, urine potassium, and urine osmolality tests.
- Obtain and report hemodynamic parameters indicating decreased CO. CO ≤4 L/min, CI ≤2.7 L/min/m², and PCWP ≥12 mm Hg.
- Obtain and report clinical findings associated with decreased CO: tachycardia, hypotension, peripheral pulses ≥+2, and capillary refill ≥3 seconds.
- Monitor intake, output, and daily weight. Report UO ≤30 mL/h or ≤0.5 mL/kg/h.
- Monitor continuous ECG to assess HR and rhythm. Document ECG rhythm strips every 2 to 4 hours when patient experiences dysrhythmias.
- Administer prescribed intravenous potassium chloride to correct hypokalemia.

■ HYPERCALCEMIA

(*For related information see Part I: Renal trauma, p. 447; Acute tubular necrosis, p. 455; Acute renal failure, p. 459. Part II: Renal transplantations, p. 491. Part III: Hemodialysis, p. 496; Peritoneal dialysis, p. 502; Continuous renal replacement therapy, p. 505.*)

Definition
Hypercalcemia is an excess of calcium in the extracellular fluid. The serum calcium can be ≥10.5 mg/100 mL.

Pathophysiology
An increase in the albumin concentration in blood or an increase in abnormal binding protein may lead to an increase in total serum concentration. Acidemia leads to increase in calcium. Hypercalcemia is classified as mild ≤12 mg/dL, moderate 12 to 15 mg/dL and severe ≥15 mg/dL.

Nursing Assessment

PRIMARY CAUSES
- Causes include vitamin D or vitamin A excess and primary hyperparathyroidism as a result of adenoma, hyperplasia, or carcinoma; secondary hyperparathyroidism resulting from renal insufficiency or malabsorption. Other causes include acromegaly, adrenal insufficiency, metastasis to bone, lymphoproliferative disease, use of thiazide diuretics, sarcoidosis, Paget's disease of bone; hypophosphatasia, or immobilization.

PHYSICAL ASSESSMENT
- Inspection: Anorexia, nausea, vomiting, constipation, polyuria, muscle weakness, tremor, fatigue, muscle hypotonicity, disorientation, loss of memory, depression, lethargy, confusion, stupor, and coma.
- Auscultation: Dysrhythmias.

DIAGNOSTIC TEST RESULTS

Standard Laboratory Tests
- Serum chemistry: Elevated calcium ≥10.5 mg/100 mL and normal or low phosphate.
- Urinalysis: Elevated urine calcium, reduced urine osmolality, and specific gravity.

ECG
- Reveals shortened QT interval and shortened ST segment.

MEDICAL AND SURGICAL MANAGEMENT

PHARMACOLOGY
- Diuretic: Intravenous furosemide is administered every 4 to 6 hours to prevent fluid volume overload and accelerate calcium excretion.
- Phosphate: Intravenous phosphate causes calcium complex formation, which rapidly lowers serum calcium. Oral phosphate can be given to patients who are not hyperphosphemic.

- Mithramycin: Mithramycin, a cytotoxic antibiotic, is used to inhibit bone absorption of calcium.
- Calcitonin: Used to decrease calcium release from bone while increasing its renal excretion (see Table 4–4).
- Glucocorticoids: Used to decrease intestinal calcium absorption and increase renal excretion.
- Ethylenediaminetetraacetic acid (EDTA): Used to lower serum calcium by chelation.

FLUID THERAPY
- Sodium chloride 0.9% or 0.45% can be infused to promote excretion of both sodium and calcium; when renal function is normal, 6 to 12 L of IV fluids can be given over 24 hours.
- Dextrose 5% can be used if the patient is hypernatremic or has congestive heart failure.

DIET
- Low-calcium diet.

DIALYSIS
- Hemodialysis with a dialysate low in calcium is used to correct serum calcium level.

NURSING MANAGEMENT: NURSING DIAGNOSES AND COLLABORATIVE PROBLEMS

Nursing Diagnoses
Common nursing goals for patients with hypercalcemia are to promote urinary elimination, prevent injury, and prevent constipation.

Altered pattern of urinary elimination related to calcium stone formation, diuretics, or renal dysfunction.

Expected Patient Outcome. Patient maintains normal voiding pattern.

- Review results of tests for serum electrolytes, blood urea nitrogen (BUN), and creatinine.

- Provide a low-calcium diet.
- Monitor clinical findings associated with a kidney stone: hematuria, intermittent pain, nausea, and vomiting.
- Measure daily weight, intake, specific gravity, and urinary output (UO). Report UO $\leq$30 mL/h or $\leq$0.5 mL/kg/h, specific gravity $\leq$1.015, and weight gain.
- Strain and monitor the urine for stones.
- Encourage patient to drink fluids such as cranberry or prune juice to decrease risk of calcium stone formation.
- Administer prescribed IV 0.9% or 0.45% sodium chloride fluid to promote hydration and renal excretion of calcium. May use two large-bore IV lines, since fluid might need to be as high as 500 mL/h.
- Administer prescribed IV phosphate to decrease calcium.
- Administer prescribed medications such as mithramycin and EDTA.
- Administer calcitonin to increase bone deposition of calcium and phosphorus or increase urinary calcium and phosphate excretion.

High risk for injury related to muscle weakness, confusion, tremors, or lethargy.

Expected Patient Outcomes. Patient displays absence of neuromuscular or sensorium alteration: weakness, confusion, tremors, or lethargy.

- Evaluate patient's level of consciousness and orientation to person, time and place.
- Monitor and report neuromuscular changes such as muscle hyperactivity, muscular weakness, and tremor.
- Monitor muscle movement, strength, and tone.
- Encourage patient to ambulate, when appropriate, to reduce the release of bone calcium.
- Initiate passive and active range of motion exercises.
- Provide appropriate environmental stimuli to increase patient's level of orientation.

- Provide safe environment when increasing patient's physical activity.
- Initiate seizure precautions.
- Protect patient as he or she stands or ambulates in room.
- Monitor continuous ECG to assess heart rate (HR) and rhythm. Document ECG rhythm strips every 2 to 4 hours in patients with dysrhythmias.
- Encourage patient to increase mobility, when realistic, to reduce bone softening.
- Instruct patient as to the reasons for muscle weakness, tremors, or confusion.

Constipation related to excess fluid loss and increased calcium.

Expected Patient Outcome. Patient maintains normal bowel habits.

- Encourage patient to eat a diet high in fiber to aid in elimination.
- Encourage patient to increase fluid intake to assist with elimination.
- Reduce calcium in diet to reduce tendency toward constipation.
- Encourage patient to increase physical activity.
- Administer prescribed IV fluids to maintain adequate hydration.
- Administer stool softeners as prescribed.

Collaborative Problem

A common collaborative goal for patients with hypercalcemia is to increase cardiac output.

Potential Complication: Decreased Cardiac Output. Decreased cardiac output related to hypertension secondary to renal dysfunction.

Expected Patient Outcomes. Patient maintains adequate cardiac output, as evidenced by cardiac output (CO) 4 to 8 L/min, central venous pressure (CVP) 2 to 6 mm Hg, pulmonary capillary wedge pressure (PCWP) 6 to 12 mm Hg, HR ≤100 bpm, respiratory rate (RR) 12 to 20 BPM, blood pressure (BP) within patient's normal range, absence of neck vein distention, absence of crackles, and UO ≥30 mL/h.

- Review results of ECG.
- Obtain and report elevated BP resulting from increased peripheral vascular resistance caused by calcium.
- Measure intake, output, specific gravity, and daily weight. Report UO ≤30 mL/h or ≥0.5 mL/kg/h.
- Monitor continuous ECG and report shortened Q-T interval and widened T wave.
- Administer prescribed intravenous phosphate.
- Administer prescribed mithramycin, calcitonin, glucocorticoids, or EDTA.
- Administer prescribed atropine should patient develop heart block.
- Should pharmacological therapy not correct the heart block, prepare patient for pacemaker.

■ HYPOCALCEMIA

(For related information see Part I: Renal trauma, p. 447; Acute tubular necrosis, p. 455; Acute renal failure, p. 459. Part II: Renal transplantations, p. 491. Part III: Hemodialysis, p. 496; Peritoneal dialysis, p. 502; Continuous renal replacement therapy, p. 505.)

Definition

Hypocalcemia is a deficit of calcium in the extracellular fluid. The serum calcium level can be ≤8.5 mg/100mL.

Pathophysiology

Pathophysiological changes can reflect inadequate calcium input into the circulation, excessive loss of calcium, or malabsorption syndrome.

Nursing Assessment

PRIMARY CAUSES

- Causes include damaged parathyroid gland, hypoproteinemia, inadequate dietary intake, osteoblastic metastases, thyroid carcinoma, alkalosis caused by vomiting, alkali ingestion, hyperventilation, chronic renal failure, chronic malabsorption because of gastrectomy, high-fat diet, small-bowel disorders, hypomagnesemia, or acute pancreatitis.

PHYSICAL ASSESSMENT

- Inspection: Muscle cramps, numbness, tetany, tingling of the extremities, carpopedal spasms, convulsions, laryngeal stridor, dyspnea, diplopia, abdominal cramps, Chvostek's sign, Trousseau's sign, vomiting, paralytic ileus, abdominal pain and tenderness, and distention.
- Auscultation: Adventitious breath sounds and wheezes.

DIAGNOSTIC TEST RESULTS

Standard Laboratory Tests

- Serum chemistry: Reduced calcium (≤ 8.5 mg/100 mL), magnesium, and albumin. Depressed ratio 0.8 to 1.0 mg calcium: 1 g of albumin.

ECG

- Includes prolonged QT interval and lengthened ST segment.

MEDICAL AND SURGICAL MANAGEMENT

PHARMACOLOGY

- Calcium gluconate: Is administered as 10 to 20 mL of 10% calcium gluconate IV, not to exceed 0.5 mL/min. Oral calcium can supplement and is begun as soon as tolerated.
- Magnesium sulfate: Hypomagnesium inhibits the release and action of parathyroid hormone (PTH). The dose is administered 1 to 2 g every 4 to 6 hours intramuscularly, depending upon the extent of hypomagnesemia.
- Vitamin D supplement: Used if vitamin D deficiency is the underlying cause of hypocalcemia.

DIET

- High-calcium and low-phosphorus diet.

NURSING MANAGEMENT: NURSING DIAGNOSES AND COLLABORATIVE PROBLEMS

Nursing Diagnoses

Common nursing goals for patients with hypocalcemia are to maintain effective breathing and prevent injury.

Ineffective breathing pattern related to tetany, convulsions, and laryngeal spasm.

Expected Patient Outcomes. Patient maintains effective breathing pattern, as evidenced by arterial blood gases within normal range, respiratory rate (RR) 12 to 20 BPM, absence of cyanosis, heart rate (HR) ≤ 100 bpm, absence of laryngeal stridor or dyspnea, normal motor nerve excitability, and absence of adventitious breath sounds.

- Review arterial blood gas or serum electrolyte results.
- Monitor clinical indicators of respiratory status: rate, depth, symmetry of chest excursion, use of accessory muscles, skin color, and presence of adventitious breath sounds.
- Obtain and report clinical findings of enhanced motor nerve excitability characterized by muscle twitching, neuromuscular irritability, paresthesia, stridor, tetany, bronchospasm, and laryngospasm.
- Monitor patient's airway status for spasm or obstruction.
- Obtain and report other clinical findings indicating ineffective breathing pattern: tachypnea, dyspnea, and cyanosis.
- Administer prescribed oxygen 2 to 4 L/min by mask or nasal cannula to enhance oxygenation.
- Should airway obstruction occur, prepare patient for intubation and ventilatory support.
- Administer prescribed calcium gluconate or magnesium sulfate to increase calcium level.

High risk of injury related to neuromuscular changes.

Expected Patient Outcome. Patient is free of injury.

- Provide foods that are high in calcium (meats, leafy vegetables, and milk) and low in phosphorus.
- Monitor and report signs of tetany: numbness and tingling in the fingers, around the mouth, and over the face.
- Obtain and report clinical findings associated with hypocalcemia: numbness and tingling of the extremities, muscle cramps, tetany, positive Chvostek's and Trousseau's signs, seizures, carpopedal spasm, laryngeal stridor, abdominal cramps, nausea, vomiting, diarrhea, and dry skin.
- Monitor continuous ECG and report changes associated with calcium level ≤ 8.5 mg/100 mL: a lengthened ST segment and prolonged QT interval.
- Check Chvostek's sign periodically by percussing the facial nerve in the face anterior to the auricle of the ear. Hypocalcemia response is unilateral twitching of the facial muscles, eyelid, and lips.
- Test for Trousseau's sign periodically by inflating a blood pressure cuff around the upper extremity for 3 to 4 minutes, which occludes blood supply to the extremity, thereby producing ischemia. Hypocalcemia is confirmed when the induced ischemia produces carpopedal spasm.
- Initiate seizure precautions.
- Provide a safe environment for the patient.
- Assist with self-care activities for patients with weakness or sensorimotor changes.
- Establish progressive exercise program as tolerated or when hypocalcemia is corrected.
- Assist patient and family to coordinate medications around dietary intake.
- Teach patient reasons for weakness, fatigue, and tetany.
- Administer prescribed IV infusion of 10% calcium gluconate undiluted at 1 mL/min for emergency replacement.
- Administer prescribed phosphate-binding antacids to reduce phosphate absorption and cause an inverse increase in calcium.
- Administer prescribed vitamin D and calcium supplements 1 hour after meals and at bedtime. This will maximize calcium absorption and utilization.

....

PART II: SURGICAL CORRECTION AND NURSING MANAGEMENT

....

■ RENAL TRANSPLANTATION

(For related information see Cardiac deviations, Part I; Shock, p. 174; Dysrhythmias, p. 184. Part I: Acute tubular necrosis, p. 455; Acute renal failure, p. 459.)

Case Management Basis
DRG: 302 Kidney transplantation
LOS: 13.90 days

Definition
Renal transplantation is used for the treatment of end-stage renal disease (ESRD). The goal is to achieve an optimal level of function and reversal of problems associated with renal failure.

Patient Selection

INDICATIONS. Chronic renal failure resulting from glomerulonephritis, pyelonephritis, multiple system disease, and multiple organ failure.

CONTRAINDICATIONS. Active infection, malignant tumors, drug abuse, advanced cardiopulmonary disease, marked obesity, and positive T cell lymphocytotoxic cross match.

Procedure

TECHNIQUE. The right iliac fossa is the position used for placement of the transplanted kidney. The most frequently used anastomosis is end-to-side, with the external iliac artery and the graft renal artery. The venotomy accommodates the diameter of the renal vein. After the arterial and venous anastomoses are completed and blood flow has been established, the kidney color becomes pink and it begins to form urine. Once revascularization of the kidney is finished, ureteral anastomosis is started. The ureter for the kidney graft is tunneled into the bladder mucosa.

Complications

Transplant rejection may include four phases: hyperactive, accelerated, acute, and chronic.

Hyperactive rejection: This occurs within minutes to hours after the surgical anastomoses are completed and is due to the reaction of preformed cytotoxic antibodies in the recipient's body with the foreign antigen.

Accelerated rejection: This can occur within 7 days after transplant and is the result of preformed antibodies.

Acute rejection: This is the common form of rejection. The inflammatory changes from this cellular immune response are reversed with immunosuppression.

Chronic rejection: This is characterized by a progressive deterioration of renal function, which may occur over months to years. Chronic rejection does not respond to treatment and eventually leads to failure of the graft.

MEDICAL AND SURGICAL MANAGEMENT

PHARMACOLOGY

- Immunosuppressive therapy: Corticosteroids (prednisone, prednisolone, and methylprednisolone) inhibit the production of interleuken-1 from the activated macrophage, which blocks the immune response and prevents graft injury. They are also used as prophylactics against rejection. The dosage range is from 1.5 to 2.0 mg/kg/min IV or PO. Azathioprine is used only as a prophylactic against rejection. Cyclosporin A blocks the production of interleukin-2 in the activated helper cells and is used as a prophylactic against rejection. It is administered IV by central or peripheral access, whereas the oral form is given in gelatin capsules or in liquid form. The dosage range is 8 to 14 mg/kg/d PO or 3 to 4 mg/kg by continuous IV infusion. Antilymphocyte globulin (ACG) is used in the early postoperative period for prophylactic use and during rejection episodes if these fail to respond to corticosteroids. ACG is an intravenous preparation in saline, administered in a prophylactic dose of 10 to 15 mg/kg IV for 5 to 10 days or, in rejection, as 10 to 15 mg/kg IV for 10 to 14 days. Muromonab-CD3 (OKT3) binds to the CD3 antigen complex on the T-cell membrane surface, preventing normal activation in response to foreign antigens. It is used to treat rejection episodes. The intravenous preparation is given by peripheral or central access as a bolus of 5 mg during a 1-minute period in the port most proximal to the vein. FK506 is being investigated as a treatment for rejection and prophylaxis.
- Calcium chloride: It is given intravenously to protect the myocardium should hyperkalemia occur (see Table 1–15, p. 129).
- Sodium polystyrene sulfonate (Kayexalate): Used if hyperkalemia occurs postoperatively (see Table 4–4).
- Antibiotics: Antibiotics are given if an infection develops in a compromised immune system (see Table 1–14, p. 122).

INDWELLING URINARY CATHETER

- An indwelling urinary catheter is used for 1 to 7 days postoperatively to decompress the bladder. The urinary catheter is checked for patency and irrigated, using sterile technique, with an antibiotic solution. The amount of irrigation used is small because the bladder may be small as a result of prolonged disuse.

FLUID THERAPY

- A dextrose solution with 0.45% saline is used to maintain volume and combat hypokalemia. Intravenous administration of glucose and regular insulin may be given if hyperkalemia occurs. This will facilitate the movement of the potassium ions into the cells.

NURSING MANAGEMENT: NURSING DIAGNOSES AND COLLABORATIVE PROBLEMS

Nursing Diagnoses

Common nursing goals for patients with renal transplantation are to maintain fluid balance, maintain normal urinary elimination, prevent infection, increase renal tissue perfusion, prevent injury, and provide knowledge.

Fluid volume excess related to fluid overhydration or renal hypoperfusion.

Expected Patient Outcomes. Patient maintains normal fluid balance, as evidenced by blood pressure (BP) within patient's normal range, urinary output (UO) $\geq$30 mL/h, specific gravity 1.015 to 1.025, central venous pressure (CVP) 2 to 6 mm Hg, heart rate (HR) $\leq$100 bpm, respiratory rate (RR) 12 to 20 BPM, absence of crackles, absence of edema, stable weight, and hemoglobin or hematocrit within normal range.

- Review results of blood urea nitrogen (BUN) and creatinine in response to graft function. A decrease in these values signifies a functioning graft. Delayed function manifests itself as oliguria or anuria, elevated BUN, and elevated creatinine.
- Review potassium, sodium, bicarbonate, chloride, calcium, magnesium, and glucose values.
- Review results of renal scan, which is done to rule out rejection or technical complications.
- Monitor patient for postoperative overhydration because of fluid volume given intraoperatively to maintain renal perfusion.
- Measure urinary volume, which initially may be 1000 mL/h because with a new graft, osmotic diuresis may occur as a result of renal tubular dysfunction, inability to fil-

ter BUN, and intraoperative overhydration. Urinary volume decreases as creatinine and BUN return to normal.

- Monitor clinical indicators of hydration: skin turgor, peripheral pulses, HR, mean arterial pressure (MAP), BP, UO, and capillary refill.
- Obtain and report clinical findings associated with fluid overload: jugular vein distention, peripheral edema, crackles, shortness of breath, and presence of a S_3 heart sound.
- Maintain CVP $\geq$7 mm Hg and systolic BP $\geq$110 mm Hg to sustain renal perfusion and prevent renal tubular damage.
- Monitor daily weight, intake, specific gravity, and UO. Report UO $\leq$30 mL/h or $\leq$0.5 mL/kg/h and weight gain $\geq$0.5 kg/d.
- Administer IV fluids to replace hourly UO. Large volumes may be required for UO $\geq$600 mL/h.
- Administer prescribed morphine in patients with peripheral edema resulting from reduced UO and fluid overload, to reduce preload from pulmonary edema, reduce anxiety, and relax the smooth airway muscle, which facilitates gas exchange.

Altered urinary pattern of elimination related to renal rejection or obstruction of the indwelling urinary catheter or cyclosporine toxicity.

Expected Patient Outcome. Patient maintains normal urinary pattern, as evidenced by UO $\geq$30 mL/h or $\geq$0.5 mL/kg/h.

- Review test results: Renogram and ultrasound imaging, BUN, creatinine, complete blood count (CBC), platelet count, and T-cell subsets.
- Maintain proper function of the large indwelling catheter, which remains in place for 1 to 7 days. It is used to decompress the bladder.
- Encourage patient to void frequently when the catheter is removed in order to reduce pressure on suture line and facilitate bladder healing.

- Monitor urine color and output. Urine color may range from clear yellow to cherry red. Report the presence of large clots or UO ≤30 mL/h or ≤0.5 mL/kg/h.
- Should the cause of decreased UO be blood clots obstructing the flow of urine, prepare to irrigate the catheter with the prescribed sterile solution. Caution is used during irrigation, since the bladder may be small because of prolonged disuse.
- Notify the physician before the catheter is changed because a stent may be sutured to the end of the catheter to prevent urethral stenosis.
- Administer prescribed oxybutynin chloride or propantheline bromide to reduce pain from bladder spasm. These agents are discontinued 24 hours before the catheter is removed (see Table 4–4).
- Teach patient that the volume of urine may be greater at night than during the day for the first 1 to 2 months after renal transplantation. Patients should awaken to void during the night.

High risk of infection related to uremia, surgical procedure, catheter vascular lines, and immunosuppressive therapy.

Expected Patient Outcomes. Patient is free of infection, as evidenced by white blood cells (WBC) ≤11,000/µL; negative cultures; no fever; and absence of redness, tenderness, swelling, or drainage from incision.

- Consult with physician about the risk of infection for the specific patient.
- Review results of WBC, renal biopsy, or cultures.
- Provide a diet low in carbohydrates, high in protein, low in sodium, and possibly low in potassium.
- Record temperature hourly and report elevation, which could be an indication of bacterial, viral, fungal, or protozoan infection.
- Record urine volume, color, appearance, and presence of odor. Cloudy, foul smelling urine, frequency of urination, and complaints of flank pain are indication of renal-urinary infection.

- Obtain and report clinical indications of infection: fever; malaise; and swelling, redness, tenderness, or drainage at catheter or vascular line.
- Obtain and report clinical findings associated with protozoan infection with *Pneumocystis carinii:* fever, malaise, dyspnea, nonproductive cough, and hypoxia.
- Auscultate the lungs for absent, abnormal, or adventitious breath sounds.
- Encourage patient to turn, cough, deep breathe, and use incentive spirometer to facilitate lung expansion and reduce stasis.
- Monitor patient for candidiasis, which is manifested as localized white plaquelike patches in the mouth.
- Use strict aseptic technique when changing all dressings.
- Provide sterile irrigation of the catheter with an antibiotic solution as prescribed.
- Administer prescribed antibiotics to treat bacterial, viral, fungal, or protozoan infection.
- Provide prescribed nystatin swishes and clotrimazole troches to relieve discomfort from candidiasis.
- Should systemic fungal infection occur, administer prescribed amphotericin B.
- Should a protozoan infection occur, administer prescribed sulfamethoxazole-trimethoprim and pentamidine (see Table 4–4).
- Teach patient to report any signs of rejection: Fever, weight gain, edema, malaise or oliguria.

Altered renal tissue perfusion related to renal artery thrombosis secondary to size mismatch at the site of the anastomosis.

Expected Patient Outcomes. Patient maintains adequate renal tissue perfusion, as evidenced by BP within patient's normal range, HR ≤100 bpm, UO ≥30 mL/h or 0.5 mL/kg/h, stable weight, absence of edema of the thigh and leg on the side of transplant, and BUN and creatinine level within normal range.

- Review results of coagulation profile, ultrasound, renal scan, and studies of serum electrolytes, serum BUN, and creatinine.

- Obtain and report clinical indicators of decreased renal tissue perfusion: hypertension and gross edema of the thigh and leg on the side of the transplant.
- Monitor intake, output, and daily weight. Report UO $\leq$ 30 mL/h or $\leq$ 0.5 mL/kg/h and weight gain $\geq$ 0.5 kg/d.
- Administer prescribed heparin to correct renal artery thrombosis.
- Should pharmacological therapy be ineffective, prepare patient for thrombectomy.
- Prepare patient for angioplasty or surgical repair.
- Instruct patient to report any weight gain, oliguria, edema, or tenderness over incision site.
- Instruct patient to avoid heavy lifting and resume driving in 3 to 6 weeks.

High risk of injury related to renal dysfunction secondary to rejection.

Expected Patient Outcomes. Patient is free of symptoms of rejection.

- Consult with nephrologist regarding the expected symptoms associated with rejection: weight gain, hypertension, edema, oliguria, fever, tenderness over surgical site and increased BUN and creatinine.
- Review results of renal biopsy, WBC, BUN, and creatinine.
- Monitor temperature and vital signs hourly.
- Obtain and report clinical findings associated with rejection: fever, rapid weight gain ($\geq$ 2 to 3 lb/24 h), decreased UO, peripheral edema, hypertension, malaise, and tenderness over graft.
- Monitor and report fever, chills, dyspnea, and malaise within the 6 hours after the first dose of muromonab-CD3.
- Obtain and report local or systemic allergic response aftre infusion of antilymphocyte globulin (ACG) and antithymocyte globulin (ATG). Administer through a central line.
- Maintain strict infection control during the treatment with antirejection therapy.
- Administer prescribed IV bolus corticosteroids for 3 to 4 days and antilymphocyte

preparation in patients experiencing accelerated acute rejection.
- Administer prescribed immunosuppressive agents (muromonab-CD3) during acute rejection. Premedicate patient before first dose with methylprednisolone and acetaminophen (see Table 1–15, p. 129).
- During pharmacological therapy with muromonab-CD3, monitor vital signs every 15 minutes for 2 hours, then every 30 minutes until the patient is stable.
- Administer prescribed ACG and ATG during acute rejection (see Table 1–15, p. 129).
- Teach patient the purpose behind taking the prescribed immunosuppressive agents.
- Instruct patient to report malaise or tenderness over graft, which might indicate rejection.

Knowledge deficit related to the surgical procedure and immunosuppressive therapy.

Expected Patient Outcome. Patient verbalizes knowledge of surgical procedure and immunosuppressive agents.

- Listen to patient's questions regarding the surgical procedure, postoperative care, and immunosuppressive agents.
- Provide patient with information regarding renal transplantation and the potential for rejection.
- Reassure patient that rejection may occur and can be reversed.
- Teach patient about the immunosuppressive agent, dose, route, side effects, and precautions.

Collaborative Problems

A common collaborative goal for patients with renal transplantation is to restore electrolyte balance.

Potential Complication: Electrolyte Imbalance. Electrolyte imbalance related to hyperkalemia secondary to renal tubular damage.

Expected Patient Outcomes. Patient maintains electrolyte balance, as evidenced by potassium 3.5 to 5.5 mEq/L.

- Review results of tests for serum electrolytes, albumin:protein ratio, BUN, creatinine, hematocrit, serum osmolality, and urine osmolality.
- Provide a low-protein low-potassium diet.
- Monitor continuous ECG to assess HR and rhythm. Document ECG rhythm strips every 2 to 4 hours in patients with dysrhythmias.
- Obtain and report clinical findings indicative of hyperkalemia: weakness, cramps, paresthesia of face, tingle in extremities, hypotension, dysrhythmias, anorexia, and abdominal distention.
- Obtain and report ECG changes associated with potassium 5.5 to 6.0 mmol/L: tall peaked symmetric T wave in the precordia leads, QT interval is normal or decreased, with occasional ST depression.
- Monitor and report ECG changes associated with potassium 6.0 to 7.0 mmol/L: prolonged PR interval and QRS duration.
- Obtain and report ECG changes associated with potassium 7.0 to 8.0 mmol/L: flattened P wave, QRS complex continues to widen with increased delays in atrioventricular conduction.
- Obtain and report ECG changes associated with potassium 8.0 to 10.0 mmol/L: irregular ventricular rhythm, absent P waves, and markedly increased QRS complexes, with the eventual merging of the complexes with the T wave.
- Obtain and report ECG changes associated with potassium 10.0 to 12.0 mmol/L: ventricular fibrillation or asystole.
- Limit potassium intake in diet to reduce plasma and total body potassium content.
- Administer sodium polystyrene sulfonate (Kayexalate), mixed in water and sorbitol and given orally, rectally or through nasogastric tube: Renin captures potassium in the bowel and eliminates it in the feces (see Table 4–4).
- In patients with serum potassium ≥ 6.5 mEq/L, administer prescribed 10% calcium gluconate, 500 mL 10% glucose with 10 units regular insulin IV over 30 minutes and sodium bicarbonate 2 to 3 ampules in 500 mL glucose IV over 1 to 2 hours. This will shift the potassium intracellularly (see Table 4–4).
- Administer prescribed IV fluids to maintain adequate hydration. Replace serum electrolytes as prescribed: 5% normal saline solution.
- Administer small doses of IV sodium bicarbonate ($NaHCO_3$) 50 to 100 mmol to increase pH≥ 7.2 and $HCO_3 \geq 15$ mM/L.
- Should pharmacological therapy be ineffective in reducing serum potassium, prepare patient for dialysis.

DISCHARGE PLANNING

The critical care nurse will provide patient and significant other(s) with verbal or written discharge notes regarding the following subjects:

1. The signs and symptoms of acute or chronic rejection that could occur months to years after transplantation.
2. The importance of taking immunosuppressive agents.

- The importance of protecting patient for infection because of immunosuppressive therapy,
- The significant symptoms of rejection that warrant immediate medical attention.
- The dose, time, and side effects of immunosuppressive agents taken by patient.
- The names of community agencies that can enhance learning and provide support.

PART III: SUPPORTIVE PROCEDURES AND NURSING MANAGEMENT

■ HEMODIALYSIS

(For related information see Part I: Renal trauma, p. 447; Acute tubular necrosis, p. 455; Acute renal failure, p. 459; Part II: Re-

nal transplantations, p. 491. Part III: Peritoneal dialysis, p. 502; Continuous renal replacement therapy, p. 505.)

Case Management Basis

DRG: 317 Admit for renal dialysis
LOS: 2.50 days

Definition

Hemodialysis is the separation of solutes by differential diffusion through a celluloid membrane positioned between the individual's blood and the dialysate solution. Hemodialysis occurs outside the patient's body.

Patient Selection

INDICATIONS. Hemodialysis is used in patients with chronic renal failure; with acute renal failure experiencing volume overload, hypertension, blood urea nitrogen (BUN) ≥ 80 to 100 mg/dL, acidosis, or symptoms of uremia; and those with drug toxicity.

CONTRAINDICATIONS. Hemodialysis is contraindicated in patients with hemodynamic instability causing severe hypertension and in patients for whom aggressive medical therapy is not appropriate.

Procedure

TECHNIQUE. Temporary hemodialysis accesses are external. The most common vascular access is the dual-lumen subclavian catheter. A shorter version of the dual-lumen catheter is available for insertion into the femoral vein. Two forms of permanent vascular access are used in patients with chronic renal failure. They consist of an internal arteriovenous (AV) fistula or a graft AV fistula. The hollow-fiber dialyzer consists of fine capillaries with a semipermeable membrane enclosed in a plastic cylinder. Blood is pumped through the capillaries, and dialysate is pumped countercurrent or crosscurrent to the blood on the outside of the capillaries. The parallel-flow plate dialyzer consists of two layers of semipermeable membrane (cellophane or Cuprophan) held together by semirigid or rigid supporting structures. Blood flows inside the two membrane layers, and dialysate flows countercurrent to the blood between the outsides of the membranes and the adjacent supporting structures.

Blood flow rate up to 330 to 400 mL/min is required during dialysis. The dialysis process consists of osmosis, hydrostatic pressure, and ultrafiltration. Osmosis is the passage of solvent across a semipermeable membrane from an area of lesser solute concentration to an area of greater solute concentration. The force that causes the solvent to move through the membrane is osmotic pressure. Excess glucose is added to dialysate to cause an osmotic gradient between the blood and dialysate. Hydrostatic pressure is the pressure that a liquid exerts against the wall of its container. A positive hydrostatic pressure is applied to the blood compartment and a negative hydrostatic pressure is applied to the dialysate compartment of the dialyzer. Transmembrane hydrostatic pressure (TMP) is the sum of the average pressure of the blood entering and leaving the dialyzer minus the average pressure of the dialysate entering and leaving the dialyzer. Ultrafiltration is the movement of water from an area of higher pressure to an area of lower pressure. The coefficient of ultrafiltration for a dialyzer is the amount of water removed from the blood during a given period and at a specified pressure and is expressed as mL/h/mmHg TMP.

EQUIPMENT. The delivery system continuously mixes dialysate concentration with treated water and warms the dialysate to body temperature. Dialysate solution can be adjusted to correct specific electrolyte imbalances in the patient's serum and is available with or without glucose and containing either acetate or bicarbonate as a buffer. The dialyzer functions as the artificial kidney. Two types of dialyzers are used: the hollow-fiber and the parallel-plate. Other equipment used consists of an AV shunt, subclavian catheter, femoral dialysis catheter, and graft. The AV shunt consists of two pieces of Silastic tubing, each connected to a sturdy Teflon tip. One tip is inserted surgically into an artery, the other into a vein. Blood flows from the artery to the vein. The subclavian catheter is a temporary access for short-term dialysis. Femoral dialysis catheters include the Shaldon catheter, which is a single-lumen catheter requiring a second access to avoid recirculation of the blood, leading to inadequate dialysis. The newer femoral catheter has a double lumen so that blood can be taken from one port and returned through the other during dialysis without mixing of dialyzed and nondialyzed blood. The graft is an anastomosis between an artery and a vein and serves as a conduit for blood flow and site of needle placement. Graft materials include bovine tissue and polytetrafluoroethylene (PTFE).

Complications

Hypotension, electrolyte imbalance, dialysis disequilibrium syndrome, hemorrhage, air embolus, blood leaks (dialyzer), chilling, and infection.

NURSING MANAGEMENT: NURSING DIAGNOSES AND COLLABORATIVE PROBLEMS

Nursing Diagnoses

Common nursing goals for patients undergoing hemodialysis are to maintain fluid balance, increase peripheral tissue perfusion, prevent infection, and provide adequate nutrition.

Fluid volume deficit related to volume loss secondary to excess fluid removed during dialysis or bleeding caused by anticoagulants.

Expected Patient Outcomes. Patient maintains adequate fluid balance, as evidenced by blood pressure (BP) within patient's normal range, heart rate (HR) ≤100 bpm, mean arterial pressure (MAP) 70 to 100 mm Hg, cardiac output (CO) 4 to 8 L/min, central venous pressure (CVP) 2 to 6 mm Hg, urinary output (UO) ≥30 mL/h, stable daily weight, absence of bleeding, normal skin turgor, and hemoglobin and hematocrit within normal range.

- Confer with physician regarding the desired intravascular fluid volume.
- Consult with physician about the maximum safe rate of ultrafiltration used (1.5 L/h) so that risk for hypotension can be anticipated.
- Consult with physician as to whether diuretics or antihypertensive agents are to be withheld.
- Review hemoglobin, hematocrit, arterial blood gas, and serum electrolyte results.
- Limit physical activity to bed rest until intravascular fluid volume stabilizes.
- Place patient in a horizontal position to maximize venous return when hypotension occurs.
- Monitor clinical indicators of perfusion: BP, MAP, HR, skin turgor, capillary refill, peripheral pulses, CVP, and UO.
- Obtain and report hemodynamic parameters indicating fluid volume deficit: CO ≤4 L/min and CVP ≤2 mm Hg.
- Obtain and report clinical findings associated with fluid volume deficit: hypotension, tachycardia, poor skin turgor, weight loss, and bleeding.
- Monitor cannula or fistula for patency and intactness.
- Monitor blood lines for separation: Clamp the arterial blood line and stop the blood pump to minimize further blood loss.
- Evaluate AV shunt, fistula, or graft for bruit and thrill each shift.
- Weigh patient daily and report UO ≥1500 mL over intake.
- Monitor sodium level of the dialysate to help prevent hypotensive episodes and muscle cramps during and after dialysis.
- Administer prescribed IV solution such as normal saline or volume expander such as albumin to maintain adequate circulating volume.
- Administer prescribed blood or packed red cells to correct hemorrhagic losses.

- Should bleeding occur as a result of heparin therapy, administer prescribed protamine sulfate.

Fluid volume excess related to high total body sodium and fluid overload secondary to renal dysfunction.

Expected Patient Outcomes. Patient maintains fluid balance, as evidenced by BP within patient's normal range, HR ≤100 bpm, respiratory rate (RR) 12 to 20 BPM, stable weight, UO ≥30 mL/h, CVP 2 to 6 mm Hg, flat neck veins, absence of dyspnea, and absence of adventitious breath sounds.

- Review results of tests of hemoglobin, hematocrit, electrolytes, BUN, creatinine, and arterial blood gases.
- Fluid restriction (1500 to 1800 mL/d) may be necessary if weight gain 1.5 to 2.0 kg/d occurs as a result of fluid retention between dialysis treatments.
- Measure intake, output, specific gravity, and daily weight. Report UO ≤30 mL/h or ≤0.5 mL/kg/h and weight gain ≥0.5 to 1.0 kg/d.
- Obtain and report clinical findings of fluid volume excess: tachycardia; crackles; peripheral, periorbital, or sacral edema; tachypnea, and dyspnea.
- Monitor BP during dialysis: Hypertension can occur as a result of renin production in response to ultrafiltration and an increase in renal ischemia; dialysis disequilibrium syndrome can also occur.
- Maintain IV and oral fluid restriction should urinary output be less than intake and daily weight exceed 0.5 to 1.0 kg/d.
- Administer hydralazine (Apresoline) if diastolic blood pressure is ≥120 mm Hg.

Altered peripheral tissue perfusion related to interruption of vascular flow secondary to thrombus in access site or a disconnected shunt.

Expected Patient Outcomes. Patient's dialysis access site maintains adequate perfusion as evidenced by palpation of thrill, visualization of blood flow, auscultation of bruit, and warmth of shunt.

- Review results of prothrombin time, activated clotting time, or whole blood partial thromboplastin time.
- Evaluate patency of access site by palpitating for a thrill and auscultating for a bruit over the shunt or AV fistula.
- Monitor the access extremity for warmth and brisk capillary refill ≤3 seconds.
- Maintain shunt tubing and report the presence of dark stains indicating clotting.
- Should the shunt not maintain its patency, prepare to administer prescribed streptokinase to save the fistula.
- Should hypotension occur, check fistula, graft, or shunt for patency.
- Administer constant infusion of prescribed heparin (10 U/mL) through subclavian or femoral line or flush with heparinized saline and cap to prevent clotting of blood in the dialyzer and blood lines. Heparin is the anticoagulant used because of its rapid onset of action and short half-life. Trisodium citrate is a new regional anticoagulant and is an alternative to heparin. Trisodium citrate functions by forming a complex with calcium, preventing normal progression of the clotting cascade.
- Keep shunt clamp or rubber band hemostat at bedside to clamp lines in the event of accidental disconnection.
- Instruct patient to report any pain in access site or sensation changes in affected extremity such as the hand.

High risk for infection related to decreased immunological response or drainage from catheter, wound, or access site.

Expected Patient Outcomes. Patient is free of infection, as evidenced by normothermia, white blood cells (WBC) ≤11,000/μL; negative cultures; dialysate free of infectious organisms; absence of redness, tenderness, swelling, or drainage at access site.

- Review results of WBC, count and culture.

- Obtain and report clinical findings associated with infection: fever; chills; tachycardia; crackles; cloudy and foul-smelling urine; redness, swelling, or drainage from access site or urethral drainage.
- Encourage patient to turn, cough, deep breathe, and ambulate to facilitate adequate ventilation.
- Monitor access site for redness, swelling, tenderness, or drainage.
- Use sterile technique when cleaning catheter site and connecting or disconnecting dialysate bags.
- Obtain culture specimens as ordered.
- Place a sterile dressing over all external access sites.
- Monitor temperature every 1 to 2 hours or as necessary.
- Protect patient with decreased immunological response from infection by appropriately suctioning, providing Foley catheter care, or changing dressings.
- Administer prescribed antibiotics should infection occur.

Altered nutrition: Less than body requirement related to dietary restriction and protein loss.

Expected Patient Outcomes. Patient maintains adequate nutrition, as evidenced by stable body weight, calorie intake 35 to 45 calories/kg, high biologic value protein 50% to 75% of patient's daily protein intake, and nitrogen intake 4 to 6 g more than nitrogen loss.

- Confer with dietitian regarding patient's dietary intake, taking into consideration patient's physiological needs and preferences.
- Maintain total caloric intake between 35 to 45 calories/kg body weight/24 h.
- Restrict the intake of protein 1.0 to 1.2 g/kg/d, sodium 80 to 100 mEq/d, and potassium 40 to 80 mEq/d. Provide nutritional supplements of amino acids and the water-soluble vitamins, since these can be depleted during hemodialysis.
- Minimize the intake of low biologic value proteins such as bread, cereals, grains, fruits, and vegetables.

- Provide caloric intake that does not contain protein or carbohydrates: Cal-Powder, Controlyte, Hycal, and Polycose.
- Weigh patient daily and report losses ≥10% of patient's normal body weight over a 1-week period.
- Teach patient to count calories consumed with each meal for a total caloric intake of 35 to 45 calories/kg/body weight/24 h.
- Instruct patient regarding the need for low protein, low sodium, and high calorie intake.

Collaborative Problems

Common collaborative goals for patients undergoing hemodialysis are to prevent dialysis disequilibrium syndrome, increase CO, correct hypotension, prevent hypoxemia, and correct dysrhythmias.

Potential Complication: Dialysis Disequilibrium Syndrome. Dialysis disequilibrium syndrome (DDS) related to cerebral edema secondary to urea being cleared more quickly from blood than from brain cells, causing an osmotic gradient and a shift of fluid into the brain.

Expected Patient Outcomes. Patient is free of signs and symptoms associated with disequilibrium: restlessness, confusion, twitching, nausea, and vomiting.

- Monitor when BUN ≥150 mg/dL, serum sodium ≥147 mEq/L, pH ≤7.35, partial pressure of arterial carbon dioxide ($PaCO_2$) ≤35 mm Hg, and bicarbonate (HCO_3) ≤22 mEq/L.
- Limit physical activity to bed rest until dialysis disequilibrium syndrome is corrected.
- Assess patient for DDS, which can appear 2 to 3 hours into treatment or after hemodialysis has been concluded.
- Obtain and report clinical indicators of DDS: headache, nausea, emesis, restlessness, muscle twitching, lethargy, blurred vision, and hypertension.
- Maintain slow dialysis during the first one or two hemodialysis treatments when patients have elevated BUN to avoid DDS.

- Administer prescribed high dialysate sodium, or hypertonic fluids such as mannitol. The fluids help to promote vascular refilling by maintaining serum osmolality during diffusion.
- Administer sedatives to prevent more serious symptoms of DDS.

Potential Complication: Decreased Cardiac Output. Decreased CO related to loss of blood into the dialyzer, dialyzer membrane incompatibility, or excess ultrafiltration.

Expected Patient Outcomes. Patient maintains adequate cardiac output, as evidenced by BP within patient's normal limit, HR ≤ 100 bpm, CVP 2 to 6 mm Hg, CO 4 to 8 L/min, peripheral pulses, $+2$, capillary refill $\leq$ seconds, normal ultrafiltration, and absence of blood loss into the dialyzer.

- Monitor for the presence of blood in the dialyzer or for dialyzer membrane incompatibility.
- Obtain and report hemodynamic parameters that indicate altered CO: CO ≤ 4 L/min and CVP ≤ 2 mm Hg.
- Obtain and report clinical indicators of reduced CO: hypotension, tachycardia, poor skin turgor, peripheral pulses $\leq +2$, and capillary refill ≥ 3 seconds.
- Administer prescribed colloidal agents, such as blood, albumin, or fresh frozen plasma, if the patient has a decreased hematocrit or serum albumin or requires clotting factors.
- Measure daily weight, intake, specific gravity, and UO. Report UO ≤ 30 mL/h or ≤ 0.5 mL/kg/h.
- Monitor the amount of dialysate solution administered and rate of ultrafiltration.

Potential Complication: Hypotension. Hypotension related to a decrease in intravascular volume secondary to ultrafiltration.

Expected Patient Outcomes. Patient maintains adequate BP within 10 mm Hg of baseline.

- Consult with physician as to the causes of hypotension: intravascular volume decreases to the extent that normal compensatory responses are unable to restore BP, vasoconstriction does not occur, or CO does not increase.
- Consult with physician about withholding antihypertensive agents for 4 to 8 hours before dialysis.
- Use prescribed dialyzer; one with a small surface area decreases the extracorporeal blood volume and provides a slow rate of diffusion to prevent rapid changes in serum osmolality.
- Should hypotension occur during dialysis, administer prescribed 100 to 250 mL bolus of saline.
- Administer prescribed hypertonic fluid such as mannitol to promote vascular refilling by maintaining serum osmolality during diffusion.
- Administer colloid products such as blood, albumin, or fresh-frozen plasma when patient has a decreased hematocrit or serum albumin or requires clotting factors.
- Employ sequential dialysis, as prescribed, which involves performing ultrafiltration alone for the initial part of the treatment to prevent the osmotic shifts that occur with diffusion.
- Administer, prescribed vasopressor agents, if necessary, to avoid volume overload and maintain BP. This also prevents continued ultrafiltration.
- Should patient's BP not respond to the above interventions, dialysis is discontinued.

Potential Complication: Electrolyte Imbalance. Electrolyte imbalance related to excess electrolyte removal.

Expected Patient Outcome. Patient maintains serum electrolytes within normal limits.

- Review results of laboratory tests such as serum sodium (135 to 145 mEq/L), potassium (3.5 to 5.0 mEq/L), HCO_3 (25 to 30 mEq/L), calcium (8.0 to 10.3 mg/dL), phosphorus (2.5 to 4.5 mg), magnesium (1.5 to 1.7 mEq/L), and arterial blood gas measurements.

- Monitor continuous ECG to assess HR and rhythm. Document ECG rhythm strips every 2 to 4 hours in patients with dysrhythmias.
- Maintain and restore electrolyte balance through dialysis and dietary control.
- Evaluate patient for muscle cramps associated with shifts in sodium and water during hemodialysis: Reduce the flow rate and ultrafiltration or supplement the serum osmolality with an intravenous medication.
- Administer hypertonic saline, sodium bicarbonate, and 50% dextrose to relieve muscle cramping.
- Maintain dialysate calcium at 3.0 to 3.5 mEq/L to prevent loss of calcium from the blood to the dialysate.
- Administer phosphate binders to control hyperphosphatemia.

Potential Complication: Dysrhythmias. Dysrhythmias related to hyperkalemia.

Expected Patient Outcomes. Patient maintains normal sinus rhythm.

- Consult with physician as to the causes of dysrhythmias in conjunction with dialysis: rapid changes in serum electrolytes and pH levels, hypoxemia, or antidysrhythmia medication in the dialysate.
- Should dysrhythmia occur, consult with physician to determine the need for a change in dialysate potassium or calcium concentration or increased oxygenation
- Review results of ECG.
- Monitor continuous ECG to assess HR and rhythm. Document ECG rhythm strips every 2 to 4 hours in patients with dysrhythmias.
- Provide prescribed oxygen 2 to 4 L/min by nasal cannula or mask to increase oxygenation
- Administer prescribed antidysrhythmic agents.

DISCHARGE PLANNING

The critical care nurse will provide patient and significant other(s) with verbal or written discharge notes regarding the following subjects:

1. The importance of keeping scheduled dialysis appointments to prevent complications.
2. Importance of daily checking the shunt for the presence of redness, swelling, tenderness, or drainage from access site.
3. Importance of care of subclavian catheter or AV shunt, keeping dressing clean, dry, and secure.
4. Importance of maintaining dietary restriction.

■ PERITONEAL DIALYSIS

(For related information see Part I: Renal trauma, p. 447; Acute tubular necrosis, p. 455; Acute renal failure, p. 459; Part II: Renal transplantations, p. 491. Part III: Hemodialysis, p. 496; Continuous renal replacement therapy, p. 505.)

Case Management Basis
DRG: 315 Other kidney and urinary tract
   O.R. procedures
LOS: 7.00 days

Definition
Peritoneal dialysis involves the introduction of sterile dialyzing fluid through an implanted catheter into the abdominal cavity. The dialysate bathes the peritoneal membrane, which covers the abdominal organs and overlies the capillary bed supporting the organs dwells for a prescribed period of time, and is drained.

Patient Selection

INDICATIONS. Preferred treatment for patients with severe cardiovascular disease; those who are hemodynamically unstable; the chronic peritoneal dialysis patient with peritonitis, fluid imbalance, or electrolyte imbalance; or small children. It offers optimal treatment for patients with diabetes, the elderly, those with poor vascular access, those who refuse blood products, and the hemodynamically stable.

CONTRAINDICATIONS. Contraindications are bowel perforation, bowel obstruction, severe respiratory disease, multiple abdominal surgeries with scarring or adheions, or pleural abdominal fistulas.

Procedure

TECHNIQUE. By the process of osmosis, diffusion, and active transport, excess fluid and solutes travel from the peritoneal capillary fluid through the capillary walls, through the peritoneal membrane, and into the dialyzing fluid. In peritoneal dialysis, dialysis solution is infused into the peritoneal cavity, dwells there for a period of time, and is drained. Flow times vary depending on the distance between the drain or infusion bag and the patient's abdomen and the inner diameter of the tubing. The in-dwelling time can be short, several minutes or 1 to 2 hours.

The types of dialysis include intermittent, continuous cycle, and continuous ambulatory. Intermittent peritoneal dialysis (IPD) uses automated equipment to provide 3 to 7 treatments per week lasting up to 10 hours. The fluid is drained and the peritoneal cavity is empty until the next treatment. Continuous cycle peritoneal dialysis (CCPD) is automated, with treatments performed each night for 8 to 10 hours. During the last exchange, the fluid is allowed to remain in the peritoneal cavity overnight. Continuous ambulatory peritoneal dialysis (CAPD) does not require automated equipment. CAPD involves a prolonged time the fluid remains in the abdomen (4 hours) during the day and 8 hours during the night. The patient may experience 4 to 5 exchanges during a day. CAPD occurs 24 hours a day.

EQUIPMENT. Automated peritoneal dialysis cycler, dialysate bags, or manifold so that several bags can be hung at the same time.

Complications

Technical complications include incomplete recovery of fluid, leakage around the catheter, or blood-tinged peritoneal fluid. Physiological complications consist of peritonitis, catheter infection, hypotension, intraperitoneal abscess, or hypokalemia.

NURSING MANAGEMENT: NURSING DIAGNOSES AND COLLABORATIVE PROBLEMS

Nursing Diagnoses

Common nursing goals for patients undergoing peritoneal dialysis are to maintain fluid balance, prevent injury, facilitate effective breathing, minimize or prevent pain, and facilitate nutritional status.

Fluid volume excess related to fluid retention or poor drainage.

Expected Patient Outcomes. Patient maintains adequate fluid balance, as evidenced by absence of abdominal distention, central venous pressure (CVP) 2 to 6 mm Hg, blood pressure (BP) within patient's normal range, heart rate (HR) $\leq$100 bpm, urinary output (UO) $\geq$30 mL/h, absence of weight gain, absence of edema, and absence of adventitious breath sounds.

- Check patency of catheter, noting difficulty in drainage. Report presence of fibrin strips or plugs.
- Observe tubing for kinks, bags and bottles for placement, and anchor catheter for good inflow and outflow.
- Elevate head of bed, turn from side to side, and apply pressure to the abdomen to enhance outflow of fluid.
- Measure daily weight, intake, specific gravity, and UO. Report UO $\leq$30 mL/h or $\leq$0.5 mL/kg/h.
- Measure and record serial weight. Weigh patient when the abdomen is empty of dialysate. Compare weight with intake and output balance. A positive fluid balance with an increase in weight indicates fluid retention.
- Obtain and report clinical findings suggesting excess fluid volume: distended neck

veins, hypertension, shortness of breath, and edema.

- Restrict the amount of oral and IV fluids given to patient.
- Administer hypertonic dialysate solution.
- Should the catheter remain patent and excess fluid volume occur, the number of dialysis cycles can be increased to aid in increasing the amount of fluid removed.

High risk of injury related to traumatic insertion of peritoneal catheter.

Expected Patient Outcomes. Patient experiences an untraumatic insertion without bowel or bladder injury.

- Anchor catheter and tubing with tape to prevent risk of trauma by manipulation of the catheter.
- Obtain and report clinical findings associated with bladder perforation: intense urge to urinate, large UO, and high urine glucose concentration.
- Obtain and report clinical findings associated with bowel perforation: fecal material in dialysate return, urge to defecate, stool mixed with large amount of fluid, hypotension, and tachycardia.
- Should peritoneal injury occur, prepare patient for surgical repair of the peritoneum.
- Cease peritoneal dialysis when bladder or bowel injury occurs.
- Administer prescribed antibiotics.
- Administer prescribed lidocaine as an intraperitoneal anesthetic should pain occur.
- Administer prescribed heparin to prevent catheter obstruction.
- Instruct patient to report bladder or bowel discomfort.

Ineffective breathing pattern related to decreased lung expansion secondary to dialysis fluid.

Expected Patient Outcomes. Patient maintains effective breathing pattern, as evidenced by respiratory rate (RR) ≤24 BPM, no shortness of breath, symmetrical chest movement, and absence of dyspnea.

- Place patient in semi-Fowler's position to facilitate respiratory excursion.
- Obtain and report clinical findings associated with ineffective breathing pattern: tachypnea, shortness of breath, dyspnea, and asymmetry of chest movement.
- Encourage patient to turn, deep breathe, and use incentive spirometer every 2 to 4 hours to prevent atelectasis when dialysate is draining.
- Ambulate patient to chair 3 to 4 hours a day if not contraindicated.
- Administer prescribed oxygen at 2 to 4 L/min by nasal cannula or mask to maintain oxygenation.
- Administer prescribed prophylactic vancomycin 1 g IV given at the time of catheter insertion. Cephalosporins are used against gram-positive organisms at 125 mg/L of dialysate. Gentamicin and tobramycin used for gram-negative organisms at a loading dose of 1.75 mg/kg of body weight with maintenance doses of 5 mg/L of dialysate.

Pain related to abdominal distention.

Expected Patient Outcome. Patient reports absence of pain.

- Listen to patient's description of pain in terms of its location, intensity, duration, and quality.
- Monitor pain that begins during inflow and continues during equilibrium period.
- Monitor for discomfort occurring at end of inflow and beginning of outflow phase. The discomfort is due to peritoneal or abdominal distention with dialysis.
- Assess for continuing pain that can be reflective of peritonitis.
- Initiate smaller dialysate volumes, in conjunction with physician, to reduce the amount of fluid in the abdomen.
- Administer prescribed lidocaine via catheter to reduce pain.

- Administer analgesics as prescribed.
- Instruct patient to report pain.
- Teach patient alternative approaches to alleviate pain: progressive relaxation, meditation, and guided imagery.

Altered nutrition: Less than body requirements related to loss of protein and water soluble vitamins secondary to peritoneal dialysis.

Expected Patient Outcome. Patient maintains adequate nutritional intake.

- Review results of serum albumin and protein tests.
- Provide diet that increases protein, vitamins, and caloric intake while maintaining blood urea nitrogen (BUN) at an acceptable level, maintaining electrolyte balance, and preventing fluid retention. Protein is lost during dialysis.
- Provide prescribed hyperalimentation or total parenteral nutrition to offset protein, vitamin, or caloric loss. The amount infused depends on the remaining kidney function and other fluid being administered to the patient.
- Fluid replacement equals the output for all body sources. Approximately 300 mL insensible loss can be added to the amount.
- Administer prescribed lipid emulsion; hypertonic dextrose can be added for calories.
- While administering hypertonic dextrose, maintain patient's RR, depth, and rhythm, since excessive carbohydrates can cause increased carbon dioxide production.
- Administer prescribed insulin to counteract the effect of total parenteral nutrition.

Collaborative Problems

A common collaborative goal for patients undergoing peritoneal dialysis is to prevent peritonitis.

Potential Complication: Peritonitis. Peritonitis related to a break in dialysis system and catheter or tunnel infection.

Expected Patient Outcomes. Patient is free from infection, as evidenced by normothermia, white blood cell (WBC) $\leq 11,000/\mu L$; negative wound culture; absence of redness, swelling, tenderness, or drainage from catheter sites.

- Review results of WBC count and cultures.
- Limit activity to bed rest while patient is febrile.
- Obtain and report clinical findings of infection at the exit site: swelling, pain, warmth, and exudate.
- Administer cephalosporins in combination with gentamicin or tobramycin, cephalosporins are effective against gram positive organisms, and gentamicin and tobramycin fight gram negative organisms. The cephalosporin dose is 125 mg/L of dialysate. Gentamicin and tobramycin have a loading dose of 1.75 mg/kg of body weight and maintenance doses of 5 mg/L of dialysate.
- Prevent infection by using aseptic technique when manipulating the catheter or dressings, performing site care, and securing the access to prevent pulling and twisting.
- Obtain and report clinical findings associated with peritonitis: cloudy effluent, abdominal pain, fever, difficulty draining, nausea, and vomiting.
- Infuse a bag of dialysate and immediately drain it to reduce irritation in patient with severe abdominal pain.
- Administer prescribed antibiotics such as cephalosporins in combination with gentamicin or tobramycin to correct peritonitis.
- Administer prescribed heparin to all bags when the dialysate effluent is cloudy.

■ CONTINUOUS RENAL REPLACEMENT THERAPY

(For related information see Part I: Renal trauma, p. 447; Acute tubular necrosis, p. 455; Acute renal failure, p. 459. Part II: Re-

nal transplantations, p. 491. Part III: Hemo-dialysis, p. 496; Peritoneal dialysis, p. 502.)

Case Management Basis
DRG: None

Definition
Continuous renal replacement (CRRT) is an extracorporeal whole blood circulation from an artery to a vein through a highly porous hemofilter. There are three variations of CRRT. Slow continuous ultrafiltration (SCUF) retains small amounts of plasma water and solutes. Continuous arteriovenous hemofiltration (CAVH) is a renal replacement therapy in which large amounts of plasma water and solutes are removed on a continuous basis. Continuous arteriovenous hemodialysis (CAVHD) combines the convective transport of CAVHD with diffusion dialysis.

Patient Selection

INDICATORS. With SCUF, fluid removal rates are between 150 and 300 mL/h; it is used for patients with azotemia or significant electrolyte imbalance. It is also useful in controlling fluid volume overload in patients with severe congestive heart failure unresponsive to diuretic therapy; and as an adjunct to hemodialysis in patients with acute renal failure (ARF) and those requiring large volumes of maintenance therapy. The CAVH removal rate is between 400 and 800 mL/h; it can be used as the primary dialysis therapy for ARF patients with mild to moderate azotemia and electrolyte imbalance. Finally, CAVHD can be used as the primary dialysis therapy in ARF, azotemia, and electrolyte imbalance. In general, patients who benefit from CRRT are those with advanced cardiac disease, recent acute myocardial infarction, coronary artery bypass graft, valve replacement, septicemia, who are resistant to diuretics, are receiving total parenteral nutrition for their medical or surgical conditions, or are suffering from renal insufficiency and end-stage renal disease.

CONTRAINDICATIONS. Patients with chronic renal failure who require peritoneal or hemodialysis.

Procedure

TECHNIQUE. The CRRT operates in a pumpless circuit as opposed to intermittent forms of dialytic therapy such as hemodialysis. In CRRT, a blood pump is not necessary because a pressure gradient is obtained with blood flow from an artery to a vein. The hydrostatic pressure exerted by the patient's mean arterial pressure and the negative pressure created by the level of the drainage bag push fluid across the hemofilter membrane. When the hydrostatic pressure exceeds the oncotic pressure, ultrafiltration occurs. CRRT uses the principles of filtration, hydrostatic pressure, convection, and diffusion. Diffusion is the removal of a solute by creating a concentration gradient on either side of a semipermeable membrane. Fluid is administered as predilutional or postdilutional replacement. In the CAVH system, when fluid is administered through the arterial side (before the filter), the urea present in the plasma is diluted. Predilution also enhances filtration. Hydrostatic pressure propels the fluid through the membrane, whereas the oncotic pressure produced by plasma proteins hold fluid back. Filtration is a function of the difference between hydrostatic pressure and oncotic pressure. Predilutional replacement lowers the concentration of plasma proteins and decreases oncotic pressure.

When postdilutional fluid replacement is used, the high concentration of protein entering the filter opposes some of the hydrostatic filtration pressure. When fluid is removed the concentration of protein increases, thereby decreasing filtration. Predilution is used more frequently than postdilution.

EQUIPMENT. Four types of hemofilters (Hospal, Gambro, Renal Systems, or Amicon) are used; vascular access; arterial and venous blood tubing; replacement fluid; heparin; and collection bag such as Foley or urometer bag.

Complications

Complications consist of problems with insertion site, bleeding, blood leak, and drop in ultrafiltration rate.

NURSING MANAGEMENT: NURSING DIAGNOSES AND COLLABORATIVE PROBLEMS

Nursing Diagnoses

Common nursing goals for patients undergoing CRRT are to maintain fluid balance, promote peripheral tissue perfusion, prevent infection, support physical mobility, prevent injury, and provide information.

Fluid volume deficit related to ultrafiltration exceeding intravascular volume requirement or bleeding.

Expected Patient Outcomes. Patient maintains adequate fluid volume, as evidenced by blood pressure (BP) within patient's normal range, mean arterial pressure (MAP) 70 to 100 mm Hg, heart rate (HR) ≤100 bpm, central venous pressure (CVP) 2 to 6 mm Hg, urinary output (UO) ≥30 mL/h, capillary refill ≤3 seconds, peripheral pulses +2, and absence of bleeding from arterial or venous tubing.

- Review results of tests of hemoglobin, hematocrit, blood urea nitrogen (BUN), creatinine, serum electrolytes, prothrombin time (PT), partial thromboplastin time (PTT), and activated clotting time (ACT).
- Provide total parenteral nutrition or fluid replacement to help patient meet nutritional requirement.
- Obtain and report hemodynamic parameters suggesting decreased fluid volume: cardiac output (CO) ≤4 L/min and CVP ≤2 mm Hg.
- Monitor clinical indicators of perfusion: BP, HR, MAP, capillary refill, skin color, and peripheral pulse.

- Report other clinical findings suggesting decreased fluid volume: hypotension, tachycardia, peripheral pulses +2, capillary refill ≥3 seconds, and MAP ≤60 mm Hg.
- Measure weights three times a day. Report weight gain or loss ≥0.5 kg/d.
- Measure all intake and output fluids: input from IV, oral, and parenteral nutrition tube feedings; output including urine, chest tube, CRRT, and gastric drain. If intake is 275 mL, output is 610 mL, and the prescribed net loss is 200 mL, the amount to be administered over the next hour is $(630-275 = 355-200 = 155$ mL/h).
- Tape and secure all connectors within the system to avoid accidental disconnection and bleeding.
- Position filter and lines close to the access extremity and secure with gauze wraps and tape to prevent traction on the connectors.
- Monitor ultrafiltrate hourly for presence of blood and check solute for blood.
- Provide prescribed replacement fluids: can be standard IV fluids, such as lactated Ringer's solution or 0.45% sodium chloride with 5% dextrose. Patient may require special fluid therapy for metabolic and nutritional replacement with 25% sodium chloride with 100 mmol sodium bicarbonate or 0.9% sodium chloride with 1 g calcium chloride. Fluids can be administered before or after dilution.
- Adjust ultrafiltration flow (UF) rate when IV fluid replacement is prescribed.
- Should hypotension resulting from fluid volume deficit continue, the UF rates can be adjusted to equal the total IV fluid intake, creating an even fluid balance, or the UF can be further decreased, thereby creating a positive balance.
- When using a vacuum suction to collect ultrafiltrate, keep suction set between 80 to 120 mm Hg.
- Should systolic BP be ≤90 mm Hg, place patient in a flat or Trendelenburg's position. Reduce the UF rate by lowering the bed, raising the collection bag, or decreasing suction.

- Administer prescribed replacement solution hourly through the arterial side (predilutional) or venous side (postdilutional) of the circuit. Replacement, usually on the predilutional, side is based on ultrafiltration.

Fluid volume excess related to volume overhydration resulting from decreased ultrafiltration secondary to clogged hemofilter or improper heparinization.

Expected Patient Outcomes. Patient maintains adequate fluid balance, as evidenced by normal ultrafiltration, BP within patient's normal range, patent hemofilter, and ACT within two to three times that of the baseline value.

- Review results of ACT test.
- Obtain and report the set rate per hour of the replacement fluid in relation to the UF amount. Should the rate of replacement fluid exceed UF amount, volume overload can occur. Decrease fluid replacement and notify physician.
- Monitor and report hypotension and MAP ≤60 to 70 mm Hg, which can reduce the ultrafiltration rate.
- Check hemofilter and blood tubing hourly for the presence of blood.
- Should clotting occur, flush hemofilter with heparinized saline as prescribed.
- Should the UF rate decrease to 20% to 50% of baseline, notify physician and check arterial and venous lines for kinking, ultrafiltrate tubing for kinking, check infusion pump for proper functioning, and check level of the pump and ultrafiltration bag.
- Draw blood from the venous port every 4 hours for PTT and ACT.
- If a Schribner shunt is used, compress the soft tubing to check for patency. If sluggish or there is no return, notify physician.
- Secure tubing to prevent stasis from kinking or compression of tubing.
- When using a gravity drainage bag, keep the bag at least 16 inches below the filter. The nurse can increase or decrease the UF rate by lowering the collection bag.

- Administer prescribed heparin to the system. The system is prepared with a heparinized 0.9% sodium chloride solution. A heparin bolus of 0 to 2000 IU can be administered in the prefilter line as the therapy is started. A continuous drip of 5 to 10 IU/kg of body weight is used to maintain patency of the hemofilter and blood lines. Often 20,000 units or 40,000 units of heparin in a liter of normal saline is standard.
- Administer prescribed vasopressin to maintain MAP ≥60 to 70 mm Hg to drive the blood through the hemofilter.

Altered peripheral tissue perfusion related to thrombus at arterial tubing site or kinked catheter.

Expected Patient Outcome. Patient has perfusion maintained distal to arterial and venous tubing insertion.

- Review results of coagulation studies.
- Monitor peripheral pulses distal to insertion of tubing. Report diminished or absent pulses, cyanosis, or coolness.
- Should a femoral access be used, the head of bed is kept at ≤30 degrees.
- Check the hemofilter frequently for clot formation after a hypotensive episode.
- Obtain and report indicators of clotting: excessive collection of small clots in the venous header of the hemofilter, darkening of the blood in the line, separation of serum in the blood lines and in the UF chamber.
- Should clotting be associated with decreased UF amount, change the system because delays may cause clotting in the access.
- Administer heparin at 500 IU/h or 1000 IU/h as prescribed should clotting occur.

High risk for infection related to access site.

Expected Patient Outcomes. Patient is free from infection, as evidenced by normothermia; white blood cells (WBC) ≤11,000/μL; negative cultures; and absence of redness, swelling, tenderness, or drainage from access site.

- Review results of WBC count and cultures.
- Monitor temperature every 2 to 4 hours or as necessary.
- Monitor catheter exit site for swelling, tenderness, redness, or drainage.
- Perform daily exit site care.
- Use strict aseptic technique when entering the system to draw blood or change tubing.
- Instruct patient to report any redness, tenderness, or drainage from the access site.

Impaired physical mobility related to movement restriction secondary to catheter access site and hemofiltration process.

Expected Patient Outcomes. Patient is able to move around in bed with assistance while not disrupting the hemofiltration.

- Should femoral access to used, elevate the head of bed to ≤30 degrees.
- Assist patient when moving the accessed limb.
- Turn and reposition patient every 2 hours while maintaining appropriate alignment of the access limb.
- Support the access limb with pillows.
- Provide comfort measures such as massage.
- Teach patient to use isometric exercises in the univolved extremity.

Knowledge deficit related to CAVH.

Expected Patient Outcome. Patient verbalizes the purposes behind ultrafiltration.

- Explain the purpose behind the vascular access.
- Explain the length of time the patient will receive ultrafiltration.
- Describe the equipment used during ultrafiltration.
- Teach patient the purpose of fluid insertion, collection of filtrate, and administration of heparin.

Collaborative Problem

Common collaborative goals for patients undergoing CRRT is to restore electrolyte balance and maintain ultrafiltration rate.

Potential Complication: Electrolyte Imbalance. Electrolyte imbalance related to incorrect replacement of fluids or incorrect dialysate secondary to CRRT.

Expected Patient Outcome. Patient maintains electrolyte balance.

- Consult with physician about clinical conditions other than CRRT that can remove or decrease potassium: metabolic alkalosis, increased gastrointestinal fluid loss, insulin therapy, or antibiotic therapy such as with gentamicin or amphotericin B.
- Review results of serum electrolyte tests.
- Replace sodium by changing base solutions of IV fluids to normal saline.
- Continuously monitor ECG to assess HR or rhythm. Document ECG rhythm strips every 2 to 4 hours in patients with hypokalemia.
- Increase the amount of sodium in the total parenteral nutrition (TPN) to 140 mEq/L.
- Add sodium as prescribed to replacement or dialysate solution.
- Administer prescribed potassium to the dialysate for stabilization.
- Should hypocalcemia occur, administer prescribed calcium supplements through TPN or with calcium boluses.

Potential Complication: Decreased Ultrafiltration Rate. Decreased ultrafiltration rate related to hypovolemia or hypotension.

Expected Patient Outcomes. Patient maintains adequate ultrafiltration rate, as evidenced by ultrafiltration flow rate (UFR) ≥10 mL/min, BP within patient's normal range, MAP ≥70 mm Hg, HR ≤100 bpm, CO 4 to 8 L/min, and hemoglobin and hematocrit within normal range.

- Review hematocrit and plasma protein levels: Increase in both results in increased viscosity of the blood in the venous side of the filter, which leads to higher resistance to blood flow through the system.
- Monitor clotting times at least every 4 hours and titrate heparin accordingly.

- Measure blood flow (mL/min) through the ultrafiltration system: Reduced blood flow leads to clot formation in the filter.
- Obtain and report hypotension, tachycardia, and MAP ≤60 to 70 mm Hg.
- Measure daily weight, intake, specific gravity, and UO.
- Monitor UFR: milliters of fluid in the collecting set after 1 minute.
- Lower collecting set to increase distance in height between the hemofilter and bag, creating a more efficient treatment.
- Determine replacement of fluids: infusion rate equals ultrafiltrate plus other losses per hour minus all fluid infused, minus net removal rate.
- Administer normal saline or lactated Ringer's solution to replace the sodium lost through ultrafiltration.
- Administer heparin based upon patient needs: 500 to 1000 IU/h.

SELECTED REFERENCES

Aaberg RA, Flaherty R, Smith RB. Renal artery occlusive disease. *Crit Care Nurs Clin North Am.* 1991;3:507–514.

Baer CL, Lancaster LE. Acute renal failure. *Crit Care Nurs Q.* 1992; 14(4):1–21.

Baer CL. Acid-base balance. In: Kinney MR, Packa DR, Dunbar SB, eds. *AACN's Clinical Reference for Critical Care Nursing,* 3rd ed. St. Louis, MO: Mosby Year Book; 1993:209–216.

Baer CL. Fluid and electrolyte balance. In: Kinney MR, Packa DR, Dunbar SB, eds. *AACN's Clinical Reference for Critical Care Nursing,* 3rd ed. St. Louis, MO: Mosby Year Book; 1993: 173–228.

Baer CL. Acute renal failure. In: Kinney MR, Packa DR, Dunbar SB, eds. *AACN's Clinical Reference for Critical Care Nursing,* 3rd ed. St. Louis, MO: Mosby Year Book; 1993:885–901.

Beckman NJ, Schell HM, Calixto P, et al. Kidney transplantation: a therapy option. *AACN Clin Issues Crit Care Nurs.* 1992;3:570–584.

Binkley, LS, Whittaker A. Erythropoietin use in the critical care setting. *AACN Clin Issues Crit Care Nurs.* 1992;3:640–649.

Blanford NL. Renal transplantation: a case study of the ideal. *Crit Care Nurse.* 1993;13(1): 46–55.

Bosworth C. SCUF/CAVH/CAVHD: critical differences. *Crit Care Nurs Q.* 1992;14(4):45–55.

Carroll PR, McAnich JW. Staging of renal trauma. *Urol Clin North Am.* 1989;16:193–201.

Chmielewski C, Zellers L, Eyer J. Continuous arteriovenous hemofiltration in the patient with hepatorenal syndrome. *Crit Care Nurs Clin North Am.* 1990;2:115–122.

Chmielewski CM. Nursing management of the patient with end-stage renal disease. In: Dolan JT, ed. *Critical Care Nursing: Clinical Management Through the Nursing Process.* Philadelphia, PA: FA Davis Co. 1991:520–534.

Cunningham N, Smith SL, Postoperative care of the renal transplant patient. *Crit Care Nurse.* 1990;10(9):74–81.

Deglin JH. Vallerand AP. Davis Drug Guide for Nurses. 4th ed. Philadelphia, PA: FA Davis Co. 1993.

Deutsch S. The patient with end-stage renal disease. *Curr Rev Post Anesth Care Nurse.* 1987; 9(11):87–92.

De Angelis R, Lessig L. Hyperkalemia. *Crit Care Nurse.* 1992;12(1):55–59.

Dolan JT, ed. *Critical Care Nursing: Clinical Management Through the Nursing Process.* Philadelphia, PA: FA Davis Co; 1991.

Douglas S. Acute tubular necrosis: diagnosis, treatment and nursing implications. *AACN Clin Issues Crit Care Nurs.* 1992;3:688–697.

Flynn JB, Bruce NB. Renal dialysis. Introduction to Critical Care Skills. St. Louis, MO: Mosby Year Book; 1993.

Glassock, RJ, Brenner BM. et al, The major glomerulonephritis. In: Petersdorf RG, Adams RD, Braunwald, E. (eds). *Harrison's Principles of Internal Medicine,* 10th ed. pp. 1632–1649, New York, NY: McGraw-Hill Book Company; 1983:1632–1649.

Govoni LE, Hayes JE, Shannon MT, et al. *Drugs and Nursing Implications,* 8th ed. Norwalk, CT: Appleton & Lange; 1995.

Guerriero WG. Etiology, classification and management of renal trauma. *Surg Clin North Am.* 1988;68:1070–1085.

Harasyko C. Kidney transplantation. *Nurs Clin North Am.* 1989;24:851–863.

Harper J. Rhabdomyolysis and myoglobinuric renal failure. *Crit Care Nurse.* 1990;10(3):32–36.

Hudak C, Gallo BM, Benz JJ. *Critical Care Nursing: A Holistic Approach,* 6th ed. Philadelphia, PA: JB Lippincott Co; 1994.

Innerarity SA. Electrolyte emergencies in the critically ill renal patient. *Crit Care Nurs Clin North Am.* 1990;2:89–99.

Innerarity SA. Hyperkalemic emergencies. *Crit Care Nurs Q.* 1992;14(4):32–39.

Kaye WA. Understanding kidney disease. *Diabetes Forecast.* 1987;40(11):24–29.

Kidd PS. Genitourinary trauma. In: Neff JA, Kidd PS, eds. *Trauma Nursing the Art and Science.* St Louis, MO: Mosby Year Book; 1993.

Kiely MA, Kiely DC. Rhabdomyolysis. *J Emerg Nurs.* 1986;2(3):153–156.

Lancaster LE. Renal and endocrine regulation of water and electrolyte balance. *Nurs Clin North Am.* 1987;22:761–772.

Loeb S. *Nurse's Handbook of Drug Therapy.* Springhouse, PA: Springhouse Publishing; 1993.

Loeb S. *Clinical Laboratory Tests.* Springhouse, PA: Springhouse Publishing; 1991.

Moore-Sylvan H, Worden JP. Lovastatin-associated rhabdomyolysis. *Heart Lung.* 1991;20:464–466.

Mudge C, Carlson L. Hepatorenal syndrome. *AACN Clin Issues Crit Care Nurs.* 1992;3: 614–632.

Paradiso C. Hemofiltration: an alternative to dialysis. *Heart Lung.* 1989;18:282–290.

Peschman P. Acute renal failure. In: Rueden KV, Walleck CA, eds. *Advanced Critical Care Nursing.* Rockville, MD: Aspen Systems Corp; 1989:251–273.

Peschman P. Acute hemodialysis: issues in the critically ill. *AACN Clin Issues Crit Care Nurs.* 1992;3:545–557.

Peterson NE. Complications of renal trauma. *Urol Clin North Am.* 1989;6:221–236.

Price CA. Continuous arteriovenous ultrafiltration: a monitoring guide for ICU nurse. *Crit Care Nurse.* 1989;9(1):12–19.

Price CA. An update on continuous renal replacement therapies. *AACN Clin Issues Crit Care Nurs.* 1992;3:597–604.

Price CA. Issues related to the care of critically ill patients with end-stage renal failure. *AACN Clin Issues Crit Care Nurs.* 1992;3:585–596.

Roberts SL. Acute renal failure. *Physiological Concepts and the Critically Ill Patient.* Engle-wood Cliffs, NJ: Prentice Hall; 1985. [out of print].

Sander RA. Genitourinary trauma: the overlooked kidney. In: Knezevich BA, ed. *Trauma Nursing Principles and Practice.* Norwalk, CT: Appleton-Century-Crofts; 1986:113–139.

Schluckebier-Murray JA, Chmielewski C. Nursing management of the renal transplant patient. In: Dolan JT, ed. *Critical Care Nursing: Clinical Management Through the Nursing Process.* Philadelphia, PA: FA Davis Co; 1991:535–545.

Smith MF. Renal trauma adult and pediatric consideration. *Crit Care Nurs Clin North Am.* 1990;2:67–77.

Smith LJ. Peritoneal dialysis in the critically ill patient. *AACN Clin Issues Crit Care Nurs.* 1992;3:558–569.

Smith J. Dialysis options in the critically ill patient. Hemodialysis, peritoneal dialysis, and continuous renal replacement therapy. *Crit Care Nurs Q.* 1992;14(4):40–44.

Stark JL. Acute tubular necrosis: differences between oliguria and nonoliguria. *Crit Care Nurs Q.* 1992;14(4):22–27.

Stark JL. Dialysis options in the critically ill patient: hemodialysis, peritoneal dialysis, and continuous renal replacement therapy. *Crit Care Nurs Q.* 1992;14(4):40–44.

Stillwell SB. *Mosby's Critical Care Nursing Reference.* St. Louis, MO: Mosby Year Book; 1992.

Strohschein BL, Caruso DM, Greene ICA. Continuous venovenous hemodialysis. American Journal of Critical Care. 1994;3(2):92–99.

Swearingen PL, Keen JH. *Manual of Critical Care,* 2nd ed. St. Louis, MO: Mosby Year Book; 1992.

Tierney LM, McPhenn SJ, Papadakis MA. *Current Medical Diagnosis and Treatment,* 33rd ed. Norwalk, CT: Appleton & Lange, 1994.

Varella L, Utermohlen V. Nutritional support for the patient with renal failure. *Crit Care Nurs Clin North Am.* 1993;5:79–96.

Whittaker A. Continuous ultrafiltration therapy. In: Clochey JM, ed. *Advanced Technology in Critical Care Nursing.* Rockville, MD: Aspen Systems Corp; 1989:143–156.

Whittaker AA. Patients with acute renal failure. In: Clochesy JM, Breu C, Cardin S. et al, eds. *Critical Care Nursing,* Philadelphia, PA: WB Saunders Co; 1993:886–904.

5

Gastrointestinal Deviations

PART 1: HEALTH PROBLEMS AND
NURSING MANAGEMENT

■ ACUTE GASTROINTESTINAL BLEEDING

(For related information see Part 1: Abdominal trauma, p. 533; Acute mesenteric ischemia, p. 538. Part III: Total parenteral nutrition, p. 551.)

Case Management Basis
DRG:174 Gastrointestinal hemorrhage with complications
LOS: 5.50 days
DRG:175 Gastrointestinal hemorrhage without complications
LOS: 3.80 days

Definitions
Acute *upper* gastrointestinal (GI) bleeding is the loss of blood from the gastrointestinal system at a site above the ligament of Treitz at the duodenojejunal junction. Acute *lower* GI bleeding or hemorrhage from the lower intestine is rare with 10% of rectal bleeds being classified as severe.

Pathophysiology
Pathophysiological changes associated with blood loss depend on the amount of hemorrhage, the time span over which the hemorrhage occurs, and the general health of the individual. A loss in volume (hemorrhage) decreases venous return to the heart, with a corresponding decrease in cardiac output. The amount of blood loss that will produce shock depends on age, size, and the rapidity of bleeding. Physiological responses to acute hemorrhage are divided into classes I to IV. Class I hemorrhage is the loss of up to 15% of the total blood volume. Class II hemorrhage involves 15% to 30% loss. Class III hemorrhage occurs with 30% to 40% loss. Finally, class IV hemorrhage involves more than a 40% volume loss.

Nursing Assessment

PRIMARY CAUSES
- Upper gastrointestinal bleeding mechanisms include peptic ulcer of the duodenum, stomach, or esophagus; esophageal varices; gastritis; Mallory-Weiss syndrome; ulcerogenic drugs such as aspirin, nonsteroidal anti-inflammatory drugs, or alcohol; an-

giodysplasia; Crohn's disease; Meckel's diverticulum; and vascular lesions.

- Lower gastrointestinal bleeding mechanisms consist of ulcerative colitis, regional enteritis, infectious diarrhea, radiation colitis, diverticulosis, hemorrhoids, angiodysplasia, bowel ischemia, colonic varices, aortic aneurysm with enteric fistula, telangiectasias, arteriovenous malformation, anticoagulant drugs, and massive upper GI bleeding.

RISK FACTORS
- History of alcohol abuse.

PHYSICAL ASSESSMENT
- Inspection: Melena, hematemesis, pallor, weakness, restlessness, apprehension, altered mentation, abdominal pain, fever, and diaphoresis.
- Palpation: Cool, clammy skin; hepatomegaly; splenomegaly; pulses weak, thready; and abdominal tenderness with guarding.
- Auscultation: Tachycardia, hyperactive or absent bowel sounds, or hypotension.

DIAGNOSTIC TEST RESULTS

Standard Laboratory Tests. (see Table 1–1, p. 3, and Table 5–1, p. 515)

- Blood studies: Reduced hematocrit and hemoglobin and increased white blood cells (WBC).
- Serum chemistry: Elevated blood uvea nitrogen (BUN), creatinine normal, elevated ammonia in liver dysfunction, and elevated platelets. Reduced clotting time, increased sodium and potassium.

Invasive GI Diagnostic Procedures. (see Table 5–2, p. 516)

- Arteriography: Selective mesenteric arteriography is used to localize the site of bleeding in patients. Blood loss must be ≥5 to 0.6 mL/min for this procedure to be useful.

- Endoscopy: Identifies the bleeding site and becomes a source of treatment. Treatment includes sclerotherapy of esophageal varices and thermal treatment of bleeding gastric or duodenal ulcer.
- Radionuclide scanning: Technetium Tc 99m red cell labeling.

Noninvasive GI Diagnostic Procedure. (see Table 5–3, p. 518)

- Abdominal films: Used to determine the presence of perforation, masses, bowel obstruction, and sign of mesenteric vascular ischemia.

MEDICAL AND SURGICAL MANAGEMENT

PHARMACOLOGY
- Histamine receptor antagonist: Histamine (H_2) receptor antagonists (cimetidine, ranitidine, famotidine, or nizatidine) are used to reduce gastric acid output and concentration. They are effective for the treatment of GI bleeding when hemorrhage is not caused by the erosion of major blood vessels (Table 5–4).
- Antacids: Antacids dissolve in gastric acid secretion, releasing anions that partially neutralize gastric hydrochloride acid. The four classifications of acids include calcium carbonate, sodium bicarbonate, magnesium hydroxide, and aluminum hydroxide (see Table 5–4).
- Sucralfate: It is an inhibitor of pepsin and an antiulcer agent. Sucralfate provides a productive barrier against hydrogen ions and pepsins. A gastric pH of 3.4 is necessary for sucralfate to be effective (1 g four or five times daily orally) (see Table 5–4).
- Prostaglandins: The E series of prostaglandins act by suppressing parietal cell activity and curtailing gastric acid secretion. Misoprostal, a synthetic prostaglandin E_1, is given at a dose of 200 μg qid orally.
- Vasopressin infusion: Vasopressin (Pitressin) acts by constricting the arteries and contracting the bowel wall. Mucosal blood

TABLE 5–1. STANDARD GASTROINTESTINAL LABORATORY TESTS

TABLE 5-1

Test	Purpose	Normal Value	Abnormal Findings
Fecal			
Leukocytes	Helps determine cause of diarrhea, confirms active inflammatory bowel disease, determines need for antibiotic therapy	Negative, absence of leukocytes	Large bowel bacterial invasion of *Shigella* or *Escherichia coli*
			Leukocytes from pus: acute or chronic ulcerative colitis, colonic or rectal abscesses, diverticulitis, Crohn's disease, rectal fistulas
			Absence of leukocytes in presence of diarrhea: viral gastroenteritis or amebiasis
Mucus in stool	Assesses mucus in stool in conditions for parasympathetic excitability	Negative	Translucent mucus: spastic constipation, mucous colitis, excessive straining at stool
			Bloody mucus: neoplasm or inflammation of the rectal canal
			Mucus with pus: ulcerative colitis, bacillary dysentery, ulcerative cancer of the colon
Occult blood tests	Detects GI bleeding and colorectal cancer	Negative: less than 2.5 mL of blood, causing a green reaction	Positive: GI bleeding with 0.50–0.75 mL blood loss
Gastrin	Diagnoses gastroma and differentiates between gastric and duodenal ulcers and pernicious anemia	Serum gastrin levels $\leq$300 pg/mL	Elevated level: Zollinger-Ellison syndrome, duodenal ulcer, extensive stomach carcinoma
Peritoneal fluid analysis	Determines cause of ascites and detects abdominal trauma	Element Gross appearance: odorless, clear to pale with scant amount, <50 mL	Milk-colored fluid: parasitic infection
			Cloudy fluid: peritonitis, ruptured bowel after trauma, infarcted intestine, or appendicitis
			Bloody fluid: benign or malignant tumor
			Bile-stained green fluid: perforated intestine or duodenal ulcer
		RBCs: None	RBC count >100/μL: neoplasm
		WBCs: $\leq$300/μL	>300/μL: bacterial peritonitis
		Protein: 0.3–4.1 g/dL	
		Glucose: 70–100 mg/dL	<60 mg/dL: tuberculosis, peritonitis, peritoneal carcinomatosis
		Amylase: 138–404 amylase units/L	>404 amylase units/L: Intestinal necrosis or intestinal strangulation
		Ammonia: <50 μg/dL	Ruptured of strangulated large and small intestines or ruptured ulcer

TABLE 5-1

TABLE 5-2

TABLE 5–1. CONTINUED

Test	Purpose	Normal Value	Abnormal Findings
Peritoneal fluid analysis (*cont.*)		Alkaline phosphatase: Men: 239 units/L; Women: 196–250 units/L	Twice normal can indicate ruptured or strangulated small intestine
		LDH: Equal to serum level	
		Cytology: No malignant cells present	
		Bacteria: None	Presence: primary peritonitis or gram-negative organisms
		Fungi: None	Positive for candidiasis or histoplasmosis
Schilling test	Indirect test of intrinsic factor deficiency	Excretion of 8% or more of test dose of cobalt-tagged vitamin B$_{12}$ in urine	0%–3% implies absence of intrinsic factor and defective absorption in the ileum
	Evaluates ability to absorb vitamin B$_{12}$ from GI tract		

GI, gastrointestinal; LDH, lactate dehydrogenase; RBC, red blood cells; WBC, white blood cells.

From Loeb S, 1991; Krumberger JM, Gastrointestinal disorders, 1993; Stillwell SB, 1992.

TABLE 5–2. INVASIVE GASTROINTESTINAL DIAGNOSTIC PROCEDURES

Test	Purpose	Normal Value	Abnormal Findings
Biopsy			
Endoscopic biopsy of GI tract	Provides direct visualization of GI tract and site that needs tissue biopsy	Normal tissue	Cancer, lymphoma, gastric ulcers, Crohn's disease, chronic ulcerative colitis, gastritis, multiple gastric polyps, colon cancer, polyps, chronic ulcerative colitis
Small bowel biopsy	Diagnoses diseases of the small bowel	Normal tissue	Suggest Whipple's disease, lymphoma, lymphangiectasia, eosinophillic enteritis, giardiasis
Endoscopic Studies			
Colonoscopy	Detects inflammatory disease, ulcerative bowel disease, colonic strictures, polyps, benign or malignant lesions	Mucosa of large intestine beyond sigmoid colon is light pink-orange	Suggest site of lower GI bleeding, diverticula, polyps, stricture, tumor, site of ulcerative colitis
	Locates origin of lower GI bleeding	Blood vessels are seen below intestinal mucosa	
Esophagogastroduodenoscopy (Gastroscopy)	Determines site and cause of bleeding, structural abnormalities, upper GI disease	Smooth mucosa of esophagus is yellow-pink, with a fine vascular network	Suggest site of upper GI bleeding, peptic ulcer, tumor, esophagitis, gastritis, duodenitis,

TABLE 5–2. CONTINUED

TABLE 5-2

Test	Purpose	Normal Value	Abnormal Findings
Esophagogastro-duodenoscopy (Gastroscopy) (cont)	Obtains a biopsy Evaluates the stomach or duodenum postoperatively Diagnoses an esophageal injury caused by the ingestion of chemicals	The mucosa of distal duodenum has circular folds and is lined with villi	diverticula, hiatal hernia
Proctosigmoidoscopy	Evaluates rectum and sigmoid colon	Normal rectum and sigmoid	Ulcerative or granulomatous colitis, inflammation of rectosigmoid area, tumors of rectosigmoid area
Gastric acid stimulation	Diagnoses duodenal ulcer or gastric carcinoma	Gastric secretion ranges from 11–21 mEq/L in women and 18–28 mEg/L in men	Increased gastric secretions: duodenal ulcer Decreased gastric secretions: gastric carcinoma
Gastric culture	Diagnoses mycobacterial infection	Negative culture specimen for mycobacteria	Pulmonary disease indistinguishable from tuberculosis
Gastrointestinal Studies			
Esophagography	Assesses pharyngeal and esophageal abnormalities	Mucosa appears smooth and regular Esophageal size, contour, and peristalsis are normal	Suggest hiatus hernia, esophageal diverticula, strictures, tumors, polyps, ulcers, esophageal spasms
Lower series	Diagnoses colorectal cancer, polyps, diverticula changes, or inflammatory disease	Uniform filling and passage of barium Normal contour, patency, and mucosal pattern	Carcinoma, diverticulitis, chronic ulcerative colitis, polyps
Upper Series	Diagnoses hiatal hernia, diverticula, varices, strictures, ulcers, tumors, or regional enteritis Detects motility disorders	Normal size and contour of the esophagus, stomach, and small intestine Normal peristalsis	Esophagus: Strictures, tumors, hiatal hernia, varices, ulcers Stomach: Regional enteritis, tumors
Gastrointestinal angiography	Determines site of bleeding	Absence of bleeding Normal anatomy and strictures	Gastrointestinal hemorrhage, presents as extravasation of contrast medium into interstitium
Tagged RBC scan (GI bleed scan)	Detects site or origin of GI bleeding	Even distribution of radioisotope throughout blood pool	Suggest site of active bleeding in the bowel

GI, gastrointestinal; RBC, red blood cells.

From Loeb S, 1991; Krumberger JM, Gastrointestinal disorders, 1993; Stillwell SB, 1992.

TABLE 5-3

TABLE 5-4

TABLE 5–3. NONINVASIVE GASTROINTESTINAL DIAGNOSTIC PROCEDURES

Test	Purpose	Normal Value	Abnormal Findings
Computerized tomographic (CT) magnetic resonance imaging (MRI) scan	Visualizes all gastrointestinal organs		Abnormal findings include tumor or mass
Radiological studies Abdominal Plain Film	Detects perforation, presence of metallic foreign substance, thickening of the gastric wall, and displacement of the gastric air bubble	Normal size and contour	Foreign bodies, existence of an extrinsic mass, intrinsic tumor
Ultrasonography	Delineates fluid, tumor, masses, fistulas, pseudocyst, or abscess Diagnoses portal hypertension		Abnormal findings include tumor, masses, fistulas, pseudocyst or abscess

From Loeb S, 1991; Krumberger JM, Gastrointestinal disorders, 1993; Stillwell SB, 1992.

TABLE 5–4. GASTROINTESTINAL-RELATED DRUGS

Medication	Route/Dose	Uses	Side Effects
Antibiotics			
Ampicillin	Systemic infections PO: 250–500 mg q 6 h IM/IV: 250 mg, 2 g q 2 h	Infections of GU, respiratory, and GI tract and skin and soft tissues	Seizures, diarrhea, nausea, vomiting, pruritus, urticaria, or anaphylactoid reaction
Cephapirin sodium (Cefadyl)	Infection IM/IV: 500 mg, 1 g q 4–6 h up to 12 g/day Renal impairment IM/IV: serum creatinine ≤5 mg/dL: 7.5–15.0 mg/kg q 12 h	Serious infections of respiratory and urinary tracts, skin and soft tissue, or endocarditis	Nausea, vomiting, diarrhea, abdominal cramps, rash, urticaria, drug fever, or anaphylaxis
Clindamycin hydrochloride	Infection PO: 150–450 mg q 6 h IM/IV: 300–900 mg q 6–8 h for a maximum 2700 mg/d	Treats serious infections when less toxic alternatives are inappropriate	Diarrhea, abdominal pain, bloating, nausea, vomiting, loss of taste, hypotension, dryness, fever, skin rashes, pruritus, or urticaria
Kanamycin (Kantrex)	Infection IM/IV:15 mg/kg/d in equally divided doses q 8–12 h Intraperitoneal: 500 mg diluted in 20 mL sterile water instilled through wound catheter	Reduces ammonia-producing bacteria in intestinal tract as adjunctive therapy of hepatic coma	Dizziness, peripheral neuritis, headache, restlessness, tremors, lethargy, convulsions, nausea, vomiting, diarrhea, abdominal discomfort, rash, urticaria, drug fever, or anaphylaxis

TABLE 5-4

TABLE 5–4. CONTINUED

Medication	Route/Dose	Uses	Side Effects
Kanamycin (Kantrex) (*cont*)	Inhalation: 250 mg diluted in 3 mL normal saline administered per nebulizer q 6–12 h Irrigation: 0.25% solution prn		
Gentamicin sulfate (Garamycin)	Infection IM/IV: 1.5–2.0 mg/kg loading dose followed by 3–5 mg/kg/d in 2–3 divided doses Bacterial endocarditis Intramuscular/Intravenous: 1.5 mg/kg 30 min before procedure, may repeat in 8 h	Treatment of GI, respiratory, and urinary tract infection	Paresthesia, headache, lethargy, tremors, muscle cramps, apnea, weakness, anorexia, nausea, vomiting, joint pain, pruritus, or nephrotoxicity
Metronidazole (Flagyl)	Anaerobic infection PO: 7.5 mg/kg q 6 h (max 4 g/d) IV: 15 mg/kg loading dose, then 7.5 mg/kg/q 6 h (max 4 g/d) Amebiasis PO: 500–750 mg tid Pseudomembranous colitis PO: 250–500 mg tid IV: 250–500 mg tid or qid	Intestinal amebiasis, amebic liver abscess, prophylaxis in colorectal surgery	Rash, urticaria, pruritus, flushing, vertigo, ataxia, headache, confusion, weakness, diarrhea, dry mouth, fatigue, bitter taste, polyuria, decreased libido, or incontinence
Neomycin sulfate (Mycifradin)	Intestinal antisepsis PO: 1 g q 1 h times 4 doses, then 1 g q 4 h times 5 doses Diarrhea PO: 50 mg/kg in 4 divided doses for 2–3 days IM: 1.3–2.6 mg/kg q 6 h	Severe diarrhea, inhibit nitrogen-forming bacteria of GI tract, or urinary tract infection	Diarrhea, nausea, vomiting, vitamin B_{12} deficiency, nephrotoxicity, or respiratory paralysis
Penicillin G sodium	Infection PO: 1.6–3.2 million U divided q 6 h IM/IV: 1.2–24.0 million U divided q 4 h	Infections caused by penicillin-sensitive microorganisms or staph infections	Hypokalemia, hypernatremia, hypersensitivity, pruritus, flushed skin, coughing, sneezing, anaphylaxis, diarrhea, abdominal cramps, edema, laryngospasm, bronchospasm, hypotension, or cardiac arrest

TABLE 5-4. CONTINUED

TABLE 5-4

Medication	Route/Dose	Uses	Side Effects
Polymixin B sulfate (Aerosporin) stride powder	Infections IV: 15,000–25,000 U/kg/d divided q 12 h IM: 25,000–30,000 U/kg/d divided q 4–6 h	Used in combination with other anti-infectives or corticosteroids for various infections Infection; urinary tract, bloodstream, or meninges	Irritability, facial flushing, vertigo, ataxia, blurred vision, generalized muscle weakness, respiratory depression, hypersensitivity, GI disturbance, or anaphylaxis
Antacid			
Aluminum hydroxide (ALternaGEL)	PO: 500–1800 mg (5–30 mL) 3–6 times/d.	Lowers phosphate level in patients with chronic renal failure Adjunct therapy in peptic, duodenal, and gastric ulcers	Constipation
Magnesium hydroxide	PO: 2.4–4.8 g (30–60 mL/d in 1 or more divided doses	Relieves GI symptoms from hyperacidity Adjunct therapy for peptic ulcer	Nausea, vomiting, abdominal cramps, diarrhea, hypotension, bradycardia, complete heart block
Calcium carbonate	PO: 1–2 g bid or tid	Relieves symptoms of hyperacidity Calcium supplement when calcium intake is reduced	Constipation, nausea, flatulence, or hypercalcemia
Antidiuretic Hormone			
Vasopressin (Pitressin)	Abdominal distention IM: 5 units initially, may increase to 10 units if needed q 3–4 h. GI bleeding IV: 0.2–0.4 U/min may be increased up to 0.9 U/min	Central diabetes insipidus or abdominal distention	Rash, dizziness, chest pain, abdominal cramps, belching, diarrhea, nausea, vomiting, heartburn, sweating, or trembling
Antiulcer			
Misoprostal (Cytotec)	PO: 200 μg four times daily with or after meals and bedtime or 400 μg twice daily (AM and bedtime)	Prevents gastric mucosal injury from NSAID	Headache, diarrhea, abdominal pain, vomiting, flatulence, dyspepsia, constipation or dysmenorrhea
Sucralfate (Carafate)	PO: 1 qid 1 hour before meals and at bedtime	Duodenal ulcer	Nausea, gastric discomfort, constipation, or diarrhea
Gastrointestinal Anti-inflammatory			
Sulfasalazine (Azulfidine)	PO: 1–2 g/d in 4 divided doses and may increase up to 8 g/d if needed	Ulcerative colitis and mild regional enteritis	Nausea, vomiting, bloody diarrhea, anorexia, rash, blood dyscrasias, or allergic reactions

TABLE 5–4. CONTINUED

TABLE 5-4

Medication	Route/Dose	Uses	Side Effects
Histamine H₂ Antagonist Antiulcer			
Cimetidine (Tagamet)	Ulcer PO: 300 mg 4 times daily or 800 mg at bedtime or 400 mg twice daily for up to 8 wk; maximum dose is 2.4 g/d IM/IV: 300 mg q 6 h; maximum 2.4 g/d	Treat active duodenal ulcer, prophylaxis of duodenal ulcer, GI hypersecretory states, or stress ulcer	Drowsiness, dizziness, confusion, headache, bradycardia, nausea, diarrhea, constipation, rashes, urticaria, muscle pain, nephritis, or aplastic anemia
	Gastric hypersecretory disease PO: 300 mg qid with meals and at bedtime; may increase up to 2400 mg/d		
	Gastrointestinal bleeding PO: 300 mg qid or 600 mg bid		
Famotidine (Pepcid)	Stress ulcers IV: 300 mg q 6 h to maintain gastric pH ≥4	Active duodenal ulcer and gastric hypersecretory states	Dizziness, headache, drowsiness, tinnitus, palpitations, diarrhea, bronchospasm, bradycardia, nausea, rash, pruritus, fever, fatigue, flushing, constipation, or abdominal cramps
	Duodenal ulcer PO: 40 mg at bedtime or 20 mg bid; maintenance dose of 20 mg at bedtime IV: 20 mg q 12 h		
Nizatidine (Axid)	Active duodenal ulcer PO: 150 mg bid or 300 mg at bedtime; maintenance therapy 150 mg at bedtime	Active duodenal ulcer and maintenance therapy	Fatigue, pruritus, sweating, dysrhythmias, urticaria, hyperuricemia
Ranitidine hydrochloride (Zantac)	Duodenal and peptic ulcer PO: 150 mg bid of 300 mg at bedtime; maintenance dose of 150 mg at bedtime IV: 50 mg q 6–8 h	Short-term treatment of duodenal ulcer and maintenance therapy after ulcer heals	Confusion, dizziness, headache, malaise, bradycardia, tachycardia, rashes, blurred vision, nausea, abdominal pain, diarrhea, hepatotoxicity, or anaphylaxis
	Hypersecretory problems PO: 150 mg bid up to 6.3 g/d IV: 50 mg q 6–8 h		
Hormone			
Glucagon	Diagnostic aid IM/IV: 0.25–2.0 U 10 min before procedure	Facilitates examination of the GI tract Management of severe hypoglycemia	Nausea, vomiting, or hypersensitivity

TABLE 5-4

TABLE 5–4. CONTINUED

Medication	Route/Dose	Uses	Side Effects
Lipid Lowering Agent			
Cholestyramine resin (Questran)	PO: 3–4 g tid or qid	Adjunct in management of hyper-cholesterolemia	Headache, dizziness, syncope, fatigue, hypersensitivity, nausea, constipation, abdominal discomfort, diarrhea, backache, arthritis, acute myocardial infarction, angina, or rash
Vasodilator			
Papaverine hydrochloride	PO: 100–300 mg 3–5 times/d; 150 mg sustained release q 8–12 h IM/IV: 30–120 mg q 3 h as needed	Relieves visceral spasm in ureteral, biliary, or GI colic	Nausea, anorexia, constipation, dizziness, drowsiness, headache, hepatotoxicity, or respiratory distress
Antisecretory			
Omeprazole (Prilosec)	Gastroesophageal reflux PO: 20 mg once/d for 4–8 wk Hypersecretory disease Oral: 60 mg once/d up to 120 mg tid	Gastroesophageal reflux disease including erosive esophagitis	Headache, dizziness, fatigue, diarrhea, abdominal pain, nausea, or rash

GI, gastrointestinal; GU, genitourinary; IM, intramuscular; IV, intravenous; NSAID, nonsteroid anti-inflammatory drug; PO, by mouth.

From Deglin, Vallerand, 1991; Govoni LE, Hayes JE, Shannon ME, et al., 1995; Loeb S, 1993.

flow is reduced and thrombus formation can occur. It is useful in treating massive GI hemorrhage (see Table 5–4).

FLUID THERAPY

- Crystalloid solution: Normal saline and lactated Ringer's are infused to replace volume during the initial phase of fluid resuscitation.
- Blood products: Packed red blood cells (PRBC) are replaced milliliter for milliliter of estimated blood loss and crystalloid solution in a 3:1 ratio. Albumin or plasmate may be used as volume expanders. Fresh frozen plasma may be received to replace clotting factors.

NASOGASTRIC INTUBATION

- Nasogastric (NG) intubation is used to obtain a gastric specimen for occult blood testing, to clear stomach for endoscopic examination, and to evacuate blood from the stomach.

ENDOSCOPIC ELECTROCOAGULATION

- Electrocoagulation can be achieved through use of a bipolar (BICAP) probe. BICAP uses an electric current that flows between two electrodes in close proximity to each other. This therapy is done using endoscopy to induce coagulation of bleeding lesions.

TRANSCATHETER EMBOLIZATION

- The angiographic modality is used in patients whose bleeding is unresponsive to vasopressin and who are poor risks for surgery. After the bleeding artery has been visualized with angiography, embolic material is injected through the catheter into the bleeding artery.

PHOTOCOAGULATION

- The use of laser for coagulation of bleeding source can be beneficial in treating ulcers and gastric erosions.

SURGICAL INTERVENTION

- Surgical treatment is indicated if healing is not accomplished with medical treatment, if ulcer recurrence becomes a problem, if malignancy is suspected, or if complication such as perforation or intractable hemorrhage occurs (see Gastric surgery, p. 547).

NURSING MANAGEMENT: NURSING DIAGNOSES AND COLLABORATIVE PROBLEMS

Nursing Diagnoses

Common nursing goals for patients with acute GI bleeding are to restore fluid balance, maintain gas exchange, prevent diarrhea, promote activity balance, reduce fatigue, and control pain.

Fluid volume deficit related to blood loss secondary to hemorrhage.

Expected Patient Outcomes. Patient maintains adequate fluid volume, as evidenced by systolic blood pressure (SBP) 90 to 100 mm Hg; mean arterial pressure (MAP) 70 to 100 mm Hg; heart rate (HR) $\leq$100 bpm; cardiac output (CO) 4 to 8 L/min; cardiac index (CI) $\geq$2.7 L/min/m^2; urinary output (UO) $\geq$30 mL/h; central venous pressure (CVP) 2 to 6 mm Hg; skin turgor normal; skin warm, dry, and pink; absence of hematemesis or melena; and hemoglobin and hematocrit within normal range.

- Review test results for BUN, creatinine, serum albumin, complete blood count (CBC), aminotranferases, albumin:globulin ratio, prothrombin time, endoscopy, and angiography.
- Limit physical activity to bed rest until bleeding ceases.
- Obtain and report hemodynamic parameters associated with fluid volume deficit: CO $\leq$4 L/min and CVP $\leq$2 mm Hg.

- Monitor clinical indicators of perfusion: BP, HR, skin turgor, capillary refill, MAP, peripheral pulses, and UO.
- Obtain and report other clinical findings associated with fluid volume deficit: hypotension; tachycardia; poor skin turgor; weakness; fatigue; capillary refill $\geq$3 seconds; skin cool, pale, or cyanotic; and peripheral pulses $\leq$+2.
- Insert NG tube to decompress the stomach, assist with endoscopy, test gastric aspirate for blood, administer antacids, and administer iced saline lavage.
- Should fresh blood or large amount of old blood be present during gastric aspiration, report and prepare patient for gastric lavage.
- Implement prescribed gastric lavage with iced saline to cause vasoconstriction of bleeding varicosities.
- Maintain patency of NG tube by irrigation with saline to minimize saline depletion and reposition if necessary.
- Implement continuous gastric suction as prescribed to minimize the amount of blood passing into the intestine, where it is metabolized to ammonia.
- Assist with the insertion of Sengstaken-Blakemore tube to control hemorrhage from esophageal and gastric varices by applying direct pressure to the bleeding blood vessels.
- Administer prescribed oxygen 2 to 4 L/min by nasal cannula or mask to promote tissue oxygenation.
- Administer prescribed normal saline, lactated Ringer's, or colloids to restore intravascular volume.
- Administer prescribed blood products such as packed red blood cells or fresh frozen plasma to restore circulating volume.
- Administer prescribed H$_2$ receptor antagonists to decrease gastric acid secretion and neutralize gastric pH (see Table 5–4).
- Administer prescribed sucralfate to prevent the development of mucosal lesion (see Table 5–4).
- Administer prescribed antacid to neutralize hydrochloric acid.

- Should pharmacological therapy be ineffective in stopping bleeding, prepare patient for endoscopic electrocoagulation.
- Should medical interventions be ineffective, prepare patient for gastric surgery (see Gastric surgery, p. 547).
- Instruct patient to report any tarry stool.

Impaired gas exchange related to compromised oxygenation secondary to reduced circulatory volume and hemoglobin.

Expected Patient Outcomes. Patient maintains adequate gas exchange, as evidenced by respiratory rate (RR) ≤24 BPM, absence of dyspnea, no shortness of breath, HR ≤100 bpm, skin warm and dry, absence of cyanosis, normal lung sounds, arterial blood gases within normal range, alertness, and hemoglobin 12 to 18 g/100 mL.

- Review results of arterial blood gas measurement and CBC.
- Obtain and report clinical findings associated with impaired gas exchange: tachypnea, dyspnea, restlessness, tachycardia, or crackles.
- Evaluate skin color, as cyanosis is a late sign of impaired gas exchange and signifies desaturation of at least 5 g/100 mL of hemoglobin.
- Continually monitor ECG to assess HR and rhythm. Document ECG rhythm strips every 2 to 4 hours or more frequently in patients with dysrhythmias.
- Encourage patient to use stress-reducing strategies such as progressive relaxation, meditation, or guided imagery.
- Encourage patient to cough, turn, deep breathe, and use incentive spirometer to facilitate lung expansion.
- Provide frequent rest periods.
- Administer oxygen 2 to 4 L/min by nasal cannula or mask to promote oxygenation.
- Administer prescribed blood or blood products to restore circulating volume.

Diarrhea related to irritated bowel from bleeding.

Expected Patient Outcome. Absence of diarrhea or melena.

- Review results of tests of stool for occult blood, hemoglobin, hematocrit, coagulation profile, and serum electrolytes.
- Keep patient on nothing by mouth status (NPO) until diarrhea or bleeding has subsided.
- Monitor patient's stool for amount, odor, consistency, and presence of blood.
- Evaluate for the presence of hyperactive or absent bowel sounds.
- Administer IV fluids as prescribed to maintain adequate hydration.
- Teach patient to report increased frequency of diarrhea or presence of blood in stool.

Pain related to irritation of the GI mucosal lining secondary to enhanced gastric acidity.

Expected Patient Outcome. Patient verbalizes pain relief.

- Evaluate patient's complaint of pain including severity, location, radiation, and duration on a scale of 1 to 10.
- Place patient in a position of comfort while experiencing pain.
- Raise gastric pH ≥4.5 by administering prescribed antacids.
- Encourage patient to inform nurse when pain occurs. Note what precipitates or aggravates the pain.
- Administer prescribed H_2 antagonist drugs to inhibit gastric acid secretion (see Table 5–4).
- Administer prescribed analgesics to reduce pain.
- Teach patient stress reduction exercises to reduce risk of increased gastric acid production.

Knowledge deficit related to causes of gastrointestinal bleeding.

Expected Patient Outcome. Patient is able to verbalize the risk factors associated with GI bleeding and its treatment.

- Consult with physician regarding the amount of information to be shared with patient.
- Using illustrations, teach patient the location of GI bleeding and the relationship of risk factors to bleeding.
- Teach patient the purpose behind eliminating irritants, changing diet, and taking the prescribed medications.
- Instruct patient to report any changes in bowel habits or abdominal epigastric pain.
- Teach patient how to use stress-reduction techniques: progressive relaxation, meditation, or guided imagery.

Activity intolerance related to weakness and fatigue.

Expected Patient Outcome. Patient is able to maintain physical activity without experiencing weakness or fatigue.

- When bleeding ceases, encourage incremental physical activity: out of bed, standing, sitting in chair, ambulating in room, and ambulating in hallway.
- Monitor BP, HR, RR, and cardiac rhythm as patient increases activity.
- Provide rest periods before and after physical activity.
- Instruct patient to report dizziness, weakness, or tachycardia while increasing activity.

Fatigue related to blood loss.

Expected Patient Outcomes. Absence of fatigue, absence of melena or hematemesis, and red blood cells (RBC) within normal limits.

- Review results of hemoglobin, hematocrit, and WBC tests.
- Encourage patient to gradually increase activity when bleeding ceases and RBC improves.
- Monitor sensorimotor function when increasing activity to avoid an injury from falling.
- Measure cardiac rhythm, skin color, HR, RR, and BP as patient begins to increase activity.

- Provide an atmosphere conducive for resting or sleeping.
- Encourage patient to rest after activity.
- Instruct patient to report any unusual feelings of fatigue.

Anxiety related to bleeding, its cause, and treatment.

Expected Patient Outcome. Patient expresses less verbalization of anxious feelings and demonstrates more relaxed behavior.

- Encourage patient to discuss concerns and fears associated with GI bleeding.
- Answer patient's questions regarding the causes of GI bleeding and its implications for his or her future.
- Include the family in patient teaching.
- Help patient to identify factors contributing to anxious feelings.

Collaborative Problems

Common collaborative goals for patients with acute gastrointestinal bleeding are to correct electrolyte imbalance and increase cardiac output.

Potential Complication: Electrolyte Imbalance. Electrolyte imbalance related to hyperkalemia or hypocalcemia secondary to blood loss and NG drainage.

Expected Patient Outcomes. Patient maintains electrolyte balance, as evidenced by absence of bleeding in emesis, stool, or NG drainage; BP within patient's normal range; MAP 70 to 100 mm Hg; HR $\leq$ 100 bpm; absence of dysrhythmias; and serum electrolytes within normal range.

- Consult with physician about causes of hyperkalemia in patient with acute GI bleeding: Hyperkalemia may occur if aging RBCs release potassium in the banked blood.
- Consult with physician about causes of hypokalemia: Hypocalcemia may result when ionized calcium in the banked blood binds to the citrate derivation used as an anticoagulant.

- Review results of serum electrolyte, BUN, and creatinine tests.
- Limit activity to bed rest to avoid exertion, increased intra-abdominal pressure, and bleeding.
- Obtain and report clinical findings indicative of hyperkalemia: weakness, cramps, paresthesia of face, tingle in extremities, hypotension, dysrhythmias, anorexia, and abdominal distention.
- Obtain and report ECG changes associated with potassium 5.5 to 6.0 mmol/L: tall, peaked, symmetric T wave in the precordial leads; QT interval is normal or decreased, with occasional ST depression.
- Monitor and report ECG changes associated with potassium 6.0 to 7.0 mmol/L: prolonged PR interval and QRS duration.
- Obtain and report ECG changes associated with potassium 7.0 to 8.0 mmol/L: flattened P wave, QRS complex continues to widen with increased delays in atrioventricular conduction.
- Obtain and report ECG changes associated with potassium 8.0 to 10.0 mmol/L: irregular ventricular rhythm, absent P waves, and markedly increased QRS complexes, with the eventual merging of the complexes with the T wave.
- Obtain and report ECG changes associated with potassium 10.0 to 12.0 mmol/L: ventricular fibrillation or asystole.
- Limit potassium intake in diet to reduce plasma and total body potassium content.
- Administer sodium polystyrene sulfonate (Kayexalate), mixed in water and sorbitol, and administered orally, rectally, or through NG tube: Renin captures potassium in the bowel and eliminates it in the feces.
- In patients with serum potassium ≥ 6.5 mEq/L, administer prescribed 10% calcium gluconate, 500 mL 10% glucose with 10 units regular insulin IV over 30 minutes, and sodium bicarbonate 2 to 3 ampules in 500 mL glucose IV over 1 to 2 hours. This will shift the potassium intracellularly.
- Administer prescribed IV fluids to maintain adequate hydration. Replace serum electrolytes as prescribed: 5% normal saline solution.
- Administer small doses of IV sodium bicarbonate (NaHCO$_3$) 50 to 100 mmol to increase pH ≥ 7.2 and HCO$_3$ ≥ 15 mM/L.
- Should pharmacological therapy be ineffective in reducing serum potassium, prepare patient for dialysis. (see Hemodialysis, p. 496, and Peritoneal dialysis, p. 502).
- Obtain and report clinical findings associated with hypocalcemia: numbness and tingling of the extremities, muscle cramps, tetany, positive Chvostek's and Trousseau's signs, seizures, carpopedal spasm, laryngeal stridor, abdominal cramps, nausea, vomiting, diarrhea, and dry skin.
- Monitor continuous ECG and report changes associated calcium level ≤ 8.5 mg/100 mL: a lengthened ST segment and prolonged QT interval.
- Check Chvostek's sign periodically by percussing the facial nerve in the face anterior to the auricle of the ear. Hypocalcemia response is unilateral twitching of the facial muscles, eyelid, and lips.
- Test for Trousseau's sign periodically by inflating a BP cuff around the upper extremity for 3 to 4 minutes, which occludes blood supply to the extremity, thereby producing ischemia. Hypocalcemia is confirmed when the induced ischemia produces carpopedal spasm.
- Provide foods that are high in calcium and low in phosphorus.
- Administer prescribed IV infusion of calcium chloride, or calcium gluconate (see Table 5–4).
- Obtain and report clinical findings associated with hypochloremia (≤ 96 mEq/L): muscle weakness, tetany, agitation, irritability, and slow, shallow respirations.
- Replace lost chloride with three fourths of the amount of the imbalance being sodium chloride and one fourth being potassium chloride. Sodium chloride or ammonium chloride is used in place of potassium chloride if serum potassium is ≥ 5.5 mEq/L.

- Insert a Levin or Salem sump gastric tube to determine the rate of bleeding, remove irritating gastric secretions, prevent gastric dilatation, and prevent accumulation of blood in the GI tract, and lavage with a solution that will decrease blood flow.
- Irrigate stomach with tepid or iced saline to prevent washing out of electrolytes and to cause vasoconstriction to decrease blood flow.

Potential Complication: Decreased Cardiac Output. Decreased CO related to blood loss secondary to bleeding.

Expected Patient Outcomes. Patient maintains adequate CO, as evidenced by CO 4 to 8 L/min, CI ≥2.7 L/min/m², MAP ≥70 mm Hg, BP within patient's normal range, HR ≤100 bpm, liver function studies and coagulation profile within normal limits, CVP 2 to 6 mm Hg, skin color normal, capillary refill ≤3 seconds, peripheral pulses +2, and UO ≥30 mL/h.

- Review results of coagulation profile.
- Limit activity to bed rest.
- Obtain and report hemodynamic parameters indicating decreased CO: CO ≤4 L/min, CI ≤2.7 L/min/m², and CVP ≤2 mm Hg.
- Evaluate clinical indicators of perfusion: BP, HR, skin color, capillary refill, and peripheral pulses.
- Report clinical findings associated with decreased CO: hypotension, tachycardia, pallor or cyanosis, peripheral pulses ≤+2, and capillary refill ≥3 seconds.
- Continuously monitor ECG to assess HR and rhythm. Document ECG rhythm strips every 2 to 4 hours or as necessary in patients with dysrhythmias.
- Measure and test urine, diarrhea, and NG drainage for occult blood.
- Measure all intake including oral, parenteral, or NG irrigations.
- Measure daily weight and report weight gain 0.5% from baseline.

- Administer prescribed oxygen 2 to 4 L/min by nasal cannula or mask to facilitate oxygen delivery to the tissues.

DISCHARGE PLANNING

Critical care nurse will provide patient and significant other(s) verbal or written discharge notes regarding the following subjects:

1. Medications, including drug name, dosage, route, purpose, schedule, and side effects.
2. The signs and symptoms suggesting GI bleeding: nausea, vomiting of blood, dark stools, and dizziness.
3. Importance of keeping all medical appointments.
4. Importance of avoiding medications that can cause gastric irritation.

■ GASTROINTESTINAL ULCERS

(For related information see Part II: Gastric surgery, p. 547. Part III: Total parenteral nutrition, p. 551.)

Case Management Basis

DRG: 176 Complicated peptic ulcer
LOS: 5.90 days
DRG: 177 Uncomplicated peptic ulcer with complications
LOS: 5.10 days
DRG: 178 Uncomplicated peptic ulcer without complications
LOS: 3.80 days
DRG: 182 Esophagitis, gastroenteritis, and miscellaneous digestive disorders, age greater than 17 with complications
LOS: 4.90 days
DRG: 183 Esophagitis, gastroenteritis, and miscellaneous digestive disorders, age greater than 17 without complications
LOS: 3.50 days

Definition

Peptic ulcer is a break in the mucosa of the duodenum or gastric area of the stomach extending through the muscularis mucosa. The ulcer crater is usually surrounded by areas of acute or chronic inflammation. Gastric ulcer refers to a break in the mucosal barrier; they are located at or near the lesser curvature and most frequently on the posterior wall. Duodenal ulcer is a chronic and recurrent disease that occurs in the duodenal bulb or cap.

Pathophysiology

Peptic ulceration depends on the defensive resistance that the mucosa has relative to the aggressive force of peptic activity. Ulceration occurs when the defensive resistance of the mucosa depends on the following: mucosal integrity and regeneration, presence of a protective mucous barrier, normal blood flow, and ability of the duodenal inhibitory mechanism to regulate secretion. There may be primary defects in gastric mucosal resistance or direct gastric mucosal injury. Serum gastrin levels are increased in some gastric ulcer patients. Regurgitation of duodenal contents, especially those containing bile, may induce gastric mucosal injury and subsequent gastric ulceration. These patients also have increased duodenogastric reflux of bile and greater concentration of bile in their stomachs. Duodenal ulcer patients secrete more acid than normal and have increased gastric secretion of pepsin and an increase in serum pepsinogen level. The ulceration varies from a few mm to 1 to 2 cm in diameter and extends through the muscularis mucosa, through to the serosa, and into the pancreas.

Nursing Assessment

PRIMARY CAUSES

- Include drugs such as cinchophen, corticosteroids, indomethacin, phenylbutazone, chemotherapeutic agents, reserpine, vasopressors, or aspirin. Also can include disease processes such as chronic renal failure, alcoholic cirrhosis, renal transplantation, hyperthyroidism, systemic mastocytosis, and chronic obstructive pulmonary disease.

RISK FACTORS

- Family history of duodenal ulcer with increased serum pepsinogen inherited as an autosomal dominant trait and life-style factors such as cigarette smoking. Also family history of peptic ulcer, chronic aspirin use, high steroid intake, caffeine-containing beverages, alcohol, diet, emotional stress, or nonsteroidal anti-inflammatory drugs.

PHYSICAL ASSESSMENT

- Inspection: Epigastic pain described as gnawing or burning sensation, nausea, vomiting, weight loss, or anorexia. With duodenal ulcer, patient experiences pain near midline in the epigastrium near xiphoid and it may radiate below the costal margins into the back or to the right shoulder.
- Palpation: Superficial or deep epigastric tenderness and involuntary muscle guarding.
- Auscultation: Tachypnea or hypotension.

DIAGNOSTIC TEST RESULTS

Standard Laboratory Tests (see Table 5–1)

- Gastric analysis: An acid pH after pentagastrin and usually the presence of low normal to normal secretin with gastric ulcer. With duodenal ulcer gastric analysis shows acid and a basal and maximal gastric hypersecretion of hydrochloric acid.
- Serum chemistry: complete blood count (CBC), serum electrolytes, creatinine, sedimentation rate, liver function, 72-hour stool for guaiac collection, acid secretory output, and fasting serum gastrin. Amylase elevated if there is posterior penetration or duodenal ulcer.
- Stool: Occult blood.

Invasive Gastrointestinal Diagnostic Procedures. (see Table 5–2)

- Cytologic examination: Biopsy
- Endoscopy: Permits direct visualization of the ulcer crater or duodenitis and provides

for documentation by photography. Also permits multiple biopsies and cytologic examination.

- Radiography: Reveals irritability of the bulb with difficulty in retaining barium there, point tenderness over the bulb, pylospasm, gastric hyperperistalsis, and hypersecretion or retained secretions.

MEDICAL AND SURGICAL MANAGEMENT

PHARMACOLOGY

- Antacids: Used to control the pH of the gastric mucosa. Antacids are administered every 1 to 2 hours initially. If necessary they may be given through the nasogastric (NG) tube. The goal is to maintain a gastric pH ≥ 5.0 (see Table 5–4).
- Histamine blockers: Histamine blockers (cimetidine, rantitidine, or famotidine) block parietal cell stimulation and secretion of hydrochloride acid (see Table 5–4).
- Omeprazole: As a new drug, it suppresses gastric acid secretion by inhibiting the proton pump mechanisms, thereby blocking acid secretion. It can be helpful to patients resistant to histamine receptor antagonists (see Table 5–4).
- Mucosal barrier agents: Prostaglandin or carbenoxolone improves the mucosal barrier and increases mucosal blood flow. Misoprostol, a prostaglandin E_1 analogue, suppresses acid secretion for 3 to 5 minutes. Sucralfate is used to treat duodenal ulcers by forming a protective barrier over the ulcer site. Colloidal bismuth binds to the ulcer base and stimulates mucus secretion, which deters further mucosal damage (see Table 5–4).

GASTRIC LAVAGE

- Although controversial, gastric lavage can be used during acute bleeding episodes. Should lavage be ordered, 1000 to 2000 mL of room-temperature normal saline is instilled via NG tube and then removed by manual or intermittent suction until the secretions are clear.

FLUID THERAPY

- Fluid replacement is initiated to prevent hypovolemia, using lactated Ringer's, normal saline, or 5% dextrose in water (D_5W).
- Blood or blood products: PRBC are used to reestablish oxygen-carrying capacity of the blood. One unit of PRBC can increase hemoglobin 1 g and hematocrit 2 to 3 g, depending on patient's intravascular volume and presence of active bleeding. Colloids can also be used.

HEMODYNAMIC MONITORING

- Used to monitor fluid status, especially when patient requires massive fluid replacement or has underlying cardiovascular disease.

ARTERIAL LINE

- Used for constant monitoring of SBP and to obtain blood for laboratory tests. A systolic blood pressure (SBP) ≤ 100 mm Hg or a postural decrease of ≤ 10 mm Hg reflects a blood loss of at least 1000 mL, or more than 25% of the total blood volume.

SCLEROTHERAPY

- Sclerotherapy controls: acute variceal bleeding in 90% to 95% of patients. Sclerosant solution is injected directly into the lumen of the varix or into the submucosa around the varix. Injection of sclerosant solution results in the contraction of the varix and cessation of bleeding. The inflammatory reaction produced by the sclerosant solution causes venous thrombosis which is eventually converted to a fibrous band.

THERMAL METHODS

- Thermal methods of endoscopic tamponade include use of the heater probe, laser photocoagulation, and electrocoagulation.

SURGICAL INTERVENTION

- Surgical therapies for peptic ulcer disease include gastric resection (antrectomy, gastrectomy, or gastroenterostomy), vagotomy, or combined surgeries such as

Billroth I or Billroth II to restore gastrointestinal continuity. An antrectomy can be used for duodenal ulcer to decrease the acidity of the duodenum by removing the gastric acid-secreting cells in the antrum.

NURSING INTERVENTIONS: NURSING DIAGNOSES AND COLLABORATIVE PROBLEMS

Nursing Diagnoses

Common nursing goals for patients with gastrointestinal ulcers are to maintain fluid balance, prevent injury, increase tissue perfusion, provide nutritional requirements, and minimize pain.

Fluid volume deficit related to abnormal fluid loss secondary to hemorrhage or perforation.

Expected Patient Outcomes. Patient maintains adequate fluid volume, as evidenced by blood pressure (BP) within patient's normal range, mean arterial pressure (MAP) $\geq$70 mm Hg, cardiac output (CO) 4 to 8 L/min, cardiac index (CI) 2.7 to 4.3 L/min/m^2, central venous pressure (CVP) 2 to 6 mm Hg, heart rate (HR) $\leq$100 bpm, respiratory rate (RR) 12 to 20 BPM, skin warm and dry, normal skin turgor, absence of epigastric pain, normal bowel sounds, stool negative for occult bleeding, coagulation profile normal, urinary output (UO) $\geq$30 mL/h, peripheral pulses +2, and capillary refill $\leq$3 seconds.

- Review test results of white blood cells (WBC), coagulation profile, creatinine, stool for occult blood, serum amylase, gastric analysis, serum electrolytes, radiography, and endoscopy.
- Maintain bed rest with the head of bed elevated to help prevent further bleeding and to decrease the risk of aspiration.
- Obtain and report hemodynamic parameters suggesting fluid volume deficit: CO $\leq$4 L/min, CI $\leq$2.7 L/min/m^2, and CVP $\leq$2 mm Hg.
- Obtain and report clinical findings associated with fluid volume deficit: hypotension,

tachycardia, peripheral pulses $\leq$+2, capillary refill $\geq$3 seconds, epigastric pain, and hyperactive bowel sounds.
- Obtain and report clinical findings associated with perforation of the gastric mucosa as a complication of peptic ulcer: abrupt onset of abdominal tenderness, abdominal rigidity, and absence of bowel sounds.
- Measure daily weight, intake, specific gravity, and UO. Report UO $\leq$30 mL/h.
- Encourage patient to avoid exertion so that intra-abdominal pressure can be decreased, thereby decreasing bleeding.
- Insert prescribed NG tube and perform gastric lavage. Avoid using iced saline, since it may free hydrochloride acid to diffuse back into the submucosa and increase bleeding.
- Collect gastric contents and obtain gastric pH for antacid administration. Irrigate the NG tube with 10 to 15 mL normal saline, clamp tube for 30 minutes, and institute suction for 30 minutes before obtaining a sample for pH analysis.
- Administer prescribed antacids orally or titrated via NG tube to maintain gastric pH $\geq$5.0.
- Administer prescribed oxygen 2 to 4 L/min by nasal cannula or mask to enhance tissue oxygenation.
- Administer prescribed lactated Ringer's, normal saline, or D$_5$W to prevent hypovolemia and blood loss between 700 and 1500 mL.
- Administer prescribed blood or blood products should blood loss be $\geq$1500 mL.
- Administer histamine H$_2$ receptor antagonists to inhibit gastric secretions: cimetidine (Tagamet) 300 mg 4 times d before meals and at bedtime or 400 mg 2 times/d; ranitidine (Zantac) PO 150 mg/12 h or 300 mg at dinnertime, IV 50 mg/6h or 8.3 mg/h by continuous infusion after an initial bolus dose of 50 mg; famotidine (Pepcid) PO 40 mg at dinnertime, IV 20 mg/12 h (see Table 5–4).
- Administer prescribed mucosal barrier agent (prostaglandin, carbenoxolone, misoprostol, sucralfate, or colloidal bismuth) to

reduce the effects of acid secretion (see Table 5–4).

- Prepare patient for sclerotherapy, which causes necrosis and sclerosis of the bleeding vessel.
- Should pharmacological therapy or endoscopic therapies be ineffective in controlling life-threatening bleeding, with a loss of 8 units of blood within 24 hours, prepare patient for surgery.
- Teach patient about the purpose of treatment or diagnostic procedures.
- Teach patient about the association of effects of alcohol, tobacco, emotional stress, and infections on the recurrence of duodenal ulcer.

Injury, high risk for damage to visceral structures or duodenum secondary to ulcer penetration through walls of viscera.

Expected Patient Outcomes. Patient is free of injury, as evidenced by absence of abdominal tenderness, absence of abdominal rigidity, normal bowel sounds, normothermia, HR ≤100 bpm, absence of pain, absence of nausea or vomiting, and RR 12 to 20 BPM.

- Review results of radiograph monitoring for free air under the diaphragm shown on comparison of supine, upright, and lateral decubitus roentgenograms.
- Review results of WBC count and abdominal roentgenograms, which may show presence of free air, confirming peritonitis resulting from perforation of the gastric mucosa.
- Monitor clinical indicators of ulcer penetration or perforation through viscera leading to peritonitis: abdominal tenderness, abdominal rigidity, and absence of bowel sounds.
- Record temperature every 1 to 2 hours when patient is febrile.
- Administer prescribed IV fluids to maintain adequate hydration.
- Administer prescribed antibiotics should peritonitis occur.

Altered tissue perfusion related to reduced blood loss or vasoconstriction secondary to bleeding.

Expected Patient Outcomes. Patient maintains adequate tissue perfusion, as evidenced by BP within patient's normal range, HR 70 to 100 bpm, absence of abdominal pain, skin warm and dry, peripheral pulses +2, capillary refill ≤3 seconds, UO ≥30 mL/h or ≥0.5 mL/kg/h, stool negative for blood, and hemoglobin and hematocrit within normal range.

- Review results of hemoglobin and hematocrit tests.
- Maintain bed rest to prevent further bleeding.
- Minimize patient's exertion because exertion increases intra-abdominal pressure and thereby increases the risk of bleeding.
- Monitor clinical indicators of tissue perfusion: BP, MAP, HR, peripheral pulses, skin color, and capillary refill.
- Report clinical findings associated with decreased tissue perfusion: hypotension, tachycardia, MAP ≤70 mm Hg, peripheral pulses ≤+2, cyanosis, and capillary refill ≥3 seconds.
- Measure intake, UO, NG tube drainage, and daily weight. Report UO ≤30 mL/h or ≤0.5 mL/kg/h.
- Test NG aspirate and stool for occult blood.
- Administer prescribed IV fluids, blood, or blood products to maintain adequate circulatory volume.
- Administer prescribed antacids, histamine blockers, or mucosal enhancers to decrease the effects of acid secretion (see Table 5–4).
- Instruct patient to report changes in the location, intensity and duration of pain.
- Teach patient regarding the association of alcohol, tobacco, emotional stress and infections on the recurrence of ulcer.

Nutrition, altered: Less than body requirements related to nausea, vomiting, or NG tube.

Expected Patient Outcome. Patient maintains adequate diet and body weight.

- Confer with nutritionist regarding the appropriate diet for patient.
- Encourage patient to begin eating the prescribed diet when bleeding subsides.
- Weigh patient daily and report weight loss 5% from baseline.
- Provide prescribed parenteral nutrition during the acute phase of bleeding.
- Teach patient the reasons for making lifestyle dietary changes, thereby avoiding foods that could contribute to ulcer formation.
- Instruct patient as to the importance of regular meals and restriction of coffee, tea, decaffeinated coffee, and alcohol.

Pain related to gastric irritation.

Expected Patient Outcome. Patient experiences absence or minimization of pain.

- Limit physical activity while patient is experiencing abdominal pain.
- Listen to patient's description of pain.
- Encourage patient to change position in bed, if not contraindicated, to reduce discomfort.
- Encourage patient to identify the origin, intensity, and duration of pain.
- Provide comfort measures until patient is ready for surgery.
- Teach patient to report any sudden change in pain: Sudden and sharp pain begins in the midepigastric area and spreads over the entire abdomen. The amount of pain depends on the amount and type of content spilled.
- Teach patient to reduce anxiety during a pain episode: meditation, progressive relaxation, or guided imagery.

Collaborative Problems

A common collaborative goal for patients with gastrointestinal ulcers is to correct gastric outlet obstruction.

Potential Complication: Gastric Outlet Obstruction.

Gastric outlet obstruction related to gastric retention, inflammation, edema, scarring and loss of chloride secondary to peptic ulcer.

Expected Patient Outcomes. Patient is free of gastric outlet syndrome, as evidenced by absence of pain, electrolytes within normal range, absence of abdominal distention and tenderness, absence of vomiting, absence of undigested food in gastric residue, absence of succession splash on pressure in the left upper quadrant, and stable body weight.

- Consult with physician as to the origin of gastric outlet syndrome: Pyloroduodenal obstruction can cause gastric dilation, gastritis, and gastric stasis.
- Review levels of serum electrolytes, blood urea nitrogen (BUN), creatinine, overnight gastric residual ≤50 mL, and serial scinti-scanning and barrium meal radiograph.
- Limit diet, since the stomach may retain undigested food.
- Obtain and report clinical findings associated with gastric outlet obstruction: vomiting late in the day, pain relieved by vomiting, anorexia, abdominal tenderness, or weight loss.
- Monitor continuous ECG to assess HR and rhythm. Document ECG rhythm strips every 2 to 4 hours or more frequently in patients with dysrhythmias.
- Evaluate patient's emesis for undigested, foul-smelling gastric contents without bile or with food that has been eaten 6 or more hours prior to vomiting episode.
- Insert NG tube to monitor the amount of residual gastric volume exceeding ≥50 mL.
- Monitor gastric contents and tolerance for NG tube clamping: absence of distention, nausea, or vomiting; normal gastric residual (60 to 120 mL); and passage of appropriate amount of fluid through stomach when 200 mL of water is given and tube is clamped (only 35 to 70 mL remain when gastric contents are aspirated at end of 2 hours).
- Monitor daily weight, intake, specific gravity, urine volume, and NG drainage.
- Evaluate patient for postprandial fullness and abdominal tenderness.

- Administer prescribed IV fluids to maintain adequate hydration and restore electrolytes.
- Administer prescribed IV H_2 receptor antagonist to reduce gastric volume and accelerate healing of active ulcers (see Table 5–4).
- Should pharmacological therapy be ineffective, prepare patient for surgery.
- Instruct patient to report postprandial fullness or abdominal distention.

DISCHARGE PLANNING

The critical care nurse will provide patient and significant other(s) verbal or written discharge notes regarding the following subjects:

1. Medications, including drug name, dosage, route, purpose, schedule, and side effects.
2. The signs and symptoms suggesting GI ulcer: nausea, vomiting, abdominal tenderness, and abdominal distention.
3. Importance of keeping all medical appointments.
4. Importance of avoiding medications that can cause gastric irritation.

■ ABDOMINAL TRAUMA

(For related information see Part I: Acute gastrointestinal bleeding, p. 513; Acute mesenteric ischemia, p. 538. Part III: Total parenteral nutrition, p. 551. See also Behavioral Deviations, Part I: p. 725).

Case Management Basis

DRG: 188 Other digestive system diagnoses, age greater than 17 with complications
LOS: 5.20 days
DRG: 189 Other digestive system diagnoses, age less than 17 without complications
LOS: 2.80 days

Definition

Abdominal trauma is attributed to blunt or penetrating injury. Blunt trauma can occur from a motor vehicle accident or physical assault and produces deceleration and compression injuries. With deceleration injuries in an automobile crash, the driver or passenger's forward motion is stopped on impact with a seat belt or other fixed structure, while the abdominal organs continue to advance within their confined space until structural impact, tear, or rupture occur. Compression injuries occur when the abdominal contents are squeezed between the vertebral column and the impacting object itself. Penetrating injuries are due to gunshot wounds and stabbings. Stab wounds to the abdomen are superficial in as many as 25% of patients and fail to penetrate the peritoneal cavity.

Pathophysiology

The abdominal wall offers very little support and protection from injury. Abdominal trauma may result in massive blood loss with subsequent hemorrhagic shock or peritoneal contamination with eventual peritonitis. There are two types of abdominal trauma, blunt and penetrating. Blunt trauma involves a crushing force that can compress the abdominal contents against the vertebral column, causing massive hemorrhage. Tearing of organs can occur as a result of deceleration in motor vehicle accidents. Damage ranging from a single organ to poly trauma can occur. Penetrating trauma of the abdomen occurs when the injury goes beyond the posterior rectus fascia or the internal oblique muscle.

Nursing Assessment

PRIMARY CAUSES
- Blunt trauma is due to seat-belt injuries, fall, motor accident, or assault with a blunt object. Penetrating trauma is caused by gunshot, stabbing, icepick, or flying missile wounds.

PHYSICAL ASSESSMENT
- Inspection: Ecchymosis, left shoulder pain (Kehr's sign) indicating splenic rupture with blood irritating the phrenic nerve,

hematomas, lacerations, abdominal or bladder distention.

- Palpation: Muscular rigidity and involuntary guarding, rebound tenderness or mass, indicating bleeding or abdominal fluid.
- Percussion: Resonance on the right flank when patient lies on left side (Ballance's sign), which indicates splenic rupture; loss of dullness over solid organs, which indicates free air; and dullness over region containing gas, which indicates presence of blood or fluid.
- Auscultation: Decreased or absent bowel sounds or bruits indicating arterial obstruction or aneurysm.

DIAGNOSTIC TEST RESULTS

Standard Laboratory Tests. (see Table 1–1, p. 3, and Table 5–1)

- Blood studies: White blood cell (WBC) count is initially elevated, with a later increase or shift to the left reflecting increased neutrophils and indicating inflammation. Reduced hemoglobin, hematocrit, and platelet levels $\leq$20,000 to 30,000 μL.
- Serum chemistry: Elevated amylase, serum glutamic-oxaloacetic transaminase (SGOT), serum glutamate pyruvate transaminase (SGPT), lactate dehydrogenase (LDH), and glucose levels.
- Stool: Occult blood.
- Urinalysis: Hematuria.

Invasive Gastrointestinal Diagnostic Procedures. (see Table 5–2)

- Angiography: Used to detect injury to spleen, liver, pancreas, duodenum, and retroperitoneal vessels.
- Computerized tomography (CT): Used in the presence of blunt trauma, since it is not sensitive to hollow viscus injuries commonly seen with penetrating trauma. CT can locate injury to the liver, spleen, and kidney as well as indicate the amount of blood present.
- Contrast duodenography: Used to diagnose stomach and duodenal injury.

- Peritoneal lavage: Used to diagnose intraperitoneal bleeding. A positive evaluation of lavage fluid is indicated by the presence of the following: amylase $\geq$100 Somogyi units/100mL. Aspiration of $\geq$10 mL gross blood; aspiration of lavage return of feces, bile, intestine, or bacteria; hematocrit $\geq$2% nonclotting blood; red blood cell (RBC) count $\geq$100,000/mm^3 (blunt trauma) or RBC $\geq$10,000/mm^3 (penetrating trauma); WBC $\geq$500/mm^3, and lavage fluid return through chest tube or Foley catheter.

Noninvasive Gastrointestinal Diagnostic Procedures. (see Table 5–3)

- Abdominal roentgenogram: Upright abdominal reveals air below the diaphragm, indicating disruption of a hollow organ, or abdominal densities associated with bleeding from solid organs. Lateral decubitus position reveals disruption of hollow organs through air along the lateral aspects of the abdomen.
- CT: Used to determine sites of bleeding and to quantify bleeding intraperitoneally and extraperitoneally.
- Sonography: Used to detect peritoneal penetration by stab wounds.
- Ultrasonography: Detects the presence of hemoperitoneum, perineal hematoma, or parenchymal injury to the liver, spleen, or kidney.

MEDICAL AND SURGICAL MANAGEMENT

PHARMACOLOGY

- Antibiotics: Abdominal trauma can cause intra-abdominal abscess, sepsis, and wound infection. Broad-spectum antibiotics can be administered postoperatively should surgery be required (see Table 1–14, p. 122).
- Analgesics: Used to alleviate pre- and postoperative pain.

FLUID THERAPY

- Crystalloids: Balanced salt solution in 0.9% normal saline (NS), lactated Ringer's is used since it traverses between the intravascular, interstitial, and intracellular spaces when membranes are intact.

- Colloids: Colloids, such as dextrose 70, hetastarch, or albumisol, exert an osmotic force to retain fluid (colloid osmotic pressure) within the intravascular space.
- Blood: Packed cells and fresh frozen plasma are used in treating traumatic shock and massive blood loss.

DIET

- Injury to the small or large intestine requires tube feedings or intraoperative placement of jejunostomy tubes.

GASTRIC INTUBATION

- NG intubation is used for gastric decompression, to assist in removal of gastric contents, to prevent accumulation of air in the GI tract, and to permit analysis of aspirated contents for blood.

AUTOINFUSION

- Autoinfusion is used to reinfuse shed blood into the patient. This allows rapid cellular and volume replacement and decreases the risk of transfusion reactions. Each autotransfusion set is used for approximately 4 hours to avoid bacterial contamination.

PNEUMATIC ANTISHOCK GARMENT

- Pneumatic antishock garment (PASG) or military antishock trousers (MAST) are used to increase external pressure, enhance venous return, increase blood volume, increase blood pressure, and splint fractures. Controversy exists regarding their efficiency, associated physiological changes, and the impact in the patient's outcome. While MAST does increase blood pressure (BP), it is not by an autotransfusion effect but rather through elevation of systemic vascular resistance.

SURGICAL INTERVENTION

- Surgical exploration and repair is required for penetrating injuries caused by stab wounds or gunshot wounds.

NURSING MANAGEMENT: NURSING DIAGNOSES AND COLLABORATIVE PROBLEMS

Nursing Diagnoses

Common nursing goals for patients with abdominal trauma are to maintain fluid balance, increase GI tissue perfusion, facilitate effective breathing pattern, promote skin integrity, foster nutritional balance, promote positive body image, minimize post-traumatic response, and reduce pain.

Fluid volume deficit related to active loss secondary to bleeding or hypovolemia resulting from injury or drainage through drainage tube.

Expected Patient Outcomes. Patient maintains adequate fluid volume, as evidenced by BP within patient's normal range, cardiac output (CO) 4 to 8 L/min, cardiac index (CI) 2.7 to 4.3 L/min/m², central venous pressure (CVP) 2 to 6 mm Hg, mean arterial pressure (MAP) ≥70 mm Hg, pulmonary capillary wedge pressure (PCWP) 6 to 12 mm Hg, heart rate (HR) ≤100 bpm, peripheral pulses +2, capillary refill ≤3 seconds, normal skin turgor, urinary output (UO) ≥30 mL/h, alertness, and normal cardiac rhythm.

- Review hemoglobin, hematocrit, serum amylase values, and CT, angiography, ultrasonography, and peritoneal lavage results.
- Limit activity to bed rest to reduce further bleeding.
- Obtain and report hemodynamic parameters associated with fluid volume deficit: CO ≤4 L/min, CI ≤2.7 L/min/m², CVP ≤2 mm Hg, and PCWP ≤6 mm Hg.
- Obtain and report clinical findings associated with fluid volume deficit: hypotension, tachycardia, pallor, peripheral pulses ≤+2, capillary refill ≥3 seconds, and poor skin turgor.
- Monitor intake, UO, NG tube drainage, blood loss, daily weight, and specific gravity. Report ≤UO 30 mL/h.
- Insert NG tube for gastric lavage.

- Measure abdominal girth for distention reflecting bleeding.
- Monitor continuous ECG to assess HR and rhythm. Document ECG rhythm strips every 2 to 4 hours or more frequently in patients with dysrhythmias.
- Document the frequency of dressing changes required by saturation with blood to estimate the amount of blood loss from wound site.
- Administer prescribed IV crystalloids 3mL/1mL blood loss or colloid or blood 1mL/1mL of blood loss, to maintain adequate circulating volume.
- Administer prescribed oxygen 2 to 4 L/min by nasal cannula or mask to provide tissue oxygenation.

Altered gastrointestinal tissue perfusion related to impaired blood flow to abdominal viscera.

Expected Patient Outcomes. Patient maintains adequate gastrointestinal tissue perfusion, as evidenced by BP within patient's normal range; MAP ≥70 mm Hg; HR ≤100 bpm; skin warm, dry, and pink; absence of visceral or organ ischemia manifested as absence of abdominal pain, normal bowel sounds, normal bowel elimination, absence of blood in gastric drainage, and flat abdomen.

- Review hematocrit, and hemoglobin values, and coagulation profile and peritoneal lavage results.
- Monitor for clinical indicators of visceral or organ ischemia: abdominal pain, abdominal distention, guarding, abdominal wall integrity, rebound tenderness, or decreased bowel sounds.
- Monitor clinical indicators of perfusion: BP, HR, MAP, skin color, peripheral pulses, or capillary refill.
- Report clinical findings associated with decreased GI tissue perfusion: hypotension, tachycardia, diaphoresis, pallor, abdominal distention, abdominal pain from peritoneal irritation, and capillary refill ≥3 seconds.

- Report absent femoral pulses, since this is indicative of aortic dissection.
- Administer prescribed IV crystalloids, colloids, or blood to maintain circulatory volume.
- Prepare patient for emergency laparotomy to determine the source of bleeding and repair the damage.
- Instruct patient to report any changes in abdominal pain.

Ineffective breathing pattern related to intrathoracic abdominal injury secondary to trauma.

Expected Patient Outcomes. Patient maintains ineffective breathing pattern, as evidenced by symmetrical chest movement, respiratory rate (RR) 12 to 20 BPM, absence of dyspnea, arterial blood gases within normal limits, absence of crackles, and HR ≤100 bpm.

- Obtain and report clinical findings associated with ineffective breathing pattern: tachycardia, tachypnea, cyanosis, asymmetrical chest movement, dyspnea, and crackles.
- Encourage patient to take deep breaths to facilitate lung expansion.
- Maintain airway patency and anticipate the necessity of ventilatory support.
- Should patient be unable to maintain effective breathing, intubate and provide ventilatory support.
- Administer prescribed oxygen 2 to 4 L/min by nasal cannula or mask to provide tissue oxygenation.

High risk of infection related to peritoneal contamination and subsequent peritonitis.

Expected Patient Outcomes. Patient is free of infection, as evidenced by normothermia; WBC ≤11,000/μL; RR 12 to 20 BPM; HR ≤100 bpm; skin dry; absence of redness, swelling, tenderness, or drainage at injury site; and wound culture negative.

- Review results of WBC count and cultures.
- Monitor temperature every 1 to 2 hours or while patient is febrile.

- Obtain and report clinical indicators of infection: tachypnea, tachycardia, fever, and diaphoresis.
- Evaluate incision, wound sites, and catheter site for redness, tenderness, swelling, or drainage.
- Obtain culture of drainage, noting its color, characteristics, and odor.
- Change dressings as prescribed, using aseptic technique. If there is more than one dressing, change separately to prevent cross contamination.
- Administer prescribed IV fluids to maintain adequate hydration.
- Administer prescribed antibiotics such as cefoxitin.
- Instruct patient to report any tenderness or drainage from wound or cannulation site.

Impaired skin integrity related to tissue disruption secondary to penetrating trauma.

Expected Patient Outcomes. Patient maintains skin integrity, as evidenced by absence of bacterial infection, proper wound healing, and intact skin.

- Provide diet high in protein or calories for tissue healing.
- Protect the skin around tubes or drains, keeping the areas clean and free from drainage.
- Should the wound become infected, remove affected tissue by irrigation or wound packing as prescribed.
- Cleanse and irrigate all open wounds following unit protocol: Irrigating removes debris and decreases bacteria causing infection.
- Inspect dressing, wound, or incision for drainage, noting the amount, color, and consistency.
- Cover sucking wound with gauze impregnated with petroleum jelly.
- Change dressing immediately when soaked with drainage or blood, using sterile technique.
- Maintain patient's body temperature, if decreased, with blankets or heated fluids.

- Prepare patient for surgical debridement if wound packing does not revitalize the tissue.

Altered nutrition: Less than body requirements related to decreased intake secondary to injured GI tract.

Expected Patient Outcome. Patient maintains adequate nutritional intake, as evidenced by stable weight within 5% of baseline.

- Consult with dietitian to estimate patient's metabolic and dietary needs.
- Review blood urea nitrogen (BUN), serum electrolyte, and serum glucose levels.
- Inspect patency of gastric or intestinal tubes to maintain decompression and healing and return bowel function.
- Change total parenteral nutrition (TPN) tubing every 48 to 72 hours.
- Record weight and maintain weight gain at ≤0.5 kg(1lb)/24 h.
- Collect urine specimens and check for glucose and acetone. If urine is 3+ or greater, obtain blood glucose via laboratory or glucometer. Report if value 200 mg/dL or greater.
- Terminate TPN gradually to prevent rebound hypoglycemia. TPN fluid can be reduced to 85 mL/h on day 1, 42 mL/h on day 2, and discontinued on day 3.
- Provide prescribed TPN to provide energy requirements of 30 to 35 kcal/kg/24 h or 2000 to 2500 kcal/24 h. The standard IV solution, 1000 mL 5% dextrose with electrolytes and water, contains 170 kcal.
- Administer prescribed insulin while patient is receiving TPN: for serum glucose (SG) 200 to 300 mg/dL administer insulin 2 U/h; for SG 300 to 400 mg/dL administer insulin 3 to 4 U/h; or SG ≥400 mg/dL administer insulin 4 to 5 U/h.

Body image disturbance related to stoma or disfiguring physical injury.

Expected Patient Outcome. Patient acknowledges body image changes.

- Consult with physician about the opportunity for patient to share with an ostomate or other individual who has had a similar experience.
- Encourage patient to express feelings, especially about the way he or she feels.
- Observe patient's reaction to the stoma or disfigurement.
- Discuss the loss or change with patient and significant others.
- Provide reliable information and reinforce information already given.
- Should loss of body part or disfigurement occur, evaluate the meaning of the loss for patient and significant others in relation to the visability of the loss and emotional investment in the affected part.
- Anticipate patient's response to the loss with denial, shock, anger, and depression.
- Assist with the resolution of a surgically created altered body image by encouraging patient to look at or touch the altered part.

Post-trauma response related to unresolved feelings about the physical trauma.

Expected Patient Outcomes. Patient verbalizes an acknowledgment of the traumatic event and begins to work through the trauma by talking about the experience.

- Consult with psychologist or psychiatric nurse clinician or specialist should patient experience severe stress reactions or depression.
- Evaluate the severity of the responses and the effects on patient's current functioning level.
- Provide a safe environment where the patient can regain control.
- Reassure patient that negative feelings are normal after experiencing a traumatic event.
- Assist patient to acknowledge the traumatic event and begin to work through the trauma by talking over the experience and expressing feelings such as fear, anger, and guilt.
- Assist individual to become involved with a support group.

Pain related to tissue or nerve damage.

Expected Patient Outcome. Absence of or reduced verbalization of pain.

- Consult with trauma physician or surgeon as to the location of damaged nerve and the expected patient response.
- Explain procedures or activities in a calm manner.
- Provide diversional activities such as conversation or concentration on breathing.
- Encourage patient to assume a position of comfort, if not contraindicated.
- Initiate back rubs to reduce discomfort.
- Encourage patient to describe the abdominal pain including type, intensity, location, and duration. Have patient evaluate pain on a scale of 1 to 10.
- Administer analgesics as prescribed.
- Instruct patient to report any changes in the location, intensity, or duration of pain.
- Teach patient stress-reduction techniques.

DISCHARGE PLANNING
The critical care nurse will provide patient and significant other(s) verbal or written discharge notes regarding the following subjects:

1. Medications, including drug name, dosage, route, purpose, schedule, and side effects.
2. Report abdominal discomfort.
3. Importance of keeping all medical appointments.
4. Importance of avoiding medications that can cause gastric irritation.

◼ ACUTE MESENTERIC ISCHEMIA

(For related information see Part I: Acute gastrointestinal bleeding, p. 513; Acute mesenteric ischemia, p. 538. Part III: Total parenteral nutrition, p. 551. Multisystem Deviations, Part I, Sepsis, p. 772)

Case Management Basis
DRG: 188 Other digestive system diagnoses, age greater than 17 with complications
LOS: 5.20 days

DRG: 189 Other digestive system diagnoses, age less than 17 without complications
LOS: 2.80 days

Definition

Acute mesenteric ischemia occurs when oxygen and nutrient supply needed to carry out essential cellular metabolic function are compromised. Injury and tissue necrosis occur at the mucosal surface and may extend to deeper layers of gastrointestinal (GI) tract tissue, which can cause complete transmural infarction and rupture.

Pathophysiology

When tissue becomes hypoxic, cellular damage and tissue necrosis occur. The damage is due to the loss of energy stores and the accumulation of toxic metabolites. The loss of blood flow leads to local tissue acidosis and anaerobic metabolism. Acidosis causes dilation of the capillaries. Increased capillary permeability causes leakage of fluid into the interstitium. The tissue swells as a result of fluid leak while mucosal cells, lacking an adequate blood supply to regenerate, slough off and expose the microvasculature to bacteria-rich intestinal content. Eventually sepsis occurs because of the increased vascular permeability and bacterial translocation. Deeper layers of the gastrointestinal tract become injured, leading to complete transmural necrosis and perforation.

Nursing Assessment

PRIMARY CAUSES

- Acute mesenteric arterial thrombosis can be due to atherosclerosis, a dissecting aortic aneurysm, or systemic vasculitis. Chronic mesenteric occlusion is caused by intestinal angina resulting from narrowing of the major splanchnic vessels, compression of blood vessels by adjacent structures, or an expanding abdominal aortic aneurysm; atherosclerotic process; anemia; and alveolar hypoventilation with reduced arterial partial pressure of oxygen (PaO_2). Nonocclusive mesenteric ischemic infarction is due to atherosclerotic changes, vasoconstriction or vasospasm of splanchnic blood vessels, vasopressors, beta-agonists, anemia, and alveolar hypoventilation with reduced PaO_2. Mesenteric venous ischemic mechanisms include idiopathic causes, appendicitis, pelvic abscess, polycythemia, carcinoma, local venous congestion or stasis of blood flow, cirrhosis, anemia, and alveolar hypoventilation with reduced PaO_2.

PHYSICAL ASSESSMENT

- Inspection: Pain is severe, cramping, and nonlocalized. Blood-tinged or bloody diarrhea or vomiting with fever can exist.
- Palpation: Abdomen may become firm. Peritoneal signs include tenderness and rigidity.
- Auscultation: Bowel sounds hyperactive, then absent.

DIAGNOSTIC TEST RESULTS

Standard Laboratory Tests. (see Cardiac Table 1–1, p. 3)

- Serum chemistry: Leukocytosis with a shift to the left, hematocrit normal or reduced, phosphate elevated, serum amylase may or may not be elevated, and lactic acid elevated.
- Serum enzymes: Elevated lactate dehydrogenase (LDH), creatine kinase (CK), serum glutamic pyruvic transaminase (SGPT) are seen late in ischemia and reflect muscle necrosis.

Invasive GI Diagnostic Procedures. (see Table 5–2, p. 516)

- Angiography: Provides direct visualization of the intestinal vasculature and can differentiate emboli, thrombi, or arterial vasospasm as the origin of ischemia.
- Barium enema: Useful in identifying ischemic injury in the large intestine. Colonic ischemia presents with thumbprint pattern, which reflects submucosal edema or hemorrhage.

- Endoscopy: Used for the early detection of colonic ischemia and provides direct visualization of the mucosal surface.
- Laparoscopy: Provides a direct inspection of the mesentery and intestinal serosal layer.
- Peritoneal fluid analysis: The appearance of white blood cells (WBC) or bacteria provides information for the diagnosis of bowel infarction.

Noninvasive GI Diagnostic Procedures. (see Table 5–3, p. 518)

- Abdominal roentgenogram: Shows a pattern suggestive of ileus or obstruction. Gas may be seen in the portal vein and is indicative of the absorption of gas-forming bacteria from the intestine into the circulation. Abdominal films may also show a pattern suggestive of ileus or obstruction.
- Computerized tomography (CT): Demonstrates superior mesenteric venous occlusion. Contrast-enhanced scans reveal a high-density vein wall surrounding a central filling defect plus associated collateral circulation.
- Tonometry: Provides an indirect measurement of intramural pH to detect acidosis secondary to GI wall changes when oxygen delivery falls below tissue need. A low pH is a metabolic reflection of intestinal ischemia in the bowel lumen. Measuring pH provides information as to the adequacy of oxygen supply related to tissue demand.
- Ultrasound: Used to examine the portal system and the inferior vena cava.

MEDICAL AND SURGICAL MANAGEMENT

PHARMACOLOGY

- Papaverine hydrochloride: A smooth-muscle relaxant that dilates arterioles and is used to improve blood flow to the mesentery. An intra-arterial catheter is placed in the area of poor perfusion under angio-graphic guidance. Papaverine is infused at 30 to 60 mg/h and continued for 12 to 48 hours (see Table 5–4).
- Thrombolytic therapy: The mesenteric arterial clot is localized by arteriography and the vessel is cannulated for selective infusion of the drug. Streptokinase is infused at a rate of 5000 U/h for up to 36 hours (see Table 1–8, p. 32).
- Anticoagulant therapy: Heparin is started to prevent new clot formation and administered after streptokinase is discontinued. Warfarin therapy can be initiated after heparin therapy is discontinued (see Table 1–8, p. 32).
- Dopamine: Used to enhance mesenteric blood flow (see Table 1–10, p. 50).
- Antibiotics: Intitiated to treat or minimize septic consequences of bacterial translocation or of perforation.

FLUID THERAPY

- Crystalloids (normal saline [NS] or lactated Ringer's) or colloids are used for fluid resuscitation.
- Dextran: Used if antiplatelet activity is desired.
- Bicarbonate therapy may be used should severe metabolic acidosis occur.

SURGICAL INTERVENTION

- The goal of surgery is revascularization of viable bowel and resection of necrotic bowel. During surgery a laser Doppler flowmeter is used to assess tissue viability. A laser is transmitted to the mucosa so that blood flow can be calculated. The technique limits the need for a second-look surgical procedure 24 to 48 hours after the initial resection. Thrombectomy and embolectomy are performed to remove vascular obstruction. Intestinal vascular bypass is likened to coronary artery bypass, in that the vascular obstruction is circumvented using native or synthetic graft material. The goal is to reestablish blood flow to the involved area.

NURSING MANAGEMENT: NURSING DIAGNOSES AND COLLABORATIVE PROBLEMS

Nursing Diagnoses

Common nursing goals for patients with acute mesenteric ischemia are to maintain fluid balance, increase GI tissue perfusion, facilitate tissue integrity, promote effective breathing pattern, and correct pain.

Fluid volume deficit related to vomiting or third spacing secondary to obstruction or increased capillary permeability.

Expected Patient Outcomes. Patient maintains adequate fluid volume, as evidenced by normal skin color and turgor; blood pressure (BP) within patient's normal range; mean arterial pressure (MAP) 70 to 100 mm Hg; heart rate (HR) ≤100 bpm; urinary output (UO) ≥30 mL/h; cardiac output (CO) 4 to 8 L/min; central venous pressure (CVP) 2 to 6 mm Hg; capillary refill ≤3 seconds; peripheral pulses +2; hemoglobin, hematocrit, and electrolytes within normal range; and normal stool.

- Review hemoglobin, hematocrit, and electrolyte values.
- Obtain and report hemodynamic parameters associated with fluid volume deficit: CO ≤4 L/min and CVP ≤2 mm Hg.
- Evaluate the adequacy of fluid therapy through specific indexes: skin temperature, UO, daily body weight, central nervous system function, blood lactate levels, and presence or absence of metabolic acidosis.
- Obtain and report other clinical findings suggestive of fluid volume deficit: hypotension, MAP ≤70 mm Hg, tachycardia, poor skin turgor, skin cool and dry, peripheral pulses ≤+2, capillary refill ≥3 seconds, and UO ≤30 mL/h or ≤0.5 mL/kg/h.
- Measure intake, output, daily weight, and specific gravity to evaluate fluid balance.
- Test stool and emesis for occult blood.

- Administer prescribed IV fluids such as crystalloids or colloids to restore circulating volume.

Altered gastrointestinal tissue perfusion related to decreased CO secondary to poor myocardial contractility.

Expected Patient Outcomes. Patient maintains adequate GI tissue perfusion, as evidenced by absence of pain, soft abdomen, positive bowel sounds, normothermia, absence of blood-tinged or bloody diarrhea, normal intraluminal fluid level, BP within patient's normal range, HR ≤100 bpm, CO 4 to 8 L/min, cardiac index (CI) 2.7 to 4.3 L/min/m², left ventricular stroke work index (LVSWI) 35 to 60 g-m/m², right ventricular stroke work index (RVSWI) 7 to 12 g-m/m², stroke index (SI) 40 to 50 mL/beat/m², and stroke volume (SV) 60 to 80 mL/beat.

- Evaluate abdomen for tenderness and distention.
- Obtain temperature every 2 hours if the patient is febrile.
- Obtain and report hemodynamic parameter contributing to decreased GI tissue perfusion: CO ≤4 L/min, CI ≤2.7 L/min/m², SV ≤60 mL/beat, LVSWI ≤35 g-m/beat/m², RVSWI ≤7.0 g-m/beat/m² and SI ≤40 mL/beat/m².
- Monitor and report other clinical findings associated with decreased GI tissue perfusion: hypotension, tachycardia, decreased or absent bowel sounds, peripheral pulses ≤+2, abdominal pain, and abdominal rigidity.
- Insert nasogastric tube to suction to relieve abdominal distention and improve intramural blood flow.
- Administer prescribed IV dextran if antiplatelet activity is desired.
- Administer prescribed oxygen 2 to 4 L/min by nasal cannula or mask to increase tissue oxygenation.
- Administer prescribed papaverine hydrochloride, a smooth muscle relaxant that dilates arterioles, is used to improve blood

flow to the mesentery. An intra-arterial catheter is positioned into the area of poor perfusion under angiographic guidance. Papaverine is infused at a rate of 30–60 mg/h for 12 to 48 hours.

- Administer prescribed concomitant anticoagulant therapy with heparin to prevent new clot formation.
- Administer prescribed thrombolytic therapy (streptokinase) to lyse clot in occluded mesenteric artery. Streptokinase can be infused via an intra-arterial catheter.
- Administer prescribed dopamine to enhance CO and subsequent mesenteric tissue perfusion.
- Should pharmacological therapy be ineffective, prepare patient for surgery such as thrombectomy, embolectomy, or intestinal vascular bypass.

Ineffective breathing pattern related to abdominal distention or abdominal pain secondary to peritoneal inflammation.

Expected Patient Outcomes. Patient maintains effective breathing pattern, as evidenced by respiratory rate (RR) 12 to 20 BPM, symmetrical chest excursion, skin warm and dry, absence of dyspnea, absence of cyanosis, HR ≤100 bpm, and arterial blood gases within normal range.

- Review arterial blood gas, hemoglobin, and hematocrit values.
- Encourage patient to assume a comfortable position when experiencing intestinal angina, to deep breathe and cough to prevent alveolar hypoventilation and stasis.
- Evaluate breathing pattern for rate, depth of excursions, symmetry of chest excursions, presence of abdominal or adventitious breath sounds, or changes in skin color.
- Report clinical findings associated with ineffective breathing pattern: tachycardia, dyspnea, shortness of breath, asymmetrical chest excursion, cyanosis, diaphoresis and tachypnea.
- Evaluate airway patency and need for ventilatory support.

- Encourage patient to turn, cough, deep breathe and use incentive spirometry to facilitate lung expansion.
- Provide prescribed oxygen 2 to 4 L/min by nasal cannula or mask to increase tissue oxygenation.

Pain related to intestinal angina.

Expected Patient Outcome. Absence of or reduced verbalization of abdominal pain.

- Place patient in a position of comfort.
- Encourage patient to describe the location, intensity, and duration of abdominal pain.
- Provide analgesics to reduce pain episode.
- Instruct patient to report changes in the intensity of pain.
- Teach patient to decrease pain through meditation, progressive relaxation, or guided imagery.

Collaborative Problems

Common collaborative goals for patients with acute mesenteric ischemia are to minimize reperfusion injury, correct dysrhythmias, and correct thromboembolism.

Potential Complication: Reperfusion Injury. Reperfusion injury related to injury to the microvascular and parenchymal tissue.

Expected Patient Outcome. Patient experiences minimal or no reperfusion injury.

- Review results of WBC count, especially polymorphonuclear leukocytes, which mediate the increased vascular permeability.
- Limit physical activity to bed rest until abdominal pain subsides.
- Monitor and report reoccurrence of abdominal cramping pain and abdominal tenderness resulting from formation of reactive oxygen metabolites. The oxidants damage tissue and cause cell lysis.
- Evaluate abdomen for tenderness, distention, or rigidity.
- Provide nasogastric suction and decompression to relieve vomiting and reduce abdominal distention.

- Administer prescribed investigational medications (allopurinal or superoxide dismutase) to eliminate reactive oxygen metabolites, thereby minimizing reperfusion injury.
- Administer investigational medications (iron chelates or monoclonal antibody 1B4) which interferes with polymorphonuclear leukocyte infiltration and adherence to the microvasculature.
- Administer prescribed antibiotics should bowel infection occur.
- Administer prescribed IV fluid to maintain hydration and adequate circulatory volume.
- Prepare patient for intestinal resection and possible second operation 6 to 24 hours after revascularization. Pure emboli in patients without atherosclerosis seldom require a second surgery; however some venous occlusions and almost all atherosclerotic thrombi require second surgery.
- Prepare patient for embolectomy, endarterectomy, or bypass grafting: used in superior mesenteric artery occlusion or nonocclusive mesenteric ischemia or infarction.

Potential Complication: Dysrhythmias. Dysrhythmias related to coronary artery disease and electrolyte imbalance.

Expected Patient Outcome. Patient maintains normal sinus rhythm.

- Review results of 12-lead ECG and serum electrolyte and serum enzyme levels.
- Monitor continuous ECG to assess HR and rhythm. Document ECG rhythm strips every 2 to 4 hours or more frequently in patients with dysrhythmias.
- Administer prescribed IV fluids and electrolytes to maintain hydration and correct electrolyte imbalance.
- Administer prescribed oxygen 2 to 4 L/min by nasal cannula or mask to increase tissue oxygenation.
- Administer prescribed antidysrhythmic agents should patient have underlying cardiac insufficiency and dysrhythmias (see Table 1–11, p. 54).

- Instruct patient to report chest pain and evaluate it on a scale of 1 to 10.

Potential Complication: Thromboembolism. Thromboembolism related to low flow secondary to a vessel lumen narrowed by arteriosclerotic disease, vasospasm, or vessel constriction.

- Review results of coagulation studies.
- Obtains and report clinical findings associated with mesenteric thromboembolism: abdominal pain, abdominal rigidity, absence of bowel sounds, and fever.
- Administer prescribed papaverine hydrochloride via intra-arterial catheter positioned in the area of poor tissue perfusion to improve blood flow to the mesentery.
- Administer prescribed concomitant anticoagulant therapy with heparin to prevent new clot formation.
- Administer prescribed thrombolytic therapy (streptokinase) to lyse clot in occluded mesenteric artery. Streptokinase can be infused via an intra-arterial catheter (see Table 1–8, p. 32).

DISCHARGE PLANNING

The critical care nurse will provide patient and significant other(s) verbal or written discharge notes regarding the following subjects:

1. Medications, including drug name, dosage, route, purpose, schedule, and side effects.
2. Importance of reporting any changes in bowel habit, abdominal pain, or abdominal distention.
3. Importance of keeping all medical appointments.
4. Importance of maintaining a postoperative activity program if not contraindicated, to minimize risk of thromboembolism.

■ PERITONITIS

(For related information see Part I: Acute gastrointestinal bleeding, p. 513); Abdominal trauma, p. 533; Acute mesenteric ischemia, p. 538. Part III: Total parenteral nutrition, p. 551).

Case Management Basis

DRG: 188 Other digestive system diagnoses, age greater than 17 with complications
LOS: 5.20 days
DRG: 189 Other digestive system diagnoses, age less than 17 without complications
LOS: 2.80 days

Definition

Peritonitis is an inflammation of the lining of the peritoneum and may be caused by bacterial invasion or chemical irritation.

Pathophysiology

The local reaction of the peritoneum to contamination involves vascular dilatation and increased capillary permeability. Polymorphonuclear leukocytes pour into the peritoneal cavity. Phagocytosis of bacteria and any foreign material is carried out by polymorphonuclear leukocytes. Peritoneal irritation is a chemical reaction from the spillage of digestive enzymes. The irritation stimulates vascular dilatation, hyperemia, and a fluid shift. Toxins and bacteria are absorbed into the bloodstream, leading to septicemia and bacteremia. A fluid shift occurs from the extracellular fluid compartment into the free peritoneal space, into the loose connective tissue, and into the lumen of the atonic gastrointestinal tract. The translocation of water, electrolytes, and protein into the peritoneal (third) space compartment depletes the circulatory blood volume.

Nursing Assessment

PRIMARY CAUSES

- Gangrene of the bowel from strangulation, obstruction, mesenteric ischemia, perforated peptic ulcer, ruptured appendix, ruptured diverticulum, penetrating abdominal trauma, *Escherichia coli,* abscess, fibrin clot, bile, pancreatitis, neoplastic disease, *Streptococcus, Staphylococcus, Pneumococcus, Pseudomnas aeruginosa,* and *Clostridium perfringens.*

RISK FACTORS

- Inflammatory processes such as diverticulitus, appendicitis, Crohn's disease, diabetes, malignancy, malnutrition, and advanced age.

PHYSICAL ASSESSMENT

- Inspection: Malaise, nausea, anorexia, vomiting, septic fever, abdominal pain, coughing, rebound tenderness, muscle rigidity, involuntary guarding, abdominal distention, fever, or chills.
- Palpation: Rigidity of abdominal wall.
- Percussion: Tenderness to light percussion over the inflamed peritoneum.
- Auscultation: Diminished to absent bowel sounds; tachycardia; shallow, rapid respiration.

DIAGNOSTIC TEST RESULTS

Standard Laboratory Tests

- Serum chemistry: Elevated leukocyte level, especially polymorphonuclear cells. Reduced electrolytes or albumin.

Invasive Gastrointestinal Diagnostic Procedures. (see Table 5–2, p. 516)

- Abdominal tap: Peritoneal paracentesis is used to obtain ascitic fluid for amylase and protein measurement, culture, and cytologic examination.
- Barium enema: Used to determine whether large bowel obstruction is present.

Noninvasive Gastrointestinal Diagnostic Procedures. (see Table 5–3, p. 518)

- Abdominal roentgenogram: Used to visualize gas and fluid collection in both the large and small bowel with generalized dilatation. Demonstrates the amount of abdominal distention, inflammation, and edema of the intestinal wall.
- Computerized tomography: Used to visualize abscesses.
- Ultrasonography: Used to locate small amounts of localized fluid.

MEDICAL AND SURGICAL MANAGEMENT

PHARMACOLOGY

- Antibiotics: Aerobic organisms can be treated with aminoglycosides. Anaerobic bacteria treatment includes clindamycin, chloramphenicol, or metronidazole. Penicillins are used for enterococcal infection (see Table 5–4, p. 518).
- Narcotic analgesics: Given cautiously to avoid alteration in gastrointestinal motility and depressed breathing.

FLUID THERAPY

- Colloids: Plasma or albumin can be used to replace decreased intravascular proteins.
- Crystalloids: Ringer's lactate and 5% dextrose in water (D_5W) are used for fluid resuscitation.

NASOGASTRIC TUBE

- Used to prevent abdominal distention secondary to fluid accumulation in the atonic bowel. Also can be used to provide enteral nutrients when bowel sounds improve.

PERITONEAL IRRIGATION

- Peritoneal irrigation can be used during surgery or postoperatively to decrease mortality and morbidity from acute diffuse peritonitis.

SURGICAL INTERVENTION

- Colostomy may be required when peritonitis is due to perforation of the colon. The procedure diverts the fecal stream. The colostomy following peritonitis is often temporary.

NURSING MANAGEMENT: NURSING DIAGNOSES AND COLLABORATIVE PROBLEMS

Nursing Diagnoses

Common nursing goals for patients with peritonitis are to restore fluid balance, promote tissue integrity, maintain normothermia, maintain adequate nutritional state, and promote activity tolerance.

Fluid volume deficit related to third spacing of fluid secondary to peritoneal inflammation.

Expected Patient Outcomes. Patient maintains adequate fluid volume, as evidenced by blood pressure (BP) within patient's normal range, central venous pressure (CVP) 2 to 6 mm Hg, mean arterial pressure (MAP) 70 to 100 mm Hg, pulmonary capillary wedge pressure (PCWP) 6 to 12 mm Hg, heart rate (HR) ≤100 bpm, respiratory rate (RR) 12 to 20 BPM, skin turgor normal, capillary refill ≤3 seconds, peripheral pulses +2, urinary output (UO) ≥30 mL/h, and serum protein within normal range.

- Review serum protein and electrolyte values.
- Place patient in a semi-Fowler's position to assist in localizing the infection.
- Obtain and report hemodynamic parameters associated with fluid volume deficit: cardiac output (CO) ≤4 L/min, cardiac index (CI) ≤2.7 L/min/m², CVP ≤2 mm Hg, and PCWP ≤6 mm Hg.
- Obtain and report other clinical findings associated with fluid volume deficit: hypotension, tachycardia, tachypnea, poor skin turgor, MAP ≤70 mm Hg, peripheral pulses ≤+2, and capillary refill ≤3 seconds.
- Measure or estimate all fluid loss: oral, parenteral IV, or irrigation intake; and output from urine, tube drainage, catheters, and drains.
- Measure daily weight to evaluate balance between intake and output.
- Provide oxygen by Venturi mask or nasal cannula at the prescribed amount: Oxygen can help to decrease intestinal anoxia and facilitate diffusion of nitrogen from the intestine to the blood.
- Administer prescribed IV crystalloids or colloids to maintain adequate circulatory volume.

Impaired tissue integrity related to abscess formation in pelvis, subphrenic space, and in the abdomen.

Expected Patient Outcomes. Patient maintains tissue integrity, as evidenced by no abscess formation, absence of nausea or vomiting, normothermia, flat abdomen, and negative cultures.

- Consult with physician regarding potential formation of a peritoneal abscess.
- Review results of white blood cell (WBC) count; cultures; serum albumin, hemoglobin, hematocrit, and electrolyte values; or CT scan.
- Limit physical activity to bed rest in semi-Fowler's position while patient is febrile and complaining of abdominal pain in order to localize the infection.
- Monitor and report clinical indicators of abscess: fever, chills, pain, abdominal distention, elevated and fixed diaphragm in right subphrenic abscess.
- Monitor temperature every 2 to 4 hours while patient is febrile.
- Prepare patient for the surgical drainage of abscess.
- Administer IV fluids as prescribed to maintain adequate hydration.
- Administer antibiotics as prescribed.

Hyperthermia related to peritoneal inflammation, gastroduodenal perforation, or abscess.

Expected Patient Outcome. Patient is afebrile.

- Review results of WBC count and cultures.
- Inspect skin that comes in contact with the hypothermic blanket every 2 hours for evidence of tissue damage caused by local vasoconstriction.
- While using hypothermic blanket, evaluate patient's temperature frequently to anticipate a sudden decrease leading to shivering, increase in metabolic rate, and a subsequent rise in temperature.
- Check all wounds, tubes, catheters, and drains for redness, swelling, tenderness, or unusual drainage.
- Pack open wounds using sterile technique.
- Provide prescribed continuous irrigation of the peritoneal cavity using sterile technique.

- When not using hypothermic blanket, turn patient to facilitate gravity drainage from drains.
- Insert nasogastric tube to alleviate abdominal distention should paralytic ileus develop.
- Provide prescribed hypothermic blanket, if necessary, when temperature ≥38.9°C (102°F) and patient is unresponsive to antipyretics.
- Administer IV fluids and electrolytes to maintain hydration and electrolyte balance.
- Administer prescribed antipyretics for temperature ≥38.9°C (102°F).
- Administer prescribed antibiotics such as penicillin, sulfonamides, kanamycin, neomycin, polymyxin, and chloramphenicol (see Table 5–4).
- Teach patient the reasons for elevated temperature and need for hypothermic blanket.

Altered nutrition: Less than body requirement related to nausea, vomiting, or paralytic ileus.

Expected Patient Outcome. Patient maintains normal body weight and normal nitrogen balance on nitrogen studies.

- Consult with dietitian regarding patient's diet.
- Review serum electrolyte, albumin, blood urea nitrogen (BUN), and creatinine values.
- Insert nasogastric tube to maintain nothing by mouth (NPO) status until patient is able to tolerate gradual advancement in foods.
- Measure abdominal girth should abdominal distention as a result of ileus.
- Monitor bowel sounds every 1 to 8 hours and report any sudden absence or return.
- Ensure that the nasogastric, intestinal, and other GI drainage tubes are patent.
- Evaluate output from drainage tubes for occult blood.
- When peritonitis subsides and bowel sounds return, prepare patient for enteral feedings.
- Should gastric ulcers be the cause of peritonitis, administer prescribed antacids and

histamine H_2 antagonist to decrease gastric acid secretion.

- Assist with the insertion of Miller-Abbott tube: In paralytic ileus, the intestinal tract is decompressed through use of a long intestinal tube.
- Administer antacids and histamine H_2 antagonists to reduce the corrosiveness of gastric acid (see Table 5–4).

Activity intolerance related to pain or weakness.

Expected Patient Outcome. Patient tolerates gradual increases in activity.

- Encourage gradual increases in physical activity when patient is afebrile and free of abdominal pain.
- Monitor BP, HR, RR, cardiac rhythm, and presence of abdominal pain while gradually increasing physical activity.
- Provide rest period before and after gradual increase in physical activity: out of bed, sit in chair, ambulate in room, and ambulate in hallway.
- Instruct patient to report any weakness or abdominal pain while increasing physical activity.

Collaborative Problem

A common collaborative goal for patients with peritonitis is to restore electrolyte balance.

Potential Complication: Electrolyte Imbalance. Electrolyte imbalance related to vomiting, nasogastric suction, or transudation of fluid.

Expected Patient Outcome. Patient maintains electrolyte balance, as evidenced by normal sinus rhythm, absence of abdominal distention, and serum electrolytes within normal range.

- Review results of serum electrolytes.
- Obtain and report clinical findings associated with electrolyte imbalance resulting from translocation of fluid into the peritoneal space: abdominal pain, abdominal distention, tachycardia, and jugular vein distention.
- Monitor continuous ECG to assess HR and rhythm in patients who may experience hypokalemia.
- Measure daily weight, intake, nasogastric output, and urinary output.
- Administer prescribed IV crystalloids or colloids to maintain adequate hydration and reduce translocation of fluids into the peritoneal space.
- Administer prescribed parenteral electrolytes to replace electrolytes lost in the peritoneal space.

DISCHARGE PLANNING

The critical care nurse will provide patient and significant other(s) verbal or written discharge notes regarding the following subjects:

1. Medications, including drug name, dosage, route, purpose, schedule, and side effects.
2. Signs and symptoms associated with infection: fever; drainage from surgical site; and swelling, tenderness, or redness surrounding surgical incision.
3. Importance of keeping all medical appointments.
4. Importance of seeking medical attention should signs and symptoms associated with adhesions occur: pain, persistent vomiting, or abdominal distention.

PART II: SURGICAL CORRECTION AND NURSING MANAGEMENT

■ GASTRIC SURGERY

(For related information see Part I: Acute gastrointestinal bleeding, p. 513; Gastrointestinal ulcers, p. 527. Part III: Total parenteral nutrition, p. 551.)

Case Management Basis
DRG: 148 Major small and large bowel procedures with complications
LOS: 13.50 days
DRG: 149 Major small and large bowel procedures without complications
LOS: 8.90 days

Definition
Gastric surgery is considered for patients who have massive bleeding despite the use of medical therapy. Surgical options include gastric oversew, antrectomy, vagotomy, pyloroplasty, Billroth I, and Billroth II.

Patient Selection

INDICATIONS. Gastric surgery is used in patients when medical therapy does not heal the ulcer, when ulcer recurrence becomes a problem, when a malignancy is suspected, or when complications occur.

CONTRAINDICATIONS. If patient is a poor surgical risk.

Procedure

TECHNIQUE. Gastric oversew involves suture ligation of the bleeding vessel and closure of the ulcer crater. The procedure is used for a subcardial gastric ulcer. Antrectomy is performed for duodenal ulcers to decrease the acidity of the duodenum by removing the gastric-acid–secreting cells in the antrum. The antrum of the stomach is removed and the remaining portion of the stomach is anastomosed to the duodenum. A vagotomy decreases acid secreting cells in the stomach by dividing the vagus nerve along the esophagus. There are three types of vagotomies: (1) Truncal vagotomy denervates stomach, upper abdominal organs, and intestine to the left flexure of the colon. (2) Selective gastric vagotomy denervates the stomach only and weakens motility of the antrum. (3) Proximal cell vagotomy denervates only the proximal, acid-producing portion of the stomach, while innervation and motility of the antrum are undisturbed. A pyloroplasty can be performed with a vagotomy to prevent stomach atony. Resection is achieved by either a Billroth I or Billroth II operation. In the Billroth I procedure, the distal portion of the stomach is removed with an anastomosis of the proximal portion to the duodenum (gastroduodenostomy). The Billroth II procedure consists of removing the lower portion of the stomach, with anastomosis to the jejunum (gastrojejunostomy). Billroth II is used to treat duodenal ulcer.

Complications
Postoperative complications include wound infection, dehiscence and evisceration, hemorrhage, peritonitis, pancreatitis, anastomotic leak, duodenal stump leak, afferent loop syndrome, stomach wall necrosis, postoperative enteritis or necrosis, subphrenetic and subhepatic abscesses, postoperative jaundice, or gastric retention.

NURSING MANAGEMENT: NURSING DIAGNOSES AND COLLABORATIVE PROBLEMS

Nursing Diagnoses
Common nursing goals for patients undergoing gastric surgery are to restore fluid balance, maintain adequate nutrition, prevent infection, maintain skin integrity, and reduce pain.

Fluid volume deficit related to anastomotic leak secondary to a clogged nasogastric (NG) tube increasing pressure at the site of the anastomosis.

Expected Patient Outcomes. Patient maintains adequate fluid volume, as evidenced by blood pressure (BP) within patient's normal range, mean arterial pressure (MAP) 70 to 100 mm Hg, heart rate (HR) ≤ 100 bpm, respiratory rate (RR) 12 to 20 BPM, central venous pressure (CVP) 2 to 6 mm Hg, urinary output (UO) ≥ 30 mL/h, skin turgor normal, capillary refill ≤3 seconds, peripheral pulses ≤+2, absence of blood in gastrointestinal (GI) drainage, and hemoglobin and hematocrit within normal limits.

- Confer with physician about the amount and type of NG drainage postoperatively. Gastric drainage can be bright red immediately postoperatively; drainage is dark-red within 12 hours postoperatively; and green-yellow within 24 to 36 hours postoperatively.
- Review hemoglobin, hematocrit, serum electrolyte, and serum albumin values.
- Obtain and report clinical findings associated with fluid volume deficit: tachycardia, hypotension, peripheral pulses ≤+2, capillary refill ≥3 seconds, poor skin turgor, or ≥300 mL bloody NG tube drainage within 24 hours.
- Obtain and report changes in NG tube drainage such as ≥300 mL bloody drainage/ 24 h or failure of drainage to occur, signifying a clogged tube.
- Measure intake, output, and daily weight to determine fluid balance.
- Maintain patency of the tube to prevent undue pressure on the suture line. Do not manipulate or irrigate tubes without a physician's order.
- Measure daily weight, as a change in weight of 1 kg reflects a fluid loss or gain of 1 liter.
- Administer prescribed crystalloids or blood products to correct intravascular volume and replace blood loss.
- Administer prescribed vitamin B₁₂ supplements to patients undergoing a total gastrectomy to prevent pernicious anemia.
- Administer prescribed antiemetics to prevent vomiting and maintain suture line.
- Should an anastomotic leak occur, report clinical findings of sudden pain, fever, chills, and tachycardia.
- Should an anastomotic leak, peritonitis, cellulitis, or abscess develop, prepare patient for surgery.
- Instruct patient to report any bleeding from incision site.

Altered nutrition: Less than body requirement related to nutritional deficiency or fluid restriction.

Expected Patient Outcome. Patient maintains adequate nutritional intake, as evidenced by daily weight within 5% of baseline and nitrogen balance.

- Consult with physician about patient's daily nutritional requirements.
- Consult with a dietitian, when appropriate, regarding patient's dietary program.
- Review blood urea nitrogen (BUN) and creatinine levels.
- Provide prescribed enteral nutrition.
- Evaluate bowel sounds and passage of flatus every 4 to 8 hours.
- Insert prescribed NG tube to decompress the stomach, to prevent undue pressure on the suture line, or to test gastric contents for blood and pH. The NG tube is not manipulated or irrigated unless ordered.
- Administer small amount of water via NG tube as prescribed when bowel sounds return, indicating the return of peristalsis.
- Aspirate stomach 2 hours after last feeding. Report contents ≥100 mL, pain, distention, or nausea.
- Initiate prescribed oral fluids by offering 5 to 10 mL of water, then gradually increase the amount until 90 to 120 mL is tolerated by patient.
- Discontinue feeding and report if pain, nausea, distention, or vomiting occur.
- Obtain and report clinical findings associated with dumping syndrome secondary to rapid passage of a hypertonic bolus of food into the jejunum, causing an osmotic shift of fluid into the bowel: abdominal distention, vertigo, palpitations, sweating, and diarrhea. One to 3 hours later patients may experience diaphoresis, vertigo, and headache.
- Measure all intake.
- Progress diet, as prescribed, to small, frequent meals of soft foods. Avoid milk as it can cause dumping syndrome.
- Administer IV fluids as prescribed to maintain adequate fluid volume: Dumping syndrome can lead to the withdrawal of fluid

from the extracellular fluid compartment into the lumen of the bowel, thus decreasing plasma volume.

- Administer prescribed vitamin supplements in gastric resection patients, since the absorption of vitamins can lead to pernicious anemia. Administer prescribed iron, folic acid, calcium, and vitamins D and B_{12}.
- Teach patient the intestinal manifestation of dumping syndrome: epigastric fullness, distention, discomfort, abdominal cramping, nausea, or vomiting.
- Teach patient to eat small, frequent meals.
- Instruct patient to avoid high-carbohydrate foods, restrict fluids with meals, and rest after meals.

Infection, high risk for related to incision or cannulation site.

Expected Patient Outcomes. Patient is free of infection, as evidenced by normothermia, negative cultures, white blood cell (WBC) count ≤11,000/μL, or absence of drainage from incision from stomal or cannulation site.

- Review results of WBC count and cultures.
- Monitor temperature every 2 to 4 hours or as necessary while the patient is febrile.
- Monitor and report clinical findings associated with infection: redness, swelling, tenderness, or drainage from incison, stoma, or cannulation site.
- Use sterile technique when manipulating GI tubes, surgical dressings, and indwelling lines.
- Palpate patient's abdomen for tenderness, rigidity, or distention that could indicate the presence of peritonitis.
- Administer IV fluids at the prescribed amount to maintain adequate hydration.
- Administer prescribed antipyretics when patient is febrile.
- Administer prescribed antibiotics should infection occur.
- Instruct patient to report any drainage for incision or pain.

Impaired skin integrity related to stomal drainage.

Expected Patient Outcome. Integrity of patient's skin maintained.

- Check dressings and incision for drainage every 4 hours. Reinforce and change dressing as needed.
- Protect the integrity of the skin during frequent dressing changes by using Montgomery straps. Use an abdominal binder to protect the wound.
- Evaluate skin around stoma for edema and swelling.
- Clean peristomal skin with soap and water, with an appropriate skin barrier film applied before a pouch is applied.
- Measure contents of pouch and drain when it is one third full to minimize the chance of leakage.
- Use sterile technique when changing dressings.
- Assess the incision for redness, swelling, tenderness, or drainage.
- Obtain prescribed culture of wound drainage.
- Administer prescribed IV fluids to maintain adequate hydration.
- Administer prescribed antipyretic agents should patient become febrile.
- Administer prescribed antibiotics to treat infection.
- Instruct patient to note any redness or swelling of the skin or stoma.

Pain related to incision.

Expected Patient Outcomes. Absence of or diminished verbalization of pain.

- Encourage patient to describe the location, intensity, and duration of pain.
- Administer analgesics as prescribed.
- Teach patient alternative strategies to cope with any pain: meditation, progression relaxation, or guided imagery.

Collaborative Problems

Common collaborative goals for patients undergoing gastric surgery are to improve gastric function and prevent afferent loop syndrome.

Potential Complication: Impaired Gastric Function. Impaired gastric function related to acute gastric distention and delayed gastric emptying.

Expected Patient Outcomes. Patient maintains adequate gastric function, as evidenced by absence of epigastric pain, HR $\leq$100 bpm, BP within patient's normal range, absence of rebound tenderness or rigidity, absence of fullness or hiccups, electrolytes and total protein within normal range.

- Review serum electrolytes and protein values.
- Obtain and report clinical findings associated with acute gastric dilatation: epigastric pain, tachycardia, hypotension, feelings of fullness, hiccups, or gagging.
- Insert prescribed NG tube or clear plugged tube to correct distention of the stomach or edema at the anastomosis or adhesions obstructing the distal loop.
- Evaluate patient's respirations for rate and depth: Gastric dilatation can occur when patient swallows inspired air, causing the stomach to become distended. This can affect the paitent's respiratory rate and depth.
- Monitor patient with potential gastric dilatation fluid status as fluid may accumulate in stomach, leading to dehydration and a decrease in plasma volume: BP, skin turgor, MAP, HR, UO, and capillary refill.
- Administer prescribed IV fluids to maintain adequate hydration and circulatory volume.
- Instruct patient to report epigastric pain or feelings of fullness.

Potential Complication: Afferent Loop Syndrome. Afferent loop syndrome related to pancreatic secretion and bile filling the afferent loop of the duodenum secondary to obstruction or stress of the afferent loop.

Expected Patient Outcome. Patient is free from afferent loop distention.

- Obtain and report clinical findings associated with afferent loop syndrome: vomiting, feeling of fullness, epigastric pain, and diarrhea if the condition persists.

- Provide prescribed low-fat diet.
- Place patient in position of comfort to reduce feelings of fullness.
- Measure the amount and content of emesis.
- Should afferent loop syndrome not improve with low-fat diet, prepare patient for surgery.

DISCHARGE PLANNING

The critical care nurse will provide patient and significant other(s) verbal or written discharge notes regarding the following subjects:

1. Medications, including drug name, dosage, route, purpose, schedule, and side effects.
2. Signs and symptoms associated with infection: fever, drainage from surgical site, and swelling, tenderness, or redness surrounding surgical incision.
3. Importance of eating small, frequent meals at regular intervals; avoiding high-fiber foods, sugar, salt, caffeine, alcohol, milk, and tobacco; taking fluids between meals, not with meals.
4. Measuring weight every 2 to 4 days.
5. Signs and symptoms of dumping syndrome: epigastric pain, weakness, nausea, vomiting after eating.
6. Importance of keeping all medical appointments.
7. Importance of adequate rest and exercise with planned rest periods.

....

PART III: SUPPORTIVE PROCEDURES AND NURSING MANAGEMENT

....

■ TOTAL PARENTERAL NUTRITION

(For related information see Part I: Acute gastrointestinal bleeding, p. 513; Abdominal trauma, p. 533; Acute mesenteric ischemia, p. 538; Peritonitis, p. 543. Part II: Gastric surgery, p. 547.)

Definition

Total parenteral nutrition (TPN) or hyperalimentation is the intravenous administration of varying combinations of hypertonic glucose, amino acids, lipids, electrolytes, vitamins, and trace elements.

Patient Selection

INDICATIONS. Patients with burns, multisystem trauma, extensive surgery, sepsis, diseases of the small intestine, radiation enteritis, severe diarrhea, intractable vomiting, high-dose chemotherapy, pancreatitis, enterocutaneous fistula, inflammatory bowel disease, inflammatory adhesions with small-bowel obstruction, or malnutrition.

CONTRAINDICATIONS. When TPN is required for ≤ 5 days, a functional and stable gastrointestinal (GI) tract capable of absorption of adequate nutrition, a prognosis that does not warrant aggressive nutritional support, or when aggressive nutritional support is not wanted by the individual or legal guardian.

Procedure

TECHNIQUE. The TPN solution can have an osmolality of 1700 to 2200 µmol/L. The concentrated solution can be administered by the central venous route into a high-flow vessel to reduce the threat of venous irritation or clinical phlebitis. The catheter is usually inserted into the right subclavian or internal jugular vein and threaded into the superior vena cava outside the right atrium. Other veins used for central venous insertion sites include the external jugular, and the cephalic and basilic veins. Peripheral parenteral nutrition (PPN) is used when patients are receiving suboptimal oral nutrition for short-term requirements. To prevent thrombophlebitis, concentration of glucose does not exceed 10% to 12.5%.

EQUIPMENT. Central venous tunneled catheters such as Hickman, Boviac, or Hickman-Broviac catheter; peripherally inserted central catheter (PICC): such as 1 long-line catheter; or implanted venous access ports such as Medi-Port, Port-a-Cath, Infuse-a-Port or Groshong catheter.

Complications

Metabolic complications include hypoglycemia, rebound hypoglycemia, protein intolerance, and hyperchloremic metabolic acidosis. Electrolyte imbalance complications are hyperkalemia, hypokalemia, hypermagnesemia, hypomagnesemia, hypercalcemia, hypocalcemia, hyperphosphatemia, hypophosphatemia, allergy to fat emulsions, hypervolemia, hypovolemia, or excessive weight gain. Septic complications consist of bacteremia, candidemia, catheter entrance site infection, solution-related sepsis, or septic thrombosis.

NURSING MANAGEMENT: NURSING DIAGNOSES AND COLLABORATIVE PROBLEMS

Nursing Diagnoses

Common nursing goals for patients receiving TPN are to maintain adequate nutrition, prevent infection, and prevent injury.

Altered nutrition: less than body requirements related to inability to ingest or absorb nutrients.

Expected Patient Outcomes. Patient maintains adequate nutrition, as evidenced by weight change 0.50 kg (1 lb) or less/24 h, serum albumin 3.5 to 5.5 g/dL, prealbumin 15.7 to 29.6 mg/mL, transferrin 250 to 300 mg/dL, serum creatinine 0.6 to 1.6 mg/dL, 24-hour urinary creatinine 500 to 1200 mg/d, 24-hour urinary urea nitrogen ≤ 5 g/d, retinol-binding protein 40 to 50 µg/mL, nitrogen balance, blood urea nitrogen (BUN) 8 to 23 mg/dL, and total lymphocyte count $\leq 1500/mm^3$.

- Consult with physician about the amount of TPN to be given each day, depending on patient's needs.
- Review values for serum albumin, prealbumin, transferrin, serum creatinine, retinol-

binding protein, BUN, total lymphocytes, 24-hour urinary creatinine, and 24-hour urinary urea nitrogen.

- Regulate the prescribed volume and concentration of TPN and increase gradually according to fluid and glucose tolerance.
- Collect urine specimen and check for glucose and acetone every 6 hours or more frequently depending on the TPN calories infused. Report if urine is 3+ or greater and blood glucose is ≥200 mg/dL.
- Should patient receive high-calorie (3300) TPN infusion because of massive trauma or burns, larger doses of insulin may be required.
- Record weight and maintain weight gain at ≤0.5 kg (1 lb)/24 h.
- Change TPN containers every 24 hours or according to unit protocol.
- Change TPN administration tubing every 48 to 72 hours or according to unit protocol.
- Terminate TPN, as prescribed, gradually to prevent rebound hypoglycemia. This occurs when patient is taking adequate enteral nutrition (two thirds of maintenance calories).
- Reduce prescribed TPN fluids to 5 mL/h on day 1, 42 mL/h on day 2, and discontinue on day 3.
- Obtain and report clinical findings associated with lipid infusions: chest or back pain, fever, shaking, chills, dyspnea, palpitations, and cyanosis.
- Use indirect calorimetry, if available, for the calculation of heat production through the measurement of oxygen consumption and carbon dioxide production. An individual's resting energy expenditure (REE) is calculated on the basis of respiratory gas exchange and can be used as a guide to caloric replacement for patient. The values for the volume of oxygen and carbon dioxide, V_{O_2} and V_{CO_2}, enable the calculation of the respiratory quotient (RQ): $RQ = V_{CO_2}/V_{O_2}$. Normally RQ is 0.67 to 1.25. A RQ ≤0.70 is found in ketosis with ketonuria. RQ ≥1.0 reflects lipogenesis seen in patients receiving glucose loads in excess of energy expenditure.

- Administer prescribed intravenous fat emulsions to provide essential fatty acids as a source of calories. Administration of lipids continuously provides continual oxidation of lipids, thereby minimizing carbohydrate utilization. Fat emulsion may not exceed 60% of the caloric intake as fat or exceed 2.5 g/kg/24 h.
- Administer prescribed continuous insulin infusion (CII) which is titrated to keep serum glucose (SG) in the range of 120 to 250 mg/dL with no glycosuria.

Infection related to invasive procedure or solution-related sepsis.

Expected Patient Outcomes. Patient is free of infection, as evidenced by normothermia; white blood cell (WBC) count ≤11,000/μL; negative cultures; and absence of redness, drainage, tenderness, swelling, or warmth at the catheter site.

- Review results of WBC count and cultures.
- Monitor and report temperature elevation; redness, swelling, tenderness, or drainage around catheter sites or wounds.
- Maintain aseptic system including all lumens of multilumen catheters.
- Change transparent, semipermeable, polyurethane film dressing (Op-Site) every 72 hours or according to unit protocol.
- Clean catheter hub connector sites to prevent infectious organisms gaining entry through line connectors.
- Change all TPN administration tubing, filters, and extension sets every 48 to 72 hours.
- Send cultures of urine, wounds, sputum, and peripheral and central blood samples for bacterial, fungal, or viral cultures as ordered.
- Administer prescribed antibiotics should patient develop an infection.
- Administer prescribed antipyretics should patient become febrile.

High risk of injury related to occlusion of central venous access device secondary to fibrin or clot formation.

Expected Patient Outcome. Patient's central venous access device (VAD) remains patent.

- Review results of coagulation studies.
- Obtain chest roentgenogram, as prescribed, to determine the position of the catheter tip before using urokinase.
- Monitor continual patency of VAD, since an occlusion can lead to infection, occlusive vascular thrombosis, or pulmonary emboli.
- Should VAD be occluded, administer prescribed urokinase to dissolve catheter clots.
- If unable to flush VAD, remove dressing and observe for kink or obstruction of catheter by sutures.
- Have patient cough, turn side to side, or raise arm over head of the affected side.
- If unable to instill flush, attempt to aspirate 3 mL to check for a blood return.
- Clamp catheter and attach 5-mL syringe with 4-mL (10 U/mL) heparin flush solution. Unclamp catheter and instill heparin.

Collaborative Problems

Common collaborative goals for patients receiving TPN are to maintain glucose balance and prevent thromboembolism.

Potential Complication: Hyperglycemia. Hyperglycemia related to hormonal changes secondary to stress, injury, or excess glucose administration.

Expected Patient Outcomes. Patient maintains glucose balance, as evidenced by absence of thirst, malaise, dry mouth, flushed skin, nausea, vomiting, or polyuria.

- Review results of serum glucose tests.
- Test urine for sugar and acetone every 6 hours.
- Obtain and report clinical findings associated with hyperglycemia: thirst, malaise, dry mouth, flushed skin, nausea, vomiting, and polyuria.
- Administer prescribed CII, which is titrated to attempt to keep the SG in the range of 120 to 250 mg/dL with no glycosuria. CII rates are administered according to the following schedule: SG 200 to 300 mg/dL, administer insulin 2 U/h; for SG 300 to 400 mg/dL, administer insulin 3 to 4 U/h; and for SG $\geq$400 mg/dL, administer insulin 4 to 5 U/h.
- Instruct patient to report signs associated with hypoglycemia.

Potential Complication: Thromboembolism. Thromboembolism related to hypertonic solution irritating the veins secondary to increased osmolarity.

Expected Patient Outcome. Patient is free of thromboembolism when PPN is used.

- Assess insertion site when PPN is used on patients receiving suboptimal oral nutrition or when it is not possible to use a subclavian vein catheter.
- Rotate peripheral infusion site every 24 to 48 hours.
- Monitor osmolarity of TPN, noting that phlebitis can occur if the infusate is $\geq$500 mOsm or if the potassium is $\geq$6.0 mEq/L.
- Monitor insertion site for inflammation and swelling, which can indicate infiltration and phlebitis.
- Inspect infusion site for redness and swelling.
- Remove catheter as ordered.
- Apply heat, as ordered, to the infusion site.
- Administer prescribed PPN, not to exceed 10% to 12.5%.
- Add prescribed lipids to PPN solutions to provide a calorie source without increasing the osmolarity of the solution. Using fats, dextrose, and proteins, supply a maximum energy of 2500 kcal/24 h through PPN.

■ ENTERAL NUTRITION

For related information see Part I: Acute gastrointestinal bleeding, p. 513; Abdominal trauma, p. 533; Acute mesenteric ischemia, p. 538; Peritonitis, p. 543. Part II: Gastric surgery, p. 547.)

Definition

Enteral feedings, or enteral nutrition, are the administration of liquid formula taken by mouth or delivered into the gastrointestinal tract through nasogastric, nasoenteric, esophagostomy, gastrostomy, or jejunostomy tube.

Patient Selection

INDICATIONS. Used in patients with protein-caloric malnutrition, major full-thickness burns, dysphagia, massive small bowel resection, in combination with TPN, radiation therapy, major trauma, liver failure, or serum renal dysfunction.

CONTRAINDICATIONS. Severe diarrhea, complete mechanical intestinal obstruction, ileus or intestinal hypomotility, high output external fistula, shock, acute pancreatitis, or patient does not desire aggressive nutritional support.

Procedure

TECHNIQUE. The enteral route includes the use of an oral-nasal gastric feeding tube, a jejunostomy tube or, for long-term use, a gastrostomy tube. A soft Silastic tube in a small French size is used.

Complications

Complications consist of aspiration, diarrhea, abdominal distention, impaired gastrointestinal (GI) motility, hypokalemia, hyponatremia, or hyperglycemia hyperosmolar nonketotic coma.

NURSING MANAGEMENT: NURSING DIAGNOSES AND COLLABORATIVE PROBLEMS

Nursing Diagnoses

Common nursing goals for patients receiving enteral feedings are to maintain fluid balance, prevent aspiration, and correct diarrhea.

Fluid volume deficit related to diarrhea or inadequate fluid volume secondary to enteral feeding.

Expected Patient Outcomes. Patient maintains adequate fluid volume, as evidenced by blood pressure (BP) within patient's normal range, heart rate (HR) ≤ 100 bpm, respiratory rate (RR) 12 to 20 BPM, urinary output (UO) ≥ 30 mL/h or ≥ 0.5 mL/kg/h, central venous pressure (CVP) 2 to 6 mm Hg, cardiac output (CO) 4 to 8 L/min, specific gravity 1.003 to 1.030, weight change ≤ 1 kg (2 lbs)/24 hours, moist mucous membranes, normal skin turgor, peripheral pulses +2, and capillary refill ≤ 3 seconds.

- Review hematocrit, serum electrolyte, blood glucose, blood urea nitrogen (BUN), creatinine values and liver function tests and nitrogen balance.
- Obtain and report hemodynamic parameters associated with fluid volume deficit: CO ≤ 4 L/min and central venous pressure (CVP) ≤ 2 mm Hg.
- Obtain and report clinical findings associated with fluid volume deficit: hypotension, tachycardia, tachypnea, weight loss, dry mucous membranes, poor skin turgor, peripheral pulses $\leq +2$, and capillary refill ≥ 3 seconds.
- Monitor oxygen consumption (Vo_2) derived from hemodynamic findings, which can be used to estimate metabolic expenditure using the formula: calorie (24 hours = $7.0 \times Vo_2$ (mL/min).
- Check UO, specific gravity, sugar, acetone, and daily weight. Report UO ≤ 30 mL/h or ≤ 0.5 mL/kg/h, specific gravity ≤ 1.003, and weight loss ≥ 0.5 to 1.0 kg/24 h.
- Monitor continuous ECG to assess HR and rhythm. Document ECG rhythm strips every 2 to 4 hours or more frequently in patients with dysrhythmias.
- Measure fluid losses through drains, emesis, and loose stools when calculating patient's fluid requirement.
- Use, if available, indirect calorimetry to estimate resting energy expenditure (REE),

use of energy substrate, protein requirements, and the respiratory quotient (RQ). Indirect calorimetry measures oxygen consumption (Vo_2) and carbon dioxide production (Vco_2). The RQ reflects the oxidation of a mixed fuel (fat, carbohydrate, and amino acids). It also reflects whether patient is well nourished (0.85), starved (0.7), or overfed (≥ 1.0).

- Provide prescribed enteral formulas, which can be classified into two main categories: modular and nutritionally complete. Modular formulas consist of one major macronutrient such as carbohydrate, protein, or fat. Nutritionally complete formula contain all the necessary macronutrients plus vitamins, minerals, and trace elements. Nutritionally complete formulas are also classified into either polymeric, predigested, or disease-specific formulas. Most enteral formulas are isotonic and provide approximately 45 g/L of protein. Some formulas used are high-fiber, low-residue, or supplements that provide extra calories.
- Monitor IV flow rates and volumes to ensure that patient is receiving the prescribed amount of calories.
- Provide recommended intake of water, 1 mL of free water for each calorie provided if not contraindicated. The usual fluid requirements are 1500 mL/m^2 or 35 mL/kg/24 h.
- Administer prescribed free water supplement to prevent dehydration. Patient may receive as much as 0.5 mL for every 1 mL of feeding.

High risk of aspiration related to intragastric administration of enteral feedings secondary to decreased gastrointestinal motility.

Expected Patient Outcome. Patient does not aspirate gastric contents.

- Review chest roentgenogram and arterial blood gas results.
- Maintain head of bed at 30 to 40-degree angle.
- Monitor the amount of gastric retention by checking for gastric residuals every 4 hours or at the beginning of each intermittent feeding. Note where the volume of aspirate does not exceed 50% of the previous feeding for intermittent feedings or 50% of the hourly infusion rate for continuous feeding.
- Use glucose oxidase reagent strips to detect presence of glucose in pulmonary secretions. Secretion ≥ 130 mg/dL of glucose is enough to discontinue the feeding.
- Auscultate breath sounds every hour and report clinical findings associated with aspiration: coughing, dyspnea, wheezing, restlessness, tachycardia, tachypnea, crackles, and fever.
- Evaluate the cuff pressure of patients with artificial airways and ensure the cuff is inflated to minimum occlusion volume of 20 to 25 cm H_2O or 15 to 18 mm Hg.
- Monitor RQ for excess carbon dioxide production. This is shown as RQ ≥ 0.8.
- Initiate small bowel feedings at 50 mL/h with full-strength isotonic solution. Gradually increase the rate, usually 25 mL every 8 hours and increase the strength of the formula.
- Initiate prescribed intragastric feedings and tube feedings with an isotonic formula. The nutrient requirement is achieved by increasing the rate over 1 to 2 days.
- Should respiratory distress occur during tube feeding, discontinue gastric feedings.
- Obtain and report gastric residuals ≥ 100 mL in continuous feedings and ≥ 150 mL in intermittent feedings.
- Irrigate the feeding tube with 50 to 150 mL of water before and after each intermittent feeding.
- Administer prescribed metoclopramide (Reglan) to increase gastric motility.

Diarrhea related to enteral feedings.

Expected Patient Outcome. Patient's stools are of normal consistency.

- Evaluate patient's tolerance to rate, osmolality, and nutrient composition of formula.
- Evaluate gastrointestinal tolerance to enteral feedings and report nausea, vomiting,

diarrhea, cramping, abdominal distention, or absence of bowel sounds.

- Monitor for presence of hyperactive bowel sounds and report passage of ≥4 bowel movements per day or a large (≥200 g) liquid stool.
- Record the consistency and number of stools per shift.
- Check small-bore tubes for gastric retention by observing for distention, palpitating for tautness of abdomen, and measuring abdominal girth every 8 hours.
- Administer prescribed IV fluids to maintain hydration in patients with diarrhea.

SELECTED REFERENCES

Bezaarro ER. Changing perspectives of H_2 antagonists for stress ulcer prophylaxis. *Crit Care Nurs Clin North Am.* 1993;5:325–331.

Boyd CR, Tolson MA. Mechanisms of abdominal trauma: implications for initial care. *Emerg Care Q.* 1988;3:22–35.

Bennington S. Surgical treatment of ulcerative colitis. *Can O R Nurs J.* 1988;6(2):20–31.

Breesler MJ. Computed tomography vs peritoneal lavage in blunt abdominal trauma. *Topics Emerg Med.* 1988;10(1):59–73.

Bruce NP. Total parenteral nutrition. In: Flynn JB, Bruce NP, eds. *Introduction to Critical Care Skills.* St. Louis, MO: Mosby Year Book; 1993:340–365.

Bruce NP. Enteral feeding. In: Flynn JB, Bruce NP, eds. *Introduction to Critical Care Skills.* St. Louis, MO: Mosby Year Book; 1993:366–387.

Busby HC. Acute gastrointestinal bleeding. In: Hudak CM, Gallo BM, Benz JJ, eds. *Critical Care Nursing: A Holistic Approach,* 6th ed. Philadelphia, PA: JB Lippincott Co; 1994:838–847.

Clearfield HR, Wright RA. Update on peptic ulcer disease. *Patient Care.* 1990;24(3):28–40.

Debas HT, Mulholland MW. Drug therapy in peptic ulcer disease. *Curr Probl Surg.* 1989; 26(1):1–54.

Deglin JH. Vallerand AH. Davis's Drug Guide For Nurses, 4th ed, Philadelphia, PA: FA Davis Co; 1993.

Dolan JT. Nursing management of the patient with acute upper gastrointestinal hemorrhage. *Critical Care Nursing Clinical Management Through the Nursing Process.* Philadelphia, PA: FA Davis Co; 1991:1042–1065.

Dolan JT. Nursing management of the patient with gastrointestinal dysfunction: intestinal ischemia, acute inflammatory bowel disease and intestinal obstruction. *Critical Care Nursing Clinical Management Through the Nursing Process.* Philadelphia, PA: FA Davis Co; 1991: 1109–1124.

Englert DM, Ruppert SD. Patients with gastrointestinal bleeding. In: Clochesy JM, Breu C, Cardin S, eds. *Critical Care Nursing.* Philadelphia, PA: WB Saunders Co; 1993:945–969.

Friedman G. Peptic ulcer disease. *Clin Symp.* 1988; 40(5):2–32.

Friedman LS, Knauer C. Liver, biliary tract and pancreas. In: Tierney LM, McPhee SJ, Papadakis MA, eds. *Current Medical Diagnosis and Treatment,* 33rd ed. Norwalk, CT: Appleton & Lange; 1994:528–562.

Govoni LE, Hayes JE, Shannon MT, et al. *Drugs and Nursing Implications,* 8th ed. Norwalk, CT: Appleton & Lange; 1995.

Grove KL, Klofas ES. Acute gastrointestinal hemorrhage. *Topics Emerg Med.* 1990; 12(2):9–16.

Hennessy K. Nutritional support and gastrointestinal disease. *Nurs Clin North Am.* 1989;24: 373–382.

Hoffman J, Lanng C, Amiri-Shokouh MH. Peritoneal lavage in the diagnosis of acute peritonitis. *Am J Surg.* 1988;155:359–360.

Jacobs BB, Jacobs LM. *Assessment of the abdomen. Emerg Care Q* 1988;3(4):12–21.

Jagelman DG. Surgical alternatives for ulcerative colitis. *Med Clin North Am.* 1990;74(1): 155–167.

Keithley JK, Eisenberg P. The significance of enteral nutrition in the intensive care unit patient. *Crit Care Nurs Clin North Am.* 1993;3:23–29.

Kerr RM. Acute abdominal pain. *Physician Assist* 1988;12(9):51–56.

Knodell RG, Garjian P, Schreiber JB. Newer agents available for treatment of stress-related upper gastrointestinal tract mucosal damage. JAMA. 1987;83(suppl 6A):36–40.

Krumberger JM. (1993) Gastrointestinal data acquisition. In: Kinney MR, Packa DR, Dunbar SB, eds. *AACN's Clinical Reference for Critical Care Nursing,* 3rd ed., St. Louis, MO: Mosby Year Book, 1993:1129–1140.

Krumberger JM. Gastrointestinal disorders. In: Kinney MR, Packa DR, Dunbar SB, eds.

AACN's Clinical Reference for Critical Care Nursing, 3rd ed. St. Louis, MO: Mosby Year Book; 1993:1141–1185.

Lawrence DM. Gastrointestinal trauma. Critical Care Nursing Clinics of North America. 1993; 5(1):127–140.

Loeb S. *Clinical Laboratory Tests.* Springhouse, PA: Springhouse Corp; 1991.

Loeb S. *Nurse's Handbook of Drug Therapy.* Springhouse, PA: Springhouse Corp; 1993.

McQuaid KH, Knauer CM. (1994). Alimentary tract and liver. In: Tierney LM, McPhee SJ, Papadakis MA, eds. *Current Medical Diagnosis and Treatment,* 33rd ed. Norwalk, Conn.: Appleton & Lange; 1994:467–527.

Maddaus MA, Ahrenholz D, Simmons RL. The biology of peritonitis and implications for treatment. *Surg Clin North Am.* 1988;68:431–443.

McConnel EA. Fluid and electrolyte concerns in intestinal surgical procedures. *Nurs Clin North Am.* 1987;22:843–860.

Meredith JW, Trunkey DD. CT scanning in acute abdominal injuries. *Surg Clin North Am.* 1988; 68:255–268.

Peterson WL. (1988). Obscure gastrointestinal bleeding. *Med Clin North America.* 1988; 72:1169–1176.

Phillips MC, Olson LR. The immunologic role of the gastrointestinal tract. Critical Care Nursing Clinics of North America. 1993;5(1):107–120.

Quinn A. Acute mesenteric ischemia. *Crit Care Nurs Clin North Am.* 1993;5:171–175.

Rao SSC, Read NW, Brown C, et al. Studies in the mechanism of bowel disturbance in ulcerative colitis. *Gastroenterol.* 1987;93:934–940.

Reddy S, Jeejecbhoy KN. Acute complications of Crohn's disease. *Crit Care Med* 1988;16: 557–561.

Roberts SL. Acute pancreatitis. *Physiological Concepts of the Critically Ill Patient.* Englewood Cliffs, NJ: Prentice-Hall; 1985. [out of print]

Ruderman WB. Newer pharmacologic agents for the therapy of inflammatory bowel disease. *Med Clin North Am.* 1990;74:133–153.

Schoffel U, Zeller T, Lausen M, et al. Monitoring of the inflammatory response in early peritonitis. *Am J Surg.* 1989;157:567–572.

Shaff MI, Tarr RW, Partain CL, et al. Computed tomography and magnetic resonance imaging of the acute abdomen. *Surg Clin North Am.* 1988; 68:233–254.

Sirlin SM, Benkov KJ, LeLeiko NS. Inflammatory bowel disease. *Physician Assist.* 1988; 12(3): 24–25, 29–32, 43, 36, 38, 43–46, 50–51.

Stillwell SB. *Mosby's Critical Care Nursing Reference.* St. Louis, Mo: Mosby Year Book; 1992.

Swearingen P, Keen JH. *Manual of Critical Care.* St. Louis, Mo: Mosby Year Book; 1992.

Weir DG. Peptic ulceration. *Br Med J.* 1988;290: 195–200.

Williams LF. Mesenteric ischemia. *Surg Clin North Am.* 1988;68:331–353.

Worthington PH, Wagner BA. Total parenteral nutrition. *Nurs Clin North Am.* 1989;24:355–371.

Liver and Pancreas Deviations

6

PART I: HEALTH PROBLEMS AND
NURSING MANAGEMENT

■ HEPATIC FAILURE

(For related information see Part I: Hepatic encephalopathy, p. 571; Portal hypertension, p. 575; Hepatorenal syndrome, p. 581. Part II: Shunt surgery, p. 594; Liver transplantation, p. 597. See also Behavioral Deviations, Part I, p. 725; Anxiety, p. 725; Body image disturbance, p. 730; Ineffective individual coping: Anger, p. 731; Ineffective individual coping: Depression, p. 733; Ineffective individual copying: Loss, p. 735; Denial, ineffective, p. 737; Fear, p. 740; Hopelessness, p. 740; Thought process altered: Confusion, p. 747).

Case Management Basis
DRG: 205 Disorders of liver except malignancy, cirrhosis, and alcoholic hepatitis with complications
LOS: 6.70 days
DRG: 206 Disorders of liver except malignancy, cirrhosis, and alcoholic hepatitis without complications

LOS: 3.70 days

Definition
Hepatic failure involves the structural changes or derangement of one or all of the functioning units of the liver. Hepatic or liver failure may develop within 6 months after the onset of detectable liver disease and may in certain cases of acute poisoning progress within days from asymptomatic to stage IV encephalopathy.

Pathophysiology
Hepatic failure involves a rapid, progressive deterioration and degeneration of liver parenchyma, frequently with massive hepatocellular necrosis, resulting in severe hepatic dysfunction. The underlying disease process may precipitate hepatic failure within 4–8 weeks of the onset of symptoms in an individual with normal liver function. More specifically, in hepatic failure, the liver is unable to metabolize carbohydrates, fats, proteins, and vitamins to conjugate ammonia. Increased amounts of ammonia (NH_4) with dissociation of NH_3 and $H+$ result in acidosis and elevated ammonia levels, which interfere with normal brain metabolism.

Nursing Assessment

PRIMARY CAUSES. General causes of hepatic failure include shock states, viral hepatitis, gallbladder disease, biliary obstruction, neoplasms, anesthesia, antibiotics, chemotherapeutic agents, portal caval shunt surgery, severe dehydration, or fever. Congenital causes consist of Wilson's disease, glycogen storage disease, or homozygous familial hypercholia. Other causes are Budd-Chiari syndrome, metastatic cancer, schistosomiasis, veno-occlusive disease, extrahepatic vein thrombosis, tularemia, and cryptogenic hepatic failure. Causes associated with cirrhosis include alcoholic liver disease, biliary disease, hepatitis, exposure to toxins, liver trauma, upper gastrointestinal (GI) bleeding, nutritional deficiencies, congestive heart failure, cancer, or rheumatic heart disease.

RISK FACTORS
- Life-style factors include alcohol abuse.

PHYSICAL ASSESSMENT
- Inspection: Dyspepsia, palmar erythema, testicular atrophy, gynecomastia, ascites, peripheral edema, asterixis, tremor, fector hepaticus, tachypnea, fever, epistaxis, purpura, ecchymosis, weakness, fatigability, weight loss, slowness of mentation, absent corneal reflex, confusion, anorexia, nausea, vomiting, diarrhea, constipation, spider nevi, distended neck veins, elevated and laterally displaced cardiac apex.
- Palpation: Hepatomegaly, spleenomegaly, abdominal pain, abdominal tenderness, or distended abdomen.
- Percussion: Shifting dullness to percussion and positive fluid wave.
- Auscultation: Tachycardia, hypotension, or crackles.

DIAGNOSTIC TEST RESULTS

Standard Laboratory Tests. (see Table 6–1)
- Serum chemistry: Reduced hemoglobin, hematocrit, white blood cell (WBC) count, serum albumin and protein, platelets, blood urea nitrogen (BUN), fibrinogen level, serum glucose, potassium, and sodium. Elevated serum glutamic-oxaloacetic transaminase (SGOT) and serum glutamate pyruvate transaminase (SGPT), alkaline phosphatase, bilirubin, gamma globulin, serum ammonia, and prothrombin time.
- HBsAg and anti-HAV antigen testing: Used to assess for the presence of active viral hepatitis.

Invasive Liver Diagnostic Procedures. (see Table 6–2)
- Arteriography: Evaluate the patency of the portal vein and splenic vein.
- Barium study: Upper GI tract may show the presence of esophageal or gastric varices.
- Esophagogastroscopy: Demonstrates the presence of varices and detects specific causes of bleeding in the esophagus, stomach, and proximal duodenum.
- Hepatic scanning: Uses technetium 99 mTc sulfur colloid to document splenomegaly.
- Liver biopsy: Used to diagnose the extent of hepatic cellular damage and show cirrhosis by detecting fatty infiltrates, fibrosis, or destruction of hepatic tissues.
- Lumbar puncture: Performed if central nervous system infection is suspected.
- Peritoneoscopy: Used to evaluate the type of cirrhosis present.
- Splenoportography: Evaluates the patency of the portal and splenic veins.

Noninvasive Liver Diagnostic Procedures. (see Table 6–3)
- Abdominal ultrasound: Used if biliary obstruction is suspected.
- Abdominal roentgenography: Reveals hepatic or splenic enlargement.
- Computerized tomography (CT): Used to visualize the liver to determine its size and configuration and the presence of abnormal tissue or tumors.

TABLE 6-1

TABLE 6–1. STANDARD LIVER AND PANCREATIC FUNCTION TESTS

Test	Purpose	Normal Value	Abnormal Findings
Liver Function Tests			
Serum chemistry			
Albumin	Reflects capacity to synthesize protein	3.5–5.0 g≠dL	Hypoalbuminemia: Cirrhosis, tumors, malnutrition, protein wasting, renal or gastrointestinal diseases, burns, acute or chronic infections
Ammonia	Evaluate metabolism Evaluate progress of liver disease Evaluate liver's ability to remove ammonia from portal vein blood flow Evaluate liver's ability to convert ammonia to urea	11–35 μg≠dL	Elevated levels: Liver disease, hepatic coma, portal hypertension, esophageal varices, severe heart failure, azotemia, cor pulmonale, pulmonary emphysema, pericarditis, acute bronchitis
Bilirubin	Evaluate liver function Increase in free-flowing bilirubin found in dysfunction or blockage of liver.	Total: 1.0 mg/dL Direct: 0.5 mg/dL Indirect: 0.5 mg/dL	Elevated: Viral hepatitis or cirrhosis Elevated direct bilirubin: Cancer of head of pancreas, choledocholithiasis Elevated indirect bilirubin: Hemolytic anemias, trauma with large hematomas, hemorrhagic pulmonary infarcts
Prothrombin time	Measures clotting time to determine activity of prothrombin and fibrinogen	≤3 s over control	Elevated: Vitamin K deficiency, abnormal bleeding
Total protein	Measures albumin and globulins in blood	6.0–8.4 g/100mL	Reduced: Long-standing hepatocellular dysfunction
Urea	Evaluate renal function	8–20 mg/dL	Reduced: Severe liver disease
Alkaline phosphatase (ALP)	Index of liver disease (excretion of enzyme impaired by obstruction in biliary tract)	20–90 IU/L (SMA 1260) 30–120 U/L 1.5–4.0 U/dL (Bodansky) 4.0–13.5 U/dL (Icing-Armstrong) 0.8–2.5 U/dL (Bessey-Lowry)	Elevated: Space-occupying lesions from cancer or abscesses, hepatocellular cirrhosis, biliary cirrhosis. Reduced: Malnutrition, hypothyroidism, hypophosphatasia
Alkaline phosphatase isoenzymes	Distinguish between bone and liver origin of alkaline phosphatase	AP-1, Alpha; AP-2, Beta 1; AP-3, Beta 2	>25%: Liver disease, such as cancer and biliary obstruction

TABLE 6-1

TABLE 6–1. CONTINUED

Test	Purpose	Normal Value	Abnormal Findings
Gamma glutamyl transpeptidase (SGGT)	Measure enzyme activity in liver, biliary tract, pancreas, kidney tubules Used with alkaline phosphatase to suggest source of elevated alkaline phosphatase levels	Men: 10–48 U/L Women: 6–29 U/L	Elevated SGGT: Chronic liver disease associated with chronic alcohol abuse, liver metastasis, or acute pancreatitis
Glutamic-oxaloacetic transaminase (SGOT/AST)	Assist in diagnoses of acute hepatic disease	10–40 U/mL	Elevated: Acute viral hepatitis, skeletal muscle trauma, drug-induced hepatic injury, passive liver congestion
Glutamate pyruvic transaminase (SGPT/ALT)	Detect and evaluate treatment of acute hepatic disease (hepatitis, cirrhosis without jaundice)	10–32 U/L	Elevated findings: Acute hepatocellular injury such as cirrhosis and drug-induced or alcoholic hepatitis
Lactate dehydrogenase (LDH)	Differentiate diagnoses of liver diseases	Total LHD 60–120 U/mL; LDH4 (6%–16%) liver, skeletal muscle, brain, or kidneys; LDH5 (2%–13%) liver, skeletal muscle, brain, or kidneys	Abnormal findings: Liver, skeletal muscle, brain, or kidney disease
HBsAg	Hepatitis B surface antigen found within 30 days of exposure and persists up to 3 months after jaundice, unless a carrier state occurs		Indicates hepatitis is infectious
Anti-HAV	Antibody to hepatitis A virus (HAV) Detectable at beginning of disease before jaundice	Negative	Confirms lifelong immunity Elevated: Suggests hemolytic jaundice
Stool			
Bile	Determines presence and degree of biliary tract obstruction in patient with jaundice	30–200 mg/100 g of feces	Elevated: Associated with hemolytic anemias Reduced: Associated with severe liver disease
Urobilinogen	Assess pressure of liver disease where flow of bilirubin to the intestine reduced, with decreased fecal excretion of urobilinogen	60–200 mg/24 hrs 30–130 IU/L	Elevated levels: Associated with Chronic pancreatitis, obstruction of the pancreatic duct
Pancreatic Function Tests			
Amylase	Diagnose and monitor treatment of acute pancreatitis	0–1 U/mL 4–24 IU/dL	Elevated: Suggest acute pancreatitis, may be high when amylase levels normal

TABLE 6-1

TABLE 6-2

TABLE 6–1. CONTINUED

Test	Purpose	Normal Value	Abnormal Findings
Lipase	Diagnose pancreatitis Differentiate pancreatitis from acute surgical abdominal injury	32–80 U/L	Reduced: Suggest pancreatitis, obstruction of pancreatic duct, pancreatic carcinoma, cirrhosis

From et al., Ford RD, 1987; Loeb S, 1991; Smith, 1993.

TABLE 6–2. PARTIAL LIST OF INVASIVE LIVER AND PANCREATIC DIAGNOSTIC PROCEDURES

Test	Purpose	Normal Value	Abnormal Findings
Abdominal Plain Films	Visualize size, shape, and position of liver	Normal abdominal structures	Accumulation of gas or ascites in gastrointestinal tract
Liver Diagnostic Procedures			
Liver biopsy	Diagnose hepatic parenchymal disease, malignancy, granulomatous infections	Healthy liver consists of sheets of hepatocytes supported by a reticulin framework	Diffuse hepatic disease, such as cirrhosis or hepatitis
Liver cell function scan	Determine functions and anatomy of liver cells, gallbladder, and upper intestine.	Normal size of cardiac impression on liver and normally functioning liver	A diffuse nodular pattern of decreased uptake: cirrhosis, hepatitis, or diffuse cancer A solitary filling pattern: Primary or metastatic tumor, cyst, or perihepatic abscess
Liver scan (blood vessel structural scan)	Detect structural defects of the liver Used to evaluate the size, shape, and position of liver and spleen	Normal size, shape, and position of liver; no evidence of filling defects	Cysts, tumors, abscesses, high portal pressure, cirrhosis, or hepatitis
Pancreatic diagnostic Procedures			
Endoscopic retrograde cholangiopancre-atography (ERCP)	Diagnose cancer of the pancreas and the biliary ducts Locate calculi and stenosis in the pancreatic ducts and hepatobiliary tree	Pancreatic and hepatobiliary ducts are patent and separate orifices are sometimes present Contrast medium uniformly fills the pancreatic duct	Suggest pancreatic cysts, pancreatic pseudocysts, pancreatic tumor, carcinoma of the head of the pancreas, chronic pancreatitis, pancreatic fibrosis
Pancreas scan	Rule out cancer of pancreas and determine progress of pancreatitis Differentiate obstructive jaundice from tumors of the head of the pancreas	Normal size and position of pancreas.	Inability to visualize pancreas may suggest pancreatic disease

From et al Ford RD, Loeb S, 1991; Smith, 1993.

TABLE 6-3

TABLE 6–3. NONINVASIVE LIVER AND PANCREATIC DIAGNOSTIC PROCEDURES

Test	Purpose	Normal Value	Abnormal Findings
Liver Diagnostic Procedures			
Liver computed tomography	Detect intrahepatic tumors, abscesses, subphrenic and subhepatic abscesses, cysts, hematomas	Liver has uniform density that is greater than pancreas, kidneys, and spleen	Primary hepatic neoplasms, metastatic hepatic neoplasms, hepatic abscesses, hepatic cysts, hepatic hematomas
Liver sonogram	Screen or detect hepatocellular disease or hepatic metastases or hematomas Defines cold spots as tumors, abscesses, or cysts	Normal size, shape and position of liver	Metastasis to liver, cirrhosis, necrotic tumor, intrahepatic abscesses, cysts, hematomas
Pancreatic Diagnostic Procedures			
Pancreatic computed tomography	Detect pancreatic carcinoma, pseudocysts, pancreatitis Distinguish between pancreatic disorders and disorders of retroperitoneum	Pancreas is normal in size, shape and position	Acute pancreatitis, chronic pancreatitis, pancreatic carcinoma, benign pancreatic tumor, pancreatic abscess, pancreatic pseudocysts

From et al, Ford RD, 1987; Loeb S, 1991; Smith, 1993.

MEDICAL AND SURGICAL MANAGEMENT

PHARMACOLOGY

- Diuretics: Used to inhibit renal sodium conservation mechanisms. Spironolactone (Aldactone) and triamterene are used for initial control of ascites. Furosemide and mannitol can also be used (see Table 1–13, p. 75).
- Neomycin: A broad-spectrum antibiotic that destroys normal gut flora and decreases protein breakdown and ammonia production (see Table 5–4, p. 518).
- Lactulose: Creates an acidotic environment in the bowel. This causes ammonia to leave the bloodstream and to enter the colon, where it is trapped. Lactulose has a laxative effect. The initial dose of 30 to 45 mL/h may be administered orally or by nasogastric (NG) tube three to four times daily until two or three soft stools are produced daily. The maintenance dose is 30 to 45 mL 3 to 4 times per day (see Table 6–4).

DIET

- Sodium restriction: Sodium may be restricted from 0.5 to 2.0 g/d.
- A high-calorie, 80- to 100-gram protein diet of high biologic value is used to repair tissue. Caloric intake is 2500 to 3000/d.

FLUID THERAPY

- Crystalloids and electrolytes: Used to restore fluid volume and electrolyte balance.
- Salt-poor albumin: Administered to increase colloid osmotic pressure in the peritoneum and to prevent rapid reaccumulation of ascites.
- Restriction of fluid intake.

PHYSICAL ACTIVITY

- Bed-rest in semi-Fowler's position helps to initiate diuresis and allows for free diaphragmatic movement.

TABLE 6-4

TABLE 6–4: LIVER-AND PANCREAS-RELATED DRUGS

Medication	Route/Dose	Uses/Effects	Side Effects
Lactulose (Cephulac)	Acute portal-systemic encephalopathy Oral: 30– 45 mL tid or qid adjusted to produce 2 or 3 soft stools/d Rectal: 300 mL diluted with 700 mL water given via rectal balloon catheter and retained for 30–60 min; may repeat in 4–6 h if necessary or until patient can take oral	Prevent and treat protal-systemic encephalopathy (PSE) including stages of hepatic precoma and coma	Flatulence, belching, abdominal cramps, nausea, vomiting, or hypernatremia
Diazepam (Valium)	Oral: 2–10 mg tid or qid or 15–30 mg of extended release capsule/d	Treat tension or anxiety	Drowsiness, lethargy, fainting, slurred speech, blurred vision, nausea, vomiting, rash, urticaria
Regular Insulin	Diabetes mellitus Subcutaneous: 5–10 U 15–30 min after meals and bedtime; dose based on blood glucose levels Ketoacidosis Intravenous: 2.4–7.2 U loading dose; followed by 2.4–7.2 U/h continuous infusion Maintenance therapy: Subcutaneous 50 U/d or less of intermediate-acting insulin	Treat diabetic ketoacidosis, coma, and initiate therapy in insulin-dependent diabetes mellitus	Profuse sweating, hunger, headache, nausea, tremors, pallor, palpitations, paresthesias, loss of consciousness, irritability, ataxia, apprehension, coma

From Deglin, Vallerand R, 1995; Loeb S, 1993; Shannon MJ, Wilson BA, 1992.

PARACENTESIS

- Paracentesis may be indicated for removal of ascites when it is compromising effective breathing, eating, or moderate physical activities.

SURGICAL INTERVENTION

- Peritoneovenous shunting: This is a surgical procedure to relieve ascites that is resistant to medical therapies. Two shunts are the LeVeen or Denver shunts. The LeVeen shunt, or valve, is inserted with the distal end of a tube under the peritoneum and the other end tunneled under the skin into the jugular vein or superior vena cava. A valve opens and closes according to the pressure gradient, which allows ascitic fluid to flow into the vessel. The Denver shunt includes a pump that is used in addition to the peripheral catheter. Ascitic fluid is allowed to flow through the pump at a uniform rate or can be squeezed to increase flow.

NURSING MANAGEMENT: NURSING DIAGNOSIS AND COLLABORATIVE PROBLEMS

Nursing Diagnoses

Common nursing goals for patients with hepatic failure are to maintain fluid balance, promote effective breathing pattern, enhance normal thought process, maintain adequate nutrition, prevent infection, and promote adequate adjustment.

Fluid volume deficit related to fluid sequestration secondary to hypoalbuminemia, bleeding, or diuretic therapy.

Expected Patient Outcomes. Patient maintains adequate fluid volume, as evidenced by heart rate (HR) ≤100 bpm, blood pressure (BP) within 10 mm Hg of baseline, mean arterial pressure (MAP) 70 to 100 mm Hg, cardiac output (CO) 4 to 8 L/min, central venous pressure (CVP) 2 to 6 mm Hg, pulmonary artery pressure (PAP) systolic 15 to 30 mm Hg or PAP diastolic 5 to 15 mm Hg, pulmonary capillary wedge pressure (PCWP) 6 to 12 mm Hg, body weight within 5% of baseline, serum albumin 3.5 to 5.0 mg/dL, hemoglobin ≥12 g/dL, hematocrit ≥35%, red blood cell (RBC) count ≥4.7 to 5.9 million/μL, platelet count ≥150,000 mm³, serum osmolality 285 to 295 mOsm/kg, electrolytes within normal limits, urinary output (UO) ≥30 mL/h, normal skin turgor, peripheral pulses +2, and capillary refill ≤3 seconds.

- Consult with physician regarding the potential for bleeding.
- Review levels of serum electrolytes, serum albumin, serum osmolality, hemoglobin, hematocrit, RBC count, and platelet count.
- Limit physical activity to bed rest if patient is actively bleeding as a result of GI bleeding or esophageal varices.
- Obtain and report hemodynamic parameters associated with fluid volume deficit: CO ≤4 L/min, CVP ≤2 mm Hg, PAP systolic ≤15 mm Hg or diastolic ≤5 mm Hg, and PCWP ≤6 mm Hg.
- Obtain and report other clinical findings associated with fluid volume deficit: hypotension, tachycardia, MAP ≤70 mm Hg, poor skin turgor, peripheral pulses ≤+2, capillary refill ≥3 seconds, and pallor.
- Monitor intake, output, and specific gravity as a reflection of diuretic therapy. Report UO ≤30 mL/h.
- Measure daily weight and report changes 0.5 to 1.0 kg/d indicating fluid imbalance.

- Monitor and report petechiae or bleeding from gums, puncture site, urine, stool, and gastric aspirate.
- Monitor continuous ECG to assess HR and rhythm. Document ECG rhythm strips every 2 to 4 hours or more frequently in patients with dysrhythmias.
- Restrict sodium to 0.5 g/d to reduce fluid retention and enhance mobilization of excessive fluids from the tissue.
- Restrict fluid to 1000 mL/d to decrease generalized edema.
- Administer prescribed crystalloids, such as dextrose, to minimize risk of hypoglycemia and colloids to increase oncotic pressure, which can pull osmotic fluid into the intravascular space.
- Administer prescribed blood and blood products to replace RBCs and clotting factors.
- Administer prescribed diuretics (spironolactone, triamterene, or furosemide) to decrease edema.
- Administer prescribed potassium to replace that lost from diuretics or liver disease.
- Administer prescribed protein supplement to restore intravascular colloidal osmotic pressure and enhance movement of edema fluid into the intravascular space, leading to diuresis.
- Should pharmacological therapy and sodium restriction be ineffective in controlling abdominal distention from ascites, prepare patient for shunt surgery (see Shunt surgery, p. 594).

Ineffective breathing pattern related to elevation of diaphragm secondary to ascites.

Expected Patient Outcomes. Patient maintains effective breathing pattern, as evidenced by respiratory rate (RR) 12 to 20 BPM, arterial blood gases (ABG) within normal limits, absence of crackles, symmetrical chest movement, absence of dyspnea or shortness of breath, HR ≤100 bpm, absence of cyanosis, and hemoglobin within normal limits.

- Review ABG and hemoglobin values.
- Place patient in a semi-Fowler's position to allow for maximal respiratory excursion and lung expansion.
- Obtain and report clinical findings associated with ineffective breathing pattern: tachypnea, crackles, asymmetry of chest movement, diaphragmatic excursion, dyspnea, shortness of breath, and tachycardia.
- Evaluate tidal volume $\geq$5 to 7 mL and vital capacity $\geq$ 12 to 15 mL/kg as a reflection of ventilatory effectiveness.
- Monitor intake, output, specific gravity, and daily weight.
- Encourage patient to cough, deep breathe, and use incentive spirometer.
- Administer prescribed oxygen 2 to 4 L/min to enhance tissue oxygenation.
- Should patient's ABGs fail to improve with oxygen therapy, prepare patient for ventilatory support.

Altered thought processes related to increased ammonia level secondary to increased protein load resulting from GI bleeding or dehydration.

Expected Patient Outcomes. Patient maintains normal thought process, as evidenced by intact memory; orientation to person, place, and time; absence of asterixis; and serum ammonia 12 to 55 umol/L.

- Review serum ammonia levels.
- Restrict dietary protein intake to reduce ammonia production and subsequent increase in serum ammonia level.
- Provide prescribed high-carbohydrate diet (1400 calories) or intravenous infusion of 10% glucose to provide the primary source of energy for cerebral tissue.
- Initiate prescribed NG intubation to reduce absorption of protein breakdown products.
- Monitor level of consciousness using Glasgow coma scale.
- Report clinical findings associated with altered thought process: confusion, agitation, memory lapses, combativeness, and asterixis.

- Administer prescribed lactulose, which favors the conversion of ammonia to a minimum for the colon to evacuate.
- Monitor serum glucose in patients receiving lactulose because it creates galactose and glucose.
- Administer prescribed antibiotic therapy (neomycin and kanamycin) to reduce intestinal bacterial flora, which reduces bacterial ammonia production (see Table 5–4).
- Administer stool softener as prescribed.
- Maintain safe environment by removing hazardous objects from the bedside.
- Reorient patient to person, place, and time.
- Explain all procedures and reinforce what patient already knows.
- Encourage patient to ask questions about the illness, risk factors, and treatment.
- Evaluate patient for altered thought process: short attention span, inattentiveness, irritability, confusion, or stupor.
- Provide continuity of care so that subtle behavioral changes can be identified.
- Avoid use of narcotics or sedatives since they may not be metabolized quickly, thereby causing a cumulative effect.

Altered nutrition: less than body requirements related to anorexia, nausea, vomiting, or malnutrition.

Expected Patient Outcomes. Patient maintains body weight within 5% baseline; nitrogen balance and serum glucose level are within normal range.

- Consult with dietitian regarding patient's diet.
- Review serum BUN, creatinine, albumin, hemoglobin, and hematocrit values.
- Provide bed rest or rest periods to conserve patient's energy, thereby reducing metabolic demand.
- Restrict protein to 20 to 60 g/d depending on patient's level of consciousness.
- Restrict sodium to 250 to 500 g/d because of sodium and water retention resulting from secondary hyperaldosteronism.

- Provide carbohydrates so total caloric intake is 200 to 3000/d to help prevent catabolism, to maintain weight, and to prevent the use of dietary protein for energy needs.
- Provide soft foods if patient has esophageal varices.
- Restrict fluids to 1000 mL/d depending on the degree of third-spacing.
- Monitor intake, output, and daily weight.
- Encourage visit by family at mealtime if patient desires.
- Administer prescribed vitamin supplements such as A, D, E, K, vitamin B_{12}, and thiamine.
- Administer prescribed enteral feedings to patients who are unable to ingest food normally.
- Teach patient the reason behind dietary restriction.

High risk for infection related to impaired immunity or invasive procedures.

Expected Patient Outcomes. Patient is free of infection, as evidenced by normothermia; WBC count ≤11,000/μL; negative cultures; and absence of redness, tenderness, swelling, or drainage from incision or cannulation site.

- Review results of WBC count and cultures.
- Limit activity to bed rest while patient is febrile.
- Obtain and report clinical findings indicating infection: fever, redness, tenderness, swelling, or drainage from cannulation site or incision.
- Use aseptic technique when changing dressings.
- Assess patient's environment for infection risks since the immune system can be depressed in patients with liver disease.
- Administer prescribed IV fluids to maintain adequate hydration.
- Administer prescribed antibiotic therapy.
- Instruct patient to report any tenderness or drainage from cannulation or incision site.

Impaired adjustment related to the inability to cease using alcohol.

Expected Patient Outcomes. Patient adjusts to his or her circumstances or agrees to seek counseling in an attempt to cease using alcohol.

- Consult with physician regarding the need for psychiatric counseling.
- Support patient as he or she attempts to adjust to ceasing alcohol intake.
- Listen to patient's concerns or fears regarding the cessation of alcohol.
- Encourage patient and family to discuss how they can support each other through the recovery phase.

Collaborative Problems

Common collaborative goals for patients with hepatic failure are to reduce peritoneal fluid accumulation, correct electrolyte imbalance, maintain oxygenation, and prevent hepatorenal syndrome.

Potential Complication: Ascites. Ascites related to hypoalbuminemia or sodium retention secondary to increased intraperitoneal pressure.

Expected Patient Outcomes. Patient is free of abnormal accumulation of fluid in the peritoneum, as evidenced by absence of abdominal distention, absence of abdominal discomfort, absence of jugular vein distention, CVP 2 to 6 mm Hg, absence of dyspnea, RR 12 to 20 bpm, HR ≤100 bpm, UO ≥30 mL/h or 0.5 mL/kg/h, PCWP ≤12 mm Hg, serum osmolality 285 to 295 mOsm/kg, and serum albumin 3.5 to 5.5 g/100 mL.

- Consult with physician regarding the need for paracentesis or peritonovenous shunt surgery.
- Review levels of serum electrolytes, serum osmolality, and serum albumin.
- Place patient in a high Fowler's position to promote lung expansion.
- Place patient on a low-protein, high-caloric diet.
- Restrict sodium intake to 300 to 500 mg/d to reduce fluid retention and enhance mobilization of excess fluid from the tissues.

- Restrict fluid intake to 1000 to 1500 mL/d to decrease ascites and generalized edema.
- Measure abdominal girth daily to determine the status of ascites. Ascites is evident after ≥1500 mL of ascites fluid has accumulated.
- Measure daily weight to evaluate total body fluid volume. Report UO ≤30 mL/h.
- Obtain and report clinical findings suggesting ascites: increased abdominal girth, skin tautness, shifting dullness on percussion, palpable fluid wave, dyspnea, abdominal distention, neck vein distention, new striae, and fatigue.
- Administer prescribed protein supplementation to restore intravascular colloidal osmotic pressure and enhance the movement of edema fluid into the intravascular space, thereby promoting diuresis.
- Assist with abdominal paracentesis to relieve dyspnea and compromised respiratory excursion.
- Assess paracentesis insertion site for bleeding or infection.
- Monitor BP while the prescribed fluid is being removed. Fluid removal in excess of 1 to 1.5 L can lead to hypotension.
- Administer prescribed IV fluids to maintain circulatory volume.
- Should pharmacological therapy or sodium restriction be ineffective, prepare patient for peritinoneovenous shunt such as Le-Veen valve.
- Enhance flow through shunt using abdominal binder and teach patient to perform breathing exercises, which stimulate the shunt, thereby causing fluid to flow from the peritoneal cavity into the thoracic veins.

Potential Complication: Electrolyte Imbalance.
Electrolyte imbalance related to hypokalemia and hyponatremia secondary to hormonal imbalance such as increased aldosterone and diuretic therapy.

Expected Patient Outcomes. Patient maintains adequate electrolyte balance, as evidenced by serum sodium 135 to 148 mEq/L, potassium 3.5 to 5.5 mEq/L, stable body weight, and absence of dysrhythmias.

- Review serum electrolyte values.
- Monitor continuous ECG to assess HR and rhythm. Report ECG changes suggesting hypokalemia: flat T waves, U waves, peaked P waves, and ST depression.
- Obtain and report clinical findings associated with hypokalemia: hypoactive reflexes, cramps, weakness, apathy, tremors, tachycardia, hypotension, shallow respirations, and GI irritability and distention.
- Monitor daily weight and report weight loss in nonedematous ascitic patient ≥1.0 to 1.5 lb/d.
- Obtain and report clinical findings associated with dilutional hyponatremia: malaise, edema, flushed skin, crackles, dyspnea, headache, confusion, irritability, abdominal cramps, or nausea.
- Administer prescribed IV fluids to maintain adequate hydration.
- Administer prescribed intravenous potassium not to exceed 20 mEq/100mL/h to replace potassium.
- Administer prescribed diuretics to reduce volume and correct dilutional hyponatremia.

Potential Complication: Hypoxemia.
Hypoxemia related to intrapulmonary shunting or hypoventilation secondary to ascites.

Expected Patient Outcomes. Patient maintains adequate oxygenation, as evidenced by ABGs within normal range, RR 12 to 20 BPM, HR ≤100 bpm, hemoglobin and hematocrit within normal range, ventilation-perfusion scan normal, absence of crackles, normal skin color, CO 4 to 8 L/min, cardiac index (CI) 2.7 to 4.3 L/min/m², arterial oxygen saturation (Sao_2) 95 to 97.5%, and mixed venous oxygen saturation ($S\bar{v}o_2$) 60% to 80%.

- Review of hemoglobin, hematocrit, ABG, and chest roentgenogram results.
- Place patient in position of comfort to facilitate oxygenation: Sitting rather than supine may reduce hypoxemia.

- Continually monitor oxygen saturation with pulse oximetry and report $SpO_2 \leq 90\%$.
- Evaluate ventilation:perfusion ($\dot{V}:\dot{Q}$) ratio: Arterial hypoxemia in cirrhosis may result from an increased perfusion to lung units with a lower than normal $\dot{V}A:\dot{Q}$ ratios, whereas in others there may be a increased $\dot{V}A:\dot{Q}$ when position is changed from supine to sitting, indicating that the abnormal vessels in the lower lobes may dilate under increased hydrostatic pressure in the erect position.
- Assess clinical indicators of respiratory status: rate, rhythm, symmetry of chest movement, presence of cyanosis, and crackles.
- Obtain and report clinical findings associated with hypoxemia: restlessness, tachypnea, tachycardia, and labored breathing.
- Encourage patient to cough, turn, deep breathe, and use incentive spirometer to facilitate aeration and increase lung expansion.
- Administer prescribed oxygen 2 to 4 L/min to enhance tissue oxygenation.
- Administer prescribed IV fluids to maintain adequate hydration.
- Should supplementary oxygen support be ineffective, prepare patient for ventilatory support.
- Teach patient to cough, turn, and deep breathe.

Potential Complication: Hepatorenal Syndrome.
Hepatorenal syndrome related to renal hypoperfusion secondary to decreased effective plasma volume.

Expected Patient Outcomes. Patient maintains normal hepatorenal function, as evidenced by UO ≥ 30 mL/h or 0.5 mL/kg/h; absence of weakness, nausea, or vomiting; specific gravity 1.010 to 1.030; and BUN and creatinine within normal limits.

- Review values for BUN, creatinine, and creatinine clearance.
- Provide a diet low in protein to minimize uremia and high in carbohydrates to minimize protein breakdown.

- Obtain and report clinical findings associated with hepatorenal syndrome: weakness, nausea, vomiting, UO ≤ 30 mL/h or ≤ 0.5 mL/kg/h, and specific gravity ≤ 1.010.
- Measure intake, output, and specific gravity to assess fluid balance.
- Measure daily weight to evaluate whether fluid balance is being achieved.
- Restrict fluid intake as necessary to maintain fluid balance.
- Administer prescribed colloidal fluids or blood products to restore effective plasma volume.
- Prepare patient for dialysis while waiting for liver transplantation.

Potential Complication: Increased Intra-abdominal Pressure.
Increased intra-abdominal pressure related to peritoneal ascites.

Expected Patient Outcomes. Patient maintains normal intra-abdominal pressure, as evidenced by intra-abdominal pressure of ≤ 25 cm H_2O and absence of abdominal distention.

- Consult with physician regarding intra-abdominal pressure and its relationship to other hemodynamic pressures.
- Review intra-abdominal pressure levels.
- Place patient in position of comfort should abdominal distention occur.
- Measure abdominal girth.
- Prepare patient for paracentesis when intra-abdominal pressure ≥ 25 cm H_2O to decrease the pressure by at least 10 cm H_2O.

DISCHARGE PLANNING
The critical care nurse will provide patient and significant other(s) verbal or written discharge notes regarding the following areas:

1. Medications, including drug name, dosage, route, purpose, schedule, and side effects.
2. Importance of maintaining sodium restriction should ascites occur.
3. Importance of avoiding alcohol ingestion.
4. The signs and symptoms of unusual bleeding: bruising, petechia, or dark stools.

5. Importance of keeping all medical appointments.
6. Importance of avoiding medications that can cause gastric irritation.
7. Importance of adhering to prescribed diet and obtaining adequate rest.
8. Importance of taking daily weight and reporting significant gain or loss.
9. Names and phone numbers of support groups.

■ HEPATIC ENCEPHALOPATHY

(For related information see Part I: Hepatic failure, p. 559; Portal hypertension, p. 575; Hepatorenal syndrome, p. 581. Part II: Shunt surgery, p. 594; Liver transplantation, p. 597. See also Behavioral Deviations Part I, p. 725) Anxiety, p. 725; Body image disturbance, p. 730; Ineffective individual coping: Anger, p. 731; Ineffective individual coping: Depression, p. 733; Ineffective individual coping: Loss, p. 735; Denial, ineffective, p. 737; Fear, p. 740; Hopelessness, p. 740; Thought process altered: Confusion, p. 747).

Case Management Basis
DRG: 205 Disorders of liver except malignancy, cirrhosis, and alcoholic hepatitis with complications
LOS: 6.70 days
DRG: 206 Disorders of liver except malignancy, cirrhosis, and alcoholic hepatitis without complications
LOS: 3.70 days

Definition
Hepatic encephalopathy (HE) is a neuropsychiatric dysfunction resulting from liver disease and failure. It is characterized by a deterioration in intellectual function, personal behavior, and level of consciousness. Encephalopathy is also referred to as portal-systemic encephalopathy (PSE).

Pathophysiology
Normally the liver plays a vital role in the metabolism, transformation, and detoxification of both exogenous and endogenous substances. In portal-systemic encephalopathy, almost all the portal circulation can be diverted away from the liver by collaterals. Exogenous and endogenous toxins deprived of hepatic filtration may accumulate in the systemic circulation. Their toxic effect involves alteration in brain energy metabolism, alteration in neuronal membrane physiology or derangement in neurosynaptic transmission. Ammonia intoxication is identified with hepatic encephalopathy. Ammonia originates in the gastrointestinal tract where it is diverted from metabolism of ingested proteins, breakdown of blood or degradation of urea secreted into the colon. When the ammonia bypasses the liver and is not detoxified as in portal-systemic shunting, it accumulates in the blood and transverses the blood-brain barrier where fragile brain tissue becomes exposed to high ammonia concentration.

Nursing Assessment

PRIMARY CAUSES
• Include infection and fluid and electrolyte disturbances such as acidosis, alkalosis, hypokalemia, or hypovolemia. Nitrogen overload causes include constipation, gastrointestinal bleeding, high protein intake, increased BUN, shunting of blood around diseased liver, portal-systemic bypass of liver, or transfusion with stored blood. Pharmacological causes include analgesics, diuretics, hyponotics, narcotics, or sedatives. Other causes are diarrhea, vomiting, hypoglycemia, hypoxia, anemia, hypotension, abdominal paracentesis, dehydration, or azotemia.

RISK FACTORS
• History of alcohol abuse.

PHYSICAL ASSESSMENT
• Inspection: Grade I HE shows total orientation, with progression to confusion and disorientation, forgetfulness, restlessness, irritability, apathy, depression, lack of mus-

cular coordination, and yawning. Grade II HE consists of decreased level of consciousness (LOC), disorientation as to time and place, severe confusion, amnesia, decreased inhibitions, lethargy, apathy, hypoactive reflexes, asterixis, or slurred speech. Grade III HE involves complete disorientation when aroused, inability to make computations, apathy, Babinski's sign, clonus, rigidity, or seizures. Grade IV HE describes coma, seizures, rigidity progressing to flaccidity, or dilated pupils.

- Auscultation: Tachypnea, hyperventilation or tachycardia.

DIAGNOSTIC TEST RESULTS

Standard Laboratory Tests. (see Table 6–1)

- Sulfobromophthalein sodium (Bromsulphalein) excretion: Increased retention.
- Cephalin-cholesterol flocculation test: Positive indicates active liver cell damage.
- Serum chemistry: Decreased albumin; increased alkaline phosphatase, ammonia, bilirubin, globulins, serum glutamic-oxaloacetic transaminase (SGOT) and serum glutamate pyruvate transaminase (SGPT).
- Stool: Decreased fecal urobilinogen in obstructive liver disease.
- Urine: Increased urine bilirubin and urobilinogen.

MEDICAL AND SURGICAL MANAGEMENT

PHARMACOLOGY

- Neomycin: Used against ureolytic gram-negative organisms. It reduces biotransformation of nitrogenous substances in the intestine and induces regular bowel movement. Neomycin is administered up to 4 to 6 g/d in divided doses (see Table 5–4, p. 518).
- Lactulose: A saline laxative that is converted in the gut to lactic acid and acetic acid. Ammonia in the intestine remains in the ionized form and cannot cross the intestinal membrane into the systemic circulation. Lactulose also decreases fecal pH

(5.0), which inhibits growth of ammonia-forming bacteria.

- Potassium: Given as a supplement if patient has received loop diuretics (see Table 6–4).
- Mannitol: An osmotic diuretic that is used to reduce intracranial pressure and is effective when the intracranial pressure (ICP) is ≤60 mm Hg. An ICP volume ≥60 mm Hg is not responsive to mannitol. If serum osmolality is ≥320 mOsm/kg, mannitol is contraindicated.
- Diazepam: Used in doses of 2 to 10 mg IV to treat seizures (see Table 6–4).
- Lasix: Used when renal function is adequate.
- Antidysrhythmia agents: Used to correct dysrhythmias resulting from acid-base imbalance, hypoxia, and hypotension (see Table 1–11, p. 54).

FLUID THERAPY

- Intravenous infusions of glucose 10% are administered. Ringer's lactate solution is avoided in hepatic failure since this is likely to cause lactic acidosis.
- Fresh frozen plasma is used to treat active bleeding.

DIET

- Dietary protein is restricted.
- A 1200 caloric diet with 3 to 6 g of essential amino acids and a high carbohydrate content is provided.

NURSING MANAGEMENT: NURSING DIAGNOSES AND COLLABORATIVE PROBLEMS

Nursing Diagnoses

Common nursing goals for patients with HE are to maintain fluid volume, support normal thought process, prevent infection, and prevent injury.

Fluid volume deficit related to bleeding secondary to coagulopathy problem.

Expected Patient Outcomes. Patient maintains adequate fluid volume, as evidenced by central venous pressure (CVP) 2 to 6 mm Hg,

blood pressure (BP) within patient's normal range, mean arterial pressure (MAP) ≥70 mm Hg, heart rate (HR) ≤100 bpm, respiratory rate (RR) 12 to 20 BPM, capillary refill ≤3 seconds, peripheralpulses +2, urinary output (UO) ≥30 mL/h, absence of cyanosis, cardiac output (CO) 4 to 8 L/min, pulmonary artery pressure (PAP) 20 to 30/8 to 15 mm Hg, pulmonary capillary wedge pressure (PCWP) 6 to 12 mm Hg, and coagulation studies within normal range.

- Consult with physician regarding the presence of any bleeding.
- Review results of coagulation profile.
- Obtain and report hemodynamic parameters associated with fluid volume deficit: CO ≤4 L/min, CVP ≤2 mm Hg, PAP ≤20/8 mm Hg, and PCWP ≤6 mm Hg.
- Obtain and report clinical findings reflecting fluid volume deficit: hypotension, tachycardia, tachypnea, ecchymosis, bleeding, peripheral pulses ≤+2, capillary refill ≥3 seconds, and MAP ≤70 mm Hg.
- Test patient's stool and urine for occult blood.
- Measure intake, output, specific gravity, and body weight to evaluate fluid balance. Report UO ≤30 mL/h.
- Administer prescribed blood products, albumin, or crystalloids to correct hypotension resulting from bleeding or fluid volume deficit.
- Administer prescribed vitamin K to ensure that a deficiency does not contribute to decreased levels of clotting factors.
- Administer prescribed fresh frozen plasma to treat active bleeding.
- Administer prescribed cytoprotective sucralfate, H_2 receptor-antagonists, and antacids as prophylaxis for gastrointestinal bleeding.

Altered thought processes related to increased ammonia.

Expected Patient Outcomes. Patient maintain normal thought processes and ammonia level within normal range.

- Consult with physician regarding the relationship between central nervous system activity and ammonia level.
- Review serum creatinine, electrolytes, albumin, and blood urea nitrogen (BUN) values.
- Provide a low protein and high carbohydrate diet (1400 calories).
- Provide IV infusion of 10% glucose: Glucose provides energy for cerebral tissues and prevents gluconeogenesis.
- Monitor patient for clinical indicators of altered mentation: memory lapses, shortened attention span, confusion, agitation, combativeness, incoherence, drowsiness, lethargy, or personality changes.
- Monitor patient's neurological status indicating HE: asterixis, tremors, unresponsiveness to painful stimuli, oculocephalic reflexes, decorticate or decerebrate posturing, hyperactive deep tendon reflexes, or bilateral Babinski's sign.
- Insert nasogastric tube to decompress and provide iced gastric lavage for patients with gastrointestinal bleeding.
- Assist with the insertion of Sengstaken-Blakemore tube to control esophageal and variceal bleeding.
- Assist with selective angiography with continuous vasopressin (Pitressin) infusion.
- Monitor UO and number of stools per day.
- Monitor for the presence of lactulose side effects: abdominal cramping, abdominal bloating, diarrhea, nausea, vomiting, and fluid electrolyte imbalance.
- Prepare patient with secondary hepatorenal syndrome, azotemia, or acute tubular necrosis for peritoneal dialysis.
- Initiate therapy to reduce gastric acidity: combination of parenteral ranitidine or cimetidine (H_2 antagonists) and antacid therapy via nasogastric tube.
- Administer lactulose (Cephuliac) therapy to create an acid environment in the bowel, which causes ammonia to leave the blood and move into the colon, or to create a laxative effect to facilitate the elimination of ammonia: oral syrup 20 to 30 g (30 to 45

mL) three or four times a day or retention enema of 200 g of lactulose (300 mL syrup) diluted in 1000 mL of water every 4 to 6 hours (see Table 6–4).

- Administer antibiotic therapy: aminoglycosides such as neomycin and kanamycin to reduce intestinal bacterial flora and subsequent bacterial ammonia production.
- Administer, if appropriate, branched-chain amino acids to improve the nutritional status of HE patients.
- Administer levodopa when HE is thought to be related to defective neurotransmitters.

Infection, high risk for related to impaired host defenses.

Expected Patient Outcomes. Patient is free of infection, as evidenced by normothermia, white blood cell (WBC) count ≤11,000/μL; culture negative; or absence of redness, tenderness, swelling, or drainage.

- Review results of WBC count and cultures.
- Obtain and report clinical findings associated with infection: fever, swelling, tenderness, redness, or drainage from wound or catheter site.
- Measure temperature every 2 to 4 hours when patient is febrile.
- Use strict aseptic technique while changing tubing or dressings.
- Obtain cultures of sputum, blood, urine, or wound drainage as ordered.
- Administer prescribed antibiotic therapy should infection occur.
- Administer prescribed IV fluids to maintain adequate hydration.

High risk of injury related to seizures secondary to elevated ammonia or cerebral edema.

Expected Patient Outcomes. Patient is free of seizure activity.

- Monitor and report seizure activity.
- Provide a safe environment to protect patient from injury during seizure.

- Protect patient from aspiration during seizure by maintaining a patent airway.
- Initiate seizure precaution.
- Reorient patient to person, place, and time.
- Initiate physical restrictions, if not contraindicated, to protect patient from harm should patient become restless and delirious.
- Administer prescribed IV diazepam, in doses of 2 to 10 mg to treat seizures.

(For additional nursing diagnoses see Hepatic Failure: **Altered thought process** related to increased ammonia level, p. 567).

Collaborative Problems

Common collaborative goals for patients with HE are to reduce ICP, restore electrolyte balance, correct dysrhythmias, and correct hypoglycemia.

Potential Complication: Increased ICP. Increased ICP related to cerebral edema secondary to portal hypertension or increased ammonia.

Expected Patient Outcomes. Patient maintains normal ICP, as evidenced by ICP 0 to 15 mm Hg; cerebral perfusion pressure (CPP) 70 to 90 mm Hg; alterness; absence of confusion; absence of decerebrate posturing; pupils reactive; absence of drowsiness, headache, or lethargy; RR 12 to 20 BPM; BP within patient's normal range; arterial blood gases (ABGs) within normal limit; and serum ammonia within normal range.

- Review ABG, serum ammonia, and serum osmolality levels.
- Position patient with head and upper trunk elevated 30 to 40 degrees to the horizontal, because ICP is affected by posture.
- Obtain and report ICP 20 to 25 mm Hg and sustained CCP ≤70 mm Hg.
- Obtain and report clinical findings associated with increased ICP secondary to cerebral edema: lethargy, confusion, decerebrate posturing, drowsiness, dilated pupils, hyperventilation, and hypotension.

- Avoid extreme flexion, rotation, or extension of the patient's head, thereby reducing potential increase in ICP during movement.
- Administer prescribed mannitol to reduce ICP. Mannitol is effective when ICP is ≤60 mm Hg. Values ≥60 mm Hg do not respond well to mannitol, and it is contraindicated if serum osmolality is ≥300 mOsm/kg.

Potential Complication: Metabolic Acidosis. Metabolic acidosis related to hepatic necrosis, hypotension, or hypoxemia.

Expected Patient Outcomes. ABGs and ammonia within normal range.

- Review serum ammonia and ABG levels.
- Monitor clinical indicators of metabolic acidosis: shortness of breath, weakness, tachypnea, restlessness, headache, drowsiness, confusion, nausea, anorexia, dysrhythmias, or hypotension.
- Evaluate sensory-perceptual status while patient is gradually increasing physical activity.
- Measure daily weight, intake, specific gravity, and UO.
- Administer IV fluids and electrolytes to maintain adequate hydration and electrolyte balance.
- Administer sodium bicarbonate for metabolic acidosis.

Potential Complication: Hypoglycemia. Hypoglycemia related to increased plasma insulin level or liver necrosis causing impaired hepatic glucose release.

Expected Patient Outcomes. Patient maintains normal serum glucose level.

- Review serum glucose levels.
- Obtain and report clinical findings associated with mild hypoglycemia: pallor, diaphoresis, tachycardia, palpitations, hunger, paresthesia, and shakiness.
- Obtain and report clinical findings associated with moderate hypoglycemia: inability

to concentrate, confusion, irrational behavior, slurred speech, blurred vision, fatigue, or somnolence.

- Provide a minimum of 1400 calories/d as carbohydrates.
- Institute seizure precautions, such as padded side rails.
- Administer prescribed IV infusion 10% to 50% dextrose.
- Administer prescribed IV fluids with 5% to 10% glucose solution.

(For an additional collaborative problem see Hepatic Failure: Electrolyte Imbalance, p. 569.)

DISCHARGE PLANNING
(See Hepatic Failure, p. 00.)

■ PORTAL HYPERTENSION

(For related information see Part I: Hepatic failure, p. 559; Hepatic encephalopathy, p. 571; Hepatorenal syndrome, p. 581. Part II: Shunt surgery, p. 594; Liver transplantation, p. 597. See also Behavioral Deviations, Part I, p. 725.)

Case Management Basis
DRG: 205 Disorders of liver except malignancy, cirrhosis, and alcoholic hepatitis with complications
LOS: 6.70 days
DRG: 206 Disorders of liver except malignancy, cirrhosis and alcoholic hepatitis without complications
LOS: 3.70 days

Definition
Portal hypertension is increased hydrostatic pressure within the portal venous system. It is a portal venous pressure ≥5 to 10 mm Hg. Esophageal varices develop as a result of hypertension.

Pathophysiology
Portal pressure is increased by obstruction of blood flow through the liver. The obstruc-

tion can be in one of the following three areas: in the portal vein before the emptying of blood into the sinusoids (presinusoidal), within the hepatic tissue itself (intrahepatic), or in the hepatic outflow channels (suprahepatic). Three pathophysiological changes include splenomegaly, formation of collateral channels, and ascites. Splenomegaly involves increased portal venous pressure, which delays blood flow through the splanchnic bed, causing the spleen to become congested and enlarged. When collateral channels are formed, perfusion through the liver is blocked and portal venous pressure is increased; collateral channels develop as a compensatory mechanism. The collateral channels redirect portal venous blood into systemic venous beds of lower resistance to avoid the blockage. Ascites leads to increased pressure within the portal system and increases the hydrostatic pressure inside the vessel, leading to the movement of fluid into the peritoneal cavity.

Nursing Assessment

PRIMARY CAUSES

- Prehepatic mechanisms include splenic vein thrombosis, portal vein thrombosis, or cavernomatosis of the portal vein. Intrahepatic causes consist of partial nodular transformation, nodular regenerative hyperplasia, congenital hepatic fibrosis, polycystic disease, idiopathic portal hypertension, sarcoidosis, amyloidosis, mastocytosis, Rendu-Osler-Weber disease, hematologic liver disease, severe viral hepatitis, chronic active hepatitis, hepatocellular carcinoma, nonalcoholic liver cirrhosis, alcoholic cirrhosis, acute alcoholic hepatitis, or veno-occlusive disease. Posthepatic mechanisms include Budd-Chiari syndrome, congenital malformations, thrombosis of the inferior vena cava, constrictive pericarditis, or tricuspid valve disease.

PHYSICAL ASSESSMENT

- Inspection: Lethargy, weight loss, telangiectasis, palmar erythema, testicular atrophy, abdominal distention, ascites, rectal bleeding, pedal edema, jaundice, or caput medusa.
- Palpation: Spleenomegaly, hepatomegaly, and pitting edema.
- Auscultation: Tachycardia or hypotension.

DIAGNOSTIC TEST RESULTS

Standard Laboratory Tests. (see Table 6–1)

- Serum chemistry: Elevated bilirubin, globulin, alkaline phosphatase, SGOT/SGPT, prothrombin, and ammonia; reduced albumin, esterified cholesterol levels, and platelet count.

Invasive Liver Diagnostic Procedures. (see Table 6–2)

- Azygos blood flow: Signifies an index of blood flow through the gastroesophageal collaterals and esophageal varices in portal hypertension; normal value 0.15 to 0.25 L/min.
- Endoscopy: Used to show pressure of variceal bleeding and grade variceal size on a I to IV scale; endoscopic pressure-sensitive gauges allow the measurement of variceal pressure without puncturing the varices.
- Esophagoscopy: Used to evaluate the presence of varices.
- Fiberoptic esophagogastroduodenoscopy: Used to visualize the bleeding area; must be performed within 8 hours of the hemorrhage.
- Portal venous pressure: Value: 10 mm Hg; gradient between portal pressure and inferior vena cava (IVC) pressure ≥ 2 to 6 mm Hg. May be achieved by surgical catheterization of the portal vein, percutaneous transhepatic puncture and catherization of the portal vein, transjugular portal vein catheterization, hepatic vein catheterization, or splenic pulp puncture.
- Splenic venography: Used to visualize the portal system and collaterals. The portal pressure can also be measured through the splenic needle.

- Visceral angiography: Visualizes the hepatic arterial system and allows space-filling lesions in the liver to be identified.
- Portal pressures: Normal portal pressure is 9 mm Hg and normal inferior vena cava pressure is 2 to 6 mm Hg. A persistent portal pressure ≥12 mm Hg increases one gradient between portal venous pressure and inferior vena cava pressure when one gradient between portal venous pressure and inferior vena cava pressure ≥10 mm Hg portal venous blood is directed away from the liver into low pressure bed.

NONINVASIVE LIVER DIAGNOSTIC PROCEDURES.
(See Table 6–3)

- Ultrasound: Used to visualize the portal vein at the hilum of the liver. A normal portal vein is visualized, while an incompetent or recanalizing vein is irregular and reduced in diameter, and a thrombosed vein is not detected.

MEDICAL AND SURGICAL MANAGEMENT

PHARMACOLOGY

- Vasopressin (Pitressin): Vasopressin is a vasoconstrictor that lowers portal pressure by reducing blood flow in the splanchnic arterial bed. An IV loading dose of 20 U in 50 mL of 5% dextrose is administered over 30 minutes, followed by a maintenance infusion of 0.1 to 0.5 U/min. Infusion rate is not to exceed 0.6 U/min (see Table 5–4, p. 518).
- Nitroglycerin (NTG): Used to minimize the undesirable effects of vasopressin, NTG improves coronary artery blood flow and reduces myocardial work by decreasing preload and systemic vascular resistance. Portal venous resistance is reduced. An initial NTG dose of 50 µg/min is followed by increases of 50 µg/min every 15 minutes while maintaining systolic blood pressure (SBP) ≥100 mm Hg. A maximum dose is 400 µg/min (see Table 1–4, p. 20).
- Propranolol: This is used to decrease heart rate (HR), cardiac output (CO), and hepatic

venous pressure. The dosage of propranolol can be 40 to 280 mg/d (see Table 1–10, p. 50).

FLUID THERAPY

- Crystalloids: Normal saline is used for isotonic fluid replacement. The patient is monitored for hypernatremia, peripheral edema, and increased ascites.
- Packed red blood cells (RBC): RBC are administered to keep the hematocrit at 30%. The patient is monitored for portal hypertension and variceal rupture from over-transfusion.
- Fresh frozen plasma, vitamin K, and platelets: These are administered to improve coagulation.

ENDOSCOPIC INJECTION SCLEROTHERAPY

- Scleropathy controls acute variceal bleeding. It is accomplished by using a modified fiberoptic endoscope with an injection port through which a flexible cable injector is inserted. Sclerosant solution is injected directly into the lumen of the varix or into the submucosa around the varix. The sclerosant solution causes contraction of the varix and cessation of bleeding. A venous thrombosis occurs and is converted to a fibrous band.

ESOPHAGOGASTRIC BALLOON TAMPONADE

- An esophagogastric tamponade tube applies local pressure to the bleeding site, usually at the cardioesophageal junction. The goal is to decrease blood flow to the bleeding esophageal varices and directly compress gastric varices.
- Two types of tubes: The Sengstaken-Blakemore tube has three lumens: two are used to inflate the gastric and esophageal balloons, while the third lumen is used for gastric aspiration. A small nasogastric tube can be positioned above the esophageal balloon to permit aspiration of esophageal and pharyngeal secretions. The Minnesota tube is a four-lumen tube that is similar to the Sengstaken-Blakemore. The fourth lumen is for esophageal aspiration. The balloon is

maintained in position with balanced traction (1 to 2 lb) or secured to the faceguard of a football helmet. Pressure (20 to 45 mm Hg) is placed on the varices at the cardioesophageal junction.

TRANSJUGULAR INTRAHEPATIC PORTOSYSTEMIC SHUNT (TIPS)

- TIPS is a nonsurgical technique that uses the normal vascular anatomy of the liver to create a shunt between the portal and systemic venous system entirely within the liver, using a metallic stent, thereby relieving portal hypertension.

SURGICAL INTERVENTION

- Shunt surgery: Used for decompression of the varices and is categorized as nonselective and selective. With nonselective shunt surgery, all the portal blood flow enters the systemic circulation without first passing through the liver. Portal blood flow is shunted around the liver. In selective shunts, portal venous flow through the liver is preserved (see Shunt surgery, p. 594).
- Liver transplant: Used to correct portal pressure, control bleeding, and restore normal liver function (see Liver transplantation, p. 597).

NURSING MANAGEMENT: NURSING DIAGNOSES AND COLLABORATIVE PROBLEMS

Nursing Diagnoses

Common nursing goals for patients with portal hypertension are to maintain fluid volume, increase esophageal tissue perfusion, facilitate effective breathing pattern, and promote self-concept.

Fluid volume deficit related to visceral hemorrhage secondary to portal hypertension.

Expected Patient Outcomes. Patient maintains adequate fluid volume, as evidenced by CO 4 to 8 L/min, cardiac index (CI) 2.7 to 4.3 L/min/m², blood pressure (BP) within pa-

tient's normal range, HR ≤100 bpm, respiratory rate (RR) 121 to 20 BPM, capillary refill ≤3 seconds, peripheral pulses +2, absence of cyanosis, absence of bleeding, serum albumin 3.5 to 5.0 mg/dL, hemoglobin ≥12 g/dL, hematocrit ≥35%, RBC count ≥4.7 to 5.9 million/μL, platelet count ≥150,000 mm³, and serum osmolality 285 to 295 mOsm/kg.

- Review levels of hematocrit, hemoglobin, serum osmolality, serum albumin, serum creatinine, blood urea nitrogen (BUN), RBC, and platelet count.
- Review results of BUN:serum creatinine ratio, which ranges from 10 to 20:1. If the BUN increases as creatinine stays unchanged, thereby increasing the BUN:creatinine ratio, decreased intravascular volume may be the cause.
- Maintain head of bed 30 to 45 degrees to prevent reflux into the esophagus.
- Place patient with an esophageal tube in low or semi-Fowler's position, which allows best ventilation and prevents gastric acid reflux.
- Initiate prescribed nasogastric tube with low, intermittent suction to prevent pooling of blood and secretions, which could be aspirated.
- Obtain and report hemodynamic parameters associated with fluid volume deficit: CO ≤4 L/min, CI ≤2.7 L/min/m², and CVP ≤2 mm Hg.
- Obtain and report clinical findings associated with fluid volume deficit: hypotension, tachycardia, tachypnea, mean arterial pressure (MAP) ≤70 mm Hg, poor skin turgor, peripheral pulses ≤+2, skin cool, pallor, and capillary refill ≥3 seconds.
- Measure intake, output, and specific gravity to evaluate fluid balance, renal perfusion, or glomerular filtration rate. Report UO ≤30 mL/h.
- Measure daily weight to evaluate total body fluid volume.
- Monitor coronary perfusion pressure and BP while patient receives vasopressin. Vasopressin reduces coronary blood flow and

increases BP, thereby creating an imbalance between myocardial oxygen supply and oxygen demand.

- Monitor continuous ECG to assess HR and rhythm. Document ECG rhythm strips every 2 to 4 hours or more frequently in patients with dysrhythmias.
- Obtain and report clinical findings associated with bowel ischemia resulting from vasoconstriction of the mesenteric artery from vasopressor: pain in the periumbilical area, abdominal distention, paralytic ileus, nausea, and diarrhea.
- Assist with endotracheal intubation to protect the airway.
- Administer prescribed IV fluids, blood, or blood products to maintain hydration, maintain circulatory volume, and improve coagulation.
- Administer prescribed vasopressin to reduce portal pressure by reducing blood flow in the splanchnic arterial bed.
- Should pharmacological therapy be ineffective in controlling bleeding, prepare patient for endoscopic injection sclerotherapy (EJS) (see EJS, p. 601).
- Prepare patient for esophagogastric balloon tamponade or TIPS (see TIPS, p. 603).
- Should nonsurgical methods be ineffective in controlling bleeding, prepare patient for shunt surgery (see Shunt surgery, p. 594).

Altered esophageal tissue perfusion related to esophageal erosion or necrosis secondary to balloon tamponade.

Expected Patient Outcomes. Patient maintains adequate esophageal tissue perfusion, as evidenced by balloon pressure 20 to 45 mm Hg. Absence of esophageal pain, capillary venous pressure 10 to 15 mm Hg, capillary arterial pressure 30 to 40 mm Hg, and absence of bleeding.

- Elevate head of bed 30 to 45 degrees to prevent reflux into the esophagus.
- Maintain balloon in position with balanced traction (1 to 2 lb) or secured to the faceguard of a football helmet.

- Maintain pressure monitoring outlet for the esophageal balloon and inflation to a pressure of 20 to 45 mm Hg. A pressure ≥45 mm Hg exceeds arterial-side capillary closing pressure and puts patients at risk for esophageal necrosis and perforation.
- Check esophageal balloon pressure every 1 to 2 hours to ensure adequate tamponade pressure.
- Deflate esophageal balloon, as ordered, for 5 minutes every 6 hours to reduce the risk of esophageal necrosis.
- Obtain and report clinical findings associated with esophageal perforation: substernal pain aggravated by respiration, upper abdominal or back pain, and hypotension.
- Limit esophageal inflation to 24 to 36 hours.
- Assess patient for airway obstruction from esophageal balloon migration. The gastric balloon is not deflated while the esophageal balloon is inflated.
- Keep scissors at bedside to be used should the balloon migrate proximally and occlude the upper airway. The lumens are cut to facilitate removal of the tube.
- Apply suction above the most proximally inflated balloon to help prevent pulmonary aspiration.
- Label each lumen of the tube to prevent accidental deflation of the gastric balloon.

Ineffective breathing pattern related to elevated diaphragm secondary to ascites.

Expected Patient Outcomes. Patient maintains effective breathing pattern, as evidenced by RR 12 to 20 BPM, HR ≤100 bpm, symmetry of chest movement, absence of dyspnea, absence crackles, absence of cyanosis, and arterial blood gases within normal range.

- Review arterial blood gas levels and chest roentgenogram.
- Position patient in semi-Fowler's position to provide maximal respiratory excursion and lung expansion.
- Assess the clinical indicators of respiratory status: rate, depth, symmetry of chest, skin

color and warmth, presence or absence of adventitious breath sounds.

- Obtain and report clinical findings associated with ineffective breathing pattern: tachypnea, tachycardia, asymmetry of chest movement, dyspnea, and crackles.
- Encourage patient to deep breathe and use incentive spirometer to facilitate lung expansion.
- Administer prescribed oxygen 2 to 4 L/min to provide tissue oxygenation.
- Administer prescribed diuretic to reduce intra-abdominal volume.
- Assist with paracentesis to remove intraperitoneal fluid and reduce pressure on the diaphragm.

Self-concept disturbance related to altered physical appearance secondary to ascites or jaundice.

Expected Patient Outcomes. Patient is able to express feelings about self, participate in decision-making process, or initiate self-care.

- Allow patient to discuss feelings about self in relation to the disease process.
- Explain all procedures and allow patient to participate in procedures when realistic.
- Evaluate patient's readiness for learning about the disease, treatment, and prognosis.
- Encourage patient to talk about the illness and its impact on self and the family.
- Assist patient and family to identify their strengths, weaknesses, and coping strategies.
- Encourage patient to discuss feelings about life-style changes that may be required.
- Identify areas of improvement in patient's illness and prognosis.
- Teach patient that the jaundice, edema, and ascites are temporary.

Collaborative Problems

Common collaborative problems for patients with portal hypertension are to decrease portal pressure and increase cardiac output.

Potential Complication: Increased Portal Pressure. Increased portal pressure related to increased vascular resistance secondary to increased portal blood flow.

Expected Patient Outcomes. Patient maintains normal portal pressure, as evidenced by approximately 1500 mL/min of blood perfusing the liver, BP within patient's normal range, capillary arterial pressure 30 to 40 mm Hg, and azygos blood flow 0.15 to 0.25 L/min.

- Consult with physician about the desired hemodynamic flow to liver: Flow (F) is determined by pressure (P) over resistance (R): F=P/R.
- Consult with physician to validate expected patient outcomes used to evaluate whether normal portal pressure has been achieved.
- Review test results: PVP, WHVP, free hepatic venous pressure (FHVP), azygos blood flow, splenic venography, visceral angiography, ultrasound, and serum bilirubin, globulin, alkaline phosphatase, prothrombin, albumin, and ammonia.
- Monitor esophageal balloon pressure ≤45 mm Hg so not to exceed arterial-side capillary closing pressure (30 to 45 mm Hg), which places the patient at risk for esophageal necrosis and perforation.
- Evaluate clinical indicators of portal hypertension: PVP ≥12 mm Hg, azygos blood flow 0.65 L/min, and WHVP equal to PVP at 10 to 12 mm Hg.
- Administer a continuous IV infusion of vasopressin (0.4 U/min) for a maximum of 2 hours, or the drug can be administered through the superior mesenteric artery.
- Administer vasopressor and beta-adrenergic blocking drugs to reduce portal pressure: 20 to 40 units of vasopressin can be infused in 100 to 200 mL of 5% dextrose in water over a 10 to 40 minute period IV.
- Administer propranolol to reduce portal pressures: 20 to 180 mg twice a day or in a dosage to reduce the resting HR by 25%.
- Prepare patient for shunt surgery: end-to-end portocaval shunt, side-to-side or double portocaval shunt, mesocaval shunt,

splenorenal shunt, renoportal shunts, or central or distal splenorenal shunt (see Shunt surgery, p. 594).

- Should a nonsurgical approach be needed to reduce variceal bleeding resulting from portal hypertension, prepare patient for TIPS with stent (see TIPS, p. 603).

Potential Complication: Decreased Cardiac Output. Decreased CO related to blood loss or vasoconstriction secondary to varices or vasopressor therapy.

Expected Patient Outcomes. Patient maintains adequate CO, as evidenced by CO 4 to 8 L/min, CI 2.7 to 4.3 L/min/m², central venous pressure (CVP) 2 to 6 mm Hg, HR ≤100 bpm, BP within patient's own range, mean arterial pressure (MAP) ≥70 mm Hg, peripheral pulses +2, capillary refill ≤3 seconds, absence of cyanosis, systemic vascular resistance (SVR) 900 to 1200 dynes/s/cm⁻⁵, systemic vascular resistance index (SVRI) 1970 to 2390 dynes/s/cm⁻⁵/m², mixed venous oxygen saturation (S$\bar{v}$o₂) 60% to 80%, and absence of cyanosis.

- Place patient in semi-Fowler's position to optimize lung expansion.
- Obtain and report hemodynamic parameters associated with decreased CO. CO ≤4 L/min, CI ≤2.7 L/min/m², CVP ≤2 mm Hg, SVR ≥1200 dynes/s/cm⁻⁵, and SVRI ≥2390 dynes/s/cm⁻⁵/m².
- Obtain and report clinical findings associated with peripheral vasoconstriction: skin cool and cyanotic, peripheral pulses ≤+2, and capillary refill ≥3 seconds.
- Monitor continuous ECG to assess HR and rhythm. Document ECG rhythm strips every 2 to 4 hours in patients experiencing dysrhythmias associated with vasopressor therapy.
- Administer prescribed IV fluids to maintain adequate circulatory volume.

(For an additional collaborative problem see Hepatic Failure: Ascites, p. 568).

DISCHARGE PLANNING
(See Hepatic Failure, p. 570.)

■ HEPATORENAL SYNDROME

(For related information see Part I: Hepatic failure, p. 559; Hepatic encephalopathy, p. 571; Portal hypertension, p. 575. Part II: Shunt surgery, p. 594; Liver transplantation, p. 597. See also Behavioral Deviations, Part I, p. 725.)

Case Management Basis
DRG: 205 Disorders of liver except malignancy, cirrhosis, and alcoholic hepatitis with complications
LOS: 6.70 days
DRG 206: Disorders of liver except malignancy, cirrhosis, and alcoholic hepatitis without complications
LOS: 3.70 days

Definition
Hepatorenal syndrome (HRS) is sudden renal failure that is associated with progressive liver disease in patients with prior normal renal function. It develops in the presence of end-stage liver disease without obvious cause or clinical, laboratory, or anatomic evidence of other known causes of renal failure.

Pathophysiology
HRS is associated with severe renal hypoperfusion with vasomotor instability. Renal hypoperfusion has an effect on the renal cortex, causing decreased filtration because the cortical nephrons participate in the filtration process within the kidney. Renal vasomotor instability is revealed as an increase in renal vascular resistance that has an affinity for the interlobular arteries and afferent arterioles. Overall there is a decrease in renal perfusion with cortical ischemia, increased renal vascular resistance in the interlobular arteries and afferent arterioles, and reduction in the glomerular filtration rate (GFR).

Nursing Assessment

PRIMARY CAUSES

- The HRS can be due to development of shunts in the kidney that divert blood away from the renal cortex to the medulla, thus decreasing GFR; decrease in blood volume causing the release of renin, renal vasoconstriction, and a decrease in urinary output; renal damage resulting from circulating endotoxins not removed from the blood by the liver; or production of a vasoconstriction substance that causes decreased renal perfusion. Other causes include abdominal paracentesis, iatrogenic loss of fluids secondary to excessive diuresis, hemorrhage, and alcoholic cirrhosis.

RISK FACTORS

- History of alcoholic cirrhosis.

PHYSICAL ASSESSMENT

- Inspection: Oliguria, anorexia, nausea, vomiting, fatigue, thirst, weakness, and drowsiness.
- Auscultation: Hypotension.

DIAGNOSTIC TEST RESULTS

Standard Laboratory Tests. (see Table 6–1)

- Serum chemistry: Elevated blood urea nitrogen (BUN) $\geq$50 mg/dL and creatinine$\geq$2.5 mg/dL. Reduced sodium.
- Urinalysis: Urine sodium concentration $\leq$5 to 10 mmol/L, fractional excretion of sodium $\leq$1, urine:plasma creatinine ratio $\geq$30:1, urine osmolality $\geq$400 mOsm/kg H_2O, specific gravity $\geq$1.025, proteinuria, hematuria, and granular casts.

MEDICAL AND SURGICAL MANAGEMENT

PHARMACOLOGY

- Calcium antagonists: Can have a beneficial effect on the kidney and liver. Calcium antagonists are only currently used as renal dilators in the setting of renal transplant.

These drugs may overcome the intense renal vasoconstriction associated with HRS.
- Spironolactone: The goal is to attain a slow and gradual diuresis that does not exceed the body's capacity to mobilize ascitic fluid. Spironoloctone accomplishes this goal when given as 25 mg/d. The recommended diuresis is 300 to 600 mL/d (see Table 1–13, p. 76).

DIET

- Restrict sodium to 250 mg/d or 10 to 15 mmol/d.

PARACENTESIS

- Used in treating refractory ascites and to temporarily improve renal function by decreasing intraperitoneal pressure. This leads to increased inferior vena cava blood flow, venous return, cardiac output (CO), and renal blood flow.

PERITONEOVENOUS SHUNT

- Used to increase fluid distribution by mobilizing fluid from the peritoneal cavity to the central circulation (see Shunt surgery, p. 594).

HEMODIALYSIS

- Hemodialysis can benefit lost renal function by correcting fluid, electrolyte, and acid-base imbalance, correcting platelet defect of uremia, and removing toxic metabolites. Used only in patients with reversible acute liver disease.

CONTINUOUS RENAL REPLACEMENT THERAPY

- Used to maintain slow, controlled fluid volume removal and initiate continuous arterial venous hemofiltration with dialysis.

WATER IMMERSION

- This is an experimental technique used to redistribute body fluid from the peripheral to the central circulation. The patient is immersed in a tank of isothermic water for 5 hours and exposed to a pressure gradient that increases at the rate of 22.4 mm Hg/ft from the surface to the bottom of the tank. Body fluid is translocated from the lower extremities and buttocks to the central circulation.

SURGICAL INTERVENTION

- With liver transplantation, the diseased liver is removed, thereby allowing renal failure to reverse.

NURSING MANAGEMENT: NURSING DIAGNOSES AND COLLABORATIVE PROBLEMS

Nursing Diagnoses

Common nursing goals for patients with hepatorenal syndrome are to increase renal tissue perfusion, maintain fluid balance, and provide nutritional requirements.

Altered tissue perfusion renal related to vasoconstriction secondary to increased intrarenal renin.

Expected Patient Outcomes. Patient maintains adequate renal perfusion, as evidenced by urinary output (UO) $\geq$30 mL/h or $\geq$0.5 mL/kg/h, specific gravity 1.010 to 1.025, absence of edema, serum BUN 8 to 23 mg/dL, creatinine 0.6 to 1.6 mg/dL, and osmolality and sodium within normal range.

- Review serum BUN, creatinine, and electrolyte values.
- Restrict sodium intake to 250 mg/d or 10 to 15 mmol/d.
- Obtain and report clinical findings associated with decreased renal tissue perfusion: UO $\leq$30 mL/h or $\leq$0.5 mL/kg/h, specific gravity $\geq$1.025, and peripheral edema.
- Measure intake, output, specific gravity, and daily weight as indicators of fluid balance and effectiveness of sodium restriction or diuretic therapy.
- Treat gastrointestinal bleeding, as prescribed, in a timely manner to restore adequate circulatory volume and maintain renal perfusion.
- Limit the frequency of abdominal paracentesis to restrict the volume of fluid removed.

- Should large-volume paracentesis occur, administer prescribed IV colloid solution such as albumin.
- Should lactulose be used to decrease blood ammonia circulation, administer cautiously to avoid massive diarrhea and subsequent hypovolemia and decreased renal blood flow.
- Administer prescribed IV fluids to maintain adequate circulatory volume.
- Administer prescribed diuretic (spironolactone) to provide a gradual mobilization of ascitic fluid and diuresis. Maintain a diuresis of 300 to 600 mL/d with an upper limit of 700 to 900 mL/d (see Table 1–13, p. 76).
- Assist with paracentesis, which decreases intraperitoneal pressure, increasing CO and renal blood flow.
- Should pharmacological therapy and paracentesis be ineffective in increasing effective fluid distribution and mobilizing fluid from the peritoneal cavity, prepare patient for shunt surgery (see Shunt surgery, p. 594).
- Prepare patient for hemodialysis or continuous renal replacement therapy to regulate fluids, maintain electrolyte balance, and remove toxic waste products from the body (see Hemodialysis, p. 496, and Continuous renal replacement therapy, p. 505).

Fluid volume deficit related to extracellular fluid translocation or accumulation of fluid into interstitial compartment.

Expected Patient Outcomes. Patient maintains adequate fluid volume, as evidenced by blood pressure (BP) within patient's normal range; mean arterial pressure (MAP) $\geq$70 mm Hg; heart rate (HR) $\leq$100 bpm; CO 4 to 8 L/min; cardiac index (CI) 2.7 to 4.3 L/min/m^2; central venous pressure (CVP) 2 to 6 mm Hg; peripheral pulses +2; capillary refill $\leq$3 seconds; good skin turgor; skin warm and dry; UO $\geq$30 mL/h or $\geq$0.5 mL/kg/h; stable weight; and serum osmolality, hematocrit, and electrolytes within normal limits.

- Review serum osmolality, hematocrit, and electrolyte levels.

- Obtain and report hemodynamic parameters associated with fluid volume deficit: CO $\leq$4 L/min, CI $\leq$2.7 L/min/m², and CVP $\leq$2 mm Hg.
- Obtain and report clinical findings associated with fluid volume deficit: hypotension, tachycardia, poor skin turgor, pallor, peripheral pulses $\leq$2, and capillary refill $\geq$3 seconds.
- Monitor hourly intake and output to determine changes in fluid status. Report UO $\leq$30 mL/h or $\leq$0.5 mL/kg/h.
- Measure daily weight, which can be an indicator of fluid status and changes. Report weight gain $\geq$5% of baseline.
- Monitor specific gravity every 2 to 4 hours and report $\geq$1.025, which can indicate increased urine concentration and renal tubular failure.
- Administer prescribed IV fluids to increase circulatory volume.
- Administer prescribed diuretics to mobilize ascitic fluid into the vasculature.
- Administer prescribed IV colloid fluids during paracentesis to minimize protein loss during the procedure.

Altered nutrition: Less than body requirements related to anorexia or fatigue secondary to HRS.

Expected Patient Outcomes. Patient maintains adequate nutritional intake.

- Consult with dietitian to individualize patient's diet based on nutritional requirements.
- Review results of serum albumin and electrolytes tests.
- Restrict sodium intake to 250 mg/d or 10 to 15 mmol/d.
- Monitor the amount of patient's dietary intake.
- Assist patient with feedings as needed to ensure dietary intake.
- Encourage rest before and after meals.
- Measure mid-arm circumference and tricep skinfold as an indicator of protein and fat stores.

- Should patient have a nasogastric tube, provide prescribed enteral feedings.
- Administer prescribed IV fluids to maintain adequate hydration.

DISCHARGE PLANNING
The critical care nurse will provide patient and significant other(s) verbal or written discharge notes regarding the following subjects:

1. Medications, including drug name, dosage, route, purpose, schedule, and side effects.
2. Importance of reporting any significant changes in urinary elimination.
3. Importance of keeping all medical appointments.
4. Importance of taking daily weight and reporting significant gain or loss.

■ ACUTE HEPATITIS

(For related information see Part I: Hepatic failure, p. 559; Hepatic encephalopathy, p. 571; Portal hypertension, p. 575. Part II: Shunt surgery, p. 594; Liver transplantation, p. 597. Part III: Esophagogastric balloon tamponade, p. 603.)

Case Management Basis
DRG: 202 Cirrhosis and alcohol hepatitis
LOS: 7.20 days

Definition
Hepatitis is an acute inflammation of the entire liver, characterized by centrilobular necrosis and infiltration of the portal tracts by leukocytes.

Pathophysiology
There is general accumulation of inflammatory cells and edema in hepatitis. The inflammatory cells consist of Kupffer's cells, lymphocytes, and monocytes. Initially there can be local, spotty, or single-cell necrosis. As hepatitis progresses, the liver's normal lobular pattern is distorted by inflammation,

necrosis, and degeneration and regeneration of liver cells. Eventually, portal venous pressure increases and damaged liver cells are removed by phagocytes.

Nursing Assessment

PRIMARY CAUSES

- Hepatitis A virus (HAV), in which the virus is spread by the fecal-oral route by oral ingestion of fecal contaminants. The sources of infection include contaminated food, contaminated water, and shellfish caught in contaminated water. The incubation period is from 2 to 6 weeks.
- Hepatitis B virus (HBV), in which the HBV is spread by blood, blood products, semen, and saliva. The sources of infection include percutaneous, through mucous membranes, or direct contact with infected fluids and contaminated inanimate objects. The incubation period is 6 to 12 weeks. Delta hepatitis is associated with a coexistent HBV infection. Delta virus and HBV may coinfect, a delta virus hepatitis may be superimposed on HBV carrier states.
- Hepatitis C virus (HCV), a single-stranded linear RNA virus similar to flavivirus. People at risk are IV drug users, heterosexuals with multiple sexual partners or an infected partner, hemophiliacs, chronic hemodialysis patients, and health care personnel exposed to blood and blood products.
- Hepatitis E virus, also called enterically transmitted NANB hepatitis, epidemic NANB hepatitis, and fecal-oral NANB hepatitis.

PHYSICAL ASSESSMENT

- Inspection: Malaise, myalgia, arthralgia, diarrhea, constipation, fever, fatigability, anorexia, nausea, vomiting, jaundice, chills, irritability, depression, or palmar erythema.
- Palpation: Abdominal pain or liver tenderness in the upper right quadrant or right epigastrium, hepatomegaly, splenomegaly, or enlarged lymph nodes in the cervical or epitrochlear areas.

DIAGNOSTIC TEXT RESULTS

Standard Laboratory Tests. (see Table 6–1)

- Serum chemistry: Hepatitis A is serum positive for IgM class antibody to HAV (IgM anti-HAV). Hepatitis B is serum positive for hepatitis B surface antigen (HBsAg) and hepatitis B core antibody (anti-HBc). Other findings include reduced white blood cell (WBC) count, atypical lymphocytes, elevated serum glutamic-oxaloacetic transaminase (SGOT), lactate dehydrogenase (LDH), serum glutamate pyruvate transaminase (SGPT), alkaline phosphatase, and direct indirect bilirubin.
- Stool: Clay-colored.
- Urinalysis: Proteinuria, hematuria, bilirubinuria, and elevated urobilinogen.

INVASIVE LIVER DIAGNOSTIC PROCEDURE. (see Table 6–2)

- Liver biopsy: Used to define the extent of liver necrosis.

MEDICAL AND SURGICAL MANAGEMENT

PHARMACOLOGY

- Corticosteroids: Corticosteroids may not alter the course of acute hepatitis but they can slow the progression of the disease.

DIET

- A high-carbohydrate and low-fat diet.

PHYSICAL ACTIVITY

- Bed rest is initiated to decrease metabolic demands on the liver.

NURSING MANAGEMENT: NURSING DIAGNOSES AND COLLABORATIVE PROBLEMS

Nursing Diagnoses

Common nursing goals for patients with acute hepatitis are to provide adequate nutrition, prevent infection, promote physical mobility, limit fatigue, and minimize pain.

Altered nutrition: Less than body requirement related to anorexia, nausea, or vomiting.

Expected Patient Outcomes. Patient maintains adequate nutrition, as evidenced by body weight within 5% of baseline body weight, nitrogen balance tests, blood glucose 100 to 160 mg/dL, serum albumin 3.5 to 5.5 g/dL, retinol-binding protein 40 to 50 μg/mL, and thyroxine-binding prealbumin 200 to 300 μg/mL.

- Consult with physician and dietitian to determine patient's nutritional needs and individual preferences.
- Review results of tests of nitrogen balance, blood glucose, serum albumin, retinol-binding protein, and thyroxine-binding prealbumin.
- Provide a high-carbohydrate diet (4 g/kg) and avoid foods high in fat.
- Measure all intake and output.
- Measure daily weight and report loss ≥5% of baseline weight.
- Obtain and report clinical findings contributing to reduced nutritional intake: nausea, anorexia, or vomiting.
- Provide small, frequent meals when patient is anorexic.
- Encourage fluids to 3000 mL/24 h if not contraindicated and include fruit juices or carbonated beverages.
- Restrict protein intake should severe hepatic disease occur.
- Administer prescribed vitamin B complex, vitamin C, and other dietary supplements to aid in the healing process.
- Administer prescribed IV fluids when nausea and vomiting are serious.
- Teach patient to avoid alcohol intake to reduce risk of hepatic irritation and prolonged recovery.
- Instruct patient to maintain adequate dietary and fluid intake.
- Instruct patient to wash hands after going to the bathroom.

High risk of infection related to loss of liver cell function secondary to phagocytic barrier.

Expected Patient Outcomes. Patient is free of infection, as evidenced by WBC count ≤11,000 /μL; absence of redness, swelling, tenderness, or drainage from catheter site; normothermia; or negative sputum and wound cultures.

- Review results of WBC count and cultures.
- Obtain cultures of all suspicious drainage from tubes or catheters.
- Assess and report redness, swelling, or tenderness around IV or central lines.
- Use strict aseptic technique when changing dressings or invasive lines.
- Maintain strict use of universal precautions or of body substance isolation procedures.
- Administer prescribed corticosteroids to slow the progression of the disease and lessen symptoms.
- Administer prescribed antibiotics should an infection occur.

Impaired physical mobility related to decreased strength and endocrine activity secondary to decreased energy metabolism by the liver.

Expected Patient Outcomes. Patient maintains physical mobility, as evidenced by increasing strength and endurance.

- Promote bed rest to reduce energy requirement.
- Encourage patient to change position frequently to promote respiratory function and minimize pressure areas when on bed rest.
- Provide a quiet environment conducive to rest and relaxation.
- Prepare increased activity as tolerated when serum enzymes decline.
- Explain reasons why reduced physical activity is necessary early in the course of hepatitis.
- Teach patient relaxation strategies such as guided imagery and meditation to reduce stress.

Fatigue related to liver cell inflammation and reduced energy.

Expected Patient Outcomes. Patient experiences reduced level of fatigue with incremental increases in physical activity when bed rest is discontinued.

- Encourage patient to rest before and after incremental increases in activity.
- Assess patient's tolerance of activity: blood pressure (BP), heart rate (HR), respiratory rate (RR), cardiac rhythm, and presence of weakness.
- Report clinical findings associated with activity intolerance caused by fatigue: tiredness, tachycardia, dyspnea, and weakness.
- Provide a quiet environment that promotes rest and relaxation.
- Limit the number of visitors while patient is fatigued.
- Provide adequate diet and supplements to meet energy requirements.
- Teach patient the factors causing fatigue and diversional strategies to minimize boredom.

Pain related to liver tenderness.

Expected Patient Outcomes. Decrease or absence of liver tenderness.

- Listen to patient's expression of pain and reassure him or her it will subside.
- Explain the origin of abdominal tenderness and reason why sedation, analgesics, or narcotics may not be administered.
- Provide patient with diversional activities: TV, radio, book, or magazine.
- Instruct patient to report any changes in abdominal discomfort.
- Teach patient alternative strategies to cope with discomfort: progressive relaxation, meditation, or guided imagery.

DISCHARGE PLANNING

The critical care nurse will provide patient and significant other(s) verbal or written discharge notes regarding the following subjects:

1. Medications, including drug name, dosage, route, purpose, schedule, and side effects.

2. Importance of infection control such as HBV prophylaxis for sexual partners and significant others living in the same house. Importance of avoiding sharing toothbrush or razor as precautions.
3. Importance of avoiding secondary infections, especially if patient is debilitated.
4. Importance of avoiding alcohol ingestion.
5. Importance of keeping all medical appointments for assessment and laboratory tests.
5. Importance of adhering to prescribed diet and obtaining adequate rest.

■ ACUTE PANCREATITIS

(For related information see Cardiac Deviation, Part I: Shock, p. 174; Behavioral Deviations, Part I, p. 725.)

Case Management Basis
DRG: 204 Disorders of pancreas except malignancy
LOS: 6.10 days

Definition
Acute pancreatitis is an inflammatory and autodigestive disease in which the pancreas is damaged by the enzymes it produces. Pancreatitis consists of edematous interstitial pancreatitis and hemorrhagic necrotizing pancreatitis. Edematous interstitial pancreatitis is characterized by interstitial edema, exudation of small numbers of polymorphonuclear leukocytes, engorgement of capillaries, and dilation of lymphatic vessels. Necrotic pancreatic tissue is characterized by an inflammatory process that extends beyond the pancreas, thereby causing retroperitoneal and peritoneal fat necrosis.

Pathophysiology
Activation of the complement and kinin system, mediated by activated C3 and bradykinin, causes vasodilation and increased permeability of the vasculature. The complement factor activates polymorphonuclear

leukocytes and forms intravascular micro-aggregates. Increased polymorphonuclear leukocytes, recruited to the site, cause further membrane damage and increased vascular permeability. The change in capillary permeability can lead to sequestration of fluid and subsequent depressed cardiac function and pulmonary edema. The kallikrein-kallidin-bradykinin system leads to edema, vasodilation with increased capillary permeability, infiltration of inflammatory cells, and pain. Pancreatitis is classified as edematous or hemorrhagic. In edematous pancreatitis, the pancreas becomes edematous and enzymes escape into the nearby tissues and the peritoneal cavity. In hemorrhagic necrotic pancreatitis, the proteolytic enzymes accumulate within the pancreas and digest it and blood escapes into the pancreatic tissue and into the retroperitoneum. In addition, there is hemorrhage, thrombosis, peripancreatic fat necrosis, and possible pseudocyst and abscess formation.

Nursing Assessment

PRIMARY CAUSES
- Causes include biliary tract disease, alcohol abuse, peptic ulcer, duodenal disease, pancreatic tumors, hypertriglyceridemia, trauma, surgery, third trimester pregnancy, infectious agents, hypercalcemia, and vascular insufficiency. Additional causes are drugs such as thiazide diuretics, furosemide, estrogens, azathioprine, methyldopa, sulfanilamide, pentamidine sulfa antibiotics, procainamide, tetracycline, mercaptopurine, and excessive vitamin D.

RISK FACTORS
- Heredity; history of alcohol abuse.

PHYSICAL ASSESSMENT
- Inspection: Fever; confusion; agitation; restlessness; distress; apprehension; vomiting; nausea; abdominal distention; abdominal guarding; tachypnea; skin pale, mottled, jaundiced, or edematous; Turner's sign

(blue-green-brown discoloration in the flanks resulting from blood accumulation); Cullen's signs (similar discoloration around the umbilicus); or coarse tremors.
- Palpation: Upper abdomen guarding, distention, rebound, palpable abdominal mass, skin is cold and moist.
- Auscultation: Bowel sounds decreased or absent as a result of reduced peristalsis or ileus, hypertension, tachycardia, or basilar crackles.

DIAGNOSTIC TEST RESULTS

Standard Laboratory Tests. (see Table 6–1)

- Arterial blood gases: Hypoxemia and hypercarbia.
- Serum chemistry: Elevated amylase, blood urea nitrogen (BUN), lipase, bilirubin, alkaline phosphatase, triglycerides, lactate dehydrogenase (LDH), (SGOT), and glucose levels. Reduced levels of albumin, protein, calcium, potassium, and prolonged prothrombin time.
- Blood studies: Elevated white blood cell (WBC) count and hematocrit.
- Stool: Increased fat content.
- Urinalysis: Increased amylase, hematuria, and proteinuria.

Invasive Pancreatic Diagnostic Procedures. (see Table 5–2 and Table 6–2)

- Barium studies: Findings include regional or localized ileus, sentinel loop, presence of pancreatic pseudocyst, blurring of the renal outline and left margin, elevation of the diaphragm, pleural effusion, pericardial effusion, and pulmonary edema. Barium studies are helpful only when the head of the pancreas is inflamed.

Noninvasive Pancreatic Diagnostic Procedures. (see Table 6–3)

- Abdominal roentgenogram: Identifies gallstones, sentinel loop (segment of air-filled small intestine in the left upper quadrant), colon cutoff sign (gas-filled segment of transverse colon abruptly ending at the area of pancreatic inflammation), or linear focal atelectasis of the left lower lobe of the lungs with or without pleural effusion.

- Chest roentgenogram x-ray: Pleural effusion.
- Computed tomography (CT): Provides imaging of the pancreas and abdominal cavity. Estimates the size of the pancreas, aids in evaluating cystic lesions and in identifying fluid collections, abscesses, or mass lesions.
- Ultrasound: Used to identify areas of enlargement or distention of the common bile duct, pancreatic mass, pseudocyst, or accumulation of fluid in the abdominal cavity. It can also be used to localize a cyst for percutaneous drainage.

ECG
- Reveals ST-T wave changes.

MEDICAL AND SURGICAL MANAGEMENT

PHARMACOLOGY
- Nonopiate analgesics: Meperidine hydrochloride (Demerol), levorphanal tartrate, and fentanyl citrate are used because they do not cause spasm of the sphincter of Oddi. Patient-controlled analgesic (PCA) is effective in relieving patient's pain, since it allows self-administration of the analgesic.
- Anticholinergic agents: Atropine is used to decrease the stimulation of the pancreas.
- Histamine (H_2) receptor antagonists: Cimetidine or ranitidine can be used to reduce risk of stress ulcers in patients with acute pancreatitis (see Table 5–4, p. 518).
- Dopamine: Low-to-moderate dose ranges (2 to 10 μg/kg/min) support myocardial contractility without vasoconstriction effects. It can also reduce pancreatic inflammation by reducing pancreatic ductal or microvascular permeability through stimulation of beta-adrenergic receptors (see Table 1–10, p. 50).

- Insulin: Is used in patients receiving total parenteral nutrition (TPN) in order to manage complications of glucose metabolism.
- Antibiotics: Are used to treat established infections in patients with acute pancreatitis.

FLUID THERAPY
- Colloid and Ringer's lactate: Are used to replace plasma volume.
- Fresh frozen plasma: Is used to replenish plasma fibronectin.

NUTRITIONAL SUPPORT
- TPN: The goal of TPN is to provide adequate amounts of calories and protein to meet patient's needs and to promote anabolism without stimulating the pancreas. The solution can be a mixture of 29% to 30% hypertonic dextrose and 5% to 12% crystalline amino acids.
- Supplemental vitamins and minerals: These are indicated for patients with pancreatitis.
- Enteral feedings: These are used to supply nutrients if pancreatitis stimulation is bypassed by infusing feeding distal to the duodenum. Intrajejunal feeding is the method used for enteral feeding.

SUPPLEMENTAL OXYGEN
- Oxygen supplement: Is used to maintain normal partial pressure of arterial oxygen (PaO_2).

NASOGASTRIC INTUBATION
- Nasogastric (NG) intubation: NG intubation rests the pancreas by halting the secretion of pancreatic enzymes. Nausea, vomiting, and abdominal distention can be decreased with NG intubation and intermittent suction.

PERITONEAL LAVAGE
- The goal is to remove the vasoactive substances released by the damaged pancreas into the peritoneal fluid.
- The technique involves the placement of a percutaneous peritoneal dialysis catheter

and infusion of 1 to 2 L of isotonic solution continuously.

SURGICAL INTERVENTION

- Pancreatic drainage: The surgical intervention is used to drain the pancreatic bed and to reduce stimulation of the gland by the placement of sump drains.
- Pancreatic resection: The removal of devitalized or necrotic tissue is performed in patients with severe disease or infected pancreatic necrosis or abscess. Once the devitalized liver is removed, Penrose and soft sump drains are placed in the head, body, and tail of the pancreas to evacuate infected material.
- Cholecystectomy: This operation is used in patients with pancreatitis caused by biliary stones.

NURSING MANAGEMENT: NURSING DIAGNOSES AND COLLABORATIVE PROBLEMS

Nursing Diagnoses

Common nursing goals for patients with acute pancreatitis are to maintain fluid balance, promote oxygenation, prevent infection, maintain adequate nutrition, and minimize pain.

Fluid volume deficit related to fluid translocation into the peritoneal cavity secondary to vasodilation and increased permeability of the vasculature.

Expected Patient Outcomes. Patient maintains adequate fluid volume, as evidenced by cardiac output (CO) 4 to 8 L/min, cardiac index (CI) 2.7 to 4.3 L/min/m^2, central venous pressure (CVP) 2 to 6 mm Hg, blood pressure (BP) within patient's normal range, mean arterial pressure (MAP) 70 to 100 mm Hg, heart rate (HR) ≤100 bpm, capillary refill ≤3 seconds, normal skin turgor, urinary output (UO) ≥30 mL/h, peripheral pulses +2, serum protein 6 to 8 g/dL, serum electrolytes within normal limits, hemoglobin ≥10 g/dL, and hematocrit ≥30%.

- Consult with physician regarding patient's volume status and causes of any deficit: Hypovolemia may be due to loss of circulating blood volume from increased capillary endothelial permeability and decreased peripheral resistance.
- Consult with physician to validate expected patient outcomes used to evaluate adequate fluid status.
- Review levels of hemoglobin, hematocrit, albumin, and electrolytes.
- Obtain and report hemodynamic parameters associated with fluid volume deficit: CO ≤4 L/min, CI ≤2.7 L/min/m^2, and CVP ≤2 mm Hg.
- Obtain and report clinical findings associated with fluid volume deficit: hypotension, tachycardia, tachypnea, poor skin turgor, pallor, diaphoresis, peripheral pulses +2, and capillary refill ≤3 seconds.
- Measure intake, output, and daily weight to evaluate patient's fluid balance. Report UO ≤30 mL/h or a daily weight gain 0.5 to 1.0 kg/d, suggesting sequestering of fluid.
- Continuously monitor ECG to assess HR and rhythm. Document ECG rhythm strips ever 2 to 4 hours or more frequently in patients with dysrhythmias or electrolyte imbalance.
- Measure abdominal girth if ascites is present. Fluid, 4 to 12 L, can be sequestered in the peritoneal cavity.
- Evaluate the amount, color, and characteristics of gastric drainage since fluid loss in gastric secretions can be ≥2 L/d.
- Administer prescribed colloids and Ringer's lactate, since saline solution and albumin can promote mobilization of fluid back into the vascular space.
- Administer prescribed fresh frozen plasma to replenish plasma fibronectin.
- Administer prescribed low-to-moderate dopamine if hypotension continues despite fluid resuscitation.
- Prepare the patient for surgery: proximal and distal ligation of the bleeding vessel with possible drainage procedures for pseudocysts.

- Prepare patient for more aggressive surgery, such as distal pancreatectomy with splenectomy, if necessary.

Impaired gas exchange related to damaged pulmonary microvasculature secondary to trypsin causing vasoconstriction, bronchoconstriction, and ventilation-perfusion imbalance.

Expected Patient Outcomes. Patient maintains adequate gas exchange, as evidenced by respiratory rate (RR) 12 to 20 BPM, absence of dyspnea, lung sounds clear, HR $\leq$100 bpm, arterial oxygen saturation (SaO$_2$) $\geq$90%, PaO$_2$ 60 to 100 mm Hg, partial pressure of arterial carbon dioxide (PaCO$_2$) 35 to 45 mm Hg, pH 7.35 to 7.45, and symmetrical chest excursion.

- Review levels of arterial blood gases and the chest roentgenogram.
- Place patient in semi- to high Fowler's position to facilitate lung expansion, thereby improving diaphragmatic excursion.
- Reposition patient every 2 hours to prevent atelectasis.
- Assist patient to assume a position of comfort.
- Monitor and report clinical findings associated with impaired gas exchange: tachypnea, tachycardia, dyspnea, crackles, and cyanosis.
- Continuously monitor oxygen saturation and report SaO$_2$ $\leq$90%.
- Encourage patient to deep breathe, cough, change position, and use incentive spirometer to facilitate lung expansion and prevent atelectasis.
- Measure abdominal girth when abdominal distress occurs to monitor increasing distention and impairment of diaphragmatic excursion.
- Administer prescribed supplementary oxygen by nasal cannula, mask, or ventilatory support to improve oxygenation.

High risk of infection related to pancreatic abscess and infected pancreatic necrosis.

Expected Patient Outcomes. Patient is free from infection, as evidenced by WBC count $\leq$11,000/μL; normothermia; absence of redness, swelling, tenderness, or drainage from wound or drains; and negative cultures.

- Review results of WBC count and cultures.
- Monitor temperature every 2 to 4 hours while patient is febrile.
- Use strict aseptic technique when changing dressings, invasive lines, indwelling catheter, or tubes and drains.
- Change soiled dressings one at a time to prevent cross contamination.
- Obtain culture of blood, wound, urine, sputum, or pancreatic aspirate.
- Monitor invasive lines, indwelling catheter, tubes, or drains for swelling, redness, tenderness, or drainage.
- Assist with peritoneal lavage to remove vasoactive substances. One to 2 liters of isotonic solution is infused continuously through a percutaneous peritoneal dialysis catheter.
- Evaluate aspirated peritoneal fluid as an indicator of severity of the disease: dark-colored free fluid, mid-straw colored lavage return fluid, and $\geq$2 ml of free fluid regardless of color.
- Administer prescribed antibiotics such as gentamicin or tobramycin to treat sepsis.
- Prepare patient for surgery such as pancreatic drainage for a pancreatic infection.

Altered nutrition: Less than body requirements related to nausea, vomiting, or abdominal pain.

Expected Patient Outcomes. Patient maintains adequate nutrition, as evidenced by body weight within 5% of baseline body weight, nitrogen balance tests, blood glucose 100 to 160 mg/dL, serum albumin 3.5 to 5.5 g/dL, retinol-binding protein 40 to 50 μg/mL, and thyroxine-binding prealbumin 200 to 300 μg/mL.

- Consult with physician and dietitian to individualize patient's diet while including his or her preferences.

- Consult with physician about the decreased concentration of plasma total protein and albumin, which is maintained at ≥ 6.5 g/dL and 3.5 g/dL.
- Review levels of serum albumin, glucose, retinol-binding protein, and thyroxine-binding prealbumin.
- Obtain and record intake, output, and caloric intake while patient is ingesting food and fluids.
- Measure daily weights to determine if the ideal body weight is being achieved.
- Insert NG tube to reduce vomiting and abdominal distention.
- Provide enteral feedings if the process of pancreatic stimulation is bypassed by infusion feeding distal to the duodenum.
- Resume oral intake with clear liquids and administer diet slowly to provide high protein and high carbohydrate, if not contraindicated. Oral fluids are given for 3 to 6 days, then regular diet by day 5 to 7.
- Administer prescribed TPN solutions to meet nutritional requirements.
- Administer prescribed supplemental elements, such as vitamins and minerals.
- Provide prescribed insulin when using TPN to control glucose levels.
- Administer prescribed H_2 blockers to reduce gastric acidity and pancreatic juices (see Table 5–4, p. 518).

Pain related to increased pancreatic secretory activity.

Expected Patient Outcomes. Patient is free of pain.

- Keep patient on nothing by mouth (NPO) status to rest gastrointestinal tract and halt pancreatic enzyme excretion.
- Limit activity to bed rest and to reduce patient's metabolic rate.
- Assist patient to assume a knee-to-chest, or fetal, position to promote comfort.
- Initiate comfort measure by massaging patient's back.
- Provide a quiet, relaxed environment conducive to rest.

- Administer prescribed nonopiate analgesics such as meperidine hydrochloride, levorphoral tartrate, or fentanyl citrate because they do not cause spasm of the sphincter of Oddi.
- Instruct patient to described pain using a pain rating scale of 1 to 10. Continued severe pain can indicate progression of the inflammatory process.

Collaborative Goals

Common collaborative goals for patients with acute pancreatitis are to decrease pancreatic secretion, increase cardiac output, correct hyperglycemia, and restore electrolyte balance.

Potential Complication: Increased Pancreatic Secretion. Increased pancreatic secretion related to inflammation resulting in activation of pancreatic enzymes secondary to mechanical, metabolic, or miscellaneous causes.

Expected Patient Outcomes. Patient maintains normal pancreatic secretion without experiencing inflammation or pain.

- Review of serum amylase levels.
- Place patient on bed rest to decrease basal metabolic rate and decrease pancreatic secretion stimulation.
- Initiate NG suction to rest the pancreas by suppressing pancreatic exocrine secretion and preventing the release of secretin in the duodenum.
- Monitor Ranson's criteria and clinical indicators for severity of acute pancreatitis: hemotocrit decrease $\geq 10\%$, BUN ≥ 5 mg/dL, serum calcium ≤ 8 mg/dL, arterial Pao_2 ≤ 60 mm Hg, base deficit ≥ 4 mEq/L, and estimated fluid sequestration ≥ 6 L.
- Assess patient for reduced nausea, vomiting, and abdominal pain when NG tube is connected to intermittent suction.
- Halt oral intake until abdominal pain subsides and serum amylase levels return to normal.
- Initiate oral fluids as prescribed within 3 days to 1 week with slow advancement of solid food.

- Administer prescribed anticholinergic agents: Glucagon, cimetidine, and calcitonin can be used to block stimulation of gastrointestinal function and pancreatic secretion.
- Administer prescribed somatostatin to decrease interstitial motility and reduce endocrine and exocrine secretion.

Potential Complication: Decreased Cardiac Output. Decreased CO related to altered preload, afterload and contractility secondary third spacing of fluids.

Expected Patient Outcomes. Patient is able to maintain CO, as evidenced by CO 4 to 8 L/min, CI 2.7 to 4.3 L/min/m², CVP 2 to 6 mm Hg, pulmonary capillary wedge pressure (PCWP) 6 to 12 mm Hg, BP within patient's normal range HR≤100 bpm, RR 12 to 20 BPM, absence of dysrhythmias, peripheral pulses +2, capillary refill ≤3 seconds, systemic vascular resistance (SVR) 900 to 1200 dynes/s/cm⁻⁵, (SVRI) 1970 to 2390 dynes/s/cm⁻⁵/m², UO ≥30 mL/h, skin warm and dry, and absence of cyanosis.

- Obtain and report hemodynamic findings associated with decreased CO: CO ≤4 L/min, CI ≤2.7 L/min/m², CVP ≤2 mm Hg, PCWP ≤6 mm Hg, SVR ≥1200 dynes/s/cm⁻⁵, and SVRI ≥2390 dynes/s/cm⁻⁵/m².
- Obtain and report other clinical findings associated with decreased CO: hypotension, tachycardia, dysrhythmias, peripheral pulses +2, capillary refill ≥3 seconds, poor skin turgor, pallor or cyanosis, diaphoresis.
- Continuously monitor ECG to assess HR and rhythm. document ECG strips every 2 to 4 hours or more frequently in patients with dysrhythmias or electrolyte imbalance.
- Measure intake and output to evaluate the patient's fluid balance. Report UO ≤30 mL/h.
- Measure daily weight to determine if patient is retaining fluids more than 0.5 to 1.0 kg/d.
- Provide oxygen by nasal cannula, mask, or mechanical ventilation.

- Administer prescribed IV fluids to maintain adequate circulatory volume.
- Administer prescribed low-to-moderate dopamine to support myocardial contractility without vasoconstrictor effects and to decrease pancreatic inflammation (see Table 1–10 p. 50).

Potential Complication: Hyperglycemia. Hyperglycemia related to damaged islet cells secondary to disease process.

Expected Patient Outcomes. Patient's serum amylase and glucose are within normal range.

- Review levels of serum amylase and glucose.
- Test urine for glucose and report findings.
- Obtain and clinical findings associated with hyperglycemia: dehydration, loose or dry skin, hypotension, and tachycardia.
- Measure daily weight, intake, specific gravity, and UO.
- Administer isotonic saline and electrolytes IV to expand extracellular fluid volume.
- Administer hyposmolar solution, such as 0.45% saline, slowly to allow for diffusion and equilibration of water and osmolality, once hyperosmolality is determined.
- Provide low-dose insulin when serum glucose is ≥250 mg/dL.

Potential Complication: Electrolyte Imbalance. electrolyte imbalance related to hypokalemia and hypocalcemia secondary to decreased calcium binding with proteins in the plasma or loss of potassium into the peritoneal cavity.

Expected Patient Outcomes. Patient's serum electrolytes are within normal range.

- Review levels of serum electrolytes.
- Evaluate serum calcium in relation to serum albumin: Hypoalbuminemia seen in acute pancreatitis may account for decreased calcium, as calcium is bound to albumin.
- Obtain and report clinical findings associated with hypokalemia: cardiac dysrhythmias, headache, lethargy, hypotension,

weakness, fatigue, nausea, vomiting, muscle weakness, paresthesia, or hyporeflexia.

- Obtain and report clinical findings associated with hypocalcemia: tremors, paresthesia, tetany, laryngospasm, seizures, positive Chvostek's and Trousseau's signs.
- Measure daily weight, intake, specific gravity, UO or NG drainage.
- Continuously monitor ECG to assess HR and rhythm. Document and report lengthening Q-T, signifying hypocalemia, or ventricular dysrhythmias reflective of hypokalemia.
- Initiate seizure precautions.
- Administer IV fluids or blood products to restore intravascular volume, thereby improving tissue perfusion and oxygenation.
- Administer albumin if necessary, to replace plasma protein lost from intravascular space and causing a disruption of colloidal osmotic pressure and subsequent interstitial edema.
- Administer prescribed calcium replacement via a central line, since peripheral infiltration can cause tissue necrosis.
- Administer prescribed potassium, since potassium is lost with fluid leakage into the peritoneal cavity.
- Administer calcium gluconate IV when patient experiences hypokalemia.

DISCHARGE PLANNING
The critical care nurse will provide patient and significant other(s) verbal or written discharge notes regarding the following subjects:

1. Medications, including drug name, dosage, route, purpose, schedule, and side effects.
2. Importance of avoiding alcohol ingestion.
3. Importance of keeping all medical appointments.
4. Reporting signs and symptoms of infection such as fever, drainage from surgical site, redness around surgical site, or pain.
5. Importance if adhering to prescribed low-fat diet and obtaining adequate rest.

PART II: SURGICAL CORRECTIONS AND NURSING MANAGEMENT

■ SHUNT SURGERY

(For related information see Part I: Hepatic failure, p. 559; Hepatic encephalopathy, p. 571; Portal hypertension, p. 575. Part II: Liver transplantation, p. 597.)

Case Management Basis
DRG: 191 Major pancreas, liver, and shunt procedures with complications
LOS: 15.50 days
DRG: 192 Major pancreas, liver, and shunt procedures without complications
LOS: 8.50 days

Definition
Shunt surgery is used for decompression of varices. It lowers venous pressure and diverts portal blood flow from the gastroesophageal area. Shunt surgery consists of two categories: nonselective and selective. With nonselective shunt surgery, all the portal blood flow enters the systemic circulation without first circulating through the liver. In selective shunts, portal venous flow through the liver is preserved.

Patient Selection

INDICATIONS. Candidates are patients who have no ascites, jaundice, or portal systemic encephalopathy; the patient who has experienced previous episodes of gastrointestinal bleeding; who are under age 50; with serum albumin ≥ 3 g/dL, serum bilirubin ≤ 2.5 mg/dL and prothrombin time $\geq 50\%$ of normal.

CONTRAINDICATIONS. Patient with poorly controlled sepsis and uncontrollable coagulopathies

Procedure

TECHNIQUE. Nonselective shunt surgeries include end-to-end portacaval shunt and side-to-side portacaval shunt. End-to-end portacaval shunt is a procedure that divides the portal vein at its bifurcation before it enters the liver at the porta hepatis. The access of the portal vein to the liver is tied off. The proximal transected portal vein is anastomosed to the side of the infrahepatic inferior vena cava (IVC). Side-to-side portacaval shunt involves the anastomosis of a side of the portal vein to the side of the vena cava. The liver and splanchnic bed are decompressed. Variceal bleeding is prevented and postoperative ascites is inhibited. Mesocaval shunt consists of positioning a prosthetic graft to divert portal blood flow from the liver to the vena cava.

Selective shunt surgeries involve distal splenorenal shunt (DSRS), which is a low-pressure, high-flow shunt that lowers esophagogastric and splenic variceal pressure and controls bleeding. Venous blood supply from the left upper quadrant of the abdomen is shunted from the portal circulation. Portal-system encephalopathy is reduced by maintaining superior mesenteric blood flow to the liver.

Transjugular intrahepatic portosystemic shunt (TIPS) is a new alternative nonsurgical approach to treating variceal bleeding caused by portal hypertension. The normal vascular anatomy of the liver is used to create a shunt between the portal and systemic venous system within the liver. This is accomplished by using a metallic stent to relieve portal hypertension. The technique involves catheterization of the hepatic vein using a jugular vein approach. A needle is directed fluoroscopically from the hepatic vein into the branch of the portal vein along an intrahepatic tract. The intrahepatic tract is then dilated and kept open with a metallic stent delivered on a balloon catheter. The goal during the TIPS procedure is to reduce the pressure gradient to 10 mm Hg.

Complications

Ascites, esophageal varices, portal hypertension, or portal systemic encephalopathy.

NURSING MANAGEMENT: NURSING DIAGNOSES AND COLLABORATIVE PROBLEMS

Nursing Diagnoses

Common nursing goals for patients undergoing shunt surgery are to maintain fluid volume, prevent infection, support effective breathing pattern, promote sleep, and minimize pain.

Fluid volume deficit related to bleeding secondary to altered coagulation.

Expected Patient Outcomes. Patient maintains adequate fluid volume, as evidenced by absence of bleeding, coagulation profile within normal limits, blood pressure (BP) within patient's normal range, heart rate HR $\leq$ 100 bpm, central venous pressure (CVP) 2 to 6 mm Hg, respiratory rate (RR) 12 to 20 BPM, capillary refill $\leq$ 3 seconds, peripheral pulse +2, stable weight, urinary output (UO) $\geq$ 30 mL/h, and absence of cyanosis.

- Review serum albumin levels and coagulation studies.
- Obtain and report clinical findings associated with fluid volume deficit: hypotension, tachycardia, tachypnea, pallor or cyanosis, skin cool, peripheral pulses $\leq$ +2, and capillary refill $\geq$ 3 seconds.
- Measure intake and output. Report UO $\leq$ 30 mL/h or $\leq$ 0.5 mL/kg/h.
- Measure daily weight and report loss $\geq$ 0.5 to 1.0 kg/d.
- Assess dressings and drainage from tubes or drains for bleeding. Test drainage, urine, sputum, or stool for occult blood.
- Monitor systolic BP (SBP) continuously to protect the integrity of the graft from hypertension and prevent thrombosis secondary to hypotension.
- Report clinical indicators of bleeding, since shunt thrombosis is a primary cause of rebleeding after a DSRS.

- Administer prescribed fresh frozen plasma to replace clotting factors and osmotic proteins.
- Administer prescribed crystalloids and 5% dextrose to maintain adequate circulatory volume.

High risk for infection related to incisional or cannulation site inflammation.

Expected Patient Outcomes. Patient is free from infection, as evidenced by normothermia; negative cultures; white blood cell (WBC) count ≤11,000/μL; and absence of redness, swelling, tenderness, or drainage from incision or cannulation site.

- Review results of WBC count and cultures.
- Evaluate incision, dressing, or cannulation site for redness, tenderness, swelling, or drainage.
- Change dressing and tubing using aseptic technique.
- Monitor temperature every 2 to 4 hours while patient is febrile.
- Should drainage occur from a catheter or drain, assess the color and odor to determine whether patient is at risk of infection. Report and send specimen to the laboratory.
- Administer IV fluid as prescribed to maintain adequate hydration.
- Administer antibiotics as prescribed.

Ineffective breathing pattern related to elevated diaphragm secondary to abdominal distention resulting from ascites.

Expected Patient Outcomes. Patient maintains effective breathing pattern, as evidenced by RR 12 to 20 BPM, HR ≤100 BPM, absence of crackles, symmetry of chest movement, warm and dry skin, absence of cyanosis, absence of shortness of breath or dyspnea, and arterial blood gases within normal range.

- Review arterial blood gas levels and chest roentgenogram.
- Monitor clinical indicators of respiratory status: RR and depth, symmetry of chest movement, use of accessory muscles, skin color, and lung sounds.

- Report clinical findings associated with ineffective breathing pattern: tachycardia, tachypnea, dyspnea, shortness of breath, cyanosis, and crackles.
- Continuously monitor ECG to assess HR and rhythm. Document ECG rhythm strip every 1 to 2 hours if patient experiences dysrhythmias as a result of hypoxemia.
- Encourage patient to sit in a semi-Fowler's position to facilitate lung expansion.
- Assist patient to change position as tolerated to prevent atelectasis.
- Encourage patient to cough, turn, deep breathe, and use incentive spirometer to enhance lung expansion.
- Initiate prescribed nasogastric (NG) tube for gastric decompression and to decrease abdominal distention.
- Provide prescribed oxygen by nasal cannula or mask to increase tissue oxygenation.

Sleep pattern disturbance related to discomfort secondary to surgical incision.

Expected Patient Outcomes. Patient is able to use techniques that promote sleep.

- Provide a calm, quiet environment conducive to sleep.
- Assist patient to assume a position of comfort, which facilitates rest.
- Provide rest measures by massaging patient's back.
- Reduce environmental noise.
- Encourage patient to use sleep-inducing strategies such as progressive relaxation, reading, or meditation.
- Listen to patient's description of bedtime routine such as time, hygiene measures, or rituals such as reading.
- Explain to patient or family the causes of sleep and rest disturbance and possible ways to avoid them.

Pain related to incision.

Expected Patient Outcomes. Absence of or decreased verbalization of pain.

- Maintain bed rest in a quiet environment.
- Evaluate patient's pain on a scale of 1 to 10.

- Change patient's position to assist in reducing discomfort.
- Assist patient with passive or active range of motion exercises every 4 hours during bed rest.
- Administer analgesics when appropriate and as prescribed.
- Instruct patient to report any changes in type of pain.
- Instruct patient to use alternative stress-reducing strategies: progressive relaxation, meditation, or guided imagery

DISCHARGE PLANNING

The critical care nurse will provide patient and significant other(s) verbal or written discharge notes regarding the following subjects:

1. Medications, including drug name, dosage, route, purpose, schedule, and side effects.
2. Importance of keeping all medical appointments.
3. Reporting signs and symptoms of infection, such as fever, drainage from surgical site, redness around surgical site, or pain.

■ LIVER TRANSPLANTATION

(For related information see Part I: Hepatic failure, p. 559; Hepatic encephalopathy, p. 571; Portal hypertension, p. 575.)

Case Management Basis

DRG: 201 Other hepatobiliary or pancreas
   O.R. procedure
LOS: 8.80 days

Definition

Liver transplantation is a surgical alternative to the conservative medical management of end-stage chronic liver disease or acute hepatic failure.

Patient Selection

INDICATIONS. Indications are advanced cirrhosis secondary to cholestatic syndrome or hepatic disease, hepatocellular disease, metabolic liver disease, acute fulminant hepatic failure, cryptogenic cirrhosis, primary biliary cirrhosis, primary sclerosing cholangitis, Budd-Chiari syndrome, and refractory variceal bleeding.

CONTRAINDICATIONS. Contraindications are active hepatitis (positive serology for hepatitis B surface antigen [HBsAg] or hepatitis Beantigen [HBeAg]), active alcohol or drug abuse, hepatic malignancy, and portal vein thrombosis.

Procedure

TECHNIQUES. The orthotopic procedure involves the following four vascular anastomoses: suprahepatic inferior vena cava, infrahepatic inferior vena cava, portal vein, and hepatic artery. There is also a biliary anastomosis. An autologous transfuser or cell saver device is used to decrease the amount of donor red blood cells used. Blood is drained from the infrahepatic vena cava and the portal vein to a centrifugal pump that returns blood to the ipsilateral axillary and internal jugular vein. Once the four vascular anastomoses are completed, the biliary anastomoses can be achieved via a choledochocholedochostomy (end-to-end donor to recipient) or a choledochojejunostomy, (end-to-side donor common duct to Roux-en-Y limb of recipient jejunum. A choledochocholedochostomy is stented with a T tube and the choledochojejunostomy is not usually stented but may be.

NURSING MANAGEMENT: NURSING DIAGNOSES AND COLLABORATIVE PROBLEMS

Nursing Diagnoses

Common nursing diagnoses for patients experiencing liver transplantation are to maintain fluid balance, promote oxygenation, support urinary elimination, facilitate normal thought process, and prevent injury.

Fluid volume deficit related to bleeding secondary to coagulation problems or rupture of an anastomosis.

Expected Patient Outcomes. Patient maintains adequate fluid volume, as evidenced by cardiac output (CO) 4 to 8 L/min; cardiac index (CI) 2.7 to 4.3 L/min/m²; central venous pressure CVP 2 to 6 mm Hg, blood pressure (BP) within patient's normal range, heart rate (HR) ≤100 bpm, respiratory rate (RR) 12 to 20 BPM; normal skin turgor; skin warm and dry; absence of pallor or cyanosis; peripheral pulses +2; capillary refill ≤3 seconds; urinary output (UO) ≥30 mL/h or ≥0.5 mL/kg/h, coagulation studies, serum electrolytes, and serum albumin within normal limits.

- Review coagulation studies and serum electrolyte, serum albumin, and hematocrit levels.
- Obtain and report hemodynamic parameters associated with fluid volume deficit: CO ≤4 L/min, CI ≤2.7 L/min/m², and CVP ≤2 mm Hg.
- Assess clinical indicators of hydration: BP, HR, skin turgor, skin warmth and color, peripheral pulses, and capillary refill.
- Report clinical findings associated with fluid volume deficit: hypotension, tachycardia, poor skin turgor, pallor or cyanosis, peripheral pulses ≥+2 and capillary refill ≥3 seconds.
- Assess fluid volume status by measuring all intake and output hourly. Compare results to previous hour and report UO ≤30 mL/h or ≤0.5 mL/kg/h.
- Report sudden change in systolic blood pressure (SBP) and mean arterial pressure (MAP), which can signify ruptured anastomoses.
- Monitor abdominal drainage from sump drains that are connected to continuous suction at 90 to 110 mm Hg: 250 to 500 mL/8 h, with the total being 500 to 750 mL/24 h.
- Irrigate sump drain with 20 to 30 mL normal saline three times a day while using sterile technique.

- Administer prescribed IV crystalloids or colloids to maintain adequate circulatory volume.
- Administer prescribed IV blood products to replace clotting factors.
- Should an anastomosis rupture, prepare patient for surgery.

Impaired gas exchange related to atelectasis or ventilation-perfusion imbalance secondary to diaphragmatic insult, anesthesia, or pain.

Expected Patient Outcomes. Patient maintains adequate gas exchange, as evidenced by RR 12 to 20 BPM, lungs clear, skin warm and dry, symmetry of chest movement, absence of dyspnea, absence of shortness of breath, arterial blood gases within normal range.

- Review results of chest roentgenogram and arterial blood gas measurement.
- Place patient in a semi-Fowler's position, if not contraindicated, to facilitate lung expansion.
- Monitor clinical indicators of respiratory status: RR and depth, symmetry of chest wall movement, use of accessory muscles, skin color, and lung sounds.
- Report clinical findings associated with impaired gas exchange: tachypnea, dyspnea, shortness of breath, crackles, cyanosis, and asymmetry of chest movement.
- Maintain a patient airway by suctioning patient according to unit protocol.
- Assist patient to turn every 2 hours to avoid atelectasis.
- Encourage patient to cough, deep breathe, and use incentive spirometer, if not contraindicated, to facilitate lung expansion.
- Assist with the removal of secretions by suctioning as needed.
- Assess patient's incisional pain, which could cause splinting and shallow breathing.
- Administer prescribed oxygen by nasal cannula, mask, or mechanical ventilation to enhance tissue oxygenation.
- Administer prescribed IV fluids to maintain adequate hydration.

Altered pattern of urinary elimination related to oliguria secondary to intraoperative hypotension, sepsis, or use of immunosuppressive agent.

Expected Patient Outcomes. Patient maintains normal pattern of urinary elimination, as evidenced by UO $\geq$30 mL/h or $\geq$0.5 mL/kg/h, serum blood urea nitrogen (BUN) 8 to 23 mg, serum creatinine 0.6 to 1.2 mg, creatinine clearance 120 to 130 mL/min, serum potassium 3.5 to 5.0 mEq/L, BP within patient's normal range, absence of edema, and specific gravity 1.010 to 1.025.

- Consult with physician and pharmacist about the blood's concentration level of cyclosporine (400 to 600 ng/mL), which can cause nephrotoxicity.
- Review levels of serum creatinine, potassium, and BUN and creatinine clearance.
- Obtain and report clinical findings associated with altered pattern of urinary elimination: oliguria, specific gravity $\leq$1.010, edema, and weight gain.
- Monitor continuous ECG to assess HR and rhythm. Document ECG rhythm strips every 2 hours or more frequently in patients with electrolyte imbalance.
- Monitor fluid volume status by accurately measuring intake, output, and weight.
- Administer prescribed IV plasma expanders to maintain adequate circulatory volume.
- Should patient receiving cyclosporine experience UO $\leq$30 mL/h, report and discontinue drug as ordered.
- Should UO fail to improve, prepare patient for hemodialysis.

High risk of injury related to seizure secondary to cyclosporine or electrolyte imbalance.

Expected Patient Outcomes. Patient is free from seizure activity.

- Consult with physician about potential causes of seizure activity in liver transplantation patient.

- Review arterial blood gas and serum sodium levels.
- Monitor and report seizure activity.
- Provide a safe environment to protect patient from injury during seizure.
- Protect patient from aspiration during seizure by maintaining a patent airway.
- Initiate seizure precaution.
- Reorient patient to person, place, and time.
- Initiate, physical restrictions if not contraindicated, to protect patient from harm in case of restlessness and delirium.
- Administer prescribed IV diazepam in doses of 2 to 10 mg to treat seizures.

Collaborative Problems

Common collaborative goals for patients experiencing liver transplantation are to minimize immunodeficiency, prevent allograft rejection, and prevent thrombophlebitis.

Potential Complication: Immunodeficiency. Immunodeficiency related to the use of immunosuppressive therapy.

Expected Patient Outcomes. Patient's immune system function normally.

- Consult with physician about the type of immunosuppressive agents used and potential complications specific to individual patient.
- Provide adequate nutritional support as determined by consultation with the dietitian and physician.
- Review results of serum white blood cell (WBC) count coagulation studies; albumin, bilirubin, alkaline phosphatase, and amino transferase levels, hematocrit; hemoglobin; radioimmunoassay (RIA) or high-pressure liquid chromatography (HPLC).
- Assess and report elevated temperature and redness, swelling, tenderness, or drainage from catheter site or incision.
- Change all dressings, lines or catheters using strict aseptic techniques.
- Maintain patient in protective or reverse isolation.

- Limit the number of invasive devices to reduce the risk of infection.
- Cleanse the incision line and drain sites with half-strength hydrogen peroxide and normal saline every 8 hours.
- Administer prescribed cyclosporine, antilymphocyte globulins, and OKT3 to suppress the T-lymphocyte response (see Table 1–15, p. 129).
- Administer prescribed corticosteroids to decrease serum levels of lymphocyte and monocyte by moving them from the peripheral circulation and may inhibit serum IgG levels.
- Should patient experience rejection, prepare patient for liver biopsy.

Potential Complication: Allograft Rejection. Allograft rejection related to graft-vs-host reaction.

Expected Patient Outcomes. Patient is free from allograft rejection, as evidenced by serum bilirubin total ≤1.3 mg/dL, direct ≤0.4 mg/dL, serum glutamic oxaloacetic transaminase (SGOT) ≤36 IU/L, serum glutamate pyruvate transaminase (SGPT) ≤24 IU/L, alkaline phosphatase ≤90 IU/L, amylase ≤130 IU/L, prothrombin time (PT) ≤16 seconds, partial thromboplastin time (PTT) ≤45 seconds, normothermia, HR ≤100 bpm, and golden bile drainage.

- Review serum bilirubin, alkaline phosphatase, and aminotransferase levels.
- Monitor patient and report clinical indicators of acute rejection: malaise, fever, abdominal pain, change in color of bile resulting from decreased biliary bilirubin excretion, and a decrease in bile output from the T-tube.
- Change dressings or tubes using strict aseptic technique.
- Should acute rejection be suspected, prepare patient for liver biopsy.
- Evaluate for the presence of pain in upper right quadrant or flank.
- Inspect bile drainage hourly, noticing the amount and color.

- Obtain daily cyclosporine levels to minimize risk of nephrotoxicity.
- Administer prescribed corticosteroids such as methylprednisolone (1 g bolus IV) with a maintenance dose to treat acute rejection.
- Administer prescribed immunosuppressants, single or in combination, to alter immune responses in order to prevent rejection: azathioprine, cyclosporine, antilymphocyte globulin, antithymocyte globulin, and OKT3 (see Table 1–15, p. 129).
- Teach patient the common side effects of immunosuppressive agents.

Potential Complication: Thrombophlebitis. Thrombophlebitis related to vascular insufficiency secondary to venovenous bypass.

Expected Patient Outcomes. Patient is free from thrombophlebitis in left upper and lower extremities.

- Review results of coagulation studies.
- Reposition patient hourly to prevent pressure areas and maintain skin integrity.
- Assess clinical indicators of peripheral perfusion: peripheral pulses, capillary refill, skin color, skin temperature, and sensorimotor function.
- Report clinical findings associated with altered peripheral perfusion resulting from thrombophlebitis: peripheral pulses ≤+2, capillary refill ≥3 seconds, skin warm and swelling, pallor or cyanosis, and loss of sensorimotor function.
- Auscultate for bruit in any area of suspected vascular insufficiency.
- Instruct patient to report any changes in sensorimotor sensation.

DISCHARGE PLANNING
The critical care nurse will provide patient and significant other(s) verbal or written discharge notes regarding the following subjects:

1. Medications, including drug name, dosage, route, purpose, schedule, and side effects.

2. Importance of keeping all medical appointments.
3. Reporting signs and symptoms of rejection: low-grade temperature, malaise, skin color changes, and tiredness.
4. Importance of taking immunosuppressive drugs and reporting any significant side effects.
5. Importance of avoiding secondary infections.
6. Eating appropriate diet and maintaining adequate rest periods.

PART III: SUPPORTIVE PROCEDURES AND NURSING MANAGEMENT

■ ENDOSCOPIC INJECTION SCLEROTHERAPY

Definition

Endoscopic injection sclerotherapy (EIS) is the injection of a sclerosing or coagulating substance into the varices to stop or decrease the risk of bleeding. The technique is an alternative to surgery.

Patient Selection

INDICATIONS. Used in patients who have had at least one variceal hemorrhage.

Procedure

TECHNIQUE. The endoscope is inserted through the esophagus to the gastroesophageal junction, and an injector with a 23 or 25 gauge retractable needle is inserted via the biopsy channel. As the esophagus is insufflated, the varices are localized and the needle is inserted into a varix. A sclerosing agent is used (0.5 to 4.0 mL of sclerosing agent per varix for a total of 15 to 25 mL sclerosant per session). Injection can be paravariceal or intravariceal. Paravariceal injection is made into the tissue surrounding the varix. This process causes the formation of fibrous tissue around the varix, which ceases bleeding. Intravariceal injection is made directly into the lumen of the varix. This process causes thrombus formation in the vein and obliterates bleeding. The patient is placed on his or her left side with the head of bed elevated 30 degrees to prevent aspiration.

EQUIPMENT. Sclerosing agents such as sodium tetradecyl sulfate (1.5% or 3%).

Complications

Esophageal ulcerations, esophageal stricture, esophageal perforation, mucosal sloughing, venous embolism, fever, retrosternal burning pain, bacteremia sepsis, aspiration pneumonia, pleural effusion, bradycardia, and dysphagia.

NURSING MANAGEMENT: NURSING DIAGNOSES AND COLLABORATIVE PROBLEMS

Impaired tissue integrity related to esophageal ulceration or mucosal sloughing.

Expected Patient Outcome. Patient's esophageal tissue remains intact or is healing appropriately.

- Consult with physician regarding the presence of esophageal ulceration or mucosal sloughing.
- Review results of white blood cell (WBC), count and hemoglobin and hematocrit levels.
- Elevate the head of bed 30 degrees to prevent risk of aspiration.
- Evaluate for the presence of esophageal ulceration, manifested as bleeding, which may occur in the first 1 to 2 weeks after EIS.
- Obtain and report clinical findings associated with esophageal rebleeding: hypotension, tachycardia, nausea, bloody emesis, and pain.

- Instruct patient as to the cause of esophageal ulceration should it occur.

Hyperthermia related to contaminants in the sclerosant or the inflammatory process produced within the vein.

Expected Patient Outcomes. Patient's temperature within normal range.

- Review results of WBC count.
- Monitor temperature every 2 to 4 hours while patient is febrile.
- Administer antipyretic agents as prescribed.
- Instruct patient that febrile reactions are common and can subside within 48 hours.

Impaired gas exchange related to aspiration pneumonia or pleural effusion.

Expected Patient Outcomes. Patient maintains adequate gas exchange, as evidenced by arterial blood gases within normal range, respiratory rate (RR) 12 to 20 BPM, absence of cyanosis, arterial oxygen saturation (Sao_2) 95% to 97.5%, and absence of adventitious breath sounds.

- Review arterial blood gas, hemoglobin and hematocrit levels, WBC count, and chest roentgenogram.
- Place patient in a position of comfort to enhance ventilation and oxygenation.
- Monitor the clinical indicators of respiratory status: rate, depth, symmetry of chest wall movement, use of accessory muscles, skin color and temperature, and presence of adventitious breath sounds.
- Report clinical findings associated with impaired gas exchange: tachypnea, dyspnea, cough, tachycardia, and cyanosis.
- Suction patient as necessary using unit protocol.
- Encourage patient to cough, turn, and deep breathe.
- Provide oxygen by nasal cannula or Venturi mask at the prescribed amount.
- Administer antibiotics as prescribed.

Swallowing impaired related to esophageal narrowing.

Expected Patient Outcomes. Patient is able to swallow without distress.

- Evaluate patient for evidence of swallowing difficulties.
- Encourage patient to report any difficulty swallowing after EIS.
- Prepare for esophageal dilation if necessary.
- Instruct patient that impaired swallowing will improve within a few days.

High risk for infection related to esophageal perforation, abscess, or diffuse mediastinitis.

Expected Patient Outcomes. Patient is free from infection, as evidenced by WBC count ≤11,000/μL, normothermia, and absence of esophageal perforation.

- Review results of WBC count.
- Monitor temperature every 2 to 4 hours while patient is febrile.
- Administer IV fluids as prescribed to maintain adequate hydration while the patient is permitted nothing by mouth (NPO) and is febrile.
- Administer parenteral hyperalimentation, if necessary, to maintain adequate nutritional intake.
- Administer antibiotics as prescribed.

Pain related to sclerosing agent causing retrosternal burning.

Expected Patient Outcome. Absence of or decreased verbalization of pain.

- Place patient in position of comfort to minimize pain.
- Encourage patient to describe pain and rate it on a scale of 1 to 10.
- Administer analgesics: Meperidine (Demerol) or acetaminophen.
- Teach patient the origin of pain, since it may mimic myocardial pain.

ESOPHAGOGASTRIC BALLOON TAMPONADE

Definition

Esophagogastric balloon tamponade is accomplished with a Sengstaken-Blakemore (SB) tube. The SB tube is a triple-lumen, double-balloon catheter used to control bleeding from esophageal and gastric varices. The goal is to cause balloon tamponade of the bleeding varices.

Patient Selection

INDICATIONS. Patients with hemorrhaging from esophageal and gastric varices.

Procedure

TECHNIQUE. The most basic device (one Linton tube) contains just one balloon which is inflated in the stomach and drawn upward to the esophagogastric junction. A distal suction port is used to decompress the stomach, while an esophageal port aids in the prevention of aspiration. The Sengstaken-Blakemore tube has an esophageal and a stomach balloon, with only a gastric suction port. The Minnesota tube has two balloons and two suction ports. The balloons may be placed transorally or transnasally. The inflated balloon creates a tamponading effect on the bleeding varices located in the proximal gastric and gastro-esophageal junction mucosa. The gastric aspiration port is connected to low, intermittent suction. Traction is maintained by pulling the tube taut and attaching it to a face bar or football helmet.

EQUIPMENT

- Three-lumen tube: One lumen is for gastric decompression, the second lumen for inflation of the gastric balloon, and third lumen for the esophageal balloon.
- Maintenance: The gastric tube is irrigated every 30 to 60 minutes with iced saline and water until returns are clear. The gastric lumen is attached to continuous intermittent suction and the patient evaluated for bleeding.

Complications

Complications consist of pulmonary aspiration, rupture of the esophagus, and rupture or dilation of the balloon.

NURSING MANAGEMENT: NURSING DIAGNOSES AND COLLABORATIVE PROBLEMS

Nursing Diagnoses

Common nursing goals for patients undergoing esophagogastric balloon tamponade are to prevent injury and reduce the risk of aspiration.

High risk of injury related to esophageal ulceration or necrosis secondary to balloon tamponade.

Expected Patient Outcomes. Patient is free from esophageal injury.

- Consult with physician about the specific pressure used to inflate the esophageal balloon.
- Report clinical findings associated with esophageal rupture, which is manifested as a sudden onset of upper abdominal or back pain and a sudden decrease in systolic blood pressure (SBP).
- Place patient in a semi-Fowler's position.
- Inflate the gastric balloon, as prescribed, with 300 to 500 mL of air and double-clamp the port with rubber clamp.
- Should gastric balloon inflation fail to stop bleeding, inflate esophageal balloon, as prescribed, to 25 to 40 mm Hg and double clamp the esophageal lumen with rubber clamp.
- Check esophageal balloon every 30 to 60 minutes.
- Deflate and inflate esophageal balloon as prescribed.

- Deflate balloon for a period of 12 hours before to its removal and monitor patient for evidence of bleeding.
- Maintain esophageal pressure for up to 48 hours, since longer use could cause esophageal tissue injury, necrosis, and perforation.
- Maintain tube's traction with a football helmet.

High risk for aspiration related to pooling of secretions in the esophagus above the inflated balloon.

Expected Patient Outcomes. Patient is able to handle secretions and does not experience aspiration.

- Maintain patient in a semi-Fowler's position.
- Place patient on complete bed rest, avoiding exertion such as coughing or straining, which can increase intra-abdominal pressure.
- Keep scissors at the bedside should the gastric balloon rupture and cause tube to move out of the esophagus or cause obstruction injury. Cut through the entire tube and remove it.
- Irrigate gastric tube every 30 to 60 minutes with iced saline or water until the returns are clear.
- Connect gastric lumen to continuous intermittent suction and monitor returns.
- Assess patient for persistent bleeding, since erosive gastritis may occur.
- Obtain and report clinical findings associated with pulmonary aspiration: tachypnea, tachycardia, dyspnea, shortness of breath, restlessness, cough, and agitation.
- Initiate suctioning to remove excess secretions.
- Insert a nasogastric tube, as prescribed, to the level of gastroesophageal junction and connect to low, intermittent suction. This will help to reduce the risk of pulmonary aspiration.
- Instruct patient to report any difficulty breathing.

REFERENCES

Adams L, Soulen MC. TIPS: a new alternative for the variceal bleeder. *Am J Crit Care* 1993;2: 196–201.

Adinaro D. Liver failure and pancreatitis. *Nurs Clin North Am.* 1987;22:843–852.

Agusti A, Roca J, Roisin-Rodriguez R, et al. Pulmonary hemodynamics and gas exchange during exercise in liver cirrhosis. *Am Rev Resp Dis.* 1989;139:485–491.

Babb R, Jackman R. Needle biopsy of the liver. *West J Med.* 1989;50:39–42.

Beckermann S, Galloway S. Elective resection of the liver: nursing care. *Crit Care Nurse* 1989; 9(10):40–47.

Berger HG. Surgical management of necrotizing pancreatitis. *Surg Clin North Am.* 1989;69: 529–549.

Bongard FS, Sue DY. Current Critical Care Diagnosis and Treatment. Norwalk, Conn: Appleton & Lange;1994.

Bosch J, Navasa M, Pagan-Garcia JC, et al. Portal hypertension. *Med Clin North Am.* 1989;73: 931–953.

Bradley EL. Complications of chronic pancreatitis. *Surg Clin North Am* 1989;69:481–497.

Brown A. Acute pancreatitis: pathophysiology, nursing diagnoses, and collaborative problems. *Focus Crit Care.* 1991;18(2):121–130.

Bruckstein AH. Chronic hepatitis. *Postgrad Med.* 1989;85(7):67–74.

Bruns SM, Martin MJ. VP/NTG therapy in the patient with variceal bleeding. *Crit Care Nurse.* 1990;10(9):42–49.

Busby HC. Hepatic disorders. In: Hudak CM, Gallo BM, Benz JJ, eds. *Critical Care Nursing,* 6th Ed. Philadelphia, Pa: JB Lippincott Co; 1994:848–858.

Covington H. (1993). Nursing care of patients with alcoholic liver disease. *Crit Care Nurse.* 1993; 13(3):47–57.

Deglin JH, Vallerand AH. Davis's Drug Guide For Nurses 4th Ed. Philadelphia, FA Davis, Co; 1995.

Dolan JT. Nursing management of the patient with hepatic failure and hepatic encephalopathy. *Crit Care Nurs.* Philadelphia, Pa: FA Davis Co; 1991:1066–1092.

Edell ES, Cortese DA, Krowka MJ. et al. Severe hypoxemia and liver disease. *Am Rev Resp Dis.* 1989; 140:1631–1635.

Fain JA, Vealey-Amato E. Acute pancreatitis: a gastrointestinal emergency. *Crit Care Nurse.* 1988;8(5):47–60.

Ford RD. Diagnostic Test Handbook. Springhouse, Pa: Springhouse Corporation; 1987.

Foster JH. Liver resection techniques. *Surg Clin North Am.* 1989;69:235–249.

Gammal SH, Jones AE. Hepatic encephalopathy. *Med Clin North Am.* 1989;73:793–813.

Garcia G, Gentry KR. Chronic viral hepatitis. *Med Clin North Am.* 1989;73:971–983.

Hennessy K. Patients with acute pancreatitis. In: Clochesy JM, Breu C, Cardin S, et al, eds. *Critical Care Nursing.* Philadelphia, Pa: WB Saunders Co, 1993:970–1008.

Holm A, Halpern N, Aldrete JS. Peritoneovenous shunt for intractable ascites of hepatic, nephrogenic, and malignant causes. *Am J Surg.* 1989; 158:162–166.

Jeffres C. Complications of acute pancreatitis. *Crit Care Nurse*; 1989;9(4):38–48.

Jenkins RL, Fairchild RB. The role of transplantation in liver disease. *Surg Clin North Am.* 1989; 69:371–382.

Kaplan MM. Chronic liver disease: current therapeutic options. *Hosp Prac.* 1989;24(3):111–130.

Katelaris PH, Jones DB. Fulminant hepatic failure. *Med Clin North Am.* 1989;73:955–970.

Keith JS. Hepatic failure: etiologies, manifestations, and management. *Crit Care Nurse.* 1985; 5(1):60–86.

Kerber K. The adult with bleeding esophageal varices. *Crit Care Nurs Clin North Am.* 1993; 5:153–162.

Kigerl K. Patients with disorders of glucose metabolism. In: Clochesy JM, Breu C, Cardin S, et al, eds. *Critical Care Nursing.* Philadelphia, Pa: WB Saunders Co; 1993: 1029–1036.

Krumberger JM. Acute pancreatitis. *Crit Care Nurs Clin North Am.* 1993;5:185–202.

Kucharski SA. Fulminant hepatic failure. *Crit Care Nurs Clin North Am.* 1993;5:141–151.

Lee SS. Cardiac abnormalities in liver cirrhosis. *West J Med.* 1989;151:530–535.

Loeb S. Clinical Laboratory Test. Springhouse, Pa: Springhouse Corp; 1991.

Loriaux TC, Dras JA. Endocrine and diabetic disorders. In: Kinney MR, Packa DR, Dunbar SB, eds. *AACN'S Clinical Reference for Critical Care Nursing,* 3rd ed. St. Louis, Mo: Mosby Year Book; 1993:927–959.

Melot C, Naeije R, Dechamps P, et al. Pulmonary and extrapulmonary contributors to hypoxemia in liver cirrhosis. *Am Rev Resp Dis.* 1989; 139:632–640.

Miller HD. Liver transplantation: postoperative ICU care. *Crit Care Nurse.* 1988;8(6):19–31.

Moorhouse MF, Geissler AC, Doenges ME. Acute pancreatitis. *J Emerg Nurs.* 1988;14: 387–391.

Mudge C, Carlson L. Hepatorenal syndrome. *AACN Clin Issues Crit Care Nurs.* 1992;3: 614–632.

Munoz SJ, Friedman, LS. Liver transplantation. *Med Clin North Am.* 1989;73:1011–1039.

Otero-Moreno R, Melman-Lister M, Jones EA. Pulmonary biliary cirrhosis. *Med Clin North Am.* 1989;73:911–929.

Peck SN, Griffith D. Reducing portal hypertension and variceal bleeding. *Dimensions Crit Care Nurs.* 1988;7:269–278.

Pierce JD, Wilkerson E, Griffiths SA. Acute esophageal bleeding and endoscopic injection sclerotherapy. *Crit Care Nurse.* 1990;10(9): 67–72.

Potts JR. Acute pancreatitis. *Surg Clin North Am.* 1988;68:281–299.

Rector WG, Hossack KF. Pathogenesis of sodium retention complicating cirrhosis: is there room for diminished effective arterial blood volume? *Gastroenterol.* 1988;95: 1648–1657.

Roberts SL. Acute pancreatitis. *Physiological Concepts and the Critically Ill Patient.* Englewood Cliffs, NJ: Prentice-Hall; 1985:310–339. [out of print]

Roberts SL. Hepatic encephalopathy. *Physiological Concepts and the Critically Ill Patient.* Englewood Cliffs, NJ: Prentice-Hall; 1985:245–280. [out of print]

Root RK. Fulminant hepatic failure. *Wes J Med.* 1988;149:586–591.

Runyon BA, Antillon MR, Montano AA. Effect of diuresis versus therapeutic paracentesis on ascitic fluid opsonic activity and serum complement. *Gastroenterol.* 1989;97:158–162.

Rustgi AK, Saini S, Schapiro RH. Hepatic imaging and advanced endoscopic techniques. *Med Clin North Am.* 1989;73:895–909.

Savino JA, Cerabona T, Agarwal N, et al. Manipulation of ascitic fluid pressure in cirrhosis to optimize hemodynamic and renal function. *Ann Surg.* 1988;208:504–511.

Shannon MT, Wilson BA. Govoni & Hayes Drugs and Nursing Implications. 7th ed. Norwalk, Conn: Appleton Lange; 1992.

Smith SL. Patients with liver dysfunction. In: Clochesy JM, Breu C, Cardin S, et al, eds. *Critical Care Nursing*. Philadelphia, Pa: WB Saunders Co; 1993:970–1008.

Smith SL, Ciferni M. Liver transplantation for acute heart failure: a review of clinical experience and management. *Am J Crit Care*. 1993; 2:137–144.

Steer ML. Classification and pathogenesis of pancreatitis. *Surg Clin North Am*. 1989;69:467–480.

Stillwell SB. *Mosby's Critical Care Nursing Reference*. St. Louis, Mo: Mosby Year Book; 1992.

Swearingen PL, Keen JH. *Manual of Critical Care,* 2nd. ed. St. Louis, Mo: Mosby Year Book; 1992.

Toto KH. Endocrine physiology: a comprehensive review. *Crit Care Nurs Clin North Am*. 1994; 6:637–660.

Toto KH. Regulation of plasma osmolality. *Crit Care Nurs Clin North Am*. 1994;6:661–674.

Vuji CI. Vascular complications of pancreatitis. *Radiol Clin North Am*. 1989;27:81–91.

7

Neurological Deviations

■ CEREBRAL HEMORRHAGE

*(For related information, see Part I: Acute
head injury, p. 620; Cerebrovascular accident,
p. 630; Status epilepticus, p. 636. Part II: Craniotomy, p. 664. Part III: Intracranial pressure
monitoring, p. 671; Barbiturate coma, p. 674;
and Cerebral balloon angioplasty, p. 674. See
also Behavioral Deviations Part I, p. 725.)*

Case Management Basis

DRG: 34 Other disorders of nervous system
   with complications
LOS: 5.90 days
DRG: 35 Other disorders of nervous system
   without complications
LOS: 3.70 days

Definition

Cerebral aneurysm is a localized dilatation or
ballooning of a cerebral artery caused by
weakness in the vessel wall. Aneurysms are
classified according to their configuration as
saccular, fusiform, or dissecting. Subarachnoid hemorrhage (SAH) is due to a cerebral
vessel that has leaked or ruptured, thereby allowing blood to flow into the subarachnoid
space. Intracerebral hemorrhage (ICH) results
from bleeding into the brain parenchyma.

Pathophysiology

Saccular or berry aneurysms form at the place
of arterial bifurcation in the anterior cerebral
circulation of the circle of Willis. Saccular
aneurysms have a narrow neck that extends
from the parent vessel and expands into a
broader dome. Fusiform aneurysms are spin-
dle-shaped dilatations of an artery with a tapering end found in the vertebrobasilar artery.
Dissecting aneurysms form a tear in the endothelium, which creates a false channel.
With SAH, several responses occur that alter
regional cerebral blood flow. The responses
include loss of cerebral autoregulation, decreased cerebral perfusion pressure, increased
intracranial pressure, and arterial vasospasm.
The overall consequence is cerebral ischemia
and infarction. ICH can develop gradually as
a result of the low pressure of arterioles and
capillaries. Most ICHs occur in the cerebral
hemisphere within the putamen, thalamus,

and lobar regions, while a small percentage occurs in the cerebellum and pons.

Nursing Assessment

PRIMARY CAUSES

- Aneurysms occur at bifurcation sites of major arteries at one base of the brain and usually point in the direction of blood flow. At these bifurcation sites a defect in the medial elastic lumina is believed to occur. Aneurysms occur in patients with hypertension, coarctation of the aorta, Ehlers-Danles syndrome, pseudoxanthoma, elasticum and cerebral anteriovenous malformations.
- SAH is due to a ruptured cerebral aneurysm and, less commonly, to arteriovenous malformations, head injury, or blood dyscrasias.
- ICH is caused by hypertension, with vascular malformations a nonhypertensive cause.

PHYSICAL ASSESSMENT

Aneurysm

- Inspection: Explosive headache with or without loss of consciousness, nuchal rigidity, nausea, vomiting, neck pain, lethargy, altered mentation, confusion, disorientation, seizures, photophobia, diplopia, and vertigo.
- Auscultation: Tachycardia-bradycardia or hypotension.

SAH

- Inspection: Headache, confusion, apathy, restlessness, irritability, nuchal rigidity, fever, nausea, vomiting, motor weakness, sensory disturbance, speech disorders, seizures, visual disturbances, and diplopia.

DIAGNOSTIC TEST RESULTS

Standard Laboratory Tests. (Table 7–1)

- Serum chemistry: Elevated white blood cell (WBC) count.
- Urine chemistry: Transient glycosuria.

Invasive Neurological Diagnostic Procedures. (Table 7–2)

- Cerebral angiography: Used to locate aneurysm and the degree of vasospasm.
- Lumbar puncture: The cerebrospinal fluid (CSF) or SAH contains frank blood that does not clear. Fluid that is xanthochromic (deep yellow) is due to the presence of blood breakdown products. Other CSF examination includes opening pressure, protein and glucose levels.

NONINVASIVE NEUROLOGICAL DIAGNOSTIC PROCEDURE

- Computerized tomography (CT): Used to detect and determine the extent of acute bleeding and size of an aneurysm.
- EEG: Can be used to indicate the site or sites of hemorrhage but usually shows only a diffuse abnormality.
- Transcranial Doppler (TCD): Used to diagnose and monitor vasospasm in the middle and anterior cerebral arteries. The TCD can also detect increased blood velocity secondary to a narrowed vessel lumen that may suggest symptomatic vasospasm.
- Magnetic resonance imaging (MRI): ICH and its relationship to the surrounding brain are visualized on MRI. MRI is effective in identifying small vascular lesions.

ECG

- Used to detect myocardial changes and dysrhythmias caused by hypothalamic dysfunction.

MEDICAL AND SURGICAL MANAGEMENT

PHARMACOLOGY

- Anticonvulsants: Agents such as diazepam, larazepam, phenytoin, and phenobarbital are administered in an attempt to control seizure activity by inhibiting either the initiation of the epileptic discharge or its spread (Table 7–4).
- Diuretics: Mannitol increases the osmotic pull of the intravascular space, leading to a

TABLE

7-1

TABLE 7–1. STANDARD LABORATORY TESTS

Test	Purpose	Normal Value	Abnormal Findings
Lumbar puncture	Measure CSF pressure, sample CSF, or inject medication or contrast media		
Pressure	Assess pressure in jugular and vertebral veins that connect with intracranial dural sinuses and spinal dura	50–180 mm H_2O	Elevated: Intracranial tumors, hemorrhage, edema caused by trauma
Albumin and IgG	Evaluate integrity and permeability of blood-CSF barrier Evaluate synthesis of IgG within CNS Diagnose multiple myeloma	Albumin ≤43.2 mg/dL IgG ≤8.3 mg/dL	Elevated: Infectious disease, multiple sclerosis, chronic phases of CNS infections, meningitis, Guillain-Barré syndrome, neurosyphilis
Chloride	Diagnosis of tuberculous meningitis	118–132 mEq/L	≤118 mEq/L: Tuberculous or bacterial meningitis
Glucose	Determine whether transport of glucose from plasma to CSF impaired Assess increased use of glucose by CNS, leukocytes, and microorganisms	45–85 mg/dL	Elevated: Bacterial or fungal infection, meningitis, or SAH Reduced: Lymphomas with meningeal spread, leukemia with meningeal spread, hypoglycemia
Glutamine	Determine pressure of hepatic encephalopathy Determine CSF acidosis	6–20 mg/dL	Elevated: Hepatic encephalopathies, hepatic coma, cirrhosis, hypercapnia, Reye's syndrome
Lactic acid	Used to detect central nervous system disease and differentiate bacterial meningitis versus viral meningitis.	24 mg/dL	Elevated: Bacterial meningitis, hypocapnia, brain abscess, cerebral ischemia, traumatic brain injury, idiopathic seizures, respiratory alkalosis, cerebral infarct, cancer of the CNS
LDH	Differentiate between bacterial and viral meningitis.	0.10 value of serum	Elevated: Bacterial meningitis, viral meningitis, SAH, lymphoma or metastatic carcinoma of the CNS
Protein	Evaluate presence of protein in CSF.	15–45 mg/dL (lumbar) 15–25 mg/dL (cisternal) 5–15 mg/dL (ventricular)	Elevated: Increased permeability of the blood-CSF barrier, obstructions in circulation of CSF, increased synthesis of protein within CNS, tissue degeneration as in Guillain-Barré syndrome and brain tumors

TABLE 7-1

TABLE 7-2

TABLE 7–1. CONTINUED

Test	Purpose	Normal Value	Abnormal Findings
Total cell count	Assess presence of WBCs or tumor cells	0–5/mm^3	Elevated: Viral infections, syphilis of CNS, tuberculous meningitis, tumor or abscess, bacterial meningitis, multiple sclerosis, encephalopathy, Guillain-Barré syndrome, sarcoidosis, periarteritis of CNS
Queckenstedt's test	Detect subarachnoid obstruction from spinal tumor or vertebral compression fracture used in conjunction with lumbar puncture	Manual compression of jugular vein for 10 s produces rapid rise in CSF pressure and fall to normal on release	Little or no change in CSF pressure: Block in vertebral canal

CNS, central nervous system; CST, cerebrospinal fluid; IgG, immunoglobulin G; LDH, lactate dehydrogenase; SAH, subarachnoid hemorrhage; WBC, white blood cells.

From Corbett, 1992; Dolan, 1991; Ford RD, 1987; Mitchell, 1993; Loeb S, 1991.

TABLE 7–2. INVASIVE NEUROLOGICAL DIAGNOSTIC PROCEDURES

Test	Purpose	Normal Value	Abnormal Findings
Brain scan	Detect intracranial mass or vascular lesion. Locate areas of ischemia, vascular lesions, cerebral infarction, ICH	Normal barrier between bloodstream brain substance	Increased uptake: Metastatic lesions, cerebral infarction, cerebritis, subdural hematomas. Decreased uptake: Brain abscess, infection
Cerebral angiography	Visualize lumen of vessels to provide information about patency, size, irregularities, or occlusion	Normal cerebral blood flow	Cerebrovascular abnormalities: Aneurysm, vessel thrombosis, stenosis, occlusion. Vascular changes associated with hematoma formation, cyst, edema, arterial spasm
CBF studies	Measure amount of blood flow overall or in regions of the brain to detect areas of increased or decreased cerebral circulation. Evaluate cerebral vasospasm after subarachnoid hemorrhage, CBF during operative procedures requiring hypotension (aneurysm clipping), changes in CBF after cerebral vascular surgery (carotid endarterectomy, cerebral revascularization)	50–55 mL/100 g of cerebral tissue per minute	Altered CBF after operative procedures or cerebral vascular surgery

TABLE 7-2

TABLE 7–2. CONTINUED

Test	Purpose	Normal Value	Abnormal Findings
Digital subtraction angiography (DSA)	Provides images of extracranial vasculature including vessel size, patency, degree of stenosis or occlusion Evaluate carotid or renal artery disease, thrombotic or embolic disease of great vessels, aneurysms	Normal carotid and vertebral arteries	Stenosis of arteries, large aneurysms, large jugular tumors and masses, total occlusion of arteries
Jugular venous oxygen saturation (SjVo$_2$)	Detect cerebral ischemia after traumatic brain injury		
Myelography	Visualize spinal canal, subarachnoid space around spinal cord, and spinal nerve roots through use of radiograph Detect neoplasms, ruptured intravertebral disks, other intraspinal pathology	Normal lumbar or cervial myelogram	Ruptured intervertebral disk, compression of spinal cord, level of intravertebral tumors, obstruction of spinal cord, avulsion of nerve roots
Positron-emission tomography (PET)	Measure metabolism of CBF Detect structural abnormalities such as vascular disorders, tumors	Normal cellular metabolism and CBF	Vascular disorders, tumors
Single photon emission tomography (SPET)	Measure rCBF (Since blood flow linked to metabolism, can be indirect measure of brain metabolism activity)		Abnormal changes in rCBF
Pneumoencephalogram (PEG)	Diagnose intracranial lesions by change in size, shape, and position of ventricles Procedure contraindicated should ICP be suspected	Ventricles appear normal	
Ventriculogram	Withdraw CSF for examination CSF removed is replaced with gas directly into ventricle Relieve ICP	Normal CSF characteristics and normal ICP	

CBF, cerebral blood flow; ICH, intracranial hemorrhage; ICP, intracranial pressure; rCBF, regional cerebral blood flow.

From Corbett, 1992; Dolan, 1991, Ford RD, 1987; Loeb S, 1991; Mason PB, 1992; Mitchell, 1993.

TABLE 7-3

TABLE 7–3. NONINVASIVE NEUROLOGICAL DIAGNOSTIC PROCEDURES

Test	Purpose	Normal Value	Abnormal Findings
Brain sonogram (Echo-encephalogram)	Assess position of midline structure of brain, shift in midline of brain from space-occupying intracranial lesions, size of ventricle	Ventricles normal size Midline structure of brain in normal position	Shift in midline structure, ventricles of abnormal size (dilated ventricles) posterior fossa abnormalities
Computerized axial tomography (CAT) scan	Assess cerebral neoplasms, inflammation, hematomas, infarctions, infections, cerebral edema	No evidence of tumor or pathological activity	Increased density: Hematoma, multiple aneurysm, craniocerebral trauma Tissue with decreased density are associated with infarctions, infection, necrosis in malignant tumors, cyst formation, degenerative processes, or edema.
Electromyography (EMG)	Localize lesions Differentiate primary disease of muscle fibers or neuromuscular junction from lower motor neuron disease	Normal muscle, at rest, exhibits electrical activity	Muscular dystrophies, minimal amyotrophic lateral sclerosis, myasthenia gravis, peripheral denervation conditions
Magnetic resonance imaging (MRI)	Identify areas of cerebral infarct, cerebral edema, hemorrhage, blood vessels Differentiate small tumors by tissue densities different from those of surrounding cells	Normal anatomical and biochemical tissue details in any plane	Cerebral edema, multiple sclerosis, plaque formation, infarctions, tumors, blood clots, hemorrhage, abscesses
Neurophysiologic Studies			
Electroencepha-lography (EEG)	Help diagnose epilepsy Identify brain tumor, abscesses, subdural hematomas Diagnose cerebrovascular diseases (cerebral infarcts, intracranial hemorrhages)	Normal symmetrical pattern of alpha activity	Generalized seizures, brain abscesses, cerebrovascular accidents, head injury
Somatosensory evoked potential or (SEP)	Visual evoked potentials (responses) Aid in evaluating post-traumatic injury Auditory evoked potentials (responses) Aid in localizing auditory lesions; evaluating integrity of brain stem and sequential auditory pathways located therein	Senses normal responses to visual, auditory, or somatosensory (tactile) stimuli	Auditory evoked potentials (responses): Posterior fossa lesions, multiple sclerosis, potential for reversibility of coma Somatosensory evoked potential: Demyelinating disease

TABLE 7–3. CONTINUED

Test	Purpose	Normal Value	Abnormal Findings
Somatosensory evoked potential or (SEP) (*cont.*)	Somatosensory evoked potentials (responses) Aid in diagnosing peripheral nerve disease and lesions in brain and spinal cord Monitor for neurological injury before, during, and after surgery involving nerve tissue		
Skull roentgenogram	Identify fractures, anomalies, tumors	Normal structure	Skull fracture, abnormalities of cranial vault, intracranial calcification, dense vascular markings, or increased ICP
Carotid artery imaging	Doppler and B-mode scanner Ultrasound waves are reflected off RBCs, vessel walls, muscles surrounding vessels Measures the velocity of blood flow from sound waves reflecting from RBC		Doppler and B-mode scanner: May show variation in velocity, indicating whether arteries narrowed or patent Transcranial Doppler: Can detect vasospasm in SAH patient
Nerve conduction studies	Record speed of conduction of motor and sensory fibers in peripheral nerves	Nerve conduction 50–60 m/s for ulnar and median nerves; 45–55 m/s for lateral popliteal nerve	Value ≤40 m/s: neuropathy Abnormal conduction studies are found in patients with neuropathy of diabetes, alcoholism, metabolic and nutritional disorders. Compression or trauma to nerves
Spinal roentgenogram	Identify vertebral fracture or dislocation that might impinge on spinal cord or its nerve roots	Normal spinal cord	Spinal fracture, spinal dislocation
Spinal computed tomography (CT)	Diagnose spinal lesions and abnormalities Assess effects of spinal surgery or therapy	Normal density, size, shape, and position of spinal structures	Spinal tumors, herniated intervertebral disks, paraspinal cysts, vascular malformation
Transcranial Doppler ultrasound (TOU)	Predict vasospasm, auto-regulation, increased ICP	Normal blood flow velocity in a cerebral vessel	Vasospasm or changes in ICP

ICP, intracranial pressure; RBC, red blood cells; SAH, subarachnoid hemorrhage.

Corbett JV, 1992; Dolan JT, 1991; Ford RD, 1987; Loeb S, 1991; Mason PB, 1992; Mitchell, 1993.

TABLE 7-3

TABLE 7-4

TABLE 7–4. NEUROLOGICAL-RELATED DRUGS

Drug	Route/Dose	Uses/Effects	Side Effects
Aminocaproic acid (Amicar)	PO/IV: 4–5 g during first hour, then 1–1.25 g q h for 8 h until bleeding is controlled; maximum: 30 g/24 h	Control excess bleeding, prevent recurrence of SAH	Dizziness, malaise, headache, thromboses, nausea, vomiting, diarrhea, rash, acute renal failure.
Carbamazepine Tegretol (Epitol)	Anticonvulsant PO: 200 mg bid, increase by 200 mg/d; therapeutic range is 800–1200 mg/d in divided doses q 6–8 h	Treat tonic-clonic, mixed, complex-partial seizures	Drowsiness, fatigue, ataxia, blurred vision, pneumonitis, hypotension, syncope, hypertension, rashes, heart block, urticaria
	Antidiuretic PO: 300–400 mg/d in 3–4 divided doses	Manage pain of trigeminal neuralgia	
Clonazepam (Klonopin)	PO: 1.5 mg/d in 3 divided doses; increased by 0.5–1.0 mg q 3 d until seizures are controlled; maximum dose: 20 mg/d	Treat petit mal, petit mal variant, myoclonic seizures	Drowsiness, ataxia, coma, bradycardia, increased secretions, respiratory depression, anorexia, constipation, diarrhea, nocturia, skin rash
Chlorpropamide (Diabinese)	Antidiuretic PO: 100–250 mg/d; may adjust q 2–3 d up to 500 mg/d	Treat neurogenic diabetes insipidus	Drowsiness, muscle cramps, weakness, anorexia, diarrhea, constipation, rash, pruritus, hypoglycemia
Diazepam (Valium)	PO: 8–30 mg/d	Treat status epilepticus	Drowsiness, ataxia, respiratory depression, hypotension
Ethosuximide (Zarontin)	PO: 250 mg bid, may increase by 250 mg/d q 4–7 d up to 1.5 g/d in divided dose; maximum: 20 mg/kg d	Manage petit mal, myoclonic seizures, akinetic epilepsy	Drowsiness, headache, dizziness, anorexia, nausea, vomiting, weight loss, diarrhea, urticaria, blurred vision, epigastric distress, cramping
Fentanyl (Sublimaze)	General anesthesia IV: Up to 150 μg/kg as required Postoperative pain IM: 50– 100 μg q 1–2 h as needed	Narcotic supplement in general and regional anesthesia	Sedation, dizziness, diaphoresis, delirium, hypotension, bradycardia, cardiac arrest, blurred vision, nausea, vomiting, layngospasm, respiratory depression or arrest
Lidocaine	IV: Loading dose of 1.5–3.0 mg/kg, followed by infusion of 3–10 mg/kg/h	Treat status epilepticus unresponsive to other therapies	Dysrhythmias
Lorazepam (Ativan)	PO: 2–6 mg/d in divided doses; maximum dose: 10 mg/d	Manage anxiety and status epilepticus	Drowsiness, sedation, dizziness, weakness, restlessness, confusion, disorientation, blurred vision, nausea, vomiting, abdominal discomfort

TABLE 7-4

TABLE 7–4. CONTINUED

Drug	Route/Dose	Uses/Effects	Side Effects
Papaverine hydrochloride	Cerebral/peripheral ischemia PO: 100–300 mg 3–4 times/d; 150-mg sustained release q 8–12 h IM/IV: 30–120 mg q 3 h as needed	Relieve cerebral and peripheral ischemia from arterial spasm, MI complicated by dysrhythmias	Nausea, anorexia, constipation, diarrhea, dizziness, headache, hepatotoxicity, respiratory depression, fatal apnea
Phenobarbital (Luminal)	Anticonvulsant PO: 60–250 mg/d single dose or 2–3 divided doses (total of 600 mg/24 h) IV: 200–600 mg. Maximum 600 mg/24 h Status epilepticus IV: 10–20 mg/kg, may be repeated	Treat tonic-clonic, partial, febrile seizures	Drowsiness, vertigo, depression, respiratory depression, hypotension, nausea, vomiting, rashes, diarrhea, constipation, urticaria, photosensitivity
Phenytoin (Dilantin)	PO: 15–18 mg/kg; then 300 mg/d in 1–3 divided doses; then increased by 100 mg/w IV: 15–18 mg/kg or 1 g loading dose; then 100 mg tid	Treat tonic-clonic (grand mal) seizures and nonepileptic seizures (after head trauma)	Drowsiness, dizziness, confusion, tremors, bradycardia, hypotension, ventricular fibrillation, nausea, vomiting, constipation, weight loss, weight gain, fever, edema, rash, aplastic anemia
Primidone (Mysoline)	PO: Initial dose of 100–125 mg at bedtime for 3 d, then 100–125 mg bid for 3 d, then 100–125 mg tid for 3 d; maintenance dose: 250 mg 2–4 times daily; maximum: 2g/d	Management of tonic-clonic, complex, partial, and focal seizures	Drowsiness, ataxia, vertigo, lethargy, edema, nausea, dyspnea, anorexia, vomiting, rashes, blood dyscrasias
Sulfinpyrazone (Anturane)	PO: 200 mg tid or qid	Inhibit platelet aggregation Prevent TIAs and stroke should platelet aggregation occur	Nausea, vomiting, diarrhea, epigastric pain, blood loss, dizziness, vertigo, edema, labored respirations, skin rash
Valproic acid	PO: 15 mg/kg/d in divided doses when total daily dose ≥250 mg; increase at 1 wk intervals by 5–10 mg/kg/d; maximum: 60 mg/kg/d	Treat simple and complex absence seizures	Drowsiness, sedation, headache, dizziness, ataxia, confusion, nausea, vomiting, indigestion, anorexia, diarrhea, constipation, prolonged bleeding time

IM, intramuscular; IV, intravenous; MI, myocardial infarction; PO, by mouth; SAH, subarachnoid hemorrhage; TIA, transient ischemic attack.

From Deglin JH, Vallerand AH, 1995; Govoni LE, Hayes JE, Shannon MT, et al., 1995; Loeb S, 1993; Rose BA, 1993.

net flow of fluid from the intracellular and transcellular spaces into the vascular system. The increased vascular volume leads to diuresis and reduces tissue edema. Furosemide (Lasix) used alone or in combination with albumin produces decreases in intracranial pressure (ICP) equal to that of mannitol (see Table 1–13, p. 76).

- Corticosteroids: Dexamethasone (Decadron) at a dose of 10 mg four times a day is used to treat brain edema resulting from tumors or trauma (see Table 1–15, p. 129).
- Calcium channel blockers: Nifedipine can preserve cerebral blood flow despite lowered cerebral perfusion pressure and increased ICP, possibly as a result of overriding cerebral autoregulation. Nimodipine decreases cerebrovascular spasm and increases flow beyond the areas of obstruction or spasm, thereby preserving perfusion to ischemic tissues (see Table 1–6, p. 28).
- Antifibrinolytics: Antifibrinolytics such as aminocaproic acid (Amicar) or tranexamic acid (Cyklokapron) are used to prevent the bleeding from a ruptured intracranial aneurysm. The drugs prevent the lysis of thrombus on the surface of an aneurysm (see Table 7–4).
- Antipyretics: Acetaminophen is used to control fever.
- Stool softener: Docusate sodium (Colace) is administered to reduce straining during bowel movement.

FLUID THERAPY

- Blood or blood products: Used to expand intravascular volume and create a positive fluid balance by maintaining central venous pressure (CVP) 10 to 12 mm Hg and pulmonary capillary wedge pressure (PCWP) 15 to 20 mm Hg.
- Crystalloids: Used to maintain normal serum electrolytes.

PHYSICAL ACTIVITY

- Activity is limited to bed rest to decrease ICP. Passive range-of-motion exercise prevents formation of thrombi with potential for pulmonary emboli.

- Head of bed (HOB): HOB is elevated 30 degrees to aid venous drainage.

SURGICAL INTERVENTION

- Metal clip: In surgical treatment of saccular aneurysms, a metal clip is placed across the base of the lesion at the point where it comes from the parent vessel. Surgery within the initial 48 hours can eliminate the risk of aneurysmal rebleeding and reduce vasospasm by recovering the subarachnoid clot.
- Embolization: The procedure is used to obliterate inoperable vascular malformations, including aneurysms. Catheterization and angiography are used to deliver the embolizing material.

NURSING MANAGEMENT: NURSING DIAGNOSES AND COLLABORATIVE PROBLEMS

Nursing Diagnoses

Common nursing goals for patients with cerebral hemorrhage are to restore cerebral tissue perfusion, maintain effective breathing pattern, support sensory-perceptual activity, and promote effective thermoregulation.

Altered cerebral tissue perfusion related to rupture of cerebral artery or vasospasm secondary to vasoconstriction of cerebral vessels caused by blood.

Expected Patient Outcomes. Patient maintains adequate cerebral tissue perfusion, as evidenced by cerebral perfusion pressure (CPP) 60 to 100 mm Hg; ICP 0 to 15 mm Hg; CSF pressure 10 mg Hg; systolic blood pressure (SBP) 90 to 140 mm Hg; mean arterial pressure (MAP) 70 to 100 mm Hg; heart rate (HR) ≤100 bpm; normothermia; pupils equal and reactive; normal sensorimotor function; being alert and oriented to person, place, and time; absence of headache; and absence of seizure.

- Review results of CT scans, cerebral angiography, MRI, transcranial Doppler, CSF studies and arterial blood gas measurement.

- Maintain complete bed rest to decrease ICP.
- Elevate HOB 15 to 45 degrees or as prescribed to promote cerebral venous outflow.
- Limit fluid restriction to 1500 to 1800 mL daily or as ordered.
- Assess clinical indicators of neurological status: reflexes, respiratory rate (RR), pupillary reaction, HR, temperature, BP, level of consciousness, and sensorimotor function.
- Report clinical findings associated with decreased cerebral tissue perfusion: SBP $\geq$140 mm Hg, tachycardia-bradycardia, MAP $\geq$160 mm Hg, headache, hemiparesis, sensory defect, motor weakness, deteriorating level of consciousness, and elevated temperature.
- Measure CPP (CPP = mean systolic arterial pressure $-$ ICP) and report $\leq$30 mm Hg.
- Measure ICP pressure, analyze ICP wave form every hours, and report ICP $\geq$15 mm Hg.
- Perform feeding, bathing, or shaving activities for patient to prevent elevated ICP.
- Maintain patient airway and assist with intubation and ventilatory support.
- Administer prescribed oxygen by nasal cannula, mask, or mechanical ventilation.
- Administer prescribed antihypertensive (hydralazine hydrochloride) to control elevated SBP.
- Administer prescribed IV fluids 5% dextrose in water (D_5W) or normal saline (NS) to maintain adequate circulatory volume.
- Administer prescribed low-dose dopamine (2 to 5 μg/kg/min), which dilates cerebral arteries, causing an increase in cerebral perfusion, and dobutamine, which can indirectly increase cerebral blood flow by its inotropic effects (see Table 1–10, p. 50).
- Administer prescribed calcium channel blockers (nifedipine or nimodipine) to preserve cerebral blood flow (see Table 1–6, p. 28).
- Administer prescribed antifibrinolytics, such as aminocaproic acid 5 g in an IV bolus, followed by a continuous infusion of 24 to 36 g/d for 10 to 14 days unless sur-

gery is attempted. Another agent is tranexamic acid. These agents prevent rebleeding from a ruptured intracranial aneurysm (see Table 7–4).
- Teach patient to avoid a Valsalva's maneuver or straining, since these activities can increase ICP and decrease cerebral tissue perfusion.

Ineffective breathing pattern related to altered level of consciousness secondary to hypothalamic dysfunction.

Expected Patient Outcomes. Patient maintains effective breathing pattern, as evidenced by RR 12 to 20 BPM, symmetry of chest wall movement, color normal skin, clear lungs, HR$\leq$100 bpm, and arterial blood gases within normal limits.

- Review levels of arterial blood gas.
- Elevate HOB 30 degrees to decrease ICP.
- Assess clinical indicators of respiratory status: rate, depth, symmetry of chest wall movement, skin color, use of accessory muscles, and lung sounds.
- Report clinical findings associated with ineffective breathing pattern: tachypnea, tachycardia, cyanosis, asymmetrical chest wall movement, and crackles.
- Maintain patient airway and suction using unit protocol. Continuously monitor ICP while suctioning. Should ICP increase, cease suctioning.
- Assist patient to change positions to enhance lung expansion. Any pronounced angulation of the neck can obstruct venous return from the brain and increase ICP.
- Provide a warm, relaxed environment.
- Provide prescribed oxygen by nasal cannula, mask, or mechanical ventilation.
- Teach patient to take deep breaths in order to minimize the risk of atelectasis.

Sensory-perceptual alterations related to weakness or seizure secondary to cerebral ischemia or infarction.

Expected Patient Outcomes. Patient maintains sensory-perceptual function, as evidenced by orientation to person, place and time, ability to concentrate, and absence of weakness.

- Evaluate environmental factors that contribute to patient's sensory-perceptual alteration, such as excessive noise, constant and monotonous noise, or restricted environment because of immobility.
- Provide meaningful sensory stimulation by providing a radio or tape recordings of family and significant others.
- Protect patient from injury during seizure activity.
- Obtain and report clinical findings associated with sensory-perceptual alterations: confusion, disorientation, weakness, and short attention span.
- Explain the purpose behind routines, procedures, and equipment using simple explanations.
- Evaluate patient's sleep-rest pattern to determine its contribution to sensory-perceptual disorder.

Ineffective thermoregulation related to meningeal irritation secondary to the hematoma or bleeding.

Expected Patient Outcome. Patient maintains normothermia.

- Obtain and record temperature every 2 hours while patient is febrile.
- Obtain specimens, as prescribed, for blood, urine, and sputum cultures to rule out infection.
- Report clinical findings associated with hyperthermia: temperature $\geq 38°C$ (101°F), pallor, absence of perspiration, and warm skin.
- Assess wounds for evidence of infection such as erythema, tenderness, purulent drainage, or swelling.
- Should the patient be hyperthermic, administer tepid bath, hypothermic blanket, or ice bags to axilla or groin.
- Administer prescribed antipyretics when patient is febrile.

- Administer prescribed chlorpromazine to treat or prevent shivering, which can increase ICP.

Collaborative Problems
Common collaborative goals for patients with cerebral hemorrhage are to decrease ICP, minimize seizures, and prevent cerebral vasospasm.

Potential Complication: Increased ICP. Increased ICP related to intravascular bleeding secondary to aneurysm or SAH.

Expected Patient Outcomes. Patient maintains normal ICP, as evidenced by ICP 0 to 15 mm Hg, CPP 60 to 100 mm Hg, alertness, equal and normoreactive pupils, BP within patient's normal range, HR ≤ 100 bpm, RR 12 to 20 BPM, normal respiratory pattern, normal sensorimotor function, absence of headache, absence of papilledema, and absence of vomiting.

- Consult with physician about factors contributing to sustained spikes in ICP: hypercapnia, hypoxemia, Valsalva's maneuver, certain body position, isometric muscle contraction, coughing or sneezing, or arousal from sleep.
- Review arterial blood gas valves.
- Maintain patient in semi-Fowler's position with head elevated 30 degrees. Avoid the prone position and exaggerated neck flexion to decrease intrathoracic pressure, promote drainage from the venous vessels from the head and brain, and decrease ICP.
- Restrict fluid intake to 1500 to 1800 mL/ 24 h to decrease extracellular fluid of body tissue, thereby decreasing ICP.
- Assess clinical indicators of neurological status: level of consciousness (LOC), sensorimotor function, RR and pattern, pupils, and vital signs.
- Report clinical findings associated with increased ICP: deterioration of LOC, pupillary dilatation or constriction, increased SBP, widening pulse pressure, bradycardia,

altered respiratory pattern, loss of sensori-motor function, papilledema, headache, and vomiting.

- Monitor ICP continuously for pressure 0 to 15 mm Hg and three pressure waves, A, B, and C. Report ICP ≤15 mm Hg and presence of A wave. The A, or plateau, waves are sudden, transient waves lasting 5 to 20 minutes and they begin from a baseline of already elevated ICP. The A waves cause cerebral ischemia. The B waves are seen in relation to fluctuations of respiratory pattern such as Cheyne-Stokes respirations.
- Assess respiratory pattern and report changes such as Cheyne-Stokes respiration, central neurogenic hyperventilation, apneustic breathing, cluster breathing, and ataxic breathing.
- Measure CPP every hour and report ≤30 mm Hg.
- Measure intake and output to evaluate the amount of diuresis and urinary dilution.
- Apply antiembolic elastic stockings to prevent risk of thrombophlebitis.
- Administer prescribed broad-spectrum antibiotics if patient is on ventricular drainage or continuous ICP monitoring.
- Administer prescribed mannitol (0.5 to 2.0 g/kg over a period of 20 to 30 minutes), which results in diureses, reduces tissue edema, and induces cerebral arterial vasoconstriction, which diminishes the size of the cerebrovascular components of ICP.
- Administer prescribed furosemide (0.1 to 2.0 mg/kg) to reduce ICP. When used in combination with albumin or mannitol, the dose is 1.0 mg/kg.
- Administer prescribed corticosteroids (dexamethasone) at a dose of 10 mg four times a day to reduce cerebral edema and bring about subsequent decrease in ICP (see Table 1–15, p. 129).
- Administer prescribed barbiturate (phenobarbital) at a loading dose of 6 to 8 mg/kg or as a single dose (60 mg/min) to reduce cerebral blood flow in patients with increased ICP (see Table 7–4).

- Administer prescribed antipyretic agents such as acetaminophen alone or in combination with a hypothermia blanket to control elevated temperature.
- Should pharmacological therapy be unable to control spikes in ICP, prepare patient for ventriculostomy and ventricular drainage. Drainage catheters are inserted into a cerebral ventricle to drain excess CSF.
- Monitor the amount of drainage in the collection container.
- Prepare patient for prescribed barbiturate therapy (3 to 5 mg/kg at slow IV push) to control increased ICP by causing cerebral vasoconstriction, which decreases cerebral blood flow and blood volume, decreases cerebral metabolism, and reduces ICP to ≤10 mm Hg within 10 to 15 minutes. Monitor BP and ICP throughout the entire process.
- Should barbiturate therapy be initiated, monitor for loss of the following neurological parameters: pupillary, oculocephalic, oculovestibular, coroneal, gag, and swallowing reflexes.

Potential Complication: Seizures. Seizures related to an underlying structural abnormality secondary to an acute cerebral injury.

Expected Patient Outcomes. Patient's seizures will be prevented or controlled.

- Review results of electroencephalogram (EEG), CT scan, serum glucose and arterial blood gas measurements.
- Maintain patient airway to ensure adequate oxygenation.
- Monitor temperature and in case of hyperthermia provide external cooling measure.
- Provide a quiet, calm environment with subdued lighting.
- Pad bed rails and keep rails up when patient is in bed.
- Monitor continuous ECG to assess HR and rhythm. Document ECG rhythm strips every 2 hours in patients with dysrhythmias resulting from loss of the sodium-to-potassium gradient, leading to cellular edema.

Liberation of intracellular potassium can cause dysrhythmias.

- Protect patient from aspiration of gastric content during status epilepticus.
- Administer prescribed anticonvulsants such as diazepam (Valium) at an initial-dose up to 40 mg and phenytoin (Dilantin) 18 to 20 mg/kg. If seizure is not terminated, provide phenobarbital at a dose of 20 mg/kg (see Table 7–4).
- Administer prescribed oxygen by nasal cannula, mask, or intubation. Hyperventilate patient with 100% oxygen during status epilepticus, which increases cerebral and systemic metabolic rates by 200% to 300%.
- Administer prescribed antipyretic agents when patient is febrile.

Potential Complication: Cerebral Vasospasm. Cerebral vasospasm related to abnormal narrowing of an artery secondary to SAH as a result of rupture of sacular aneurysm.

Expected Patient Outcomes. Consult with physician about causes of cerebral vasospasm and time frame in which it might occur (4 to 12 days post SAH).

- Review results of cerebral angiography and CT scan.
- Obtain and report clinical findings associated with cerebral vasospasm: deterioration of LOC, hemiparesis, visual disturbance, and seizure activity.
- Restrict fluid intake to 1500 to 1800 mL/24 h to assist in reduction of brain swelling.
- Measure CPP, ICP, and MAP (CPP = MAP−ICP). The goal is to keep ICP no greater than 25 mm Hg, CPP no less than 50 mm Hg, and MAP preferably in the range of 70 to 100 mm HG to facilitate cerebral circulation.
- Reduce ICP if pressure ≥15 to 25 mm Hg, as prescribed, with ventricular drainage and osmotic diuresis.
- Continuously monitor ECG to assess HR and rhythm. Report bradycardia, since the use of fluid expansion and induced hypertension to increase the CPP, may cause autoregulatory reflex bradycardia.

- Administer prescribed intravascular volume expanders with crystalloids and colloids to maintain PCWP 18 to 20 mm Hg with recommended hematocrit of 30% to 40%.
- Should neurological status not improve, controlled hypertension is induced, as prescribed, with vasopressors. The goal is to raise the SBP in the range of 180 to 200 mm Hg, which improves neurological status.
- Should raising SBP cause bradycardia, administer prescribed atropine to maintain HR 80 to 100 bpm.
- Administer prescribed plasma volume expanders to minimize cerebral vasospasm by increasing cerebral perfusion. This creates a positive fluid balance as measured by CVP 10 to 12 mm Hg and PCWP 15 to 20 mm Hg.

DISCHARGE PLANNING

The critical care nurse will provide patient and significant other(s) verbal or written discharge notes regarding the following subjects:

1. Medications, including drug name, dosage, route, purpose, schedule, and side effects.
2. Importance of keeping all medical appointments.
3. Referrals to physical, speech, and occupational therapist, depending upon the severity of patient's problem.
4. Signs and symptoms of rebleeding and need to report changes to the physician.
5. Referral to social services and community nursing services.
6. Referral to family support groups.
7. An activity schedule that is dependent upon patient's neurological deficit and need for assistive devices resulting from sensorimotor alterations.

■ ACUTE HEAD INJURY

(For related information see Part I: Cerebral hemorrhage, p. 607; Cerebrovascular accident, p. 630; Status epilepticus, p. 636. Part II: Craniotomy, p. 664. Part III: Intracranial pressure monitoring, p. 671; Barbiturate coma,

p. 674; Cerebral balloon angioplasty, p. 676.
See also Behavioral Deviations Part I, p. 00.)

Case Management Basis

DRG: 31 Concussion age ≥17 with compli-
   cation
LOS: 4.30 days
DRG: 32 Concussion age ≥17 without com-
   plication
LOS: 2.60 days

Definition

Acute head injury refers to any injury of the
scalp, skull, or brain. Primary head injury involves the actual brain damage resulting from
the initial force or impact of the injury. Secondary injury signifies the pathophysiological consequences of the initial damage as the
body responds to the injury.

Pathophysiology

MECHANISMS OF INJURY. Acceleration and
deceleration can occur with head injury. As
the skull hits or is hit by a force, the semisolid
substance of the brain continues to move and
the brain tissue hits the skull, reverses direction, and hits the other side of the skull. Coup
injuries occur directly at the site of the impact. The contrecoup injury, or laceration, occurs at the opposite pole of impact as the brain
rebounds and strikes other parts of the skull.

PRIMARY HEAD INJURY. Primary injury is one
that occurs at the time of the impact. Loss of
autoregulation and increased permeability of
the blood-brain barrier occur. These dysfunc-
tions can lead to increased blood volume,
vasodilation of cerebral vessels, and increase
in the extracellular fluid space. The overall
consequence is increased intracranial pressure. Primary head injuries include concussion, cerebral contusion, cerebral laceration,
and intracranial hemorrhage. A concussion is
a transient period of unconsciousness caused
by acceleration-deceleration and rotational
motion of the head. A cerebral contusion is an
actual bruising of the brain, with edema and
capillary hemorrhage in the affected areas of

the brain. Contusions most frequently occur
at the base of the frontal and temporal lobes.
Cerebral laceration is a tear in brain tissue associated with shearing forces, which causes
the brain to strike irregular surfaces at the
base of the cranial vault. Intracranial hemorrhage or hematomas are due to a mass lesion
and cause increased intracranial pressure.
There are three types of hematomas: epidural
and subdural, which are located outside the
brain tissue and produce injury by displacement of intracranial contents; and intracerebral, which directly damages neural tissue as
well as producing injury from pressure and
displacement of intracranial contents.

SECONDARY HEAD INJURY. Secondary head
injuries occur as a consequence of the primary injury and include hypoxia, hypoxemia,
hypotension, cerebral edema, and intracranial
hypertension. Secondary injuries can also
contribute to herniation.

Nursing Assessment

PRIMARY CAUSES
- Causes include motor vehicle accidents,
  falls, assaults, and motorcycle accidents.

PHYSICAL ASSESSMENT
- Inspection: Verbal response is slurred, confusion, repetitive or no response.
- Palpation: Appropriate-inappropriate response to tactile or painful stimulation and
  warm skin.
- Auscultation: Bradycardia-tachycardia;
  widening pulse pressure; increased systolic
  blood pressure (SBP); normal diastolic
  blood pressure (DBP), apnea alternating
  with hyperventilation; normal, decreased,
  or absent breath sounds.

DIAGNOSTIC TEST RESULTS

Standard Laboratory Tests
- Arterial blood gases: Show ventilation or
  oxygenation problems. Arterial partial pressure of carbon dioxide ($PaCO_2$) is 27 to 33
  mm Hg with mandatory hyperventilation.

- Blood studies: White blood cell (WBC) count, hemoglobin, hematocrit, and coagulation profile may be altered as a result of infection or bleeding.
- Serum chemistry: Serum electrolytes and serum osmolality may be altered.
- Urinalysis: Urine osmolality, electrolytes, and specific gravity are used to evaluate fluid balance.

Invasive Neurological Diagnostic Procedures. (see Table 7–2)

- Cerebral arteriography: Used to detect aneurysm, occlusions, hematomas, tumors, and other lesions large enough to destroy cerebral vessels.
- Cerebrospinal fluid (CSF): Used to diagnose subarachnoid hemorrhage.
- Continuous cerebral blood flow: This involves the continuous monitoring of cerebral circulation. The technology uses radiologically tagged xenon gas, delivered by a computerized ventilator that monitors xenon uptake as a reflection of cerebral blood flow. The study is helpful in determining the effect of brain injury on blood flow and monitoring the effects of treatment to improve blood flow in ischemic areas.
- Pneumoencephalography: Involves the removal of CSF and the injection of air to visualize the ventricular system. Used to diagnose hydrocephalus, tumors, and cerebral palsy.
- Ventriculography: The procedure provides information the patency of the ventricular system, localization of the intracranial masses, and detection of the cerebral atrophy.

Noninvasive Neurological Diagnostic Procedures. (see Table 7–3)

- Computerized tomography (CT): Used to identify space-occupying lesions, contusions, hemorrhage, or edematous areas in the brain.
- Electroencephalography (EEG): Used to evaluate status of comatose patient and pro-

vides a comparison in case of subsequent extension of an injury.
- Evoked potential studies (EPS): The EPS reflects the brain's response to specific sensory stimulation. The test can be used in patients who are untestable or are in a comatose state because of the influence of central nervous system (CNS) depressants or barbiturate-induced coma.
- Magnetic resonance imaging (MRI): MRI differentiates between gray and white matter and can detect small hemorrhages in diffuse axomal injury.

MEDICAL AND SURGICAL MANAGEMENT

PHARMACOLOGY

- Corticosteroids: Dexamethasone and methylprednisolone can be used to improve neuronal function by improving cerebral blood flow and restoring autoregulation (see Table 1–15, p. 129).
- Diuretics: Mannitol is given as an IV bolus or continuous infusion in doses of 0.5 to 2.0 g/kg of body weight. Furosemide as a loop diuretic reduces intracranial pressure (ICP) by decreasing sodium transport within the brain, reducing systemic fluid volume, and inhibiting CSF production (see Table 1–13, p. 76).
- Barbiturate: Pentobarbital or thiopental are used to reduce increased ICP and protect against cerebral hypoxia and ischemia. High doses produce superimposed coma, which reduces cerebral metabolisms and cerebral blood flow (see Table 7–4).
- Pancuronium bromide (Pavulon): Used to keep patient synchronized with the ventilator (see Table 3–5, p. 388).
- Narcotic sedation: Can be used as an alternative to barbiturate therapy to control agitation and ICP. Fentanyl can be administered intravenously in doses of 1 to 5 mL (see Table 7–4).
- Investigational agents: Used to manage ICP. Alfaxalone, an intravenous steroid anesthetic, has properties similar to barbiturates with no systemic hypotension. Dimethyl

sulfoxide (DMSO) is used in experimental treatment of acute head injury and spinal cord injury. The drug causes vasodilation, osmotic diuresis, decreased ICP, and decreased cellular oxygen consumption.

- Lidocaine can be used to suppress the cough reflex and minimize the risk of arterial hypertension with endotracheal intubation. Lidocaine can be used in doses of 50 to 100 mg administered over 2 minutes before suctioning to reduce sudden increases in ICP.
- Phenytoin, an anticonvulsant, is used to decrease cerebral oxygen consumption.
- Alkaylating agents: Buffering agents such as tromethamine (THAM) and superoxide dismutase (SOD) are used experimentally in acute head injury to counteract acidosis.

ICP MONITORING
- Used to monitor patient's ICP and response to therapy.

VENTILATORY SUPPORT
- Hyperventilation therapy is used to maintain the $Paco_2$ 25 to 30 mm Hg and the arterial partial pressure of oxygen $(PaO_2) \geq 80$ mm Hg, thereby preventing hypercapnia and hypoxemia. Each millimeter of mercury decrease in $Paco_2$ leads to a cerebral blow flow reduction of 2 to 3 mL/100g of tissue per minute.
- Oxygenation: High levels of supplemental oxygen are provided to ensure adequate cerebral oxygenation. The goal is to keep PaO_2 80 to 100 mm Hg.

ARTERIAL PRESSURE LINE
- Used to monitor patient's systemic blood pressure (BP) and pulse pressure and facilitate close monitoring of cerebral perfusion pressure (CPP) in relation to ICP.

PULMONARY ARTERY CATHETER
- Used to assess and maintain patient's fluid state. In patients with cerebral edema, the goal is slight dehydration.

FLUID THERAPY
- Hyperosmotic (dextran or mannitol) and hypertonic (7.5% saline) solutions improve systemic hemodynamics and cerebral blood flow while decreasing ICP and cerebral water content.

PHYSICAL ACTIVITY
- Head of bed (HOB) is elevated to 30 degrees and the head kept in a neutral plane to the body to maximize venous drainage from the brain.

MAINTENANCE OF NORMOTHERMIA
- Hyperthermia is controlled with antipyretic or cooling blanket in an attempt to decrease the metabolic activity of the brain and carbon dioxide production.

SURGICAL INTERVENTION
- Craniotomy: Performed to remove a hematoma to relieve ICP and prevent herniation (see Part II: Craniotomy, p. 664).

NURSING MANAGEMENT: NURSING DIAGNOSES AND COLLABORATIVE PROBLEMS

Nursing Diagnoses
Common nursing goals for patients with acute head injury are to maintain adequate cerebral tissue perfusion, promote oxygenation, maintain fluid balance, support physical mobility, enhance cognitive function, encourage family coping, prevent disuse syndrome, and encourage adjustment.

Decreased cerebral tissue perfusion related to cerebral edema or intracranial bleeding secondary to cerebral injury.

Expected Patient Outcomes.
Patient maintains adequate cerebral tissue perfusion as evidenced by CPP ≥ 50 mm Hg, ICP ≤ 15 mm Hg, mean arterial pressure (MAP) 80 mm Hg, Glasgow Coma Scale (GCS) within normal range, and BP within patient's normal range.

- Review levels of arterial blood gases, serum electrolytes, serum osmolality, hemoglobin, hematocrit, coagulation studies, urine osmolality, lumbar puncture, CT, or MRI.
- Maintain HOB 30 to 45 degrees to facilitate venous drainage and maintain the head and neck in a neutral position to increase cerebral tissue perfusion by decreasing ICP.
- Assess neurological status hourly using GCS for level of consciousness (LOC), pupillary reflexes, and motor function.
- Monitor ICP trends continuously every hour or more often if patient's condition changes. Evaluate ICP wave form and calculate CPP every 30 to 60 minutes. Report ICP ≥ 15 mm Hg and CPP ≤ 60 mm Hg leading to decreased cerebral blood flow (CBF).
- Report clinical findings associated with decreasing cerebral tissue perfusion: progressive deterioration in LOC, deterioration in motor function, changes in respiratory pattern, ipsilateral pupil dilation, and pupils sluggish or nonreactive to light.
- Obtain and report changes in reflexes that may indicate injury at midbrain or brain stem. The changes include loss of corneal reflex (nerves V and VII) signifying damage to the pons and medulla; absence of cough and gag reflexes (nerves IX and X) reflecting damage to medulla; and presence of positive Babinski's sign indicating injury along the pyramidal pathway.
- Organize nursing activities to provide rest between activities to maintain cerebral perfusion by reducing ICP.
- Log-roll patient, when turning, to prevent the possibility of turning the head and obstructing the jugular veins.
- Administer prescribed oxygen by nasal cannula, mask, or mechanical support to maximize tissue oxygenation.
- Prepare patient for craniotomy to evacuate the hematoma.
- Instruct patient as to the purpose behind evaluating CPP.

Impaired gas exchange related to neurogenic pulmonary edema or hypoventilation secondary to cerebral injury.

Expected Patient Outcomes. Patient maintains adequate gas exchange, as evidenced by arterial blood gases within normal range, respiratory rate (RR) 12 to 20 BPM; heart rate (HR) ≤ 100 bpm; arterial oxygen saturation (SaO$_2$) 95% to 97.5%; absence of cyanosis; BP within patient's normal range; absence of dyspnea, restlessness, or anxiety; and absence of adventitious breath sounds.

- Review arterial blood gas, hemoglobin, hematocrit levels, and chest roentgenogram.
- Place patient on bed rest and elevate HOB 30 to 45 degrees to promote venous return and ventilation.
- Monitor clinical indicators of respiratory status: rate, depth, symmetry of chest wall movement, use of accessory muscles, skin color, and presence of adventitious breath sounds.
- Assess respiratory pattern for changes such as Cheyne-Stokes respirations resulting from hemispheric compression; central neurogenic hyperventilation indicates lesions in the lower midbrain and upper pons; apneustic breathing indicates injury in the mid and lower pons; cluster breathing can occur with involvement of lower pons and upper medulla; and ataxic breathing involves lesions of the medulla.
- Report clinical findings associated with impaired gas exchange related to neurogenic pulmonary edema: tachypnea, tachycardia, crackles, dyspnea, restlessness, anxiety, cold and clammy skin, expectoration of mucus, and cyanotic skin color.
- Obtain and report clinical findings associated with hypoxia: changes in LOC, restlessness, and irritability.
- Calculate arteriovenous oxygen difference (C[a−v]o$_2$) to estimate whether CBF is altered. Report value ≤ 4 mL/100 mL, indicating poor tissue utilization of oxygen.
- Monitor oxygen consumption (Vo$_2$) and oxygen consumption index (Vo$_2$I). Report Vo$_2 \geq 250$ mL/min or Vo$_2$I ≥ 165 mL/min/m^2, since increased values produces significant hypoxemia in the presence of a ventilation:perfusion ($\dot{V}/\dot{Q}$) mismatch.

- Maintain controlled hyperventilation to keep $Paco_2$ 27 to 35 mm Hg, as prescribed. This will cause cerebral vasoconstriction, correct brain tissue acidosis, improve autoregulation, and decrease ICP.
- Hyperoxygenate before and after suctioning, since suctioning can aggravate hypoxia, produce vasoconstriction, and affect cerebral perfusion.
- Provide supplemental oxygenation by nasal cannula, mask, or ventilatory support to ensure adequate cerebral oxygenation and maintain Pao_2 ≥70 mm Hg.
- Provide prescribed ventilatory support and positive end-expiratory pressure (PEEP) to prevent collapse of the alveoli at the end of expiration and to improve gas exchange.
- Administer prescribed lidocaine, sedatives, and neuromuscular blockers to prevent increased ICP, assisted with endotracheal suctioning.
- Should PEEP be required, elevate HOB to 30 degrees to reduce the effect of PEEP on ICP.

Fluid volume deficit related to diabetes insipidus secondary to disturbance of the posterior lobe of the pituitary gland, which produces antidiuretic hormone.

Expected Patient Outcomes. Patient maintains adequate fluid volume, as evidenced BP within patient's normal range, HR ≤100 bpm, urinary output (UO) ≥30 mL/h and ≤200 mL/h, specific gravity 1.010 to 1.025, peripheral pulses +2, capillary refill ≤3 seconds, daily weight within 5% of baseline, good skin turgor, MAP 80 to 100 mm Hg, and serum electrolytes within normal range.

- Review levels of serum electrolytes and osmolality.
- Obtain and report clinical findings associated with decreased fluid volume: thirst, tachycardia, poor skin turgor, peripheral pulses ≤+2, capillary refill ≥3 seconds, altered LOC, and hypotension.
- Obtain and report clinical findings associated with diabetes insipidus: polyuria, polydipsia, specific gravity ≤1.005, hypotension, and tachycardia.
- Measure intake, output, specific gravity, and body weight to determine fluid balance. Report UO ≥200 mL/h for 2 consecutive hours, specific gravity 1.010 to 1.025, and weight loss.
- Encourage fluid intake, if not contraindicated, to maintain circulatory fluid volume and CPP.
- Administer prescribed IV fluids to minimize fluctuations in vascular load and maintain adequate hydration.
- Administer prescribed vasopressin (Pitressin) IV or subcutaneously at a dose of 10 mg to correct diabetes insipidus by promoting water absorption (see Table 5–4, p. 518).

Impaired physical mobility related to altered state of consciousness or restricted activity associated with increased ICP secondary to neuromuscular impairment.

Expected Patient Outcomes. Patient maintains full range of motion and mobility.

- Consult with physical therapist about an individualized activity program that takes into account patient's neurological and musculoskeletal status.
- Implement measures to improve mobility as appropriate.
- Assist with passive range of motion (ROM) exercises to prevent pooling of blood in the extremities.
- Perform passive ROM exercises every 4 hours in all extremities while monitoring ICP.
- Obtain and report changes in neuromuscular function: limitations in ROM, incoordination of movement, and sensorimotor dysfunction.
- Assess the effect of body position, turning, suctioning, Valsalva's maneuver when using the bedpan on ICP. The nursing care activities may increase ventricular drainage and increase ICP.
- Provide rest periods between nursing care activities.
- Teach patient the reasons behind restricted activity.

Altered thought process related to cerebral ischemia or sedation secondary to cerebral injury.

Expected Patient Outcome. Patient attains maximal cognitive functioning.

- Should patient be in a deep sleep, unresponsive to stimuli; react inconsistently and nonpurposefully to stimuli in a nonspecific manner; or react specifically but inconsistently to stimuli, provide only low-level stimulation of all senses.
- Provide soft increases in auditory stimulation.
- Stimulate one sense at a time to avoid confusion.
- Assess LOC, orientation, memory, attentiveness, and ability to solve problems.
- Report restlessness, irritability, reduced attentiveness, impaired memory, confusion, and inability to solve problems. Disruption in thought process can suggest hemispheric lesions, while altered arousal and cognition can reflect disruption of reticular activating system.
- Reorient patient to person, place, and time.
- Orient patient to the immediate critical care environment while minimizing excess stimulation.
- Repeat instructions and information while allowing patient enough time to process the data and ask questions.
- Encourage patient and family to ask questions.
- Provide praise and encouragement when patient makes positive gains in cognitive functioning.
- Provide patient with realistic decision-making options and support his or her choices.

Ineffective family coping related to a head injury of a family member.

Expected Patient Outcomes. Patient and family are able to cope with the situation, as evidenced by their positive adaptation to limitations.

- Listen to patient and family's description of limitations in terms of fear, feeling of helplessness, and loss of control.
- Assist family in identifying care activities such as exercises they can perform that help to promote recovery and progress.
- Encourage family to talk about their needs and problems so they can be incorporated into the nurse's care.
- Encourage family to reminisce about patient's background and accomplishments.
- Instruct family about support services available through the National Head Injury Foundation, Inc.

High risk for disuse syndrome related to immobility.

Expected Patient Outcomes. Body systems remain intact through therapy.

- Consult with physical therapist regarding exercise program to prevent disuse syndrome.
- Provide ROM exercises if not contraindicated.
- Position patient to reduce ICP and maintain proper alignment.
- Evaluate situation contributing to disuse syndrome: paralysis, mechanical immobilization, prescribed immobilization, pain, or altered LOC.
- Provide antithromboembolic stockings as prescribed.

Adjustment impaired related to neurological dysfunction or dependency on others.

Expected Patient Outcome. Patient is able to adjust to changes.

- Confer with physical therapist as to exercise or therapy program designed to assist patient to strengthen muscular function.
- Listen to patient's concerns about the progress of his or her adjustment to changes and potential dependency on others.
- Encourage patient, when realistic, to become physically independent so his or her dependency on others is reduced.

- Encourage patient's family to share their concerns about potential long-term physiological changes and their role in supporting patient through the changes.

Collaborative Problems

Common collaborative goals for patients with acute head injury are to reduce cerebral edema, minimize intracranial hypertension, reduce CPP, correct electrolyte imbalance, correct dysrhythmias, and prevent thromboembolism.

Potential Complication: Cerebral Edema. Cerebral edema related to movement of fluid into the cerebral tissue secondary to localized loss of autoregulatory mechanisms, increase of blood flow, and dilation of focal bleed vessels.

Expected Patient Outcomes. Patient is free of cerebral edema, as evidenced by normal mentation, adequate arousal, alert and oriented behavior, ICP ≤15 mm Hg, and CPP 60 to 100 mm Hg.

- Review serum osmolality and serum electrolyte values.
- Review results of serum tests, since hyperglycemia is induced by corticosteriod therapy.
- Assess clinical indicators of neurological status: LOC, sensorimotor function, RR and pattern, pupils, and vital signs.
- Report clinical findings associated with increased ICP: deterioration of LOC, pupillary dilatation or constriction, increased SBP, widening pulse pressure, bradycardia, altered respiratory pattern, loss of sensorimotor function, papilledema, headache, and vomiting.
- Monitor ICP continuously for pressure 0 to 15 mm Hg and three pressure waves, A, B, and C. Report ICP ≥15 mm Hg and presence of A wave. The A, or plateau, waves are sudden, transient waves lasting 5 to 20 minutes, which begin from a baseline of already elevated ICP. The A waves

cause cerebral ischemia. The B waves are seen in relation to fluctuations of respiratory pattern such as Cheyne-Stokes respiration.

- Assist with removal of CSF to reduce cerebral edema and ICP. Document the amount of drainage, time interval for drainage, color, clarity, consistency, and amount of fluid drained.
- Continuously monitor and report CPP ≤30 mm Hg.
- Assess cranial nerve and pupillary reaction.
- Restrict fluid intake to 1200 to 1500 mL/d, which decreases intracellular fluid volume, thereby minimizing or preventing cerebral edema formation by keeping patient slightly dehydrated.
- Administer prescribed hypertonic solution to reduce cerebral edema.
- Administer prescribed hyperosmolar agents (mannitol), which increase the osmolality of circulating blood, thereby causing fluid to move down the concentration gradient from the brain interstitium into the intravascular compartment.
- Administer prescribed furosemide to reduce cerebral edema.
- Administer prescribed glucocorticosteroids (dexamethasone [Decadron] and methylprednisolone sodium succinate [Solu-Medrol]) to relieve cerebral edema, thereby reestablishing and maintaining the integrity of the blood-brain barrier (see Table 1–15, p. 129).

Potential Complication: Intracranial Hypertension. Intracranial hypertension related to hypoxia or hypotension secondary to brain injury.

Expected Patient Outcomes. Patient is free from intracranial hypertension, as evidenced by ICP 0 to 15 mm hg, PaO_2 80 to 100 mm Hg, BP within patient's normal range, and CPP ≤50 mm Hg.

- Review levels of arterial blood gases.
- Place patient in a semi-Fowler's position with HOB elevated 30 degrees to help drain

blood and CSF from the cranial vault via gravity.

- Align patient's body in a midline position with the head maintained in a neutral position. Avoid neck flexion and head rotation, since this position can impair outflow of blood and CSF from the cranial vault.
- Continuously monitor ICP and CPP. Report repeated increases in resting ICP ≥ 20 mm Hg, resting CPP ≤ 50 mm Hg, wide-amplitude ICP tracing, or ICP ≥ 10 mm Hg response to nursing care activities lasting more than 3 minutes.
- Minimize fluctuations in SBP and maintain SBP between 80 to 100 mm Hg. Elevated SBP increases intracranial blood volume and CBF, causing increased ICP.
- Suction with extreme caution to minimize coughing, which can increase intracerebral hypertension.
- Continuously monitor and report SBP ≤ 70 mm Hg and MAP ≤ 70 mm Hg, since hypotension can contribute to cerebral hypoperfusion and intracranial hypertension.
- Avoid loud noises and sudden tactile stimuli to reduce intracerebral hypertension resulting from increased ICP.
- Provide undisturbed rest periods.
- Reduce environmental noise and encourage stress reduction through progressive relaxation and guided imagery.
- Assist with the removal of CSF to reduce ICP as ordered to increase intracranial adaptive capacity.
- Maintain $Paco_2$ ≤ 30 to 35 mm Hg to cause cerebral vasodilation, which decreases cerebral blood volumes, and maintain ICP within 0 to 15 mm Hg.
- Suction when patient is at rest and ICP is at baseline to reduce risk of increased ICP.
- Prior to suctioning, hyperventilate with 100% oxygen using a hand-held resuscitator to reduce risk of hypoxemia and dysrhythmias.
- Provide controlled hyperventilation, as prescribed, to maintain $Paco_2$ 25 to 30 mm Hg and a Pao_2 ≥ 80 mm Hg. Maintain a slow rate (10 to 12 BPM) and a high tidal volume (15 mL/kg) to attain the expected carbon dioxide and oxygen tension.

- Administer prescribed IV isotonic crystalloid and colloid to optimize intravascular volume and correct hypotension without increasing cerebral edema.
- Administer prescribed osmotic diuresis with mannitol to increase adaptive capacity and decrease ICP.
- Administer prescribed oxygen by nasal cannula, mask, or mechanical support to provide adequate oxygenation.
- Administer prescribed pancuronium bromide (Pavulon) to control RR and tidal volume and to keep patient in pace with the ventilator (see Table 3–5, p. 338).
- Administer prescribed furosemide to decrease cerebral edema.
- Administer prescribed barbiturate to cause cerebral vasoconstriction, reduce the cerebral blood volume, and reduce cerebral BP, which helps to decrease cerebral edema. Titrate 3 to 5 mg/dL according to ICP measurements.

Potential Complication: Increased Cerebral Perfusion Pressure. Increased CPP related to cerebral edema secondary to cerebral trauma.

Expected Patient Outcomes. Patient maintains adequate CPP, as evidenced by CPP 60 to 100 mm Hg, ICP ≤ 15 mm Hg, MAP ≥ 70 mm Hg, intact LOC and mentation, and normal sensorimotor function.

- Assess the clinical indicators of neurological status: LOC, mentation, RR and pattern, pupillary size and reactivity, BP, HR, and sensorimotor function.
- Report clinical findings associated with increased CPP. Deterioration in LOC, pupillary dilation or constriction, confusion, increased SBP, widening pulse pressure, bradycardia, altered respiratory pattern, altered sensorimotor function, or papilledema.
- Monitor ICP continuously and CPP hourly. Report a sustained increase in ICP ≥ 25 to

30 mm Hg for more than 15 to 30 minutes, which can compromise CPP.

- Maintain a closed ICP monitoring system to reduce the risk of infection.
- Maintain proper positioning and keep HOB elevated 30 degrees to facilitate venous drainage and decrease ICP.
- Maintain controlled hyperventilation and oxygenation, since hypercapnia can cause cerebral vasodilation, thereby increasing intracerebral blood flow and CPP.
- Restrict fluid intake to reduce extracellular fluid volume.
- Assess patient for the presence of pressure waves on the ICP tracing, signifying reduced cerebral compliance. Compliance is an index of the volume-pressure relationship within the skull. When cerebral compliance is reduced, increase CPP to 90 to 100 mm Hg.
- Improve CPP by increasing MAP and decreasing CSF volume.
- Continuously monitor arterial BP to determine CPP and to evaluate hemodynamic function.
- Administer prescribed osmotic diuretic (mannitol) to decrease cerebral edema, thereby improving CPP.
- Administer prescribed agents such as dopamine and phenylephrine to increase arterial BP.
- Titrate prescribed labetalol with phenylephrine and dopamine to facilitate adequate MAP without exceeding SBP of 180 mm Hg.
- Drain CSF via a ventricular catheter, as prescribed, to improve CPP.

Potential Complication: Electrolyte Imbalance. Electrolyte imbalance related to diuretic therapy or diabetes insipidus secondary to cerebral injury.

Expected Patient Outcomes. Patient maintains normal electrolyte balance.

- Review levels of serum electrolytes.
- Obtain and report clinical findings associated with electrolyte imbalance resulting from diabetes insipidus: polyuria, polydipsia, and specific gravity ≤ 1.005.
- Monitor ECG continuously to assess HR and rhythm. Document ECG rhythm strips every 2 to 4 hours or more frequently in patients with dysrhythmias resulting from hypokalemia.
- Measure intake, output, specific gravity, and daily weight to evaluate fluid balance.
- Administer prescribed IV therapy to maintain adequate hydration and restore electrolytes.
- Administer prescribed vasopressin replacement therapy such as chlorpropamide or carbamazepine (see Table 7–4).
- Administer prescribed potassium should hypokalemia occur.

Potential Complication: Dysrhythmias. Dysrhythmias related to tachycardia-bradycardia secondary to hypothalamic dysfunction.

Expected Patient Outcomes. Patient maintain regular sinus rhythm.

- Review results of 12-lead ECG.
- Obtain and report ECG dysrhythmias such as progressive bradycardia, junctional escape rhythm, and idioventricular rhythm, which can occur with cerebral hemorrhage and increased ICP.
- Monitor and report ECG dysrhythmias such as atrial and ventricular ectopy and conduction defects, which can signify acute subdural hematoma.
- Monitor ECG rhythm continuously. Document and report ST and T wave changes resulting from cerebral ischemia caused by acute head injury and increased ICP. Inverted T waves with increased amplitude and duration are associated with neurological pathology.
- Reduce ICP to minimize dysrhythmias.
- Administer prescribed antidysrhythmic agents.

Potential Complication: Thromboembolism. Thromboembolism related to venostasis secondary to immobility.

Expected Patient Outcomes. Patient is free from thromboembolism in lower extremities.

• Assess lower extremity circumference daily and report increases ≥2 cm.
• Provide ROM exercises every 4 hours, if not contraindicated, to promote venous return.
• Apply antiembolic hose or alternating pneumatic pressure devices on the legs, as ordered, to facilitate venous return.
• Elevate the entire lower extremity 10 to 15 degrees, thereby preventing venostasis.
• Assist with early mobilization, if not contraindicated.

DISCHARGE PLANNING

The critical care nurse will provide patient and significant other(s) verbal or written discharge notes regarding the following subjects:

1. Medications, including drug name, dosage, route, purpose, schedule, and side effects.
2. Importance of keeping all medical appointments.
3. Referrals to physical, speech, and occupational therapist depending on the severity of patient's problem.
4. Referrals to vocational rehabilitation agencies and cognitive retraining specialists.
5. Signs and symptoms of rebleeding and need to report changes to the physician.
6. Referral to family support groups.
7. Name and phone number of national support group such as National Head Injury Foundation.

■ CEREBROVASCULAR ACCIDENT

(For related information see Respiratory Deviations, Part I: Pneumonia, p. 375; Pulmonary edema, p. 346; Respiratory acidosis, p. 412. Part III: Pulse oximetry, p. 426; Mechanical ventilation, p. 428; Capnography, p. 439. Part I: Cerebral hemorrhage, p. 607; Acute head injury, p. 620; Status epilepticus, p. 636. Part II: Craniotomy, p. 664. See also Behavioral Deviations, Part I, p. 725.)

Case Management Basis
DRG: 14 Specific cerebrovascular disorders except transient ischemic attack (TIA)
LOS: 7.20 days

Definition
A cardiovascular accident (CVA) is the alteration or disruption of the cerebral circulation, which predisposes the individual to cerebral ischemia, injury, and neuronal death from infarction.

Pathophysiology
Disruption of cerebral blood flow to any part of the brain can cause cerebral ischemia and subsequently cerebral infarction. When the integrity of plasma membrane is altered, cerebral edema occurs. An increase in cerebral edema causes the capillaries to become compressed, thereby impairing cerebral perfusion and leading to cerebral tissue ischemia. Thrombosis and embolism are two mechanisms that contribute to strokes. The pathological mechanism behind arterial thrombosis is atherosclerosis. In atherosclerosis, damage involves the endothelial lining and sublying intima of the vessel wall. There is proliferation of smooth muscle cells with accompanying atheromatous plaque. Simultaneously the intima becomes thin and fibrous. Ultimately arteries lose their distensibility and are easily ruptured. Thrombosis occurs in atheromatous vessels with a narrowed lumen.

Cerebral embolism can result from embolic material from a thrombus within the heart, most frequently they lodge within the middle cerebral artery and its branches. Cerebral infarction produced by cerebral emboli is more extensive than that associated with cerebral thrombosis.

Nursing Assessment

PRIMARY CAUSES
• Thrombosis associated with sepsis, lupus erythematosis, polyarteritis nodosa, prolonged vasospasm associated with subarachnoid hemorrhage, shock, hypercoagulability syn-

dromes, dissecting aortic aneurysm, carotid artery trauma, or postradiation necrosis. Embolism can occur from extracranial atheromatous plaque or thrombosis from carotid, aortic, or vertebral arteries; presence of foreign substances or tumor in the circulatory blood; or alterations in the coagulable state.

RISK FACTORS

- History of hypertension, diabetes mellitus, or heart disease. Other factors include age ≥ 65 and use of oral contraceptives. Lifestyle factors include cigarette smoking, obesity, sedentary life-style, and genetic predisposition.

PHYSICAL ASSESSMENT

- Inspection: Pupil deviation is toward the lesion in hemispheric abnormalities and away from the lesion in brain-stem abnormalities, nuchal rigidity, hemiplegia, hemianesthesia, speech disturbance, facial weakness, confusion, disorientation, dizziness, numbness, visual defects in one or both fields, or dysphagia.
- Auscultation: Cheyne-Stokes respiration or jugular bruits.

DIAGNOSTIC TEST RESULTS

Standard Laboratory Tests. (see Table 7–1)

- Cerebrospinal fluid (CSP): Used to assess the presence of blood in CSF.
- Serum chemistry: Reduced hemoglobin; elevated white blood cells (WBC), glucose, and lipids.
- Urinalysis: Elevated blood urea nitrogen (BUN), glycosuria, albumin, and casts.

Invasive Neurological Diagnostic Procedures. (see Tables 7–1 and 7–2)

- Angiography: Performed if an intracranial hemorrhage is suspected, if the patient is deteriorating neurologically, or if the patient has a suspected acute carotid occlusion.

- Lumbar puncture: Pressure is normal in cerebral thrombosis, embolism, and transient ischemic attack (TIA) and the fluid is clear. The pressure is elevated and the fluid is bloody in subarachnoid and intracerebral hemorrhage. With thrombosis resulting from the inflammatory process, CSF reveals elevated total protein level.

Noninvasive Neurological Diagnostic Procedures. (See Table 7–3)

- Computerized tomography (CT): CT scan can be useful in differentiating between cerebrovascular lesions and nonvascular lesions.
- Electroencephalogram (EEG): Useful in locating the damaged area in the brain.
- Skull roentgenogram: May reveal shift of pineal gland to the opposite side from the expanding mass, and calcifications of the internal carotid may be visible in cerebral thrombosis.

ECG

- Atrial fibrillation.

MEDICAL AND SURGICAL MANAGEMENT

PHARMACOLOGY

- Vasopressor: Low-dose dopamine can be used to dilate cerebral arteries, leading to increases in cerebral perfusion (see Table 1–10, p. 50).
- Antihypertensives: Diazoxide is used to maintain blood pressure at preexisting levels (see Table 1–16, p. 146).
- Anticoagulant therapy: Used to restore or improve cerebral circulation and prevent further occlusion of the compromised cerebral vasculature. Heparin can be administered as a bolus followed by continuous intravenous infusion or by serial subcutaneous route. Warfarin (Coumadin) is a mainstay of oral anticoagulation therapy (see Table 1–8, p. 32).
- Antiplatelet therapy: Dipyridamole (Persantine), sulfinpyrazone (Anturane), and

acetylsalicyclic acid (aspirin) can be used to reduce platelet adhesiveness and reduce risk of recurrent thrombosis or embolism.

• Cerebral vasodilatory therapy: Papaverine (Pavabid) is used to increase blood flow to areas of brain compromised by occlusion or vasospasm (see Table 7–4).

OXYGEN THERAPY

• Supplemental humidified oxygen therapy is given by fraction of inspired oxygen (FIO_2) 24% to 28% via Venturi mask or 2 to 3 L via nasal cannula to maintain optimal arterial oxygen tension.

SURGICAL INTERVENTION

• Extracranial-intracranial bypass surgery has been used to improve cerebral blood flow in patients with inaccessible stenosis or occlusion of the carotid, middle cerebral, or basilar arteries.

NURSING MANAGEMENT: NURSING DIAGNOSES AND COLLABORATIVE PROBLEMS

Nursing Diagnoses

Common nursing goals for patients with CVA are to provide effective breathing pattern, support effective airway clearance, maintain normothermia, support physical mobility, maintain swallowing, enhance cognitive function, provide communication strategies, and support sensory-perceptual function.

Ineffective breathing pattern related to brain-stem compression or impaired chest excursion secondary to hemorrhage, cerebral edema, or hemiparesis.

Expected Patient Outcomes. Patient maintains adequate breathing pattern, as evidenced by respiratory rate (RR) 12 to 20 BPM, adequate alveolar ventilation partial pressure of arterial carbon dioxide ($PaCO_2$) $\leq$30 to 35 mm Hg or partial pressure of arterial oxygen (PaO_2) $\geq$80 mm Hg, tidal volume $\geq$7 to 10 mL/kg, vital capacity $\geq$12 to 15 mL/kg, absence of rales or wheezes, respiratory pattern synchro-

nized, absence of adventitious breath sounds, and skin color normal.

• Consult with physician about the desired arterial blood gas values, tidal volume, and vital capacity.

• Review arterial blood gas values.

• Maintain patient in semi-Fowler's position to permit maximal chest excursion and drainage of blood and CSF from the cranial vault via gravity.

• Assess clinical indicators of respiratory status: rate, depth, rhythm, use of accessory muscles, symmetry of chest movement, skin color, and lung sounds.

• Report clinical findings associated with ineffective breathing pattern: tachycardia, tachypnea, dyspnea, crackles, cyanosis, and hyper- or hypoventilation.

• Maintain nasogastric decompression as indicated to prevent abdominal distention, which can compromise diaphragmatic excursion, and to reduce risk of aspiration.

• Maintain mechanical ventilation via endotracheal intubation in patient with compromised protective mechanisms such as cough, gag, and epiglottal closure.

• Administer prescribed IV fluids to maintain adequate hydration.

• Administer prescribed oxygen 2 to 4 L by means of nasal cannula, Venturi mask, or mechanical ventilation to maintain PaO_2 $\geq$80 mm Hg and $PaCO_2$ 35 to 45 mm Hg.

• Instruct patient to deep breathe and cough when cerebral perfusion pressure (CPP) and intracranial pressure (ICP) have stabilized.

Ineffective airway clearance related to compromised cough or inability to handle tracheobronchial secretions secondary to dysphagia or inability to cough.

Expected Product Outcomes. Patient maintains effective airway clearance, as evidenced by patent airway with normal breath sounds, and demonstrates secretion-clearing cough.

• Consult with physician about patient's protective mechanisms: gag reflex, cough reflex, or epiglottal closure.

- Reposition patient hourly to prevent pooling of secretions (unless contraindicated by increased ICP): side-lying position to allow drainage of secretion from mouth and drainage of secretion from lung segments.
- Obtain and report clinical findings associated with ineffective airway clearance: loss of gag reflex, loss of cough reflex, dyspnea, tachypnea, restlessness, and cyanosis.
- Auscultate the lungs every 2 hours for presence of crackles, wheezes, or rhonchi, which indicate increased pulmonary secretions.
- Initiate suctioning of tracheobronchial secretions when necessary and assess its effect on ICP.
- Follow unit protocol regarding suctioning: Reduce suctioning time and hyperventilate with 100% oxygen to reduce risk of hypercapnia or hypoxemia.
- Administer prescribed IV fluids to maintain adequate hydration.
- Administer prescribed humidified oxygen 2 to 4 L by means of nasal cannula or Venturi mask.

High risk for ineffective thermoregulation related to cerebral edema with altered hypothalamic function or infection.

Expected Patient Outcomes. Patient maintains normal body temperature.

- Review results of WBC count, chest roentgenogram, and culture and sensitivity tests.
- Monitor body temperature every 1 to 2 hours while patient is febrile.
- Inspect all invasive sites or wounds for signs of infection: redness, warmth, swelling, tenderness, and amount and color of drainage.
- Measure intake and output. Encourage fluid intake to maintain adequate hydration and avoid dehydration.
- Apply cooling measures should patient experience elevated temperature.
- Initiate measure to reduce high body temperature: hypothermia blanket.
- Administer prescribed antipyretic to reduce temperature.
- Administer prescribed antibiotics should infection occur.

Mobility, impaired physical related to impaired neurophysiological function secondary to decreased cerebral blood flow and ischemia.

Expected Pateint Outcomes. Patient maintains full range of motion.

- Consult with physical therapist regarding exercise program to maintain or strengthen muscles.
- Consult with physician to determine musculoskeletal status.
- Position patient to maintain optimal body alignment by supporting the affected extremity in a functional position.
- Encourage the use of range-of-motion exercises to maintain muscle tone, prevent atrophy, and stimulate circulation.
- Initiate a gradual exercise program, as prescribed, by assisting patient to dangle legs over the side of the bed and transfer to a chair.
- Maintain optimal body alignment by supporting the affected extremities in a functional position to avoid dependent edema.
- Encourage patient to perform basic activities of daily living (ADL), unless contraindicated, using the unaffected side (bathing, brushing teeth, combing hair, and eating).
- Provide antiembolic stockings to avoid thromboembolism.
- Assist with progressive physical activity: sitting position and transfer from bed to chair. These activities will assist patient to regain his or her positional sense.
- Teach patient to turn, cough, and deep breathe every 2 to 4 hours. This will facilitate chest and lung expansion, prevent atelectasis, and mobilize excess secretions.
- Teach patient to use supportive devices such as an overhead trapeze.
- Instruct patient to use the involved side when possible.

Swallowing, impaired related to altered consciousness, absent gag reflex, or decreased strength of muscles used in mastication.

Expected Patient Outcome. Patient swallows without impairment.

- Consult with Physical Therapy regarding an eating program that encompasses any alteration in swallowing.
- Consult with speech therapist interested in dysphagia to teach techniques, such as compensatory head and neck posture, pharyngeal icing, sucking exercises, tongue manipulation exercises, supraglottic cough, and dry-cough sequencing technique.
- Review results of videofluroscopy, which can document how patient is handling lights, pudding, or cookies coated with barium.
- Provide patient, when ready, with a pureed diet, which is easier to swallow than liquids.
- Provide patient, when ready, with a high-fiber diet of 40 to 70 g of fiber per day to avoid constipation.
- Assess the adequacy of fluid and calorie intake through urine specific gravity or the presence of ketouria without glycosuria as indicator of negative nitrogen balance.
- Begin nasogastric feedings when patient is unable to take adequate fluid and calories by mouth: Use small-volume feedings, elevate head of bed 30 degrees for 2 hours, and check tube placement before and after each feeding.
- Administer docusate sodium (Colace) or psyllium (Metamucil) to help prevent constipation.

Altered thought process related to confusion secondary to cerebral ischemia or medication.

Expected Patient Outcomes. Patient is oriented to time and person, with improved memory and improved attentiveness.

- Assess cognitive parameters: state of awareness, ability to concentrate, memory, and ability to solve problems.
- Observe and report clinical findings indicating altered thought process: disorientation, impaired memory, restlessness, and impaired attentiveness.

- Provide patient with quiet, structured rest periods midmorning and midafternoon. The time allows for a reduction in stress levels and promotes effective sleep pattern.
- Provide a sense of security through a structured routine, familiar staff, and a familiar environment.
- Keep routines simple and choices limited so patient doesn't become further confused.
- Encourage problem solving by providing patient with solvable problems in gradual increments.
- Reorient patient, when necessary, to person, place, and time.
- Provide information in increments that can be understood and internalized.
- Provide encouragement and feedback regarding patient's progress, including positive accomplishments.
- Use verbal and nonverbal messages to communicate acceptance to the confused CVA patient.
- Instruct family as to the need to keep patient oriented and reduce frustration when not understood.

Impaired verbal communication related to dysarthria, dysphasia, or aphasia secondary to frontal or left cerebral hemisphere dysfunction.

Expected Patient Outcomes. Patient appropriately uses language to verbalize or communicate needs.

- Consult with speech therapist about patient's specific communication deficits and develop a care plan.
- Assess for the presence of alteration in communication skills, articulation, comprehension, or verbalization.
- Encourage patient to attempt communication verbally or in writing with a picture, felt board, or slateboard.
- Provide clear communication to patient: Speak slowly and clearly; report questions or directions as needed; minimize distractions; and offer encouragement.

- Minimize distractions while talking with patient to encourage concentration on his or her communication skills.
- Involve family in patient's speech program.
- Reassure patient when attempting to communicate so feelings of frustration can be minimized.

Powerlessness related to loss of mobility (sensorimotor function) and changes in life-style.

Expected Patient Outcomes. Patient expresses feelings of control over self-care, illness experience, or future change in life-style.

- Listen to patient's concerns over physical limitations that may require dependency on others.
- Create an immediate environment that contains personal items.
- Provide decisional control, when realistic, by allowing patient to decide when to bathe or get out of bed.
- Instruct patient as to risk factors associated with CVA and need for compliance with therapy and treatment schedule.
- Instruct patient stress reduction techniques: progressive relaxation, meditation, or guided imagery.

Altered sensory-perceptual function related to impaired neurological function secondary to cerebral perfusion.

Expected Patient Outcomes. Patient maintains a level of sensory-perceptual function, as evidenced by adequate perception of external stimuli, sounds, lights, sensations such as pain, pressure, temperature, and absence of visual loss.

- Consult with physician about the desired activity program that takes into consideration existing sensory-perceptual alterations.
- Assess patient's sensory awareness by measuring response to hot and cold, dull and sharp pain, awareness of motor function and location of body position.

- Arrange the environment to compensate for any neurological deficits.
- Orient and reorient patient time, place, and events while conscious to reduce confusion.
- Talk to patient while providing care to facilitate auditory stimulation and reduce feelings of sensory deprivation.
- Establish with patient and family a means of communication: call bell, Magic Slate, wordboard, symbols, and gestures, and one-word commands.
- Provide meaningful tactile stimulation to reassure patient.
- Provide range-of-motion (ROM) exercises to all body joints every 2 to 4 hours.
- Teach patient the importance of beginning activity as soon as realistic.
- Teach patient the need for regular exercise program to maintain mobility.

Collaborative Problems

A common collaborative goal for patients with CVA is to maintain normal CPP.

Potential Complication: Altered Cerebral Perfusion Pressure. Altered CPP related to decreased systemic arterial pressure secondary to intracranial hemorrhage.

Expected Patient Outcomes. Patient maintains adequate CPP, as evidenced by CPP 60 to 100 mm Hg, blood pressure (BP) within patient's normal limits, mean arterial pressure (MAP) 70 to 100 mm Hg, ICP $\leq$15 mm Hg, cerebral spinal pressure 130 mm H_2O (10 mm Hg), orientation to time and place, heart rate (HR) $\leq$100 bpm, cardiac rhythm normal, neurological signs normal, and arterial blood gases within normal limits.

- Consult with physician to validate expected patient outcomes used to evaluate CPP.
- Review results of CT scan, EEG, skull roentgenogram, and lumbar puncture.
- Limit physical activity to bed rest and elevate head of bed to 30 to 45 degrees: Allows for optimal venous drainage via gravity and prevents compromise of cerebral blood flow.

- Obtain and report clinical findings associated with altered CPP: CPP ≤60 mm Hg, altered level of consciousness (LOC), loss of sensation and reflexes, generalized weakness, pupil inequality, elevated BP, and altered motor function.
- Monitor continuous ECG to assess HR and rhythm. Document ECG rhythm strips every 4 hours in patients with dysrhythmias.
- Maintain a normal CPP through controlled hyperventilation, $Paco_2$ 25 to 35 mm Hg and Pao_2 ≥80 mm Hg: Reduced $Paco_2$ causes cerebral vasoconstriction and lowers cerebral blood volume.
- Measure specific gravity, intake and output. Dehydration causes hemoconcentration and may decrease cerebral blood flow.
- Administer prescribed IV fluids to maintain adequate hydration.
- Administer prescribed oxygen 2 to 4 L by means of nasal cannula or Venturi mask to maintain normal arterial blood gases.
- Administer prescribed antihypertensive agents (diazoxide), in prestroke hypertensive patient.
- Administer prescribed diuretics to maintain urinary output (UO) ≥30 mL/h or ≥0.5 mL/kg/h.
- Administer prescribed corticosteriods to decrease cerebral edema and increase cerebral perfusion.
- Administer prescribed anticoagulants to restore or improve cerebral circulation and prevent further occlusion of the compromised cerebral vasculature.
- Administer antiplatelet aggregation therapeutic agent (dipyridamole, sulfinpyrazone, and aspirin) to reduce platelet adhesiveness and risk of recurrent thrombosis or emboli (see Table 1–8, pp. 32).
- Should pharmacological therapy be ineffective, prepare patient for surgery: carotid endarterectomy to improve cerebral blood flow; extracranial-intracranial bypass surgery in patients with inaccessible stenosis or occlusion of the carotid, middle cerebral, or basilar arteries. The surgery involves the anastomosis of the superior temporal artery with the middle cerebral artery.
- Administer cerebral vasodilator (papaverine) to increase blood flow to areas of brain compromised by occlusion or vasospasm (see Table 7–4).
- Teach alert patient to avoid excessive coughing or straining: These activities increase intrathoracic and intra-abdominal pressures, which impede outflow of blood from the cranium.

DISCHARGE PLANNING

The critical care nurse will provide patient and significant other(s) verbal or written discharge notes regarding the following subjects:

1. The signs and symptoms that warrant immediate medical attention: sensorimotor changes, confusion, and disorientation.
2. Importance of family to encourage independent activities as realistic.
3. Importance of keeping follow-up visits and laboratory studies appointments.
4. Common side effects of diuretics.
5. Importance of continuation of exercise program.
6. Names of community agencies that could support patient and family.

■ STATUS EPILEPTICUS

(For related information see Part I: Acute head injury, p. 620; Cerebral hemorrhage, p. 607; Cerebrovascular accident, p. 630. Part II: Craniotomy, p. 664. Part III: Intracranial pressure monitoring, p. 671; Barbiturate coma, p. 674; Cerebral balloon angioplasty, p. 676. See also Behavioral Deviations Part I, pp. 725.)

Case Management Basis
DRG: 24 Seizure and headache, age greater 17 with complication
LOS: 5.30 days
DRG: 25 Seizure and headache, age greater than 17 without complication
LOS: 3.50 days

Definition

Seizures are a symptom of central nervous system irritability characterized by abnormal neuronal discharge. Epilepsy is a chronic seizure disorder of the cerebral tissue characterized by recurrent paroxysmal discharge resulting in disturbed motor, sensory, and behavioral alterations and loss of consciousness. Epilepsy is a syndrome rather than a disease.

Pathophysiology

GENERAL. A seizure involves an autonomous paroxysmal discharge of electrical activity that is enhanced or minimized depending on the neurotransmitter that is active on the post-synaptic membrane. During seizure activity, cerebral oxygen consumption increases, while there is also an increase in blood flow to meet metabolic demands. In status epilepticus there is a rapid depletion of oxygen and nutrient stores, which leads to hypoxemia, hypercapnia, and hypoglycemia.

CLASSIFICATION OF SEIZURES. Partial (focal) seizures are unilateral and involve a localized or focal area of the brain. These seizures occur without loss of consciousness and involve sensory or motor symptoms. Simple partial seizure involves clonic movements of a single muscle group and may spread to involve contiguous regions of the motor cortex, as in jacksonian march, for example. With a complex partial seizure, consciousness is impaired but not lost and seizure discharge arises from the temporal lobe or medial frontal lobe. Generalized (unlocalized) seizure involves both the cerebral hemispheres and connections with the subcortical nuclei. The patient's consciousness is always impaired. The two generalized seizures are petit mal and tonic-clonic seizure. Petit mal seizure is characterized by short lapses of consciousness lasting a few seconds, vacant stare, or brief pause in conversation. Tonic seizure is characterized by continuing muscle contraction, fixation of the limbs, deviation of the head and eyes to one side, loss of consciousness, and absence of clonic phase. Clonic seizure is characterized by repetitive clonic jerking associated with loss of consciousness. The tonic-clonic seizure consists of four phases: preictal or aura phase, tonic phase, clonic phase, and postictal phase.

Nursing Assessment

PRIMARY CAUSES

- Idiopathic epilepsy, head trauma, stroke, subarachnoid hemorrhage, vasospasm, brain abscess, central nervous system (CNS) mass lesion, cerebral hypoperfusion or hypoxia, meningitis, encephalitis, hyponatremia, hypoglycemia, hyperosmolar nonketotic hyperglycemia, hypocalcemia, hypertensive encephalopathy, eclampsia, porphyria, hypercapnia, cerebral thrombosis, cerebral embolization, noncompliance with prescribed anticonvulsant therapy, or hyperthermia.

RISK FACTORS

- Family history of epilepsy, drug or alcohol abuse, recent head trauma, or infection.

PHYSICAL ASSESSMENT

- Inspection: Loss of consciousness, restlessness, irritability, confusion, nausea, visual disturbances, generalized contraction of muscles, cyanosis, dilated pupils, incontinence, sweating, clonic jerking movements, headache, or muscle aches.
- Auscultation: Stertorous respirations, tachycardia, or bradycardia.

DIAGNOSTIC TEST RESULTS

Standard Laboratory Tests

- Serum chemistry: Glucose, electrolytes, hepatic studies, blood urea nitrogen (BUN), creatinine, platelet count, sedimentation rate; serological or immunological tests are obtained to rule out metabolic or other disease processes.

Invasive Neurological Diagnostic Procedure. (see Table 7–2)

- Lumbar puncture: Can reveal cerebrospinal fluid (CSF) with an increased cell count, which indicates infection as the cause of seizures. The CSF pressure ≥ 180 mm H_2O may indicate a tumor or other problems causing increased intracranial pressure (ICP) and subsequent seizures.

Noninvasive Neurological Diagnostic Procedures. (see Table 7–3)

- Computerized tomographic (CT) scan: Used to visualize tumor, aneurysm, cerebral edema, infarct, congenital lesion, hemorrhage, cerebral arteriovenous malformation, or ventricular enlargement.
- Electroencephalogram (EEG): Used to diagnose the type of seizure and may also isolate the epileptogenic focus through its abnormal neuronal activity. Petite mal seizures show a 3-second spiked wave complex seen in all leads. High-voltage spikes are seen with tonic-clonic seizures. Square-topped spike complexes represent temporal lobe, psychomotor, or complex partial seizures. Lastly, delta waves can be associated with necrotic brain tissue caused by infarction, tumor, or abscess.

MEDICAL AND SURGICAL INTERVENTIONS

PHARMACOLOGY

- Carbamazepine (Tegretol): Used to treat simple and complex partial, secondary generalized, and tonic-clonic primary generalized seizures at daily maintenance dose of 10 to 20 mg/kg (see Table 7–4).
- Clonazepam (Klonopin): Used to treat myoclonic and atonic primary generalized seizures at a daily maintenance dose of 0.05 to 0.2 mg/kg (see Table 7–4).
- Ethosuximide (Zarontin): Used to treat petit mal and atonic seizures at a daily maintenance dose of 20 to 40 mg/kg (see Table 7–4).
- Phenobarbital: Used to treat simple and complex partial, secondary generalized, and tonic-clonic primary generalized seizures at a daily maintenance dose of 3 to 5 mg/kg (see Table 7–4).
- Phenytoin sodium (Dilantin): Used to treat simple and complex partial, secondary generalized, and tonic-clonic primary generalized seizures at a daily maintenance dose of 10 to 25 mg/kg (see Table 7–4).
- Primidone (Mysoline): Used to treat simple and complex partial and secondary generalized seizures at a daily maintenance dose of 3 to 5 mg/kg (see Table 7–4).
- Valproic acid and derivatives (Depakene, Depakote): Used to treat primary generalized seizures at a daily maintenance dose of 15 to 30 mg/kg monotherapy and 30 to 45 mg/kg combination therapy (see Table 7–4).
- Diazepam (Valium): Used to treat status epilepticus at 5 to 10 mg over 5 to 10 minutes. This is repeated at 15-minute intervals, not to exceed a total of 30 mg (see Table 7–4).
- Lorazepam (Ativan): Used to treat status epilepticus. The drug is administered at 4 to 8 mg IV over 2 minutes and can be repeated in 10 minutes (see Table 7–4).

SURGICAL INTERVENTION

- Surgical ablation of the epileptogenic focus is performed in patients who fail to respond to drug therapy

NURSING MANAGEMENT: NURSING DIAGNOSES AND COLLABORATIVE PROBLEMS

Nursing Diagnoses

Common nursing goals in patients with status epilepticus are to prevent injury, maintain cerebral tissue perfusion, improve oxygenation, maintain normothermia, enhance knowledge, minimize fatigue, and encourage compliance.

High risk of injury related to trauma secondary to seizure activity.

Expected Patient Outcomes. Patient is protected from injury and seizure activity is controlled.

- Obtain serum levels of antiepilepsy agents to determine whether their therapeutic levels have been achieved or exceeded.
- Identify and avoid precipatory factors contributing to seizure activity.
- Initiate seizure precautions such as keeping padded side rails up and keeping airway at bedside in order to minimize injury.
- Initiate suctioning during and after seizures to maintain airway and prevent aspiration when salivation is excessive.
- Assess baseline and neurological status during the postictal phase for confusion, lethargy, weakness, and changes in speech every 15 minutes for 1 hour, then every 30 minutes for 2 hours.
- Monitor blood pressure after seizure every 5 minutes, then every 15 minutes.
- Position patient on side to facilitate drainage of oral secretions. Be careful not to bend neck, thereby interfering with venous return and increasing ICP.
- Remain with patient during seizure to assess its type and location.
- After seizure, reorient and reassure patient.
- Measure intake and output, since myoglobinuria can occur with prolonged skeletal activity, leading to risk of renal failure.
- Administer prescribed antiepileptic agents: diazepam up to 40 mg and phenytoin 18 to 20 mg/kg. Should the seizure not be terminated, add phenobarbital 20 mg/kg, followed by paraldehyde rectally (see Table 7–4).
- Administer prescribed oxygen with ambu bag to increase availability of oxygen during seizure activity and limit hypoxia.
- Instruct patient about the cause of seizure and need for precautions to avoid injury.

Altered cerebral tissue perfusion related to increased cerebral blood flow secondary to metabolic demands from continuous seizure activity.

Expected Patient Outcomes. Patient maintains adequate cerebral tissue perfusion, as evidenced by cerebral perfusion pressure (CPP) 60 to 100 mm Hg, systolic blood pressure (SBP) 90 to 140 mm Hg, heart rate (HR) ≤ 100 bpm, being alert and oriented, equal and normoreactive pupils, normal sensorimotor function, respiratory rate (RR) 12 to 20 BPM, mean arterial pressure (MAP) 70 to 100 mm Hg, and normothermia.

- Review results of EEG, CT scan, lumbar puncture, and arterial blood gas measurement.
- Obtain and report clinical findings associated with altered cerebral tissue perfusion: SBP ≥ 140 mm Hg, tachycardia, tachypnea, altered level of consciousness (LOC), pupils unequal and dilated, sensorimotor dysfunction, and elevated temperature.
- Calculate CPP every hour, since cerebral blood flow to the brain is increased approximately 250% during a seizure to increase oxygen.
- Administer prescribed fraction of inspired oxygen (FIO_2) 100% during seizure activity to enhance tissue oxygenation, since cerebral oxygen consumption can be increased by as much as 60%.

Impaired gas exchange related to obstruction of airway or hypoxemia secondary to increased metabolic activity.

Expected Patient Outcomes. Patient maintains adequate gas exchange, as evidenced by RR 12 to 20 BPM, symmetrical chest wall movement, absence of cyanosis, HR ≤ 100 bpm, and absence of adventitious breath sounds, arterial oxygen saturation SaO_2 95% to 97.5%, arterial partial pressure of oxygen (PaO_2) ≥ 80 mm Hg, arterial partial pressure of carbon dioxide ($PaCO_2$) 35 to 45 mm Hg, and pH 7.35 to 7.45.

- Review results of arterial blood gas measurement.
- Position patient on his or her side, if not contraindicated, to facilitate drainage of oral secretions.
- Assess clinical indicators of respiratory status: rate and depth of respirations, symmetry of chest movement, use of accessory muscles, lung sounds, and skin color.

- Report clinical findings associated with impaired gas exchange: tachycardia, tachypnea, dyspnea, use of accessory muscles, assymetry of chest movement, crackles, and cyanosis.
- Monitor for clinical indicators of hypoxemia: cyanosis, restlessness, confusion, tachypnea, tachycardia, hypertension, arrhythmias, tremor, $PaO_2 \geq 60$ mm Hg, and $SaO_2 \geq 90\%$.
- Insert an oral airway to maintain airway control and maximize delivery of oxygen to the brain cells.
- Suction patient as necessary to remove excess secretions.
- Insert nasogastric (NG) tube, as ordered, to prevent vomiting and risk of aspiration.
- Assess effects of antiepilepsy agents on respiratory status since the patient's respiratory system can become depressed.
- Administer prescribed FIO_2 to maintain adequate tissue oxygenation.
- Administer prescribed antiepilepsy medication to control seizure activity.

High risk of hyperthermia related to increased metabolic activity secondary to status epilepticus.

Expected Patient Outcomes. Patient maintains normothermia.

- Obtain temperature every 30 minutes to hourly during the postictal phase of the seizure.
- Should patient become febrile, initiate cooling measures as prescribed: apply cool bath, ice bags to groin and auxillary regions, or cooling blanket.
- Administer prescribed antipyretic agents when cooling measures fail to adequately reduce patient's temperature.
- Administer prescribed IV fluids to maintain adequate hydration.
- Teach patient that change in temperature is a normal response to status epilepticus.

Knowledge deficit related to disease process and medication therapy.

Expected Patient Outcomes. Patient and family are able to verbalize an understanding of the disease process causing seizures and rationale for therapy.

- Encourage patient and family to adopt a positive attitude toward patient's life and treatments.
- Explain the need to identify and avoid stimuli that can stimulate the onset of seizure activity.
- Explain to patient the importance of maintaining a well-balanced diet and avoidance of excessive alcohol intake.
- Teach patient and family to recognize and treat seizure activity.
- Instruct patient about the need for medications to control seizure activity, including the need for continuous therapy to ensure adequate blood levels of medication.
- Teach patient the schedule and potential side effects for the prescribed medication.
- Teach patient to avoid excessive physical and emotional excitement or stress.

Fatigue related to postseizure muscle weakness.

Expected Patient Outcomes. Patient resumes activity level without verbalization of fatigue.

- Evaluate patient for muscle weakness while gradually increasing physical activity after a seizure episode.
- Allow patient to rest after a seizure episode.
- Listen to patient's verbalization of fatigue and reassure him or her this is normal after a seizure.
- Provide an environment that promotes rest by limiting the number of interventions or family visits.

Noncompliance related to taking medications.

Expected Patient Outcome. Patient maintains compliance to taking medications.

- Encourage patient to discuss why he or she did not comply with medication orders.

- Evaluate patient's knowledge of epilepsy and medication treatment.
- Refer patient to epilepsy support group.
- Listen to patient's and family's discussion of epilepsy, impact on their life-style.
- Teach patient the importance of taking medications and maintaining a daily schedule of therapy.

Collaborative Problems

Common collaborative goals for patients with status epilepticus are to correct hypoglycemia and correct dysrhythmias.

Potential Complication: Hypoglycemia. Hypoglycemia related to increased metabolic activity in contracting skeletal muscles secondary to seizure activity.

Expected Patient Outcomes. Patient maintains serum glucose with normal limits 80 to 120 mg/dL and serum ketones are negative.

- Review results of serum glucose and serum ketone tests.
- Obtain and report clinical findings associated with hypoglycemia: inability to concentrate, confusion, irrational behavior, slurred speech, blurred vision, fatigue, somnolence or seizure, tachycardia, and shallow respirations.
- Assess glucose with finger stick for quick evaluation of level hourly during initial treatment. In patients with serum glucose ≤50 mg/dL, raise to 100 mg/dL.
- Administer prescribed 10% to 50% dextrose IV or IV therapy with 5% to 10% glucose solution to restore serum glucose level.
- Teach patient the reasons for feelings of detachment and weakness associated with hypoglycemia.

Potential Complication: Dysrhythmias. Dysrhythmias related to increased intracellular potassium.

Expected Patient Outcome. Patient maintains regular sinus rhythm.

- Review results of 12-lead ECG and arterial blood gas measurement.
- Monitor dysrhythmias continuously to assess HR and rhythm. Document rhythm strips every 2 to 4 hours noting flat T waves, U waves, peaked P waves, and ST depression associated with altered potassium levels.
- Administer prescribed potassium IV at a rate not to exceed 20 mEq/100 mL/h.
- Administer prescribed IV fluids to maintain adequate circulatory volume.
- Provide oxygen by nasal cannula or Venturi mask at 24% to 28% oxygen at 4 to 6 L/min as prescribed.
- Administer antidysrhythmia medications as prescribed.

DISCHARGE PLANNING

The critical care nurse will provide patient and significant other(s) verbal or written discharge notes regarding the following subjects:

1. The signs and symptoms that warrant immediate medical attention: sensorimotor changes, confusion, and disorientation.
2. Names of available agencies for use such as Epilepsy Foundation of America.
3. Importance of possible limitations or restrictions of driving privileges.
4. Importance of keeping follow-up visits and laboratory studies appointments.
5. Importance of taking medications on schedule.

■ MENINGITIS

(For related information see Part I: Status epilepticus, p. 636. See also Behavioral Deviations Part I, pp. 725.)

Case Management Basis
DRG: 21 Viral meningitis
LOS: 4.40 days

Definition

Meningitis is an infectious process causing acute inflammation of the meningeal coverings of the brain and spinal cord. Once in the subarachnoid space, the infectious process can extend and spread throughout the subarachnoid space to the ventricles of the brain.

Pathophysiology

There are two types of meningitis. Suppurative meningitis is associated with infections of bacterial origin and may occur as a result of upper respiratory infection. The cerebrospinal fluid is turbid in appearance, with high leukocytosis and neutrophils, increased protein, and low to normal glucose content. Nonsuppurative meningitis is viral in origin and usually self-limiting, with complete recovery. The cerebrospinal fluid is clear, leukocyte count is low in lymphocytes, protein is increased, and the glucose is within normal limits.

CATEGORIES OF MENINGITIS. Categories consist of bacterial, viral, tuberculous, and fungal. Bacterial meningitis is a purulent infection involving the piarachnoid layers of the meninges and the subarachnoid space, including the cerebrospinal fluid (CSF). Neutrophils migrate into the subarachnoid space and engulf the bacteria. The phagocytic cells degenerate, combining with the exudate from tissue destruction to form purulent material, which increases over the base of the brain into the sheaths of cranial and spinal nerves. The cortical vessels become dilated and congested. Should inflammation occur through the walls of the veins, thrombosis or necrosis with risk of hemorrhage develops. The irritation from the bacteria and toxins causes swelling and an increase in endothelial cells. Viral meningitis is also known as acute benign lymphocytic meningitis and acute aseptic meningitis. There is an inflammatory meningeal reaction mediated by lymphocytes. With tuberculous meningitis, the infectious process reaches the CNS by the blood stream. There is a basal meningeal exudate containing mainly mononuclear cells. Tubercles may be seen on the meninges and surface of the brain. Fungal meningitis can occur by hematogenous trans-

fer from the lungs, heart, gastrointestinal or genitourinary tract, or skin.

Nursing Assessment

PRIMARY CAUSES
- Bacterial meningitis is due to *Staphylococcus aureus, Escherichia coli,* systemic or parameningeal infection, head trauma, anatomic defects involving the meninges, cancer, alcoholism, and other immunodeficiency states, *Streptococcus pneumoniae,* or *Haemophilus influenzae.*
- Tuberculous meningitis is caused by pulmonary tuberculosis, alcoholism, corticosteroid treatment, latent infection with *Mycobacterium tuberculosis,* or primary infection acquired by inhaling bacillus-containing droplets.
- Viral meningitis is due to echoviruses, mumps, coxsackie A, coxsackie B, herpes simplex type 2, lymphocytic choriomeningitis, hepatitis viruses, or Epstein-Barr virus.
- Fungal meningitis is caused by *Cryptococcus neoformans, Coccidioides immitis, Candida* species, *Aspergillus* species, *Mucor* species, *Histoplasma capsulatum, Blastomyces dermatitidis,* or *Nocardia* species.

PHYSICAL ASSESSMENT

Bacterial Meningitis
- Inspection: Fever, confusion, deterioration of level of consciousness (LOC), irritability, restlessness, agitation, hypersensitivity, photophobia, vomiting, headache, neck stiffness, petechial rash, and seizure. Positive Kernig's sign, which is the presence of pain and spasm of the hamstrings when an attempt is made to extend the knee. The pain is due to inflammation of the meninges and spinal roots. Brudzinski's sign is positive when both upper legs at the hips and the lower legs at the knees are flexed in response to passive flexion of the neck and head on the chest.
- Auscultation: Tachycardia and hypotension.

Tuberculosus Meningitis

- Inspection: Fever, lethargy, confusion, headache, weight loss, vomiting, neck stiffness, diplopia, focal weakness, seizures, papilledema, ocular palsies, hemiparesis, positive Kernig's and Brudzinski's signs.
- Auscultation: Tachycardia and hypotension.

Viral Meningitis

- Inspection: Fever, headache, neck stiffness, photophobia, drowsiness, malaise, nausea, vomiting, skin rash, pleuritis, jaundice, diarrhea, or orchitis.
- Palpation: Lymphadenopathy or organomegaly.

Fungal Meningitis

- Inspection: Headache, lethargy, confusion, nausea, vomiting, visual loss, seizures, focal weakness, papilledema, ocular or cranial nerve palsies, or hemiparesis.
- Palpation: Spine tenderness or parethesia, loss of sensation over the legs and trunk.

DIAGNOSTIC TEST RESULTS

Standard Laboratory Tests

- Blood studies: Elevated or reduced white blood cells (WBC).
- Purified protein derivative (PPD) skin test: Positive in tuberculosis.
- Serum chemistry: Amylase elevated in mumps and abnormal liver function test with hepatitis.

Invasive Neurological Diagnostic Procedures.
(see Tables 7–1 and 7–2)

Bacterial

- CSF pressure ≥180 mm H_2O; turbid to purulent; WBC 1000 to 20,000/μL consisting of polymorphonuclear leukocytes; elevated lactate dehydrogenase (LDH); creatine kinase (CK), and acid phosphate; protein concentration 100 to 500 mg/dL, and glucose level ≤40 mg/dL.

Tuberculous

- Lumbar puncture: CSF pressure is increased; fluid is clear and colorless; fluid clots on standing, lymphocytes and mononuclear cell pleocytosis of 50 to 500 cells/μL; protein ≥100 mg/dL and can exceed 500 mg/dL; glucose level ≤20 mg/dL; decreased chloride; and culture tuberculosis bacilli from CSF.

Viral

- CSF pressure is normal or increased; lymphocytic or monocytic pleocytosis ≤1000 μL; protein normal or slightly increased 80 to 200 mg/dL; glucose normal or decreased; and CSF protein electrophoresis abnormalities.

Fungal

- CSF pressure normal or elevated; fluid is clear; lymphocytic pleocytosis of up to 1000 cells/μL; protein not in exceeding 200 mg/dL; glucose is normal or decreased, rarely ≤10 mg/dL.

Noninvasive Neurological Diagnostic Procedures.
(see Table 7–3)

- Computerized tomographic (CT) scan: Demonstrates enhancement of the cerebral convexities, the base of the brain, ventricular ependyma, basal cisterns, cortical meninges, or hydrocephalus.
- Countercurrent immunoelectrophoresis (CIE): Detects bacteria responsible for meningitis.
- Electroencephalogram (EEG): Slowed and focal abnormalities suggest focal cerebritis, abscess formation, or scarring.
- Roentgenogram: Chest, sinuses, or mastoid bones to determine primary site of infection.

MEDICAL AND SURGICAL MANAGEMENT

PHARMACOLOGY

- Antibiotics: Penicillins such as ampicillin and penicillin G; methicillin; nafcillin;

aminoglycosides such as gentamicin; streptomycin; and amphotericin B. Chloramphenicol is used because it penetrates the
blood-brain barrier (Table 1–14, p. 122).
- Corticosteroids: Dexamethasone (Decadron) can be used to decrease intracranial
pressure (ICP) (see Table 1–15, p. 129).
- Analgesics: Non-narcotic agents are used to
treat headache and pain.
- Antipyretic: Used to control fever.
- Antiepilepsy agents: Used to control
seizure activity (see Table 7–4).

DIET
- Total parenteral nutrition (TPN) is given
should patient be unable to tolerate oral intake because of reduced LOC or intake is
not sufficient.
- Nasogastric (NG) tube feedings can be begun after TPN and before patient can tolerate an oral diet.

NURSING MANAGEMENT: NURSING DIAGNOSES AND COLLABORATIVE PROBLEMS

Nursing Diagnoses
Common nursing goals in patients with
meningitis are to maintain cerebral tissue
perfusion, prevent injury, maintain normothermia, support effective breathing pattern,
support cognitive functioning, and reduce pain.

Altered cerebral tissue perfusion related
to increased ICP secondary to inflammatory
process and cerebral edema.

Expected Patient Outcomes. Patient maintains
adequate cerebral tissue perfusion, as evidenced by cerebral perfusion pressure (CPP)
60 to 100 mm Hg, blood pressure (BP) within
patient's normal range, systolic blood pressure (SBP) 90 to 140 mm Hg, normal pulse
pressure, being alert, and heart rate (HR)
≤100 bpm.

- Elevated head of bed 30 degrees and maintain alignment of neck to facilitate venous
drainage.

- Assess clinical indicators of neurological
status: LOC, pupillary size and reaction,
sensorimotor function, reflexes, and vital
signs.
- Report clinical findings associated with altered cerebral tissue perfusion: confusion,
restlessness, lethargy, dilated pupil(s),
hemiparesis, hemiplegia, tachycardia-
bradycardia, altered cranial nerve responses, and hypertension.
- Measure CPP, BP, and pulse pressure
hourly.
- Limit fluid intake to avoid overhydration
and subsequent cerebral edema.
- Measure intake, output, and specific gravity
to determine fluid balance.
- Administer prescribed oxygen by nasal
cannula, mask, or ventilatory support to optimize cerebral oxygenation.
- Administer prescribed corticosteroids to reduce cerebral edema.
- Administer prescribed antibiotics specific
to the type of meningitis to correct inflammatory response and subsequent cerebral
edema.

High risk of injury related to meningeal irritation and seizure activity.

Expected Patient Outcomes. Patient is free from
injury and seizures are controlled.

- Monitor for clinical indicators of meningeal
irritation: increased restlessness, presence
of positive Kernig's or Brudzinski's signs,
fever, headache, photophobia, nuchal rigidity, lethargy, or seizure.
- Evaluate neurological status through Glasgow coma scale (GCS): LOC, pupillary reaction, and motor function.
- Provide a quiet environment in a darkened
room because patient might be hypersensi-
tive to environmental stimuli such as noise
or lights.
- Consolidate nursing care activities to avoid
needless stimulation.
- Keep side rails padded and up.
- Initiate nasopharyngeal suction to remove
excess secretions.

- Maintain a patent airway to ensure adequate ventilation.
- Remain with patient if he or she is restless or confused.
- Administer prescribed anticonvulsant drugs should seizure occur.
- Administer antipyretic agents to control fever.

Hyperthermia related to infection.

Expected Patient Outcome. Patient maintains normothermia.

- Obtain temperature every 2 hours. Report temperature 38°C to 39.5°C (101°F to 103°F) since hyperthermia can increase ICP and need for oxygen.
- Maintain a cool environment by removing unnecessary equipment or darkening the room.
- Remove excess bed covers.
- Use external cooling measures such as a tepid or alcohol sponge bath or cooling blanket to reduce temperature.
- Provide frequent oral hygiene, since hyperthermia can dry mucous membranes.
- Administer prescribed antipyretic drugs such as acetaminophen (Tylenol) to reduce temperature.
- Administer prescribed IV fluids to maintain adequate hydration.
- Administer prescribed antibiotics depending on the cause of meningitis.

Ineffective breathing pattern related to increased ICP or depressed cerebral function secondary to compression of the brain stem from cerebral edema.

Expected Patient Outcomes. Patient maintains effective breathing pattern, as evidenced by respiratory rate (RR) 12 to 20 BPM, symmetry of chest movement, absence of cyanosis, HR ≤100 bpm, arterial blood gases within normal limits, and normal lung sounds.

- Review results of arterial blood gas measurement.
- Assess clinical indicators of respiratory status: RR and rhythm, symmetry of chest movement, use of accessory muscles, lung sounds, and skin color.
- Report clinical findings associated with ineffective breathing pattern: tachypnea, use of accessory muscles, asymmetry of chest movement, crackles, and cyanosis.
- Maintain patient airway through proper positioning and suctioning.
- Change patient's position every 2 hours, if not contraindicated, to prevent pooling of secretions and atelectasis.
- Administer prescribed corticosteroids to decrease cerebral edema.

Altered thought processes related to changes in LOC secondary to inflammatory process and meningeal irritation.

Expected Patient Outcomes. Patient maintains normal cognitive functioning.

- Assess clinical indicators of cognition: LOC; attention span; memory; and orientation to time, place, and person.
- Report clinical findings associated with altered thought process: disorientation, restlessness, combativeness, shortened attention span, difficulty following commands, and poor memory.
- Assess patient's responsiveness to painful stimuli.
- Assist patient to interpret environmental stimuli.
- Provide a quiet, dark environment since meningitis may cause hypersensitivity to environmental noises and light.
- Avoid needless stimulation of patient by consolidating nursing care activities.
- Evaluate patient's readiness for incremental increases in information.
- Reassure patient that confusion, lapse of memory, or inattentiveness is temporary and will subside when the infection is controlled.
- Instruct family as to causes of patient's altered LOC.

Pain related to headache and photophobia secondary to meningeal irritation.

Expected Patient Outcomes. Patient verbalizes reduction of or absence of pain.

- Provide a dark, quiet environment for patient when he or she experiences headache or photophobia.
- Teach and encourage patient to describe pain on a scale of 1 to 10.
- Elevate head of bed (HOB) 30 degrees to relieve headache.
- Provide rest periods before and after treatments or invasive procedures.
- Organize nursing care activities so patient can have uninterrupted rest periods.
- Avoid overstimulation, since this can increase SBP and aggravate patient's headache.
- Administer analgesics to control pain.

Collaborative Problem

A common collaborative goal for patients with meningitis is to reduce ICP.

Potential Complication: Increased Intracranial Pressure. Increased ICP related to cerebral inflammation or edema secondary to meningeal infection.

Expected Patient Outcomes. Patient maintains normal ICP, as evidenced by ICP 0 to 15 mm Hg, CSF pressure $\leq$180 mm H_2O, CSF findings normal, and normal GCS.

- Review results of lumbar puncture.
- Elevate HOB 30 to 45 degrees to promote venous drainage and decrease ICP.
- Monitor ICP continuously and report $\geq$15 mm Hg, since an elevated volume resulting from cerebral edema can decrease cerebral tissue perfusion.
- Obtain and report clinical findings associated with increased ICP: widening pulse pressure, bradycardia, ataxic respirations, vomiting, elevated BP, deterioration in LOC, pupillary dilation or constriction, decreased sensory function, loss of motor function, and headache.
- Monitor temperature every 2 hours while patient is febrile.

- Monitor for the presence of seizure activity, evaluate the type of seizure, and protect patient from injury.
- Maintain fluid restriction to minimize cerebral edema.
- Provide prescribed TPN with Intralipid should patient be unable to eat.
- Administer prescribed IV fluids to maintain adequate circulatory volume and hydration.
- Administer prescribed antibiotic therapy to correct specific causes of meningitis.
- Provide mechanical ventilation, as prescribed, to hyperventilate patient, thereby creating cerebral vasoconstriction and reduced ICP.
- Administer antipyretic agents for hyperthermia: aspirin or acetaminophen.
- Teach the patient to avoid straining or coughing in an attempt not to increase ICP.

DISCHARGE PLANNING

The critical care nurse will provide patient and significant other(s) verbal or written discharge notes regarding the following subjects:

1. The signs and symptoms that warrant immediate medical attention: sensorimotor changes, confusion, and disorientation.
2. Importance of keeping follow-up visits and laboratory studies appointments.
3. Importance of taking medications on schedule.

■ GUILLAIN-BARRÉ SYNDROME

(For related information see Respiratory Deviations, Part III: Mechanical ventilation, p. 428. See also Behavioral Deviations, Part 1, p. 725.)

Case Management Basis

DRG: 18 Cranial and peripheral nerve disorders with complications
LOS: 5.90 days
DRG: 19 Cranial and peripheral nerve disorders without complications
LOS: 3.90 days

DRG: 34 Other disorders of nervous system with complications
LOS: 5.90 days
DRG: 35 Other disorders of nervous system without complications
LOS: 3.70 days

Definition

Guillain-Barré Syndrome (GBS) is an inflammatory syndrome, also referred to as polyradiculoneuritis and acute idiopathic polyradiculopathy, that involves the peripheral nervous system. It is characterized by a demyelination and degeneration of the myelin sheath of peripheral nerves, including cranial and spinal nerves, dorsal root ganglia, and ventral and dorsal spinal roots.

Pathophysiology

In Guillian-Barré syndrome, there is a disruption of Schwann's cells and destruction of myelin that involves the peripheral nerves. The demyelination process affects both motor and sensory neurons, with sensory neurons affected to a lesser degree. Loss of myelin abolishes the transmission of nerve impulses by saltatory conduction, causing muscle weakness and paralysis.

GBS is divided into three phases: progression, plateau, and recovery. The progressive phase involves muscle weakness and paralysis that increases in severity. The phase can last from a few hours to 1 month. The plateau phase occurs when there is no further development of weakness or paralysis. The recovery phase begins 2 to 4 weeks after plateau and is characterized by a slow return of muscular strength.

Nursing Assessment

PRIMARY CAUSES

- The primary cause of GBS is unknown, but a preceding or triggering event can be a viral infection such as a cold, sore throat, flu, viral hepatitis, or infectious mononucleosis. Immunosuppressive states such as pregnancy or immunosuppressive therapy for malignant neoplasms and organ transplantation can initiate GBS.

PHYSICAL ASSESSMENT

- Inspection: Paresthesia; muscular aches; cramps; hyperesthesias; bilateral muscle weakness beginning distally and progressing in an ascending manner; facial muscle weakness; dysphagia; inability to talk or blink eyelids; numbness, tingling, prickling, or burning sensations in the lower extremities.
- Palpation: Deep tendon reflexes may be depressed or absent.
- Auscultation: Autonomic dysfunction includes orthostatic hypotension, hypertension, bradycardia, heart block, or asystole.

DIAGNOSTIC TEST RESULTS

Standard Laboratory Tests

- Serum chemistry: Elevated complete blood count (CBC) levels.

Invasive Neurological Diagnostic Procedures.
(see Tables 7–1, 7–3)

- Lumbar puncture: Shows a normal protein initially that is elevated in the 4th to 6th week.
- Nerve conduction studies: Tests the velocity at which nerve impulses are conducted. These are significantly reduced with the demyelinating process of the disease.

Noninvasive Neurological Diagnostic Procedures.
(see Table 3–2, p. 334)

- Respiratory function tests: A tidal volume (V_T) of ≤ 5 mL/kg and a vital capacity (VC) ≤ 12 to 15 mL/kg signify the onset of respiratory failure.

MEDICAL AND SURGICAL MANAGEMENT

PHARMACOLOGY

- Corticosteroids: Although their use is controversial, corticosteriods are used to decrease the inflammatory process.

- Vasopressors: Dopamine may be necessary to maintain adequate systemic perfusion should hypotension occur as a result of autonomic nervous system dysfunction.
- Analgesics: These are used to control pain.
- Antibiotics: These are used to treat infection to prevent sepsis.

PLASMAPHERESIS
- Plasmapheresis involves plasma exchanges or washes that remove the antibodies causing the GBS (see Multisystem Deviations, Plasmapheresis, p. 790).

DIET
- Nasogastric (NG) tube feedings: They are initiated in patients experiencing dysphagia. Supplemental feedings can maintain sufficient caloric intake for energy, positive nitrogen balance, and fluid electrolyte balance.
- Total parenteral nutrition (TPN): Adequate nutritional support can also be provided by TPN.

OXYGEN THERAPY
- Intubation and mechanical ventilatory support: Intubation and mechanical ventilation are recommended when VC is 1 liter or less or is 30% or less of predicted value for patient, when negative inspiratory force is 20 cm H_2O or less, and pharyngeal paralysis and inability to clear oral secretions are present.

NURSING MANAGEMENT: NURSING DIAGNOSES AND COLLABORATIVE PROBLEMS

Nursing Diagnoses
Common nursing goals in patients with GBS are to support effective breathing pattern, prevent aspiration, promote physical mobility, reduce pain, maintain adequate nutritional intake, reduce fear, support verbal communication, and promote hopefulness.

Ineffective breathing pattern related to compromised respiratory musculature secondary to GBS.

Expected Patient Outcomes. Patient maintains effective breathing pattern, as evidenced by respiratory rate (RR) 12 to 20 BPM, respiratory function tests within normal range, arterial blood gases within normal range arterial oxygen saturation (SaO_2) 95% to 97.5%, absence of cyanosis, and absence of adventitious breath sounds.

- Consult with physical therapist to develop an individualized plan that trains respiratory muscles while preparing for successful weaning off the mechanical ventilator.
- Review arterial blood gas, hemoglobin, hematocrit values and results of respiratory function tests.
- Place patient in a position that maintains body alignment, enhances drainage of secretions, and fosters oxygenation.
- Place patient in Roto-Kinetic bed, as ordered, to help prevent pooling of tracheobronchial secretions.
- Assess clinical indicators of respiratory status: rate, depth, symmetry of chest wall movement, skin color, use of accessory muscles, and presence of adventitious breath sounds.
- Report clinical findings associated with ineffective breathing pattern: tachypnea, dyspnea, use of accessory muscles, cyanosis, and crackles.
- Maintain patent airway and note loss of gag, swallow, or cough reflexes. Loss of muscle strength and function may lead to ineffective airway clearance and poor ventilation.
- Suction patient every 2 hours using unit protocol to mobilize excess secretions.
- Assist with intubation and mechanical ventilation when patient's VC, V_T, and inspiratory force are significantly reduced while partial pressure of arterial carbon dioxide ($PaCO_2$) is elevated.
- Assist with breathing exercises, chest percussion, vibrations, or postural drainage to enhance ventilation and reduce risk of atelectasis by promoting expansion of alveoli.
- Administer prescribed oxygen and humidification by nasal cannula, mask, or me-

chanical ventilation to help enhance tissue oxygenation and loosen secretions while keeping the mucous membranes moist.

- Administer prescribed IV fluids to maintain adequate hydration.
- Initiate weaning from mechanical ventilation, as prescribed, once respiratory muscle strength returns as shown by a VC exceeding 30% of the predicted value for patient and a negative inspiratory force of 20 cm H_2O or greater.
- Prepare patient for tracheostomy should the duration of intubation exceed 10 days.

High risk for aspiration related to dysphagia, compromised cough, and compromised gag reflex.

Expected Patient Outcomes. Patient is able to cough and handle oral secretions without aspiration.

- Review results of arterial blood gas measurement.
- Elevate head of bed 60 to 90 degrees if patient is hypotensive to maintain a patent airway and enhance lung expansion.
- Assess patient's ability to gag, cough effectively, and clear secretions. Dysphagia may manifest itself as increased oral secretions.
- Obtain and report clinical findings associated with aspiration: agitation, abnormal breath sounds, dyspnea, tachycardia, and tachypnea.
- Encourage patient to cough every 2 hours.
- Initiate oropharyngeal suctioning to remove excess secretions, thereby preventing atelectasis.
- Assist with intubation at the first indication of dysphagia to prevent aspiration.
- Insert NG tube to prevent gastric inspiration and provide feeding for the patient with dysphagia.
- Teach patient to report any difficulty swallowing or coughing.

Impaired physical mobility related to muscle weakness or paralysis secondary to bulbar nerve involvement.

Expected Patient Outcomes. Patient's physical mobility is maintained or improved as evidenced by improved muscle strength.

- Consult with physical therapist regarding exercise program for patient.
- Maintain good body alignment.
- Turn patient every 2 hours to maintain skin integrity and enhance ventilation.
- Support extremities and joints in functional position to prevent contractures and loss of joint function.
- Assess clinical indicators of peripheral neurological function: bilateral muscle symmetry; bilateral muscle strength; deep tendon reflexes of achilles, patellar, biceps, triceps, and brachioradial; presence of paresthesia; or change in sensory response.
- Report increasing muscle weakness, paresthesia, and decreasing deep tendon reflexes.
- Avoid active exercises during the progressive phase of GBS since active exercise may precipitate autonomic dysfunction or exacerbate GBS.
- Apply antithromboembolic stockings or pneumatic stockings on lower extremities if necessary and as prescribed.

Pain related to paresthesia or a hyperesthesia secondary to sensorimotor dysfunction.

Expected Patient Outcome. Patient verbalizes reduced pain.

- Place patient in a position of comfort.
- Assess and report painful sensations such as paresthesia, muscular aches and cramps, and hyperesthesias.
- Minimize environmental stimuli including touching of patients with hyperesthesia.
- Encourage patient to describe, verbally or nonverbally, the location, quality, and intensity of pain on a scale of 1 to 10.
- Encourage patient to share what nursing care activities increase or relieve the pain.
- Provide nursing care activities to manage pain by passive range of motion exercises, massage, distraction, ice, heat, cutaneous stimulation, and transcutaneous electrical nerve stimulation (TENS).

- Use communication aids such as letter boards, picture boards, or writing devices that allow patient to describe the location or intensity of the pain when patient on a ventilator.
- Administer prescribed narcotics to reduce pain while patient is intubated and on a ventilator.
- Administer prescribed analgesic to reduce pain.
- Teach patient that the pain may be worse at night and may occur mostly in the buttocks, quadriceps, and hamstrings.
- Teach patient to use meditation or guided imagery when in pain or feeling stressed.

Alteration in nutrition: less than body requirement related to decreased gastrointestinal mobility, dysphagia, or anorexia.

Expected Patient Outcomes. Patient maintains adequate nutritional intake by supplemental feedings.

- Consult with dietitian about the family bringing in home-cooked foods.
- Review results of serum albumin and total lymphocyte counts to determine nutritional status.
- Provide prescribed semisolid to solid foods for patient with mild dysphagia. Place patient in an upright position.
- Avoid liquids, since these are easily aspirated.
- Monitor continuously patient's ability to chew and shallow, since increasing muscle weakness may indicate the need for alternative methods of feeding.
- Record patient's calorie intake to determine any nutrient deficiencies.
- Monitor daily weight and report a weight loss $\geq 5\%$.
- Assess patient with NG feedings for excessive gastric residual ≥ 50 mL in 2 hours for continuous feedings and ≥ 100 mL for every 4 hour feeding.
- Administer prescribed enteral or parenteral nutrition to patients with moderate to severe dysphagia.

Fear related to loss of sensorimotor function, dependence upon supportive devices, and changes in life-style.

Expected Patient Outcomes. Patient is able to identify situations that cause fear and is comfortable with his or her situation.

- Consult with physician as to the type or amount of realistic information to be given to patient.
- Provide sensory information for painful or uncomfortable procedures.
- Listen to patient or family's misconceptions of distorted perception and clarify as appropriate.
- Provide a quiet environment so patient can sleep, since fear may be exacerbated by lack of sleep.
- Allow patient control in establishing daily schedule.
- Encourage former GBS patient to visit during the plateau or recovery phase.
- Evaluate patient and family's fears and coping strategies used to alleviate their fear.
- Encourage patient to verbalize questions, fears, or concerns even when it may be necessary to use communication aids.
- Administer prescribed hypnotics, if not contraindicated, to promote rest.
- Inform patient of the prognosis that spontaneous recovery occurs over time.
- Teach patient and family the signs and symptoms, clinical course, and prognosis of GBS.
- Teach patient why it is necessary to perform frequent neurological assessments.
- Teach patient about the GBS support group to share feelings, hope, and practical information on coping strategies.

Impaired verbal communication related to intubation or muscle paralysis.

Expected Patient Outcomes. Patient maintains optimal communication level or uses alternative means of communication.

- Encourage use of exaggerated lip movements and articulation of key words with patients with little or no facial muscle weakness.

- Use letter or picture boards with patients who have facial paralysis.
- Utilize a talk trach with air vents below the vocal cords for patients who do not have vocal cord paralysis. When the talk trach is connected to 4 to 6 L of air flow, the patient is able to speak.
- Explore the use of mechanical communication devices. A Sip-n-Puff call system works well if the patient cannot use a pressure-sensitive plate.
- Constantly reassure patient that his or her needs will be met.
- Teach patient and family how to use alternative methods of communication.
- Inform patient and family that verbal communication will return when muscle function returns and patient is extubated.

Hopelessness related to muscular weakness and dependence upon others.

Expected Patient Outcomes. Patient is able to verbalize feelings of hopelessness or becomes hopeful as muscle strength returns.

- Convey empathy to encourage verbalization of fears, concerns, and feelings of hopelessness.
- Encourage patient to verbalize what situations tend to cause feelings of hopelessness.
- Assist patient to understand that he or she can handle the temporary hopeless aspects of GBS by separating them from the hopeful aspects, such as less pain or increased peripheral sensation.
- Assist patient and family to facilitate short- or long-term goals.
- Assist patient to identify sources of hope.
- Teach patient to identify small accomplishments.

Collaborative Problems

Common collaborative goals for patients with GBS are to correct dysrhythmias and prevent orthostatic hypotension.

Potential Complication: Dysrhythmias. Dysrhythmia related to autonomic dysfunction secondary to lesions in the affected limb of the baroreflex arc or postganglionic sympathetic fibers of the spinal nerves.

Expected Patient Outcomes. Patient maintains regular sinus rhythm.

- Consult with physician regarding expected dysrhythmias.
- Review results of ECG.
- Monitor continuous ECG to assess heart rhythm and rate. Report dysrhythmias resulting from abnormal vagal responses, such as bradycardia, heart block, and asystole.
- Obtain and report clinical findings associated with dysrhythmias resulting from autonomic dysfunction: bradycardia, hypotension, syncope, and seizure activity.
- Prepare patient for pacemaker should heart block and asystole occur.
- Administer prescribed epinephrine at dose 1:10,000, 0.5 to 1.0 mg IV push or atropine at dose 1 mg IV push repeated in 5 minutes for patient with asystole following advanced cardiac life support (ACLS) protocol.

Potential Complication: Orthostatic Hypotension. Orthostatic hypotension related to autonomic dysfunction secondary to GBS.

Expected Patient Outcomes. Patient maintains systolic blood pressure (SBP) 80 to 140 mm Hg.

- Elevate head of bed (HOB) 30 degrees at night to enhance renin secretion, causing sodium retention and increased blood volume. The result is a reduction in orthostatic hypotension.
- Continuously monitor blood pressure whenever patient's head is elevated.
- Provide elastic support stockings to upper legs to provide compression, thereby decreasing venous pooling and decreasing orthostasis.
- Continually monitor ECG to assess heart rate and rhythm. Document ECG rhythm strips every 2 hours or more frequently

when patient experiences an unstable autonomic nervous system and orthostatic hypotension.

- Teach patient the reason for slowly elevating the HOB.
- Instruct patient to report dizziness when HOB being elevated.

DISCHARGE PLANNING

The critical care nurse will provide patient and significant other(s) verbal or written discharge notes regarding the following subjects:

1. The signs and symptoms that warrant immediate medical attention.
2. Importance of keeping follow-up visits and laboratory studies appointments.
3. Importance of taking medications on schedule.
4. Referrals to physical, speech, and occupational therapist, depending on the severity of any residual problem.
5. Referral to social services and community nursing services.
6. Referral to family support groups.
7. Following an activity schedule that is dependent on any neurological deficit.

■ SPINAL CORD INJURY

(For related information see Respiratory Deviations, Part I: Pneumonia, p. 375; Part III: Mechanical ventilation, p. 428. See also Behavioral Deviations, Part I, p. 725.)

Case Management Basis
DRG: 9 Spinal disorders and injuries
LOS: 7.10 days

Definition
Spinal cord injury is an acute insult to the spinal cord that interrupts sensory and motor communication within the central nervous system (CNS) and between the CNS and the peripheral nervous system. Primary injuries result from the initial mechanical trauma to the spinal cord nervous tissue, which causes

irreversible damage. Neurological damage can occur from secondary mechanisms, which include hemodynamic instabilities and mechanical reinjuries.

Pathophysiology

GENERAL. Hemodynamically, autoregulation is lost during the acute phase of injury, profoundly decreasing blood flow and causing ischemic injury to the cord. There are also changes in the tissue oxygen tension that affect metabolic function. Free radicals are released from ischemic areas when perfusion is compromised. This leads to increased damage at the original injury as a result of increased ischemia, vasospasm, and hypoxia.

LEVELS OF INJURY. C-1 to C-3: Lack of spontaneous respirations, respiratory quadriplegia, loss of bowel and bladder control, at risk for urinary tract infection, and loss of intercostal muscle function.

- C-4: Same as with C-1 and C-3 but some shoulder movement, some diaphragm control, and shoulder shrugs.
- C-5: Complete control of head, neck, and shoulders; elbow flexion; quadriplegia complete; phrenic nerve intact; no intercostal muscle function; poor pulmonary capacity and reserve; independence with electric wheelchair.
- C-5 to C-6: Full elbow flexion, some wrist extension, bend wrist up, quadriplegia possibly incomplete, thumb and index finger function, phrenic nerve intact, no intercostal muscle function, independent respiratory function but poor pulmonary capacity and reserve, independence with adaptive equipment, independence on feeding and grooming, help to dress self, and dependent for transfer.
- C-6 to C-7: Elbow extension with some finger control, quadriplegia incomplete, middle and part of ring finger sensory function, phrenic nerve intact, no intercostal muscle function, independent respiratory function,

bend elbow, make a fist, apposite thumb to each fingertip, independence of activities of daily living (ADL), use of wrist extensor splint to induce finger flexion, some assistance in transfer, and may be able to drive.

- C7−T1: Motor function is same as moderate to full control of arm, wrist, and fingers; full sensation of entire hand and medical aspects of upper and lower arm; respiratory function; bladder and bowel function and movement requested of patient same as above; independent in transfers with adaptive equipment; can grasp and release hands voluntarily, independent in ADL.
- T-1 to T-3: Full control of upper extremities; some intercostal function; sensation intact to midchest including upper extremities; pulmonary capacities within physiological limits; independent with adaptive devices; completely independent in wheelchair and ADL; at risk for postural hypotension and autonomic dysreflexia.
- T-2 to T-12: Full control of abdominal and trunk muscles; hip rotation and some hip flexion; sensation below waist; some sensation to anterior and medial thigh; full control of intercostals; no interference with respiratory function; tighten abdomen; flex hip; complete abdominal, back, and respiratory control; and participate in athletic activities.
- L-1 to S-1: Knee extension; dorsiflexion of ankle; foot movement; knee flexion; plantar flexion; sensation to upper legs, anterior, posterior, and lateral surfaces of lower leg and dorsum of foot; independent with or without adaptive devices; flex hip; straighten leg; bend and straighten toes; and optimal use of leg braces.
- L-1 to S-4: Some foot control; reflex centers for bowel, bladder, and sexual function; lumbar nerves innervate part of lower legs and feet; sacral nerves innervate lower legs, feet, and perineum; tighten anal sphincter around examining finger; sensorimotor assessment of perineal area is critical to determine extent of function; independent with or without short leg braces.

DEGREE OF INJURY. Complete injury involves permanent loss of all movement and sensation below the level of injury. Losses result from irreversible spinal cord damage. Incomplete injury (partial transection) results in mixed loss of motor and sensory function because some spinal cord tracts remain intact. There are five distinct patterns of neurological dysfunction with incomplete injury. Central cord syndrome occurs with hyperextension injury and is characterized by hemorrhage and edema in the central gray matter of the cord. There is upper extremity motor weakness and sensory and bladder dysfunction.

MECHANISM OF INJURY. Flexion injury is a traumatic injury caused by diving or motor vehicle accident whereby the spine is hyperflexed. There may also be a fractured vertebral body that damages the cord by an unstable vertebra resulting from ligament or disk injury. Extension injuries occur when the spine is hyperextended as a result of motor vehicle accident or fall. This injury can cause a fracture of the posterior elements of the spine and ligament. A compression injury occurs when the spine is compressed as a result of a fall or diving injury. The injury can cause a burst fracture or simple compression fracture. A penetrating injury is due to a bullet or knife injury. A rotational injury is caused by an involuntary twisting of the body. This can occur when the individual is hurled from a car or falls down a stairway.

Nursing Assessment

PRIMARY CAUSES
- Motor vehicle accidents, falls, sports injuries, penetrating injuries such as gunshot or stab wounds, or blunt trauma.

Physical Assessment
- Inspection: Motor function reveals flaccid or total paralysis of skeletal muscles below the level of injury, absence of deep tendon reflexes. Sensory function includes loss of tactile sensation, vibration, proprioception,

pain, temperature, and loss of somatic or visceral sensation below the level of the lesion; and autonomic function changes show loss of perspiration below the level of injury, paralytic ileus, absence of visceral sensation, bowel and bladder dysfunction, and loss of sexual reflexes.
- Palpation: Skin warm and dry.
- Auscultation: Decreased or unstable blood pressure, or bradycardia.

DIAGNOSTIC TEST RESULTS

Standard Laboratory Tests
- Arterial blood gases: partial pressure of arterial oxygen (Pao_2) ≤ 60 mm Hg or partial pressure of arterial carbon dioxide from ($Paco_2$) ≥ 45 mm Hg can indicate ineffective gas exchange and ineffective ventilatory effort.
- Blood studies: Reduced hemoglobin and hematocrit resulting from blood loss from hemorrhage caused by internal injury.
- Serum chemistry: Baseline studies of serum electrolytes, glucose, and enzymes to be used later.
- Urinalysis: Used to detect presence of bacteria or blood resulting from bladder or kidney injury.

Invasive Neurological Diagnostic Procedure. (see Table 7–2)

- Arteriography: Selective catheterization of veretebral arteries and costal cervical trunks can be used to diagnose cervical and high thoracic spinal cord injuries.
- Cinefluoroscopy: Demonstrates instability of the upper cervical spine.
- Myelogram: Used to determine any source of pressure on the spinal cord.

Noninvasive Neurological Diagnostic Procedure. (see Table 7–3, and Table 3–2, p. 334)

- Computerized tomographic (CT) scan: Used to demonstrate fractures of the spinal column, encroachment on the spinal canal, spinal cord, cauda equina, and root injury.

- Magnetic resonance imaging (MRI): Used for the same purposes as CT scan. Also defines internal organ structures, soft tissue involvement such as spinal cord contusion and edema, and evaluates blood flow pattern and blood vessel integrity.
- Spinal roentgenogram: Anteroposterior (AP) provides a view of the uncinate process and joints of Luschka in the lateral mass region. Oblique view used to diagnose minor fractures. Lateral and AP can be used to diagnose unstable fractures of the spine.
- Somatosensory evoked potential (SEP): Evoked responses reflect neural pathway function. SEPs are absent in complete spinal injury because no transmission can pass the site of injury. Incomplete spinal injury brings an altered SEP response.
- Respiratory function tests: Tidal volume and vital capacity measure maximum volume of inspiration and expiration in spinal cord injury (SCI) patients with cervical lesions with possible phrenic nerve involvement.

MEDICAL AND SURGICAL MANAGEMENT

PHARMACOLOGY
- Corticosteroids: Methylprednisolone can be started within 8 hours of the injury as a bolus of 30 mg/kg, followed by 5.4 mg/kg/hr for 23 hours (see Table 1–15, p. 129).
- Inotropic agents: Dopamine at a dose of 3 to 5 mg/kg/min can be supplemented with dobutamine in low doses to maintain arterial blood pressure of 80 to 90 mm Hg with increased cardiac output (see Table 1–5, p. 24).
- Atropine: Is used to treat bradydysrhythmias with a bolus dose of 0.60 mg.
- Anticoagulant therapy: Low-dose heparin (5000 to 7000 U/12 h) may be used in high-risk patients, such as those with long bone fractures, the elderly, or the obese (see Table 1–8, p. 32).
- Histamine H_2 receptor blocking agents: Ranitidine, cimetidine, or famotidine are used to prevent gastrointestinal (GI) hemorrhage (see Table 5–4, p. 518).

- Antacids: Are used to prevent GI hemorrhage.
- Experimental drugs: Naloxone hydrochloride is an endogenous opioid antagonist, which reduces secondary ischemic injury from opioids that decrease microcirculatory blood flow. Thyrotropin-releasing hormone (TRH) is a partial physiological antagonist of endogenous opioids. TRH blocks the release of leukotrienes and other substances thought to be involved in secondary ischemic injury and enhances spinal blood flow.
- Antihypertensive agents: Ganglionic blocking agents may be required to disrupt the hyperreflexic state. Hydralazine hydrochloride and diazoxide are used to treat hypertension.
- Stool softners: Glycerine suppositories are used to prevent fecal impaction.

IMMOBILIZATION OF SPINAL CORD

- Skeletal cervical traction: Used in patients with upper level SCI to realign the spinal column and relieve the spinal cord pressure from the displaced bony fragment. The traction devices are Crutchfield tongs, Vinke tongs, Gardner-Wells, and Halobrace. Weight is applied to the traction based on the 5-lb/interspace formula (C_{5-6} injury may require 25 to 30 lb of traction).

OXYGENATION

- Oral airway: Used to reestablish and maintain airway patency without hyperextending the neck.
- Supplemental oxygen: Ventilation via bag-mask resuscitation is initiated with oxygen concentration of 8 to 12 L/min.
- Intubation and ventilation: Intubation requires the use of the jaw-thrust maneuver to prevent hyperextension of the neck. Use of nasotracheal intubation is preferred. When attempts at nasotracheal intubation fail, a cricothyrotomy is performed.
- Tracheostomy: A tracheostomy is used in patients with high cervical lesions in whom weaning from a ventilator is difficult.

NASOGASTRIC TUBE

- A nasogastric (NG) or sump tube is placed to decompress the stomach, which helps prevent vomiting, aspiration, and respiratory compromise associated with gastric dilatation and ileus. NG tubes remove hydrochloric acid and permit monitoring gastric pH at frequent intervals.

DIET

- Total parenteral nutrition (TPN): TPN is administered to ensure caloric intake of 2000 calories per 24 hours.
- NG feedings: Initiated when GI function returns or patient has a patent airway. Patient can be started with clear fluids at a rate of 25 to 50 mL/h. If no residual is present, fluids can be gradually increased. Food intake may begin when patient tolerates 75 to 150 mL of fluid/h.

URINARY CATHETERIZATION

- Indwelling catheter: Used when patient is receiving IV fluids, remobilization of sequestered fluids from the interstitium, or inability to control fluid output.
- Intermittent catheterization: Fluid intake is restricted to 200 mL/2 h and the catheter is inserted every 4 hours. The patient is taught to void by Valsalva or any method that triggers voiding prior to catheterization. Residual volumes determine the need for catheterization.

PACEMAKERS

- Temporary transvenous or transcutaneous pacing is used should prolonged treatment be required for bradydysrhythmias (see Cardiac Deviations, Pacemakers, p. 270).

EXPERIMENTAL THERAPIES

- A small pad is positioned surgically on the epidural layer of the injured spinal cord. Cooled saline is circulated through the pad for 3 to 4 hours. The goal is to produce local vasoconstriction and decrease edema formation.

- Hyperbaric oxygen therapy: The procedure is thought to reduce ischemia and cord destruction by enhancing oxygen diffusion.

SURGICAL INTERVENTION

- Indications: Surgical interventions can be used to manage unstable injuries, especially if cord transection is incomplete, there is open injury of the cord, or progressive neurological dysfunction occurs.
- Surgical stabilization: Surgical technique consists of surgical wiring, Harrington rods, laminectomy with fusion, and anterior corpectomy (removal of the vertebral body) and fusion.

NURSING MANAGEMENT: NURSING DIAGNOSES AND COLLABORATIVE PROBLEMS

Nursing Diagnoses

Common nursing goals for patients with SCI are to maintain fluid balance, increase spinal cord tissue perfusion, restore physical mobility, promote effective breathing pattern, enhance airway clearance, maintain thermoregulation, strengthen urinary elimination, eliminate constipation, provide adequate nutritional intake, maintain skin integrity, enhance feelings of powerfulness, and encourage socialization.

Fluid volume deficit related to hypovolemia secondary to hemorrhage.

Expected Patient Outcomes. Patient maintains adequate fluid volume, as evidenced by heart rate (HR) 60 to 100 bpm, blood pressure (BP) within patient's normal range, central venous pressure (CVP) 2 to 6 mm Hg, skin warm and dry, absence of bleeding, regular sinus rhythm, being alert, and urinary output (UO) ≥30 mL/h.

- Review results of coagulation studies, hemoglobin, and hematocrit levels, and urine, stool, and gastric drainage negative for blood.
- Obtain and report clinical findings associated with hypovolemia resulting from

bleeding: hypotension, tachycardia, weak and thready pulse, capillary refill ≤3 seconds, pallor, skin cool and moist, weakness, and confusion.
- Measure intake, output, specific gravity, and daily weight to evaluate fluid volume. Report weight loss ≥5% of baseline and UO ≤30 mL/h.
- Elevate lower extremities, if not contraindicated, to improve venous return of peripheral blood causing hypovolemia.
- Provide Trendelenburg positioning, if not contraindicated, to improve venous return.
- Administer IV crystalloids, plasma expanders, and blood to replenish the intravascular volume and maintain systolic blood pressure (SBP) ≥80 mm Hg.
- Teach patient to use alternative strategies to reduce stress: meditation, progressive relaxation, and guided imagery.

Impaired physical mobility related to loss of motor function secondary to spinal shock.

Expected Patient Outcomes. Patient does not have further injury or maintains physical mobility.

- Assess motor function using a five-point motor scoring system to grade muscle function (5 = normal movement, 3 = movement against gravity, 0 = total paralysis) every 4 hours. The patient is asked to flex, extend, abduct, and adduct each extremity in order to evaluate muscle groups.
- Assess sensory function including proprioception (position sense), temperature, and pain.
- Report clinical findings associated with impaired physical mobility: decreased motor function, altered proprioception, hypothermia, and decreased pain sensation.
- Assist with cervical immobilization and continuous traction by use of skull tongs, such as Gardner-Wells and Crutchfield tongs. Skeletal traction can provide reduction and immobilization of the fracture or dislocation.

- Maintain spinal stability with the use of prescribed mechanical bed such as Stryker frame, which turns from supine to prone position, and kinetic therapy beds, which constantly rotate in a 60 to 60 degree arc.
- Check traction to ensure that the frames are secure and weights are hanging free. Provide weights (10 to 20 lb) depending on patient's size and amount of cervical reduction needed to maintain the vertebrae in the appropriate position.
- Assist with halo immobilization brace to achieve cervical immobilization, traction, positioning, and alignment.
- Move patient and halo immobilization brace as a unit to avoid stress on any one part.
- Clean pin site areas twice daily with normal saline and hydrogen peroxide, followed by application of povidone-iodine ointment.
- Examine pin sites for evidence of inflammation: pain, redness, swelling, drainage, and increased temperature.
- Turn patient every 2 hours, if not contraindicated, to prevent skin breakdown and excess pressure on the pin site.
- Provide passive range of motion (ROM) exercises every 4 hours to prevent contractions.
- Maintain correct body position by using adjunctive devices such as antirotation boots, antidrop foot splints, trochanter rolls, and wrist splints.
- Position arms at 90 degree angle every 4 hours to prevent frozen shoulder contraction.
- Apply antiembolic hose to reduce pooling of blood in the lower extremities, thereby decreasing the risk of thrombus formation.
- Administer prescribed corticosteroids such as dexamethasone (Decadron) or methyprednisolone sodium succinate (Solu-Medrol) to reduce spinal cord edema and improve spinal cord perfusion (see Table 1–15, p. 129).
- Prepare patient for surgical stabilization of the spinal cord.
- Teach patient and family to perform ROM exercises to prevent risk of contraction of nonparalyzed areas.

Ineffective breathing pattern related to paralysis of intercostal and abdominal muscles or limited diaphragmatic excursion secondary to upper SCI at C-1 to C-4.

Expected Patient Outcomes. Patient maintains effective breathing pattern, as evidenced by respiratory rate (RR) $\leq$25 BPM, normal lung sounds, symmetry of chest movement, arterial blood gases within normal range, absence of cyanosis, arterial oxygen saturation (Sao_2) 95% to 97.5%, tidal volume $\geq$7 to 10 mL/kg, and vital capacity $\geq$15 to 20 mL/kg.

- Review results of arterial blood gas measurement.
- Assess clinical indicators of respiratory status: rate, depth, symmetry of chest wall movement, skin color, use of accessory muscles, nasal flaring, and presence of adventitious breath sounds.
- Report clinical findings associated with ineffective breathing pattern: tachypnea, shallow respirations, use of accessory muscles (C-2 to C-3 intact), and diaphragmatic breathing with minimal movement of the chest wall and passive movement of the flaccid abdominal wall.
- Should injury to C-5 occur and vital capacity be $\leq$500 mL on spirometry, prepare patient for intubation and ventilatory support.
- Use pulse oximetry to measure oxygen saturation and as an indirect parameter of Pao_2.
- Perform nasotracheal suctioning to maintain a patent airway.
- Preoxygenate patient prior to suctioning and administer prescribed IV atropine to provide parasympathetic blockade.
- Continuously monitor ECG, while patient is suctioned, for the presence of heart block.
- Apply abdominal binder to provide external support of abdominal muscles so breathing and coughing can be enhanced.
- Administered prescribed supplemental oxygen to minimize hypoxic effects.

Ineffective airway clearance related to ineffective cough secondary to paralysis of the abdominal and intercostal muscles.

Expected Patient Outcomes. Patient is able to effectively maintain a patent airway, as evidenced by clear lung sound, sustaining a secretion-clearing cough, arterial blood gases within normal range, and absence of paradoxical respirations.

- Review results of arterial blood gas measurement and chest roentgenogram.
- Monitor respirations: When injury is below C-4, patient can develop diaphragmatic fatigue in 48 to 72 hours, which may require ventilation.
- Assess clinical indicators of respiratory status: rate, depth, symmetry of chest wall movement, skin color, use of accessory muscles, and presence of adventitious breath sounds.
- Report paradoxical respirations in which the rib cage collapses passively in inspiration while the diaphragm descends and expands on expiration as the diaphragm ascends.
- Report loss of intercostal muscle use (T-2 to L-1), which reduces necessary expansion of the rib cage, decreases alveolar ventilation by 60%, and causes rapid shallow respiration.
- Determine patient's ability to cough and clear secretions. Coughing is dependent on use of intercostal and abdominal muscles, which may be lost with SCI.
- Report a moist-sounding but unproductive cough, which could signify retention and pooling of pulmonary secretions.
- Assist patient with quad-assist cough hourly to augment the abdominal muscles during the expiratory phase of a cough. The nurse places a fist between the xiphoid process and umbilicus and applies a thrust during the coughing effort.
- Turn and position patient frequently, with a mechanical bed, to prevent stasis of secretions.
- Provide prescribed humidified oxygen to keep secretions moist.
- Utilize chest physiotherapy, if not contraindicated, to mobilize secretions.

- Initiate incentive spirometry to maintain expansion of alveoli, performed every 1 to 2 hours.
- Provide mechanical ventilation via endotracheal tube as prescribed for patients with injury above C-4.
- Administer prescribed IV fluids to maintain adequate hydration and keep secretions moist.
- Teach patient breathing exercises in the postacute phase.
- Teach patient and family quad-assist technique.

Ineffective thermoregulation related to autonomic dysfunction secondary to SCI.

Expected Patient Outcomes. Patient maintains a normal body temperature.

- Monitor rectal temperature every 4 hours for the first hours post injury.
- Assess for the presence of perspiration, since an inability to perspire in areas of the body below the lesion prevents normal loss of body heat when body temperature is elevated.
- Since patient's body temperature fluctuates with that of room temperature, minimize fluctuations of body and room temperatures.
- Avoid drafts, which can cause an episode of autonomic dysreflexia in patients with injury above C-7 to T-1.
- Place an extra blanket on patient when the environment is cool.
- Report hyperthermia resulting from infection and hypothermia resulting from injury to T-1 and above.
- Should patient experience hyperthermia, initiate cooling measures such as tepid bath and hypothermia blanket.
- Should patient be hyperthermic, administer prescribed antipyretic agents to lower temperature.

Altered pattern in urinary elimination related to disruption of normal neurological bladder innervation secondary to SCI.

Expected Patient Outcomes. Patient maintains UO $\geq$30 mL/h or $\geq$0.5 mL/kg/h.

- Consult with physician about the criteria used to determine when intermittent catheterization should be initiated: negative urine cultures, no use of diuretics, and tolerance of fluid restriction to 1800 to 2200 mL/24 h.
- Palpate bladder for distention, since an injury above L-2 results in bladder dysfunction as of a result of loss of bladder contraction.
- Insert Foley catheter, if prescribed, to avoid an overdistended bladder.
- Provide aseptic catheter care to minimize the risk of infection.
- Determine the need for catheterization, which is based upon the amount of urine obtained from each 4-hour catheterization.
- Initiate intermittent catheterization to minimize renal or urinary complication resulting from infection.
- Measure hourly fluid intake and limit fluid after the evening meal.
- Teach patient and family the reasons behind intermittent catheterization.

Alteration in bowel elimination: constipation related to atonic bowel secondary to spinal shock.

Expected Patient Outcome. Patient is able to pass a formed stool every other day without straining.

- Consult with dietitian to develop or individualize a diet plan for the patient.
- Obtain and report clinical findings associated with GI dysfunction: absent bowel sounds, abdominal distention, and altered elimination (reflex defecation in nonsacral injuries and fecal retention and oozing of stool with sacral cord injury).
- Measure abdominal girth in patients exhibiting abdominal distention.
- Monitor and report constipation: dull sound over descending colon on percussion and palpation of hard, rigid stool over areas of bowel.

- Initiate bowel regimen, as ordered, when peristalsis returns: pysllium hydrophilic mucilloid and stool softener daily, and cup of warm fluid every other day to stimulate the gastrocolic or duodenocolic reflex.
- Should the above bowel regimen be ineffective, insert prescribed glycerin suppository and employ digital stimulation of the internal anal sphincter.
- Avoid use of enemas, which can dilate the rectum and sigmoid colon.
- Provide TPN as prescribed to ensure patient receives the necessary calories.
- Administer prescribed IV fluids to maintain adequate hydration.

Alteration in nutrition: less than body requirements related to nothing by mouth, weakened cough or gag reflexes, or anorexia secondary to SCI.

Expected Patient Outcomes. Patient maintains adequate nutritional intake, as evidenced by body weight within 5% of baseline; triceps skinfold measurement maintained within baseline range; blood urea nitrogen (BUN), creatinine, and total protein albumin within normal range.

- Review BUN, creatinine, and total protein albumin results.
- Consult with dietitian to develop an individualized diet that incorporates patient's likes and maintains a positive nitrogen balance.
- Maintain accurate intake and output records.
- Weigh daily and report weight loss of $\geq$5% baseline.
- Initiate clear liquid diet at 25 to 50 mL/hour when enteral feedings are tolerated and patient is able to maintain airway clearance.
- Provide prescribed TPN during period of spinal shock and paralytic ileus.
- Administer prescribed enteral feelings when bowel sounds return and check residuals every 2 hours.

Impaired skin integrity related to loss of mobility and sensation, impaired circulation, and inadequate nutrition.

Expected Patient Outcome. Patient's skin remains intact.

- Assess clinical situations that could alter skin integrity such as loss of mobility and sensation, impaired circulation, and inadequate nutrition, which could increase the risk of skin breakdown.
- Monitor areas at risk for skin breakdown such as weight-bearing bony prominences, depending on the position assumed.
- Report clinical findings associated with altered skin integrity such as balancing, redness, swelling, and ulceration.
- Assess halo and tong insertion sites and cleanse using unit protocol. Report any redness, swelling, or skin breakdown.
- Reposition frequently by using a turning frame or kinetic bed.
- Provide ROM exercises with dorsoflexion of feet to prevent foot drop.
- Administer lotion to bony and reddened areas to stimulate circulation.

Powerlessness related to loss of physical control and independence.

Expected Patient Outcome. Patient maintains feeling of control.

- Listen to patient's verbalization of when he or she feels powerless.
- Encourage patient to participate in care decisions, thereby increasing decisional control.
- Help patient identify positive aspects of the injury that can be incorporated into future goals.
- Encourage patient to participate in physical therapy and ROM exercises, which promote feelings of control.

Social isolation related to immobility and depression.

Expected Patient Outcomes. Patient interacts with others and maintains relationships.

- Confer with Occupational Therapy regarding development of diversional program.
- Evaluate patient's ability to interact with others.
- Encourage patient to use diversional activities: TV, radio, or reading.
- Monitor for clinical indicators of social isolation: loneliness, flat affect, depression, withdrawal, or preoccupation.
- Encourage patient to verbalize when he or she feels socially isolated.
- Assist family with patient's reintegration into social encounters.

Collaborative Problems

Common collaborative goals for patients with SCI are to minimize spinal shock, minimize autonomic dysreflexia, promote oxygenation, correct dysrhythmias, prevent thromboembolism, and increase cardiac output.

Potential Complication: Spinal Shock. Spinal shock related to interruption of all neurological function below the level of the lesion with SCI at the level T-4 to T-6 and above secondary to spinal compression or trauma.

Expected Patient Outcome. Patient experiences minimal spinal shock.

- Obtain and report clinical findings associated with interruption of all neurological function below the level of the lesion causing spinal shock: falccid, total paralysis of all skeletal muscles, loss of spinal reflexes, loss of sensation such as pain, proprioception, touch, temperature and pressure, and bowel and bladder dysfunction.
- Obtain and report other clinical findings associated with neurogenic shock: unstable hypotension SBP ≤90 mm Hg, bradycardia (HR ≤50 bpm), and hypothermia (≤37°C or ≤98.6°F).
- Monitor arterial blood pressure and MAP hourly since loss of vasomotor tone results in vasodilation of the systemic vasculature.
- Apply antiembolism hose to increase venous reurn and decrease pooling of blood in the lower extremities.

- Monitor skin temperature since vasodilation can cause warm, dry skin and hypothermia since body heat is lost through the dilated peripheral blood vessels.
- Monitor continuously ECG to assess heart rate and rhythm. Report bradycardia which may occur as a result of unopposed parasympathetic innervation of the heat by the vagus nerve.
- Elevated the patient's lower extremities to decrease venous pooling and increase venous return to the heart.

Potential Complication: Autonomic Dysreflexia. Autonomic dysreflexia related to uninhibited response of the sympathetic nervous system secondary to SCI at T-4 to T-6 level or above.

Expected Patient Outcome. Patient will experience minimal injury associated with autonomic dysreflexia.

- Consult with physician about the stimuli causing autonomic dysreflexia: overdistended bladder, infection, skin stimulation, pain, sudden changes in environmental temperature, and a full rectrum.
- Obtain and report clinical findings associated with autonomic dysreflexia: severe headache, hypertension (240 to 300 mm Hg/150 mm Hg), bradycardia, tachycardia, profuse diaphoresis, flushing above the level of injury, pallor and coolness below the level of injury, nasal stuffiness, and apprehension.
- Using a kinetic bed, elevate head of bed (HOB) to lower BP by creating orthostatic hypotension.
- Monitor BP and HR every 5 minutes. Report SBP $\geq$240 mm Hg.
- Assist patient to avoid urinary retention and bladder distention by monitoring intake and output, avoiding overhydration, maintaining patency of indwelling catheter, and observing for bladder spasm.
- Avoid bowel retention or fecal impaction by maintaining strict adherence to bowel regimen, using Nupercainal for digital examination, and providing appropriate diet and fluid intake.
- Assess skin for pressure areas and impaired integrity.
- Provide a calm, quiet environment, since anxiety can increase catecholamine secretion, which enhances the risk of a sympathetic response.
- Remain with patient and family to provide emotional support.
- Administer prescribed antihypertensive medications such as diazoxide (Hyperstat) and hydralazine (Apresoline).
- Teach patient and family the causes of autonomic dysreflexia.

Potential Complication: Hypoxemia. Hypoxemia related to hypoventilation, diffusion defects, shunting or ventilation-perfusion imbalance secondary to respiratory dysfunction following SCI.

Expected Patient Outcomes. Patient maintains adequate oxygenation, as evidenced by RR 12 to 20 BPM, HR 60 to 100 bpm, being alert and oriented, SaO_2 $\geq$90%, arterial blood gases within normal range, BP within patient's normal range, lungs clear, vital capacity 15 mL/kg, tidal volume $\geq$5 mL/kg, and absence of cyanosis.

- Review results of arterial blood gas measurement.
- Assess clinical indicators of respiratory status: RR and rhythm, symmetry of chest movement, use of accessory muscles, inspiratory effort, skin color, and lung sounds.
- Report clinical findings associated with impaired oxygenation, depending on the site of injury: tachypnea, diminished chest mobility, prominent use of accessory muscles, reduced inspiratory ability, paradoxical breathing patterns, shortness of breath, cyanosis, and crackles.
- Continually monitor oxygen saturation with pulse oximetry.
- Obtain and report respiratory function, which suggests intercostal and abdominal muscle motion and strength: tidal volume

≤1000 mL, negative inspiratory force (NIF) ≤ -20 cm H_2O, and vital capacity ≤15 mL/kg.

- Assess patient for difficulty swallowing or coughing, which may indicate ascending cord edema.
- Should halo vest be used, monitor patient for reduced chest expansion.
- When the spinal cord is immobilized, initiate preventive nursing care measures such as positioning, coughing, deep breathing, and incentive spirometry every 2 hours.
- Utilize a kinetic bed, as ordered, to mobilize secretions.
- Suction patient as necessary. Hyperventilate patient prior to suction and limit the catheter pass to 15 seconds or less to minimize desaturation and bradycardia.
- Assist with intubation and mechanical ventilation in patients with cervical injury C-3 to C-6 and above.
- Check patency of NG tube 2 to 4 hours, since abdominal distention can impair diaphragmatic breathing.
- Monitor continuous ECG rhythm for bradycardia during suctioning.
- Administer prescribed IV atropine should bradycardia occur during suctioning.
- Administer prescribed humidified oxygen by nasal cannula, mask, or ventilator to enhance tissue oxygenation and loosen secretions.
- Administer prescribed IV fluids to maintain adequate hydration.

Potential Complication: Dysrhythmias. Dysrhythmia related to spinal cord shock or suctioning secondary to stimulation of vagus nerve.

Expected Patient Outcomes. Patient maintains regular sinus rhythm.

- Consult with physician as to the expected rhythm of spinal shock, which is bradycardia (≤60 bpm).
- Review result of 12-lead ECG.
- Monitor continuous ECG to assess HR and rhythm. Document ECG rhythm every 2 to 4 hours or while patient is being suctioned.

- Monitor ECG for bradycardia when patient is in the prone position on a Stryker frame.
- Administer prescribed bolus of atropine at dose of 0.60 mg when bradydysrhythmia occurs.
- Should bradycardia be caused by suctioning, administer prophylactic atropine.
- Should atropine be ineffective in treating bradydysrhythmias, administer prescribed isoprotenerol.
- If pharmacological therapy is ineffective in correcting bradycardia or prolonged therapy is required, prepare patient for temporary transvenous or transcutaneous pacing.
- Teach patient the causes of bradydysrhythmias and rationale for measures taken to correct the problem.

Potential Complication: Thromboembolism. Thromboembolism related to venostasis secondary to immobility.

Expected Patient Outcome. Patient is free of thromboembolism.

- Consult with physician about causes of thromboembolism in SCI patient. These include vasomotor paralysis with pooling and stasis of blood, skeletal muscle paralysis, and immobilization.
- Measure circumference of the lower extremities daily. Report a slowly increasing circumference, which is suggestive of underlying venous thrombosis.
- Assess clinical indicators of perfusion: BP, HR, peripheral pulses +2, capillary refill ≤3 seconds, skin color, and temperature.
- Report clinical findings associated with venous thrombosis of lower extremities: a bluish-red color of the skin, warm temperature, and increasing circumference.
- Report clinical findings associated with pulmonary embolism: tachypnea, dyspnea, cough with hemoptysis, tachycardia, hypotension, cyanosis, restlessness, lethargy, and confusion.
- Apply antiembolic stockings to lower extremities to decrease venous stasis.

- Apply alternating pneumatic pressure devices, as ordered, to decrease peripheral pooling by increasing venous return.
- Assist with passive ROM exercises with dorsiflexion of each foot to minimize the risk of deep venous thrombosis.
- Elevate the entire lower extremity 10 to 15 minutes, if not contraindicated, to prevent venostasis.
- Provide kinetic bed, as ordered, to promote circulation.
- Encourage patient to deep breathe each hour, if realistic, to expand the lungs and prevent atelectasis.
- Administer prescribed low-dose heparin prophylactically to prevent thromboembolism formation and clot dispersion.
- Administer prescribed oxygen by nasal cannula, mask, or ventilator to increase tissue oxygenation.

Potential Complication: Decreased Cardiac Output.
Decreased cardiac output related to decreased venous return secondary to spinal shock or autonomic dysfunction.

Expected Patient Outcomes. Patient maintains adequate cardiac output, as evidenced by BP within patient's normal range; HR ≤100 bpm; cardiac output (CO) 4 to 8 L/min; pulmonary artery pressure (PAP) 20 to 30/8 to 15 mm Hg; pulmonary capillary wedge pressure (PCWP) 12 to 15 mm Hg, which is optimal for SCI; CVP 2 to 6 mm Hg; skin warm and dry; peripheral pulses +2; capillary refill ≤3 seconds; systemic vascular resistance (SVR) 900 to 1200 dynes/s/cm^{-5}; and absence of cyanosis.

- Consult with physical therapist about techniques used to progress patient from a supine to an upright position using a tilt table or kinetic bed.
- Gradually elevate HOB until patient tolerates a high Fowler's position, if not contraindicated, to avoid hypotension and syncope: movement from supine to vertical position causes redistribution of blood, as much as 500 mL may pool in the extremities.

- Obtain and report hemodynamic parameters indicating decreased CO: CO ≤4 L/min, PAP ≤20/8 mm Hg, PCWP ≤12 mm Hg, CVP ≤2 mm Hg, and SVR ≤900 dynes/s/cm^{-5}.
- Obtain and report other clinical findings associated with decreased CO: hypotension, tachycardia, light-headedness, confusion, peripheral pulse ≤+2, capillary refill ≤3 seconds, and cyanosis.
- Monitor continuous ECG to assess HR rhythm. Document and report bradydysrhythmias and sinus pauses.
- Continuously monitor arterial BP, since hypotension can occur in response to spinal shock or autonomous dysreflexia, which can subsequently decrease CO.
- Measure intake, output, specific gravity, and daily weight. Report UO ≤30 mL/h or ≤0.5 mL/kg/h for 2 consecutive hours, which can reflect renal tissue hypoperfusion.
- Initiate measures to optimize venous return, thereby reducing the risk of reduced CO. Apply antiembolic stockings, perform passive ROM exercises every 2 hours, apply abdominal binder, and elevate lower extremities to support BP and CO.
- Administer prescribed crystalloids such as lactated Ringer's or 5% dextrose in water (D$_5$W) or normal saline at rate of 75 to 100 mL/h to maintain SBP 100 mm Hg, hydration, and circulatory volume.
- Administer prescribed dopamine or dobutamine to support CO.
- Administer prescribed atropine to treat bradydysrhythmias.

DISCHARGE PLANNING
The critical care nurse will provide patient and significant other(s) verbal or written discharge notes regarding the following subjects:

1. Importance of keeping all postdischarge medical appointments.
2. Referrals to rehabilitation center to continue supportive and strengthening exercises under supervision.

3. Medications, including their purpose, dose, route, schedule, and side effects.
4. Bladder and bowel retraining programs individualized for patient and family.
5. Signs and symptoms associated with autonomic dysreflexia: severe headache, hypertension (240 to 300 mm Hg/150 mm Hg), bradycardia, tachycardia, profuse diaphoresis, flushing above the level of injury, pallor and coolness below the level of injury, nasal stuffiness, and apprehension.
6. Referrals to social service agency to help with financial concerns resulting from the spinal injury.
7. Name of organizations that might provide supportive care: National Spinal Cord Injury Association and American Spinal Injury Association.

....

PART II: RELATED SURGICAL CORRECTIONS AND NURSING MANAGEMENT

....

■ CRANIOTOMY

(For related information see Part I: Acute head injury, p. 620. Cerebral hemorrhage, Part III: Intracranial pressure monitoring, p. 671; Barbiturate coma, p. 674. See also Respiratory Deviations, Part III: Pulse oximetry, p. 426; Mechanical ventilation, p. 428. See also Behavioral Deviations, Part I, p. 725.)

Case Management Basis
DRG: 1 Craniotomy without complications for trauma
LOS: 12.20 days
DRG: 2 Craniotomy with complications for trauma age ≥17
LOS: 11.30 days

Definition
Craniotomies can be classified as supratentorial or infratentorial. Supratentorial cran-

iotomy refers to all neurosurgical procedures in the cranium above the level of the tentorium, which allows access to the cerebral hemispheres or midbrain. Infratentorial craniotomy refers to all neurosurgical procedures in the cranium below the tentorium and provides access to the cerebellum, medulla, or pons. The transsphenoidal approach is used to gain access to the pituitary gland. Stereotaxis involves the use of three-dimensional coordinates from a special frame and allows targeting of a lesion deep within the brain with minimal trauma to brain tissue. Laser surgery is used to focus precisely on a specific tissue.

Patient Selection

INDICATIONS
• Trans-sphenoidal craniotomy: Used to resect pituitary adenomas, control metastatic bone pain via hypophysectomy, or aid in the removal of craniopharyngiomas.
• Stereotaxic craniotomy: Used to resect or biopsy small subcortical neoplasms deep within the brain; aspirate intracranial hematomas, abscesses, and cystic lesions; control chronic pain through placement of an electrode; place radiotherapeutic agents in the area of a neoplasm; and treat extrapyramidal symptoms with ablation procedure. Laser surgery allows the neurosurgeon to use microsurgical techniques to identify and apply the laser to tissues requiring resection with minimal disruption of surrounding tissues.

CONTRAINDICATIONS. Poor surgical risk.

Procedure

TECHNIQUE. Burr holes alone can be used to evacuate a hematoma, control superficial hemorrhage, perform a biopsy, drain an abscess, or place an intraventricular shunt. Once the craniotomy is done, the underlying dura is incised to allow access to the underlying brain. When the operation is completed, the dura is sutured closed, and the cranial bone is replaced and held in place with sutures pass-

ing through small holes drilled in the surrounding bone and the flap. Open (Penrose) or closed drainage systems with a plastic reservoir may be used.

With the transsphenoidal surgery, the incision is made through the upper gum and extended into both sides of the nasal system. Posterior dissection leads to the floor of the sphenoid sinuses, which can be removed, thereby allowing access to the sella turcica and dura. Microinstruments are used with a microscope to perform the surgery.

Stereotaxic surgery uses special three-dimensional coordinates to identify and target areas pinpointed with computerized tomographic (CT) scan. The surgeon then guides an electrode or microinstrument to the target tissue.

Complications

Cerebral edema, intracranial or intracordal bleeding, increased intracranial pressure, ventilatory insufficiency, cerebrovascular accident, seizure, infection, diabetes insipidus, hyperthermia, or dysrhythmias.

NURSING MANAGEMENT: NURSING DIAGNOSES AND COLLABORATIVE PROBLEMS

Nursing Diagnoses

Common nursing goals for patients undergoing cranial surgery are to maintain fluid balance, ensure cerebral tissue perfusion, support effective breathing, prevent injury, prevent infection, support cognitive function, and minimize pain.

Fluid volume excess related to increased intravascular fluid volume secondary to inappropriate secretion of antidiuretic hormone (SIADH).

Expected Patient Outcomes. Patient maintains adequate fluid balance, as evidenced by blood pressure (BP) within patient's normal range, mean arterial pressure (MAP) 70 to 100 mm Hg, respiratory rate (RR) 12 to 20 BPM, pulmonary capillary wedge pressure (PCWP) 6 to 12 mm Hg, central venous pressure (CVP)

2 to 6 mm Hg, body weight within patient's normal range, alertness, absence of edema, lungs clear, urinary output (UO) $\geq$30 mL/h or $\geq$0.5 mL/kg/h, specific gravity 1.010 to 1.030, serum sodium 137 to 147 mEq/L, urine osmolality 300 to 1090 mOsm/kg, and serum osmolality 275 to 300 mOsm/kg.

- Review results of serum sodium, serum osmolality, and urine osmolality.
- Elevate head of bed 10 to 20 degrees to enhance venous return and reduce ADH production.
- Obtain and report hemodynamic parameters that indicate fluid volume excess: CVP $\geq$6 mm Hg and PCWP $\geq$12 mm Hg.
- Obtain and report clinical findings associated with fluid volume excess: hypertension, decreasing level of consciousness (LOC), tachycardia, peripheral edema, crackles, and weight gain.
- Obtain and report clinical findings associated with SIADH: headache, confusion, disorientation, lethargy, muscle cramps, anorexia, nausea, weight gain, restlessness, irritability, abdominal cramps, twitching, decreased deep tendon reflexes, seizures, and coma.
- Assess patient for clinical findings associated with water retention and dilutional hyponatremia in SIADH: headache, somnolence, lethargy, and confusion.
- Measure intake, output, and specific gravity to determine fluid balance. Report UO $\leq$30 mL/h or $\leq$0.5 mL/kg/h.
- Maintain fluid restriction to minimize circulatory overload.
- Initiate seizure precaution to prevent injury to patient should seizure occur secondary to cerebral edema.
- Administer prescribed 0.9% or hypertonic 3% sodium chloride should patient experience hyponatremia.
- Administer prescribed lithium or demeclocycline to inhibit action of ADH on the distal renal tubules to enhance water excretion.

Fluid volume deficit related to decreased intravascular fluid volume secondary to diabetes insipidus.

Expected Patient Outcomes. Patient maintains adequate fluid volume, as evidenced by BP within patient's normal range, heart rate (HR) ≤100 bpm, CVP 2 to 6 mm Hg, PCWP 6 to 12 mm Hg, UO ≥30 mL/h and ≤200 mL/h, specific gravity 1.010 to 1.025, MAP 80 to 100 mm Hg, normal skin turgor, urine osmolality ≥200 mOsm/kg, and serum electrolytes within normal range.

- Review results of serum sodium, serum osmolality, and urine osmolality.
- Obtain and report hemodynamic parameters that indicate fluid volume deficit: CVP ≤2 mm Hg and PCWP ≤6 mm Hg.
- Obtain and report clinical findings associated with fluid volume deficit: polyuria, dilute urine, polydipsia, specific gravity ≤1.005, thirst, poor skin turgor, and dry mucous membranes.
- Obtain and report clinical findings associated with diabetes insipidus: polyuria, polydipsia, specific gravity ≤1.005, hypotension, and tachycardia.
- Measure daily weight, intake, specific gravity, and UO. Report UO ≥200 mL/h and weight loss of ≥0.5 lb/d.
- Replace fluid as prescribed by providing patient's favorite liquids or by administering hypotonic solution of 1 mL/V fluid for each 1 mL of UO.
- Provide prescribed vasopressor replacement therapy (chlorpropamide or carbamazepine) to enhance ADH secretion in patients with diabetes insipidus (see Table 7–4).

Altered cerebral tissue perfusion related to increased intracranial pressure (ICP) secondary to cerebral edema, cerebral vasospasm, or intracranial hemorrhage.

Expected Patient Outcomes. Patient maintains cerebral tissue perfusion, as evidenced by cerebral perfusion pressure (CPP) 60 to 100 mm Hg, ICP 0 to 15 mm Hg, MAP 70 to 100 mm Hg, BP within the patient's normal range, HR ≤100 bpm, pupils equal and normoreactive, normal sensorimotor function, RR 12 to 20 BPM, and normal pulse pressure.

- Monitor ICP and CPP hourly. Report ICP ≥15 mm Hg and CPP ≤60 mm Hg.
- Obtain and report clinical findings associated with decreased cerebral tissue perfusion: elevated systolic blood pressure (SBP), widening pulse pressure, bradycardia, pupils unequal, sensorimotor dysfunction, tachypnea, decreased LOC, and confusion.
- Assess patient for clinical findings associated with cerebral vasospasm, which may occur 4 to 10 days after a closed head trauma: slight change in the patient's LOC, headache, aphasia, drift of an extremity, hemiparesis, or decerebration.
- Monitor ECG rhythm for bradycardia: The use of fluid expansion and induced hypertension to increase the CPP may lead to an autoregulatory reflex bradycardia and subsequent increase in ICP.
- Create an environment conductive to rest.
- Provide quiet music and therapeutic touch to reduce stress.
- Measure intake, output, specific gravity, and daily weights to determine fluid balance. Fluid intake in excess of output might further increase ICP.
- Prevent or control situations that can increase ICP and reduce CPP: Valsalva's maneuver, pain, hypercapnia, or suctioning.
- Administer prescribed IV fluids to maintain circulatory volume.
- Provide prescribed oxygen by nasal cannula or mask.
- Administer prescribed calcium channel blocker (nifedipine or nimodipine) in patients who have experienced aneurysmal clipping to reduce risk of cerebral vasospasm (see Table 1–6, p. 28).
- Administer prescribed dopamine or dobutamine to maintain cardiac output and CPP.

Ineffective breathing pattern related to brainstem compression or respiratory depression secondary to cerebral edema or anesthesia.

Expected Patient Outcomes. Patient maintains effective breathing pattern, as evidenced by

RR 12 to 20 BPM, symmetry of chest movement, absence of dyspnea, normal skin color, absence of crackles, tidal volume ≥ 7 to 10 mL/kg, vital capacity ≥ 12 to 15 mL/kg, partial pressure of arterial carbon dioxide ($Paco_2$) ≤ 30 to 35 mm Hg, and partial pressure of arterial oxygen (Pao_2) ≥ 80 mm Hg.

- Review results of arterial blood gas measurements.
- Maintain patient in semi-Fowler's position to enhance maximal chest excursion and facilitate drainage of blood and cerebrospinal fluid (CSF) from the cranial vault via gravity.
- Assess clinical indicators of respiratory status: RR and rhythm, symmetry of chest movement, use of accessory muscles, lung sounds, and skin color.
- Report clinical findings associated with ineffective breathing pattern: tachypnea, dyspnea, cyanosis, and crackles.
- Insert nasogastric (NG) tube as ordered to prevent abdominal distention and minimize risk of aspiration and compromise of diaphragmatic excursion.
- Encourage patient to deep breathe and use incentive spirometer to enhance lung expansion.
- Initiate suctioning only when necessary to remove excess secretions so not to increase ICP. Limit suctioning time and hyperventilate with 100% oxygen before each pass and after suctioning.
- Provide prescribed humidified oxygen by nasal cannula or mask to enhance tissue oxygenation.
- Should tidal volume be ≤ 7 mL/kg and vital capacity ≤ 12 mL/kg, prepare patient for intubation and ventilatory support.

High risk for injury related to seizures secondary to cerebral ischemia or injury.

Expected Patient Outcomes. Patient is free from seizure and cranial nerve dysfunction.

- Elevate head of bed 30 degrees to promote venous drainage.

- Assess characteristics of seizure activity such as onset, type of movement, associated changes in LOC, pupillary size and reactivity, extraocular movement, vomiting, or incontinence.
- Implement measures to prevent seizure-inducing activity such as headache, anxiety, hypoxia, hyperventilation, urinary retention, fecal impaction, or hyperpyrexia.
- Initiate seizure precaution measures should seizure occur. These include maintaining a safe environment, remaining with patient, and maintaining patent airway.
- Evaluate pupil size, equality, and reactivity; extraocular movements; and presence of changes which are reflective of oculomotor (III), trochlear (IV), and abducens (VI) cranial nerves.
- Evaluate trigeminal (V) by monitoring facial sensation and corneal reflex bilaterally.
- Insert protective eye drops or lubricants and tape eyelid shut on the affected side, if necessary.
- Assess facial cranial nerve (VIII): facial weakness or asymmetry; ability to chew; speech; and facial droop causing drooling.
- Monitor glossopharyngeal (IX) and vagus (X): presence and quality of gag, cough, swallowing reflexes and ability to handle secretions.
- Assist patient with eating and encourage patient to chew on the unaffected side.
- Provide alternative communication aides.
- Suction patient if he or she is unable to handle own secretions.
- Evaluate tongue position, strength and deviation, which is reflective of hypoglossal (XII) cranial nerve.
- Monitor patient's ability to shrug shoulders, turn head, or bend forward, which reflect function of spinal accessory (XI).
- Administer prescribed anticonvulsant agents such as phenytoin or phenobarbital to prevent seizures in the postoperative patient (see Table 7–4).

High risk of infection related to invasive procedures or immunosuppression.

Expected Patient Outcomes. Patient is free of infection, as evidenced by white blood cell (WBC) count ≤11,000/μL; normothermia; absence of redness, swelling, tenderness, or drainage from incision or ventriculostomy site; and negative cultures.

- Review results of WBC count and cultures.
- Obtain and report clinical findings of redness, swelling, tenderness, or drainage from incision or ventriculostomy site.
- Utilize strict aseptic technique when changing dressings or lines.
- Obtain and record temperature every 1 to 2 hours while patient is febrile.
- Administer prescribed antipyretic when patient is febrile.
- Administer prescribed antibiotics to control infection.

Pain related to surgical incision.

Expected Patient Outcome. Patient's incisional pain is minimal or absent.

- Assess patient for nonverbal indicators of pain such as restlessness, movement of hands toward the incision site, and grimacing.
- Obtain and report clinical findings associated with pain: tachycardia, tachypnea, elevated BP, and elevated ICP.
- Position patient to relieve muscle tension and pressure on bony prominences.
- Provide a quiet environment by dimming lights, reducing noise level, and restricting visitors.
- Teach patient diversional and comfort measures such as soft music, back rub, and passive exercises.
- Teach patient stress-reduction techniques such as progressive relaxation or guided imagery.

Collaborative Problems

Common collaborative goals for patients undergoing craniotomy are to decrease ICP, reduce cerebral edema, and prevent or control seizure activity.

Potential Complication: Increased Intracranial Pressure. Increased ICP related to hematoma formation and cerebral edema.

Expected Patient Outcomes. Patient maintains normal ICP, as evidenced by ICP 0 to 15 mm Hg, CPP 60 to 100 mm Hg, alertness, equal and normoreactive pupils, BP within patient's normal range, HR ≤100 bpm, RR 12 to 20 BPM, normal respiratory pattern, normal sensorimotor function, absence of headache, absence of papilledema, and absence of vomiting.

- Consult with physician about factors contributing to sustained spikes in ICP: hypercapnia, hypoxemia, Valsalva's maneuver, certain body positions, isometric muscle contraction, coughing or sneezing, or arousal from sleep.
- Review arterial blood gas measurements.
- Maintain patient in semi-Fowler's position with head elevated 30 degrees. Avoid the prone position and exaggerated neck flexion to decrease intrathoracic pressure, promote drainage from the venous vessels from the head and brain, and decrease ICP.
- Restrict fluid intake to 1500 to 1800 mL/24 h to decrease extracellular fluid of body tissue thereby decreasing ICP.
- Assess clinical indicators of neurological status: LOC, sensorimotor function, RR and pattern, pupils, and vital signs.
- Report clinical findings associated with increased ICP: deterioration of LOC, pupillary dilatation or constriction, increased SBP, widening pulse pressure, bradycardia, altered respiratory pattern, loss of sensorimotor function, papilledema, headache, and vomiting.
- Monitor ICP continuously for pressure 0 to 15 mm Hg and three pressure waves (A, B and C). Report ICP ≥15 mm Hg and presence of A wave. The A, or plateau, waves are sudden, transient waves lasting 5 to 20 minutes and beginning from a baseline of already elevated ICP. The A waves cause

cerebral ischemia. The B waves are seen in relation to fluctuation of respiratory pattern such as Cheyne-Stokes respirations.

- Assess for the presence of Cushing's triad with a rising ICP: hypertension, bradycardia, and irregular respirations. The changes may be associated with irreversible brainstem damage.
- Monitor temperature, as hyperthermia can increase cerebral metabolic rate, thereby increasing ICP.
- Assess respiratory pattern and report changes such as Cheyne-Stokes respirations, central neurogenic hyperventilation, apneustic breathing, cluster breathing, and ataxic breathing.
- Measure CPP every hour and report ≤30 mm Hg.
- Measure intake and output to evaluate the amount of diuresis and urinary dilution.
- Apply antiembolic elastic stockings to prevent risk of thrombophlebitis.
- Administer prescribed broad-spectrum antibiotics if patient is on ventricular drainage or continuous ICP monitoring.
- Administer prescribed mannitol (0.5 to 2.0 g/kg over a period of 20 to 30 minutes) which results in diuresis, reduces tissue edema, and induces cerebral arterial vasoconstriction, which lessens the size of the cerebrovascular components of ICP.
- Administer prescribed furosemide (0.1 to 2.0 mg/kg) to reduce ICP. When used in combination with albumin or mannitol, the dose is 1.0 mg/kg.
- Administer prescribed corticosteroids (Decadron) at a dose of 10 mg four times daily to reduce cerebral edema and thus a subsequent decrease in ICP.
- Administer prescribed barbiturate (phenobarbital) at a loading dose of 6 to 8 mg/kg or as a single dose (60 mg/min) to reduce cerebral blood flow in patients with increased ICP.
- Administer prescribed antipyretic agents such as acetaminophen alone or in combination with a hypothermia blanket to control elevated temperature.

- Should pharmacological therapy be unable to control spikes in ICP, prepare patient for ventriculostomy and ventricular drainage. Drainage catheters are inserted into a cerebral ventricle to drain excess CSF. Measure the amount of drainage in the collection container.
- Prepare patient for prescribed barbiturate therapy (3 to 5 mg/kg at slow IV push) to control increased ICP by causing cerebral vasoconstriction, which decreases cerebral blood flow and blood volume, decreases cerebral metabolism, and reduces ICP to ≤10 mm Hg within 10 to 15 minutes. Monitor BP and ICP throughout the entire process.
- Should barbiturate therapy be initiated, monitor the following neurological reflex parameters for loss: pupillary, oculocephalic, oculovestibular, coroneal, gag, and swallowing.

Potential Complication: Cerebral Edema. Cerebral edema related to movement of fluid into the cerebral tissue secondary to localized loss of autoregulatory mechanisms, increase of blood flow, and dilation of focal bleed vessels.

Expected Patient Outcomes. Patient is free of cerebral edema, as evidenced by normal mentation, adequate arousal, being alert and oriented, ICP ≤15 mm Hg, and CPP 60 to 100 mm Hg.

- Review serum osmolality and serum electrolyte values.
- Review results of serum glucose test, since hyperglycemia is induced by corticosteroid therapy.
- Assess clinical indicators of neurological status: LOC, sensorimotor function, RR and pattern, pupils, and vital signs.
- Report clinical findings associated with increased ICP: deterioration of LOC, pupillary dilatation or constriction, increased SBP, widening pulse pressure, bradycardia, altered respiratory pattern, loss of sensori-

motor function, papilledema, headache, and vomiting.

- Monitor ICP continuously for pressure 0 to 15 mm Hg and three pressure waves (A, B and C). Report ICP $\geq$15 mm Hg and presence of A wave. The A, or plateau, waves are sudden, transient waves lasting 5 to 20 minutes and beginning from a baseline of already elevated ICP. The A waves cause cerebral ischemia. The B waves are seen in relation to fluctuation of respiratory pattern such as Cheyne-Stokes respirations.
- Assist with removal of CSF to reduce cerebral edema and ICP. Document the amount of drainage, time interval for drainage, color, clarity, and consistency.
- Continuously monitor and report CPP $\leq$30 mm Hg.
- Assess cranial nerve and pupillary reaction.
- Restrict fluid intake to 1200 to 1500 mL/d, which decreases intracellular fluid volume, thereby minimizing or preventing cerebral edema formation by keeping patient slightly dehydrated.
- Administer prescribed hypertonic solution to reduce cerebral edema.
- Administer prescribed hyperosmolar agents (mannitol), which increases the osmolality of circulating blood, thereby causing fluid to move down the concentration gradient from the brain interstitium into the intravascular compartment.
- Administer prescribed furosemide to reduce cerebral edema.
- Administer prescribed glucocorticosteroids, dexamethasone (Decadron) and methylprednisolone (Solu-Medrol) to relieve cerebral edema, thereby reestablishing and maintaining the integrity of the blood-brain barrier (see Table 1–15, p. 129).

Potential Complication: Seizures. Seizures related to an underlying structural abnormality secondary to an acute cerebral injury.

Expected Patient Outcomes. Patient's seizures will be prevented or controlled.

- Review results of EEG, CT scan, serum glucose and arterial blood gas measurements.
- Maintain patent airway to ensure adequate oxygenation.
- Monitor temperature and when hyperthermic, provide external cooling measures.
- Provide a quiet, calm environment with subdued lighting.
- Pad bed rails and keep rails up when patient is in bed.
- Monitor continuous ECG to assess HR and rhythm. Document ECG rhythm strips every 2 hours in patients with dysrhythmias caused by loss of the sodium and potassium gradient, leading to cellular edema. Liberation of intracellular potassium can cause dysrhythmias.
- Protect patient from aspiration of gastric content during status epilepticus.
- Administer prescribed anticonvulsants such as diazepam (Valium) at an initial dose up to 40 mg and phenytoin (Dilantin) 18 to 20 mg/kg. If seizure is not terminated, provide phenobarbital at a dose of 20 mg/kg.
- Administer prescribed oxygen by nasal cannula, mask, or intubation. Hyperventilate patient with 100% oxygen during status epilepticus, which increases cerebral and systemic metabolic rates by 200% to 300%.
- Administer prescribed antipyretic agents when patient is febrile.

Potential Complication: Dysrhythmias. Dysrhythmias related to increased ICP, vagal stimulation, or brain-stem edema.

Expected Patient Outcome. Patient maintains regular sinus rhythm.

- Review results of 12-lead ECG and serum enzymes.
- Monitor continuous ECG to assess HR and rhythm. Document ECG rhythm strips every 2 to 4 hours or more frequently in patients with dysrhythmias.
- Avoid vagal stimulation such as Valsalva's maneuver and neck vein compression.

- Administer antidysrhythmias agent, if necessary. (see Table 1–11, p. 54).

Potential Complication: Electrolyte Imbalance. Electrolyte imbalance related to diuretic therapy and diabetes insipidus.

Expected Patient Outcomes. Serum electrolytes within normal range.

- Review results of 12-lead ECG and tests for serum electrolytes and osmolality and urine sodium and osmolality.
- Assess and report clinical findings associated with decreased ADH: hypernatremia, hyperosmolality, dehydration, polyruia, polydipsia, altered LOC, hyperactive reflexes, muscle twitching, and convulsion.
- Assess and report for clinical findings associated with increased ADH: hyponatremia, hypo-osmolality, overhydration, water retention, nausea, vomiting, apathy, muscle twitching, irritability, or disorientation.
- Administer IV fluids and electrolytes as prescribed.
- Administer vasopressin replacement therapy to enhance ADH secretion: chlorpropamide or carbamazepine.

DISCHARGE PLANNING

The critical care nurse will provide patient and significant other(s) verbal or written discharge notes regarding the following subjects:

1. Importance of keeping all postdischarge medical appointments.
2. Referrals to physical, speech, or occupational therapist.
3. Medications, including purpose, dose, route, schedule, and side effects.
4. Referral to professional nursing services should patient require care in an extended care facility or home care.
5. Referrals to social support services, if necessary, should financial support be needed because of the illness or injury.

PART III: SUPPORTIVE PROCEDURES AND NURSING MANAGEMENT

■ INTRACRANIAL PRESSURE MONITORING

Case Management Basis
DRG: None

Definition
Intracranial pressure is the force or pressure exerted within the rigid confines of the skull by the brain, blood, and the cerebrospinal fluid (CSF). Intracranial hypertension (ICH) results when the volume within the rigid skull exceeds the space allowed and exists with ICP ≥15 to 20 mm Hg.

Patient Selection

INDICATIONS. Criteria for intracranial pressure (ICP) monitoring are head injury, intracerebral hematoma, subarachnoid hemorrhage, space-occupying lesions, central nervous system infection, metabolic encephalopathies, cerebral edema, near drowning, Glasgow coma scale score ≤8, paralytic agents, high-dose barbiturate, and general anesthesia.

CONTRAINDICATIONS. None.

Procedure

TECHNIQUE

Intraventricular Method. A catheter is introduced via a burr hole through the skull and positioned within the anterior or occipital horn of the ventricle.

- Devices: Ventricular catheter with multiple lateral openings at the proximal end or modified intraventricular two-lumen catheter, one lumen in the ventricular space and the other lumen leading to a balloon to assess volume-pressure responses.

- Use: For intermittent or large-volume CSF drainage. Drainage is done slowly against a pressure of 15 to 20 mm Hg to avoid ventricular collapse.

Subarachnoid Method. A subarachnoid screw is inserted by a burr hole in the skull so that the tip is positioned in the subarachnoid space. The pressures generated by CSF are then directly measured.

- Devices: Richmand screw that has a patent fluid-filled lumen in contact with CSF; modified Richard screw that accommodates different skull thickness; Philly bolt, which rests against the skull and enhances stability; Leeds screw, which is a large, two-lumen screw with an end plate and four lateral holes; subdural cup catheter, which is a Silastic ribbon with a central lumen and indented cup with an opening near the distal end.

Epidural Method. The monitor is implanted between the skull and the dura through a burr hole.

- Devices: Pressure Pill, involving a sensor that is an air-filled, compressible balloon of silicone rubber with a solid metal backing. The balloon contains a mirror, which senses pressure changes, and activated bellows to readjust to ICP from an electrical photocell signal; Long-Term Epidural Monitor involves a sensor containing a passive electrical circuit and bellows filled with nitrogen gas. There is a thin diaphragm next to the dura that is deflected from increased pressure in silicone oil to compress gas-filled bellows; Pneumatic Flow Sensor and Monitor, in which air enters sensor at 40 mL/min and pressure build up against a diaphragm-type membrane until air pressure equals ICP; Telemetric ICP Monitor is a ventricular catheter connected to a chamber with a diaphragm, which bulges outward against scalp with increased CSF pressure; or the Extradural Screw connected to a microconducer, with the screw lumen and dome filled with sterile normal saline.

Pressure Wave Forms

- A waves: These are plateau waves and are associated with cerebral ischemia. The waves may occur in patients with a ICP baseline ≥15 to 20 mm Hg. Amplitude of the plateau waves and pulse pressure may range between 50 to 100 mm Hg with a duration of 5 to 20 minutes. They are correlated with increased ICP, which leads to cerebral ischemia, cellular hypoxia, or infarction. Plateau waves signify that compensatory and autoregulatory mechanisms are ineffective in controlling ICP and subsequent loss of compliance.
- B waves: They occur in sawtooth pattern and reach an amplitude of 50 mm Hg; may occur as frequently as 1/2 to 2 minutes. The fluctuations reflect respiratory and cardiovascular alterations, and they represent a decrease in intracranial compliance.
- C waves: These are known as Traube-Hering-May waves and are rapid waves with an amplitude of 20 mm Hg and occur every 4 to 8 minutes.

EQUIPMENT. Catheters, bolt or screw, and fiberoptic monitoring devices.

Complications
Complications associated with increased ICP include hemorrhage, hematoma formation, acute overdrainage of CSF, and infection.

NURSING MANAGEMENT: NURSING DIAGNOSES AND COLLABORATIVE PROBLEMS

Nursing Diagnoses
Common nursing goals for patients with ICP monitoring are to reduce the risk of infection, maintain fluid balance, minimize pain, and reduce anxiety.

High risk for infection related to invasive ICP monitoring device.

Expected Patient Outcomes. Patient experiences normothermia; white blood cell (WBC) count ≤11,000/μL; negative cultures; and absence of swelling, tenderness, redness, or drainage from ICP monitoring site.

- Consult with physician about factors that contribute to infection. These include type of ICP monitor, those such as ventricular catheters fluid-coupled to an external transducer have the highest infection and length of ICP monitoring greater than 5 days.
- Assess and report redness, swelling, tenderness, or drainage around ICP monitoring catheter site.
- Monitor temperature every 2 hours should patient be febrile.
- Initiate prescribed flush solution in fluid-coupled ICP monitoring systems: intermittent flushes every 2 to 3 hours with 0.1 to 0.3 mL of sterile saline or an antibiotic flush solution such as bacitracin or gentamicin to prevent occlusion. Maintain a closed system to reduce the risk of infection caused by flushing.
- Maintain aseptic technique with routine use of the system and sterile technique whenever the system is opened.
- Avoid contaminating the stopcock by using a T-piece connection or rubber sampling port that is routinely cleaned with bactericidal solution before the system is entered.
- Obtain CSF sample, as prescribed, from a ventriculostomy for culture and sensitivity testing, glucose and protein and cell counts for evidence of infection.
- Obtain and report neurological clinical findings associated with infection: decreased LOC, irritability, photophobia, nuchal rigidity, and seizure activity.

Fluid volume deficit related to overdrainage of CSF.

Expected Patient Outcomes. Patient experiences the appropriate amount of CSF drainage.

- Monitor ICP continuously and report ≥15 mm Hg. Report consistent elevation.
- Initiate drainage when there is a consistent, not transient, elevation in ICP.
- Monitor the drainage, which depends on the level of ICP, rapidity of CSF drainage, and patient's condition. Should overdraining occur, the ventricles can collapse, causing the brain to pull away from the dura, leading to subdural hematoma.
- Pin or tape the drainage system to a prescribed predetermined height or patient's bed to prevent a change between patient's head and the drainage system.
- Monitor or color and consistence of CSF drainage.

Pain related to ventriculostomy.

Expected Patient Outcomes. Patient experiences minimal or no pain.

- Assess patient for nonverbal indicators of pain such as restlessness, movement of hands toward the incision site, and grimacing.
- Obtain and report clinical findings associated with pain: tachycardia, tachypnea, elevated BP, and elevated ICP.
- Position patient to relieve muscle tension and pressure on bony prominences.
- Provide a quiet environment by dimming lights, reducing noise level, and restricting visitors.
- Teach patient diversional and comfort measures such as soft music, back rub, and passive exercises.
- Teach patient stress-reduction techniques such as progressive relaxation or guided imagery.

Anxiety related to invasive procedure.

Expected Patient Outcome. Patient verbalizes decreased anxiety.

- Provide a calm, relaxed environment to reduce stress.
- Encourage patient to express concerns or needs.

- Help patient to identify situation leading to increased anxiety.
- Explain the purposes behind ICP monitoring.
- Teach patient factors that can have a negative effect upon ICP: coughing, turning, Valsalva's maneuver, or suctioning.
- Teach patient alternative strategies to reduce stress: progressive relaxation, meditation, or guided imagery if not contraindicated.

Collaborative Problems

A common collaborative goal for patients with ICP monitoring is to maintain cerebral compliance.

Potential Complication: Decreased Cerebral Compliance.

Decreased cerebral compliance related to increased ICP secondary to fluid accumulation.

Expected Patient Outcomes.

Patient maintains adequate cerebral compliance, as evidenced by ICP 0 to 15 mm Hg, cerebral perfusion pressure (CPP) 60 to 100 mm Hg, mean arterial pressure (MAP) 70 to 100 mm Hg, volume-pressure response (VPR) ≤2mm Hg/mL and volume pressure index (VPI) 25 mL of fluid required to produce increased ICP.

- Consult with physician about compliance (C), which is the ratio of the change (B) on volume (V) to the resulting change in pressure (P). High compliance means larger volume changes can occur without an increase in ICP. Low compliance means any increase in volume leads to increased ICP.
- Assess ICP, MAP, and CPP continuously. Report ICP ≥15 mm Hg, MAP ≤70 mm Hg, and CPP ≤60 mm Hg. When ICP equals mean arterial BP, CPP is 0 and cerebral blood flow ceases. When ICP is 20 mm Hg and CPP is 50 mm Hg, rapid intervention is required.
- Monitor volume-pressure response (VPR), which is the change in ICP after injection or removal of 1 mL of CSF during a period of 1 second. Report VPR ≥5 mm Hg/mL, since there is a decrease in the volume-

buffering capacity of the brain. Adequate compliance is VPR ≤2 mm Hg; the brain can adapt to increase in ICP.

- Monitor volume pressure index which is the volume of fluid injected to produce a 10 mm Hg increase in ICP. Normally, .25 mL of fluid is required. When the amount is ≤10 mL, a state of decreased compliance occurs.
- Continuously monitor and interpret ICP wave forms. The wave form is a reflection of systemic hemodynamics reflected into the intracranial cavity. The configuration of the wave form at normal pressures is P_1 (percussion wave), which is distinct and highest followed by the lower P_2 (tidal wave) and P_3 (dicrotic notch). As ICP elevates, P_2 may exceed P_1 in height. An elevated P_2 is reflective of decreased intracranial compliance.
- Report when the systolic peak of the ICP wave forms are more peaked and ICP follows systemic BP because this signifies lost autoregulation.
- Monitor ICP wave forms for a 5 to 10 minute time period to determine whether an elevated ICP exists.

■ BARBITURATE COMA

Case Management Basis
DRG: None

Definition
High doses of barbiturate, enough to induce a barbiturate coma, stabilize cell membranes and produce superimposed coma, which reduces cerebral metabolism and cerebral blood flow. The overall goal is to control intracranial hypertension, which is an intracranial pressure (ICP) ≥25 mm Hg.

Patient Selection

INDICATIONS. Used in acute head injury patients with intracranial hypertension, intractable seizures, sagittal sinus thrombosis, Reye's syndrome, and ischemic stroke.

CONTRAINDICATIONS. Those patients whose ICP is normal. Also contraindicated in patient who responds to CSF drainage, hyperventilation, or osmotic therapy. In addition, patients with cardiac disease such as heart failure who might experience myocardial depression from barbiturates.

Procedure

TECHNIQUE. A loading dose of 3 to 5 mg/kg of phenobarbital sodium can be administered. The maintenance goal is 1 to 3 mg/kg/h to keep a barbiturate level of 2.5 to 3.5 mg/dL. A barbiturate coma serves the purpose of reducing cerebral blood flow, reducing oxygen demand, and reducing cerebral metabolism.

NURSING MANAGEMENT: NURSING DIAGNOSES AND COLLABORATIVE PROBLEMS

Nursing Diagnoses

Common nursing goals for patients undergoing barbiturate coma are to maintain oxygenation and maintain cerebral tissue perfusion.

Impaired gas exchange related to hypostatic pneumonia secondary to alveolar congestion or stasis.

Expected Patient Outcomes. Patient maintains adequate gas exchange, as evidenced by respiratory rate (RR) 12 to 20 BPM, blood pressure (BP) within patient's normal range, symmetrical chest movement, normothermia, arterial blood gases within normal range, absence of cyanosis, arterial oxygen saturation (SaO_2) 95% to 97.5%, and absence of adventitious breath sounds.

- Review results arterial blood gas measurements and chest roentgenogram.
- Assess clinical indicators of respiratory status: RR, symmetry of chest movement, use

of accessory muscles, skin color, and lung sounds.
- Report clinical findings associated with impaired gas exchange: tachypnea, assymetry of chest movement, use of accessory muscles, cyanosis, or crackles.
- Continuously monitor oxygen saturation with pulse oximeter and end-tidal partial pressure of carbon dioxide ($PETCO_2$) with capnometry to determine if oxygenation is adequate.
- Assist with intubation and mechanical ventilation because barbiturates can depress the respiratory system.
- Suction patient according to unit protocol since the cough reflex is abolished.
- Insert nasogastric (NG) tube to maintain gastric decompression and prevent risk of aspiration.
- Administer prescribed IV fluids to maintain adequate circulatory volume.
- Administer prescribed oxygen by mechanical ventilation to maintain adequate oxygenation.

Altered cerebral tissue perfusion related to hypotension secondary to barbiturate coma.

Expected Patient Outcomes. Patient maintains adequate cerebral tissue perfusion, as evidenced by cerebral perfusion pressure (CPP) 60 to 100 mm Hg, ICP ≤15 mm Hg, blood pressure (BP) within patient's normal range, heart rate (HR) 60 to 100 bpm, and SaO_2 ≥95%.

- Review results of serum barbiturate level.
- Continuously monitor and report ICP unresponsive to barbiturate administration, CPP ≤60 mm Hg and hypotension.
- Measure intake, output, and cerebrospinal fluid (CSF) drainage.
- Monitor arterial BP continuously to note the pressure of barbiturate-induced hypotension and tachycardia.
- Use a portable electroencephalogram (EEG) monitor or compressed spectral analysis (CSA) to evaluate patient's response to loading and maintenance dose of barbiturate.

- Monitor CSF drainage as prescribed for ICP control during barbiturate coma.
- Provide prescribed loading dose of pentobarbital at a dose 5 to 10 mg/kg IV at a rate no faster than 100 mg/min to maintain SBP ≥90 mm Hg and CPP ≥60 mm Hg.
- Administer prescribed pentobarbital maintenance dose of 3 to 5 mg/kg/h as a bolus of a constant infusion.
- Administer IV fluids 75 to 100 mL/h to maintain systolic blood pressure (SBP) 100 mm Hg.

Collaborative Problems

A common collaborative goal for patients undergoing barbiturate coma is to maintain cardiac output.

Potential Complication: Decreased Cardiac Output.

Decreased cardiac output related to hypotension secondary to barbiturate coma.

Expected Patient Outcomes. Patient maintains adequate cardiac output, as evidenced by cardiac output (CO) 4 to 8 L/min, cardiac index (CI) 2.7 to 4.3 L/min/m^2, CPP ≥60 mm Hg, central venous pressure (CVP) 2 to 6 mm Hg, pulmonary capillary wedge pressure (PCWP) 6 to 12 mm Hg, BP within patient's normal range, HR ≤100 bpm, skin warm and dry, urinary output (UO) ≥30 mL/h, peripheral pulse +2, and capillary refill ≤3 seconds.

- Consult with physician about clinical indicators requiring temporary stoppage of barbiturate therapy: ICP unresponsive to barbiturate therapy, hypotension, unilateral change in pupil size, SaO_2 ≤95%, CPP ≤60 mm Hg, and hypothermia.
- Obtain and report hemodynamic parameters indicating decreased CO: CO ≤4 L/min, CI ≤2.7 L/min/m^2, CVP ≤2 mm Hg, and PCWP ≤6 mm Hg.
- Obtain and report clinical findings associated with decreased CO: hypotension, tachycardia, peripheral pulses ≤+2, and capillary refill ≥3 seconds.

- Measure intake, output, and CSF drainage to determine fluid and ICP balance. Report UO ≤30 mL/h.
- Provide antithromboembolic stockings to prevent pooling of blood.
- Continuously monitor and maintain SBP ≥90 mm Hg and CPP ≥60 mm Hg.
- Continuously monitor ECG to assess HR and rhythm. Document and report tachydysrhythmias while pentobarbital is ordered.
- Insert NG tube to maintain gastric decompression and prevent vomiting in the comatose patient.
- Administer prescribed dopamine to increase CO.
- Should barbiturate-induced hypotension occur, administer prescribed phenylephrine hydrochloride 50 mg/250 mL 5% dextrose in water to correct hypotension.
- Administer prescribed IV fluids to maintain adequate circulatory volume.
- Instruct family regarding the purpose of barbiturate coma.

■ CEREBRAL BALLOON ANGIOPLASTY

Case Management Basis
DRG: None

Definition
Cerebral balloon angioplasty is the use of a balloon catheter to dilate cerebral arteries narrowed by vasospasm resulting from subarachnoid hemorrhage. Cerebral vasospasm can be related to the amount of blood and clots in the subarachnoid space.

Patient Selection

INDICATIONS. General selection criteria are failure of the neurological patient to respond to conventional medical and pharmacological therapy, angiographic evidence of vasospasm that might cause ischemic deficit, or computerized tomographic (CT) or magnetic resonance imaging (MRI) evidence that infarction has not developed in the vascular distribution of spasm.

Procedure

TECHNIQUE. The patient is anesthetized by local or general anesthesia or neurological analgesia (mixture of a narcotic analgesia such as meperidine, morphine, or fentanyl and an antipsychotic such as droperidol). A catheter is threaded up the femoral artery to the aorta. There are two approaches, depending on the location of the vasospasm. For a vasospasm in the posterior circulation, the catheter is directed into the vertebral artery, right or left, and either into the basilar artery or further on into the posterior cerebral artery. For a vasospasm in the anterior circulation, the catheter is directed up the carotid artery, right or left, and then into either the anterior cerebral or the middle cerebral artery. Once the catheter is positioned in the area of the vasospasm, the balloon is dilated slowly to correct narrowing of the artery.

Complications

Complications consist of hemorrhage at the puncture site, rupture of the balloon, injury of the vessel including intimal perforation or rupture, cerebral artery thrombosis or embolism, recurrence of stenosis, or worsening of neurological deficits.

NURSING MANAGEMENT: NURSING DIAGNOSES AND COLLABORATIVE PROBLEMS

Nursing Diagnoses

Common nursing goals for patients experiencing cerebral balloon angioplasty are to prevent injury and increase cerebral artery perfusion.

High risk of injury related to vessel trauma secondary to intimal perforation or rupture.

Expected Patient Outcomes. Patient is free of intimal injury, as evidenced by blood pressure (BP) within patient's normal range, heart rate (HR) 60 to 100 bpm, absence of headache, alertness, normal sensorimotor function, absence of vomiting, and respiratory rate (RR) 12 to 20 BPM.

- Review results of angiography to determine the site of the vasospasm; CT scan to rule out other causes of neurological deterioration; and transcranial Doppler ultrasound to record changes in blood flow velocity induced by alteration in vessel caliber and increases in blood viscosity.
- Obtain and report clinical findings associated with vessel rupture: hypotension, tachycardia, tachypnea, disorientation, and motor weakness.
- Administer prescribed IV fluids to maintain adequate circulatory blood volume.
- Should vessel perforation or rupture occur and patient experience worsening neurological deficits, prepare patient for surgery.

Altered cerebral tissue perfusion related to interrupted blood flow secondary to thrombosis or embolism.

Expected Patient Outcomes. Patient maintains adequate cerebral tissue perfusion, as evidenced by BP within patient's normal range; orientation to person, place and location; HR 60 to 100 bpm; normal sensorimotor function; pupils equal and normoreactive; normothermia; absence of headache; RR 12 to 20 BPM; mean arterial pressure (MAP) 70 to 100 mm Hg; normal speech pattern; and cerebral perfusion pressure (CPP) 60 to 100 mm Hg.

- Review results of angiography, MRI, CT, and transcranial Doppler ultrasound.
- Assess clinical indicators of neurological status: level of consciousness, vital signs, sensorimotor function, reflexes, and pupillary reaction.
- Report clinical findings associated with altered cerebral tissue perfusion as a result of vasospasm: lethargy, changes in sensorium, confusion and disorientation, motor weakness, visual deficits, labile blood pressure,

bradydysrhythmias-tachydysrhythmias, seizures, headache, and low-grade fever.

- Monitor CPP continuously and report ≤60 mm Hg.
- Monitor intake, output, and specific gravity to evaluate fluid balance.
- Administer prescribed oxygen by nasal cannula or mask to maintain partial pressure of arterial oxygen (Pao_2) ≥90 mm Hg, thereby oxygenating the blood.
- Administer prescribed dopamine to induce hypertension 40 to 60 mm Hg above normal to maintain CPP. Note this may be contraindicated in patients whose aneurysm has not been clipped, since rebleeding can occur (see Table 1–10, p. 50).
- Administer prescribed calcium channel blockers (nifedipine) to prevent influx of calcium into vascular smooth muscle and inhibition of contraction (see Table 1–6, p. 28).
- Provide prescribed hypovolemic hemodilution to decrease blood viscosity by intravascular volume expansion. Volume expanders (dextran and albumin) can be used, thereby increasing cerebral blood flow.

SELECTED REFERENCES

Ammons AM. Cerebral injuries and intracranial hemorrhages as a result of trauma. *Nurs Clin North Am.* 1990; 25:23–33.

Bell J. Understanding and managing myasthenia gravis. *Focus Crit Care.* 1989; 16(1): 57–65.

Bell TN. Diabetes insipidus. *Crit Care Nurs Clin North Am.* 1994; 6:675–686.

Blissitt PA. Nutrition in acute spinal cord injury. *Crit Care Nurs Clin North Am.* 1990; 2:375–384.

Coburn K. Traumatic brain injury: the silent epidemic. *AACN Clin Issues Crit Care Nurs.* 1992; 3(1):9–18.

Coen SD. Spinal cord injury: preventing secondary injury. *AACN Clin Issues Crit Care Nurs.* 1992; 3(1):44–54.

Corbett JV. Laboratory Tests and Diagnostic Procedures with Nursing Diagnoses, 3rd ed. Norwalk, Conn: Appleton & Lange; 1992.

Darby-Mahon J, Renshaw-Ketchik B, Richmond TS, et al. Powerlessness in cervical spinal cord injury patients. *Dimensions Crit Care Nurs.* 1988; 7:346–355.

Deglin JH, Vallerand AH. Davis's Drug Guide For Nurses, 4th ed., Philadelphia, Pa: FA Davis; 1995.

DeLoach PB. Intracranial pressure monitoring, seizure control, and cervical spine traction. In: Flynn, JB, Bruce, NP, eds. *Introduction to Critical Care Skills.* St. Louis, Mo: Mosby Year Book; 1993:277–307.

Dipalma JR. Nimodipine in subarachnoid hemorrhage. *Am Fam Physician.* 1989; 40(6):143–145.

Dodson WE, Leppik JE, Pedley TA. Are you up-to-date on seizures? *Patient Care.* 1991; 162–190.

Dolan JT. *Critical Care Nursing Clinical Management Through the Nursing Process.* Philadelphia, Pa: FA Davis Co; 1991.

Ford RD. Diagnostic Tests Handbook. Springhouse, Pa: Springhouse Corp; 1987.

Fridlund-Hollingsworth P, Vos H, Daily EK. Use of fiber-optic pressure transducer for intracranial pressure measurements: a preliminary report. *Heart Lung.* 1988; 17:111–118.

Germon K. Interpretation of ICP pulse waves to determine intracerebral compliance. *J Neurosci Nurs.* 1988; 20:344–351.

Gilliam EE. Intracranial hypertension: advances in intracranial pressure monitoring. *Crit Care Clin North Am.* 1990; 2:21–37.

Govoni LE, Hayes JE, Shannon MT, et al. *Drugs and Nursing Implications.* 8th ed. Norwalk, Conn: Appleton & Lange; 1995.

Greenberg DA, Simon RP, Aminoff MJ. *Clinical Neurology.* Norwalk, Conn: Appleton & Lange; 1989.

Grimes CM. Cerebral balloon angioplasty for treatment of vasospasm after subarachnoid hemorrhage. *Heart Lung.* 1991; 20:431–435.

Halm MA. Elimination concerns with acute spinal cord trauma. *Crit Care Nurs Clin North Am.* 1990; 2:385–398.

Hahn, SM. Current concepts in bacterial meningitis. *West J Med.* 1988; 151:180–186.

Hayman, LA, Pagan JJ, Kirpatrick JB, et al. Pathophysiology of acute intracerebral and subarachnoid hemorrhage. *Am J Roentgenology.* 1989; 153:132–139.

Hickey JC. *The Clinical Practice of Neurological and Neurosurgical Nursing.* Philadelphia, Pa: JB Lippincott Co; 1992.

Hickle J. Nursing care of patients with minor head injury. *J Neurosci Nurs.* 1988; 20(1): 8–14.

Hilton G, Frei J. High-dose methylprednisolone in the treatment of spinal cord injuries. *Heart Lung.* 1991; 20:675–680.

Hugo, M. Alleviating the effects of care on the intracranial pressure (ICP) of head injured patient by manipulating nursing care activities. *Intensive Care Nurs.* 1987; 3(2):78–82.

Jastremski CA. Traumatic brain injury: assessment and treatment. *Crit Care Nurs Clin North Am.* 1994; 6:473–481.

Johanson BC, Wells SJ, Dungca CV, et al. *Standards for Critical Care.* 3rd ed. St. Louis, Mo: CV Mosby; 1988.

Johnson SM, Omery A, Nikas D. Effects of conversation on intracranial pressure in comatose patients. *Heart Lung.* 1989; 18:56–63.

Kidd PS. Emergency management of spinal cord injuries. *Crit Care Nurs Clin North Am.* 1990; 2:349–356.

Kocan MJ. Pulmonary consideration in the critical care phase. *Crit Care Nurs Clin North Am.* 1990; 2:369–374.

Kraay CR. Intracranial pressure monitoring. In: Clochesy JM, Breu C, Cardin S, et al., eds. *Critical Care Nursing.* Philadelphia, Pa: WB Saunders Co; 1993:208–226.

Latham-Pollack CL. Intracranial pressure monitoring: part II patient care. *Crit Care Nurse.* 1987; 7(6):53–72.

Loeb S. *Clinical Laboratory Tests.* Springhouse, Pa: Springhouse Publications; 1991.

Loeb S. *Nurse's Handbook of Drug Therapy.* Springhouse, Pa: Springhouse Publications, 1993.

Mason PB. Neurodiagnostic testing in critically injured adults. *Crit Care Nurse.* 1992; 12(6):64–75.

McSherry JA. Cognitive impairment after head injury. *Am Fam Physician.* 1989; 40(1):186–190.

Mitchell PH. Neurological data acquisition. In: Kinney MR, Packa DR, Dunbar SB, eds. *AACN's Clinical Reference for Critical Care Nursing,* 3rd ed. St. Louis, Mo: Mosby Year Book, 1993:781–802.

Mitchell PH. Neurological disorders. In: Kinney MR, Packa DR, Dunbar SB, eds. *AACN's Clinical Reference for Critical Care Nursing,* 3rd ed. St. Louis, Mo: Mosby Year Book; 1993: 803–853.

Murphy MD, Batnitzky S, Bramble JM. Diagnostic imaging of spinal trauma. *Radiol Clin North Am.* 1989; 27:855–872.

Palmer M, Wyness MA. Positioning and handling: important considerations in the care of the severely head-injured patient. *J Neurosci Nurs.* 1988; 20(1):42–49.

Rainbolt-Whitney CM. Patients with cerebral vascular disorders. In Clochesy JM, Breu C, Cardin S, et al, eds. *Critical Care Nursing.* Philadelphia, Pa: WB Saunders Co; 1993:708–736.

Rea JB, Dunbar SB. Neurogenic electrocardiographic abnormalities in subarachnoid hemorrhage. *Focus Crit Care* 1992; 19(1):50–54.

Richmond, TS. Sinal cord injury. *Nurs Clin North Amer* 1990; 25:57–69.

Richmond, TS. Intracranial pressure monitoring. *AACN Clin Issues Crit Care Nurs.* 1993; 4(1): 148–160.

Roberts SL. Acute head injury. *Physiological Concepts and the Critically Ill Patient.* Englewood Cliffs, NJ: Prentice-Hall; 1985; 448–498. [out of print]

Rose BA. Neurologic therapies in critical care. *Crit Care Nurs Clin North Am.* 1993; 5:237–246.

Rudy EB, Turner BS, Baun M, et al. Endotracheal suctioning in adults with head injury. *Heart Lung.* 1991; 20:667–674.

Schwenker D. Cardiovascular considerations in the critical care phase. *Crit Care Nurs Clin North Am.* 1990; 2:363–367.

Segatore M. Hyponatremia after aneurysmal subarachnoid hemorrhage. *J Neurosci Nurs.* 1993; 25:92–97.

Segatore, M, Villenueve M. Spinal cord testing: development of a screening tool. *J Neurosci Nurs.* 1988; 20(1): 30–33.

Smith JR, Flanigin HF, King DW, Gallagher BB, et al. Surgical management of epilepsy. *South Med J.* 1989; 82:736–742.

Strampfer MJ, Domenico P, Cuntia BA. Laboratory aids in the diagnosis of bacterial meningitis. *Heart Lung* 1988; 17:605–607.

Stillwell SB. *Mosby's Critical Care Nursing Reference.* St. Louis, Mo: Mosby Year Book; 1992.

Susi EA, Walls SK. Traumatic cerebral vasospasms and secondary head injury. *Crit Care Nurs Clin North Am.* 1990; 2:15–20.

Swearingen PL, Keen JH. *Manual of Critical Care,* 2nd ed. St. Louis, Mo: Mosby Year Book; 1992.

Walleck CA. Subarachnoid hemorrhage. In: Von Rueden KT, Walleck CA, eds. *Advanced Critical Care Nursing.* Rockville, Md: Aspen Publications; 1989:145–159.

Walleck CA. Closed head injury. In: Von Rueden KT, Walleck CA, eds. *Advanced Critical Care Nursing*. Rockville, Md: Aspen Publications; 1989:161–180.

Walleck CA. Spinal cord injury. In: Von Rueden KT, Walleck CA, eds. *Advanced Critical Care Nursing*. Rockville, Md: Aspen Publications; 1989:181–203.

Walleck CA. Neurologic considerations in the critical care phase. *Crit Care Nurs Clin North Am*. 1990; 2:357–361.

Walleck CA. Preventing secondary brain injury. *AACN Clin Issues Crit Care Nurs*. 1992; 3(1): 19–38.

Walleck CA. Patients with head injury and brain dysfunction. In: Clochesy JM, Breu C, Cardin S, et al, eds. *Critical Care Nursing*. Philadelphia, Pa: WB Saunders Co; 1993:677–705.

Walleck CA. Patients with spinal cord injury. In: Clochesy JM, Breu C, Cardin S, et al, eds. *Critical Care Nursing*. Philadelphia, Pa: WB Saunders Co; 1993:744–765.

8

Endocrine Deviations

◼ DIABETES INSIPIDUS

(For related information see Neurological Deviations, Part I: Cerebral hemorrhage, p. 607; Acute head injury, p. 620. Part II: Craniotomy, p. 664.)

Case Management Basis
DRG: 300 Endocrine disorders with complications
LOS: 6.90 days
DRG: 301 Endocrine disorders without complications
LOS: 4.10 days

Definition
The clinical syndrome resulting from a deficiency of antidiuretic hormone (ADH) production or release is known as neurogenic or central diabetes insipidus (DI); that occurring from renal unresponsiveness to the action of ADH is known as nephrogenic DI.

Pathophysiology
Diabetes insipidus can be classified as central or nephrogenic and may be permanent or temporary, with either partial or complete deficiency of ADH. General DI can develop when the hypothalamus or posterior pituitary gland becomes dysfunctional. Neurogenic diabetes insipidus results from damage to the hypothalamic-neurohypophysial system. Loss of approximately 75% of the ADH secretory neurons occurs before polyuria develops. Initially there is paralysis of vasopressin-producing cells, followed by cell degeneration and a massive release of the intracellular vasopressor pool, with an eventual permanent loss of vasopressor production.

Neurogenic DI occurs when the kidney is resistant to the effect of ADH. The renal tubules and collecting duct do not respond to the pressure of ADH, so water is not reabsorbed (primary nephrogenic DI), or there is chronic medullary disease associated with multiple myeloma, sickle cell anemia, or cystic fibrosis (secondary nephrogenic DI).

Nursing Assessment

PRIMARY CAUSES
- Central DI: Primary causes are idiopathic or familial. Secondary causes include post-traumatic events, hypothalamic and pituitary disruption, neurosurgical operations, craniopharyngioma, pituitary tumors and other metastases, infections such as meningitis and encephalitis, vascular lesions such as aneurysms, Sheehan's syndrome, and granulomatous disease.
- Nephrogenic DI: Primary cause is familial. Secondary causes include renal diseases, chronic hypokalemia or hypocalcemia, sickle cell disease, multiple myeloma, and drugs such as lithium carbonate, demeclocycline, amphotericin B, and methoxyflurane.

PHYSICAL ASSESSMENT
- Inspection: Polyuria, polydipsia, weight loss, sunken eyeballs, poor skin turgor, weakness, listlessness, fatigue, confusion, lethargy, seizures, coma, or muscle pain.
- Palpation: Cool skin; pulse weak, thready; decreased skin turgor; or hypothermia.
- Auscultation: Tachycardia and postural hypotension.

DIAGNOSTIC TEST RESULTS

Standard Laboratory Tests. (see Table 8–1).
- Serum chemistry: Increased serum osmolality ≥295 mOsm/kg and increased serum sodium ≥148 mEq/L.
- Urinalysis: Decreased urine osmolality 50 to 100 mOsm/kg, decreased urine sodium ≥20 mEq/L, specific gravity 1.005, and urine volume ≥6 L/d.
- Vasopressin test: Differentiates central DI from nephrogenic DI by administration of 5 units of aqueous vasopressin subcutaneously. Patient with central DI shows a decreased urine volume and increased urine concentration, whereas nephrogenic DI patients do not respond to the presence of the vasopressin.

Noninvasive Endocrine Diagnostic Procedure. (see Table 8–1).
- Computerized tomographic (CT) scan: Used to assess pituitary hypothalamic area for tumor.
- Skull roentgenogram: Used to assess pituitary hypothalamic area for tumor.
- Water deprivation test: Used to determine if patient responds to a hyperosmotic stimulus with increasing ADH release. Water intake is restricted, while changes in urine volume and plasma concentration are measured for 6 to 8 hours. The DI patient shows the following: dilute urine with urine osmolality ≤100 mOsm/kg, specific gravity of ≤1.005, and serum osmolality ≥300 mOsm/kg.

MEDICAL AND SURGICAL MANAGEMENT

PHARMACOLOGY
- Desmopressin (DDAVP): Desmopressin has a high antidiuretic affect and decreased vasopressor effect. It can be administered intranasally at a dose of 5 to 20 μg. The drug's daily dose is adjusted according to urine output achieved with IV fluid replacement minus insensible losses (Table 8–2).
- Chlorpropamide (Diabinese): Can enhance the release of ADH or augment its effects on the renal tubules.
- Carbamazepine: Used to enhance the release of ADH or augment its effects on the renal tubules (see Table 8–2).
- Thiazide diuretics: Can be used to reduce polyuria or nephrogenic and central DI by reducing urine output. This is caused by sodium depletion. The thiazides are effective in conjunction with dietary salt restriction (see Table 1–13, p. 76).
- Aqueous vasopressin: Administered subcutaneously or intramuscularly at a dose of 5 to 10 U when a short-acting agent (4 to 6 hours) is required (see Table 8–2).

TABLE 8-1

TABLE 8–1. STANDARD ADH LABORATORY TESTS

Test	Purpose	Normal Value	Abnormal Findings
ADH (serum)	Differentiates diagnoses of pituitary diabetes insipidus, nephrogenic diabetes insipidus (SIADH)	1–5 pg/mL	Elevated value: SIADH, hyperthyroidism, adrenal insufficiency, hemorrhage or shock, stress, pain Reduced value: Diabetes insipidus
Osmolality (serum)	Evaluates diluting and concentrating ability of kidneys Assists in differential diagnosis of syndrome of SIADH	Range: 50–1,400 mOsm/kg Average: 300–800 mOsm/kg	Elevated value: Diabetes insipidus, ketotic and nonketonic hyperglycemic states, Addison's disease, hypercalcemia Reduced value: is caused by water diuresis, inhibition of ADH, diabetes insipidus, thyroid hormone release
Water deprivation test (urine)	To diagnose diabetes insipidus	Urine flow decreased to ≤0.5 mL/min Urine osmolality ≥800 mOsm/L	Elevated value: Diabetes insipidus or decreased concentration ability
Vasopressin test	Differentiates diagnosis of pituitary diabetes insipidus, nephrogenic diabetes insipidus, and SIADH	1–5 pg/mL (ng/L)	Elevated level: May indicate SIADH as a result of hypothyroidism, Addison's disease, cirrhosis of the liver, infectious hepatitis, severe hemorrhage, or circulatory problems Reduced level: Pituitary diabetes insipidus resulting from hypothalamic tumor, viral infection, metastatic disease, sarcoidosis, head trauma, or neurosurgical procedures

ADH, antidiuretic hormone; SIADH, syndrome of inappropriate antidiuretic hormone.
Dolan JT, 1991; Ford RD, 1987; Loeb S, 1991.

TABLE 8-2

TABLE 8–2. DRUGS ACTING ON THE ENDOCRINE SYSTEM

Drug	Route/Dose	Purpose	Side Effects
Antihypertensive			
Prazosin hydrochloride (Minipress)	PO: Start with 1 mg at bedtime, then 1 mg bid or tid; may increase to 20 mg/d in divided doses	Treats hypertension	Dizziness, headache, vertigo, depression, edema, dyspnea, palpitations, tachycardia, angina, blurred vision, nausea, vomiting, diarrhea, urinary frequency, rash, pruritus, diaphoresis
Guanethidine sulfate	PO: 10 mg/d and may be increased by 10 mg q 5–7 d up to 300 mg/d	Treats moderate to severe hypertension	Marked orthostatic and exertional hypotension with dizziness, edema with weight gain, blurred vision, bradycardia, severe diarrhea, nausea, vomiting, urinary retention, dry mouth

TABLE 8-2

TABLE 8–2. CONTINUED

Drug	Route/Dose	Purpose	Side Effects
Phenoxybenzamine hydrochloride	PO: 5–10 mg bid; may increase by 10 mg/d at 4-d intervals to desired response; usual range 20–60 mg/d in 2–3 divided doses	Treats pheochromo-cytoma	Nasal congestion, postural hypotension, tachycardia, dizziness, fainting, drowsiness, weakness, lethargy, confusion, headache, vomiting, shock
Antidiuretics			
Desmopressin acetate	DI Intranasal: 0.1–0.4 mL in 1–3 divided doses IV/SC: 2–4 μg in two divided doses	Controls and prevents complications of central DI	Transient headache, drowsiness, nausea, listlessness, nasal irritation, mild abdominal cramps, shortness of breath, slight increase in blood pressure
Vasopressin (Pitressin)	DI: IM/SC 5–10 U aqueous solution 2–4 times/d (5–60 U/d) Intranasal: Apply as transient intranasal spray	Antidiuretic agent to treat DI Treats polyuria from ADH deficiency	Rash, tremor, nausea, vomiting, anaphylaxis, pounding in head, cardiac arrest, water intoxication, sweating, bronchoconstriction
Antithyroid Agent			
Methimazole	Hyperthyroidism PO: 5–15 mg q 8 h	Treats hyperthyroidism and before surgery or radiotherapy of thyroid	
Potassium Iodide (SSKI)	Reduce thyroid vascularity PO: 50–250 mg tid for 10–14 d before surgery Adjunct to manage thyroid crisis IV: 500 mg q 6 h	Treats hyperthyroidism or in conjunction with antithyroid agents	Diarrhea, nausea, vomiting, angioneurotic edema, fever, frontal headache, hypothyroidism, irregular heartbeat, confusion, weakness, productive cough
Propylthiouracil (PTU)	Hyperthyroidism PO: 300–450 mg/d divided q 8 h; might initially need 600–1200 mg/d	Treats hyperthyroidism, hyperthyroidism associated with thyroiditis, and iodine-induced thyrotoxicosis	Headache, vertigo, drowsiness, nausea, vomiting, diarrhea, loss of taste, enlarged thyroid, dizziness, unusual weight gain, skin rash, urticaria, pruritus
Corticosteroid			
Dexamethasone (Decadron)	Allergies or inflammation PO: 0.25–4 mg bid to qid IM: 8–16 mg q 1–3 wk or 0.8–1.6 mg q 1–3 wk Cerebral edema IV: 10 mg followed by 4 mg q 4 h, reduce dose after 2–4 d, then can be tapered over 5–7 d	Treats adrenal insufficiency, cerebral edema, or addisonian shock	Nasal irritation, dryness, epistaxis, euphoria, vertigo, headache, edema, hyperglycemia, heartburn, bowel perforation, oral candidiasis, impaired wound healing, petechiae, diaphoresis

TABLE 8-2

TABLE 8–2. CONTINUED

Drug	Route/Dose	Purpose	Side Effects
Dexamethasone (*cont.*)	Shock IV: 1–6 mg/kg as a single dose or 40 mg repeated q 2–6 h if needed		
Hydrocortisone (Cortisol)	Adrenal insufficiency PO: 10–320 mg/d in 3–4 divided doses MV: 15–800 mg/d in 3–4 divided doses up to 2 g/d	Replacement therapy in adrenocortical insufficiency, remission in nonadrenal disease, and block ACTH production in diagnostic tests	Vertigo, headache, syncopal episodes, palpitation, tachycardia, hyperglycemia, blurred vision, sodium and fluid retention, nausea, increased appetite, osteoporosis, acne, impaired wound healing, masking of infections, hypersensitivity
Fludrocortisone acetate (Florinef Acetate)	Adrenocortical insufficiency PO: 0.1 mg/d; may range from 0.1 mg 3 times/wk to 0.2 mg/d	Partial replacement therapy for adrenocortical insufficiency	Vertigo, headache, mental disturbances, insomnia, syncopal episodes, thromboembolism, palpitation, tachycardia, hyperglycemia, blurred vision, sodium and fluid retention, nausea, increased appetite, hypersensitivity reactions, malaise, weight gain, easy bruising
Enzyme Inhibitor			
Metyrosine (Demser)	Pheochromocytoma PO: 250 mg qid and may increase to 2–3 g/d in divided doses for a maximum of 4 g/d	Short-term management until surgery is performed or in patients with malignant pheochromocytoma	Sedation, fatigue, tremors, confusion, headache, diarrhea, nausea, rash, oliguria, peripheral edema
Lipid Lowering Agent			
Clofibrate (Claripex)	DI PO: 1.5–2.0 g/d in 2–4 divided doses	Treats DI	Drowsiness, dizziness, headache, dysrhythmias, nausea, diarrhea, flatulence, abdominal distress, skin rash, tremor, diaphoresis
Radiopharmaceutical			
Sodium iodide I131 (Iodotope I131)	Hyperthyroidism PO: 4–10 MCi as a single dose, second dose if needed after 6 wk	Treats hyperthyroidism and thyrotoxicosis and suppresses neoplastic disease of thyroid	Primary hypothyroidism, angioedema, petechiae, transient thyroiditis, alopecia, or thyroid nodules

TABLE 8-2

TABLE 8–2. CONTINUED

Drug	Route/Dose	Purpose	Side Effects
Thyroid Agent			
Levothyroxine sodium (Synthroid)	Thyroid replacement PO: 25–50 μg/d and gradually increase by 50–100 μg q 1–4 wk to a dose of 100–400 μg/d IV: 1/2 of normal oral dose Myxedema crisis IV: 250–500 μg IV stat, then 100–300 μg after 24 h if necessary; then 50–200 μg/d until stability achieved and oral intake possible	Replacement therapy for reduced or absent thyroid function resulting from atrophy, surgery, or anti-thyroid drugs, to mention a few uses	Irritability, nervousness, insomnia, headache, tremors, palpitations, tachycardia, angina pectoris, hypertension, nausea, diarrhea

ACTH, Corticotropin (formerly adrenocorticotropic hormone); DI, diabetes insipidus, IM, intramuscularly; IV, intravenously; PO, by mouth, SC, subcutaneously.

Deglin JH and Vallerand AH, 1993; Loeb S, 1993; Shannon MT and Wilson BA, 1992.

FLUID THERAPY

- Hypotonic saline: Hypotonic saline, such as quarter-strength or half-strength saline, are titrated to hourly urine output. The titration may be: 500 mL urine output for 1 hour is replaced by a 500 mL IV fluid bolus the next hour.

NURSING MANAGEMENT: NURSING DIAGNOSES AND COLLABORATIVE PROBLEMS

Nursing Diagnoses

Common nursing goals for patients with DI are to restore fluid volume, prevent injury, maintain skin integrity, and prevent fatigue.

Fluid volume deficit related to abnormal urinary fluid loss secondary to increased ADH.

Expected Patient Outcomes. Patient maintains adequate fluid volume, as evidenced by blood pressure (BP) within patient's normal range, mean arterial pressure (MAP) 70 to 100 mm Hg, urinary output (UO) ≥30 mL/h and ≤200 mL/h, body weight within 5% of baseline, normal skin turgor, serum osmolality 285 to 295 mOsm/kg, specific gravity 1.010 to 1.025, heart rate (HR) ≤100 bpm, central venous pressure (CVP) 2 to 6 mm Hg, and capillary refill ≤3 seconds.

- Consult with physician to validate expected patient outcomes used to evaluate fluid balance.
- Review values for serum osmolality, sodium, potassium; urine sodium, osmolality, and specific gravity.
- Provide prescribed diets with low sodium and no excess protein.
- Obtain and report hemodynamic parameters indicating decreased fluid volume: CVP ≤2 mm Hg and pulmonary capillary wedge pressure (PCWP) ≤6 mm Hg.
- Obtain and report clinical findings associated with fluid volume deficit: hypotension, tachycardia, poor skin turgor, dry mucous membrane, cool skin, and confusion.
- Measure intake, output, specific gravity, and daily weight for fluid balance. Report intake 4 to 6 L/24 h, UO 4 to 6 L/24 h, specific gravity ≤1.003, and weight loss.
- Monitor continuous ECG to assess HR and rhythm. Document ECG rhythm strips every 2 to 4 hours or more frequently in patients with dysrhythmias.
- Evaluate patient for ADH replacement side effects: diaphoresis, tremor, headache, nau-

sea, abdominal or uterine cramps, diarrhea, hypotension, or angina.
- Prepare patient for surgery: transsphenoidal hypophysectomy.
- Provide IV fluids and electrolytes to restore fluid balance, correct dehydration, and maintain electrolyte balance.
- Administer ADH replacement therapy: Desmopressin acetate intranasally 5 to 10 μg once or twice a day; or vasopressin (Pitressin) 0.5 to 1 mL intramuscularly.
- Administer hydrochlorothiazide (Hydro-DIURIL) 50 to 100 mg/d with potassium chloride to reduce the urine volume in nephrogenic DI.
- Administer chlorpropamide (Diabinese) to foster ADH's activity on the renal tubule: initial dose 250 mg twice a day and maintained as 125 to 250 mg/d.
- Administer other drugs with antidiuretic activity if not contraindicated: clofibrate or carbamazepine (see Table 8–12).

High risk for injury related to thromboembolism secondary to hemoconcentration.

Expected Patient Outcomes. Patient is free of thromboembolism injury, as evidenced by normal coagulation studies; absence of calf pain, tenderness, or swelling; good peripheral skin color and warmth; palpable peripheral pulses +2; respiratory rate (RR) 12 to 20 BPM and HR ≤100 bpm.

- Consult with physician to validate expected patient outcomes used to evaluate for the presence of thromboembolism.
- Review results of coagulation studies, chest roentgenogram, and arterial blood gas measurements.
- Obtain and report clinical findings associated with thromboembolism: tachycardia, tachypnea, cyanosis, extremity pain and swelling, peripheral pulses ≤+2, and capillary refill ≥3 seconds.
- Encourage patient to change position frequently to avoid stasis of circulation.
- Encourage patient to drink iced fluids to assist in maintaining adequate hydration.

- Measure intake, output, specific gravity, and daily weight to determine fluid balance.
- Assist with range-of-motion (ROM) exercises, if appropriate, for 5 to 10 minutes every 1 to 2 hours to increase venous return and decrease venous pooling in the extremities.
- Provide antithromboembolic stockings.
- Administer prescribed IV hypotonic saline solutions to maintain adequate hydration and circulatory volume.
- Administer prescribed hormone replacement such as lysine vasopressin nasal spray at dose of 5 to 20 U several times per day; desmopressin at dose of 10 to 20 μg; or aqueous pitressin at dose of 2 to 4 U.
- Administer prescribed nonhormonal agents: chlorpropamide (250 to 500 mg daily); carbamazepine (400 to 600 mg daily) or clofibrate (500 mg) in patients with partial central DI, some residual ADH function, or nephrogenic DI (see Table 8–2).
- Administer prescribed nonhormonal agents for nephrogenic DI: thiazide diuretics (50 to 100 mg daily).
- Teach patient the purpose of changing position and avoiding crossing legs.

Impaired skin integrity related to dehydration.

Expected Patient Outcome. Patient's skin remains intact.

- Maintain adequate protein intake as prescribed.
- Encourage patient to frequently change position to avoid skin breakdown.
- Massage bony prominences to ensure circulation and maintain skin integrity.
- Provide supplemental padding for bony pressure points.
- Provide ice chips if patient is alert or swab patient's mouth with them or lubricant.
- Evaluate skin for presence of redness, breakdown, turgor, dryness, color, or warmth.
- Assist with ROM exercises to increase venous return.

Fatigue related to excess fluid loss or electrolyte imbalance.

Expected Patient Outcomes. Absence of fatigue and serum electrolytes within normal range.

- Review serum electrolyte, hemoglobin, and hematocrit values.
- Provide rest before and after activity.
- Encourage patient to gradually increase activity while assessing his or her own fatigue level.
- Cluster interventions to avoid fatigue.
- Teach patient to identify when he or she experiences fatigue.

Collaborative Problems

Common collaborative goals for patients with DI are to correct electrolyte imbalance and increase cardiac output.

Potential Complication: Electrolyte Imbalance.
Electrolyte imbalance related to hypernatremia secondary to excess water loss.

Expected Patient Outcomes. Patient maintains electrolyte balance, as evidenced by serum sodium 135 to 148 mEq/L, urinary sodium 80 to 180 mEq/L, absence of fatigue, normal skin color, HR ≤100 bpm, BP within patient's normal range, normothermia, flat neck veins, and UO ≥30 mL/h or ≤200 mL/h.

- Review results serum sodium and osmolality.
- Obtain and report clinical findings associated with hypernatremia: lethargy, fatigue, hypotension, tachycardia, poor skin turgor, flushed skin, thirst, and low-grade fever.
- Measure intake, output, specific gravity, and body weight. Report UO ≤30 mL/h or ≥200 mL/h and a rapid decrease in weight (0.5 to 1.0 kg/d).
- Encourage fluids low in sodium such as distilled water, coffee, tea, and orange juice.
- Assist patient with position changes or ambulation because orthostatic changes can occur while patient is volume-depleted.
- Administer prescribed IV hypotonic saline to replace pure water deficit.
- Teach patient to report signs and symptoms of hypernatremia.

Potential Complication: Decreased Cardiac Output.
Cardiac output decreased related to excess volume loss.

Expected Patient Outcomes. Patient maintains adequate cardiac output (CO), as evidenced by CO 4 to 8 L/min, cardiac index (CI) 2.7 to 4.3 L/min/m², CVP 2 to 6 mm Hg, BP within patient's normal range, HR ≤100 bpm, peripheral pulses +2, capillary refill ≥3 seconds, UO ≥30 mL/h and ≤200 mL/h, and PCWP 6 to 12 mm Hg.

- Consult with physician to validate expected patient outcomes used to evaluate CO.
- Limit physical activity to bed rest while hemodynamics are labile.
- Assess clinical indicators of perfusion: BP, HR, cardiac rhythm, MAP, capillary refill, skin color and warmth, and peripheral pulses.
- Report clinical findings associated with decreased CO: tachycardia, hypotension, peripheral pulses ≤+2, capillary refill ≥3 seconds, pallor or cyanosis, and poor skin turgor.
- Obtain and report hemodynamic parameters indicating decreased CO: CO ≤4 L/min, CI ≤2.7 L/min/m², CVP ≤2 mm Hg, and PCWP ≤6 mm Hg.
- Measure daily weight, intake, specific gravity, or UO to determine fluid balance.
- Monitor continuous ECG to assess HR and rhythm. Document ECG rhythm strips every 2 to 4 hours or more frequently in patients with dysrhythmias.
- Administer IV hypotonic saline solution to maintain adequate hydration and circulatory volume.

DISCHARGE PLANNING

The critical care nurse will provide patient and significant other(s) with verbal or written discharge notes regarding the following subjects:

1. Importance of keeping all postdischarge medical appointments.
2. Signs and symptoms of diabetes insipidus that need to be reported to physician:

polyuria, polydipsia, specific gravity ≤1.005, hypotension, and tachycardia.
3. Medications, including their purpose, dose, route, schedule, and side effects.
4. Importance of adhering to medication regimen and necessity of wearing a Medic Alert identification bracelet.

■ SYNDROME OF INAPPROPRIATE ADH SECRETION

(For related information see Respiratory, Part I: Emphysema, p. 352. Renal, Part I: Hypokalemia, p. 485 and Hypocalcemia, p. 489. Neurological, Part I: Cerebral hemorrhage, p. 607).

Case Management Basis
DRG: 300 Endocrine disorders with complications
LOS: 6.90 days
DRG: 301 Endocrine disorders without complications
LOS: 4.10 days

Definition
Syndrome of inappropriate antidiuretic hormone (ADH) (SIADH) is due to the oversecretion of ADH despite low serum osmolality and expanded extracellular fluid volume.

Pathophysiology
In SIADH there is a failure in the negative feedback mechanisms that regulate the release and inhibition of ADH. The kidneys respond by reabsorbing water in the tubules and excreting sodium. Water retention occurs to the point of hyponatremic expansion of the extracellular fluid volume with secondary natriuresis.

Nursing Assessment

PRIMARY CAUSES
• Ectopic ADH occurs from malignancies such as oat cell type, lymphoid tissue, or gastrointestinal tract. Causal central nervous system disorders include brain tumors, hemorrhagic state, cerebral atrophy, head trauma, infectious meningitis, encephalitis, or brain abscess. Guillain-Barré syndrome, and lupus erythematosus. Causative nonmalignant pulmonary conditions are viral pneumonia, tuberculosis, chronic obstructive pulmonary disease, and lung abscesses. Drugs such as nicotine, carbamazepine, chlorpropamide, barbiturates, analgesics, antineoplastic drugs, anesthetics, or tricyclic antidepressants can cause SIADH.

PHYSICAL ASSESSMENT
• Inspection: Headache, irritability, lethargy, confusion, seizure, dulled sensorium, disorientation, muscle cramps, anorexia, nausea, vomiting, impaired taste, weight gain, diarrhea, abdominal cramps, weakness, twitching, hypothermia, coma.
• Percussion: Diminished deep tendon reflex.

DIAGNOSTIC TEST RESULTS

Standard Laboratory Tests
• Serum chemistry: Hypososmolality ≤275 mOsm/kg, potassium ≤3.8 mEq/L, calcium ≤8.5 mg/dL, and reduced blood urea nitrogen (BUN) and albumin.
• Urinalysis: Urine osmolality is normal or greater (≥900 mOsm/kg) than serum osmolality, urine sodium increased, (≥200 mEq/L), and specific gravity increased (≥1.030).
• Water Load Test: To prevent side effects from the fluid load, the patient must have a sodium level greater than 125 mmol/L and must not display any symptoms of hyponatremia. Patient is given a fluid challenge (20 mL/kg) and urinary output is measured over the next 5 to 6 hrs. In SIADH, less than 40 percent of water load is excreted and urine sodium is increased.
• Plasma arginine vasopressin: Levels are elevated or high normal but are inappropriate for plasma osmolality.

MEDICAL AND SURGICAL MANAGEMENT

PHARMACOLOGY
• Phenytoin: Used to reduce ADH secretion (see Table 7–4, p. 614).

- Demeclocycline or lithium: Used to decrease renal responsiveness to ADH. Oral demeclocycline is administered at a dose of 600 to 1200 mg/d, which can restore serum sodium levels within 2 weeks.
- Furosemide (Lasix): This potent loop diuretic is used to decrease the tubular reabsorption of sodium, thereby increasing the urinary excretion of sodium and water (see Table 1–13, p. 76).
- Potassium supplement: Used to correct hypokalemia.

FLUID THERAPY

- Fluid intake is restricted to 800 to 1000 mL/d. Fluid intake is not to exceed the urine output until the serum sodium levels are normal.
- In patients with hyponatremia, a 250 to 500 mL infusion of a hypertonic solution (3% sodium chloride) is used during a 2 to 4 hour period.

NURSING MANAGEMENT: NURSING DIAGNOSES AND COLLABORATIVE PROBLEMS

Nursing Diagnoses

Common nursing goals for patients with SIADH are to maintain fluid balance, prevent injury, support cognitive function, and increase urinary elimination.

Fluid volume excess related to compromised regulatory mechanism secondary to excessive ADH secretion.

Expected Patient Outcomes. Patient maintains adequate fluid volume, as evidenced by urinary output (UO) ≤30 mL/h, specific gravity 1.003 to 1.035, heart rate (HR) ≤100 bpm, blood pressure (BP) within patient's normal range, central venous pressure (CVP) 2 to 6 mm Hg, pulmonary capillary wedge pressure (PCWP) 6 to 12 mm Hg, alertness, normal deep tendon reflexes, serum electrolytes and osmolality within normal range, and absence of edema.

- Consult with physician to validate expected patient outcomes used to determine the presence of fluid balance in patients with SIADH.
- Review values of serum electrolytes, osmolality, hemoglobin, hematocrit, urine sodium and osmolality.
- Obtain and report hemodynamic parameters indicating fluid volume excess: CVP ≥6 mm Hg and PCWP ≥12 mm Hg.
- Obtain and report neurological clinical findings associated with fluid volume excess: confusion, irritability, sense of impending doom, restlessness, sluggish deep tendon reflexes, or seizures.
- Obtain and report other clinical findings associated with fluid volume excess: tachycardia, nausea, vomiting, and minimal postural or orthostatic hypotension.
- Measure intake, urine output, and specific gravity for fluid balance every 8 hours. Report fluctuation in UO and serial weight gain 0.5 to 1.0 kg/d.
- Continuously monitor ECG to assess HR and rhythm. Document ECG rhythm strips every 2 to 4 hours in patients with dysrhythmias.
- Restrict fluids as prescribed ≤500 mL/d in severe cases and 800 to 1000 mL/d in moderate SIADH.
- Provide chilled beverages when fluids are restricted. Distribute fluids throughout the day.
- Encourage patient to select fluids high in sodium content such as milk, tomato juice, beef or chicken broth.
- Provide frequent mouth care and oral rinsing without swallowing.
- Encourage patient to change position frequently and deep breathe to prevent atelectasis.
- Administer prescribed phenytoin or demeclocycline to inhibit renal response to ADH.
- Administer prescribed furosemide followed by infusion of hypertonic saline (3% saline). Furosemide decreases the tubular reabsorption of sodium and replacement of sodium losses with hypertonic saline leads to a net loss of free water.

High risk for injury related to seizure activity secondary to severe hyponatremia.

Expected Patient Outcomes. Patient is free of injury, as evidenced by absence of seizure activity, being alert and oriented to person, place and time; and serum sodium 135 to 145 mEq/L.

- Review serum electrolyte values. Seizures and irreversible brain damage can occur when the serum sodium level ≤110 to 115 mmol/L.
- Assess clinical indicators of neurological status: level of consciousness; orientation to time, place, and person; or sensorimotor activity.
- Initiate seizure precautions if necessary.
- Institute safety measures by keeping side rails up and padded should hyponatremia be severe.
- Evaluate patient's immediate environment for factors that could cause injury during seizure activity.
- Monitor volume status and sodium level to avoid potential seizure activity.
- Maintain patent airway during seizure episode.
- Assist patient to remove excess oral secretions after seizure episode.
- Administer anticonvulsant agents as prescribed.

Altered thought processes related to water intoxication, hyponatremia, and cerebral swelling.

Expected Patient Outcome. Patient alert, with memory intact and confusion absent.

- Assess clinical indicators of neurological status: level of consciousness (LOC), memory, reasoning, and attention span.
- Report clinical findings associated with altered thought process as a result of water intoxication and hyponatremia: confusion, irritability, restlessness, short attention span, fatigue, headache, nausea, vomiting, and decreased LOC.
- Encourage patient to ask questions or verbalize concerns about feelings of confusion.
- Provide explanations of illness, manifestations, or treatment in a clear and concise manner.

- Instruct patient and family as to temporary causes of altered thought process.

Altered pattern of urinary elimination related to increased ADH secretion.

Expected Patient Outcome. Patient maintains adequate urinary elimination, as evidenced by UO ≥30 mL/h or ≥0.5 mL/kg/h and specific gravity 1.003 to 1.025.

- Review levels of serum electrolytes, BUN, creatinine, osmolality, and urine sodium and osmolality.
- Measure intake, output, specific gravity, and daily weight. Report UO ≤30 mL/h, specific gravity ≤1.003, and weight gain ≥0.5 to 1.0 lb/d.
- Restrict fluid intake as prescribed to ≤500 mg/d in severe cases or 800 to 1000 mL/d in moderate cases.
- Administer volume-reducing agents (furosemide).

Collaborative Problems
- A common collaborative goal for patients with SIADH is to prevent electrolyte imbalance.

Potential Complication: Electrolyte Imbalance. Electrolyte imbalance related to hyponatremia, hypokalemia, and hypocalcemia secondary to water intoxication.

Expected Patient Outcomes. Patient maintains electrolyte balance, as evidenced by serum potassium 3.5 to 5.0 mEq/L, serum sodium 135 to 145 mEq/L, and serum calcium 4.5 to 5.5 mg/dL.

- Review levels of serum potassium, calcium, and sodium.
- Obtain and report clinical findings associated with hypocalcemia: hyperflexia, tetany, altered peripheral sensation, disorientation, tachycardia, seizure, labored breathing, carpal and pedal spasm, numbness, twitching, and abdominal cramps.
- Monitor continuous ECG to assess HR and rhythm in patients with hypocalcemia: prolonged QT interval and palpitation.

- Initiate seizure precautions by padding side rails, minimizing stimulation, and assisting patient with all activities.
- Administer prescribed 10% calcium gluconate for symptomatic hypocalcemia at a rate of 1 mL/min for replacement.
- Obtain and report clinical findings associated with hypokalemia: shortness of breath, hypoactive reflexes, numbness, cramps, weakness, paralysis, gastrointestinal irritability or distention.
- Monitor continuous ECG to assess HR and rhythm in patient with hypokalemia: flat T waves, U waves, peaked P waves, ST segments, or dysrhythmias.
- Administer prescribed IV potassium at a rate not to exceed 20 mEq/100 mL/h.
- Obtain and report clinical findings associated with hyponatremia: irritability, lethargy, confusion, malaise, edema, flushed skin, bounding pulse, crackles, dyspnea, headache, abdominal cramps, nausea, and seizure.
- Measure daily weight within 2% to 5% of baseline, intake, specific gravity 1.030, and UO.
- Administer prescribed IV 3% saline, 0.45 normal saline (NS) or 0.9 NS solution.

DISCHARGE PLANNING

The critical care nurse will provide patient and significant other(s) with verbal or written discharge notes regarding the following subjects:

1. Importance of keeping all postdischarge medical appointments.
2. Signs and symptoms associated with altered thought process caused by water intoxication and hyponatremia: confusion, irritability, restlessness, short attention span, fatigue, headache, nausea, vomiting, and decreased LOC.
3. Importance of having a kit of hydrocortisone to be used in an emergency. Teach patient and family the proper administration technique.
4. Significance of taking daily weight as an indicator of fluid status.

5. Medications, including their purpose, dose, route, schedule, and side effects.
6. Importance of maintaining adequate salt and potassium in diet, especially if diuretics are prescribed.
7. Importance of adhering to medication regimen and necessity of wearing a Medic Alert identification bracelet.

■ DIABETIC KETOACIDOSIS

(*For related information see Part I: Hyperglycemic hyperosmolar nonketotic coma (HHNK), p. 698. See also Psychosocial Deviations, Part I, p. 725.*)

Case Management Basis
DRG: 294 Diabetes, age greater than 35
LOS: 5.80 days
DRG: 295 Diabetes, age 0–35
LOS: 4.40 days

Definition
- Diabetic ketoacidosis (DKA) is an acute metabolic disorder in which an underlying pathophysiological process is attributed to an absolute or relative lack of insulin. DKA is associated with hyperglycemia, ketonemia, fluid and electrolyte imbalance, and a negative nitrogen balance.

Pathophysiology
The primary metabolic abnormalities involved in DKA are reduced glucose uptake by muscle cells, accelerated glucose production in the liver, and increased metabolism of free fatty acids into ketone bodies within the liver. The kidneys attempt to neutralize the ketone anions by excreting ketones in the urine (ketonuria). Respiratory compensation for acidosis leads to deep, accelerated respiration (Kussmaul's respiration). The elevated blood glucose levels and subsequent serum hyperosmolality cause osmotic fluid shifts, osmotic diuresis, and intracellular and extracellular dehydration. Electrolyte imbalance and metabolic acidosis occur.

Nursing Management

PRIMARY CAUSES

- Insulin-dependent diabetes mellitus (IDDM), physical and emotional stress, autoimmune destruction of beta islet cells, or genetic susceptibility; pregnancy can potentiate DKA, and medication can interfere with insulin secretion (thiazide diuretics, phenytoin, glucocorticoids, and sympathomimetics).

PHYSICAL ASSESSMENT

- Inspection: Polyuria, polydipsia, weakness, nausea, anorexia, vomiting, drowsiness, fatigue, headache, fruity odor to breath, transient hemiparesis, or flushed skin.
- Palpation: Poor skin turgor, abdominal pain and tenderness, or cool skin from hypothermia.
- Percussion: Diminished deep tendon reflexes.
- Auscultation: Tachycardia, hypotension, or tachypnea.

DIAGNOSTIC TEST RESULTS

Hemodynamic Parameters

- Alterations include central venous pressure (CVP) ≤2 mm Hg and pulmonary capillary wedge pressure (PCWP) ≤6 mm Hg.

Standard Laboratory Tests

- Arterial blood gases: pH ≤7.20 and bicarbonate (HCO_3) ≤10 mEq/L.
- Cultures: Throat, sputum, blood, urine, stool, or invasive sites.
- Serum chemistry: Glucose 350 to 750 mg/dL, hypercalcemia, hyponatremia, hypophosphatemia ≤1.0 mg/100mL, elevated amylase, hypomagnesemia, hyperkalemia, blood urea nitrogen (BUN), hematocrit, ketonemia, and fatty acids; osmolality ≤330 mOsm/kg; leukocytosis ≤25,000/μL; and anion gap ≥15 mmol/L.
- Urinalysis: Glycosuria +4, elevated acetone, ketonuria, trace sodium, reduced chloride and specific gravity ≥1.025.

EKG

- Reveals hyperkalemia: Peaked T waves, widened QRS, prolonged P-R intervals, flattened to absent P wave.
- Hypokalemia: Flat or inverted T waves, depressed ST segments or increased ventricular dysrhythmias.

MEDICAL AND SURGICAL MANAGEMENT

PHARMACOLOGY

- Regular insulin: Regular insulin is used to lower the severe hyperglycemia of DKA. It is administered first by bolus dose of 0.1 to 0.2 U/kg body weight, followed by continuous infusion at a dose of 0.1 to 0.2 U/kg until the blood glucose level is ≤300 mg/dL. When serum glucose is ≤300 mg/dL and pH ≥7.2, insulin infusion rate is reduced by 50%, and 5% or 10% dextrose is added to the infusion to maintain blood glucose at 250 mg/dL for first 12 to 24 hours. Normally blood glucose levels decrease at a rate of 100 mg/dL/h (see Table 6–4, p. 565).
- Potassium: Potassium chloride is added to IV fluids in amounts ranging from 0.5 mEq/kg/h for serum potassium ≤3 mEq/L to 0.1 to 0.2 mEq/Kg/h if serum potassium is 5 to 6 mEq/L. Potassium phosphate can be administered in limited amounts should hypophosphatemia occur.
- Bicarbonate: Bicarbonate is given in severe acidosis (pH ≤7.0), especially when hypotension and dysrhythmias are also present. It is administered as an infusion of 1 to 2 mEq/kg over 2 hours. The amount is not to exceed 3 mEq/kg over 12 hours.

FLUID THERAPY

- Isotonic saline is administered at a rate of 500 to 1000 mL/h for the first 2 to 4 hours. Infusion rates are slowed to 250 to 500 mL/h and 0.45% normal saline can be administered. IV fluid should be changed to 5% dextrose or 10% dextrose when the serum glucose decrease to 250 mg/dL, which permits continued insulin infusion without hyperglycemia.

NURSING MANAGEMENT: NURSING DIAGNOSES AND COLLABORATIVE PROBLEMS

Nursing Diagnoses

Common nursing goals for patients with DKA are to restore fluid balance, promote oxygenation, prevent injury, promote effective breathing pattern, maintain adequate nutrition, and support cognitive function.

Fluid volume deficit related to intravascular volume loss secondary to osmotic diuresis or failure of regulatory mechanism.

Expected Patient Outcomes. Patient maintains adequate fluid balance, as evidenced by urinary output (UO) $\geq$30 mL/h or $\leq$200 mL/h, specific gravity 1.003 to 1.035, blood pressure (BP) within patient's normal range, respiratory rate (RR) 12 to 20 BPM, heart rate (HR) $\leq$100 bpm, cardiac output (CO) 4 to 8 L/min, cardiac index (CI) 2.7 to 4.3 L/min/m^2, CVP 2 to 6 mm Hg, pulmonary artery systolic (PAS) pressure 15 to 30 mm Hg, pulmonary artery diastolic (PAD) 5 to 15 mm Hg, absence of diaphoresis, skin turgor normal, serum glucose 150 to 250 mg/dL, serum osmolality 285 to 295 mOsm/kg, serum sodium 135 to 145 mEq/L, and serum potassium 3.5 to 5.5 mEq/L.

- Consult with physician to validate expected patient outcomes used to determine fluid volume status.
- Review values of serum osmolality, electrolytes, glucose, hemoglobin, hematocrit, and urine ketones.
- Obtain and report hemodynamic parameters indicating fluid volume deficit: CO $\leq$4 L/min, CI $\leq$2.7 L/min/m^2, CVP $\leq$2 mm Hg, PAS $\leq$15 mm Hg, and PAD $\leq$5 mm Hg.
- Assess clinical indicators of hydration: BP, HR, skin turgor, peripheral pulses +2, capillary refill $\leq$3 seconds, and stable body weight.
- Report clinical findings associated with dehydration: hypotension, tachycardia, poor skin turgor, dry skin and mucous mem-branes, parched and cracked mucous membranes, extreme thirst, and weight loss.
- Monitor continuous ECG to assess HR and rhythm. Document ECG rhythm strips every 2 to 4 hours or more frequently in patients with dysrhythmias.
- Measure intake, output, specific gravity, and daily weight. Report water deficit of 6 L and weight loss $\geq$0.5 to 1.0 kg/d.
- Provide frequent oral hygiene, since dehydration can cause drying of the mucous membranes.
- Administer prescribed IV crystalloids at rate of 1000 mL/h until the patient's BP is stable and UO $\geq$60 mL/h, to correct dehydration.
- Administer prescribed regular insulin when serum glucose is $\geq$250 to 800 mg/dL.

Impaired gas exchange related to altered oxygen supply secondary to tachypnea or hyperventilation.

Expected Patient Outcomes. Patient maintains adequate gas exchange, as evidenced by RR 12 to 20 BPM, HR $\leq$100 bpm, arterial oxygen saturation (Sao$_2$, 95% to 97.5%, arterial blood gases within normal range, absence of cyanosis, capillary refill $\leq$3 seconds, and absence of adventitious breath sounds.

- Review results of arterial blood gas measurements.
- Limit physical activity to bed rest to reduce oxygen demands.
- Assess clinical indicators of respiratory status: rate, depth, symmetry of chest wall movement, skin color, lung sounds, and use of accessory muscles.
- Report clinical findings associated with impaired gas exchange: tachypnea, tachycardia, Kussmaul's respiration, acetone breath, dyspnea, cyanosis, use of accessory muscles and crackles.
- Encourage patient to turn, cough, deep breathe, and use incentive spirometer to facilitate lung expansion.
- Administer prescribed oxygen 2 to 4 L/min to maintain Sao$_2$ $\geq$95%.

- Administer prescribed IV fluids to maintain adequate hydration.
- Provide mechanical support if prescribed and based on patient's inability to remove secretions, ineffective breathing pattern, or altered level of consciousness.
- Teach patient to take deep breaths and turn frequently.

Injury, high risk for thromboembolism related to hemoconcentration or hypercoagulation.

Expected Patient Outcomes. Patient is free of injury, as evidenced by absence of calf pain, tenderness, or swelling; normal peripheral skin color and warmth; palpable peripheral pulses +2; and hemoglobin or hematocrit within normal range.

- Review results of coagulation studies.
- Assess and report for clinical findings associated with venous thrombosis: tenderness, warmth, pain, swelling, or presence of cyanosis; capillary refill ≥3 seconds; and peripheral pulses ≤+2.
- Encourage patient to change position frequently.
- Provide antithromboembolic stockings.
- Assist with range of motion (ROM) exercises for 5 to 10 minutes every 1 to 2 hours to increase venous return and decrease venous pooling in the extremities.
- Administer IV fluids as prescribed to maintain adequate hydration, thereby preventing stasis.
- Teach patient the purpose of changing position and avoiding crossing legs.

Ineffective breathing pattern related to hyperventilation secondary to ketonemia and acidemia.

Expected Patient Outcomes. Patient maintains effective breathing pattern, as evidenced by RR 12 to 20 BPM, absence of dyspnea or Kussmaul's breathing, absence of cyanosis, tidal volume ≥5 to 7 mL/kg, arterial blood gases within normal range, and vital capacity ≥15 mL/kg.

- Consult with physician to validate expected patient outcomes used to evaluate effective breathing pattern.
- Review results of arterial blood gas measurement.
- Place patient in a position of comfort.
- Assess clinical indicators of respiratory status: rate, depth, symmetry of chest wall movement, skin color, lung sounds, and use of accessory muscles.
- Evaluate tidal volume and vital capacity in relation to patient's breathing pattern and need for ventilatory support.
- Provide oxygen by nasal cannula or Venturi mask at the prescribed amount.
- Administer IV fluids at the prescribed amount to maintain adequate hydration.

Alterated nutrition: less than body requirements related to impaired glucose utilization secondary to insulin deficiency.

Expected Patient Outcomes. Patient maintains adequate nutritional intake, as evidenced by stable weight, serum glucose ≤250 mg/dL, and positive nitrogen balance.

- Consult with dietitian regarding patient's specific nutritional needs.
- Review results of serum glucose, ketones, electrolyte, and arterial blood gas measurement.
- Provide prescribed diet to keep serum glucose between 250 and 300 mg/dL or less with no ketones in the urine.
- Measure intake, output, specific gravity, and daily weight. Report UO ≤30 mL/h or ≥200 mL/h and weight loss ≥0.5 to 1.0 kg/d.
- Perform prescribed finger-stick glucose monitoring to obtain a bedside analysis of serum glucose.
- Administer prescribed IV dextrose 5% in 0.45 normal saline infusion when serum glucose drops to 250 mg/dL in the presence of insulin therapy.
- Administer prescribed insulin by continuous or intermittent IV infusion.
- Teach patient the relationship between diet, exercise, and insulin therapy.

Altered thought processes related to impaired cerebral cellular glucose utilization secondary to hyperglycemia.

Expected Patient Outcomes. Patient maintains normal thought process, as evidenced by serum glucose 150 to 250 mg/dL; alertness; oriented to person, time, and place; and absence of serum ketones.

- Review levels of serum glucose and ketones and urine ketones.
- Assess clinical indicators of neurological status: level of consciousness, orientation, sensorimotor function, deep tendon reflexes, ability to concentrate, ability to make decisions.
- Report clinical findings associated with neurological changes related to hyperglycemia: headache, lethargy, irritability, disorientation, and sensorimotor dysfunction.
- Insert nasogastric (NG) tube to reduce risk of vomiting and aspiration in patients with altered level of consciousness.
- Orient patient to person, time, and place.
- Listen to patient's verbalization of fears and concerns.
- Evaluate patient's readiness for learning.
- Keep explanations simple, clear, and concise.
- Encourage patient to cough, turn and deep breathe to lessen the risk of pulmonary stasis and atelectasis.
- Reposition the unconscious patient every 1 to 2 hours.
- Assist with intubation and mechanical ventilation in patients who are unable to maintain a patent airway, handle excess secretions, or maintain gas exchange.
- Suction patient as necessary following unit protocol.
- Administer prescribed regular insulin at dose of 10 U by IV bolus, followed by continuous insulin infusion of 100 U/100 mL normal saline (NS) infused at 5 to 10 U/hr (0.1 U/kg) to keep serum glucose $\leq$250 mg/dL. Serum glucose levels should decrease 40 to 80 mg/dL/h.

- Administer prescribed dextrose (D_5W) infused at 5 to 20 g/h when serum glucose is 250 to 300 mg/dL, urine ketones are absent, and pH is $\geq$7.2.

Collaborative Problems

Common collaborative goals for patients with DKA are to correct electrolyte imbalance, prevent metabolic acidosis, correct dysrhythmias, correct hyperglycemia, and increase cardiac output.

Potential Complication: Electrolyte Imbalance. Electrolyte imbalance related to electrolyte shift secondary to profound osmotic diuresis.

Expected Patient Outcomes. Patient maintains electrolyte balance, as evidenced by being oriented to person, time, and place; body weight within 5% baseline; UO $\geq$30mL/h and $\leq$200mL/h; serum electrolytes within normal range; serum osmolality 285 to 295 mOsm/kg; serum glucose 70 to 110 mg/100 mL; urine sodium 80 to 180 mEq/L; specific gravity 1.010 to 1.025; and urine negative for glucose and acetone.

- Review levels of serum electrolytes, osmolality, glucose, and urine sodium, urine, acetone, and osmolality.
- Continuously monitor ECG for changes associated with hyperkalemia: flattened P waves, tented T waves, a widened QRS interval, and a prolonged PR internal. Document ECG changes associated with hypokalemia, which include peaked P waves, flattened T waves, prominent U waves, and ST depression.
- Obtain and report clinical findings associated with hyperkalemia, which occurs in the presence of hyponatremia and acidosis (for every 0.1 decrease in pH while serum potassium increases by 0.6 mEq/L): weak, slow, and irregular pulse; irritability; restlessness; anxiety, abdominal cramps; weakness; nausea; and vomiting.
- Obtain and report clinical findings associated with hypokalemia when fluid re-

placement and insulin therapy have been initiated: muscular weakness, hypotension, anorexia, fatigue, abdominal distention, hypoactive reflexes, dizziness, and paresthesia.

- Obtain and report clinical findings associated with hypophosphatemia occurring after implementation of fluid and insulin therapy.
- Measure intake, output, specific gravity, and body weight. Report output ≤30 mL/h or ≥200 mL/h and body weight change 0.5 to 1.0 kg/d.
- Administer prescribed IV isotonic saline 0.9 NS and 5% dextrose in 0.45 NS, which are given when serum glucose is 250 mg/100 mL.
- Withhold potassium therapy until serum potassium level returns to normal.
- Administer prescribed IV potassium replacement of 20 to 40 mEq/L.
- Administer sodium bicarbonate 1 to 2 ampules (44 mEq/50mL) added to bottle of hypotonic saline when serum pH is ≤7.0 or blood bicarbonate is ≤9 mEq/L.
- Administer phosphate replacement therapy in conjunction with potassium therapy.
- Teach patient signs and symptoms of electrolyte imbalance.

Potential Complication: Metabolic Acidosis.
Metabolic acidosis related to ketoacidosis secondary to insulin deficiency.

Expected Patient Outcomes. Patient maintains normal acid-base balance, as evidenced by arterial blood gases within normal range and anion gap ≤15 mmol/L.

- Review results of arterial blood gas and anion gap measurement.
- Obtain and report clinical findings associated with metabolic acidosis: shortness of breath, weakness, tachypnea, restlessness, impaired consciousness, or coma.
- Calculate patient's anion gap, which is determined by the following formula: Na − (Cl + HCO₃). Report anion gap ≥15 mmol/L, which indicates the presence of additional

anions such as ketones, acetoacetic and beta-hydroxybutyric acids, and acetone.
- Administer prescribed 1 ampule of sodium bicarbonate (44.6 mEq/L) when pH is ≤7.0.

Potential Complication: Dysrhythmias. Dysrhythmia related to electrolyte imbalance.

Expected Patient Outcome. Patient maintains regular sinus rhythm.

- Review results of 12-lead EKG and serum electrolyte measurement.
- Obtain and report clinical findings indicative of hyperkalemia: weakness, cramps, paresthesia of face, tingle in extremities, hypotension, dysrhythmias, anorexia, and abdominal distention.
- Obtain and report ECG changes associated with potassium 5.5 to 6.0 mmol/L: tall, peaked symmetric T wave in the precordial leads; QT interval is normal or decreased, with occasional ST depression.
- Monitor and report ECG changes associated with potassium 6.0 to 7.0 mmol/L: prolonged PR interval and QRS duration.
- Obtain and report ECG changes associated with potassium 7.0 to 8.0 mmol/L: flattened P wave; QRS complex continues to widen with increased delays in atrioventricular conduction.
- Obtain and report ECG changes associated with potassium 8.0 to 10.0 mmol/L: irregular ventricular rhythm, absent P waves, and markedly increased QRS complexes, with the eventual merging of the complexes with the T wave.
- Obtain and report ECG changes associated with potassium 10.0 to 12.0 mmol/L: ventricular fibrillation or asystole.
- Limit potassium intake in diet to reduce plasma and total body potassium content.
- Administer sodium polystyrene sulfonate (Kayexalate), mixed in water and sorbitol and given orally, rectally, or through NG tube: Renin captures potassium in the bowel and eliminates it in the feces.

- Obtain and report clinical findings associated with hypokalemia: drowsiness, confusion, apathy, irritability, muscle weakness, paresthesia, muscle pain, muscle cramps, hyporeflexia, paralysis, hypoventilation, nausea, vomiting, abdominal distention, abdominal cramps, polyurea, or nocturia.
- Monitor continuous ECG and report changes associated with hypokalemia ≤ 3.5 mEq/L, which include a depressed ST segment; flattened, inverted T wave; and U wave.
- Provide high-potassium foods or potassium supplement; liquid potassium should be well diluted to decrease gastrointestinal irritation.
- Administer prescribed IV potassium chloride in severe hypokalemia. Administer in a peripheral vein at 10 to 20 mEq/h using a concentration of 40 mEq/L.
- Obtain and report serum phosphorus level of ≤ 1.0 mg/100mL, which can cause muscle weakness and depressed myocardial contractility.
- Administer prescribed IV fluids to maintain adequate hydration.
- Administer prescribed electrolytes to correct dysrhythmias.
- Administer antiarrhythmia medications as prescribed.

Potential Complication: Decreased Cardiac Output. Decreased CO related to dehydration secondary to volume loss.

Expected Patient Outcomes. Patient maintains adequate CO, as evidenced by CO 4 to 8 L/min, CI 2.7 to 4.3 L/min/m², CVP 2 to 6 mm Hg, peripheral pulses +2, capillary refill ≤ 3 seconds, HR ≤ 100 bpm, absence of cyanosis, daily weight maintained within 5% of baseline, and BP within patient's normal range.

- Consult with physician to validate expected patient outcomes used to evaluate CO.
- Obtain and report hemodynamic parameters associated with decreased CO: CO ≤ 4 L/min, CI ≤ 2.7 L/min/m², and CVP ≤ 2 mm Hg.

- Measure intake, output, specific gravity, and daily weight. Report UO ≤ 30 mL/h and weight loss ≥ 0.5 to 1.0 kg/d.
- Monitor continuous ECG to assess HR and rhythm. Document ECG rhythm strips every 1 to 4 hours in patients with dysrhythmias.
- Administer prescribed IV fluids to maintain adequate hydration and restore circulatory volume.
- Provide oxygen by nasal cannula or Venturi mask at the prescribed amount.

DISCHARGE PLANNING

The critical care nurse will provide patient and significant other(s) with verbal or written discharge notes regarding the following subjects:

1. Importance of keeping all postdischarge medical appointments.
2. Teaching the causes of DKA, including the relationship of illness, infection, and stress to DKA.
3. Importance of consistently monitoring blood glucose and of urine ketone testing.
4. Importance of maintaining a diabetic program that includes diet, insulin, and exercise.
5. Signs and symptoms of hypoglycemia and hyperglycemia.
6. Importance of meetings between dietitian and physical therapist before patient is discharged to review diet and exercise schedule.
7. Name of community diabetic support groups.

■ HYPEROSMOLAR HYPERGLYCEMIC NONKETOTIC SYNDROME

(*For related information see Part I: Diabetic ketoacidosis, p. 692.*)

Case Management Basis
DRG: 294 Diabetes, age greater than 35
LOS: 5.80 days
DRG: 295 Diabetes, age 0–35
LOS: 4.40 days

Definition

Hyperglycemic hyperosmolar nonketotic syndrome (HHNK) is characterized by severe hyperglycemia, with a blood sugar $\geq$600 mg/dL, serum osmolality $\geq$330 mOsm/kg, serum bicarbonate $\geq$20 mEq/L, and moderate mental alterations.

Pathophysiology

With HHNK there is undetected hyperglycemia and reduced peripheral glucose intake. There is an imbalance in the amount of glucose produced versus the amount used by the body. When serum osmolality increases, water osmotically diffuses from the intracellular space into the extracellular space. Water loss can exceed 8012 L. High serum osmolality can depress cerebral functioning and impair the thirst center in the hypothalamus. As water loss continues, the reduced circulating volume decreases the kidneys' ability to remove glucose, thereby increasing hyperglycemia. Glycosuria occurs when the amount of glucose in the proximal renal tubule is $\geq$225 mg/min. Eventually osmotic diuresis causes increased loss of electrolytes, such as calcium, phosphate, magnesium, and potassium. The subsequent serum hyperosmolality and dehydration can cause mild or moderate lactic acidosis.

Nursing Assessment

PRIMARY CAUSES
- Causes include massive fluid loss, infection, myocardial infarction, gastrointestinal hemorrhage, uremia, hypertonic feedings, pharmacological agents, inadequate or limited access to fluids, or surgery.

PHYSICAL ASSESSMENT
- Inspection: Weakness, polyuria, polydipsia, lethargy, confusion, visual hallucination, seizure, or coma.
- Palpation: Poor skin turgor and cool skin.
- Auscultation: Tachycardia, hypotension, or tachypnea.

DIAGNOSTIC TEST RESULTS

Standard Laboratory Tests
- Arterial blood gases: pH $\geq$7.20 and HCO_3 $\geq$10mEq/L.
- Cultures: Throat, sputum, blood, urine, stool, or cannulation sites.
- Serum chemistry: Glucose $\geq$1000 mg/dL, hypokalemia, sodium $\geq$140 mEq/L, osmolality $\geq$350 mOsm/kg with mean 405 mOsm/kg, hypophosphatemia, hypomagnesemia, hypercalcemia, blood urea nitrogen (BUN) $\geq$80 mg/100mL, BUN:creatinine ratio $\geq$1.10, anion gap $\leq$15 mmol/L, and ketonemia normal. Elevated hematocrit, white blood cell (WBC) count, and fatty acids.
- Urinalysis: Glycosuria, acetone normal, slight trace proteinuria, and specific gravity $\geq$1.025. Reduced sodium and chloride.

ECG
- Shows S-T segment and T wave alterations.

MEDICAL AND SURGICAL MANAGEMENT

PHARMACOLOGY
- Insulin: Intravenous bolus is administered at dose of 0.15 U/kg of regular U100 insulin, followed by an IV infusion at a rate of 0.1 U/kg/h (5 to 10 U/h). The infusion rate will steadily be reduced by 50%, 5%, or 10% dextrose added to the infusion when serum glucose reaches 250 to 300 mg/dL.
- Potassium: Potassium is replaced as 20 to 40 mmol in each liter of IV fluid. If serum potassium is $\leq$3 mEq/L, 60 mEq is infused over 1 hour.
- Magnesium replacement: In severe magnesium deficit, 500 mL of 20% magnesium sulfate can be infused over 4 to 6 hours. Should hypomagnesemia be less urgent, magnesium is routinely administered in doses of 0.05 to 0.1 mL of 20% magnesium sulfate per kilogram.
- Calcium replacement: Hypocalcemia can be treated with 10 mEq of calcium by IV bolus infusion.

FLUID REPLACEMENT

- A hypotonic electrolyte solution or 0.9% normal saline is administered at a rate of 1500 mL/h for the first hour; then 1000 mL/h for 2 hours; then 500 to 750 mL/h for 1 hour.
- Crystalloid solution: Is administered when large volumes are needed.
- When blood glucose decreases to 250 to 300 mg/dL, 5% dextrose in water (D_5W) is administered to permit continued insulin infusion without hyperglycemia.

NURSING MANAGEMENT: NURSING DIAGNOSES AND COLLABORATIVE PROBLEMS

Nursing Diagnoses

Common nursing goals for patients with HHNK are to maintain fluid balance, prevent injury, provide knowledge, and reduce anxiety.

Fluid volume deficit related to osmotic diuresis secondary to hyperglycemia.

Expected Patient Outcomes. Patient maintains adequate fluid balance, as evidenced by cardiac output (CO) 4 to 8 L/min, cardiac index (CI) 2.7 to 4.3 L/min/m², central venous pressure (CVP) 2 to 6 mm Hg, pulmonary capillary wedge pressure (PCWP) 6 to 12 mm Hg, pulmonary artery systolic (PAS) pressure 15 to 30 mm Hg, pulmonary artery diastolic (PAD) pressure 5 to 15 mm Hg, blood pressure (BP) within patient's normal range, mean arterial pressure (MAP) 70 to 100 mm Hg, heart rate (HR) ≤100 bpm, respiratory rate (RR) 12 to 20 bpm, peripheral pulses +2, capillary refill ≤3 seconds, normal skin turgor, moist buccal membrane, urinary output (UO) ≥30 mL/h, and serum osmolality 280 to 300 mOsm/kg.

- Consult with physician to validate expected patient outcomes used to evaluate fluid balance.
- Review serum electrolyte, osmolality, hemoglobin, and hematocrit values.

- Obtain and report hemodynamic parameters associated with fluid volume deficit: CO ≤4 L/min, CI ≤2.7 L/min/m², CVP ≤2 mm Hg, PCWP ≤4 mm Hg, PAS ≤15 mm Hg, and PAD ≤8 mm Hg.
- Obtain and report other clinical findings associated with fluid volume deficit: hypotension, tachycardia, tachypnea, confusion, disorientation, peripheral pulses ≤+2, and capillary refill ≥3 seconds.
- Measure intake, output, specific gravity, and body weight. Report UO ≤30 mL/h or ≥200 mL/h, specific gravity ≥1.022, and weight loss of ≥0.5 to 1.0 kg/d.
- Administer prescribed IV of 0.9 normal saline when serum sodium is ≤130 mEq/L or plasma osmolality ≤330 mOsm/L.
- Administer prescribed IV of 0.45 normal saline when serum sodium is ≥145 mEq/L.
- Add prescribed IV 5% dextrose to the infusion when serum glucose is 250 to 300 mg/dL to prevent rapid lowering of serum osmolality.
- Administer prescribed IV plasma expanders should isotonic solutes fail to improve intravascular volume.
- Administer prescribed potassium supplements should hypokalemia occur.
- Administer prescribed prophylactic low-dose heparin therapy to prevent clotting associated with increased blood viscosity resulting from profound diuresis.

High risk for injury related to seizure activity secondary to fluid, electrolyte, and metabolic abnormalities.

Expected Patient Outcome. Patient is free from seizure activity.

- Identify and avoid precipatory factors contributing to seizure activity.
- Initiate seizure precautions, such as keeping padded side rails up and keeping airway at bedside to minimize injury.
- Initiate suctioning during and after seizures to maintain airway and prevent aspiration when salivation is excessive.

- Assess baseline and neurological status during the postictal phase for confusion, lethargy, weakness, and changes in speech every 15 minutes for 1 hour, then every 30 minutes for 2 hours.
- Monitor BP after seizure every 5 minutes, then every 15 minutes.
- Position patient on side to facilitate drainage of oral secretions.
- Remain with patient during seizure to assess its type and location.
- After seizure, reorient and reassure patient.
- Measure intake and output, since myoglobinuria can occur with prolonged skeletal activity, leading to risk of renal failure.
- Avoid use of anticonvulsant drugs, since they are ineffective with HHNK and may inhibit insulin release.
- Administer prescribed oxygen with ambu bag to increase availability of oxygen during seizure activity and limit hypoxia.
- Instruct patient about the cause of seizure and need for precautions to avoid injury.

Knowledge deficit related to the causes of HHNK and proper insulin administration.

Expected Patient Outcome. Patient is able to verbalize the causes, treatment, and prognosis of HHNK.

- Listen to patient's concerns and questions.
- Include family or significant others in any teaching program.
- Teach patient the relationship of HHNK to diet, exercise, and insulin therapy, using visual aids.
- Teach patient the importance of maintaining a regular diet, exercise program, and rest periods.
- Instruct patient regarding insulin dosage, time, and site in relation to serum glucose and urine sugar and acetone testing.
- Teach patient to monitor blood glucose levels four times a day when ill and monitor ketone levels when blood glucose is ≥240 mg/dL if prone to ketosis.

- Teach patient the signs and symptoms of hypoglycemia and hypoglycemia.

Anxiety related to HHNK crisis.

Expected Patient Outcome. Absence of or decrease in verbalization of anxiety.

- Identify when patient becomes anxious.
- Encourage patient to verbalize anxious feelings.
- Instruct patient to note feelings of irritability, which may reflect hypoglycemia.
- Teach patient alternative strategies to decrease anxiety: progressive relaxation, meditation, or guided imagery.

DISCHARGE PLANNING

The critical care nurse will provide patient and significant other(s) with verbal or written discharge notes regarding the following subjects:

1. Importance of keeping all postdischarge medical appointments.
2. The causes, prevention, and treatment of HHNK.
3. Importance of daily monitoring of blood glucose and urine acetone levels as prescribed.
4. Importance of reporting a positive urine specimen for acetone or blood glucose ≥200 mg/dL.
5. Importance of maintaining regular diet, exercise, and avoiding infections.
6. Importance of taking prescribed oral hypoglycemic medications.

■ HYPOTHYROIDISM

(For related information see Part I: Hyperthyroidism, p. 706.)

Case Management Basis
DRG: 300 Endocrine disorders with complications
LOS: 6.90 days
DRG: 301 Endocrine disorders without complications

LOS: 4.10 days

Definition

Hypothyroidism or myxedema is the condition that results when the levels of circulating triiodothyronine (T_3) and thyroxine (T_4) are inadequate.

Pathophysiology

Destruction of the thyroid gland may be attributed to an autoimmune inflammatory process and inadequate secretion of thyrotropin-releasing hormone (TRH) by the hypothalamus, which can predispose to decreased thyrotropin (TSH) secretion. The myxedematous state involves the interstitial accumulation of mucopolysaccharides, which attract water, leading to edema. The types of hypothyroidism include primary and secondary. Primary hypothyroidism refers to diseases of the thyroid gland. Secondary hypothyroidism refers to abnormalities in the pituitary or hypothalamus.

Nursing Management

PRIMARY CAUSES

- Primary causes may be thyroid gland dysfunction such as Hashimoto's thyroiditis, autoimmune thyroiditis, ablative therapy for hyperthyroidism, and endemic iodine deficiency. Secondary causes may be pituitary disease and lack of TSH.

PHYSICAL ASSESSMENT

- Inspection: Weakness, fatigue, muscle cramps, cold intolerance, dry skin, lethargy, headache, thinning of hair, pallor, absence of sweating, weight gain, constipation, hoarsenesss, muscle cramps, dyspnea, paresthesis, anorexia, or periorbital edema.
- Palpation: Thick and dry skin, poor turgor, abdominal distention, and peripheral edema.
- Percussion: Hypoactive deep tendon reflexes.
- Auscultation: Bradycardia, decreased pulse pressure, hypertension, distant heart sounds, decreased peristalsis, or hypoactive bowel sounds.

DIAGNOSTIC TEST RESULTS

Standard Laboratory Tests. (Table 8–3).

- Antithyroid antibody titers: Elevated in thyroiditis and idiopathic myxedema.
- Serum chemistry: T_4 ≤3.3 µg/dL and free T_4≤0.8 µg/dL. Reduced hemoglobin, potassium, osmolality, and glucose. Elevated cholesterol and triglyceride levels. Elevated CPK, SGOT and LDH.
- Triiodothyronine resin uptake (T_3 RU): Reduced level ≤0.1 in hypothyroidism.
- Triiodothyronine T_3: Reduced in hypothyroidism ≤90 mg/dL.

Noninvasive Thyroid Diagnostic Procedures. (see Table 8–3)

- Radioimmunoassay of TSH: Elevated in primary hypothyroidism and decreased in pituitary hypothyroidism.
- Radioactive T_3 renin uptake: Reduced.

ECG

- Reveals sinus bradycardia, prolonged Q-T interval, and low voltage.

MEDICAL AND SURGICAL MANAGEMENT

PHARMACOLOGY

- T_4. Levothyroxine (Synthroid) is used for thyroid replacement at dose of 2 µg/kg of body weight IV. With myxedemic coma, levothyroxine is administered as 200 to 500 µg IV, then 50 µg daily until oral dosage can be tolerated.
- Hydrocortisone: Is administered as 100 to 300 mg IV if necessary to support impaired adrenocorticotropin hormone production.

MECHANICAL VENTILATION

- Ventilatory support and intubation may be used to correct respiratory acidosis and hypercarbia.

FLUID REPLACEMENT

- Glucose-containing fluids are administered IV based upon the serum glucose level.

TABLE 8–3. STANDARD THYROID LABORATORY TESTS

TABLE 8.3

Test	Purpose	Normal Value	Abnormal Findings
Antithyroid antibodies	Detects circulating antithyroglobulin antibodies in presence of clinical evidence of Graves' disease or other thyroid diseases	Antithyroglobulin titer: ≤1:20 Antimicrosomal titer: ≤1:100	High titers: Hashimoto's thyroiditis Reduced titers: Thyroid dysfunction, myxedema
Thyrotropin (formerly thyroid-stimulating hormone (TSH)	Distinguishes between primary and secondary hypothyroidism Confirms diagnosis of primary hypothyroidism Monitors effects of drug therapy in primary hypothyroidism	Standard assay: 0–6 μU/mL (mU/L) Hypersensitive assay: 0.25–3.5 μU/mL (mU/L)	Elevated value: Primary hypothyroidism Reduced value: hyperthyroidism or thyroiditis
Thyroid-stimulating immunoglobulin	Assists in diagnosing thyrotoxicosis; evaluates treatment	TSH not present	Elevated TSH levels: Exophthalmos, Grave's disease, recurrence of hyperthyroidism
TSH-sensitive assay	Assists in diagnosing primary hypothyroidism and hyperthyroidism Monitors therapy in hypothyroidism or thyroid cancer	0.4–6.0 μ/U/mL(U/L)	Elevated values: Hypothyroidism Reduced value: Primary hyperthyroidism
Thyroxine-binding globulin (TBG)	Evaluates abnormal thyrometabolic conditions not correlating with T_3 or T_4 values Assists in identifying TBG abnormalities	Electrophoresis range 10–26 μg T_4 (binding capacity)/100 mL (130–340 nmol/L) to 16–24 μg T_4 (binding capacity)/100 mL (200–310 nmol/L) Radioimmunoassay 1.3–2.0 mg/100 mL (13–20 mg/L)	Elevated TBG values: Hypothyroidism, some forms hepatic disease Reduced TBG values: Hyperthyroid, active acromegaly, nephrotic syndrome, malnutrition with hypoproteinemia, surgical stress
Thyroxine (T_4)	Evaluates thyroid function Confirms diagnosis of hyper- or hypothyroidism Monitors antithyroid medication treatment in hyperthyroidism Monitors replacement therapy in hypothyroidism	Total T_4 level: 5.0–13.5 μg/dL (64–174 nmol/L) Free T_4 level: 1–3 ng/dL (13–39 pmol/L)	Elevated value: Thyrotoxicosis, acute thyroiditis, pregnancy Reduced value: primary or secondary hypothyroidism, hypoparathyroidism, chronic debilitating illness
Triiodothyronine (T_3) thyroid suppression test	Assists in determining cause of excessive iodine uptake by thyroid gland	Administered T_3 suppresses uptake to ≥50% of baseline	Failure to suppress RAIU by 50%: suggests autonomous thyroid hyperfunction caused by Graves' disease or toxic thyroid nodule

TABLE 8-3

TABLE 8–3. CONTINUED

Test	Purpose	Normal Value	Abnormal Findings
Triiodothyronine resin uptake (T_3RU)	Aids diagnosis of hypothyroidism and hyperthyroidism when thyroxine-binding globulin (TBG) is abnormal	T_3 RU 0.1 to 1.35	A high resin uptake indicate hyperthyroidism Low resin uptake percentage, together with low T_4 levels indicate hypothyroidism
Triiodothyronine (T_3)	Aids diagnosis of hypothyroidism and hyperthyroidism	T_3 level range from 90 to 250 nq/dL (1.5 to 3.5 mmol/L)	Low T_3 level can indicate hypothyroidism while high T_3 level indicates hyperthyroidism
Water load test	Aids in the diagnosis of syndrome of inappropriate ADH secretin	Excrete 80%	Less than 40% water load excreted in SIADH

From Ford, 1987; Loeb S, 1993.

NURSING MANAGEMENT: NURSING DIAGNOSES AND COLLABORATIVE PROBLEMS

Nursing Diagnoses

Common nursing goals for patients with hypothyroidism are to maintain fluid balance, promote oxygenation, prevent hypothermia, and enhance activity tolerance.

Fluid volume excess related to abnormal extravascular volume excess secondary to interstitial accumulation of mucopolysaccharides, which attract water.

Expected Patient Outcomes. Patient maintains adequate fluid volume, as evidenced by central venous pressure (CVP) 2 to 6 mm Hg, pulmonary capillary wedge pressure (PCWP) 6 to 12 mm Hg, heart rate (HR) ≤ 100 bpm, blood pressure (BP) within patient's normal range, mean arterial pressure (MAP) 70 to 100 mm Hg, flat neck veins, normal lung sounds, absence of edema, specific gravity 1.010 to 1.030, stable weight, and urinary output (UO) ≥ 30 mL/h or 0.5 mL/kg/h.

- Review values for serum electrolytes, hemoglobin, hematocrit, osmolality, and total albumin, urine sodium and osmolality.

- Obtain and report hemodynamic parameters that indicate fluid volume excess: CVP ≥ 6 mm Hg and PCWP ≥ 12 mm Hg.
- Obtain and report other clinical findings associated with water intoxication resulting from fluid volume excess: headache, fatigue, weakness, deteriorating level of consciousness (LOC), sluggish deep tendon reflexes, confusion, agitation, and restlessness.
- Measure intake, output, specific gravity, and daily weight. Report UO ≤ 30 mL/h, specific gravity ≤ 1.010, and weight gain ≥ 0.5–1.0 kg/d.
- Restrict fluid intake to avoid volume excess.
- Provide prescribed low-calorie diet and food high in fiber when patient's condition improves.
- Initiate seizure precautions if severe hyponatremia occurs.
- Administer prescribed isotonic saline fluids IV should sodium be ≤ 120 mEq/L.
- Administer prescribed hydrocortisone 100 mg IV every 6 to 8 hours until myxedema is corrected.
- Administer prescribed T_4 with a loading dose of 300 to 500 μg followed by a daily dose of 75 to 100 μg.
- Teach patient the reasons behind fluid restriction.

Impaired gas exchange related to decreased ventilatory capacity secondary to respiratory muscle weakness and intraalveolar congestion.

Expected Patient Outcomes. Patient maintains adequate gas exchange, as evidenced by respiratory rate (RR) 12 to 20 BPM, absence of cyanosis, normal lung sounds, alertness, arterial blood gases within normal limits, and arterial oxygen saturation (SaO_2) $\geq 95\%$.

- Review results of arterial blood gas measurement and chest roentgenogram.
- Place patient in a position of comfort to facilitate ventilation and improve oxygenation.
- Assess clinical indicators of respiratory status: Respiratory rate and rhythm, lung sounds, skin color, symmetry of chest movement, and use of accessory muscles.
- Report clinical findings associated with impaired gas exchange: tachypnea, crackles, cyanosis, asymmetry of chest movement, and use of accessory muscles.
- Monitor oxygen saturation continuously with pulse oximetry (SpO_2).
- Continuously monitor ECG to assess HR and rhythm. Document ECG rhythm strips every 2 to 4 hours in patients with dysrhythmias.
- Encourage patient to cough, turn, and deep breathe.
- Suction patient, as necessary, to avoid pulmonary complications.
- Administer prescribed oxygen 2 to 4 L/min to maintain SaO_2 $\geq 95\%$.
- Instruct patient to use incentive spirometry to facilitate deep breathing and minimize atelectasis.

Hypothermia related to decreased metabolic rate.

Expected Patient Outcome. Patient maintains normothermia.

- Continuously monitor core temperature.
- Gradually raise patient's temperature by increasing room temperature, applying extra blankets or thermal blanket, and using warming lights.

- Administer prescribed T_4 at a loading dose of 300 to 500 μg followed by a daily dose of 75 to 100 μg.

Activity intolerance related to fatigue or weakness.

Expected Patient Outcome. Patient verbalizes decreased fatigue or weakness.

- Encourage patient to identify when he or she experiences feelings of fatigue or weakness.
- Provide rest periods before and after physical activity.
- Monitor patient's tolerance of incremental increases in physical activity: cardiac rhythm, HR, BP, and RR.
- Evaluate patient's sensorimotor function for presence of muscle cramps, weakness, or paresthesia.
- Monitor patient's incremental increases in physical mobility.
- Assist with range-of-motion (ROM) exercises.
- Teach patient the relationship between hypothyroidism or myxedema crisis and fatigue or weakness.
- Instruct patient to exercise legs during muscle cramps.

Collaborative Problems

A common collaborative goal for patients with hypothyroidism is to increase cardiac output.

Potential Complication: Decreased Cardiac Output. Decreased cardiac output related to depressed myocardial function secondary to reduced thyroid hormone.

Expected Patient Outcomes. Patient maintains adequate cardiac output (CO), as evidenced by CO 4 to 8 L/min, cardiac index (CI) 2.7–4.3 L/min/m², CVP 2 to 6 mm Hg, BP within patient's normal range, HR ≤ 100 bpm, UO ≥ 30 mL/h, capillary refill ≤ 3 seconds, peripheral pulses +2, and absence of cyanosis.

- Review results of serum hemoglobin, hematocrit, and thyroid studies.

- Obtain and report hemodynamic parameters associated with decreased CO: CO $\leq$4 L/min, CI $\leq$2.7 L/min/m^2, and CVP $\leq$2 mm Hg.
- Assess clinical indicators of perfusion: BP, HR, MAP, peripheral pulses, skin color and warmth, and capillary refill.
- Report other clinical findings associated with decreased CO: hypotension, tachycardia, MAP $\leq$70 mm Hg, peripheral pulses $\leq$+2, capillary refill $\leq$3 seconds, and cyanosis.
- Continuously monitor ECG to assess HR and rhythm. Document ECG rhythm strips every 2 to 4 hours in patients with hypothyroidism. The ECG may show low voltage and prolonged of QT interval.
- Measure intake, output, specific gravity, and daily weight to evaluate fluid balance. Report UO $\leq$30 mL/h and weight change 0.5 to 1.0 kg/d.
- Administer prescribed IV fluids to maintain systolic BP (SBP) $\geq$90 mm Hg.
- Administer thyroid therapy as prescribed: T$_3$ as rapid-response liothyronine sodium (Cytomel) 5 μg initially and increase slowly; or mixtures of T$_4$ and T$_3$ in a ratio of 4:1 as liotrix (Euthroid, Thyrolar) as complete replacement therapy.
- Administer emergency thyroid replacement for myxedemic coma: T$_3$ 10 to 25 μg or more by nasogastric tube every 8 hours or levothyroxine sodium 200 to 400 μg IV as a single injection and repeated once in a dose of 100 to 200 μg in 12 hours with the addition of hydrocortisone 100 mg every 8 hours.
- Administer prescribed glucocorticoid therapy should patient be hypotensive.

DISCHARGE PLANNING

The critical care nurse will provide patient and significant other(s) with verbal or written discharge notes regarding the following subjects:

1. Importance of keeping postdischarge appointments and maintaining laboratory testing.
2. Importance of taking prescribed medications.

3. The purpose, dose, and side effects of prescribed medication.
4. Signs and symptoms of hypothyroidism.

■ HYPERTHYROIDISM

(For related information see Part I: Hypothyroidism, p. 701.)

Case Management Basis
DRG: 300 Endocrine disorders with complications
LOS: 6.90 days
DRG: 301 Endocrine disorders without complications
LOS: 4.10 days

Definition
Hyperthyroidism is characterized by excessive secretion of the thyroid hormones, thyroxine (T$_4$) and triiodothyronine (T$_3$).

Pathophysiology
Thyroid hormones stimulate synthesis of beta receptors and may increase the sensitivity of these receptors to catecholamines. The increased sympathetic response and increased levels of circulating thyroid hormones can contribute to hyperthyroid crisis. A reduction in serum protein may increase the availability of free thyroid hormones. The excess free circulating thyroid hormones can react with tissues, causing an increase in metabolic reactions.

Nursing Assessment

PRIMARY CAUSES
- Hyperthyroidism is caused by Graves' disease, toxic multinodular goiter, a solitary toxic nodule, iodine-induced thyrotoxicosis. Less common causes of hyperthyroidism include toxic nodular goiter, hyperfunctioning state, and adenoma of the thyroid gland. Rare causes include thyroiditis, metastatic thyroid carcinoma, and overtreatment for hypothyroidism. Thyrotoxicosis can be due to infections, thyroid ablations from

surgery or radioiodine, trauma, myocardial infarction, pulmonary embolus, or medication overdose.

PHYSICAL ASSESSMENT

- Inspection: Hyperpyrexia, weight loss, increased appetite, nausea, vomiting, diarrhea, weakness, fatigue, jaundice, periorbital edema, weight loss, spider angiomas, heat intolerance, hyperthermia, excessive sweating, convulsions, restlessness, agitation, disorientation, dyspnea, tremors, and muscle cramps.
- Palpation: Hepatomegaly, splenomegaly, abdominal pain, and peripheral edema.
- Auscultation: Tachycardia, premature ventricular contraction, atrial fibrillation, hypotension, adventitious breath sounds, thrill or bruit over nodular goiter, or increased bowel sounds.

DIAGNOSTIC TEST RESULTS

Standard Laboratory Tests. (see Table 8–3)

- Serum chemistry: Reduced cholesterol, lymphocytosis, hypercalcemia, elevated phosphate, elevated serum alkaline phosphastase, elevated T_3 resin uptake and T_3, reduced TSH, radioimmunoassay and (RIA), and abnormal liver function tests.
- Urinalysis: Increased creatinine, increased calcium, and increased phosphate.

Noninvasive Thyroid Diagnostic Procedures. (Tables 8–4, 8–5)

- Imaging: Hypertropic osteoarthropathy and swelling of the extraocular muscles.

Invasive Thyroid Diagnostic Procedure. (see Table 8–5)

- Thyroid biopsy: cancer of thyroid.
- Thyroid scan: Enlarged thyroid.

ECG

- Reveals tachycardia, atrial fibrillation, supraventricular tachycardia, or P and T wave changes.

MEDICAL AND SURGICAL MANAGEMENT

PHARMACOLOGY

- Thionamides: Are used to block synthesis of thyroid hormones. Propylthiouracil (PTU) is administered orally at a dose of 200 mg daily and methimazole orally at a dose of 90 to 120 mg daily and reduced gradually to 40 mg daily (see Table 8–2).
- Iodine: Is used to block release of thyroid hormone. Saturated solution of potassium iodide (SSKI) contains about 50 mg of iodine per drop. In crisis states it is administered orally, 10 drops every 8 hours, initiated shortly after the first dose of PTU. Sodium iodide, an alternative, can be given 1 to 2 g/d IV (see Table 8–2).
- Beta-adrenergic blockers: Are used to inhibit the conversion of T_4 to the more physiologically active T_3. Propranolol (2 to 10 mg IV every 4 hours; 20 to 80 mg orally every 4 to 6 hours) is administered unless there is a history of asthma or congestive heart failure (see Table 1–5, p. 24).
- Reserpine and guanethidine: Reserpine (1 to 5 mg intramuscularly) and guanethidine (2 to 10 mg every 4 hours) are used to deplete catecholamine (see Table 1–16, p. 116).
- Radioactive iodine: Used in malignant thyroid disease.

DIET

- High-caloric diet is recommended.

FLUID THERAPY

- Dextrose-containing IV fluids are infused to correct fluid and glucose deficit.

SURGICAL INTERVENTION

- Surgical ablation is usually the treatment of choice for thyroid malignancies.

NURSING MANAGEMENT: NURSING DIAGNOSES AND COLLABORATIVE PROBLEMS

Nursing Diagnoses

Common nursing goals for patients with hyperthyroidism are to maintain fluid balance,

TABLE 8-4

TABLE 8-5

TABLE 8–4. NONINVASIVE THYROID DIAGNOSTIC PROCEDURES

Test	Purpose	Normal Value	Abnormal Findings
Thyroid ultrasonography	Evaluates thyroid structure Differentiates between cyst and tumor Determines dimension of thyroid nodules	Normal size and shape of thyroid gland	Cysts, tumors, thyroid nodules

From Ford RD, 1987; Loeb S, 1993.

TABLE 8–5. INVASIVE THYROID DIAGNOSTIC PROCEDURES

Test	Purpose	Normal Value	Abnormal Findings
Thyroid biopsy	Differentiates between benign and malignant thyroid disease Assists in diagnosis of Hashimoto's thyroidism, subacute granulomatous thyroiditis, hyperthyroidism, nontoxic nodular goiter	Fibrous networks dividing the gland into Pseudolobules including the follicle walls and contains the protein thyroglobulin which stress serum triiodothyronine (T_3) and serum thyroxine (T_4)	Malignant tumors such as papillary carcinoma or follicular carcinoma Benign tumors such as nontoxic nodular goiter
Thyroid scan	Evaluates size, structure, position of thyroid gland Evaluates thyroid function in relation to specific thyroid uptake studies	Normal size, shape, position, function of thyroid with uniform uptake of radioisotope	Hot spots: Hyperfunctioning nodules Cold spots: Hypofunctioning nodules

From Ford RD, 1987; Loeb S, 1993.

maintain normothermia, provide adequate nutritional intake, support activity tolerance, promote sleep, and assist with sensory-perceptual function.

Fluid volume deficit related intravascular volume loss secondary to increased temperature, and excessive sweating, diarrhea, and vomiting secondary to hypermetabolic state.

Expected Patient Outcomes. Patient maintains adequate fluid volume, as evidenced by serum osmolality 285 to 295 mOsm/kg; urinary output (UO) ≥30 mL/h or 0.5 mL/kg/h; serum electrolytes within normal range; blood pressure (BP) within patient's normal range; neurological status intact; normothermia; good skin turgor; absence of excessive sweating, diarrhea, or vomiting; and no fever.

- Review values of serum electrolytes, osmolality, blood urea nitrogen (BUN), creatinine, hemoglobin, hematocrit, total protein, urine sodium and osmolality.
- Place patient in a position of comfort and avoid strenuous exercise.
- Provide diet high in calories, proteins, and vitamins.
- Assess clinical indicators of hydration: skin color and temperature, skin turgor, capillary refill, UO, and peripheral pulses.
- Report clinical findings associated with dehydration: sunken eyeballs, poor skin turgor, dry skin and mucous membranes, tachycardia, hypotension, and flat neck veins.
- Measure daily weight, intake, specific gravity, and UO to evaluate fluid balance. Report UO ≤30 mL/h and weight loss ≥0.5–1.0 kg/d.

- Administer prescribed IV fluids and volume expanders as required to maintain adequate hydration.
- Administer prescribed antithyroid agents to block synthesis of thyroid hormone.
- Prepare patient for subtotal thyroidectomy: thiouracil drugs such as PTU, methimazole, or carbimazole; iodine; combined PTU-iodine therapy; or propranolol.
- Prepare patient for administration of radioiodine to destroy overfunctioning thyroid tissue (diffuse or toxic nodular goiter).

Hyperthermia related to hypermetabolic rate.

Expected Patient Outcome. Patient remains at normal temperature 36° to 37.5°C (97.8° to 99.4°F).

- Limit activity to bed rest in an attempt to reduce metabolic activity.
- Continually monitor temperature every 2 to 4 hours while patient febrile and evaluate the effectiveness of therapy.
- Obtain and report clinical findings associated with hyperthermia: shivering, chills, and diaphoresis.
- Measure intake, output, specific gravity to evaluate fluid balance.
- Provide cooling measures such as hypothermia blankets, tepid bath, fan, and ice packs over major vessels. The cooling methods are tapered at 38°C (100.4°F).
- Administer prescribed oxygen 2 to 4 L/min, since hypermetabolic state can cause increased oxygen demand and compliance.
- Administer prescribed antithyroid agents: PTU at a loading dose of 600 to 1000 mg, then 150 to 200 mg three to four times a day; methimazole at a loading dose of 60 to 100 mg, then 10 to 20 mg three times a day; or potassium iodide (SSKI) 10 drops every 12 hours or sodium iodide 500 to 1000 mg every 12 hours (see Table 8–2).
- Administer prescribed antipyretic agents such as acetaminophen to reduce fever.
- Administer prescribed IV fluids to maintain adequate hydration.

High risk of altered nutrition: less than body requirements related to hypermetabolism.

Expected Patient Outcomes. Patient maintains nutritional balance, as evidenced by body weight within 5% of baseline, serum proteins maintained within normal range of 6.0 to 8.4 g/100 mL, serum glucose 70 to 110 mg/100 mL, and urine negative for glucose and acetone.

- Consult with nutritionist about alteration in patient's nutrition caused by hypermetabolic state.
- Obtain and report clinical findings associated with catabolism: muscle weakness; muscle wasting; soft, fine hair; fragile nails.
- Provide prescribed diet that is high in protein, calories, and carbohydrates.
- Obtain and report clinical findings associated with hyperglycemia secondary to increased glycogenolysis, impaired insulin secretion, and insulin resistance: polydipsia, glycosuria, polyuria, nocturia, weakness, fatigue, visual disturbance, muscle cramping, and lethargy.
- Minimize energy expenditure by consolidating both patient and nursing care activities as well as providing rest periods.
- Administer prescribed electrolytes and soluble vitamin B complex and vitamin C supplements.
- Administer prescribed insulin therapy to control hyperglycemia.
- Teach patient to avoid foods such as coffee, tea, and cola, which increase peristalsis.

Activity intolerance related to tremors and muscle cramps.

Expected Patient Outcome. Absence of tremors and muscle cramps.

- Evaluate sensorimotor function: tremors, muscle cramps, or fatigue.
- Encourage patient to identify when he or she experiences muscle cramps.
- Assist patient experiencing tremors with eating.

- Assess patient's tolerance of incremental increases in physical activity: cardiac rhythm, heart rate (HR), BP, and respiratory rate (RR).
- Teach patient the relationship between hyperthyroidism and tremors or muscle cramps.

Sleep pattern disturbance related to increased metabolic rate and insomnia.

Expected Patient Outcome. Patient maintains normal sleep pattern.

- Minimize fatigue by providing uninterrupted rest periods.
- Evaluate patient's prehospital sleep history.
- Provide an environment in which unnecessary noise is minimized.
- Organize nursing care activities to provide the fewest number of disturbances during sleep.
- Explain to patient and significant others the causes of sleep and rest disturbance and ways to achieve rest.
- Encourage patient to describe factors affecting his or her sleep.
- Provide diversional activities that help to channel some of the energy associated with an overwhelming adrenergic response.
- Initiate relaxation exercises when patient's condition stabilizes.
- Assist patient to identify an unusual sleep pattern caused by illness or hospitalization.
- Administer prescribed sedative if necessary to facilitate sleepfulness.

Sensory-perceptual alterations related to ophthalmopathy or lid retraction and lag.

Expected Patient Outcome. Eye function remains normal.

- Minimize external stimuli to avoid distraction and confusion.
- Provide position of comfort.
- Assess patient's sensory-perceptual function: mental status, cranial nerves, and motor function.

- Report changes in mental status, cranial nerve function, and sensorimotor dysfunction.
- Protect patient's eyes from injury with dark glasses or eye shields.
- Maintain a safe environment if patient has visual problems.
- Assist patient with ambulation to avoid potential injury.
- Administer methylcellulose solution (1%) as prescribed to prevent drying of eyes.

Collaborative Problems

Common collaborative goals for patients with hyperthyroidism are to correct electrolyte imbalance and increase cardiac output.

Potential Complication: Electrolyte Imbalance. Electrolyte imbalance related to dehydration and hemoconcentration.

Expected Patient Outcomes. Patient maintains electrolyte balance, as evidenced by serum osmolality 285 to 295 mOsm/kg, serum sodium $\geq$135 mEq/L and $\leq$148 mEq/L, and serum potassium $\geq$3.5 mEq/L and $\leq$5.5 mEq/L, serum electrolytes and osmolality within normal range.

- Review levels of serum electrolytes and osmolality, urine sodium and osmolality.
- Obtain and report clinical findings associated with hyponatremia: headache, faintness, muscle cramps, confusion, or convulsions.
- Monitor cardiac rhythm for presence of tachycardia or atrial fibrillation associated with thyrotoxicosis and changes in configuration such as presence of U wave in hyperkalemia.
- Monitor for clinical indicators of hypokalemia: malaise, fatigue, anorexia, nausea, vomiting, diarrhea, abdominal cramps, muscle weakness, hyporeflexia, hypotension, restlessness, and irritability.
- Monitor for clinical indicators of hypercalcemia: drowsiness, fatigue, anorexia, thirst, nausea, vomiting, constipation, neuromuscular changes such as hypotonicity of muscles with weakness, deep bone pain, depression, and lethargy.

- Monitor ECG rhythm continuously for changes reflecting hypercalcemia such as shortened QT interval, and hypokalemia such as U wave.
- Administer prescribed IV saline to promote renal excretion of calcium.
- Administer IV potassium as prescribed to avoid cardiac dysrhythmias.
- Administer IV or oral phosphates, glucocorticoids, and sodium bicarbonate as prescribed: Phosphate can cause calcium excretion, glucocorticoids may inhibit calcium absorption, and sodium bicarbonate increases the fraction of calcium bound in protein.
- Administer propranolol for tachycardia as prescribed.
- Teach patient the relationship between dysrhythmias and electrolyte imbalance.

Potential Complication: Decreased Cardiac Output.

Decreased cardiac output related to increased cardiac work secondary to increased adrenergic activity.

Expected Patient Outcomes. Patient maintains adequate cardiac output (CO), as evidenced by CO 4 to 8 L/min, cardiac index (CI) 2.7 to 4.3 L/min/m^2, central venous pressure (CVP) 2 to 6 mm Hg, pulmonary artery systolic (PAS) pressure 15 to 30 mm Hg, pulmonary artery diastolic (PAD) pressure 8 to 15 mm Hg, pulmonary capillary wedge pressure (PCWP) 6 to 12 mm Hg, UO $\geq$30 mL/h, HR $\leq$100 bpm, RR 12 to 20 BPM, absence of dysrhythmias, capillary refill $\leq$3 seconds, peripheral pulses +2, absence of cyanosis, blood pressure (BP) within patient's normal range, and alertness.

- Consult with physician to validate expected patient outcomes used to evaluate whether adequate cardiac output has been achieved.
- Review levels of serum electrolytes, osmolality, hemoglobin, hematocrit, BUN, creatinine, total protein, T$_4$, and urine sodium and osmolality.

- Place patient on bed rest to reduce physical activity.
- Obtain and report hemodynamic parameters associated with decreased CO: CO $\leq$4 L/min, CI $\leq$2.7 L/min/m^2, CVP $\leq$2 mm Hg, PAS $\leq$15 mm Hg, PAD $\leq$8 mm Hg, and PCWP $\leq$4 mm Hg.
- Assess clinical indicators of perfusion: BP, HR, mean arterial pressure (MAP), skin color, UO, capillary refill, and peripheral pulses.
- Report clinical findings associated with decreased CO: hypotension, tachycardia, capillary refill $\geq$3 seconds, peripheral pulses $\leq$+2, and cyanosis.
- Measure intake, output, specific gravity, and daily weight. Report UO $\leq$30 mL/h and weight change 0.5 to 1.0 kg/d.
- Monitor ECG continuously to assess HR and rhythm. Document ECG and report dysrhythmias such as supraventricular tachyarrhythmias and ventricular dysrhythmias.
- Provide prescribed oxygen 2 to 4 L/min to maintain adequate oxygenation during hypermetabolism or increased metabolic demand.
- Administer prescribed IV fluids to maintain adequate circulatory volume.
- Administer prescribed antidysrhythmic agents to correct dysrhythmias resulting from hyperthyroid crisis.
- Administer prescribed antithyroid agents: propylthiouracil, which blocks thyroid hormone synthesis, or sodium iodide to block thyroid secretion.
- Monitor for clinical indicators of improvement after antithyroid hormone therapy: alertness, reduced temperature, decreased HR, stable BP, decreased palpitations, and decreased nervousness and diaphoresis.
- Administer prescribed beta$_2$-adrenergic blocker (propranolol) to inhibit adrenergic overactivity, thereby reducing the effects of excessive thyroid hormone.
- Administer prescribed glucocorticosteroid therapy (dexamethasone or hydrocortisone) to inhibit peripheral conversion of T$_4$ to T$_3$.

DISCHARGE PLANNING

The critical care nurse will provide patient and significant other(s) with verbal or written discharge notes regarding the following subjects:

1. The purpose, dose, and side effects of medications.
2. Importance of keeping all postdischarge appointments and evaluation of laboratory studies.
3. Signs and symptoms associated with hyperthyroidism.

■ ADRENOCORTICAL INSUFFICIENCY

(For related information see Part II: Adrenalectomy, p. 721.)

Case Management Basis
DRG: 300 Endocrine disorders with complications
LOS: 6.90 days
DRG: 301 Endocrine disorders without complications
LOS: 4.10 days

Definition
Adrenal insufficiency (AI) is characterized by the absence or deficiency of adrenocortical hormones such as glucocorticoids and mineralocorticoids. Hypoadrenalism is classified as primary AI (Addison's disease) or secondary AI (hyposecretion of corticotropin [ACTH]).

Pathophysiology
In general, if the cortisol level decreases, the hypothalamus secretes corticotropin-releasing hormone into the hypothalamic pituitary capillary system. The coricotropin-releasing hormone stimulates the pituitary gland to secrete ACTH (corticotropin, formerly called adrenocorticotropic hormone). The adrenal glands, responding to secretion of ACTH, increase secretion of cortisol and corticotropin-releasing hormone. Overall, renin-angiotensin-aldosterone controls the secretion of aldosterone. In AI, the renin-angiotensin-aldosterone mechanism is disrupted, thereby diminishing or ceasing cortisol and aldosterone secretion.

Nursing Assessment

PRIMARY CAUSES
- Primary AI causes include autoimmune disease, idiopathic atrophy, tuberculosis; fungal infections such as histoplasmosis, coccidiodomycosis; blastomycosis; cytomegalovirus; metastatic carcinoma; infiltrative diseases such as sarcoidosis or amyloidosis; adrenal hemorrhage from anticoagulation therapy; or adrenalectomy.
- Secondary AI is due to conditions associated with deficiencies in hypothalamic pituitary function affecting ACTH secretion. These conditions include diminished pituitary ACTH secretion, pituitary tumors and infarctions, hypophysectomy, irradiation of the pituitary gland, and infection.

RISK FACTORS
- Primary AI: Risk factors include a coagulopathy associated with a steep drop in hemoglobin level, fever, abdominal or back pain, history of thromboembolic disease, recent surgery or heparization.
- Secondary AI: Risk factors include iatrogenic causes such as resection of a ACTH-secreting tumor.

PHYSICAL ASSESSMENT
- Inspection: Muscular discomfort, weakness, fatigue, weight loss, skin and mucosal hyperpigmentation, diarrhea, anorexia, depression, apathy, joint pain, and vitiligo.
- Palpation: Abdominal pain and poor skin turgor.
- Auscultation: Tachycardia, tachypnea, and orthostatic hypotension.

DIAGNOSTIC TEST RESULTS

Standard Laboratory Tests. (see Table 8–6)
- Metyrapone test: Is used to determine the presence of secondary AI.

TABLE 8–6. STANDARD ADRENAL LABORATORY TESTS

Test	Purpose	Normal Value	Abnormal Findings
Adrenocortical Function			
ACTH	Assists in diagnosing Addison's disease	8 AM: <140 pg/mL 4 PM: 10–50 pg/mL	Elevated value: Primary adrenal insufficiency or stress
	Distinguishes functional hypopituitarism from organic disease of adrenal cortex		Reduced value: Hypopituitarism or adrenal hypofunction
ACTH stimulation test (25 U via IV bolus)		Cortisol 1–20 μg/dL 30–45 min after bolus	Reduced value: Possible adrenal insufficiency
Aldosterone (serum)	Assists in diagnosing primary and secondary aldosteronism	AM Supine: 5–10 ng/dL AM Upright: 9–60 ng/dL	Elevated value: Primary and secondary hyperaldosteronism, nephrotic syndrome
	Diagnoses adrenal hyperplasia, such as hypoaldosteronism		Reduced value: Salt-losing syndrome, Addison's disease, renin deficiency, hypokalemia
Aldosterone (urine)	Assists in diagnosing primary or secondary aldosteronism	3–19 μg/24 h	Elevated value: Primary or secondary aldosteronism
			Reduced value: Addison's disease, salt-losing syndrome, toxemia of pregnancy
Cortisol	Aids in diagnosing Cushing's disease, Cushing's syndrome, Addison's disease, secondary adrenal insufficiency	8 AM 8–20 μg/dL 4 AM 4–10 μg/dL	Elevated value: Adrenocortical hyperfunction in Cushing's disease, Cushing's syndrome, stress, pregnancy
			Reduced value: Adrenocortical hypofunction (Addison's disease), secondary adrenal insufficiency (hypophysectomy, chromophobe adenoma)
Dexamethasone suppression test (DST)	Measures elevated cortisol activity	Overnight screening DST (single dose): plasma cortisol ≤5 μg/dL	Reduced value can suggest Cushing's syndrome or depression
	Differentiates Cushing's syndrome		
17-Hydrocorticosteroids (urine)	Assesses adrenocortical function	Men: 4.5–12 mg/24 h Women: 2.5–10 mg/24 h	Elevated value: Adrenal hyperfunction, hyperthyroidism
			Reduced value: Adrenal hypofunction, hypopituitarism, hypothyroid

TABLE 8-6

TABLE 8-6

TABLE 8–6. CONTINUED

Test	Purpose	Normal Value	Abnormal Findings
Urinary free cortisol (UFC)		Men: 10–85 μg/dL Women: 10–90 μg/dL	Elevated value: Possible Cushing's syndrome
Adrenomedullary Evaluation			
Catecholamines (serum)	Rules out adrenal medullary or extra-adrenal pheochromocytoma in patients with hypertension	Supine, resting Epinephrine: 0–150 μg/L Norepinephrine: 100–200 μg/L	Elevated value: Pheochromocytoma, thyroid disorder, shock from hemorrhage, endotoxins, or anaphylaxis
Vanillylmandelic acid (VMH) (urine)	Assists in diagnosing pheochromocytoma Evaluates function of adrenal medulla	VMA ranges from 0.7–6.8 mg/24 h	Elevated value: Pheochromocytoma

From Ford RD, 1987; Loeb S, 1993.

- Plasma ACTH immunoassay: Baseline cortisol value of ≤ 10 μg/100mL together with an ACTH ≥ 250 μg/mL.
- Prolonged ACTH stimulation test: Is used to distinguish between primary and secondary AI. Patients with primary AI do not respond to the infusion. Patients with secondary AI have a blunted response on day 1 of the test, followed by an increasing response throughout the test.
- Rapid ACTH stimulation test: Is used to assess adrenal response to excessive ACTH stimulation. If steroid precursors are elevated, adrenal enzyme alteration may be present. If the response is blunted or absent, AI is confirmed.
- Serum chemistry: Elevated potassium, calcium, blood urea nitrogen (BUN), eosinophil count, and ACTH level ≥ 88 pmol/L (400 pg/mL). Reduced sodium, glucose, 17-ketosteroids, and 17-hydroxysteroids, and cortisol ≤ 276 nmol/L (10 μg/dL).
- Urinalysis: Reduced levels of 17-ketosteroids and 17-hydroxysteroids.

ECG. Changes include peaked T waves, widening QRS complex, prolonged PR interval, and diminished P wave amplitude.

MEDICAL AND NURSING MANAGEMENT

PHARMACOLOGY
- Hydrocortisone: Administered to patients with AI as a dose of 100 mg IV bolus. A maintenance dose of 100 mg is given every 6 to 8 hours as an IV bolus or continuous infusion.
- Dexamethasone: Administered to patients with adrenocortical failure as an alternate corticosteroid together with fluid support. A dose of 4 mg is infused IV with a maintenance dose administered every 8 hours as a bolus or a continuous infusion (see Table 8–2).
- Fluidrocortisone acetate: Used for mineralocorticoid replacement in patients with chronic AI at a dose ranging between 0.05 to 0.2 mg daily (see Table 8–2).

FLUID THERAPY
- Normal saline with 5% dextrose is administered to reverse the hypoglycemia and dehydration. Patient may require 3 L over 3 hours.

HEMODYNAMIC MONITORING
- Pulmonary artery wedge pressure, central venous pressure (CVP), and cardiac out-

put (CO) are used to assess hemodynamic status, fluid imbalance, and electrolyte imbalance.

NURSING MANAGEMENT: COLLABORATIVE PROBLEMS AND NURSING DIAGNOSES

Nursing Diagnoses

Common nursing goals for patients with AI are to maintain fluid volume, increase tissue perfusion, prevent infection, and support activity tolerance.

Fluid volume deficit related to abnormal sodium and water losses secondary to adrenocorticoid deficiency.

Expected Patient Outcomes. Patient maintains adequate fluid volume, as evidenced by CO 4 to 7 L/min, cardiac index (CI) 2.5 to 4.0 L/min/m^2, CVP 2 to 6 mm Hg, pulmonary artery systolic (PAS) pressure 15 to 30 mm Hg or pulmonary artery diastolic (PAD) pressure 8 to 15 mm Hg, pulmonary capillary wedge pressure (PCWP) 6 to 12 mm Hg, urinary output (UO) $\geq$30 mL/h or $\leq$200 mL/h, blood pressure (BP) within patient's normal range, heart rate (HR) $\leq$100 bpm, respiratory rate (RR) 12 to 20 BPM, peripheral pulses +2, capillary refill $\leq$3 seconds, absence of diaphoresis, skin turgor normal, serum osmolality 285 to 295 mOsm/kg, serum sodium 135 to 145 mEq/L, stable weight, and specific gravity 1.010 to 1.025.

- Consult with physician to validate expected patient outcomes used to evaluate fluid balance.
- Monitor serum osmolality 285 to 295 mOsm/kg, sodium 135 to 145 mEq/L, potassium 3.5 to 5.0 mEq/L, chloride 100 to 106 mEq/L, calcium 8.5 to 10.5 mg/100mL, phosphorus 3.0 to 4.5 mg/100mL, glucose 70 to 110mg/100mL, hemoglobin, hematocrit, BUN, creatinine, urine sodium 80 to 180 mEq/L, and urine negative for glucose and acetone.

- Obtain and report hemodynamic parameters associated with fluid volume deficit: CO $\leq$4 L/min, CO $\leq$2.7 L/min/m^2, CVP $\leq$2 mm Hg, PAS $\leq$15 mm Hg or PAD $\leq$8 mm Hg, and PCWP $\leq$4 mm Hg.
- Assess clinical indicators of hydration: skin turgor and warmth, peripheral pulses, and capillary refill.
- Obtain and report clinical findings associated with fluid volume deficit: hypotension, tachycardia, poor skin turgor, peripheral pulses $\leq$+2 and capillary refill $\geq$3 seconds.
- Measure intake, output, specific gravity. Report UO $\leq$30 mL/h or $\leq$0.5 mL/kg/h and weight loss 0.5 to 1.0 kg/d suggesting weight loss.
- Encourage patient to drink fluids high in sodium content to compensate for sodium loss.
- Administer prescribed IV 5% dextrose normal saline (D$_5$NS) to maintain hydration, maintain circulating volume, and provide a glucose source.
- Administer prescribed hydrocortisone (100 mg IV every 6 hours, then taper to 20 mg orally and 10 mg PM). Long-term replacement therapy may include prednisone, methylprednisolone, or hydrocortisone.
- Administer prescribed dopamine should fluids and hormone replacement fail to improve intravascular volume.
- Administer prescribed fluidrocortisone in primary AI to maintain sodium and potassium balance and control postural hypotension.

Altered cardiovascular tissue perfusion related to fluid volume deficit.

Expected Patient Outcomes. Patient maintains adequate cardiovascular tissue perfusion, as evidenced by orientation to person, place, and time; alertness; BP within patient's normal range, mean arterial pressure (MAP) 70 to 100 mm Hg, HR $\leq$100 bpm, RR 12 to 20 BPM, capillary refill $\leq$3 seconds, peripheral pulses +2, UO $\geq$30 mL/h, absence of dysrhythmias, and absence of cyanosis.

- Review results of 12-lead ECG and serum electrolyte levels.
- Assess clinical indicators of perfusion: BP, HR; skin color, peripheral pulses, capillary refill, and level of consciousness.
- Report clinical findings associated with perfusion reflecting hypovolemia: tachycardia; hypotension; weak and thready peripheral pulses; altered level of consciousness; UO ≤30 mL/h; skin cool, clammy, and mottled; and capillary refill ≥3 seconds.
- Measure intake, output, specific gravity, and daily weight. Report UO ≤30 mL/h or ≤0.5 mL/kg/h and weight loss ≥0.5 to 1.0 kg/d.
- Administer prescribed oxygen 2 to 4 L/min to maintain tissue oxygenation.
- Administer prescribed IV D_5NS to maintain adequate circulatory volume.

High risk for infection related to corticosteroid therapy or compromised immune system.

Expected Patient Outcomes. Patient is free from infection, as evidenced by normothermia; white blood cell (WBC) count ≤11,000/µL; negative cultures; and absence of redness, swelling, tenderness, or drainage from cannulation site.

- Review results of WBC count and cultures of sputum, blood, urine, or wound.
- Monitor temperature every 2 to 4 hours while patient is febrile.
- Assess all invasive line sites for redness, pain, swelling, or damage.
- Culture catheter tips according to unit protocol.
- Encourage patient to change position frequently, cough, deep breathe, and use incentive spirometer to prevent atelectasis and risk of pulmonary infection.
- Encourage patient to drink fluids to maintain adequate hydration.
- Administer prescribed IV fluids to maintain adequate hydration.
- Use sterile technique while changing tubing or dressings.

- Teach patient to report any pain, swelling, or drainage from catheter site.

Activity intolerance related to vertigo, tinnitus, or muscular weakness.

Expected Patient Outcomes. Patient maintains activity tolerance, as evidenced by absence of vertigo, tinnitus, or muscular weakness.

- Assess and report changes in sensorimotor function: tremors, muscle cramps, or fatigue.
- Encourage patient to identify when he or she experiences muscle cramps.
- Assist patient experiencing tremors with eating.
- Monitor patient's tolerance of incremental increases in physical activity: cardiac rhythm, HR, BP, and RR.
- Teach patient the relationship between AI and tremors or muscle cramps.

Collaborative Problems

Common collaborative goals for patients with AI are to correct electrolyte imbalance, increase CO, and correct dysrhythmias.

Potential Complication: Electrolyte Imbalance. Electrolyte imbalance related to hyponatremia and hyperkalemia secondary to glucocorticoid and mineralocorticoid deficiency.

Expected Patient Outcomes. Patient maintains adequate electrolyte balance, as evidenced by serum sodium ≥135 mmol/L and ≤148 mEq/L, serum potassium ≥3.5 mEq/L and ≤5.5 mEq/L, serum osmolality 285 to 295 mOsm/kg, UO ≥30 mL/h, specific gravity 1.010 to 1.025, and alertness.

- Review levels of serum sodium, potassium, and osmolality.
- Obtain and report clinical findings associated with hyperkalemia: weakness, flaccid paralysis, abdominal distention, diarrhea, and bradycardia.
- Monitor cardiac rhythm for changes associated with hyperkalemia: peak T waves of

increased amplitude, widening of the QRS and biphasic QRS-T complexes.
- Obtain and report clinical findings associated with hyponatremia: headache, nausea, vomiting, abdominal cramps, weakness, stupor, coma, and convulsion.
- Measure daily weight, intake, specific gravity, and UO.
- Provide a calm, quiet environment.
- Administer IV fluids and electrolytes to maintain adequate hydration and replenish electrolytes.
- Teach patient stress-reduction techniques.

Potential Complication: Decreased Cardiac Output.
Decreased CO related to decreased preload secondary to reduced venous return.

Expected Patient Outcomes. Patient maintains adequate CO, as evidenced by pulmonary artery pressure (PAP) 20 to 30/8 to 15 mm Hg, PCWP 6 to 12 mm Hg, CO 4 to 8 L/min, CI 2.7 to 4.3 L/min/m², HR ≤100 bpm, BP within patient's normal range, absence of adventitious breath sounds, RR 12 to 20 BPM, UO ≥30 mL/h, capillary refill ≤3 seconds, absence of cyanosis, and peripheral pulses +2.

- Consult with physician to validate expected patient outcomes used to evaluate CO.
- Place patient on bed rest to reduce myocardial work load.
- Obtain and report hemodynamic parameters associated with decreased CO: CO ≤4 L/min, CI ≤2.7 L/min/m², CVP ≤2 mm Hg, PAS ≤15 mm Hg or PAD ≤8 mm Hg, and PCWP ≤6 mm Hg.
- Obtain and report other clinical findings associated with decreased CO: hypotension, tachycardia, tachypnea, cyanosis, peripheral pulses ≤ +2, and capillary refill ≥3 seconds.
- Measure daily weight, intake, specific gravity, and UO. Report UO ≤30 mL/h.
- Continuously monitor ECG to assess HR and rhythm. Document ECG rhythm strips every 2 to 4 hours in patients with dysrhythmias.

- Administer prescribed D₅NS or plasma expanders to maintain circulatory volume.
- Administer prescribed dopamine to relieve risk of severe hypotension.
- Administer prescribed cortisol at a dose of 100 mg IV over 10 to 20 minutes.

Potential Complication: Dysrhythmias.
Dysrhythmia related to hyperkalemia secondary to hyposecretion of aldosterone and cortisol.

Expected Patient Outcomes. Patient maintains regular sinus rhythm and serum potassium 3.5 to 5.5 mEq/L.

- Review results of 12-lead ECG and serum electrolyte levels.
- Continuously monitor ECG for changes associated with hyperkalemia: flattened P waves, tented T waves, a widened QRS interval, and a prolonged PR internal. Document ECG changes associated with hypokalemia, which include peaked P waves, flattened T waves, prominent U waves, and ST depression.
- Obtain and report clinical findings associated with hyperkalemia, which occurs in the presence of hyponatremia and acidosis (for every 0.1 decrease in pH, serum potassium increases by 0.6 mEq/L): weak, slow, and irregular pulse; irritability; restlessness; anxiety; abdominal cramps; weakness; nausea; and vomiting.
- Administer IV fluids and electrolytes to maintain adequate hydration and replace potassium.
- Administer antiarrhythmia medications as prescribed.

DISCHARGE PLANNING
The critical care nurse will provide patient and significant other(s) with verbal or written discharge notes regarding the following subjects:

1. Importance of keeping all postdischarge appointments and regular laboratory studies.
2. The purpose, dose, and side effects of prescribed medications.
3. Signs and symptoms associated with AI.

■ PHEOCHROMOCYTOMA

(For related information see Cardiac Part I: acute hypertensive crisis, p. 141 and Dysrhythmias, p. 184. Neurological Part I: Status epilepticus, p. 636)

Case Management Basis
DRG: 300 Endocrine disorders with complications
LOS: 6.90 days
DRG: 301 Endocrine disorders without complications
LOS: 4.10 days

Definition
A pheochromocytoma is a chromaffin tissue tumor that secretes epinephrine and norepinephrine. The chromaffin tissue can be found in the adrenal medulla and paraspinous ganglionic regions of the abdomen and pelvis. Large amounts of catecholamines (epinephrine and norepinephrine) are released.

Pathophysiology
Pheochromocytomas are highly vascular tumors containing cystic or hemorrhagic areas whose secretions have high concentrations of norepinephrine and epinephrine. Catecholamines produce excitatory responses at some receptor locations (alpha-adrenergic) and inhibitory responses at other receptor locations (beta-adrenergic). Norepinephrine excites alpha-adrenergic receptors causing arteriolar constriction and vasoconstriction) within the skeletal muscle. There is also increased peripheral vascular resistance, persistent or paroxysmal hypertension, perspiration, decreased blood flow to intestines, impaired gastrointestinal motility, pupil dilation, and hyperglycemia. Epinephrine is a beta-adrenergic agonist, which causes increased heart rate, myocardial contractility, and oxygen consumption. Epinephrine also causes vasodilation of skeletal vessels, leading to hypotension, increased metabolic rate, weight loss, and heat intolerance.

Nursing Management

PRIMARY CAUSES
- Can be inherited as an autosomal-dominant trait. Pheochromocytoma may also be attributed to type IIA multiple endocrine neoplasia (MEN), or Sipple's syndrome, which combines pheochromocytoma with medullary carcinoma of the thyroid and hyperparathyroidism. Type IIB MEN combines pheochromocytoma with medullary carcinoma of the thyroid, multiple neuromas, ganglioneuromas, marfanoid habitus, and hypertrophic corneal nerves.

PHYSICAL ASSESSMENT
- Inspection: Severe headache, profuse sweating, pallor, flushing of face or extremities, precordial or abdominal pain, nausea, vomiting, visual disturbances, aphasia, nervousness, irritability, increased appetite, dyspnea, loss of weight, tremor, or increased temperature.
- Auscultation: Hypertension either paroxysmal or sustained, postural tachycardia ≥ 120 bpm, and postural hypotension.

DIAGNOSTIC TEST RESULTS

Standard Laboratory Tests. (see Table 8–6)

- Dexamethasone suppression test: Phentolamine, an adrenergic blocking drug, can cause a positive response by decreasing blood pressure 25 to 35 mm Hg. Clonidine causes hypotension, bradycardia, and somnolence in normal patients and in patients with pheochromocytoma. It does not decrease circulatory catecholamines.
- Serum chemistry: Thyroxine (T_4) and free T_4 are normal and catecholamine concentration ≥ 2000 pg/mL.
- Urinalysis: Glycosuria; catecholamines in urine: metanephrines 0 to 1 mg/24 h, vanillylmandelic acid 2 to 10 mg/24 h, norepinephrine 11 to 86 μg/24 h, and epinephrine 0 to 13 μg/24 h.

Invasive Endocrine Diagnostic Procedures

- Vena cava catheterization: Can be used to obtain venous sampling for catecholamines.

Noninvasive Endocrine Diagnostic Procedures

- Chest roentgenogram: Reveals thoracic primary and metastatic tumors. Also provides information on cardiac size and the presence of heart failure.
- Computerized tomographic (CT) scan: Demonstrates intra-adrenal pheochromocytomas.
- Magnetic resonance imaging (MRI): Can be used to detect and localize pheochromocytomas such as during pregnancy and pheochromocytomas from other adrenal cortical lesions but not from cancer metastasized to the adrenal.
- Ultrasonography: Demonstrates adrenal or para-adrenal masses.

MEDICAL AND SURGICAL MANAGEMENT

PHARMACOLOGY

- Phenoxybenzamine: Provides alpha-adrenergic inhibition at dose of 10 mg every 12 hours. Every 2 days the dose is increased by 10 mg a day to achieve resting blood pressure (BP) within normal range and not associated with symptomatic postural hypotension. Can be used to prevent hypotension as a major complication of tumor resection. It is administered before surgery in increasing doses to prevent side effects of orthostatic hypotension (see Table 8–2).
- Prazosin: An alpha-adrenergic blocking agent used to treat pheochromocytoma. It causes less prolonged postoperative hypotension and less tachycardia than dibenzyline (see Table 8–2).
- Metyrosine: Metyrosine, a norepinephrine synthesis blocker, inhibits the enzyme tyrosine hydroxylase and reduces the synthesis of norepinephrine to less than half the pretreatment rate. The dose is 250 mg twice a day up to 500 mg four times a day (see Table 8–2).

- Calcium antagonists: Nifedipine, verapamil, and nicardipine can be used to prevent catecholamine release from tumor, myocarditis, or coronary artery spasm (see Table 1–6, p. 28).
- Labetalol: An alpha-adrenergic and beta-adrenergic antagonist, labetatol can be used when hypertension is accompanied with tachycardia and dysrhythmias.

DIET

- Drinking caffeine-containing substances such as coffee, tea, or cola, which can promote catecholamine discharge from pheochromocytomas, should be avoided.
- Diet includes increased caloric intake to reverse the effects of catabolism.

NURSING MANAGEMENT: NURSING DIAGNOSES AND COLLABORATIVE PROBLEMS

Nursing Diagnoses

Common nursing goals for patients with pheochromocytoma are to increase tissue perfusion, promote activity tolerance, provide nutritional balance, and reduce anxiety.

Altered peripheral, myocardial, and cerebral tissue perfusion related to catecholamine effect.

Expected Patient Outcomes. Patient maintains adequate tissue perfusion, as evidenced by heart rate (HR) ≤100 bpm, BP within patient's normal range, capillary refill ≤3 seconds, absence of cyanosis, skin warm and dry, absence of dysrhythmias, absence of chest pain, alertness, normal sensorimotor function, and peripheral pulses +2.

- Assess clinical indicators of perfusion: BP, HR, skin color, mean arterial pressure (MAP), capillary refill, urinary output (UO), and peripheral pulses.
- Provide a quiet environment for adequate rest periods while patient experiences a headache.

- Avoid sudden activity or positional changes that may compress the abdomen, thereby reducing the risk of stimulating catechol-amine release from pheochromocytomas.
- Administer prescribed phenoxybenzamine to provide alpha-adrenergic inhibition.
- Administer prescribed metyrosine to re-duce the synthesis of norepinephrine.
- Administer prescribed volume expanders, isotonic fluids, and blood products to main-tain circulatory volume without increasing myocardial demand.
- Should pharmacological agents be ineffec-tive in providing alpha-adrenergic inhibition and reducing synthesis of norepinephrine, prepare patient for adrenalectomy surgery.
- Teach patient to avoid smoking and drink-ing caffeine-containing substances, which can precipitate catecholamine release from pheochromocytomas.
- Teach patient to avoid Valsalval maneuver, which can precipitate tumor secretion.

Activity intolerance related to weakness.

Expected Patient Outcome. Patient maintains activity tolerance, as evidenced by decreased verbalization of fatigue or weakness.

- Organize nursing care activities to allow patient time to accomplish activities.
- Provide a calm and relaxing environment.
- Encourage patient to identify when he or she experiences feelings of fatigue or weakness.
- Provide rest periods before and after physi-cal activity.
- Encourage patient to ambulate and assist as necessary.
- Assess patient's tolerance of incremental increases in physical activity: cardiac rhythm, HR, BP, and respiratory rate (RR).
- Restrict physical activity to patient's toler-ance and for appropriateness to avoid re-lease of catecholamines.
- Teach patient the relationship between pheo-chromocytoma and fatigue or weakness.

Altered nutrition: less than body require-ments related to abdominal pain or nausea.

Expected Patient Outcome. Patient maintains adequate nutritional intake.

- Consult with dietitian to individualize a diet that includes patient's preferences.
- Encourage patient to reduce sodium and caffeine intake.
- Encourage patient to eat small meals daily when not nauseated.
- Ask patient's family to bring favorite foods from home when within therapeutic limits of the prescribed diet.
- Obtain daily weight and report weight loss ≥0.5 to 1.0 kg/d.
- Administer prescribed medication for nau-sea, if not contraindicated, 30 minutes be-fore meals.

Anxiety related to sympathetic nervous sys-tem activation by excessive catecholamine secretion.

Expected Patient Outcome. Patient experiences reduced anxious feelings.

- Provide a quiet and calm environment con-ducive to rest.
- Explain all procedures and validate pa-tient's understanding of them.
- Reduce environmental stimuli while patient is experiencing a hypertensive episode.
- Organize nursing care activities so patient can have periods of uninterrupted sleep.
- Minimize postural positions that apply ab-dominal pressure, thereby increasing cate-cholamine release from pheochromocytoma.
- Teach patient stress-reduction techniques such as meditation and guided imagery.

DISCHARGE PLANNING
The critical care nurse will provide patient and significant other(s) with verbal or written dis-charge notes regarding the following subjects:

1. Importance of keeping all postdischarge ap-pointments and regular laboratory studies.
2. The purpose, dose, and side effects of pre-scribed medications.
3. Signs and symptoms associated with pheo-chromocytoma.

PART II: SURGICAL CORRECTION AND NURSING MANAGEMENT

■ ADRENALECTOMY

Case Management Basis
DRG: 286 Adrenal and pituitary procedures
LOS: 9.50 days

Purpose
Adrenalectomy can be used to treat physiological derangements associated with Cushing's syndrome, pheochromocytoma, and primary aldosteronism.

Patient Selection

INDICATIONS. Total bilateral adrenalectomy is performed for bilateral adrenal hyperplasia. Other indications include adenoma, adrenal carcinoma, and pheochromocytoma, and Cushing's syndrome.

CONTRAINDICATIONS. Patient poor surgical risk

Procedure

TECHNIQUE

Posterior Approach. Its advantages are that it is extraperitoneal and adrenalectomy can be performed with minimal disturbance of adjacent viscera. The posterior approach is the most direct, and no major muscles are transected; therefore discomfort is reduced. The right adrenal gland lies superior in the retroperitoneum, while the left adrenal gland is approached posteriorly through the bed of the twelfth rib.

Flank Approach. Used in obese patients, it is a extraperitoneal flank incision through the bed of the eleventh or twelfth rib. On the left side, the colon is reflected medially and the pancreas upward to expose the lateral and anterior surface of the kidney, which is then retracted downward to expose the left adrenal gland. On the right side, the colon and duodenum are reflected medially, and the liver is reflected upward to expose the kidney and adrenal gland.

Lateral Approach. This is best used on patients with small unilateral tumors. On the left side, the adrenal gland is forced laterally, branches from the phrenic artery to the superior pole of the adrenal gland are ligated, and lastly the medial and the inferior vascular attachments are taken down. On the right side, the liver is identified, infrahepatic attachments mobilized, superior blood supply secured, arterial branches from the renal vessels ligated, the main adrenal vein ligated, and the adrenal gland removed.

Thoracoabdominal Approach. The patient is placed in a semioblique position. The incision is begun in the 9th intercostal space near the angle of the rib and carried across the costal margin at the midpoint of the contralateral rectus muscle just above the umbilicus. An alternative incision can be made at or above the rib. The incision is carried down through the latissimus dorsi, external oblique, internal oblique, transversus abdominis, and rectus muscles. The lung is retracted and adrenalectomy is completed.

Complications
Myocardial infarction, pancreatic fistula, biliary leak, wound infection, urinary tract infection, atelectasis, or pleural effusion.

NURSING MANAGEMENT: NURSING DIAGNOSES AND COLLABORATIVE PROBLEMS

Nursing Diagnoses
Common nursing goals for patients experiencing adrenalectomy are to maintain fluid balance, prevent infection, and reduce pain.

Fluid volume deficit related to intravascular volume loss secondary to diuresis or hemorrhage.

Expected Patient Outcomes. Patient maintains adequate fluid volume, as evidenced by urinary output (UO) $\geq$30 mL/h or 0.5 mL/kg/h, blood pressure (BP) within patient's normal range, heart rate (HR) $\leq$100 bpm, central venous pressure (CVP) 2 to 6 mm Hg, respiratory rate (RR) 12 to 20 BPM, skin warm and dry, peripheral pulses +2, capillary refill $\leq$3 seconds, and absence of cyanosis.

- Consult with physician to validate expected patient outcomes used to evaluate fluid balance.
- Monitor results of serum osmolality 285 to 295 mOsm/kg, sodium 135 to 145 mEq/L, potassium 3.5 to 5.0 mEq/L, chloride 100 to 106 mEq/L, calcium 8.5 to 10.5 mg/100mL, phosphorous 3.0 to 4.5 mg/100mL, glucose 70 to 110 mg/100mL, hemoglobin, hematocrit, blood urea nitrogen (BUN), creatinine, urine sodium 80 to 180 mEq/L, and urine negative for glucose and acetone.
- Obtain and report hemodynamic parameters associated with fluid volume deficit: cardiac output (CO) $\leq$4 L/min, cardiac index (CI) $\leq$2.7 L/min/m^2, CVP $\leq$2 mm Hg, pulmonary artery systolic pressure (PAS) $\leq$15 mm Hg or pulmonary artery dystolic (PAD) pressure $\leq$8 mm Hg, and pulmonary capillary wedge pressure (PCWP) $\leq$4 mm Hg.
- Assess clinical indicators of hydration: skin turgor and warmth, peripheral pulses, and capillary refill.
- Obtain and report clinical findings associated with fluid volume deficit: hypotension, tachycardia, poor skin turgor, peripheral pulses $\leq$+2, and capillary refill $\geq$3 seconds.
- Measure intake, output, specific gravity. Report UO $\leq$30 mL/h or $\leq$0.5 mL/kg/h and weight loss 0.5 to 1.0 kg/d suggesting fluid retention.
- Evaluate incision, drainage tubes, or cannulation site for bleeding.

- Encourage patient to drink fluids high in sodium content to compensate for sodium loss.
- Administer prescribed IV 5% Dextrose and nasal saline (D$_5$NS) to maintain hydration, maintain circulating volume and provide a glucose source.
- Administer IV fluids or volume expanders as prescribed to maintain adequate hydration.
- Administer corticosteroids as prescribed.

High risk for infection related to drainage from incision or cannulation sites.

Expected Patient Outcomes. Patient is free of infection, as evidenced by normothermia; white blood cell (WBC) count $\leq$11,000/μL; negative cultures; and absence of redness, tenderness, swelling, or drainage from incision or cannulation site.

- Review results of WBC count and cultures of blood, urine, sputum, or wound.
- Monitor temperature every 2 to 4 hours while patient is febrile.
- Monitor dressing, incision, or cannulation site for swellings, tenderness, redness, or drainage.
- Use sterile technique when changing dressings or tubings.
- Administer antibiotics as prescribed.

Pain related to incision.

Expected Patient Outcome. Patient expresses reduced or no complaints of pain.

- Assist patient in finding a position of comfort.
- Encourage patient to describe pain on a scale of 1 to 10.
- Discuss with patient situations that increase or decrease the pain experience.
- Progress ambulation as tolerated.
- Provide support of surgical incision during movement or ambulation.
- Administer analgesics as prescribed.
- Instruct patient to use alternative strategies to reduce pain: progressive relaxation, meditation, soft music, or guided imagery.

Collaborative Problems

A common collaborative goal for patients undergoing adrenalectomy is to correct dysrhythmias.

Potential Complication: Dysrhythmias. Dysrhythmias related to electrolyte imbalance secondary to use of corticosteroids.

Expected Patient Outcomes. Patient maintains regular sinus rhythm and serum electrolytes within normal range.

- Review results of 12-lead ECG and serum electrolyte levels.
- Monitor cardiac rhythm for changes in configuration and presence of dysrhythmias resulting from hyperkalemia.
- Assess for clinical indicators of hyperkalemia: weakness, flaccid paralysis, abdominal distention, diarrhea, and bradycardia.
- Measure daily weight, intake, specific gravity, and UO.
- Administer IV fluids and electrolytes to maintain adequate hydration and electrolyte balance.

DISCHARGE PLANNING

The critical care nurse will provide patient and significant other(s) with verbal or written discharge notes regarding the following subjects:

1. Importance of keeping all postdischarge appointments and regular laboratory studies.
2. The purpose, dose, and side effects of prescribed medications.
3. Signs and symptoms associated with incisional infection.
4. Importance of achieving an adequate diet and progressive exercise program.

REFERENCES

Angermeier KW, Montie JE. Perioperative complications of adrenal surgery. *Urol Clin North Am.* 1989;16:597–606.

Batcheller JC. Disorders of antidiuretic hormone secretion. *AACN Clin Issues Crit Care Nurs.* 1992;3:370–378.

Blevins LDS, Wand GS. Diabetes insipidus. *Crit Care Med* 1992;20(1):69–79.

Bloom LS, Libertino JA. Surgical management of Cushing's syndrome. *Urol Clin North Am.* 1989; 16:547–565.

Bravo EL. Primary aldosteronism. *Urol Clin North Am.* 1989;16:481–486.

Brody GM. Diabetic ketoacidosis and hyperosmolar hyperglycemic nonketotic coma. *Topics Emerg Med.* 1992;1(4):12–22.

Brown D. Patient with disorders of the thyroid and neurohypophysis. In: Clochesy, JM, Breu C, Cardin S. et al, eds. *Critical Care Nursing.* 1037–1040. Philadelphia PA: WB Saunders Co, 1993.

Butts DE. Fluid and electrolyte disorders associated with diabetic ketoacidosis and hyperglycemic hyperosmolar nonketotic coma. *Nurs Clin North Am.* 1987;22:827–837.

Clark AP. Complications and management of diabetes: a review of current research. *Crit Care Nurs Clin North Am.* 1994;6:723–734.

Coffland FJ. Endocrine disorders affecting the cardiovascular system. *Crit Care Nurs Clin North Am.* 1944;6:735–745.

Defensor-Agana A, Proch M. Pheochromocytoma: a clinical review. *AACN Clin Issues Crit Care Nurs.* 1992;3:309–318.

Deglin JH and Vallerand AH. Davis's Drug Guide for Nurses, 4th ed. Philadelphia, PA: FA Davis, 1993.

Dolan JT. *Critical Care Nursing Clinical Management Through the Nursing Process.* Philadelphia, PA: FA Davis Co; 1991.

Epstein CD. Adrenocortical insufficiency in the critically ill patient. *AACN Clin Issues Crit Care Nurs.* 1992;3:705–713.

Fitzgerald PA. Endocrine disorders. In: Tierney LM, McPhenn SJ, Papadakis MA, eds. *Current Medical Diagnosis and Treatment.* 33rd ed. Norwalk, CT: Appleton & Lange, 1994; 912–976.

Ford RD. Diagnostic Tests Handbook. Springhouse, PA: Springhouse Corp, 1987.

Graves L. Diabetic ketoacidosis and hyperosmolar hyperglycemic nonketotic coma. *Crit Care Nurs Q.* 1990;13(3):50–61.

Isley WL. Thyroid disorders. *Crit Care Nurs Q.* 1990;13(3):39–49.

Jones TL. From diabetic ketoacidosis to hyperglycemic hyperosmolar nonketotic syndrome: the spectrum of uncontrolled hyperglycemia in diabetes mellitus. *Crit Care Nurs Clin North Am.* 1994;6:703–720.

Kessler CA. Diabetes insipidus. In: Von Rueden KT, Walleck CA, eds. *Advanced Critical Care Nursing.* Rockville, MD: Aspen Publications, 1989;207–220.

Kessler CA. Acute adrenocortical insufficiency. In: Von Rueden KT, Walleck CA, eds. *Advanced Critical Care Nursing.* Rockville, MD: Aspen Publications, 1989;221–234.

Kessler CA. Hyperosmolar coma. In: Von Rueden KT, Walleck CA, eds. *Advanced Critical Care Nursing.* Rockville, MD: Aspen Publications, 1989;235–248.

Kessler CA. An overview of endocrine function and dysfunction. *AACN Clin Issues Crit Care Nurs.* 1992;3:289–299.

Kigerl K. Patients with disorders of glucose metabolism. In: Clochesy JM, Breu C, Cardin S, et al, eds. *Critical Care Nursing.* Philadelphia, PA: WB Saunders Co; 1993;1029–1036.

Kitabchi AE, Murphy MB. Diabetic ketoacidosis and hyperosmolar hyperglycemic nonketotic coma. *Med Clin North Am.* 1988;72:1545–1563.

Lee LM, Gumowski J. Adrenocortical insufficiency: a medical emergency. *AACN Clin Issues Crit Care Nurs.* 1992;3:319–330.

Loeb S. Clinical Laboratory Tests. Springhouse, PA: Springhouse Corp., 1991.

Loeb S. Nurse's Handbook of Drug Therapy. Springhouse, PA: Springhouse Corp., 1993.

Malone MJ, Libertins JA, Tsapatsaris NP, et al. Preoperative and surgical management of pheochromocytoma. *Urol Clin North Am.* 1989;16:567–582.

McMillan JY. Preventing myxedema coma in the hypothyroid patient. *Dimensions of Crit Care Nurs.* 1988;7(3):136–144.

Mulcahy K. Hypoglycemia emergencies. *AACN Clin Issues Crit Care Nurs.* 1992;3:361–369.

Novick AC. Surgery for primary hyperaldosteronism. *Urol Clin North Am.* 1989;16:535–545.

Pitts DD, Kilo KA, Pontious SL. Nutritional support for the patient with diabetes. *Crit Care Nurs Clin North Am.* 1993;51:47–56.

Reasner CA. Adrenal disorders. *Crit Care Nurs Q.* 1990;13:67–73.

Roberts SL. Diabetic ketoacidosis. *Physiological Concepts and the Critically Ill Patient.* Englewood Cliffs, NJ: Prentice-Hall, 1985;282–329. [out of print].

Sabo CE, Michael SR. Diabetic ketoacidosis: pathophysiology, nursing diagnosis, and nursing interventions. *Focus Crit Care.* 1989;16(1):21–28.

Sauve DO, Kessler CA. Hyperglycemia emergencies. *AACN Clin Issues Crit Care Nurs.* 1992;3:350–360.

Schira MG. Steroid-dependent states and adrenal insufficiency. *Nurs Clin North Am.* 1987;22:837–841.

Shannon MT, Wilson BA. Govmi & Hayes Drugs and Nursing Implications, 7th Ed. Norwalk, CT: Appleton Lange, 1992.

Sheeler LR. Cushing's syndrome. *Urol Clin North Am.* 1989;16:447–455.

Spittle L. Diagnoses in opposition: thyroid storm and myxedema coma. *AACN Clin Issues Crit Care Nurs.* 1992;3:300–308.

Stillwell SB. *Mosby's Critical Care Nursing Reference.* St. Louis, MO: Mosby Year Book, 1992.

Swearingen PL, Keen JH. *Manual of Critical Care.* 2nd ed. St. Louis, MO: Mosby Year Book; 1992.

Winer N. Pheochromocytoma. *Crit Care Nurs Q.* 1990;13(3):14–22.

9

Psychosocial Deviations

PART I: PSYCHOSOCIAL PROBLEMS AND NURSING MANAGEMENT

■ ANXIETY

Definition

Anxiety is a state of apprehension or tension within a person that occurs when an interpersonal need for security or freedom from tension is not met. Anxiety is derived from an unknown internal stimulus that is inappropriate to the reality of an external stimulus or of a concern with a future stimulus. Mild anxiety is an expected outcome of illness and can induce a coping response by increasing alertness and encouraging learning or change. Moderate anxiety may alter a patient's ability to take in information and communicate needs. Severe anxiety or panic causes the individual to narrow his or her focus of attention, be unable to take in information, be unable to solve problems, and may cause distorted percep-

tion with the result that the patient may be unable to cope.

Behavioral Pathology

Pathological anxiety is distinguished from normative response by four criteria: First, autonomy signifies suffering that has a life of its own, with a minimal basis in recognizable environmental stimuli. Second, intensity describes a level of distress such that the individual requires interventions; the individual's capacity to bear discomfort has been exceeded. Duration, the third criterion, describes persistence of the symptoms with adaptive responses, indicating a disorder requiring treatment. And fourth, behavioral changes occur when anxiety so impairs coping that normal function is disrupted. The patient may show behavior by avoiding or withdrawing. Types of anxiety are state or trait anxiety. State anxiety is a transitory emotional condition that may vary in intensity and may fluctuate over time. Trait anxiety denotes stable, individual differences in proneness to anxiety, in which the individual sees the world as dangerous or threatening, and in the frequency with which anxiety states are experienced.

Nursing Assessment

PRIMARY CAUSES
- Lack of control over events; threats to self-control; threat of illness or disease; threat of hospital environment; separation from others; role changes; sensory or motor loss; financial problems; threat of death, divorce, unemployment, forced retirement; threat of invasive procedures or supportive devices; situational or maturational crisis; loss of status; unfamiliar environmental settings; inability to comprehend the consequences of illness; obstruction of goals; dependence; lack of knowledge or loss of decision-making power.

PHYSICAL ASSESSMENT
- Inspection: Nausea, diaphoresis, muscle tension, hand tremors, insomnia, urinary frequency and urgency, apprehension, nervousness, agitation, irritability, withdrawal, anger, regression, inability to concentrate, forgetfulness, lack of initiative or motivation, escape behavior, helplessness, dilated pupils, flushing, vomiting, diarrhea, weakness, crying, worry, tension, overexcitement, and excessive verbalization.
- Palpation: Palmar sweating.
- Auscultation: Increased blood pressure, tachycardia, or tachypnea.

NURSING MANAGEMENT: NURSING DIAGNOSIS AND COLLABORATIVE PROBLEM

Anxiety

Expected Patient Outcomes. Patient's agitation eases in response to specific therapeutic relaxation interventions; patient recognizes his or her own anxiety and verbalizes anxious feelings, exhibits a reduction in anxiety as do significant others, experiences an increase in physiological comfort, initiates measures to decrease the onset of anxiety, and uses appropriate coping mechanisms in controlling anxiety.

- Administer and review tests to measure anxiety, when appropriate (Table 9–1).
- Help patient understand the role of anxiety on his or her problem.
- Encourage patient to acknowledge and verbalize when he or she feels anxious.
- Orient patients to the environment, staff, and potentially threatening procedures so they know what to expect.
- Minimize anxiety-provoking stimuli in the environment.
- Help patient establish goals, knowing that small accomplishments can promote feelings of independence and self-esteem.
- Use distraction technique to focus patient's attention on nonthreatening stimuli that counteract those eliciting anxiety.
- Encourage the use of externally oriented relaxation techniques: progressive muscle relaxation, biofeedback, or hypnosis.
- Encourage the use of internally oriented relaxation techniques: meditation or imagery.
- Encourage the use of self-monitoring and establishment of goals by having patient write he or she is anxious.
- Allow patient a degree of control in own personal care.
- Give patient positive feedback when alternative coping strategies are used to counteract feelings of anxiety.
- Encourage the use of positive self-expectations in place of self-defeating predictions of failure and monitor patient's response.
- Utilize therapeutic touch to relax patient prior to and during perceived stressful situations.
- Clarify patient's reaction to anxiety.
- Establish a reassuring interpersonal relationship with patient.
- Plan the transfer out of critical care and discuss it with patient.
- Provide music as a relaxation technique to lower patient's anxiety.

TABLE 9–1. PARTIAL LIST OF PSYCHOSOCIAL DIAGNOSTIC TESTS

Test	Purpose/Use
Anxiety	
State Trait Anxiety (STAI)*	Assesses individual's level of anxiety at that particular moment in time; anxiety defined as score of 40 or greater on STAI test
Hospital Anxiety and Depression (HAD) Scale	14-item test that provides separate measures of anxiety and depression symptoms
Gottschalk Verbal Anxiety Scale (VA)	5-minute tape recording of topic selected by subject; asked a projective question, subject is instructed to talk about any exciting or interesting life experience he/she wishes to share
Body Image Disturbance	
Body Shape Questionnaire	Self-report questionnaire measures body dissatisfaction, fear of fatness, feelings of low self-worth because of appearance, desire to lose weight
Rosenberg Self-Esteem Scale (RSE)	10-item test with a 4-point agree-disagree scale
Coping, Ineffective Individual: Anger	
Multiple Affect Adjective Check List (Zuckerman, Lubir†)	Measures anxiety, depression, and hostility
Framingham Anger Scale	Measures modes of anger expression; assesses likelihood of anger held in, taken out on others, discussed with friends, and physical symptoms
State Trait Anger Scale (STAS)	Assesses intensity anger as an emotional state and individual differences in anger proneness as personality trait
Coping, Ineffective Individual: Depression	
Beck's Depression Inventory	21-item self-report questionnaire assesses organic, behavioral, and cognitive symptoms of depression; score of 10–18 indicates mild to moderate depression; a score of 19–29 indicates moderate to severe depression; score greater than 30 indicates severe depression
Zung Self-Rating Depression Scale (SDS) (Zung & Durham, 1965‡)	20-item scale; scores range from 0–100; score ≥50 has been associated with clinical depression
Mini-Mental State Examination (MMSE)	11-item screening test assesses orientation, meaning, attention, calculation, language, praxis, and ability to copy a design; score of 24 out of 30 indicative of impaired cognitive function
Coping Responses Questionnaire (CRQ)	Measures and classifies coping tactics adopted in the face of stressful life events
Profile of Mood States (POMS)	65-item, 5-point adjective rating scale consisting of 6 mood factors: hostility, confusion, depression, vigor, tension, fatigue
Visual Analog Scale for Depression	10-cm horizontal line representing an affective continuum used to discriminate between confused and depressed patients; patients place a slash through the line at the point indicating their feelings at the moment (left end: I am not depressed; right end: I am depressed)
Coping, Ineffective Individual: Loneliness	
Oars Multidimensional Functional Assessment Questionnaire	Obtain data related to socioeconomic, disease-related, and sociological characteristics
Coping, Ineffective Individual: Loss	
Texas Revised Inventory of Grief (Faschinghauer, DeVaul, Zisook§)	

TABLE 9-1

TABLE 9-1

TABLE 9–1. CONTINUED

Test	Purpose/Use
Coping, Ineffective Individual: Stress	
Hospital Stress Rating Scale (HSRS)	Measures psychologic stress of the hospitalization experience; stress is operationalized by a list of 49 possible hospital events or situations a person can experience; stress values can range from 13≥3 to 40.6
Gleser-Gottschalk-Wood Adjective Checklist	70-item, self-report instrument for measuring subjective feelings of tenseness-anxiousness (TA), fatigue (F), and sadness-depression (S). Reliability: tenseness-anxiousness 0.89, fatigue 0.80, and sadness-depression 0.89)
Denial, Ineffective	
Defense Mechanisms (DMI) (Gleser & Ihilevich)	Measures 5 different defenses: principalization, reversal, turning against object, projection, turning against self; first two viewed as denying defenses
Levine Denial of Illness Scale (LDIS)	Semistructured interview includes questions about patient's response to his/her illness; after each section, ratings are made on a 7-point scale; high scores indicate evidence of greater denial of illness
Family Process, Altered	
Family Inventory of Life Events and Changes (FILE)	71-item self-report of all life events experienced by family (reliability: 0.71)
Norbeck Social Support Questionnaire (NSSQ)	Measures social support
	Measures affect, affirmation, aid as functional components of social support
Indices of Coping Responses	Measures active and avoidance coping by asking respondents to rate their frequency of use of 32 different coping responses on a 1 to 4 scale
Cantril Self-Anchoring Ladder	Obtains respondents' perceptions of severity of their husband's condition; scale measures minimal severity (0) to extreme severity (10)
Strain Questionnaire (SQ)	Measures physical and psychologic stress responses
	48-item scale designed to measure self-report levels of behavioral, cognitive, and physical stress complaints
Dynamic Adjustment Scale	32-item scale used to measure marital quality
	Score range is from 0 to 151, with highest score indicating the best marital quality (reliability: 0.91)
Hopelessness	
Learned Helplessness Scale (LHS)	Items were rated as being either strongly indicative of learned helplessness or orthogonal to learned helplessness; higher the score on LHS, the higher participant's degree of learned helplessness
Erickson, Post, and Paige Hope Scale	20-item, self-report instrument focuses on importance of future-oriented goals and probability of attaining those goals; each goal rated on a 7-point scale of importance
Beck Hopelessness Scale (BHS)	Measures hopelessness
	Provides measure of the construct hope in the opposite direction
Nowotny Hope Scale (NHS)	47-item test within 6 subscales based on dimension of hope
	Dimensions consist of: orients to future, active involvement, comes from within, is possible, relates to or involves others or a higher being, related to meaningful outcomes to individuals

TABLE 9-1

TABLE 9–1. CONTINUED

Test	Purpose/Use
Pain	
Categorical Rating Scales (CRS)	Rate one dimension of pain experience
Visual Analog Scale (VAS)	Rate one dimension of pain experience

Multi-dimensional scales
  Pain Descriptive Scale
  Cross Modality Matching
  Sensory Decision Theory
  McGill Pain Questionnaire
	Qualify more than one component of pain experience, such as pain threshold and pain intensity or pain intensity and pain anxiety

Behavior and Activity Scales
  Black and Chapman's SAD Index
    (Somatic input, anxiety, and
    depression)
  University of Alabama Birmingham
    Pain Behavior Scale
  Self-Rating Pain and Distress Scale
  Wisconsin Brief Pain Questionnaire
	Scales provide information on behavior and performance dimensions that may provide clues as to patient's affective and cognitive states related to painful experiences

Powerlessness	
Multidimensional Health Locus of Control Scale (MHLOC)	Consists of 3 subscales representing internal, chance, and powerful others
Internal Health Locus of Control (IHLOC)	Assesses degree to which individual believes his/her own behavior responsible for health or illness
Chance Health Locus of Control (CHLOC)	Assesses belief that individual's level of health or illness is function of luck, chance, fate, or uncontrollable factors
Powerful Others Health Locus of Control (PHLOC)	Assesses individual's belief that degree of health or illness is determined by important figures such as physician, other health professionals, parents, or friends
Sleep Pattern Disturbance: Sleep	
Dynograph R-511A (Sensor Medics, Anaheim, CA)	Four-channel recorder provides graphic display of two channels of EEG and one channel each of EOG and submental EMG
Echol's Patient's Sleep Behavior Questionnaire Tool	Four levels of cortical vigilance defined: awake, drowsy, REM, and nonREM sleep
Verran/Snyder Halpern (VSH) Sleep Scale	14-item visual analog scale based on a taxonomy of sleep characteristics: fragmentation, length, latency, depth
Thought Process Altered: Confusion	
Clinical Assessment of Confusion (CAC)	Checklist of 25 psychomotor behaviors associated with varying degrees of confusion: greater number of behaviors observed, the more severe confusion
Visual Analogue Scale for Confusion (VAS-C)	Obtains information about context of nurse-subject relationship
Mental Status Questionnaire	Evaluates orientation and long-term memory
Cognitive Capacity Screening Examination (CCSE)	Measures orientation, registration, verbal recall, verbal concept formation

EEG, electroencephalogram; EMG, electromyogram; EOG, electro-oculogram; REM, rapid eye movement.

- Provide information about threatening or stressful situations, including invasive procedures.
- Provide accurate information regarding the current illness and care outcomes.
- Administer sedative-hypnotic, beta blocker, and antidepressant agents as prescribed and monitor patient's response, noting potential side effects.
- Teach the purpose of interventions and changes in care environment briefly, simply, and at repetitive intervals.
- Teach patient to perceive his or her own responsibility for distress rather than attributing it to someone or something else.
- Teach patient externally oriented relaxation techniques such as progressive muscular relaxation, biofeedback, and therapeutic touch.
- Teach patient internally oriented relaxation technique such as autogenic training, meditation, or self-hypnosis. Autogenic training consists of suggestions to oneself about the relaxing feelings such as heaviness and warmth.
- Teach patient imagery techniques, which involve the use of images or of fantasy to reduce anxiety and pain.

■ BODY IMAGE DISTURBANCE

Definition

Body image is the picture we form in our mind of our body or it is the way we perceive that our body appears to others. Body image disturbance is the state in which one experiences or is at risk of experiencing a disruption in the way one perceives one's body image. Components of body image include body reality, body ideal, and body presentation. Body reality refers to our body as it really is: tall, short, fat, thin, spotty, or coarse. It is the body viewed and measured as objectively as possible. Body ideal consists of a norm of body contours, body size, and relative proportion. Body ideal is carried in our mind and is applied to both our own body where body reality touches on the outside environment. Body presentation refers to how an individual presents his or her body appearance to the social world.

Behavioral Pathology

Disturbance in body image can manifest itself in different ways. Primary or secondary neurological disorder involves disturbance in the body percept aspect of body image. It may consist of autotopagnosia, the failure to recognize part of the body; anosognosia, the rejection of bodily disease such as hemiplegia and blindness; finger agnosia, the inability to recognize and select particular fingers; or agraphia, acalculia, and asomatognosia, the difficulty in distinguishing left from right. Disorders occurring after acute dismemberment, such as phantom phenomenon, indicate that the configuration of the body is suddenly altered, but the perception is not modified accordingly. Negative body concept in the presence of actual physical deformity concerns psychological distress that is secondary to the deformity, while the individual's personality may be well adjusted. Disturbed or negative body concept with minimal or no actual deformity applies to patients with minimal deformity who request plastic surgery and patients who think a physical defect is noticeable to others yet are in reality normal.

Nursing Assessment

PRIMARY CAUSES

- Alteration in body integrity, including disfigurement; unrealistic mental image of patient's own appearance; inconsistency between perception of body image and reality; failure to adapt to body-image alteration; negation from others; self-negation; refusal to look at altered body parts; lack of participation in self-care; social isolation; threat of loss of body part; dissociation of body from the disfiguring event; physical immobility; or lack of knowledge

PHYSICAL ASSESSMENT

- Inspection: Anorexia, weight loss, numbness of body part, fear of rejection, anger, hostility, guilt, withdrawal, personalization of injured body part, negative expression toward supportive devices, depression, restlessness, denial of lost or altered body part, alteration in body boundaries, dependence, refusal to accept change in self, apathy, or hopelessness.

- Auscultation: Hypertension, tachycardia, or tachypnea.

NURSING MANAGEMENT: NURSING DIAGNOSIS AND COLLABORATIVE PROBLEM

Body Image Disturbance

Expected Patient Outcomes. Patient verbalizes feelings about the way he or she views self and any alteration in body image, expresses the meaning the loss has for the individual and family, matches his or her perception of body image with reality, incorporates body changes into new or altered roles, and develops coping strategies for body image disturbance.

- Administer and review tests to measure body image disturbance, when appropriate (see Table 9–1).
- Listen to patient's concerns about potential or actual alterations in body image.
- Provide patient with small, achievable, enabling goals that can build self-confidence.
- Help patient identify self-negation and limit self-negation.
- Encourage positive verbalization in patient about self.
- Assist patient to realize that all body ideals are transitory, with the process continuing even when the body image has been damaged.
- Facilitate a body presentation over which patient has maximum behavioral and decisional control.
- Help patient begin to accept a body alteration in deformity.
- Encourage patient to participate in physiotherapy focused on walking, turning, sitting, and standing to improve muscle function and to create a new, acceptable body image.
- Help patient to develop coping strategies for dealing with body image disturbance.
- Assist patient in incorporating body changes into new or altered roles.
- Provide diversional activities, such as reading, television, or music.
- Monitor patient for changes associated with medications such as chemotherapy and corticosteroids.
- Encourage patient to use a social support network such as family, friends, and significant others.
- Instruct patient about the potential need for invasive procedures, surgery, and future management.
- Provide patient with body reality intervention such as maintaining adequate body weight, preparing for invasive treatment procedures.
- Monitor patient to prevent complications further altering body image.

■ INEFFECTIVE INDIVIDUAL COPING: ANGER

Definition

Anger is an emotional syndrome (or set of responses) that occurs in a social context or transitory situation. Anger is aimed at the correction of some perceived wrong. Anger can occur on three levels. At the biological level, anger is related to aggressive system and to the capacities for cooperative social living, symbolization, and reflective self-awareness. On the psychological level, anger is aimed at the correction of some perceived wrong. At the sociocultural level, anger functions to uphold accepted standards of conduct.

Behavioral Pathology

When an individual's needs are not met, frustration and anger occur. The extreme form of anger becomes hate. There are five kinds of hate: incipient, inward, explosive, deflected, and constructive. Incipient hate is a form of anger that impels the individual to action against the frustration and is the easiest to neutralize before it develops into a more vicious emotion. Inward hate is frustration turned inward to avoid experiences of anger and potential reprisals. This repressed hate operates within the person and can lead to other disorders or anxieties. Explosive hate can burst forth without warning, engulfing everyone in its path. Deflective hate is displaced from one object to another, thereby allowing its expression without hurting the original object. Constructive hate allows the individual to appropriately channel his or her anger.

Nursing Assessment

PRIMARY CAUSES

- Anger expression inhibited or internalized: perceived threat involving blocked goal, failure of individuals to live up to patient's expectations, disappointment, blow to self-view, illness perceived to be life-threatening, physical dependence, or altered social integrity. Agent of harm located in authoritative figure, family, or self.
- Anger directly expressed or externalized: perceived threat involving obstructed goal, role changes, or financial dependence. Agent of harm located in environment or critical care team.

PHYSICAL ASSESSMENT

- Inspection: Muscle tension, perspiration, flushed skin, nausea, clenched muscles or fists, avoidance of eye contact, silence, verbal abuse, argumentativeness, or demanding behavior.
- Auscultation: Hypertension, tachycardia, or tachypnea.

NURSING MANAGEMENT: NURSING DIAGNOSIS AND COLLABORATIVE PROBLEM

Ineffective Individual Coping: Anger

Expected Patient Outcomes. Patient is able to identify situations contributing to expressions

of anger and monitors behavior leading to internalization or externalization of anger.

- Administer and review test used to measure anger, when appropriate (see Table 9–1).
- Plan and provide care with respect for privacy and patient's sense of bodily integrity and control and give ample warning and explanations of all procedures.
- Provide opportunities, when appropriate, for control and decision making.
- Facilitate patient's acceptance of the angry feelings.
- Assist patient to identify the reason for anger.
- Assist patient to use anger-related energy in a constructive manner.
- Encourage patient to learn new and more effective methods of coping with anger and to recognize the situation unique to the setting that may create an angry reaction.
- Assist patient in identifying prehospital situation contributing to expression of anger.
- Assist patient to identify situations in which he or she feels anger.
- Encourage patient to acknowledge and express feelings of anger.
- Assist patient to use alternative coping strategies.
- Assist patient to identify positive aspects of the illness or injury.
- Encourage family to accept patient's behavior without judgment.
- Encourage patient to participate in decision making and self-care.
- Provide diversional activities as a way to reduce stress.
- Explore with patient the reasons behind angry feelings.
- Explore ways in which patient's behavior can change.
- Establish a reassuring interpersonal relationship so that patient can express angry feelings.
- Teach patient to evaluate feelings that lead to either internalization or externalization of anger.
- Teach patient to use progressive relaxation technique, meditation, or guided imagery to reduce feelings of anger and hostility.

- Teach family members to participate in care.
- Teach patient to use a journal so that personal anger patterns can be identified, which will assist in self-monitoring.
- Educate family members about patient's illness, the equipment at the bedside, and the treatment, which will provide understanding and a sense of control.

■ INEFFECTIVE INDIVIDUAL COPING: DEPRESSION

Definition

A decrease in normal performance, such as slowing of psychomotor activity or reduction of intellectual functioning. Depression covers a wide range of changes in affective state, ranging in severity from the normal, everyday mood of sadness or despondency to psychotic episodes with risk of suicide.

Behavioral Pathology

Major depressive disorder (unipolar depression) is characterized by one or more episodes of major depression without episodes of mania or hypomania. The individual experiences a sad mood, or a significant loss of interest occurs. Bipolar disorders are recurrent, episodic conditions characterized by a history of at least one manic or hypomanic episode.

A depressed person may make six cognitive errors. The first arbitrary inference involves drawing a negative conclusion in the absence of supporting data. The second, selective abstraction, focuses on a detail out of context, often at the expense of more salient information. The third, overgeneralization, is the drawing of conclusions about a wide variety of things on the basis of single events. The fourth error involves magnification and minimization: making errors in evaluating the importance and implications of actions. The fifth error, personalization, is the practice of relating external (negative) events to self when there is in fact no connection. The sixth, absolutist, dichotomous thinking is thinking in polar opposites.

Nursing Assessment

PRIMARY CAUSES

- Physiological causes include cardiac and vascular disease such as arteriosclerosis, congestive heart failure, hypertension, or postmyocardial infarction; drugs such as sedatives, tranquilizers, antihypertensives, or corticosteroids; and electrolyte imbalance such as bicarbonate excess, hypercalcemia, hypomagnesium, hyperkalemia, hypokalemia, or hyponatremia.
- Psychological causes include financial loss, feeling of powerlessness, guilt, role changes, life-style changes, separation from significant others, or threat to body integrity.

PHYSICAL ASSESSMENT

- Inspection: Constipation, diarrhea, headache, indigestion, menstrual changes, muscle aches, nausea, weight loss or gain, anorexia, agitation, anger, anxiety, avoidance, boredom, confusion, crying, denial, dependence, emptiness, fatigue, fearfulness, guilt, indecisiveness, indifference, irritability, loss of interest, loss of feeling, low self-esteem, sadness, self-criticism, sleep disturbance, slow thinking, social withdrawal, tension, or tiredness.
- Auscultation: Tachycardia.

NURSING MANAGEMENT: NURSING DIAGNOSIS AND COLLABORATIVE PROBLEM

Ineffective Individual Coping: Depression

Expected Patient Outcomes. The patient verbalizes when he or she is feeling depressed, initiates measures to decrease feelings of depression, and uses appropriate coping mechanisms in controlling depression through positive view of self, positive view of experience, and positive view of future.

- Administer and review tests to measure depression, when appropriate (see Table 9–1).
- Provide meaningful communication.

- Facilitate realistic appraisal of role changes.
- Assist patient to achieve a positive view of self by facilitating accurate perception of the illness, disease, or injury.
- Encourage patient to assume decision-making control.
- Encourage patient to accomplish specific tasks that enhance his or her confidence.
- Provide patient with personal space in the technical environment.
- Encourage patient to discuss the illness, treatment, or prognosis.
- Provide patient with knowledge regarding risk factors.
- Eliminate or modify causes of depression, if possible.
- Convey to patient or family an empathetic understanding.
- Provide information with emphasis on positive aspects.
- Measure progress in small increments with emphasis on each level of accomplishment.
- Help patient identify positive changes in his or her physical status.
- Assist patient in establishing realistic goals knowing that small accomplishments can enhance positive feelings of the future.
- Help patient with role transition.
- Administer antidepressive agents and monitor patient's response, noting any potential side effects.

■ INEFFECTIVE INDIVIDUAL COPING: LONELINESS

Definition
Loneliness is an emotional state in which the individual is aware of the feeling of being apart from another or others, along with the experience of a vague feeling of need for individuals.

Behavioral Pathology
Loneliness anxiety is due to a gap between what one is and what one pretends to be. The hospitalized patient no longer has an intimate sense of relatedness to the food he eats or the shelter that houses him. The person feels a sense of alienation from the world around him or her. Loneliness anxiety can stifle any emergence of self or realization of capacities. Existential loneliness is the real loneliness of genuine experience. The real loneliness may occur out of the depths of grief, despair, and the shattering of feelings.

Nursing Assessment

PRIMARY CAUSES
- Existential loneliness or real experience can be due to threat of illness, separation from significant others, separation from one's body, separation from one's values and ideas, an environment creating feelings of isolation, inability to see future changes, or physiological pain whether it is overreacted to or ignored.
- Loneliness anxiety can be due to fear of aloneness in the present or fear of aloneness in the future.

PHYSICAL ASSESSMENT
- Inspection: Loss of appetite, weight loss, fatigue, sleeplessness, anxiety, apathy, depression, lack of interest, or withdrawal.
- Auscultation: Tachycardia.

NURSING MANAGEMENT: NURSING DIAGNOSIS AND COLLABORATIVE PROBLEM

Ineffective Individual Coping: Loneliness

Expected Patient Outcomes. Patient identifies specific tensions that exacerbate loneliness, uses adequate coping strategies so that appropriate decisions can be made, and recognizes the need for support groups or significant others.

- Administer and review test to measure loneliness, when appropriate (see Table 9–1).
- Minimize the threat of illness by providing patient with realistic, yet positive goals.

- Provide knowledge regarding the critical care environment and patient's role as a patient.
- Encourage the family or significant other to participate in patient's care.
- Assist patient in establishing the boundaries of location so that he or she can have a sense of relatedness to the critical care environment.
- Assist both patient and family to look realistically at any changes that can be made in their life-style.
- Identify the tensions that enhance loneliness.
- Encourage patient to develop and use coping strategies to make appropriate decisions regarding his or her loneliness.
- Encourage patient to focus on the positive aspects of illness in terms of what he or she has learned about self and own ability to cope or adapt.
- Motivate patient toward developing expanded, rather than constricted, boundaries of illness.
- Teach the purposes of various procedures and supportive devices.

■ INEFFECTIVE INDIVIDUAL COPING: LOSS

Definition
Loss can be the result of acute illness, injury, or disease. It can be bereavement over loss of health or the loss of a limb, a blow to a person's self-concept, or the sudden necessity of changing life-style.

Behavioral Pathology
Abnormal responses to loss attributed to illness, injury, or disease may cause a threat. Threat implies anticipation of an event over which the individual may feel there is little or no control. Eventually the threat may cause behavioral responses that motivate patient to avoid the illness episode through denial. It is possible that denial can eventually lead to feelings of anger or depression.

Nursing Assessment

PRIMARY CAUSES
- Threat of illness, injury, or disease; potential for death; removal from familiar surroundings; loss of privacy; separation from significant others; loss of control; dependence on supportive devices; lack of decision-making power; loss of relatedness to physical being; incongruent expectations of self and reality; financial reversal; obstructed future goals; or alteration in body image.

PHYSICAL ASSESSMENT
- Inspection: Nausea, abdominal cramps, crying, trembling, fighting, screaming, negativism, attacking, moaning, sighing, or inability to concentrate.
- Auscultation: Tachycardia, hypertension or tachypnea.

NURSING MANAGEMENT: NURSING DIAGNOSIS AND COLLABORATIVE PROBLEM

Ineffective Individual Coping: Loneliness

Expected Patient Outcomes. Patient is able to discuss the loss; accepts the loss of function, part, or whole; makes realistic decisions about the loss and future; and incorporates the loss into future life-style changes.

- Administer and review test to measure loss, when appropriate (see Table 9–1).
- Recognize patient's need to present a positive physical body image and help patient realize there are other aspects of the individual that permit patient to continue a positive self image.
- Help patient attain a sense of self-esteem to his or her altered identity.
- Reduce patient's anxiety, since anxiety will narrow patient's perceptual field, thereby limiting information that can be provided.
- Listen to patient's discussion of the loss.

- Help patient evaluate the loss according to its nature, extent, rate of progression, degree, and reversibility of the reduced function.
- Help patient identify life situations or risk factors that can be altered to reduce future loss.
- Encourage patient's family to discuss the loss.
- Describe the stages of anticipatory grieving with both patient and family.
- Encourage family to participate in patient's care.
- Provide support system to patient that can assist him or her through the loss experience.
- Encourage patient and family to utilize pastoral services as needed.

■ INEFFECTIVE INDIVIDUAL COPING: STRESS

Definition

Stress is an intense exertion being experienced by the individual in response to stimuli that eventually tax the physiological, psychological, or sociological systems. Stressors are situational demands that disrupt smooth functioning and interfere with understood meanings in one's life by challenging one's world view. In addition, stressors become agents or factors that challenge the adaptive capacities of an individual, thereby placing a strain upon that person, which may result in stress or disease.

Behavioral Pathology

Pathological behavioral changes include pulmonary, hematological, musculoskeletal, and cardiovascular alterations. Pulmonary ventilatory changes include bronchial inflammation leading to ulceration and stenosis; mucus and secretion retention or stasis of secretions with mucus plugs, polymorphonuclear leukocytes, neutrophils, and alveolar macrophages; alveolar dilation with hyperinflation; or acinus dilation and destruction. Pulmonary circulatory changes involve the diversion of blood away from poorly functioning alveoli, increased pulmonary artery pressure, ventilation-perfusion mismatch, or pulmonary hypertension. Hematological changes include maintenance of or mild decrease in partial pressure of arterial oxygen (Pao_2), maintenance of partial pressure of arterial carbon dioxide ($PaCO_2$), normal to increase red blood cells (RBCs) and hemoglobin, acute respiratory failure, or polycythemia. Musculoskeletal changes involve the use of intercostal and abdominal muscles for breathing, some increased use of accessory muscles, use of sternocleidomastoid muscle to increase chest inflation, or respiratory muscle exhaustion. Cardiovascular changes can involve right ventricular hypertrophy or right heart failure.

Nursing Assessment

PRIMARY CAUSES

- Threat phase of illness, in which death is possibility; unfamiliar and technical environment; threat of invasive procedures; loss of biological integrity; separation from significant others; dependence on strangers; loss of control to supportive devices; lack of decision-making power; threat of complications; excess sensory stimuli; anger; depression; loss of employment; altered life-style; financial loss; lack of knowledge; insecurity about the future; obstructed goals; perception of illness incongruent with reality; or limited external resources.

PHYSICAL ASSESSMENT

- Inspection: Dry mouth, tremor, nausea, paresthesia, numbness, blurred vision, lightheadedness, dyspnea, shortness of breath, muscle tension, palpitation, anxiety, fear, restlessness, agitation, fatigue, reduced objective thinking, sarcasm, or negativism.
- Palpation: Moist skin.
- Auscultation: Tachycardia, hypertension, or tachypnea.

NURSING MANAGEMENT: NURSING DIAGNOSIS AND COLLABORATIVE PROBLEM

Ineffective Individual Coping: Stress

Expected Patient Outcomes. The patient is able to identify stressors, utilizes coping strategies to reduce stress, shares perceived origin of stress with staff, and recognizes need to change life-style to reduce stress.

- Administer and review tests to measure stress, when appropriate (see Table 9–1).
- Minimize environmental stressors, such as noise or lights.
- Help patient to identify situational or environmental stressors.
- Help patient to identify ways to cope with the stressors.
- Eliminate or modify the causes of stress, if possible.
- Assist problem solving by reducing concerns into small parts.
- Provide patient with privacy.
- Help patient to identify alternative ways of coping with stress.
- Help patient to identify environmental or situational factors contributing to stress.
- Listen to patient's verbalization of fears and anxieties related to his or her illness or disease.
- Encourage family support and participation in care.
- Identify patient's perception of his or her illness and role as a patient.
- Clarify any misconceptions regarding illness, treatments, or progress.
- Discuss with patient his or her previous hospital and illness experiences.
- Assist patient in making realistic future goals.
- Facilitate communication between patient and his or her friends.
- Encourage interdependence and eventual independence.
- Encourage patient to participate in his or her care and decision making.

- Help patient to identify external resources.
- Instruct patient as to the effects stress has on his or her illness, injury, or disease.
- Explain the purpose behind various treatment, procedures, or supportive devices.
- Teach patient externally oriented relaxation techniques such as progressive muscular relaxation, biofeedback, and therapeutic touch.
- Teach patient internally oriented relaxation technique such as autogenic training, meditation, or self-hypnosis. Autogenic training consists of suggestions to oneself about relaxing feelings, such as heaviness and warmth.
- Teach patient imagery techniques, which involve the use of images or of fantasy to reduce anxiety and pain.

■ INEFFECTIVE DENIAL

Definition

Denial is a defense mechanism operating outside of any conscious awareness in the endeavor to resolve emotional conflict and in so doing allay anxiety. The types of denial include major, partial, or minimal. Patients with major denial state they have experienced no fear at any time throughout their hospitalization or at any time earlier in their lives. Partial denial is exhibited by an individual who initially denies being frightened but eventually admits to experiencing some fear. Minimal denial applies to patients who complain of anxiety or admit to feeling frightened.

Behavioral Pathology

Possible pathological behavioral aspects of denial consist of personal relevance, urgency, vulnerability, responsibility, affect, affect relevance, or threatening information. With denial of personal relevance, an individual will face a danger and perceive it as entirely devoid of any personal threat to himself. In denial of urgency an individual is unable to face reality without the protective veil of distortion; he may thus bias the information processing and deny the urgency of the danger. In denial of vulnerability, an individual who maintains that he or she can cope with the situation denies his or her vulnerability. In denial of responsibility by denying the ability to do something about the danger, a person may abdicate his or her responsibility for what may occur and justify not taking any action. With denial of affect, the individual who denies the affect may gain some psychological comfort. With denial of affect relevance, the individual may for some time maintain the illusion that his or her fears, worries, and anxieties relate to something other than the primary threat he or she faces. In denial of threatening information, an individual shifts information in a biased manner. Thus, those aspects of the stimulus situation that are threatening can be minimized, reduced, or even avoided altogether.

Nursing Assessment

PRIMARY CAUSES
- Potential limitations of illness, hospitalization, or environment; threat of role changes; financial concerns; physical restrictions; lack of decision-making power; stress, dependence; unrealistic perceptions; and vulnerability or potential death.

PHYSICAL ASSESSMENT
- Inspection: Arrhythmias, gastrointestinal discomfort, rationalization, displacement, magical thinking, isolation, tunnel vision, selective perceptions, or withdrawal.
- Auscultation: Tachycardia, tachypnea, and normal or increased blood pressure.

NURSING MANAGEMENT: NURSING DIAGNOSIS AND COLLABORATIVE PROBLEM

Ineffective Denial

Expected Patient Outcomes. Patient is able to recognize when he or she is denying some aspect of illness or treatment and accepts symptoms associated with an illness, injury, or disease.

- Administer and review test to measure denial, when appropriate (see Table 9–1).
- Listen to patient's reasons for denial in confronting a perceived threat or harmful agent.
- Recognize the need that denial has for patient in meeting the reality of a difficult diagnosis.
- Evaluate when denial is interfering with treatment.
- Help patient to accept his or her illness or disfigurement.
- Help patient to evaluate realistically and find meaning in forced life-style changes.
- Provide knowledge regarding illness and complications as they pertain to individual patient.
- Encourage attributional thinking or causal thinking, when realistic, whereby the individual searches for and finds a cause for life events. This may help patient to recover basic assumptions that may be altered by illness situation.
- Use attention strategies to help individual focus on the stressor and his or her reaction to it.
- Should patient be unable to cope with both stress and reaction, assist with causal thinking, which requires thinking about the precursors to that event.

■ ALTERED FAMILY PROCESS

Definition
Altered family process is the inability of the family to sustain psychological stability, leading to sharpened insecurity from blocked patterns of behavior, causing the family to engage in new behaviors fostering equilibrium. A normally supportive family experiences a stressor that challenges its previously effective functioning ability.

Behavioral Pathology
When confronted with a family member's multiple losses associated with a catastrophic critical illness necessitating hospitalization in critical care, the family may become despon-

dent. The despondent family members may lack initiative, appear sad with a flat affect, lack energy, be unable to concentrate, lose weight, or lack in appetite.

Nursing Assessment

PRIMARY CAUSES

- Illness of a family member; fear of death; separation from the sick family member; sudden onset of illness without warning; unfamiliarity of the critical care environment; unfamiliarity of the critical care team; potential financial crisis; lack of knowledge regarding illness, diagnostic procedures, and prognosis; unfamiliarity with supportive devices connected to a family member; personal external stressors; role conflict; incongruent values, goals, or beliefs; unrealistic future goals; personality conflict within the family; interpersonal conflict with the sick family member; loneliness; or hopelessness.

PHYSICAL ASSESSMENT

- Inspection: Helplessness; decreased problem-solving ability; fear, anxiety; panic; withdrawal; crying; apathy; inability to meet physical, social, emotional, or spiritual needs of family members; inability to seek or accept outside help; unrealistic expectations; altered sleep pattern; anger; despair; overprotectiveness toward the sick family member; role confusion; shortened attention span; disorganized thought process; argumentative behavior; or agitation.

NURSING MANAGEMENT: NURSING DIAGNOSIS AND COLLABORATIVE PROBLEM

Altered Family Process

Expected Patient Outcomes. Family member(s) is able to verbalize concerns or fears regarding the illness, injury, disease, and need for hospitalization; verbalize concern over potential role and financial changes; participates in patient care; recognize strengths of the patient and family unit; uses effective coping strategies; and utilizes external resources.

- Consult with physician as to the amount of information that can be provided family members.
- Administer and review tests to measure altered family processes, when appropriate (see Table 9–1).
- Provide individualized and supportive care by identifying and acknowledging the family's needs.
- Answer the family's questions honestly, when appropriate.
- Assure family that their loved one is receiving the best care possible.
- Provide family, as appropriate, with specific facts about patient's program.
- Explain the rationale behind various diagnostic and treatment procedures.
- Allow family to visit frequently through open visiting to allay their anxiety.
- Provide family with daily update about patient's progress.
- Identify a consistent contact person within the family.
- Keep personal items at patient's bedside.
- Arrange a daily meeting between the family, nurse, and physician, if possible.
- Identify and clarify the family's perception about the illness, treatment, progress, and prognosis.
- Explain the purpose behind the supportive devices used in critical care.
- Encourage the use of a spiritual support system.
- Provide the family with information by answering and reanswering their questions.
- Assist the family in identifying alternative coping behaviors.
- Foster communication between the family and the sick family member.
- Provide flexible visiting hours.
- Help the family to accept potential role changes.
- Provide information regarding community resources.

- Assist the family in making decisions for the sick family member.
- Encourage the family to participate in patient's care, when realistic.
- Prepare patient for what they will see in critical care.
- Encourage the family to participate in group education sessions with families experiencing similar situations.

■ FEAR

Definition

Fear can be defined as a feeling of dread related to an identifiable source that the individual validates and perceives as being dangerous.

Nursing Assessment

PRIMARY CAUSES

- Loss of body part or function, disability, disabling illness, hospitalization, invasive procedures, pain, unfamiliar people and environment, lack of knowledge, or loss of significant others.

PHYSICAL ASSESSMENT

- Inspection: Fright, apprehension, avoidance, compulsive mannerisms, increased verbalization, muscle tightness, fatigue, anorexia, shortness of breath, nausea, diarrhea, flush or pallor, syncope, lack of concentration, irritability, or dilated pupils.
- Palpation: Warm or moist skin or paresthesia.
- Auscultation: Tachycardia, hypertension, and tachypnea.

NURSING MANAGEMENT: NURSING DIAGNOSIS AND COLLABORATIVE PROBLEM

Fear

Expected Patient Outcomes. Patient is able to identify the source of his or her fears, identifies effective coping strategies to alleviate fears, and identifies when fears are unrealistic.

- Provide knowledge regarding the critical care environment, monitoring devices, or treatments.
- Eliminate or modify causes of fear, if possible.
- Reduce impact of fear by establishing alternative approaches, such as consistent daily routine.
- Adapt patient's environment to counteract fear through keeping lights on or providing familiar objects.
- Encourage use of open visiting hours for significant others.
- Encourage patient to identify factors or situations contributing to feelings of fear.
- Provide reassuring touch when patient needs comforting.
- Provide procedural information about what will happen and sensation information about what will be felt, which can serve as a guide to reduce fear.
- Help patient identify coping strategies to lessen episodes of fear.
- Provide simple explanations as not to overload patient.
- Teach patient fear management techniques.
- Teach patient externally oriented relaxation techniques such as progressive muscular relaxation, biofeedback, and therapeutic touch.
- Teach patient internally oriented relaxation technique such as autogenic training, meditation, or self-hypnosis. Autogenic training consists of suggestions to oneself about the relaxing feelings such as heaviness and warmth.
- Teach patient to use imagery techniques, which involve the use of images or of fantasy to reduce anxiety and pain.

■ HOPELESSNESS

Definition

Hope is a multidimensional dynamic life force, characterized by a confident yet uncertain expectation of achieving a future good that is realistically possible and personally significant. Hopelessness is an emotional state displaying the sense of impossibility, the feeling that life is too much to handle. It is a subjective state in which an individual sees limited or no alternatives or personal choices available and is unable to mobilize energy in his or her behalf.

Behavioral Pathology

Individuals who experience unrealistically high levels of hope may be immobilized in the face of crises. An individual who holds a personal schema of invulnerability based on pure faith in divine healing may not perceive a need for medical intervention and is rendered inactive by hope. On the other hand, with unjustified hopelessness, a person with no hope gives up when facing a crisis. The individual accepts a negative outcome as inevitable and perceives no reason to undergo the vicissitudes of a medical regimen. In a condition of fragile coping, the individual has cognitive awareness of uncertainty. Hope permits an assumption that the dreaded outcome will not happen, but despair is a constant threat. In chronic fear, an individual has little hope and a predominance of despair.

Nursing Assessment

PRIMARY CAUSES

- Threats to internal resources such as autonomy, self-esteem, independence, strength, integrity, or biological security; threats to perceptions of external resources such as the environment, staff, or family; abandonment; failing or deteriorating condition; or long-term stress.

PHYSICAL ASSESSMENT

- Inspection: Weight loss, appetite loss, weakness, reduced activity, decreased verbalization, lack of initiative, decreased response to stimuli, decreased affect, passivity, interference with learning, mute-

ness, closing eyes, saddened expression, or not complying with treatment regimen.

NURSING MANAGEMENT: NURSING DIAGNOSIS AND COLLABORATIVE PROBLEM

Hopelessness

Expected Patient Outcomes. The patient maintains adequate self-care, assesses situations causing feelings of hopelessness, identifies feelings of hopelessness and goals for self, and maintains relationships with significant others.

- Administer and review tests to measure hopelessness, when appropriate (see Table 9–1).
- Provide an atmosphere of realistic hope.
- Create the environment to facilitate patient's active participation in self-care.
- Help patient use attachment ideation where a patient's thought focuses on loved ones and the experiences they have shared.
- Provide patient with the appropriate pastoral services.
- Provide patient with positive feedback for successful attempt to become involved in self-care.
- Encourage patient to express feelings about self and illness by active listening and asking open-ended questions.
- Motivate patient to begin participating in his or her own care.
- Encourage physical activities that give patient a feeling of progress and hope.
- Place pictures or mementos of hope objects or reminders of factors that facilitate hope close to patient.
- Evaluate whether physical discomfort is causing patient's feeling of hopelessness.
- Encourage patient to accept help from others.
- Assist patient to identify and use alternative coping mechanisms.
- Inform patient of his or her progress with an illness, disease, or injury.
- Teach patient how to identify feelings of hopelessness.

■ PAIN

Definition

Pain is a sensation perceived and interpreted in the brain. Pain does not reside in the tissues in which it is felt but is identified and evaluated in the brain. It is reviewed as an overwhelming and motivating force that drives the individual into activity aimed at stopping pain.

Nursing Assessment

PRIMARY CAUSES

- Noxious stimuli from the disease process, trauma, or chemicals, fatigue, environmental temperature changes, invasive diagnostic procedures, invasive supportive devices, muscle tension, immobility, overactivity, sensory restriction leading to sensory deprivation, anxiety, depression, anger, resentment, threat to individual's physical or emotional integrity, perceived threat of what pain implies, loneliness, or feeling of isolation.

PHYSICAL ASSESSMENT

- Inspection: Pallor, muscular tension, nausea, vomiting, weakness, fainting, twitching of facial muscles, moaning, grimacing, rapid blinking, crying, quiet and withdrawn, clenched teeth, excitement, irritability, restlessness, immobilization of painful area, and fatigue.
- Palpation: Moist skin.
- Auscultation: Hypotension, bradycardia, or tachypnea.

NURSING MANAGEMENT: NURSING DIAGNOSIS AND COLLABORATIVE PROBLEM

Pain

Expected Patient Outcomes. Patient is free of pain; describes the location, duration, and intensity of pain; uses pain relief strategies to minimize pain; identifies factors that influence the pain experience; uses pain medication appropriately; or verbalizes comfort.

- Consult with the physician regarding patient's pain experience.
- Administer and review tests to measure pain, when appropriate (see Table 9–1).
- Inform patient of the intensity and duration of the pain experience.
- Eliminate or modify causes if possible.
- Develop an individualized pain management plan for patient.
- Position patient to facilitate pain relief.
- Schedule medication for maximum coverage of pain control.
- Support patient through a painful experience.
- Reduce noxious stimulation.
- Encourage patient to verbalize concerns, fears, and anxieties.
- Encourage family to participate in pain-reduction strategies.
- Evaluate nonverbal cues for pain: facial grimace, tachycardia, tachypnea, and hypertension.
- Provide distraction to decrease the intensity of pain and to increase patient's tolerance to it.
- Encourage physical mobility.
- Encourage patient to change his or her position.
- Encourage the use of distraction techniques: puzzles, games, conversation, or music.
- Provide relaxation techniques: rhythmic breathing, imagery, hypnosis, or biofeedback.
- Utilize therapeutic touch to reduced pain.
- Provide interventions to reduce peripheral transduction: aspirin, acetaminophen, and nonsteroidal anti-inflammatory (NSAIDS) drugs (for additional information see Table 1–7).
- Explain the purposes behind transcutaneous electrical nerve stimulation (TENS): stimulate the large fiber afferents, which in turn suppress pain at the spinal cord level.
- Inform patient about risk of pain before a potentially painful procedure.

■ POWERLESSNESS

Definition

Power is the potential or actual ability of an individual to influence cognition, attitude, behaviors, or emotions of him- or herself or another individual. Powerlessness is the expectancy that one's own behavior cannot determine the outcome one seeks, a lack of personal control over certain events or situations.

Behavioral Pathology

There are several different types of power, which can be used constructively or destructively. Exploitive power is a type of power that subjects individuals to be used by and for the interest of the one who holds power. Manipulative power is power to control another individual who may originally may have ceded that power through anxiety; it involves little choice for the individual. Rational power is power to express directly what one feels and thinks and to act and participate according to one's feelings and thoughts. Nonrational power is when an individual structures his or her behavior in ways that cover or hide feelings and thoughts. Reward power involves the use of rewards or sanctions, such as recognition. Coercive power is the ability to inflict punishment or withhold reward for certain behaviors. Legitimate power is based on general agreement and evidence that there exist broad, general norms about what sorts of behavior, beliefs, options, and attitudes are appropriate and proper. Referent power is power an individual derives by identification with similarity with another individual. Informational power is power socially independent of the source. Competitive power can be power directed against another individual.

Nursing Assessment

PRIMARY CAUSES

- Sensory or motor loss, inability to communicate, inability to perform roles, lack of knowledge, lack of privacy, social isolation, inability to control personal care, separation from significant others, loss of control to others, lack of decision-making control, fear of pain.

PHYSICAL ASSESSMENT

- Inspection: Tiredness, fatigue, dizziness, headache, nausea, apathy, withdrawal, resignation, empty feeling, feeling of lack of control, fatalism, lack of knowledge of illness, anxiety, acting out behavior, restlessness, sleeplessness, lack of decision making, aggressiveness, anger, dependence on others, passivity.

NURSING MANAGEMENT: NURSING DIAGNOSIS AND COLLABORATIVE PROBLEM

Powerlessness

Expected Patient Outcomes. Patient identifies situations causing feelings of powerlessness; exhibits control over the illness and care; experiences an increase in physiological control; engages in problem-solving and decision-making behaviors; seeks information regarding the illness, treatment, and prognosis; and establishes realistic goals that foster an increased sense of control.

- Encourage patients to identify situations in which they feel powerless.
- Enhance effective communication between patient, family, and health care team.
- Eliminate or modify the causes of powerlessness.
- Provide patient with control or choices when possible or realistic.
- Provide information regarding the illness, treatment, and prognosis.
- Encourage patient to express feelings about self and illness.
- Organize care so that patient has consistent health care providers.
- Encourage patient to participate in making decisions pertaining to self-care.

- Encourage patient to ask questions and seek information.
- Involve patient and family in care.
- Accept patient's feelings of anger caused by a loss of control.
- Provide the opportunity for control in establishing privacy.
- Encourage the use of progressive relaxation, meditation, and guided imagery techniques to achieve a sense of acceptance.
- Provide patient with relevant educational information.
- Provide patient with decisional options.
- Encourage the use of appropriate diversional activity, such as play.
- Assist patient in redefining the illness situation to identify positive aspects.
- Listen to patient's discussion regarding possible role changes and financial concerns.
- Teach patient sensory changes associated with invasive procedures.
- Teach patient how to maintain own progress through the use of a journal.
- Teach patient how to accept the illness and potential changes in life-style.

■ SENSORY AND PERCEPTUAL ALTERATION: SENSORY DEPRIVATION

Definition

Sensory deprivation is a reduction in the amount and intensity of meaningful sensory input. It is a generic term for a variety of complex conditions that drastically reduce the level of variability of a person's normal stimulation from, and commerce with, his or her environment for a relatively prolonged period of time.

Nursing Assessment

PRIMARY CAUSES

- Alterations in biological stability, including complications; alterations in patient's ability to receive and interpret meaningful neurological, chemical, cardiovascular, or musculoskeletal stimuli; and understimulation of senses as a result of diagnostic or treatment modalities: tracheostomy tube, endotracheal tube, nasogastric tube, arterial line, peripheral lines, intracranial pressure monitoring, traction, casts; isolation; physical immobility; lack of patterning of environmental stimuli; meaningless stimuli from supportive devices; lack of knowledge; loss of control; overload of meaningless professional jargon; unfamiliarity in a highly technical environment; or impaired communication.

PHYSICAL ASSESSMENT

- Inspection: Minor itching, feeling excessively warm or cold, numbness in fingers or toes, disoriented as to time or place, altered problem-solving ability, altered behavior or communication pattern, inaccurate evaluation of environmental stimuli, restlessness, fear, sleep pattern disturbance, anxiousness, confusion, noncompliant behavior, or visual hallucinations.
- Auscultation: Tachycardia, tachypnea, and normal or increased blood pressure.

NURSING MANAGEMENT: NURSING DIAGNOSIS AND COLLABORATIVE PROBLEM

Sensory and Perceptual Alteration: Sensory Deprivation

Expected Patient Outcomes. Patient is able to accurately interpret environmental stimuli, increase sensory input to appropriate levels when necessary, and experiences no auditory or visual hallucination.

- Describe patient's immediate environment.
- Explain unusual or excess sounds from supportive devices.
- Provide therapeutic touch to enhance meaningful sensory input.
- Schedule care to reduce sleep interruption.
- Eliminate or modify causes of sensory deprivation.

- Provide patient with frequent reorientation to time, place, and person.
- Provide meaningful stimulation with clock, calendar, radio, or television.
- Provide sensory enhancers such as glasses or hearing aide.
- Provide diversional activities such as television, radio, or tape recorder to facilitate sensory stimulation.
- Encourage patient to gradually increase physical activity, if realistic.
- Allow family and friends to visit, thereby providing meaningful sensory input.
- Encourage patient to participate in decision-making activities.
- Reduce unnecessary lights or noise.
- Teach patient about procedures or treatments before they are initiated.

■ SENSORY AND PERCEPTUAL ALTERATION: SENSORY OVERLOAD

Definition

Sensory overload implies that two or more modalities are in action simultaneously at levels of intensity greater than normal and that the combination of stimuli is usually introduced suddenly. Sensoristasis is a drive state of cortical arousal that impels the organism to strive to maintain an optimal level of sensory variation.

Nursing Assessment

PRIMARY CAUSES

- Overstimulation in a high-load environment, territorial invasion, pain, medications, lack of space, minimal privacy, excessive noise, inability to reduce incoming stimuli through mobility, inability to derive meaning from professional jargon, erroneous perception of events leading to illness and hospitalization, instructional overload, unfamiliar supportive devices, alteration in patient's ability to receive and interpret meaningful stimuli, lack of physical mobility, lack of knowledge, or monotony of stimuli.

PHYSICAL ASSESSMENT

- Inspection: Fidgetiness, numbness, anorexia, motor incoordination, muscle tension, hallucinations, sound distortion, disturbed sense of time, feelings of floating in space, feelings of loss of control, sleeplessness, fatigue, irritability, apathy, decreased reasoning, anxiousness, or short attention span.
- Palpation: Sweating hands.
- Auscultation: Tachycardia or tachypnea.

NURSING MANAGEMENT: NURSING DIAGNOSIS AND COLLABORATIVE PROBLEM

Sensory and Perceptual Alteration: Sensory Overload

Expected Patient Outcomes. Patient is oriented to time, place, and person; identifies factors contributing to sensory and perceptual overload; interacts appropriately with staff, friends, or significant other; and identifies ways to reduce sensory overload.

- Eliminate or modify causes of sensory overload.
- Cluster treatments and procedures to avoid repeated intrusions into patient's territory and personal space.
- Provide meaningful therapeutic touch to avoid excessive sensory stimuli.
- Reduce unnecessary environmental noises and sounds.
- Evaluate patient's sensory modes and encourage the use of prosthetic devices: hearing aid or glasses.
- Assist the family in providing meaningful interventions.
- Encourage the use of favorite diversional activities: television or radio.
- Assist patient to identify coping patterns that can be used to alleviate stimuli associated with sensory overload.
- Provide uninterrupted sleep.
- Provide patient with earplugs to decrease excess sensory stimuli.

• Teach patient the purpose of equipment, procedures, treatments, and alarms.

■ SLEEP PATTERN DISTURBANCE: SLEEP DEPRIVATION

Definition

Sleep pattern disturbance is an alteration in the quality or quantity of sleep required by an individual so that he or she is unable to restructure the overcrowded data storage accumulated each day or to reinforce character structure. Sleep deprivation is the lack of adequate sleep or dream time, related to prior or unusual sleep patterns.

Nursing Assessment

PRIMARY CAUSES

• Excessive noise, pain, illness, immobility, environmental change, fear, medication, lack of exercise, fear of death, loneliness.

PHYSICAL ASSESSMENT

• Inspection: Lassitude, lethargy, hallucinations, disorientation, confusion, restlessness, irritability, apathy, poor judgment, hostility, inability to concentrate, frequent dozing, dark circles under eyes, or difficulty remaining asleep.
• Auscultation: Hypertension, tachycardia, or tachypnea.

NURSING MANAGEMENT: NURSING DIAGNOSIS AND COLLABORATIVE PROBLEM

Sleep Pattern Disturbance: Sleep Deprivation

Expected Patient Outcomes. Patient is able to sleep through the night, identifies techniques to help induce sleep, sleeps for 90 minute segments and feels refreshed, and displays no irritability, lethargy, or confusion.

• Administer and review tests to measure disturbances in sleep pattern, when appropriate (see Table 9–1).

• Evaluate the frequency and length of daytime naps.
• Adhere to patient's bedtime ritual.
• Eliminate extraneous stimuli such as lights, unnecessary activities, noise, and staff verbal exchange, when realistic.
• Position ventilator so that it produces the lowest decibel level for patient.
• Reduce machine alarm decibel to the lowest acceptable level.
• Turn off suction and oxygen units when they are not in use.
• Darken room at night and for naps.
• Adjust room temperature and provide blankets for comfort.
• Schedule treatments, including medications and respiratory therapy, prior to sleep.
• Provide daytime activity, such as range-of-motion exercises, sitting, standing, or walking.
• Encourage patient to increase his or her activity level during the day so that he or she can sleep at night.
• Position patient so that he or she is comfortable.
• Provide meaningful touch through back rubs.
• Evaluate and provide patient's usual sleep stimuli, such as radio or television.
• Allow patient's spouse to sleep over in patient's room.
• Provide earplugs to eliminate extraneous environmental stimuli, if necessary.

■ SPIRITUAL DISTRESS

Definition

Spiritual distress can be defined as a situation when an individual or group questions the belief or value system that provides hope and meaning to their lives.

Nursing Assessment

PRIMARY CAUSES

• Loss of function or body part, disease or illness, trauma, personal or family disasters, loss of significant others, distress related to treatments or invasive procedures, or being embarrassed by others.

PHYSICAL ASSESSMENT

- Inspection: Feeling separated or alienated from belief, questioning belief system, depression, despair, ambivalence regarding values and beliefs, sense of spiritual emptiness, feeling of perceived abandonment, feeling of hopelessness, or emotional detachment from self and others.

NURSING MANAGEMENT: NURSING DIAGNOSIS AND COLLABORATIVE PROBLEM

Spiritual Distress

Expected Patient Outcomes. Patient continues to maintain and practice spiritual beliefs, experiences decreased feelings of abandonment or guilt, is satisfied with personal events, and feels a sense of closeness to family and beliefs.

- Recognize patients own personal value and belief system.
- Refer to clergy as needed or appropriate.
- Assist patient with spiritual reading when requested.
- Provide privacy so patient can practice spiritual rituals.
- Allow patient to talk about own values and beliefs especially, when these may conflict with those of significant others.
- Help patient identify previous sources of spiritual comfort.
- Provide spiritual support resources if so desired by patient or family.
- Encourage diet with religious restrictions when not detrimental to health.
- Ask questions about patient's personal past and belief systems that can be used to help her or him get through the present crisis.
- Listen to patient's attempts to find reason for an illness, injury, or disease.
- Provide a reality base when patient attributes pain, suffering, or illness to punishment or judgment for past wrongdoing.

■ ALTERED THOUGHT PROCESS: CONFUSION

Definition

Confusion is an attention deficit. It also incorporates the individual's inability to integrate incoming stimuli.

Nursing Assessment

PRIMARY CAUSES

- Medical conditions include hypoxia; hypocarbia; pulmonary disease; congestive heart failure; electrolyte or fluid imbalance; disorders of thyroid, parathyroid, and adrenal glands; vitamin B_1 deficiency; alcoholism; avitaminosis; malnutrition, local infections such as pneumonia, septicemia, meningitis, or encephalitis; dysrhythmias; transfusions; low blood volume; or cardiac surgery.
- Surgical conditions consist of postoperative states, anesthesia, pain medications, hypothermia, postoperative anxiety, agitation, depression, severe postoperative illness, or cerebral trauma during surgery.
- Intoxication conditions include alcohol intoxication or withdrawal, opioid intoxication or withdrawal, anticholinergics, stimulants, sedatives, digitalis, vasopressors, steroids, or poisons.
- Neurological conditions consist of neurological disease, seizures, head trauma, cerebral anoxia, hypertensive encephalopathy, or intracranial neoplasm.
- Sensory-perceptual alterations resulting from prolonged immobilization or bed rest, recent vision or hearing loss, amputation, casts or traction, unrelieved pain, sensory overload, lengthy stay in ICU, or sleep deprivation.

PHYSICAL ASSESSMENT

- Inspection: Disorientation, impaired attention span, restlessness, anxiousness, apprehension, fear, agitation, incoherent speech, withdrawal, belligerence, combativeness, delusions, impaired memory, unable to recognize others, incontinence, or arrhythmias.

- Palpation: Moist skin.
- Auscultation: Tachycardia or hypertension.

NURSING MANAGEMENT: NURSING DIAGNOSIS AND COLLABORATIVE PROBLEM

Altered Thought Process: Confusion.

Expected Patient Outcomes. Patient is oriented to person, place, and time; recognizes family members; maintains appropriate responses to environmental stimuli; engages in appropriate conversation; and differentiates reality from fantasy.

- Administer and review tests to measure altered thought process, when appropriate (see Table 9–1).
- Ask questions that encourage answers that reflect reality perception.
- Protect patient from injury while confused.
- Identify situations or factors that might cause confusion.
- Listen to patient's confused statements and assist with reality orientation.
- Listen to family concerns, fears, and anxieties.
- Reassure patient that the confusion is temporary.
- Reduce the demand for cognitive functioning when patient is ill or fatigued.
- Introduce new experiences gradually.
- Reorient patient with each interaction.
- Evaluate confusion for frequency and situation.
- Orient patient to time, place, and person.
- Acknowledge patient's confusion and delusions so they can be described realistically in a safe manner.
- Teach patient about all procedures just prior to their occurrence.

SELECTED REFERENCES

Artinian NT. Stress experience of spouses of patients having coronary artery bypass during hospitalization and 6 weeks after discharge. *Heart Lung.* 1991;20:52–59.

Averill J. *Anger and Aggression: An Essay on Emotion.* New York, NY: Springer-Verlag; 1982.

Barnfather JS, Erickson HE. Construct validity of an aspect of the coping process: potential adaptation to stress. *Issues Men Health Nurs.* 1989; 10:23–40.

Belgrave FZ, Molock CD. The role of depression in hospital admission and emergency treatment of patients with COPD. *J Natl Med Assoc.* 1991; 83:777–781.

Biaggio MK. Therapeutic management of anger. *Clin Psychol Rev.* 1987;7:663–675.

Biley FC. Stress in high dependency units. *Intensive Care Nurs.* 1989;5:134–141.

Bolwerk CA. Effects of relaxing music on state anxiety in myocardial infarction patients. *Crit Care Q.* 1990;13:63–72.

Breznitz S. The denial of stress. New York: International Universities Press; 1983:254–280.

Brown P. The concept of hope: implications for care of the critically ill. *Crit Care Nurse.* 9:97–105.

Buckwalter K, Babich KS. Psychologic and physiologic aspects of depression. *Nurs Clin North Am.* 1990;25:945–954.

Bulechek GM, McCloskey JC. *Nursing Interventions.* 2nd ed. Philadelphia, PA: WB Saunders Co, 1992.

Carpenito LJ. *Handbook of Nursing Diagnosis.* 6th ed. Philadelphia, PA: JB Lippincott Co; 1995.

Christopher SB. Pain assessment. *Crit Care Nurs Clin North Am.* 1991;3:11–16.

Clark S. Psychosocial needs of critically ill patients. In: Clochesy JM, Breu C, Cardin S, et al, eds. *Critical Care Nursing.* Philadelphia, PA: WB Saunders Co; 1993:75–90.

Clark S. Nursing interventions for the depressed cardiovascular patient. *J Cardiovasc Nurs* 1990; 5(1):54–64.

Clements S, Cummings S. Helplessness and powerlessness: caring for clients in pain. *Holistic Nurs Prac.* 1991;6(1):76–85.

Copel LC. Loneliness. *J Psychosocial Nurs.* 1988; 26:14–19.

Cray L. A collaborative project: initiating a family intervention program in a medical intensive care unit. *Focus Crit Care.* 1989;16:212–218.

Dhooper SS. Identifying and mobilizing social support for the cardiac patient's family. *J Cardiovasc Nurs.* 1990;5:65–73.

Donovan MI. Acute pain relief. *Nurs Clin North Am.* 1990;25:851–861.

Doody SB, Smith C, Webb J. Nonpharmacologic interventions for pain management. *Crit Care Nurs Clin North Am*. 1991;3:69–75.

Dracup K, Clark S. Challenge in critical care nursing: helping patients and families cope. *Crit Care Nurse*. 1993; (suppl): 4–9.

Dufault K, Martocchio BC. Hope: its sphere and dimensions. *Nurs Clin North Am*. 1985;20:379–391.

Farrell M. Dying and bereavement. *Intensive Care Nurs*. 1989;5:39–45.

Field N. Physical causes of depression. *J Psychosoc Nurs Ment Health Serv*. 1985;23:7–11.

Fontaine DK. Measurement of nocturnal sleep patterns in trauma patients. *Heart Lung*. 1989;8:402–410.

Foreman MD. Confusion in the hospitalized elderly: incidence, onset, and associated factors. *Res Nurs Health*. 1989;12:21–29.

Galpin C. Body image and end-stage renal failure. *Br J Nurs*. 1992;1(1):21–23.

Gettrust KV, Ryan S, Engleman DS. *Applied Nursing Diagnosis*. New York, NY: John Wiley & Sons, 1985.

Hickey M. Psychosocial needs of families. In: Clochesy JM, Breu C, Cardin S, et al, eds. *Crit Care Nursing*. Philadelphia: WB Saunders Co; 1993:91–101.

Jarvis SL. Powerlessness and the patient under neuromuscular blockade. *J Neurosci Nurs*. 1992;24:346–349.

Kendell PC, Watson D. *Anxiety and Depression: Distinctive and Overlapping Features*. New York, NY: Academic Press Inc; 1989.

Kleiber C, Halm M, Tither M. et al. Emotional responses of family members during a critical care hospitalization. *Am J Crit Care*. 1993;3(1):70–76.

Kohlman-Carrieri V, Douglas MK, Gormley JM, et al. Desensitization and guided mastery: treatment approaches for the management of dyspnea. *Heart Lung* 1993;22:226–34.

Lacey JH, Birtchnell SA. Body image and its disturbances. *J Psychosom Res*. 1986;30:623–631.

Leidy NK. A physiologic analysis of stress and chronic illness. *J Adv Nurs*. 1989;14:868–876.

Light RW, Merrill EJ, Despairs JA, et al. Prevalence of depression and anxiety in patients in COPD. *Chest*. 1985;87:35–38.

Louie K. Empathy, anxiety and transcultural nursing. *Nurs Standards*. 1990;5:36–40.

Lowery BJ, Jacobsen BS, Cera MA, et al. Attention versus avoidance: attributional search and denial after myocardial infarction. *Heart Lung*. 1992;21:523–527.

McFarland GK, McFarlane EA. *Nursing Diagnosis and Interventions Planning for Patient Care*. St. Louis, MO: Mosby Year Book; 1993.

Minarik P, Leavitt M. (1989). The angry, demanding, hostile response. In: Riegel B, Ehrenreich D, eds. *Psychological Aspects of Critical Care Nursing*. Rockville, MD: Aspen Publications, 1989;66–91.

Mlynczak B. Assessment and management of the trauma patient in pain. *Crit Care Nurs Clin North Am*. 1989;1:55–64.

Price B. Normal body image. In: *Body Image Nursing Concept and Care*. Englewood Cliffs, NJ: Prentice Hall; 1990:3–16.

Price B. Planning a nursing intervention. In: Body Image Nursing Concept and Care. Englewood Cliffs, NJ: Prentice Hall, 1990:81–93.

Price B. A model for body image care. *J Advanced Nurs*. 1990;13:585–593.

Quinless FW, Nelson MA. Development of a measure of learned helplessness. *Nurs Res*. 1988;37:11–15.

Raine ML. The confused response. In: Riegel B, Ehrenreich D, eds. *Psychological Aspects of Critical Care Nursing*. Rockville, MD: Aspen Publications, 1989:109–131.

Roberts SL. *Behavioral Concepts and the Critically Ill Patient*. Norwalk, CT: Appleton-Century-Crofts, 1985. [out of print]

Roberts SL. Cognitive model of depression and the myocardial infarction. *Prog Cardiovasc Nurs*. 1989;4:61–70.

Roberts SL, White BS. Powerlessness and personal control model applied to the myocardial infarction patient. *Prog Cardiovasc Nurs*. 1990; 5:84–94.

Roberts SL. *Nursing Diagnosis and the Critically Ill Patient*. Norwalk, CT: Appleton & Lange, 1987. [out of print]

Robinson KR. Denial in myocardial infarction patients. *Crit Care Nurse*. 10:140–145.

Rosenbaum JE, Pollack MH. Anxiety. In: Hackett T, Cassem NH, eds. *Mass General Hospital Psychiatry Handbook*. 2nd ed. Littleton, MA: PSG Publishing Co; 1987:154–183.

Simpson T. Needs and concerns of families of critically ill adults. *Focus Crit Care*. 1990; 16:388–397.

Sims A, Smith P. The Management of Anxiety. Anxiety in Critical Practice. New York, NY: John Wiley & Sons; 1988;81–98.

Spielberger CD, Johnson EH, Russell SF, et al. In: Chesney M, Rosenman R (eds). The experience and expression of anger: construction and validation of an anger expression scale. *Anger and Hostility in Cardiovascular and Behavioral Disorders.* New York, NY: Hemisphere Publishing; 1985:5–30.

Stoner MH. Measuring hope. In: Stromborg-Frank M, ed. *Instruments for Clinical Nursing Research.* Norwalk, CT: Appleton & Lange, 1988.

Synder M. *Independent Nursing Interventions.* 2nd ed. Albany, NY: Delmar Publications Inc; 1992.

Topf M, Davis JE. Critical care unit noise and rapid eye movement (REM) sleep. *Heart Lung.* 1993; 22:252–258.

Urban N. Patient responses to the environment. In: Kinney MR, Packa DR, Dunbar SB, eds. *AACN's Clinical Reference for Critical Care Nursing.* 3rd ed. St. Louis, MO: Mosby Year Book; 1993:117–128.

White BS, Roberts SL. Powerlessness and the pulmonary alveolar edema patient. *Dimensions Crit Care Nurs.* 1993; 12(3):127–137.

Multisystem Deviations

10

PART I: HEALTH PROBLEMS AND
NURSING MANAGEMENT

■ DISSEMINATED INTRAVASCULAR COAGULATION

(For related information see Cardiac Deviations, Part I: Shock, p. 174. Dysrhythmias, p. 184. Part III: Hemodynamic monitoring, p. 219. Psychosocial Deviations, Part I, p. 725.

Case Management Basis
DRG: 397 Coagulation disorder
LOS: 5.50 days

Definition
Disseminated intravascular coagulation (DIC) is a syndrome caused by the presence of thrombin in the systemic circulation. In DIC there is a pathological overstimulation of normal coagulation processes, causing microvascular thrombi and hemorrhagic complications.

Pathophysiology
The clotting cascade involves the activation of the clotting factors and continues until thrombin is produced and a fibrin clot is formed. The fibrin clot is produced through either the intrinsic or extrinsic pathway. Both pathways eventually lead to thrombin and fibrin clot formation. The intrinsic pathway is activated when there is direct damage to red blood cells or platelets and when endothelial damage occurs. At this time blood comes in contact with the negatively charged particles of the exposed collagen of the basement membrane. The extrinsic pathway is stimulated when factor III, tissue factor (tissue thromboplastin), is released into the circulation from damaged tissues. Once factor VII is activated for either the intrinsic or extrinsic pathway, factor X emerges as the final common pathway. When factor X is activated, there is conversion of prothrombin (factor II) to thrombin (factor IIa). Thrombin cleaves fibrinogen into fibrin. Finally the fibrinolytic system is stimulated to control clot development and clot breakdown so normal blood flow can be restored. The pathophysiological processes of DIC can be divided into three major groups: endothelial damage, release of tissue factor, and platelet aggregation. Disruption of endothelium permits thrombogenic endothelial activity to dominate. Vascular endothelium is damaged by endotoxins, shock, acidosis, and hypoxia.

Tissue factor (factor III) from tissues damaged by trauma, obstetrical accident, or malignancies produces activation of the extrinsic pathway at factor VII. The tissue factor, found on the surface of monocytes and macrophages, is a decisive procoagulant material. Finally, excessive stimulation of platelet aggregation can lead to the inappropriate clotting found in DIC. Sepsis is associated with platelet aggregation. Any one of the three major groups can lead to overstimulation of the normal coagulation process, which results in a disseminated coagulation system and excessive fibrinolysis. Besides activation of the coagulation system, fibrinolysis, kallikrein-kinin, and complement are also activated. These factors produce thrombosis and hemorrhage. The kallikrein-kinin system produces bradykinin, a vasodilator, which causes hypotension, vascular permeability, and shock in DIC patients. The complement system produces anaphylatoxins causing cell lysis, increased vascular permeability, and platelet release reaction. The overall response is production of procoagulant material to perpetuate the clotting cycle. Excessive thrombin is also activated, causing excessive number of fibrin clots to be deposited in the microcirculation. The resulting microthrombi cause disrupted blood flow and widespread organ hypoperfusion. Excess thrombin can produce hemorrhage by converting more factor II into thrombin (factor IIa) thus continuing the cycle. Clotting factors are consumed and not replaced, thereby perpetuating the bleeding cycle. Thrombin production stimulates the fibrinolytic system to increase fibrinolysis. Finally, there is increased plasmin, which degrades the fibrin clot. When fibrinogen is broken down into fibrin, microthrombi are deposited in the intravascular circulation. Stable clots are prevented from forming at the sites of injury.

Nursing Assessment

PRIMARY CAUSES

- Obstetrical alterations include abruptio placentae, abortion, dead fetus syndrome, eclampsia, amniotic fluid embolism, retained placenta, toxemia, or hydatid mole. Tissue traumas consist of burns, head injury, heat stroke, fat embolism, transplant rejection, snake bite, acute glomerulonephritis, acute hemolysis, adult respiratory distress syndrome (ARDS), or mismatched transfusions. Neoplasms include solid tumors, acute leukemias, giant cavernous hemangioma, adenocarcinomas, sarcomas, polycythemia vera, or pheochromocytoma. Hematologic mechanisms include drowning, sickle cell crisis, acute hemolytic secondary infection, or immune mechanisms. Cardiovascular causes consist of acute myocardial infarction, cardiogenic shock, progressive strokes, or aortic aneurysms. Infections include bacterial, rickettsial, viral mycotic, or parasitic infections. Other mechanisms are liver disease, acute and chronic renal disease, collagen vascular disorders, hemolytic uremia, necrotizing enterocolitis, acute pancreatitis, allergic vasculitis, amyloidosis, polycythemia vera, or ulcerative colitis.

PHYSICAL ASSESSMENT

- Inspection: Dyspnea; fatigue; diaphoresis; headache; malaise; nausea; vomiting; vertigo; weakness; acrocyanosis; confusion; seizures; petechiae; cyanosis; ecchymosis; hematomas; epistaxis; irritability; tarry, bloody stools; hematemesis; extremity paresis or paralysis; or pale yellow skin.
- Palpation: Weak, thready pulses or abdominal pain.
- Auscultation: Hypotension, tachypnea, decreased pulse pressure, palpitations, and hyperactive bowel sounds.

DIAGNOSTIC TEST RESULTS

Standard Laboratory Tests. (see Table 10–1)

- Blood studies: Plasminogen reduced ≤75%, antithrombin III assay reduced ≤75%, and D-dimer assay elevated ≥200 mg/mL, prothrombin time prolonged ≥15 seconds, activated partial thromboplastin

TABLE 10-1

TABLE 10–1. STANDARD DISSEMINATED INTRAVASCULAR COAGULATION LABORATORY TESTS

Test	Normal Value	Abnormal Findings
Coagulation Studies		
Antithrombin time	80%–120% normal activity	Reduced in DIC
D-dimer assay	≤200 ng/mL	Elevated in DIC
Activated partial thromboplastin time (aPTT) or partial thromboplastic time (PTT)	See Table 1–1	Prolonged in DIC
Fibrinogen levels	See Table 1–1	Decreased in DIC
Fibrinogen/fibrin degradation products	See Table 1–1	Increased in DIC
Platelet count	See Table 1–1	Decreased in DIC
Prothrombin time (PT)	See Table 1–1	Prolonged in DIC
Thrombin time	See Table 1–1	Prolonged in DIC

From Bell TN, 1993; Ford RD, 1987; Loeb S, 1991; Tribett D, 1993.

time prolonged ≥60 to 90 seconds, thrombin time prolonged ≥15 to 20 seconds, fibrinogen level decreased ≤75 to 100 mg/dL, platelet count decreased from 75,000 to 20,000/μL, fibrin degradation products increased ≥100 μg/mL, protamine sulfate test positive, and euglobulin clot lysis time 120 minutes or less reflects increased levels of plasminogen activates or plasmin. New tests include thrombin-antithrombin III complex (TAT) elevated, plasmin–alpha$_2$-antiplasmin complex (PAP) elevated, and fibrinopeptide A elevated. Factor assays (extrinsic coagulation system) show decreased II, V, VII, and X.

Noninvasive Hematological Diagnostic Procedures

- Chest roentgenogram: Interstitial edema with diffuse deposition of microemboli in the lungs.

MEDICAL AND SURGICAL MANAGEMENT

PHARMACOLOGY. (see Table 10–2)

- Heparin: Used to enhance antithrombin III to neutralize free circulating thrombin causing decreased fibrin formation and to prevent microvascular obstruction by thrombi and platelet aggregation. The recommended dose of heparin is from 500 U/h IV to 5 to 10 U/kg IV every 4 hours to 10 to 15 U/kg/h to low subcutaneous doses (see Table 1–8, p. 32).
- Antithrombin III concentration: A newer and controversial treatment of DIC, it is used to correct coagulation abnormalities and prevent thrombotic complications.
- Gabexate mesylate: A new experimental synthetic antithrombin agent that inhibits thrombin and other reactors in the clotting cascade. This process can occur in the absence of antithrombin II.
- Tranexamic Acid: A new experimental antifibrinolytic agent with fewer side effects.

FLUID THERAPY

- Blood component replacement products: washed packed red blood cells, fresh frozen plasma, platelet concentration, cryoprecipitated antihemophilic factor, antithrombin III concentrates, and volume expanders such as albumin and hetastarch are used to treat DIC.
- Crystalloid solutions: Lactated Ringer's solution, normal saline, and albumin are used to maintain adequate blood pressure (BP), central venous pressure (CVP), pulmonary capillary wedge pressure (PCWP), and cardiac output (CO).

HEMODYNAMIC MONITORING

- A reduced CO, PCWP, cardiac index (CI), and CVP with a high systemic vascular

TABLE 10-2

TABLE 10–2. MEDICATIONS USED IN DISSEMINATED INTRAVASCULAR COAGULATION (DIC)

Medication	Route/Dose	Uses/Effects	Side Effects
Heparin	IV: Range includes 500 U/h to 5010 U/kg 4 h to 10–15 U/kg/h	Manages DIC when ischemic organ dysfunction or failure or potential loss of life or limb is due to microvascular thrombi	Exacerbation of bleeding diathesis
		Prevents microvascular obstruction by thrombi by minimizing platelet aggregation	
		Slows coagulation cycle to allow clotting factor replenishment	
Newer or experimental drugs			
Antithrombin III		Corrects coagulation abnormalities in clotting cascade that occur in absence of antithrombin III	
Gabexate mesylate		Inhibits thrombin and other reactions in clotting cascade that occur in absence of antithrombin III	
Tranexamic acid		Antifibrinolytic agent	

From Bell TN, 1993; Ford RD, 1987; Loeb S, 1991; Tribett D, 1993.

resistance (SVR) can indicate hypovolemia and hypoperfusion.
- An elevated pulmonary artery pressure can indicate pulmonary microvascular clotting.

OXYGEN THERAPY
- Used to improve tissue oxygenation.

EXCHANGE TRANSFUSION AND PLASMAPHERESIS
- Exchanging the patient's plasma removes fibrin degradation products and supplies fresh clotting components (see Plasmapheresis, p. 790).

NURSING MANAGEMENT: NURSING DIAGNOSES AND COLLABORATIVE PROBLEMS
Common nursing goals for patients with DIC are to maintain fluid balance, prevent injury, increase tissue perfusion, support physical mobility, and reduce anxiety.

Nursing Diagnoses
Fluid volume deficit related to abnormal intravascular fluid loss secondary to depleted clotting components, fibrinolysis, or hemorrhage.

Expected Patient Outcomes. Patient maintains adequate fluid volume, as evidenced by heart rate (HR) ≤ 100 bpm, BP within patient's normal range, urinary output (UO) ≥ 30 mL/h or 0.5 mL/kg/h, CO 4 to 8 L/min, CI 2.7 to 4.3 L/min/m^2, CVP 2 to 6 mm Hg, PCWP 6 to 12 mm Hg, peripheral pulses +2, capillary refill ≤ 3 seconds, skin warm and dry, absence of cyanosis, resolution of impaired coagulation, stable hematological indicators, and absence of bleeding.

- Consult with physician to validate expected patient outcomes used to evaluate the presence of fluid balance.
- Review values of serum hemoglobin, hematocrit, total protein, blood urea nitrogen (BUN), creatinine, coagulation tests, and liver function tests.
- Limit activity to bed rest.
- Obtain and report hemodynamic parameters associated with decreased fluid volume: CO $\leq$4 L/min, CI $\leq$2.7 L/min/m^2, CVP $\leq$2 mm Hg, and PCWP $\leq$6 mm Hg.
- Assess the clinical indicators of hydration and perfusion: skin turgor, skin color and temperature, BP, HR, capillary refill, and peripheral pulses.
- Report clinical findings associated with fluid volume deficit resulting from hemorrhage: hypotension, tachycardia, poor skin turgor, pallor, petechiae, cyanosis, peripheral pulses $\leq$+2, capillary refill $\geq$3 seconds, weakness, fatigue, and malaise.
- Monitor for clinical indicators of bleeding: hypotension, tachycardia, acrocyanosis, presence of jaundice, petechiae, fatigue, weakness, bone or joint pain, headache, abdominal distention or tenderness, decreased peripheral pulses, UO $\leq$30 mL/h or capillary refill $\geq$3 seconds.
- Measure intake, output, specific gravity, and daily weight. Report UO $\leq$30 mL/h or $\leq$0.5 mL/kg/h and weight loss $\geq$0.25 to 0.5 kg/d.
- Assess arterial and venipuncture sites for oozing of fresh blood.
- Obtain sequential measurement of extremity circumference and abdominal girth, since persistent oozing into the tissue can indicate increasing coagulopathy.
- Assess patient receiving blood component replacement for transfusion reaction. Report clinical findings associated with transfusion reaction such as hives, chills, fever, facial flushing, headache, palpitations, tachycardia, dyspnea, and chest pain.
- Measure all blood loss: stool, urine, sputum, nasogastric drainage, drains, or wounds.

- Provide oxygen by nasal cannula or Venturi mask at the prescribed amount.
- Administer lactated Ringer's, saline, albumin, and other plasma expanders as prescribed: Maintain intravascular volume at levels to maintain optimal CO to meet tissue needs for oxygen and nutrients.
- Administer blood component replacement as prescribed: whole blood, platelets, and fresh frozen plasma.
- Administer cryoprecipitate as prescribed to restore depletion of factors V and VIII.
- Administer prescribed heparin therapy via continuous infusion pump or intermittently (via minidose) to interfere with thrombus formation.
- Teach patient to gently brush teeth and clean mouth with cotton swabs.

High risk of injury related to tissue ischemia secondary to coagulopathy.

Expected Patient Outcomes. Patient maintains absence of tissue ischemia and maintains adequate systemic perfusion.

- Review results of coagulation tests and liver function tests.
- Limit activity to bed rest.
- Provide high-protein diet to facilitate tissue repair.
- Use indwelling arterial and venous lines to draw blood and administer medications.
- Provide care in positioning to avoid pressure areas and damage to fragile capillaries, since third-space fluid shifts promote edema, thereby leading to risk of tissue breakdown.
- Assess clinical indicators of peripheral tissue perfusion: peripheral pulses, capillary refill, skin color, skin turgor, and skin warmth.
- Report clinical findings associated with impaired peripheral tissue perfusion: peripheral pulses $\leq$+2, capillary refill $\geq$3 seconds, cyanosis, extremity coolness, and poor skin turgor.
- Monitor extremities for pulses, color, warmth, and presence of edema.

- Monitor hematopoietic function: presence of bleeding and amount of blood loss; presence of acrocyanosis, petechiae, ecchymosis, purpura, or hematoma.
- Assess skin and extremities: color, temperature, presence of abrasions, pulses, presence of ecchymosis, or presence of edema.
- Protect extremities and digits from injury.
- Avoid using a BP cuff and avoid rectal temperatures.
- Use low suction if oral or tracheal suction is necessary.
- Pad side rails to protect patient from injury.
- Use electric rather than straight razor for shaving patient.
- Avoid using needle sticks to avoid the risk of hematoma formation.
- Apply antithromboembolic stockings.
- Administer prescribed IV fluids to maintain adequate hydration and circulating volume.
- Administer heparin as prescribed.

Altered cardiopulmonary, cerebral, and renal tissue perfusion related to intravascular coagulation with thrombosis in the microcirculation and hypotension secondary to hypercoagulopathy and hypoperfusion.

Expected Patient Outcomes. Patient maintains adequate tissue perfusion, as evidenced by BP within patient's normal range, CO 4 to 8 L/min, CI 2.7 to 4.3 L/min/m², coronary artery perfusion pressure (CAPP) 60 to 80 mm Hg, mean arterial pressure (MAP) 70 to 90 mm Hg, arterial oxygen saturation (SaO_2) ≥95%, HR ≤100 bpm, absence of chest pain, normal lung sounds, skin warm and dry, normal heart sounds, capillary refill ≤3 seconds, peripheral pulses +2, absence of confusion, equal and normoreactive pupils, normal sensorimotor function, partial pressure of arterial oxygen (PaO_2) ≥80 mm Hg, partial pressure of arterial carbon dioxide ($PaCO_2$) 35 to 45 mm Hg, respiratory rate (RR) 12 to 20 BPM, UO ≥30 mL/h or ≥0.5 mL/kg/h, and specific gravity 1.010 to 1.030.

- Consult with cardiologist to validate the expected patient outcomes used to evaluate adequate tissue perfusion.
- Review results of ECG, echocardiogram, chest roentgenogram, and arterial blood/gas measurement.
- Restrict physical activity to bed rest with head of bed elevated to decrease myocardial tissue oxygen demand should there be decreased myocardial tissue perfusion.
- Provide prescribed nutritional supplements to avoid malnutrition or a negative nitrogen balance.
- Obtain and report hemodynamic parameters reflective of decreased myocardial tissue perfusion when CO is decreased: CAPP ≤60 mm Hg, CO ≤4 L/min, and CI ≤2.7 L/min/m².
- Obtain and report other clinical findings suggestive of decreased myocardial tissue perfusion: chest pain, capillary refill ≥3 seconds, pallor, diaphoresis, crackles, shortness of breath, HR ≥100 bpm, or BP ≤90 mm Hg.
- Assess, document, and report findings reflective of decreased pulmonary tissue perfusion: PaO_2 ≤80 mm Hg, $PaCO_2$ ≥45 mm Hg, SaO_2 ≤95%, mottled or cyanotic skin, shortness of breath, dyspnea, RR ≥20 BPM, and crackles.
- Encourage patient to deep breathe and cough every 2 hours.
- Assess clinical indicators of neurological status: mental status, level of consciousness, sensory function, motor function, cranial nerve function, and deep tendon reflexes.
- Report clinical findings indicating decreased cerebral tissue perfusion: confusion, disorientation as to time and place, pupils unequal, and sensorimotor dysfunction.
- Assess, document, and report clinical findings indicating decreased peripheral tissue perfusion: capillary refill ≥3 seconds; peripheral pulses weak or absent; skin cool, clammy, and cyanotic; and BP 90/60 mm Hg.
- Monitor, document, and report clinical findings reflecting decreased renal tissue

perfusion: UO $\leq$30 mL/h or $\leq$0.5 mL/kg/h, specific gravity 1.010 to 1.030, and peripheral edema.

- Monitor intake, output, and specific gravity every 1 to 2 hours should UO $\leq$30 mL/h. Note that diuretics will decrease volume and further impair ventricular filling.
- Administer prescribed oxygen 2 to 4 L/min by means of nasal cannula or mask or fraction of inspired oxygen (FIO_2) $\leq$50% to maintain SaO_2 $\geq$95%.
- Should oxygenation not improve arterial blood gases, prepare patient for intubation and mechanical ventilation.
- Institute air flotation therapy to preserve skin integrity.
- Administer prescribed blood products, colloids, or crystalloids to maintain adequate hydration, UO $\geq$30 mL/h or $\geq$0.5 mL/kg/h and specific gravity 1.010 to 1.030.
- Administer positive inotropes (dopamine or dobutamine) to maintain MAP 70 to 90 mm Hg, HR $\leq$100 bpm, BP within patient's normal range, and UO $\geq$30 mL/h.
- Teach patient to report the presence of chest pain.

Impaired physical mobility related to pain secondary to bleeding into muscle and joints.

Expected Patient Outcomes. Patient's verbalization of pain during physical activity is reduced.

- Confer with physical therapist regarding realistic postillness activity schedule.
- Evaluate patient's mobility: movement in all extremities, presence of joint or muscle pain, or presence of swelling and tenderness.
- Assist patient with incremental increases in physical activity.
- Assess and report joint or muscle pain, hemarthrosis, and joint or extremity swelling and tenderness.
- Provide a bed cradle to protect patient from further trauma.
- Provide prescribed hot or cold compresses to reduce bone or joint pain.

- Maintain proper body alignment.
- Provide gentle range-of-motion exercises.
- Use a draw sheet to lift the patient, thereby avoiding skin abrasions and risk of bleeding.

Anxiety related to fear of dying and insufficient information.

Expected Patient Outcome. Patient's verbalization of anxiety is reduced.

- Confer with physician regarding the information to be shared with patient and family.
- Confer with priest, minister, or rabbi regarding patient's unique concerns.
- Encourage patient to express feelings of concerns or fears.
- Instruct patient regarding the causes of DIC and its treatment.

Collaborative Problems

Common collaborative goals for patients with DIC are to improve oxygenation and increase CO.

Potential Complication: Ventilation-Perfusion Imbalance. Ventilation-perfusion imbalance related to intrapulmonary shunting secondary to increased pulmonary capillary membrane permeability and pulmonary edema.

Expected Patient Outcomes. Patient maintains adequate ventilation-perfusion balance, as evidenced by ventilation/perfusion ($\dot{V}/\dot{Q}$) ratio 1.0, SaO_2 97% mixed venous oxygen concentration ($S\bar{v}O_2$) 75%, alveolar-arterial oxygen gradient (P[A$-$a]O_2)$\leq$15 mm Hg on room air or 10 to 65 mm Hg on 100% oxygen, arterial-alveolar oxygen tension ratio (P[a:A]O_2) 0.75 to 0.90, static compliance (Cst) $\geq$50 mL/cm H_2O, dynamic compliance (Cdyn) $\geq$45 mL/cm H_2O, RR 12 to 20 BPM, absence of adventitious breath sounds, absence of cyanosis, absence of dyspnea, CO 4 to 8 L/min, CI 2.7 to 4.3 L/min/m^2, PCWP 4 to 12 mm Hg, MAP 70 to 100 mm Hg, BP within patient's normal range, arterial blood gases within normal range, and HR $\leq$100 bpm.

- Consult with physician to validate expected patient outcomes used to evaluate ventilation-perfusion balance.
- Confer with Respiratory Therapy regarding the appropriate ventilatory support for the DIC patient.
- Review arterial blood gas measurements, static lung compliance, dynamic lung compliance, physiological shunting, alveolar-arterial oxygen gradient, arterial-alveolar oxygen tension ratio, or ventilation-perfusion scan.
- Limit physical activity to bed rest to decrease the work of breathing.
- Obtain and report hemodynamic parameters that could affect ventilation/perfusion balance: CO $\leq$4 L/min, CI $\leq$2.7 L/min/m^2, PCWP $\leq$12 mm Hg, MAP $\leq$70 mm Hg, and S$\bar{v}$O$_2$ $\leq$60%.
- Assess clinical indicators of respiratory status: rate and rhythm, symmetry of chest wall movement, use of accessory muscles, skin color, and lung sounds.
- Obtain and report other clinical findings associated with decreased ventilation: perfusion ratio: tachypnea, cyanosis, crackles, dyspnea, and tachycardia.
- Monitor $\dot{V}/\dot{Q}$ ratio and report value $\leq$1.0, which signifies reduced alveolar ventilation. A low alveolar perfusion $\dot{V}/\dot{Q}$ ratio is referred to an intrapulmonary shunt (blood flow (Qs)/total flow (Qt)) $\geq$15% to 30%.
- Provide prescribed positive end-expiratory pressure (PEEP) and inverse ratio ventilation (IRV) for high Qs:Qt levels.
- Obtain the following information in order to measure Qs:Qt: hemoglobin level, FIO$_2$ level, arterial and mixed venous blood gas results, and arterial and mixed venous oxyhemoglobin (oxygen saturation) values.
- Monitor alveolar partial pressure of oxygen (PAO$_2$) and arterial partial pressure of oxygen (PaO$_2$), which are approximately equal. Report a diversion of PAO$_2$ from PaCO$_2$, which signifies the development of an intrapulmonary shunt.
- Estimate Qs/Qt using the following methods: PaO$_2$:FIO$_2$ ratio $\geq$286. arterial:alveolar

(a:A) ratio $\geq$0.60, alveolar-arterial (A$-$a) gradient $\leq$20 mm Hg with an FIO$_2$ of 0.21, respiratory index $\leq$1, and shunt equation $\leq$5%.
- Monitor and report PAO$_2$:FIO$_2$ $\leq$200, which is considered to be a large intrapulmonary shunt (20%). The lower the value, the more severe the $\dot{Q}$s/$\dot{Q}$t disturbance.
- Obtain and report SaO$_2$ $\leq$90%, which can signify intrapulmonary shunting.
- Evaluate the effectiveness of PEEP according to the following criteria: arterial blood gases, mixed venous oxygen tension, lung compliance, PCWP, and CO.
- Increase PEEP, as prescribed, in increments of 3 to 5 cm H$_2$O pressure until the desired PEEP is achieved to keep PAO$_2$ $\geq$60 mm Hg.
- Monitor and report complications associated with PEEP: reduced venous return, reduced CO, reduced cerebral perfusion, and barotrauma.
- Measure intake, output, specific gravity, and daily weight. Excessive fluid accumulation increases total lung water, contributing to an increase in ventilation-perfusion imbalance.
- Monitor skin color for the presence of cyanosis, which can reflect the desaturation of at least 5 g of hemoglobin and $\dot{V}/\dot{Q}$ mismatch.
- Encourage patient to deep breathe and use incentive spirometer to expand the lungs and prevent areas of atelectasis.
- Evaluate the adequacy of oxygenation: oxygen delivery $\geq$600 mL/min/m^2, CI $\geq$2.7 L/min/m^2, and oxygen consumption (VO$_2$) $\geq$156 mL/min/m^2.
- Administer prescribed humidified oxygen to keep secretions moist and easier to mobilize and PaO$_2$ $\geq$60 mm Hg.
- Administer IV fluids at the prescribed flow rate to maintain adequate hydration and to avoid excess fluid accumulation, which increases lung water causing increased $\dot{V}/\dot{Q}$ mismatch.
- Teach patient to cough, sneeze, and blow nose gently to reduce the risk of dislodging clots and causing rebleeding.

- Teach patient to avoid sudden Valsalva's maneuver.
- Teach patient how to use incentive spirometer.

Potential Complication: Decreased Cardiac Output. Decreased CO related to fluid volume deficit secondary to hemorrhage.

Expected Patient Outcomes. Patient maintains adequate CO, as evidenced by HR ≤100 bpm, CO 4 to 8 L/min, CI 2.7 to 4.3 L/min/m², Sao₂ 95% to 97.5%, BP within patient's normal range, UO ≥30 mL/h, peripheral pulses +2, CVP 2 to 6 mm Hg, flat neck veins, alertness, and capillary refill ≤3 seconds, pulmonary artery pressure (PAP) 20 to 30/6 to 12 mm Hg, PCWP 6 to 12 mm Hg, and SVR 900 to 1200 dynes/s/cm⁻⁵.

- Review levels of serum hemoglobin, hematocrit, total protein, electrolytes, BUN, and creatinine and results of coagulation tests and liver function tests.
- Limit activity to bed rest while patient is bleeding.
- Assess clinical indicators of perfusion: BP, MAP, HR, cardiac rhythm, presence of gallop rhythm or murmurs, skin color and temperature, capillary refill, presence of edema, and peripheral pulses.
- Report clinical findings associated with decreased CO: hypotension, tachycardia, pallor or cyanosis, cool skin, capillary refill ≥3 seconds, and peripheral pulses ≤+2.
- Obtain and report hemodynamic parameters associated with decreased CO: CO ≤4 L/min, CI ≤2.7 L/min/m², CVP ≤2 mm Hg, PCWP ≤6 mm Hg, and SVR ≥1200 dynes/s/cm⁻⁵.
- Use arterial line to reduce the number of peripheral sticks and subsequent thrombosis.
- Measure daily weight, intake, specific gravity, and UO. Report UO ≤30 mL/h or ≤0.5 mL/kg/h.
- Administer prescribed blood and blood products to replace coagulation components.

- Administer prescribed crystalloids (lactated Ringer's or normal saline) to enhance oxygen delivery.
- Administer vasopressors (dopamine or dobutamine) to increase myocardial contractility (see Table 1–10, p. 50).
- Administer prescribed folic acid and vitamin K to correct hemostatic deficiency.

DISCHARGE PLANNING
The critical care nurse will provide patient and significant other(s) with verbal or written discharge notes regarding the following subjects:

1. Importance of keeping follow-up appointments.
2. Importance of taking medications.
3. The purpose, dose, route, and side effects of medications.
4. Importance of gradually increasing physical activity.

■ BURNS

(For related information see Part I, sepsis, p. 772. Respiratory Deviations, Part III: Mechanical ventilation, p. 428. Psychosocial Deviations, Part I, p. 725.)

Case Management Basis
DRG: 280 Trauma to the skin, subcutaneous tissue, and breast age ≥17 with complications
LOS: 4.60 days
DRG: 281 Trauma to the skin, subcutaneous tissue, and breast age ≥17 without complications
LOS: 3.10 days

Definition
Burn injury is the energy transfer from hot water scalds, flame burns, direct contact with a heat source or chemicals. The thermal response can lead to small burn injuries with local tissue destruction or extensive burn injuries that produce systemic changes at the cellular level.

Pathophysiology

During thermal injury there is increased capillary permeability related to histamine release. Depending on the size of the burn, fluid alteration occurs, leading to the pouring of plasma and albumin through membrane pores, pulling fluid out of the vasculature. The leakage of fluid from the capillary bed to the interstitium causes the lymphatic system to be overwhelmed. The overall result is excess interstitial fluid and a deficit in intravascular plasma volume. Both processes put the patient at risk for massive pitting systemic edema. Approximately 48 hours after the initial burn injury, fluid alteration approaches normal, lymphatics accommodate the fluid load, fluid reabsorption in the interstitium occurs, and edema subsides.

CLASSIFICATION OF BURN INJURY. First-degree burns involve superficial tissue destruction in the outermost layers of the epidermis. Second-degree burns are classified as superficial and deep partial thickness injuries. Superficial partial thickness injury involves the epidermis and dermis. The tissue is red to pale ivory with the formation of moist, thin-walled blisters. Deep partial thickness burns can involve the entire dermis. The tissue has a mottled appearance, with large areas of white tissue surrounded by light-pink or red tissue. Blisters are flat, rather than the fluid-filled round ones seen with superficial partial thickness injury. In areas of deepest tissue injury, tactile and pain sensors are absent or diminished. Surrounding tissues with lesser depth of injury have intact pain and tactile sensors. Third-degree full thickness burns involve the epidermis, dermis, and underlying subcutaneous tissue. The tissue appears white, cherry red, or black. There may be deep blisters under what appears to be dehydrated skin and superficial blood vessels become coagulated by the heat of injury. Full-thickness burns are painless to touch because all nerve endings in the skin have been destroyed.

CLASSIFICATION OF EXTENT OF BURN INJURY. The American Burn Association classifies burn injury as minor, moderate, and major. Minor injury includes second-degree injury $\leq 15\%$ of body surface area (BSA) in adults or $\leq 10\%$ children and third-degree injury $\leq 2\%$ BSA not involving eyes, ears, face, and genitalia in adults and children. Moderate injury includes second-degree injury of 15% to 25% BSA in adults, 10% to 20% in children and third-degree injury of 2% to 10% of BSA in adults and children. Major injury involves second-degree injury of 25% BSA in adults and 20% in children or third-degree of at least 10% of BSA in both adults and children, involves hands, face, eyes, ears, feet, and perineum, inhalation injury, and all electrical injuries.

Nursing Assessment

PRIMARY CAUSES

- Burns are due to thermal injuries caused by hot water scalds, flame burns, and direct contact with a heat source. Chemical injuries are attributed to oxidizing agents (sodium hypochlorite, chromic acid, and potassium permanganate), reducing agents (nitric acid and hydrochloric acid), corrosive agents (phenols, white phosphorus, sodium metals, and lyes), protoplasmic poisons (tannic acid, picric acid, formic acid, oxalic acid, and hydrofluoric acid), desiccants (sulfuric acid and muriatic acid), and vesicants (cantharides, dimethyl sulfoxide, and mustard gas). Other causes include electrical, radiation, or tar injuries.

PHYSICAL ASSESSMENT

Integumentary System

- Inspection: Partial thickness reveals dry to moist blebs, absence or presence of blisters, absence or presence of edema, oozing of plasmalike fluid, or cherry red to mottled white coloration with blanch and refill. Full thickness includes dry, leathery eschar or waxy, charred skin that does not blanch.

- Palpation: Presence of very painful sensation to absence of pain.

Cardiovascular System
- Inspection: Edema, altered skin temperature, and skin color changes.
- Palpation: Decreased or absent peripheral pulses or delayed capillary refill.
- Auscultation: Tachycardia, hypotension, breathlessness, and dysrhythmias.

Respiratory System
- Inspection: Severe hoarseness, stridor, dyspnea, hacking cough, labored breathing, and altered level of consciousness.
- Auscultation: Crackles, rhonchi, and tachypnea.

Renal System
- Inspection: Oliguria ≤ 30 mL/h, dark amber urine, and high specific gravity.

Gastrointestinal System
- Inspection: Nausea, vomiting, absence of stools, and abdominal distention.
- Auscultation: Absence of bowel sounds.
- Inspection: Nausea, vomiting, absence of flatus, absence of stools, and abdominal distention.
- Palpation
- Auscultation: Absence of bowel sounds.

DIAGNOSTIC TEST RESULTS

Standard Laboratory Tests
- Arterial blood gases: Normal partial pressure of arterial oxygen (Pa_{O2}) and partial pressure of arterial carbon dioxide (Pa_{CO2}). Elevated carboxyhemoglobin in carbon monoxide poisoning. Reduced pH.
- Blood studies: Elevated white blood cell (WBC) count, hemoglobin, and hematocrit. Reduced platelets.
- Cultures: Gram-negative organisms can indicate *Pseudomnas aeruginosa, Klebsiella, Serratia, Escherichia coli,* and *Enterobacter cloacae.* Gram-positive organisms may indicate *Staphylococcus* and *Streptococcus.*

Fungal organisms (*Candida, Aspergillus*) can be present.
- Serum chemistry: Elevated blood urea nitrogen (BUN), glucose, potassium, chloride, and creatine kinase. Reduced sodium, total protein, and albumin.
- Urinalysis: Fixed specific gravity 1.008 to 1.012, protein, pH ≥ 7.0 or ≤ 6.0, glycosuria, positive acetone, abnormal color, and hemoglobinuria.

Invasive Diagnostic Procedures. (see Table 3–3, p. 335)

- Bronchoscopy and laryngscopy: Used to evaluate the status of mucosa in inhalation injuries such as the presence of edema, denudation, erythema, or blistering.

Noninvasive Diagnostic Procedures. (see Table 3–2, p. 334, and Table 3–4, p. 336)
- Chest roentgenogram: Used 24 to 48 hours after burn injury to show atelectasis, pulmonary edema, or acute respiratory failure.
- Respiratory function tests: Decreased vital capacity, tidal volume, and inspiratory force.

ECG
- Used to assess patient's baseline rhythm. The baseline can be compared to future dysrhythmias resulting from cardiopulmonary instability, acid-base imbalance, and electrolyte imbalance.

MEDICAL AND SURGICAL MANAGEMENT

PHARMACOLOGY
- Diuretics: Mannitol is used if hematuria or hemoglobinuria occurs. Furosemide is administered to restore fluid equilibrium.
- Tetanus toxoid or antitoxin: Are used prophylactically to combat *Clostridium tetani.*
- Antibiotics: Aminoglycosides such as amikacin, gentamicin, and tobramycin are used to combat severe infection.
- Analgesics: Anesthetic agents such as ketamine (Ketalar), sodium pentobarbital

(Nembutal) diazepam (Valium), and nitrous oxide are used. Narcotics such as intravenous morphine can be used as necessary to combat pain on admission.

- Vitamin and mineral supplements: Multivitamins (1 ampule IV or piggyback or 1 tablet PO daily), vitamin B_{12} weekly, vitamin C daily, and folic acid (1 mg IV daily).

WOUND THERAPY.

- Topical antibiotics: Includes antibiotics such as nitrofurazone (Furacin), gentamicin sulfate (Garamycin), neomycin sulfate, and bacitracin with polymyxin B (Table 10–3).
- Topical enzymatic debriding agents: Sutilains ointment (Travase), fibrinolysin and desoxyribonuclease combined (bovine) (Elase) (see Table 10–3).
- Miscellaneous topical agents: Silver sulfadiazine, mafenide acetate, sodium hypochlorite solution, povidone-iodine (Betadine), silver nitrate, bismuth tribromphenate (Xeroform), scarlet red and merbromin (Mercurochrome) (see Table 10–3).

FLUID THERAPY

- Parkland formula for fluid resuscitation: Ringer's lactate with one half of the calculated fluid (4 mL × percentage of burn × weight in kilograms) is administered in the first 8 hours following the burn. The remaining half is given in the next 16-hour period for a total of 24 hours. Colloids such as albumin can be administered in the third or fourth 8-hour period postburn if necessary.
- Evans formula: In first 24 hours, normal saline 1 mL/kg/% burn; colloid 1 mL/kg/% burn; and 5% dextrose in water (D_5W) 2 L, half in first 8 hours and half in second 16 hours. In second 24 hours, half of amount for first 24 hours of normal saline (NS) and colloid, D_5W 2 L.
- Modified Brooke formula: In first 24 hours, lactated Ringer's 2 mL/kg/% burn, half in first 8 hours and half in next 16 hours. During second 24 hours, colloid 0.3 to 0.5 mL/kg/% burn with D_5W as necessary.
- Hypertonic sodium solution: During first 24 hours, volume of fluid contains 250 mEq

of sodium/L and second 24 hours includes one third isotonic salt solution, administered orally up to 3500 mL limit.

- Whole blood: May be used to replace losses from bleeding during wound debridement, from hemolysis resulting from the burn injury, sepsis, or hemorrhage.
- Packed cells: Are obtained by centrifuging whole blood to draw off plasma and are administered to replace red blood cell (RBC) loss in anemia or to replace RBCs lost through marrow depression.

OXYGEN THERAPY

- Humidified oxygen is administered by mask 2 to 4 L/min at 40%. If necessary, intubation and mechanical ventilation are initiated.

Hydrotherapy

- Immersion: A plain water bath can replace chemical solutions such as povidone-iodine.
- Showering or spray therapy: Reduces the risk of sutocontamination from the infected area to another. Showering the mobilized burn patient accomplishes wound cleansing.
- Bed bath: Used for the patient who requires continuous monitoring for cardiac dysrhythmias, unstable blood pressure, Swan-Ganz catheterization, or mechanical ventilation.

DEBRIDEMENT

- Mechanical debridement: Loose skin and nonviable tissue are removed with scissors and forceps or with coarse-mesh gauze in a wiping manner. Chlorhexidine gluconate (Hibiclens), povidone-iodine (Betadine), and sodium hypochlorite (Clorox) are used together with sterile water, NS, or tap water.
- Chemical debridement: Can be accomplished by the application of proteolytic enzymes such as sutilains ointment. Silver sulfadiazine is impregnated into a fine-mesh gauze and applied over the ointment and repeated three to four times a day.

BIOLOGICAL DRESSINGS

- Homograft: Homograft or autograft is human skin harvested from cadavers and, using sterile technique, is placed with the dermal

TABLE 10-3

TABLE 10–3. PARTIAL LIST OF TOPICAL BURN AGENTS

Medication	Route/Dose	Uses/Effects	Side Effects
Antibiotics			
Bacitracin with polymyxin B	Combination bactericidal ointment effective on small burn areas	Gram-positive and gram-negative organisms	Itching, burning, or inflammation
Gentamicin sulfate (Garamycin)	Wide-spectrum antibiotic, available as cream or solution	Against many organisms such as *Pseudomonas* and those that do not respond to other topical antibiotics	Toxicity, nephrotoxicity
Neomycin sulfate (Mycifradin)	0.1%–0.5% in aqueous solution applied 1–3 times/d	Effective against most organisms Decreases organisms before debriding and grafting	Toxicity, nephrotoxicity
Nitrofurazone (Furacin)	Apply directly to area or dressing; reapply daily for second- or third-degree burns or q 4–5 days for second-degree burn with minimum exudation.	Prevents infection of skin grafts and donor sites Against *Staphylococcus aureus* and some antibiotic-resistant organisms	Irritation, sensitization, superinfections
Enzymatic Debriding Agents			
Fibrinolysin and Desoxyribonuclease (Elase)	Lytic enzymes combined in a petroleum base and applied to burn	Digests necrotic tissue, aids in debridement	Local hyperemia, itching, burning
Sutilains (Travase)	Apply tid or qid	Digests necrotic tissue, aids in debridement of second- or third-degree burns	Pain, paresthesia, bleeding, transient dermatitis
Other			
Mafenide acetate	White water-based cream	Maintains bacteriostatic action against many gram-negative and gram-positive organisms	Superinfection, rash, or pain when applied
Povidine-iodine (Betadine)	Apply to area as needed	Prevents and treats surface infection and antiseptic for burns	Systemic absorption can occur with extensive burns; rash, burning
Silver nitrate diluted to 0.5% for application	10% silver salt solution: full-thickness burns	Used with partial and full-thickness burns	Hyponatremia, hypochloremia, hypocalcemia
Silver sulfadiazine (Silvadene)	Water-based cream	Treat partial- and full-thickness thermal injuries Acts by binding to bacterial cell membranes and interfering with DNA	Rash, pruritus, burning
Sodium hypoclorite (Dakins)	Aqueous solution	Debridement of grafts	Clot lysis; clotting inhibition, skin irritation, electrolyte imbalance

Bell TN, 1993; Deglin JH and Vallerand AH, 1995; Loeb S, 1993; Tribett D, 1993.

side down. The strips are applied circumferentially around extremities and across the trunk surface to enhance adherence. Meshed autografts can include fine mesh gauze after neomycin application or soaks applied every 4 hours to prevent desiccation. Windows can be cut through the surgical dressing allowing for soak administration.

- Heterograft: Heterograft or xenograft is skin obtained from animals, usually pigs. Heterograft is supplied in a variety of forms such as rolls, sheets, meshed, unmeshed, fresh frozen, irradiated, or impregnated with silver. A light dressing can be applied to secure each biological dressing. The heterograft, when adherent, is cleaned and trimmed daily until the wound beneath heals.

- Biobrane: Biobrane is a semipermeable silicone membrane bonded to a nylon fabric that is coated with collagen. Biobrane is used for application to donor site, superficial partial thickness burns, and excised wounds. Biobrane separates spontaneously as reepithelization occurs.

DIET

- High-protein/high-caloric diet: Is used to achieve nitrogen balance for optimal wound healing. Protein provides a source of essential and nonessential amino acids required for protein synthesis. The goal for nitrogen balance during repair is 4 to 6 g daily. Approximately 20% to 25% of calories are of a protein nature; 5% to 15% of calories are provided by fat.

- Micronutrients: These include vitamins E and B_{12}, folate, zinc, iron, copper, and vitamins C and A.

NASODUODENAL TUBE FEEDING

- Tube feeding is used to suppress the intensity of the injury response by decreasing resting energy expenditure, providing positive nitrogen balance, and normalizing visceral proteins and catabolic hormones.

- The nasoduodenal feeding tube tip is passed beyond the pylorus and lessens the risk of gastroesophageal reflux, tracheobronchial aspiration, or tube dislodgment.

- Enteral nutritional therapy: Is started within the first 24 to 48 hours to decrease catabolic hormones and hypermetabolism, improve nitrogen balance, maintain mucosal integrity, and decrease risk of diarrhea. Continuous feeding with a tube feeding pump is given initially to meet one half the calculated caloric needs. Feedings can be advanced to 10 mL/h.

INDIRECT CALORIMETRY

- Energy expenditure is better quantified through the measurement of oxygen consumption and carbon dioxide production (see Respiratory Deviations, Indirect calorimetry, p. 441).

NASOGASTRIC SUCTION

- A nasogastric (NG) tube is connected to low suction while patient is fed through the nasoduodenal tube. Gastric decompression helps to prevent regurgitation of stomach contents and risk of aspiration.

SURGICAL INTERVENTION

- Tangential excision: Used to preserve viable dermis by removing the eschar. Punctate bleeding indicates viable tissue has been reached.

- Escharotomy: A surgical incision through the eschar or burned tissue.

- Fasciotomy: A surgical incision through the fascia or covering of muscle.

NEW WOUND COVERAGE TECHNIQUES

- Cultured epidermal autograft: The technique involves epithelial cells obtained in the laboratory from a biopsy of patient's unburned skin. When the cells have grown, a graft of cultured tissue is placed in a small excised area as in the procedure used during regular skin graft.

- Artificial skin: The process involves artificial skin consisting of a dermal substitute of bovine collagen, chondroitin 6-sulfate, and an epidermal layer of silicone rubber. When the burn wound is excised, artificial skin can be placed on the wound. The procedure prevents fluid loss and preserves the excised wound bed.

NURSING MANAGEMENT: NURSING DIAGNOSES AND COLLABORATIVE PROBLEMS

Nursing Diagnoses

Common nursing goals for patients with burns are to maintain fluid balance, enhance peripheral tissue perfusion, maintain tissue integrity, support oxygenation, prevent infection, prevent disuse syndrome, maintain adequate nutrition, support effective thermoregulation, minimize pain, and prevent body image disturbance.

Fluid volume deficit related to loss of plasma volume from the intravascular space into the interstitial space secondary to disruption between hydrostatic and osmotic pressure as a result of thermal injury.

Expected Patient Outcomes. Patient maintains adequate fluid volume, as evidenced by cardiac output (CO) 4 to 8 L/min, cardiac index (CI) 2.7 to 4.3 L/min/m^2, central venous pressure (CVP) 2 to 6 mm Hg, pulmonary artery (PA) systolic pressure 15 to 30 mm Hg or PA diastolic 8 to 15 mm Hg, pulmonary capillary wedge pressure (PCWP) 6 to 12 mm Hg, urinary output (UO) ≥30 mL/h or ≥0.5 mL/kg/h, specific gravity 1.010 to 1.030, stable body weight, heart rate (HR) ≤100 bpm, blood pressure (BP) within patient's normal range, mean arterial pressure (MAP) 70 to 100 mm Hg, skin turgor normal, capillary ≤3 seconds, and peripheral pulses +2.

- Consult with physician to validate expected patient outcomes used to evaluate fluid balance in burn patients.
- Review results of serum hemoglobin, hematocrit, total protein, blood urea nitrogen (BUN), creatinine, and coagulation tests.
- Place patient in a position of comfort depending on the location and severity of the burns.

- Obtain and report hemodynamic parameters associated with fluid volume deficit: CO ≤4 L/min, CI ≤2.7 L/min/m^2, CVP ≤2 mm Hg, PA systolic ≤15 mm Hg, PA diastolic ≤8 mm Hg, and PCWP ≤6 mm Hg. A PCWP ≥18 mm Hg suggests pulmonary edema.
- Assess clinical indicators of hydration: skin turgor, peripheral pulses, HR, BP, capillary refill, and level of consciousness.
- Report clinical findings associated with fluid volume deficit: tachycardia, hypotension, poor skin turgor, peripheral pulses ≤+2, confusion, and capillary refill ≥3 seconds.
- Measure hourly UO, which can be 1 mL/kg of preburn weight/h.
- Obtain the patient's preburn weight and monitor daily weight as an indicator of cardiac state. Report weight gain of 2.2 lb, which indicates 1 L of fluid retention. The total weight gained during the first few days should not be greater than 10% to 15% of patient's total body weight.
- Provide strict measurement of intake and output. Calculate daily fluid replacement based on BSA burned and insensible water loss.
- Administer prescribed IV fluid via two large-bore intravenous catheters at a rate sufficient to maintain UO ≥30 mL/h.
- Administer prescribed IV fluids using the appropriate formula and amount during the first 24 hours: crystalloids such as lactated Ringer's 1 mL/kg/% burn, 1.5 mL/kg/% burn, or 4 mL/kg/% burn; colloid albumin 1 mL/kg/% burn or 0.5 mL/kg/% burn; or D$_5$W 2000 mL.
- Administer IV fluids as prescribed for second 24 hours: crystalloids such as lactated Ringer's 0.5 mL/kg/% burn and 0.75 mL/kg/% burn; colloids such as albumin 0.5 mL/kg/% burn, 0.25 mL/kg/% burn, or 700 to 2000 mL, or D$_5$W 1500 to 2000 mL.
- Administer mannitol as prescribed to wash the renal tubules, should myoglobinuria occur.

Altered peripheral tissue perfusion related to decreased blood volume, poor myocardial function, and hemoconcentration resulting from decreased plasma volume secondary to thermal injury.

Expected Patient Outcomes. Patient maintains adequate peripheral tissue perfusion, as evidenced by absence of cyanosis, capillary refill ≤3 seconds, peripheral pulses +2, absence of edema, skin temperature warm to touch, absence of bleeding, coagulation studies within normal range, and BP within patient's normal range.

- Review results of blood studies.
- Should the extremity be burned, elevate the affected extremity at or above heart level to enhance venous return and reduce dependent edema formation.
- Assess clinical indicators of peripheral perfusion: BP, HR, skin color, peripheral pulses, skin temperature, and capillary refill.
- Report clinical findings associated with reduced peripheral tissue perfusion: hypotension, tachycardia, cyanosis in unaffected tissue, peripheral pulses ≤+2, capillary refill ≥3 seconds, coolness in unaffected extremity, and edema.
- Should full-thickness circumferential burn of the extremities have occurred, prepare patient for escharotomy or fasciotomy.
- Assess distal pulses every 15 minutes by Doppler technique.
- Report clinical findings associated with fluid accumulation causing deeper structures, including the blood vessels and nerves, to become hypoxic and necrotic: numbness, tingling, loss of motor function, aching and throbbing pain.
- After escharotomy or fasciotomy is performed, apply prescribed silver sulfadiazine and a light gauze dressing.
- Administer prescribed IV fluids to maintain adequate circulatory volume and hydration.
- Administer prescribed mannitol to flush the kidneys in patients with myoglobinuria.

Impaired tissue integrity related to cell destruction secondary to thermal injury.

Expected Patient Outcomes. Patient's thermal injuries exhibit evidence of granulation and healing by primary intention or split thickness skin grafting as appropriate.

- Consult with physician about patient's burns and individualized treatment protocol.
- Assess wound during each dressing change, noting color and appearance of the wound, especially the location of eschar versus appearance of skin buds or granulation tissue. Report odor, amount of exudate, presence of cellulitus, bleeding, and exposed tendon or bone.
- Cleanse and debride wound as prescribed using unit protocol.
- Apply prescribed topical antimicrobials using sterile technique with silver nitrate 0.5% solution, 1% silver sulfadiazine, or mafenide acetate. Inadequate coverage or prolonged exposure of an open wound to air can cause desiccation. On the other hand, excessive application of a topical ointment to a healthy or healed area can lead to increased moisture and subsequent maceration.
- Maintain immobility of the grafted site for 3 days as prescribed through positioning, splinting, light pressure, or sedation.
- Dressing applied circumferentially should be wrapped in a distal-to-proximal manner. Fingers and toes are individually wrapped so that range-of-motion exercises can be achieved.
- Prepare patient for immersion therapy or showering to debride necrotic tissue and visualize wound.
- Prepare patient for early excision method by a tangential or fascial excision technique. The excised wound is covered with a skin graft.
- Prepare patient with full-thickness thermal injuries for either autograft, tissue culture graft, homograft, or heterograft. Grafts can be meshed to increase the area of coverage at ratios from 1:1.5 to 1:3.

- Use a bed cradle to avoid contact by sheets with open graft areas.
- Monitor and report the type and amount of drainage from the wound.
- Review and follow unit protocol for care of burns involving the eyes, lips, ears, and nose.
- Apply dressings to immobilize the grafted area, since joint movement and shearing dislodge the graft. Bulky dressings are removed 4 days postoperatively.
- Assess the graft for adherence and rewrap with an outer dressing to secure it. Pink adherent autograft signifies a good graft, while loose, stringy, or dried autograft indicates areas that did not adhere. Report the latter so the autograft in the area can be removed as ordered.
- Initiate range-of-motion exercises 5 days after grafting.
- Initiate ambulation in patients with grafted lower extremities 7 days after the application of pressure wraps.
- Apply prescribed mild, nonirritating lotion to the healed skin to aid in range of motion (ROM) and reduce itching. Note the residue must be removed each day.
- Initiate prescribed chemical debridement through the application of proteolytic enzymes such as sutilains ointment. Silver sulfadiazine can be impregnated into a fine-mesh gauze and applied over the ointment. This process is repeated three to four times a day.

Impaired gas exchange related to upper airway obstruction or primary pulmonary damage secondary to thermal injury.

Expected Patient Outcomes. Patient maintains adequate gas exchange, as evidenced by respiratory rate (RR) 12 to 20 BPM, arterial blood gases within normal range, hemoglobin within normal range, absence of cyanosis, Pao_2 60 to 100 mm Hg, $Paco_2$ 35 to 45 mm Hg, pH 7.35 to 7.45, arterial oxygen saturation (Sao_2) 95% to 97.5%, pulse oximetry (SpO_2) $\geq$95%, arterial:alveolar oxygen tension ratio ($P[a:A]o_2$) $\geq$0.75, physiological shunt ($\dot{Q}s/\dot{Q}t$)

0% to 8%, absence of dyspnea, and absence of adventitious breath sounds.

- Consult with physician to validate expected patient outcomes used to evaluate adequate gas exchange.
- Review results of arterial blood gas measurement, hemoglobin, hematocrit, chest roentgenogram, respiratory function studies, and bronchoscopy.
- Place patient in position of comfort to maximize chest excursion.
- Assess clinical indicators of respiratory status: rate, depth, symmetry of chest wall movement, skin color, use of accessory muscles, and lung sounds.
- Monitor for clinical indicators of hypoxemia: dyspnea, cyanosis, restlessness, confusion, anxiety, delirium, tachypnea, tachycardia, hypertension, headache, arrhythmias, or tremor.
- Monitor for clinical indicators of carbon monoxide poisoning: headaches, nausea, vomiting, loss of manual dexterity, confusion, lethargy, ataxia, convulsion, and coma.
- Monitor for clinical indicators of smoke or chemical inhalation injury: laryngeal edema, dyspnea, tachypnea, tachycardia, wheezing, or rhonchi.
- Monitor for clinical indicators of respiratory acidosis: confusion, asterixis, coma, shortness of breath, and cyanosis.
- Continuously monitor oxygenation level with SpO_2 and report value $\leq$95%.
- Calculate $P(a:A)o_2$ and $\dot{Q}s/\dot{Q}t$ to estimate intrapulmonary shunting. Report $P(a:A)o_2$ $\leq$0.75 and $\dot{Q}s/\dot{Q}t$ $\geq$8%.
- Continually monitor ECG to assess HR and rhythm. Document ECG rhythm strips every 2 to 4 hours or more frequently in patients with dysrhythmias associated with hypoxemia or carbon monoxide.
- Review carboxyhemoglobin levels for carbon monoxide suggesting smoke inhalation. Report value $\geq$20%.
- Report clinical findings associated with changes in carboxyhemoglobin levels: 20% headache or mild dyspnea; 20% to 40%

fatigue, irritability, diminished judgment, dimmed vision, and nausea; 40% to 60% confusion, hallucination, ataxia, collapse, coma, reddened skin and mucous membranes; and 60% to 80% death.

- Maintain oral airway and administer supplemental oxygen as prescribed. Fraction of inspired oxygen (FIO_2) 100% is used to treat carbon monoxide poisoning.

- Should patient's blood gases and respiratory status fail to improve with supplemental oxygen, prepare patient for intubation and mechanical ventilation with positive end-expiratory pressure (PEEP).

- Promote pulmonary hygiene by encouraging patient to cough and deep breathe and use incentive spirometer. Suction as necessary.

- Provide humidified oxygen by nasal cannula or Venturi mask at the prescribed amount.

- Administer prescribed bronchodilators to treat bronchospasm.

- Administer prescribed IV fluids to maintain adequate hydration.

- Prepare patient with chest burns for escharotomies to improve compliance and ventilation.

High risk infection related to sepsis or immunosuppression.

Expected Patient Outcomes. Patient is free of infection, as evidenced by normothermia, wound culture negative, WBC count $\leq 11,000/\mu L$, and absence of drainage from wound.

- Review results of WBC count and cultures of sputum, urine, or wound.
- Provide a consistent turning schedule to improve capillary perfusion to the common pressure areas or immobilize patient. Unless contraindicated, use a ROHO mattress that uses flexible air cells adjusted after the patient is positioned to reduce pressure areas.
- Provide prescribed high-protein, high-calorie diet.
- Obtain and report clinical findings associated with burn wound sepsis: erythema, rapid separation of eschar, breakdown in areas of healing burns or skin graft, conversion of partial- to full-thickness injury, pus beneath eschar, or black or red hemorrhage area in eschar and in unburned adjacent skin.

- Assess the appearance of grafted site, including adhesion to burned site, appearance, and color. Report excessive edema formation, exudate, discoloration, odor, mottled red appearance to full-thickness necrosis and rapid eschar separation.

- Obtain and report clinical findings associated with sepsis: fever, chills, weakness, warm and flushed skin, nausea, vomiting, diarrhea, and diaphoresis, mild confusion, general malaise, cyanosis, skin warm, hypotension, tachycardia, or tachypnea.

- Use reverse isolation to protect patient against transmission of infection.

- Wash hands with a surgical detergent disinfectant for 10 to 15 seconds before and after physical contact with patient and patient's equipment or personal articles.

- Use sterile gloves when performing direct wound care or invasive procedures. Change gloves between handling of wounds on different areas of the body.

- Change burn dressings using strict sterile technique to avoid wound cross contamination.

- Should temperature $\geq 38.9°C$ (102°F) obtain wound, blood, sputum, and urine culture as prescribed.

- For patients with skin grafts, assess donor site for evidence of infection, purulent drainage, undefined borders, and foul odor.

- Prepare patient for quantitative biopsies of the eschar and granulation tissue, which are done three times a week to assess potential proliferation of organisms.

- Administer prescribed aminoglycoside class antibiotics, amikacin, gentamicin, and tobramycin to combat infection.

High risk of disuse syndrome related to inactivity secondary to pain, splints, or dressings.

Expected Patient Outcome. Patient retains and demonstrates ROM of all extremities.

- Confer with physical therapist regarding an individualized exercise program for the burned patient.
- Position patient to reduce the work load of the heart; reduce contracture formation; reduce incidence of phlebitis, thrombi, and emboli; promote lung expansion and drainage of pulmonary secretions; and prevent decubitus ulcers.
- Provide exercises that take patient through the full ROM once daily during hydrotherapy.
- Assess clinical factors that can decrease joint motion and increase contractures: bed rest, decreased protein, altered fluid and electrolytes, and poor circulation.
- Encourage patient to practice full ROM and self-care by brushing teeth, combing hair, and self-feeding.
- Provide prescribed splints to place the area in a position that will preserve or restore function.
- Apply prescribed pressure dressings such as elastic wraps and pressure garments such as Jobst garments to reduce the amount of scar tissue that can form over burned areas of the body.

Altered nutrition: less than body requirements related to increased calorie and protein needs for wound healing secondary to hypermetabolic states.

Expected Patient Outcomes. Patient maintains adequate nutritional intake of 80% of calculated nutritional needs, weight maintained within 85% of usual weight, diarrhea episodes controlled, constipation is alleviated, and wounds heal progressively.

- Confer with dietitian regarding patient's individual calorie and protein needs.
- Monitor for serum albumin ≥3.5 g/dL, balanced nitrogen states, thyroxine-binding prealbumin 200 to 300 μg/mL and retinol-binding protein 40 to 50 μg/mL.
- Insert NG tube, if necessary, to maintain adequate caloric intake: Burn patient may require up to 4000 calories/d.

- Provide prescribed high-protein and high-calorie diet.
- Provide small, frequent feedings and supplements per order should NG tube be unnecessary.
- Measure daily weight, intake, specific gravity, and UO. Report weight loss ≥0.5 to 1.0 kg/d.
- Monitor gastrointestional system function continually for alterations such as diarrhea or constipation.
- Assess abdominal girth and bowel sounds every 4 hours.
- Minimize patient's energy requirements by controlling pain, anxiety, providing rest, and preventing hypothermia, chilling, or shivering.
- Administer prescribed enteral nutrition via nasoduodenal feeding tube per protocol. Titrate as necessary to control diarrhea or other symptoms of intolerance (see Gastrointestinal Deviations, Enteral nutrition, p. 554).
- Administer prescribed stool softeners or antidiarrheal preparation per protocol.
- Administer hyperalimentation nutrition when patient is unable to tolerate enteral feedings.

High risk of ineffective thermoregulation related to loss of skin integrity secondary to thermal injury.

Expected Patient Outcomes. Patient maintains temperature between 38° and 39.5°C (100.4° and 103.1°F) during the acute phase for maximal comfort.

- Monitor temperature continuously, since absence of skin causes patient's body to assume the temperature of the environment.
- Hypermetabolism can increase core and skin temperature.
- Ambient temperature can affect patient's metabolic state. Cool ambient temperature requires patient to work to maintain warmth. The body resets temperature (1° to 2°C above normal) by shivering, thereby further increasing the metabolic rate.
- Provide an environment that is warm and conducive to maintaining temperature balance.

- Initiate procedures to prevent fluctuations in temperature.
- Provide heat shields or blankets as indicated by protocols.
- Monitor insensible water loss from the skin, since this can be a cause of hypermetabolic response.
- Administer prescribed IV fluids to maintain adequate hydration.

Pain related to thermal injury.

Expected Patient Outcomes. Patient's verbal and nonverbal evaluation of pain improves on the pain scale or patient has no pain.

- Confer with physician regarding patient's pain medication schedule.
- Encourage patient to describe pain on a scale of 1 to 10. Report increased intensity of pain, which may indicate risk of ischemia, whereas reduced pain may indicate sensory nerve fiber damage.
- Assess behavioral findings associated with excess pain: intensive care psychosis, complication in sleep-wake cycles, and personality disorders.
- Obtain and report clinical findings associated with pain: tachypnea, tachycardia, elevated BP, shivering, or guarded position.
- Provide a calm, relaxing environment to help patient achieve rest.
- Reposition patient frequently to promote comfort.
- Keep partial-thickness burn wound covered to avoid stimulus that can cause pain.
- Use nonpharmacological pain relief measures such as acupuncture, transcutaneous electrical nerve stimulation (TENS), and acupressure.
- Encourage patient to use other pain reducing techniques such as guided imagery, relaxation therapy, music therapy, and distraction.
- Administer prescribed narcotic (morphine) using patient-controlled analgesic (PCA) to relieve pain.
- Administer prescribed antianxiety medication (lorazepam) to promote stress reduction and subsequent pain relief.

- Administer prescribed anesthetic agent such as ketamine (Ketalar), sodium pentobarbital (Nembutal), and nitrous oxide to reduce pain.
- Teach patient the purpose behind each procedure that might cause pain.
- Instruct patient regarding the change in pain experiences: In partial-thickness injury the prostaglandins and histamines around the injured area can stimulate peripheral pain receptors and intensify central perception of discomfort; and full-thickness burns are painless until nerve endings regenerate, when pain occurs.
- Teach patient to use alternative strategies: progressive relaxation, meditation, and guided imagery.

Body image disturbance related to changes in appearance secondary to thermal injury.

Expected Patient Outcomes. Patient acknowledges body image changes and integrates the changes into his or her revised self-concept.

- Listen to patient's perception and feelings about the burn injury and circumstances surrounding the injury.
- Listen to patient's perception and feelings about life-style changes and their impact on relationships.
- Include significant other(s) in discussion of life-style changes, prognosis, and future care.
- Encourage patient to join support groups for burn patients.
- Provide patient with positive feedback when attempts are made to improve physical appearance.
- Inform patient about cosmetic aids that can help to conceal burns.

Collaborative Problems

Common collaborative goals for patients with burns are to prevent hypovolemic shock, correct compartmental syndrome, and correct hyperglycemia.

Potential Complication: Hypovolemic Shock. Hypovolemic shock related to loss of plasma from the circulatory blood volume secondary to increased capillary permeability or thermal injury.

Expected Patient Outcomes. Patient maintains adequate circulating volume, as evidenced by BP within patient's normal range, MAP 70 to 100 mm Hg, HR $\leq$100 bpm, CO 4 to 8 L/min, CI 2.7 to 4.3 L/min/m^2, CVP 2 to 6 mm Hg, coronary perfusion pressure (CPP) 60 to 80 mm Hg, absence of dysrhythmias, UO $\geq$30 mL/h or $\geq$0.5 mL/kg/h, stable body weight, capillary refill $\leq$3 seconds, and peripheral pulses +2.

- Consult with physician to validate expected patient outcomes used to evaluate whether hypovolemic shock has been resolved.
- Obtain and report hemodynamic parameters associated with hypovolemic shock: CO $\leq$4 L/min, CI $\leq$2.7 L/min/m^2, CVP $\leq$2 mm Hg, and CPP $\leq$60 mm Hg.
- Assess clinical indications of perfusion and hydration: BP, HR, skin turgor, capillary refill, pulse pressure, MAP, and level of consciousness.
- Report clinical findings associated with hypovolemic shock: hypotension, tachycardia, poor skin turgor, capillary refill $\geq$3 seconds, peripheral pulses $\leq$+2, MAP $\leq$70 mm Hg, and altered level of consciousness.
- Continuously monitor ECG rhythm strips for rate and rhythm. Document ECG strips every 2 to 4 hours or more frequently in patients experiencing dysrhythmias.
- Administer prescribed oxygen 2 to 4 L/min by mask, cannula, or endotracheal tube to maintain adequate hydration.
- Administer prescribed IV fluids to maintain adequate hydration and circulatory volume.

Potential Complication: Compartment Syndrome. Compartment syndrome related to massive swelling of the soft tissue secondary to interstitial edema.

Expected Patient Outcomes. Patient maintains adequate distal perfusion, as evidenced by a normal muscle tissue pressure, compartment pressure normal 9 to 15 mm Hg, capillary refill $\leq$3 seconds, pulse of +2, extremities warm, reduced edema, and absence of fluid extravasation from capillaries.

- Consult with physician to validate expected patient outcomes used to evaluate compartment syndrome.
- Review results of intracompartmental pressure measurement.
- Evaluate pulses on the burned extremities every 15 minutes using Doppler if necessary and evaluate capillary refill.
- Elevate the affected burned extremity to increase venous return and decrease edema.
- Obtain and report clinical findings indicating compartment syndrome: pain with passive stretch, hyperesthesia, loss of motor function, cool skin, pallor or cyanosis, palpable compartment tension, decreased or absent pulse, tingling or numbness, and high compartment tension.
- Assist with the measurement of intracompartment pressures: A wick catheter is connected to a standard pressure transducer and inserted into the appropriate muscle compartment.
- Obtain and report clinical findings associated with the need for a fasciotomy when there is injury to both arteries and veins: hypotension, massive swelling, and soft tissue damage.
- Should intracompartment pressure be $\geq$30 mm Hg, one of three types of fasciotomies can be performed to decompress the compartment. They include blind incision of the fascia with limited skin incision, open incision of the fascia with extensive skin incision, or resection of a part of the fibula with fasciotomy.
- Apply burn dressings loosely to permit for expansion with edema.
- Following fasciotomy, if appropriate, keep the exposed muscle moistened with NS quarter-strength (isotonic) povidone-iodine

soaked gauze. This procedure is maintained until secondary closure occurs if the area receives a skin graft. Report any muscle necrosis, since bone and soft tissue infection can occur.

- Should massive swelling occur, prepare patient for a split-thickness graft. A secondary skin graft may be necessary when there is excessive swelling and a wide fasciotomy has been performed.
- Prepare patient for fasciotomy, which is performed when there is increased intra-compartment pressure 30 to 40 mm Hg, signs of distal ischemia, or massive edema.
- Should muscle tissue become necrotic, prepare patient for surgical debridement.
- Administer IV fluids to maintain adequate hydration.
- Administer prescribed analgesic to relieve pain.
- Teach patient to report any changes in sensation or appearance.
- Instruct patient to report indicators of compartment syndrome: pain, paresthesia, hyperesthesia, paralysis, or coolness.

Potential Complication: Hyperglycemia. Hyperglycemia related to stress diabetes secondary to altered carbohydrate metabolism.

Expected Patient Outcomes. Patient maintains glucose balance, as evidenced by absence of thirst, malaise, dry mouth, flushed skin, nausea, vomiting, or polyuria.

- Review results of serum amylase and glucose tests.
- Test urine for sugar and acetone every 6 hours and report finding.
- Obtain and report clinical findings associated with hyperglycemia: thirst, malaise, dry mouth, flushed skin, nausea, vomiting, tachycardia, and polyuria.
- Measure daily weight, intake, specific gravity, and UO.
- Administer isotonic saline and electrolytes IV to expand extracellular fluid volume.

- Administer hyposmolar solution once hyperosmolality is determined, such as 0.45% saline slowly to allow for diffusion and equilibration of water and osmolality.
- Administer prescribed insulin drip, when serum glucose ≥250 mg/dL, at a consistent rate with infusion pump.
- Instruct patient to report signs associated with hypoglycemia.

DISCHARGE PLANNING

The critical care nurse will provide patient and significant other(s) with verbal or written discharge notes regarding the following subjects:

1. Importance of follow-up appointments with physical therapist and occupational therapist if necessary.
2. Appropriate use of splinting and exercise programs to prevent contractures and maintain strength.
3. Importance of skin care such as use of lubricating cream, dressings, or paddings and wearing of pressure garment to prevent excessive or hypertrophic scarring.
4. Importance of maintaining adequate diet that includes proteins and calories, which can be individualized by a nutritionist.
5. The purpose, dose, schedule, and side effects of medications.
6. Importance of keeping all postdischarge appointments.
7. Name and phone number of local community and support groups for both patient and family.

■ SEPSIS

(For related information see Cardiac Deviations, Part I: Acute myocardial infarction, p. 38; Shock, p. 174; Cardiac trauma, p. 167; Dysrhythmias, p. 184. Part III: Hemodynamic monitoring, p. 219; ST segment monitoring, p. 264. Vascular Deviations, Part I: Deep vein thrombosis, p. 504; Peripheral Vascular trauma, p. 308. Respiratory Deviations, Part I: Adult respiratory distress syndrome, p. 327; Acute

Case Management Basis

DRG: 416 Septicemia, age greater than 17
LOS: 7.50 days

Definition

Systemic inflammatory response syndrome (SIRS) is a diffuse inflammatory response to a variety of chemical insults. Sepsis is an acute, systemic inflammatory response to the invasion of microorganisms or to the toxins produced by the microorganisms. Severe sepsis has three characteristics: organ dysfunction, hypoperfusion, and hypotension. Severe sepsis can precede septic shock, which is characterized by hemodynamic instability, alteration in cellular metabolism, coagulation abnormalities, and organ failure syndromes. These characteristics are precipitated by the interaction between the body's own defense systems and bacterial toxins. A burn wound is a medium for bacterial growth greater than 10 colonies per gram of tissue.

Pathophysiology

The chemical mediators involved in the development of sepsis are endotoxin, oxygen radicals, interleukin-1 and interleukin-2, tumor necrosis factor, arachidonic acid cascade, complement cascade system, coagulation and fibrinolysis cascade, bradykinin, myocardial depressant factor, and beta-endorphins. Endotoxin, a lipopolysaccharide component of the gram-negative bacterial wall, is liberated during infection. Following microbial cell lysis or reperfusion of the microcirculation after ischemia, endotoxins can be liberated into the systemic circulation. As a result, endotoxins become primary instigators of the sepsis cascade. Endotoxins stimulate macrophages, monocytes, and neutrophils to produce vasoactive and biologically active mediators. These mediators stimulate the endothelium, which activates endothelium-derived relaxing factor (EDRF). EDRF contributes to vasodilation of some capillaries. Likewise, the breakdown of endothelium increases vascular permeability, resulting in systemic and pulmonary edema.

Oxygen-free radicals and proteolytic enzymes are released by macrophages. Normally the body's antioxidant system curtails the destructive reaction. However, patients with sepsis have depleted their antioxidant defense mechanism. Macrophages can also secrete a glycoprotein called interleukin-1.

Interleukin-1 (IL-1) causes chemotactic events that become responsible for facilitating the movement of white blood cells toward injured, ischemic, or infected cells. IL-1 damages cells and causes subsequent release of phospholipids. IL-1 activates production of interleukin-2 (IL-2). IL-2 is responsible for contributing to hypotension, reduced systemic vascular resistance, reduced left ventricular ejection fraction (LVEF), elevated left ventricular end-diastolic volume (preload), elevated cardiac output, and tachycardia.

Tumor necrosis factor (TNF), a macrophage-derived polypeptide hormone, is a significant contributor to the septic cascade by stimulating platelet-activating factors, including prostaglandin and IL-1 production. TNF secretion leads to sequestration of platelets, vasodilation, increased capillary permeability, and microvascular constriction.

Arachidonic acid is released after the action of phospholipase A_2 on the wall of cells injured by endotoxins, cellular agitation, or hypoxia. Arachidonic acid is metabolized by two major pathways: prostaglandin and leukotriene. Prostaglandins are vasodilators that attempt to balance vasoconstricting effects of thromboxane. Thromboxane contributes to the maldistribution of blood flow during sepsis through its vasoconstricting and platelet-aggregating effect. Hypoperfusion leading to tissue ischemia is initiated by thromboxane.

The complement system consists of proteins present in the serum in the active form. When the complement system becomes inactivated, there is an imbalance between cellular destruction and clearance. The biological effects of the complement cascade system include cell lysis, stimulation of smooth muscle contraction, mast cell degradation, neutrophil chemotaxis, and activation of phagocytosis. The complement cascade can be activated by the classic and alternative pathways, which have the potential to initiate inflammatory and lytic reactions.

The formation of fibrin is initiated by injury to the vascular endothelium. The toxic effects of chemical mediators in blood vessels and cell membranes stimulate the release of Hageman factor and tissue thromboplastin. Fibrin clot formations stabilize the site of injury, while fibrinolysis keeps the clotting under control. Sepsis causes the consumption of factors in both systems, leading to disseminated intravascular coagulation.

Bradykinin, a potent vasodilator, is released by activation of Hageman factor in the coagulation cascade or complement cascade. Fluid volume deficit is a result of bradykinin's ability to create vasodilation and capillary leak.

Myocardial depressant factor (MDF) affects tissue perfusion and is released by the ischemic pancreatic cell. MDF causes a decrease in the effectiveness of myocardial cells, which leads to decreased left and right ventricular ejection fraction, elevated pulmonary capillary wedge pressure (PCWP), reduced systemic vascular resistance, and elevated cardiac output.

Finally, beta-endorphins are precipitated by maldistribution of blood flow, vasodilation, and cellular alteration. When beta-endorphins attach to their receptor site in the central nervous system, there is inhibition of sympathomedullary transmission and excite-

ment of the parasympathetic efferent fibers of the heart. The overall result is peripheral vasodilation and reduced cardiac contractility.

Nursing Assessment

PRIMARY CAUSES
- Causes include burns, trauma, malnutrition, debilitating diseases, pregnancy, immuno-impaired state, foreign body insertion, immunosuppressives, artificial airways, urinary tract infection, surgery, and immobility.

RISK FACTORS
- Risk factors include nosocomial infection, age over 70 years, nutritional status, or drugs such as immunosuppressives, cytotoxics, and antibiotics.

PHYSICAL ASSESSMENT

Hyperdynamic Early Response (Septic Syndrome)
- Inspection: Changes in level of consciousness, anxiety, fever, flushed skin, chills, diaphoresis, and normal urinary output.
- Palpation: Strong, bounding peripheral pulses and skin warm and pink.
- Auscultation: Tachycardia, normal blood pressure, tachypnea, or crackles.

Hypodynamic Late Response (Septic Shock)
- Inspection: Decreased temperature, pale or cyanotic skin, impaired mental status, no response to verbal stimuli, weakness, or reduced urinary output.
- Palpation: Weak or absent peripheral pulses or skin cool and pale.
- Auscultation: Tachycardia; S_3; hypotension; rapid, shallow respirations; crackles; rhonchi; or wheezes.

DIAGNOSTIC TEST RESULTS

Hemodynamic Parameters. (see Table 1–9, p. 40.)
- Hyperdynamic early response: Normal or elevated cardiac output (CO) ≥ 8 L/min,

cardiac index (CI) 4.3L/min/m^2, PCWP ≤6 mm Hg, systemic vascular resistance (SVR) ≤900 dynes/s/cm^{-5}, pulse pressure (PP) widened, reduced ejection fraction (EF), and mixed venous oxygen saturation (S$\bar{v}o_2$) ≥80%.

- Hypodynamic late response: CO ≤4.0 L/min. CI ≤2.7 L/min/m^2, PCWP ≥12 mm Hg, SVR ≥1200 dynes/s/cm^{-5}, PP narrowed, and S$\bar{v}o_2$≤60%.

Standard Laboratory Tests. (see Table 3–1, p. 329)

- Arterial blood gases: partial pressure of arterial oxygen (Pao$_2$) fraction of inspired oxygen (Fio$_2$) ≤175 to 280 mm Hg and partial pressure of arterial carbon dioxide (Paco$_2$) ≤32 mm Hg. Serum lactate ≥2.5 to 5.0 mmol/L.
- Blood culture: A single culture is obtained before therapy to identify source of infection.
- Blood studies: Confirmatory test for disseminated intravascular coagulation (DIC) (FDP ≥1:40 or D-dimers ≥2.0), platelet count reduced by 25%, elevated prothrombin time, and elevated partial thromboplastin time.
- Serum chemistry: Leukocytosis (white blood cells [WBC] ≥12,000/mm^3), leukopenia (WBC 4000/mm^3) or ≥10% band forms; elevated serum creatinine; elevated liver function enzymes; serum bilirubin ≥2.0 mg/dL; and elevated blood urea nitrogen (BUN).
- Urinalysis: Urine sodium ≤40 mmol/L and specific gravity 1.025 to 1.035.

NONINVASIVE DIAGNOSTIC PROCEDURE

- Chest roentgenogram: Can reveal bilateral pulmonary infiltrate.

MEDICAL AND SURGICAL MANAGEMENT

PHARMACOLOGY

- Antimicrobial therapy: broad-spectrum cephalosporin is used in combination with aminoglycosides to treat a variety of pathogens.

- Vasopressor therapy: Is used when fluids fail to restore intravascular volume and tissue perfusion. Low-dose dopamine (2 to 4 μg/kg/min) is administered to increase renal blood flow and increase cardiac perfusion. Heart rate and contractility increase with dose of 5 to 10 μg/kg/min. Should larger doses be required to raise mean arterial pressure (MAP) ≥60 mm Hg, levarterenol (Levophed) can be infused at a rate of 2 to 8 μg/min to maintain MAP ≥70 mm Hg. Epinephrine and phenylephrine can be administered to support arterial pressure with an infusion rate of 1 to 8 μg/min and 20 to 200 μg/min (see Table 1–10, p. 50).
- Corticosteroids: Corticosteroids can be used to inhibit the complement system, prevent complement-induced neutrophil aggregation, stabilize lysosomal membrane, and inhibit prostaglandin and thromboxane synthesis (see Table 1–15, p. 129, Table 8–4, p. 708)

EXPERIMENTAL PHARMACOLOGICAL THERAPIES

- Naloxone (Narcan): Is believed to reverse the endogenous opiate-induced hypotension and reduced cardiac contractility that occurs during septic shock.
- Nonsteroidal anti-inflammatory drugs: Drugs such as aspirin, ibuprofen, indomethacin, and meclofenamate can be used to inhibit prostaglandin biosynthesis by blocking the activity of cyclooxygenase.
- Immune substrates: Antiserum cachectin, or TNF, may be used in patients at risk for sepsis and could deter the progression of consequences for sepsis. The antibody is thought to improve CO and reduce the effect of TNF in sepsis-related myocardial depression.

FLUID REPLACEMENT

- Blood: Is used as a volume expander when hematocrit is ≤30%.
- Albumin: Is given when albumin concentration is ≤2.0 g/dL at a rate of 50 to 100 g of albumin.
- Crystalloid solution: Should blood or blood products be ineffective, crystalloids are

administered to correct fluid and electrolyte imbalance.

OXYGEN THERAPY

- Ventilatory therapy with positive end-expiratory pressure (PEEP) or continuous positive airway pressure (CPAP) helps facilitate oxygenation.

DIET

- Enteral feedings: High-protein or enteral feedings can be given when feasible.
- Lipid or fat emulsions: Lipids can be limited to 10% to 15% of patient's total caloric requirements. Lipid or fat emulsions provide neutral triglycerides, unsaturated fatty acids, and glycerol.

NURSING MANAGEMENT: NURSING DIAGNOSES AND COLLABORATIVE PROBLEMS

Common nursing goals for patients with sepsis are to maintain fluid balance, facilitate tissue perfusion, provide oxygenation, reduce temperature, and provide adequate nutrition.

Nursing Diagnoses

Fluid volume deficit related to shift of intravascular fluid into the interstitial space secondary to vasodilation and increased capillary permeability as a result of bradykinin.

Expected Patient Outcomes. Patient maintains adequate fluid volume, as evidenced by blood pressure (BP) within patient's normal range, specific gravity 1.010 to 1.030, central venous pressure (CVP) 2 to 6 mm Hg, heart rate (HR) ≤ 100 bpm, pulmonary artery pressure (PAP) 20 to 30/8 to 15 mm Hg, PCWP 6 to 12 mm Hg, CO 4 to 8 L/min, CI 2.7 to 4.3 L/min/m^2, urinary output (UO) ≥ 30 mL/h, normal lung sounds, and skin turgor normal.

- Review levels of serum total protein, hemoglobin, hematocrit, BUN, and creatinine.
- Position patient so legs are elevated to increase venous return.

- Assess clinical indicators of hydration: skin turgor, BP, MAP, HR, capillary refill, and peripheral pulses.
- Report clinical findings associated with hyperdynamic septic shock: tachycardia, hypotension, strong and bounding peripheral pulses, tachypnea, crackles, dyspnea, flushed and warm skin, and changes in level of consciousness.
- Report clinical findings associated with hypodynamic septic shock: tachycardia; S$_3$, hypotension; weak or absent peripheral pulses; reduced respiratory rate; crackles or wheezes; cool, pale, or cyanotic skin; hypothermia; and altered level of consciousness.
- Obtain and report hemodynamic parameters associated with hyperdynamic septic syndrome: CO ≥ 8 L/min, CI ≥ 4.3 L/min/m^2, PCWP ≤ 6 mm Hg, S$\bar{v}$o$_2$ $\geq 80\%$, and SVR ≤ 900 dynes/s/cm^{-5}.
- Obtain and report hemodynamic parameters associated with hypodynamic septic shock: CO ≤ 4 L/min, CI ≤ 2.7 L/min/m^2, CVP ≤ 2 mm Hg, PCWP ≥ 18 mm Hg, and SVR ≥ 1200 dynes/s/cm^{-5}.
- Measure intake, output, specific gravity, and daily weight. Report UO ≤ 30 mL/h or ≤ 0.5 mL/kg/h, specific gravity ≥ 1.030 (dehydration) or specific gravity ≤ 1.010 (inadequate glomerular filtrate), and weight gain ≥ 0.5 to 1.0 kg/d (interstitial edema).
- Assess for the presence of interstitial edema as evidenced by leg, hand, sacral, or ankle edema.
- Administer prescribed crystalloid or colloid IV fluids to maintain adequate hydration and circulatory volume as evidenced by PCWP 6 to 12 mm Hg.
- Administer prescribed vasoactive agent (dopamine) to enhance CO.

Altered tissue perfusion related to vasoconstriction or microvascular occlusion secondary to release of sympathetic catecholamines, angiotensin, and thromboxane.

Expected Patient Outcomes. Patient maintains adequate tissue perfusion, as evidenced by

BP within patient's normal range, HR ≤ 100 bpm, UO ≥ 30 mL/h, CO 4 to 8 L/min, CI 2.7 to 4.3 L/min/m^2, SVR 800 to 1200 dynes/s/cm^{-5}, systemic vascular resistance index (SVRI) 1970 to 2390 dynes/s/cm^{-5}/m^2, S$\bar{v}o_2$ 60% to 80%, arterial oxygen saturation (Sao$_2$) $\geq 95\%$, peripheral pulses $+2$, absence of cyanosis, MAP 70 to 100 mm Hg, and capillary refill ≤ 3 seconds.

- Review WBC count, cultures, BUN, creatinine, hemoglobin, and hematocrit values.
- Elevate extremities to enhance venous return.
- Assess clinical indicators of perfusion: BP, HR, MAP, skin color and temperature, capillary refill, and peripheral pulses.
- Report clinical findings associated with decreased tissue perfusion: hypotension; tachycardia; cool, pale, or cyanotic skin; peripheral pulses $\leq +2$, and capillary refill ≥ 3 seconds.
- Obtain and report hemodynamic parameters associated with decreased tissue perfusion: CO ≤ 4 L/min, CI ≤ 2.7 L/min/m^2, CVP ≤ 2 mm Hg, SVR ≥ 1200 dynes/s/cm^{-5}, and MAP ≤ 70 mm Hg.
- Continuously monitor S$\bar{v}o_2$ and report a value $\leq 60\%$, which can indicate reduced CO.
- Administer colloids (albumin) and crystalloids (lactated Ringer's or normal saline) to raise preload as prescribed.
- Administer prescribed inotropes (dopamine or dobutamine) to increase oxygen transport by increasing myocardial contractility, stroke volume, CO, and BP (see Table 1–10, p. 50).
- Administer prescribed antibiotics, noting that they may not be effective for the first 48 to 72 hours.

Impaired gas exchange related to increased pulmonary interstitial edema or pulmonary microthrombi secondary to impaired alveolar-capillary permeability or bronchoconstriction.

Expected Patient Outcomes. Patient maintains adequate gas exchange, as evidenced by respiratory rate (RR) 12 to 20 BPM; HR ≤ 100 bpm; arterial blood gases within normal range; Sao$_2$ 95% to 97.5%; pulse oximetry (SpO$_2$) $\geq 95\%$; S$\bar{v}o_2$ 60% to 80%; absence of cyanosis; skin pink, warm, and dry; and absence of adventitious breath sounds.

- Review results of arterial blood gas measurement, hemoglobin, and hematocrit values.
- Position patient to enhance maximal chest excursion and comfort.
- Encourage patient to deep breathe, cough, turn, and use incentive spirometer to enhance lung expansion and minimize risk of atelectasis.
- Provide a quiet, relaxed environment to minimize oxygen demand.
- Assess clinical indicators of respiratory status: rate, depth, symmetry of chest wall movement, skin color, use of accessory muscles, and lung sounds.
- Report clinical findings associated with impaired gas exchange: tachypnea, asymmetry of chest wall movement, use of accessory muscles, crackles or wheezes, and cyanosis.
- Continuously monitor oxygenation status with SpO$_2$ and report SpO$_2$ $\leq 92\%$.
- Assess for clinical indicators necessitating the need for mechanical ventilation: RR ≥ 30 to 35, increased ventilatory effort, minute ventilation ≤ 5 L/min or ≥ 20 L/min, tidal volume ≤ 4 mL/kg, vital capacity ≤ 10 to 15 mL/kg, Paco$_2$ ≥ 40 mm Hg, P(A−a)o$_2$ ≥ 15 mm Hg on room air or ≥ 55 mm Hg or $\dot{Q}s/\dot{Q}t$ of more than 20% if CO is low.
- Provide mechanical ventilation, if necessary, and document use of Fio$_2$ and PEEP.
- Instruct patient to turn every 2 hours to enhance lung expansion.

Thermoregulation, ineffective related to leukotrienes, prostaglandins, and IL-1 secondary to the inflammatory response.

Expected Patient Outcomes. Patient maintains a temperature 36.5° to 38°C (97.7° to 100°F).

- Review results of WBC count and cultures of sputum, blood, urine, and wound.
- Continuously monitor core temperature. Report alterations of temperature $\geq 38.3°C$ (101°F) in sepsis syndrome or $\geq 35.6°C$ (96°F) in septic shock.
- Assess skin for the presence of diaphoresis.
- Apply extra blankets while patient is hypothermic or shivering.
- Provide prescribed tepid sponge bath or cooling blanket when patient is hyperthermic to decrease metabolic rate and myocardial oxygen demand.
- Administer IV fluids as prescribed to maintain adequate hydration.
- Administer fresh frozen plasma as prescribed to restore host defenses, such as complement, in patient with prolonged infection or malnutrition.
- Administer prescribed antipyretics to reduce fever.
- Administer prescribed antibiotics to reduce the risk of infection.

Altered nutrition: less than body requirements related to increased need for nutrients secondary to increased metabolic rate.

Expected Patient Outcomes. Patient maintains adequate nutrition as evidenced by stable weight, BUN 8 to 20 mg/dL, hematocrit M: 42% to 54% or W: 38% to 46%, hemoglobin M: 14 to 16.5 g/100 mL or W: 12 to 15 g/100 mL, lymphocytes 20% to 40%, serum albumin 3.3 to 4.5 g/dL, total serum protein 6.6 to 7.9 g/dL, electrolytes within normal range, and caloric intake range from 35 to 45 calories/kg of normal body weight.

- Confer with dietitian regarding patient's dietary needs: 3500 to 4500 nonprotein calories and 1.5 to 2.5 g of nitrogen per kg per day to restore immunological competence.
- Monitor levels of serum albumin 3.5 g/dL, thyroxine-binding prealbumin 200 to 300 μg/mL, retinol-binding protein 40 to 50 μg/mL, and BUN 10 to 20 mg/dL.
- Provide high-protein enteral feedings with iso-osmotic content.

- While patient is receiving enteral or oral feedings, assess bowel sounds every 2 hours. Report decreased or absent bowel sounds.
- For patients receiving continuous nasogastric (NG) tube feedings, monitor for residual feeding every 2 hours and before intermittent tube feedings. Hold feedings if residual is ≥ 100 mL, which may be one and one half times the rate of infusion.
- Should parenteral feedings be necessary, reduce glucose intake in the early phase of sepsis.
- Administer prescribed lipids and limit amount to 10% to 15% of one patient's total caloric requirements. Lipids or fat emulsions provide a source of neutral triglycerides, unsaturated fatty acids, glyceral, and egg yolk phospholipids. The concentration of fat emulsions may be crucial in preventing excessive amount of fatty acid administration from potentiating mediator release.

Collaborative Problems

Common collaborative goals for patients with sepsis are to increase cardiac output and maintain oxygen supply and demand balance.

Potential Complication: Decreased Cardiac Output.

Decreased cardiac output related to altered preload, afterload, and contractility secondary to MDF.

Expected Patient Outcomes. Patient maintains adequate CO, as evidenced by BP within patient's normal range, HR ≤ 100 bpm, UO ≥ 30 mL/h, CO 4 to 8 L/min, CI 2.7 to 4.3 L/min/m^2, CVP 2 to 6 mm Hg, pulmonary artery pressure (PAP) systolic 15 to 30 mm Hg or PAP diasystolic 8 to 15 mm Hg, PCWP 6 to 12 mm Hg, pulmonary vascular resistance (PVR) 37 to 250 dynes/s/cm^{-5}, MAP 70 to 100 mm Hg, left ventricular stroke work index (LVSWI) 38 to 85 g/m^2/beat, right ventricular stroke work index (RVSWI) 7 to 12 g/m^2/beat, SVR 800 to 1200 dynes/s/cm^{-5}/m^2, SVRI 1970 to 2390 dynes/s/cm^{-5}/m^2, peripheral pulses +2, absence of cyanosis, and capillary refill ≤ 3 seconds.

- Consult with physician to validate expected patient outcomes used to evaluate CO.

- Consult with physician to determine predicted final hemodynamic indicators in patients who can survive septic shock: HR 95 bpm, MAP 85 mm Hg, PCWP 9.6 mm Hg, CVP 4.4 mm Hg, stroke volume index (SVI) 4.1 mL/m^2, CI 4.1 L/min/m^2, SVRI 1691 dynes/s/cm^{-5}/m^2, pulmonary artery mean pressure 17 mm Hg, PVRI 150 dynes/s/cm^{-5}/m^2, LVSWI 41 g/m^2/beat and RVSWI 7.3 g/m^2/beat.
- Review results of blood studies and immunoglobin levels if albumin is administered, as their production may be reduced.
- Assess clinical indicators of perfusion: BP, HR, MAP, capillary refill, skin color and warmth, and peripheral pulses.
- Report clinical findings associated with reduced perfusion resulting from decreased CO. Hypotension, tachycardia, MAP ≤70 mm Hg, capillary refill ≥3 seconds, skin cool and cyanotic, and peripheral pulses ≤+2.
- Measure intake, output, specific gravity, and daily weight. Report UO ≤30 mL/h or ≤0.5 mL/kg/h.
- Obtain and report hemodynamic parameters associated with depressed preload: PCWP ≤6 mm Hg and CVP ≤2 mm Hg.
- Obtain and report hemodynamic parameters associated with decreased afterload: SVR ≤900 dynes/s/cm^{-5} and PVR ≤37 to 250 dynes/s/cm^{-5}.
- Obtain and report hemodynamic parameters used to infer decreased myocardial contractility early in the septic syndrome: CI ≥4.3 L/min/m^2, EF ≤60%, LVSWI ≤38 g/m^2/beat, and RVSWI ≤7 g/m^2/beat.
- Provide oxygen by nasal cannula or Venturi mask at the prescribed amount.
- Administer prescribed blood when hematocrit is ≤30% to maintain volume status and oxygen-carrying capacity of the blood.
- Administer prescribed albumin 50 to 100 g as a 25% solution when patient is hypoalbuminemic ≤2 g/dL.
- Administer prescribed crystalloids when hematocrit and albumin levels are normal to increase ventricular volume, maximize myocardial stretch, maintain CO, maintain MAP ≥60 mm Hg and PCWP 12 to 15 mm Hg.
- Administer prescribed vasopressor (dopamine) when maximum volume infusion (PCWP 15 to 18 mm Hg) does not normalize BP and organ perfusion as evidenced by MAP ≥60 mm Hg, decreased lactate levels, adequate UO, and normal organ function. Should hypotension continue, dopamine can be titrated up to a maximum of 20 μg/kg/min to keep MAP ≥60 mm Hg and optimize organ function parameters (see Table 1–10, p. 50).
- Administer prescribed levarterenol (Levophed) should dopamine exceed 20 μg/kg/min. It is infused at 2 to 10 μg/min until the MAP is ≥60 mm Hg (see Table 1–10, p. 50).
- Administer prescribed low-dose dopamine (1 to 4 μg/kg/min) in conjunction with levarterenol to increase renal perfusion.
- Should dopamine and levarterenol be ineffective in correcting hypotension, administer prescribed phenylephrine (Neo-Synephrine) to produce vasoconstriction without direct cardiac effect.
- Should sepsis-induced cardiogenic shock occur as evidenced by reduced MAP, elevated PCWP, and elevated SVR, administer dopamine in conjunction with vasodilator (nitroprusside) to maintain MAP, enhance myocardial contractility, and reduce afterload (SVR) and preload (PCWP).

Potential Complication: Oxygen Supply-Demand Imbalance. Oxygen supply-demand imbalance related to cellular effect, maldistribution of flow, impaired oxygen diffusion, or hypometabolism secondary to sepsis.

Expected Patient Outcomes. Patient maintains adequate myocardial oxygen supply, as evidenced by coronary artery perfusion pressure (CAPP) 60 to 80 mm Hg, CO 4 to 8 L/min, CI 2.7 to 4 L/min/m^2, oxygen consumption (Vo$_2$) ≥200 or ≤250 mL/min, oxygen consumption index (Vo$_2$I) ≥115 or ≤165 mL/min/m^2, oxygen delivery (Do$_2$) 900 to 1200 mL/min, oxygen delivery index (Do$_2$I) 500 to 600 mL/min/m^2, oxygen extraction ratio (O$_2$ER) of

25%, PCWP 6 to 12 mm Hg, PP 30 to 40 mm Hg, rate pressure product (RPP) $\leq$12,000, $S\bar{v}o_2$ 60% to 80%, SVR 900 to 1200 dynes/s/cm^{-5}, SVRI 1970 to 2300 dynes/s/cm^{-5}/m^2, stroke volume (SV) 60 to 130 mL/beat, SVI 45 to 85 mL/m^2/beat, BP $\geq$90/60 mm Hg or within the patient's normal range, MAP 70 to 90 mm Hg, HR $\leq$90 bpm, capillary refill $\leq$3 seconds, Sao_2 $\geq$95%, Pao_2 $\geq$80 mm Hg, UO $\geq$30 mL/h or $\geq$0.5 mL/kg/h, specific gravity 1.010 to 1.030, temperature $\leq$100°F, absence of dysrhythmias, and absence of chest pain.

- Consult with physician to determine the oxygen delivery and consumption and hemodynamic values in relation to therapeutic goals: CI 50% in excess of normal, normal BP, blood volume 500 mL greater than normal with PCWP not to exceed 20 mm Hg, oxygen delivery (Do_2) $\geq$600 mL/min/m^2, oxygen consumption (Vo_2) $\geq$170 mL/min/m^2, and PVRI $\leq$250 dynes/s/cm^{-5}/m^2.
- Review with the cardiologist the results of serum enzyme tests and serial ECG.
- Limit physical activity to the level of activity that does not increase HR and increase myocardial oxygen demand.
- Position patient with the bed elevated 20 to 30 degrees to decrease myocardial oxygen demand.
- Promote rest by decreasing environmental stimuli, assisting with or performing personal care activities, and pacing patient activities to reduce myocardial oxygen demand.
- Calculate CAPP, since a decrease leads to further myocardial ischemia and necrosis.
- Calculate Do_2 and Do_2I to evaluate the effectiveness of therapies that enhance perfusion.
- Obtain and report hemodynamic findings that indicate decreased myocardial oxygen sypply resulting from CAPP $\leq$60 mm Hg, CO $\leq$4 L/min, CI $\leq$2.7 L/min/m^2, Do_2 $\leq$900 mL/min and DO_2I $\leq$500 mL/min/m^2.
- Obtain, document, and report other findings suggestive of decreased myocardial oxygen

supply: HR $\geq$100 bpm, which decreases diastolic filling time, BP $\leq$90/60 mm Hg, capillary refill $\geq$3 seconds, peripheral pulses $\leq$2+, presence of dysrhythmia, and chest pain.
- Calculate Vo_2I to evaluate the effectiveness of therapies that decrease myocardial demand.
- Estimate myocardial oxygen consumption by calculating RPP, which is determined by multiplying HR with systolic blood pressure (SBP). The RPP correlates with myocardial oxygen consumption during rest and exercise.
- Obtain Vo_2 and Vo_2I in relation to Do_2 and Do_2I. When Vo_2 (oxygen consumption) is limited by Do_2 (oxygen delivery), the Vo_2 is thought of as being supply-dependent. The rate of oxygen consumed is limited by the rate of oxygen delivered to the tissues.
- Monitor and report factors that may cause increased myocardial oxygen demand: hypotension, hypertension, tachycardia, increased contractility, pain, anxiety, fever, anemia, and volume depletion.
- Obtain, document, and report hemodynamic parameters that indicate increased myocardial oxygen demand resulting from decreased CO: O_2ER $\geq$25%, PP $\leq$30 mm Hg, RPP $\geq$12,000, $S\bar{v}o_2$ $\geq$60%, SVR $\geq$1200 dynes/s/cm^{-5}, SVRI $\geq$2390 dynes/s/cm^{-5}/m^2, Vo_2 $\geq$250 mL/min and Vo_2I $\geq$165 mL/min/m^2.
- Obtain and report other findings suggestive of increased myocardial oxygen demand because they increase metabolic activity and subsequent myocardial work load: HR $\geq$100 bpm, temperature $\geq$100.8°F, and BP above patient's normal value.
- Continuously monitor $S\bar{v}o_2$ since a decreasing value $\leq$60% may indicate decreased CO and increased O_2ER ($\leq$25%).
- Continuously monitor temperature and report level $\leq$37°C, since this can shift the oxyhemoglobin dissociation curve to the left and impair the oxygen extraction ability of the tissues.

- Initiate continuous ECG to assess HR and rhythm. Document ECG rhythm strips every 2 to 4 hours in patients with dysrhythmias.
- Administer prescribed oxygen 2 to 4 L/min (24% to 36% oxygen) by means of nasal cannula or $FIO_2 \leq 50\%$ by mask to maintain $PaO_2 \geq 80$ mm Hg or $SaO_2 \geq 95\%$.
- Provide prescribed mechanical ventilation, if necessary, with sedation or neuromuscular blockade, which can be used to minimize tissue oxygen requirement.
- Administer prescribed IV fluids to maintain adequate hydration, $DO_2 \geq 900$ mL/min or $DO_2I \geq 500$ mL/min/m².
- Administer prescribed colloid to expand the plasma volume without excess increase in interstitial water to maintain PCWP no greater than 18 mm Hg.
- Administer prescribed inotrope (dobutamine) at a dose of 2 μg/kg/min to achieve the best CI, DO_2, and VO_2 (see Table 1–10, p. 50).
- Should MAP and SVRI be high, administer prescribed vasodilator (nitroglycerin or nitroprusside) to improve CI without causing hypotension. Keep MAP ≥ 80 mm Hg.
- Should fluid therapy, inotropes, and vasodilators be ineffective in achieving the therapeutic goals, administer prescribed vasopressor (dopamine) to maintain MAP 80 mm Hg and SBP 110 mm Hg.
- Administer prescribed acetaminophen to control fever, thereby restoring oxygen supply-demand balance. Note that antipyretics such as aspirin, which inhibit prostaglandin synthesis, can decrease renal blood flow.
- Teach patient the importance of reporting chest pain.
- Teach patient to pace activities so as not to increase HR and subsequently decrease myocardial tissue oxygen supply.
- Teach patient about the common side effects of vasodilators: headache, nausea, vomiting, or dizziness.
- Teach patient about the common side effects of positive inotropic agents.

- Teach patient to avoid behaviors that increase HR: excessive physical activity, straining at stool, anger, or irritability.
- Teach patient techniques to reduce myocardial tissue oxygen demand: guided imagery, meditation, or progressive relaxation.
- Teach patient to exhale with physical movement. This reduces the potential for increased intrathoracic pressure, which decreases venous return to the heart (decreased preload) and vagal stimulation, which causes a decrease in CO. When air is released, the intrathoracic pressure is decreased and preload is increased, causing increased work load for the heart.
- Teach patient to alleviate sources of psychological stress and use progressive muscular relaxation in order to decrease oxygen consumption.

DISCHARGE PLANNING

The critical care nurse will provide patient and significant other(s) with verbal or written discharge notes regarding the following subjects:

1. Importance of risk factors that may cause sepsis, such as chemotherapeutic agents.
2. Importance of maintaining an optimal nutritional intake.
3. Importance of keeping all postdischarge appointments.
4. Signs and symptoms associated with infection: hypertension, tachycardia, tachypnea, and fever.

■ ACQUIRED IMMUNODEFICIENCY SYNDROME

(For related information see Cardiac Deviations, Part I: Acute myocardial infarction, p. 38; Shock, p. 174; Cardiac trauma, p. 167; Dysrhythmias, p. 184. Part III: Hemodynamic monitoring, p. 219; ST segment monitoring, p. 264. Vascular Deviations, Part I: Deep vein thrombosis, p. 304; Vascular trauma, p. 308. Respiratory Deviations, Part I: Adult respiratory distress syndrome, p. 327; Acute pul-

monary edema, p. 346; Respiratory acidosis, p. 412. Part III: Pulse oximetry, p. 426; Mechanical ventilation, p. 428; Indirect calorimetry, p. 441. Renal Deviations, Part I: Acute tubular necrosis, p. 455; Acute renal failure, p. 459; Metabolic acidosis, p. 474. Part III: Hemodialysis, p. 496; Peritoneal dialysis, p. 502; Continuous renal replacement therapy, p. 505. Gastrointestinal Deviations, Part III: Total parenteral nutrition, p. 551; Enteral nutrition, p. 554. Psychosocial deviations, Part I, p. 725).

Case Management Basis

DRG: 398 Reticuloendothelial and immunity
    disorders with complications
LOS: 6.60 days
DRG: 399 Reticuloendothelial and immunity
    disorders without complications
LOS: 4.00 days

Definition

Acquired immunodeficiency syndrome (AIDS) is the dysruption of cellular immunity and subsequent development of opportunistic infections. The AIDS patient is a human immunodeficiency virus (HIV)-infected individual who has T_4 cell counts of 200 or less.

Pathophysiology

HIV is one of a category of viruses called retrovirsuses that are minus a DNA. To replicate, the virus uses the enzyme reverse transcriptase to reverse transcribe the viral RNA into DNA. The virus integrates itself into the host cell DNA. When HIV enters the body, it infects cells with the CD4 surface molecule. HIV eventually destroys human T_4 lymphocyte, thereby reducing their numbers. The target cells for HIV infection include T_4 lymphocytes, monocyte-macrophages, dendrite cells, Langerhans' cells, promyelocyte cell lines, Epstein-Barr virus transformed B cells, and microglial cells. Once infected, the target cell is infected for the lifetime of the cell and HIV production is activated by the following cofactors: herpes simplex virus (HSV), cytomegalovirus (CMV), Epstein-Barr virus (EBV), hepatitis B virus (HBV), *Myco-*

plasma, interleukin-6, tumor necrosis factor, or granulocyte macrophage.

HIV infections cause syndromes such as seroconversion, latency, AIDS, AIDS dementia complex, and AIDS wasting. Seroconversion is associated with the primary infection of HIV. Following seroconversion, HIV patients can enter a period of latency in which they can remain symptom-free for months to years. AIDS occurs when CD4 cell level drops below 200/mm^3. AIDS dementia complex is a syndrome involving progressive cognitive, behavioral, and motor deficits. Lastly, AIDS wasting is characterized by weight loss greater than 10% of baseline body weight, chronic diarrhea, or chronic weakness.

Nursing Assessment

PRIMARY CAUSES

- HIV virus is transmitted during sexual intercourse via semen and vaginal secretions, by intravenous use of blood-contaminated needles, by transfusion of HIV-contaminated blood or blood products, or from mother to baby during the perinatal period or through breast milk. Other sources of transmission include artificial insemination or organ transplantation.

RISK FACTORS

- High-risk groups are homosexuals or bisexual males; intravenous drug users; and those having unprotected heterosexual, bisexual, or homosexual intercourse with a known HIV-positive person or someone in a high-risk group.

PHYSICAL ASSESSMENT

Seroconversion

- Inspection: Rashes, fever, diaphoresis, lethargy, malaise, myalgia, poor skin turgor, tissue edema, arthralgia, headache, photophobia, diarrhea, sore throat, mood swings, desquamation of the sole of the feet and palms, pallor ecchymosis, vesicles, and maculopapular rash covering the face and trunk.

- Palpation: Lymphadenopathy of the axillary, occipital, and cervical nodes.
- Auscultation: Crackles.

AIDS

- Inspection: Purplish lesions (Kaposi's sarcoma); dyspnea; dry, unproductive cough (*Pneumocystis carinii*); irritability; depression; weakness to paralysis; seizures, watery diarrhea; memory loss; and weight loss.
- Palpation: Lymphadenopathy.

DIAGNOSTIC TEST RESULTS

Standard Laboratory Tests. (see Table 10–4)

- Blood studies: Reduced hemoglobin, white blood cells (WBCs), lymphocytes, and platelets.
- Cultures: HIV can be detected by culture through viral antigens in the blood (the p24 antigen assay) and by HIV gene amplification (polymerase chain reaction), which are used in cinical research.
- Enzyme-linked immunosorbent assay (ELISA): Is used to detect the presence of antibody to HIV. A normal result for the ELISA is nonreactive.
- Rapid-latex agglutination assay: A positive reaction (presence of HIV antibodies) consists of agglutination that is visible in bright light, whereas a negative reaction reveals no such agglutination.
- Skin testing with recall antigens: Diminished delayed hypersensitivity.
- Total T cell and B cells: Reduced T_4 (helper) lymphocytes and normal number of B lymphocytes.
- T_4:T_8 lymphocyte ratio: Decreased (≤ 1.0).
- Western blot analysis: Positive test confirms presence of AIDS. The test detects various antibodies made in response to HIV proteins of particular molecular weight.

Invasive Diagnostic Procedure. (see Table 3–3, p. 335, and Table 5–2, p. 516)

- Biopsies: Used to differentiate diagnosis of pneumonias, Kaposi's sarcoma, or other neoplasms.

- Bronchoscopy: Used with biopsy when *Pneumocystis carinii* pneumonia (PCP) or lung malignancies are suspected.
- Endoscopy: Used to detect disseminated *Candida* especially in the esophagus or Kaposi's sarcoma in the gastrointestional tract.
- Gallium scan: Diffuse pulmonary uptake can be found in PCP.

Noninvasive Diagnostic Procedure

- Chest roentgenogram: May reveal progressive interstitial infiltrates from PCP or other pulmonary problems.

MEDICAL AND SURGICAL MANAGEMENT

Pharmacology

- Zidovudine (AZT): AZT binds to reverse transcriptase, which prevents this enzyme from participating in the reverse transcription of RNA in HIV-infected cells. Its use is in HIV patients with T_4 counts of less than 500/mm^3. The drug is given orally 200 mg every 4 hours around the clock or as an IV dose of 1 to 2 mg/kg over 1 hour every 4 hours (Table 10–5).
- Dideoxyinosine (DDI): The DDI interacts with reverse transcriptase to inhibit HIV replication. It can be used in patients who are intolerant of AZT (see Table 10–5).
- Dideoxycytidine (ddCyd): Used in conjunction with AZT in patients with advanced HIV infection who have T_4 counts ≤ 300/mm^3. A dose of 0.75 mg is given orally with 200 mg of AZT every 8 hours (see Table 10–5).
- Trimethoprim-sulfamethoxazole (TMP-SMX): A prophylactic agent for PCP. It is given as one double-strength tablet once a day 7 days a week.
- Aerosolized pentamide with the Respirgard II Nebulizer: A prophylactic agent for PCP, it is given as 300 mg once a month. The treatment takes 30 to 45 minutes.
- Antiemetics: Metoclopramide hydrochloride (Reglan), prochlorperazine maleate (Compazine) or trimethobenzamide hydrochloride (Tigan) are used to reduce the incidence of vomiting.

TABLE 10-4

TABLE 10–4. STANDARD HIV-AIDS LABORATORY TESTS

Test	Purpose	Normal Values	Abnormal Findings
Lymphocyte marker assay (T and B cell surface markers, T-helper: T suppressor ratio)	Evaluates immune function by identifying specific cells involved in immune response Assists in diagnosing AIDS Assists in determining treatment for autoimmune disorders such as AIDS	Percentage T cells: 60.1%–88.1% Percentage helper T (CD4) cells: 34%–67% Percentage suppressor T (CD8) cells: 10.0%–41.9% Percentage B cells: 3.0%–20.8% Lymphocyte counts: 0.66–4.60 thousand/μL T cell count: 644–2201 cells/μL B cell count: 82–392 cells/μL Helper cell (CD4) count: 493–1191 cells/μL Suppressor T cell (CD8) count: 182–785 cells/μL CD4:CD8 ratio: ≥1.0	Reduced levels of T-cells and B-cells in autosomal or sex-linked recessive immunodeficiency
Enzyme-linked immunosorbent assay (ELISA)	Screening tool for blood donors and populations at risk for AIDS Assists in diagnosis when AIDS is suspected	Nonreactive	Antibody developed in an individual exposed to HIV, is detectable by ELISA within 3 months of exposure
HIV antigen testing p24 antigen capture assay	Used by researchers to measure amount of p24, a piece of HIV known as core antigen	Negative	Presence of p24 antigenemia may precede development of symptoms or infections; may be associated with depletion of T4 cells
Assay for HIV nucleic acid	Used as a molecular sign of infection when HIV infection process in latency, when HIV replication occurring at a slow rate, or when maternally derived HIV antibody from an infected mother is present in infant	Negative	Molecular sign of infection
Rapid latex agglutination assay	Diagnoses HIV May be used in blood transfusion and organ donation screening programs	Negative	A positive (presence of HIV antibodies) consists of agglutination that is visible in bright light

TABLE 10-4

TABLE 10-5

TABLE 10–4. CONTINUED

Test	Purpose	Normal Values	Abnormal Findings
Western blot analysis	Detects various antibodies made in response to HIV proteins of particular molecular weights	Negative	A positive on both ELISA and Western blot analysis suggests person infected and considered infectious

From Casey KM, Cave LH, 1993; Loeb S, 1993; Tribett D #1, 1993.

TABLE 10–5. PARTIAL LIST MEDICATIONS USED IN HIV-AIDS

Medication	Route/Dose	Uses/Effects	Side Effects
Dideoxycytidine (ddCyd)	PO: 0.75 mg is given with 200 mg zidovudine q 8 h	In combination with zidovudine for advanced HIV infection: T4 cell counts $\leq$300/mm^3 with clinical immunological deterioration	Pancreatitis, peripheral neuropathy
Dideoxyinosine (DDI)	PO	Interacts with reverse transcriptase to inhibit HIV replication Used in patients intolerant of zidovudine or who have immunological decline when receiving it	Pancreatitis, peripheral neuropathy; complaints of distal numbness, tingling, pain in feet and hands
Pentamidine isethionate (Pentam 300)	PO: 4 mg/kg/d	Treats PCP	Nausea, vomiting, anorexia, metallic taste in mouth, hypotension, dysrhythmias, azotemia, pancreatitis, hypoglycemia
Trimethoprim/ sulfamethoxazole (Bactrim, Septra)	PO: 75–100 mg/kg/d; 15–20 mg/kg/d	Treats PCP	Rash, fever, nausea, vomiting, anorexia, leukopenia, hyponatremia, abnormal liver function studies
Zidovudine (azidothymidine, AZT)	PO: 200 mg q 4 h; can be lowered to 100 mg q 4 h while awake for a total daily dose of 500 mg IV: 1 mg/kg with dose of 1–2 mg/kg/h, and given q 4 h	Prevents reverse transcription of RNA in HIV-infected cells HIV patients with T4 counts $\leq$500/mm	Myopathy, muscle tenderness, weakness, wasting

IV, Intravenous; PCP, *Pneumocystis carinii* pneumonia; PO, by mouth.

Casey K and Cave LH, 1993; Deglin JH and Vallerand AH, 1995; Hollander H and Katz MH, 1994.

- Antimicrobials: Trimethoprim-sulfameth-oxazole (Bactrim, Septra) used in treating PCP (see Table 10–5).
- Antidiarrheals: Diphenoxylate hydrochloride (Lomotil), loperamide hydrochloride (Imodium), and camphorated tincture of opium (paregoric) are used to decrease the amount and fluidity of stool by reducing intestinal spasm and peristalsis.

SURGICAL INTERVENTION
- Resection of tumors.

NURSING MANAGEMENT: NURSING DIAGNOSES AND COLLABORATIVE PROBLEMS

Nursing Diagnoses
Common nursing goals for patients with AIDs are to maintain fluid balance, prevent infection, improve oxygenation, correct diarrhea, maintain adequate nutritional intake, support cognitive function, minimize damage to mucous membranes, maintain skin integrity, encourage coping behavior, promote activity tolerance, and minimize body image disturbance.

Fluid volume deficit related to diarrhea, vomiting, and fever.

Expected Patient Outcomes. Patient maintains adequate fluid volume, as evidenced by blood pressure (BP) within normal range, mean arterial pressure (MAP) 70 to 100 mm Hg, moist mucous membranes, good skin turgor, skin pink, capillary refill ≤ 3 seconds, peripheral pulses +2, urinary output (UO) ≥ 30 mL/h or ≥ 0.5 mL/kg/h, specific gravity 1.001 to 1.035, central venous pressure (CVP) 2 to 6 mm Hg, stable body weight, and serum osmolality 275 to 295 mOsm/kg.

- Review levels of serum electrolytes, hematocrit, hemoglobin, and serum osmolality.
- Provide prescribed high-calorie and high-protein diet.
- Encourage patient to eat foods high in bulk, which can improve consistency of the stool.

- Provide low-fiber, lactulose-free or pectin-containing formulas, which can help to reduce diarrheal episodes.
- Assess clinical indicators of hydration: BP, heart rate, skin turgor, skin color and warmth, and mucous membranes.
- Report clinical findings associated with dehydration: hypotension, MAP ≤ 60 mm Hg, tachycardia, poor skin turgor, skin pale and dry, and dry mucous membranes.
- Obtain and report, if available, CVP ≤ 2 mm Hg to assess circulating fluid volume.
- Measure intake, output, specific gravity, and daily weight. Report UO ≤ 30 mL/h or ≤ 0.5 mL/kg/h, specific gravity ≥ 1.020, and weight loss ≤ 0.25 to 0.5 kg/d.
- Administer prescribed IV fluids and electrolytes to maintain adequate hydration and circulating volume.
- Administer prescribed antidiarrheal agents to control diarrhea.
- Administer prescribed antiemetic agents to control vomiting and reduce further loss of fluids and electrolytes.

Infection related to deficiency of immune system or malnutrition.

Expected Patient Outcomes. Patient is free of infection as evidenced by normothermia, negative culture or biopsy, and absence of purulent drainage or localized erythema.

- Review results of complete blood count (CBC) and cultures.
- Obtain and report clinical findings associated with infection: elevated temperature, positive cultures, tachycardia, or purulent drainage or erythema.
- Continuously monitor temperature.
- Maintain strict aseptic care for all invasive procedures to prevent further infection.
- Assess sites of invasive procedures for redness, tenderness, swelling, and purulent drainage.
- Use hand washing technique before and after all care contacts to reduce the risk of cross contamination.

- Wear gloves and gown during contact with secretions, excretions, or whenever there is a break in skin of the caregiver.
- Wear mask and protective eye wear during suctioning or intubation or extubation.
- Dispose of needles and sharps according to unit protocol.
- Label all blood bags, body fluid containers, soiled dressings and linens and identify for disposal per isolation protocol.
- Administer prescribed antibiotic, antifungal, or antimicrobial agents such as trimethaprim-sulfamethoxazole (Bactrum, Septra), nystatin (Mycostatin), or pentamidine (Pentam 300) to treat infection.
- Administer prescribed experimental drugs such as zidovudine (azidothymidine [AZT]) (see Table 10–5).
- Teach patient and significant other(s) to wash hands as indicated.

Impaired gas exchange related to increased pulmonary infiltrates, intrapulmonary shunting, or reduced lung compliance secondary to opportunistic pulmonary infections such as PCP.

Expected Patient Outcomes. Patient maintains adequate gas exchange, as evidenced by respiratory rate (RR) 12 to 20 BPM, absence of dyspnea, arterial blood gases within normal range, absence of cyanosis, arterial oxygen saturation (Sao_2) 95% to 97.5%, pulmonary vascular resistance (PVR) 37 to 97 dynes/s/cm^{-5}, pulmonary vascular resistance index (PVRI) 255 to 285 dynes/s/cm^{-5}/m^2, mixed venous oxygen saturation ($S\bar{v}o_2$ 60% to 80%, hemoglobin within normal range, and absence of adventitious breath sounds.

- Confer with physician regarding pulmonary complications such as PCP, CMV, Kaposi's sarcoma of the lung, or *Mycobacterium avium-intracellulare* (MAI) in relation to the patient and his or her blood gas values.
- Review results of chest roentgenogram, screening serology by enzyme immunoassay (EIA) or immunofluorescent assay (IFA), arterial blood gas measurements, WBC count, T-cell studies, or HIV tests.
- Limit activity to bed rest to reduce oxygen demands.
- Reposition patient every 2 hours to help prevent stasis of lung fields and to facilitate optimum arterial oxygenation.
- Assess clinical indicators of respiratory status: rate, rhythm, symmetry of chest wall movement, use of accessory muscles, skin color, and lung sounds.
- Monitor for clinical indicators of hypoxemia: dyspnea, cyanosis, restlessness, confusion, anxiety, delirium, tachypnea, tachycardia, use of accessory muscles, headache, and cardiac arrhythmia.
- Monitor for clinical indicators necessitating intubation and mechanical ventilation: progressive respiratory failure of uncertain diagnosis; respiratory failure related to bronchoscopy; seizure; or postoperative period; second or later episode of PCP in a patient receiving zidovudine (AZT); or bacterial sepsis.
- Measure daily weight, intake, specific gravity, and UO. Report UO $\leq$30 mL/h or $\leq$0.5 mL/kg/h.
- Encourage patient to turn, cough, deep breathe, and use incentive spirometer to facilitate lung expansion.
- Provide prescribed humidified supplemental oxygen by cannula, mask, intubation, or mechanical ventilation to maintain effective oxygenation and relieve mucous membrane irritation.
- Administer prescribed antimicrobials (trimethoprim-sulfamethoxazole) to treat PCP (see Table 10–5).
- Administer sedatives and analgesics to help prevent or minimize respiratory depression.
- Teach patient to report changes in cough or dyspnea.

Diarrhea related to medication therapy.

Expected Patient Outcome. Patient maintains normal bowel elimination and formed stool.

- Review results of stool cultures for bacterial infections such as *Entamoeba histolytica, Giardia, Salmonella, Shigella,* and *Campylobacter*; and serum osmolality levels.
- Provide diet high in potassium and sodium as prescribed.
- Should diarrhea be due to tube feedings, dilute strength or reduce rate of infusion, as either of these factors may cause diarrhea.
- Monitor the number and volume of diarrhea stools.
- Assess stool for the presence of blood, fat, and undigested material.
- Assess for clinical indicators of dehydration: weight loss, cool and clammy skin, decreased skin turgor, dry mucous membranes, tachycardia, hypotension, lethargy, weakness, and oliguria.
- Assess patient for clinical findings associated with electrolyte imbalance: confusion, muscle weakness, cramps, dysrhythmias, hypotension, and weak pulse.
- Measure UO and daily weight. Report UO ≥ 30 mL/h and weight loss of ≥ 0.25 to 0.5 kg/d.
- Apply zinc oxide to anorectal area as prescribed to prevent skin excoriation.
- Administer IV fluids and electrolytes as prescribed: hypertonic (3%) NaCl solutes or hypertonic $NaHCO_3$ only when serum sodium is ≤ 120 mg/dL.

Altered nutrition: less than body requirements related to malabsorption syndrome and infective or noninfective diarrhea.

Expected Patient Outcome. Patient maintains stable weight.

- Review results of blood urea nitrogen (BUN), glucose, liver function studies, electrolytes, proteins, and albumin.
- Confer with dietitian to develop an individualized diet program for patient.
- Provide high-calorie and high-protein diet with supplemental vitamins and minerals.
- Provide lipid-based (62% of the nonprotein caloric load) parenteral nutrition, if not con-

traindicated, to stabilize or reverse the wasting syndrome.
- Monitor for clinical indicators of malabsorption syndrome: weight loss; decrease in serum albumin level, retinol-binding protein, transferrin, iron-binding capacity; and decreased levels of vitamin B_{12} and folic acid.
- Monitor the effectiveness of enteral feedings because of malabsorption, nausea, and diarrhea.
- Measure daily weight, intake, specific gravity, and UO. Report weight loss ≥ 0.25 to 0.5 kg/d, which may indicate inadequacy of nutritional intake.
- Provide rest periods before and after eating.
- Administer prescribed total parenteral nutrition (TPN) should patient be unable to tolerate oral or enteral feedings.
- Administer prescribed vitamin supplements should patient experience a disorder of digestion and absorption.

Altered thought process related to impaired cognitive function secondary to infection or HIV dementia.

Expected Patient Outcomes. Patient maintains normal thought process, judgment, and cognitive function.

- Obtain physical therapy consultation for gait-assistive devices.
- Review results of cerebrospinal fluid (CSF) test, abnormal showing *Toxoplasma gondii* or *Cryptococcus neoformans*; computed tomography (CT) shows cerebral atrophy in subacute encephalitis or lesions with ring enhancement and edema in the cortical area with toxoplasmosis; magnetic nuclear resonance imaging (MRI) shows signal attenuation in the frontal white matter, associated with subacute encephalitis; and serologic tests reveal high antibody titer and detectable immunoglobulin M (IgM) in toxoplasmosis.
- Provide adequate rest periods.
- Assess clinical indicators of neurological status: mental status, level of conscious-

ness, motor function, sensory function, cranial nerves, and deep tendon reflexes.

- Report clinical findings associated with subacute encephalitis in AIDS patient: hallucinations, psychosis, or affective symptoms.
- Report clinical findings associated with focal cerebral syndromes: headache, fever, focal neurological deficit, seizures, and coma.
- Report clinical findings associated with meningitis: mild depression, headache, and fever.
- Reorient patient as necessary.
- Provide support, guidance for family and friends.
- Eliminate unnecessary environmental stimuli.
- Organize nursing activities to eliminate unnecessary encounters.
- Administer pyrimethamine and sulfadiazine as prescribed for focal cerebral syndromes.
- Administer amphotericin B as prescribed for cryptococcosis meningitis.

Altered oral mucous membrane related to opportunistic infection such as candidiasis.

Expected Patient Outcomes. Patient's existing oral lesions heal and there is absence of *Candida* infection.

- Review results of WBC count and cultures of sputum, blood, urine, and lesions.
- Use oral irrigation and suction if patient is unable to adequately rinse mouth.
- Assess patient's ability to swallow or handle secretions.
- Avoid irritating foods such as salty, spicy, abrasive and acidic food or drink.
- Resecure endotracheal tube twice daily to avoid the development of pressure points.
- Encourage oral intake of 2500 mL/d if not contraindicated.
- Include in oral care antifungal drug nystatin if not contraindicated.

Impaired skin integrity related to Kaposi's skin lesions, immobilization, and malnutrition.

Expected Patient Outcome. Integrity of patient's skin is maintained.

- Turn patient every 2 hours to prevent pressure points.
- Clean nondraining, noninfected open lesions; cover lightly or leave open.
- Clean open, draining, infected lesions with potassium permanganate soaks followed by normal saline rinse daily.
- Assess skin in the areas of the coccyx, perirectal area, elbows, heels, and scapula for pressure points.
- Use strips of appropriate dressing or gauze to pack deep wounds.
- Evaluate Kaposi's lesions for location, dissemination, or weeping.
- Maintain wound and skin precautions.
- Provide protective devices such as elbow and heel pads, sheepskin, egg crate foam mattress pad, or flotation-type mattress.
- Assist with range of motion (ROM) to increase circulation to the skin and tissue.
- Administer vinblastine 4 to 7 mg IV and vincristine 1 to 1.5 mg IV on a weekly basis as prescribed for Kaposi's sarcoma (see Table 10–5).
- Administer interferon alfa recombinant (Intron-A) for Kaposi's sarcoma if not contraindicated.

Ineffective individual coping, related to depression secondary to the deterioration of his or her condition and potential for death.

Expected Patient Outcome. Patient demonstrates effective coping.

- Listen to patient's expression of depression.
- Spend time with patient and family, encouraging them to express their feelings and concerns.
- Provide patient an opportunity to communicate in private with significant others.
- Help patient to identify any incremental positive changes associated with the illness and treatment.
- Identify factors that contribute to patient's feeling of depression.
- Encourage active role in planning activities or establishing realistic and attainable daily goals.

- Provide written and oral explanations of procedures and precautions to patient and significant others.

Activity intolerance related to weakness secondary to fluid and electrolyte imbalance, dyspnea, pain, and fever.

Expected Patient Outcomes. Patient tolerates activities, as evidenced by normal sinus rhythm, RR $\leq$24 BPM, heart rate (HR) $\leq$120 bpm (within 20 bpm of resting HR), BP within 20 mm Hg of patient's normal range, S$\bar{\text{v}}$o$_2$ $\geq$60%, absence of fatigue, and absence of weakness.

- Assess patient's BP, HR, RR, before and immediately after activity.
- Report clinical findings associated with activity intolerance: chest pain, tachycardia, tachypnea, BP $\geq$20 mm Hg or normal range, fatigue, weakness, and dyspnea.
- Plan rest periods between patient's scheduled activities.
- Adjust activities to reduce energy expedition.
- Assist with hygiene, grooming, and toileting. Protect patient during these activities, since weakness may make simple activities impossible.
- Establish realistic activity goals with patient.
- Encourage patient to maintain adequate nutritional intake to meet energy needs for activity.

Body image disturbance related to physical changes secondary to Kaposi's lesions and emaciation.

Expected Patient Outcome. Patient verbalizes positive feelings about self.

- Listen to patient's expression about the way he or she views or feels about self.
- Provide psychosocial and spiritual support to patient and significant others.
- Identify positive accomplishments in care or activities.
- Encourage patient to seek clergy or psychiatric care if necessary.
- Provide patient with names of AIDS support groups.

- Encourage patient to use make-up to cover over closed Kaposi's sarcoma lesions if appropriate.

DISCHARGE PLANNING

The critical care nurse will provide patient and significant other(s) with verbal or written discharge notes regarding the following subjects:

1. Importance of avoiding contact with persons who have infections.
2. Importance of maintaining medical follow-up appointments.
3. Need to maintain a balanced diet with supplemental food and vitamins.
4. Signs and symptoms, including changes in patient's condition: fever, additional weight loss, cognitive dysfunction, weakness, blurred vision or sensorimotor dysfunction.
5. Information about medications, such as dosage, route, purpose, and side effects.
6. Importance of modifying high-risk behaviors.
7. Name and importance of attending AIDS support groups.

PART II: SUPPORTIVE PROCEDURES AND NURSING MANAGEMENT

■   PLASMAPHERESIS

Definition

Plasmapheresis involves a complete exchange of plasma, with the removal of abnormal circulating antibodies that interfere with the acetylcholine receptors. The abnormal substance is replaced with equal volume of a plasmalike substance.

Patient Selection

INDICATIONS. Indications include hemolytic anemia, myasthenia gravis, renal transplant rejection syndrome, Goodpasture's syndrome, systemic lupus erythematosus, rheumatoid arthritis, multiple myeloma, biliary cirrhosis, hyperlipemia, or cancer conditions in which plasma substances interfere with patient's immune system.

CONTRAINDICATIONS

Procedure

TECHNIQUE. Blood is removed from the patient, centrifuged to remove the plasma, and the packed red cells are returned to the patient. The amount removed is between 60 to 80 mL/kg of plasma.

Complications

Hypovolemia, clotting abnormalities, hypotension, bradycardia, hypokalemia, hypocalcemia, myasthenia crisis, and cholinergic crisis.

NURSING MANAGEMENT: NURSING DIAGNOSES AND COLLABORATIVE PROBLEMS

Nursing Diagnoses

A common nursing goal for patient's undergoing plasmapheresis is to maintain fluid balance.

Fluid volume deficit related to intravascular volume deficit secondary to removal of up to 3 L of fluid during plasmapheresis.

Expected Patient Outcomes. Patient maintains adequate fluid volume, as evidenced by blood pressure (BP) within normal range, mean arterial pressure (MAP) 70 to 100 mm Hg, moist mucous membranes, good skin turgor, skin pink, capillary refill $\leq$3 seconds, peripheral pulses +2, urinary output (UO) $\geq$30 mL/h or $\geq$0.5 mL/kg/h, specific gravity 1.001 to 1.035, central venous pressure (CVP) 2 to 6 mm Hg, stable body weight, clotting factors within normal range, and serum osmolality 275 to 295 mOsm/kg.

- Review levels of serum electrolytes, hematocrit, hemoglobin, and serum osmolality.
- Maintain bed rest with side rails up while patient is dizzy.
- Assess clinical indicators of hydration: BP, heart rate, skin turgor, skin color and warmth, and mucous membranes.
- Report clinical findings associated with dehydration: hypotension, MAP $\leq$60 mm Hg, tachycardia, poor skin turgor, skin pale and dry, and dry mucous membranes.
- Obtain and report, if available, CVP $\leq$2 mm Hg to assess circulating fluid volume.
- Measure intake, output, specific gravity, and daily weight. Report UO $\leq$30 mL/h or $\leq$0.5 mL/kg/h, specific gravity $\geq$1.020, and weight loss $\leq$0.25 to 0.5 kg/d.
- Assess gastric aspirate and stools for occult blood.
- Monitor plasmapheresis: Remove plasma and return packed red cells; 3 to 4L of blood may be processed over 1 to 2 days.
- During plasmapheresis, assess and report excessive thirst, poor skin turgor, dizziness, convulsion, nausea, flattened neck veins, tachycardia, and hypotension.
- Administer IV fluid replacement as prescribed: Ringer's lactate.
- Administer blood, albumin, platelets, or platelet packs as prescribed when hemoglobin $\leq$9 g/100mL.
- Instruct patient regarding the purposes of plasmapheresis.

Collaborative Problem

A common collaborative goal for patients undergoing plasmapheresis is to correct electrolyte imbalance.

Potential Complication: Electrolyte Imbalance. Electrolyte imbalance related to plasmapheresis.

Expected Patient Outcome. Patient maintains serum electrolytes within normal range.

- Review levels of serum potassium and calcium.

- Obtain and report clinical findings associated with hypokalemia: bradycardia, fatigue, leg cramps, nausea, and paresthesia.
- Continuously monitor ECG to assess heart rate and rhythm. Report changes associated with hypokalemia: ST segment depression, flattened T wave, presence of U wave and ventricular dysrhythmias.
- Obtain and report clinical findings associated with hypocalcemia resulting from loss in plasma and calcium is inactivated by acid-citrate-dextrose (ACD): muscle cramps, tetany, convulsions, stridor, dyspnea, diplopia, abdominal cramps or positive Chvostek's and Trousseau's signs.
- Continuously monitor ECG to assess heart rate and rhythm. Report changes associated with hypocalcemia: prolonged QT interval.
- Encourage patient to drink milk before and during the plasma exchange.
- Assess patient's neurological status: mental status, level of consciousness, sensory function, motor function, cranial nerve function, and deep tendon reflexes.
- Administer prescribed antidysrhythmic agents.
- Administer IV fluids and electrolytes as prescribed.
- Administer calcium supplement as prescribed.

SELECTED REFERENCES

Allen C, Clochesy JM. Patients with sepsis. In: Clochesy JM, Breu C, Cardin S, et al, eds. *Critical Care Nursing.* Philadelphia, PA: WB Saunders Co; 1993:1245–1257.

Bailes BK. Disseminated intravascular coagulation. AORN *J.* 1992;55:517–528.

Bell TN. Disseminated intravascular coagulation. *Crit Care Nurs Clin North Am* 1993;5:389–410.

Caine RM, Lefcourt ND. Patients with burns. In: Clochesy JM, Breu C, Cardin S. et al, eds. *Critical Care Nursing.* Philadelphia, PA: WB Saunders Co; 1993:1188–1217.

Carr G. Opportunistic infections and pharmacology. *Crit Care Nurs Clin North Am.* 1992;4:395–400.

Casey K, Cave LH. Patients with HIV-related disease and AIDS. In: Clochesy JM, Breu C, Cardin S, et al, eds. *Critical Care Nursing.* Philadelphia, PA: WB Saunders Co; 1993:1135–1149.

Colletti RC, Drew RB, Goulart AE. Antiendotoxin therapy in sepsis. *Crit Care Nurs Clin North Am.* 1993;5:345–353.

Damrosch S, Abbey S, Warner A, et al. Critical care nurses' attitude toward, concerns about, and knowledge of the acquired immunodeficiency syndrome. *Heart Lung.* 1990;19: 395–400.

Deglin JH and Vallerand AH. Davis's Drug Guide for Nurses, 4th ed. Philadelphia, PA: FA Davis Co., 1995.

DiMola MA. The cutting edge in burn care. *Crit Care Nurse.* 1993;(suppl):24–26.

Dolan JT. *Critical Care Nursing Clinical Management Through the Nursing Process.* Philadelphia, PA: FA Davis Co; 1991.

Dressler, DK. Disseminated intravascular coagulation. In: Von Rueden KT, Walleck CA, eds. *Advanced Critical Care Nursing.* Rockville, MD: Aspen Publications; 1989:293–308.

Dressler, DK. Patients with coagulopathies. In: Clochesy JM, Breu C, Cardin S, et al, eds. *Critical Care Nursing.* Philadelphia, PA: WB Saunders Co; 1993:1055–1070.

Epstein C, Bakanauskas A. Clinical management of DIC: early nursing interventions. *Crit Care Nurse* 1991;2(10):42–53.

Faldmo L, Kravitz M. Management of acute burns and burn shock resuscitation. *AACN Clin Issues Crit Care Nurs.* 1993;4:351–366.

Ford RD. Diagnostic Tests Handbook. Springhouse, PA: Springhouse Corp, 1987.

Gatea, DM. Myocardial dysfunction in sepsis and multisystem organ failure. In: Huddleston VB, ed. *Multisystem Organ Failure.* St. Louis, MO: Mosby Year Book; 1992;178–203.

Guidry HM, Grimes RM. Management of HIV infection: a summary of summaries (I) Hospital Practice 1992;27(11):185–216.

Harper J. The cutting edge in immunology. *Crit Care Nurse.* 1993;(suppl):27–28.

Hazinski MF, Iberti TJ, MacIntyre NR, et al. Epidemiology, pathophysiology and clinical presentations of gram-negative sepsis. *Am J Crit Care.* 1993;2(3):224–237.

Hollander H, Katz MH. HIV infection. In: Tierney LM, McPhenn SJ, Papadakis MA, eds. *Current Medical Diagnosis and Treatment.*

33rd. Norwalk, CT: Appleton & Lange; 1994: 1074–1097.

Linker CA. Blood. In: Tierney LM, McPhenn SJ, Papadakis MA, eds. *Current Medical Diagnosis and Treatment.* 33rd ed. Norwalk, CT: Appleton & Lange, 1994:415–466.

Loeb S. Clinical Laboratory Tests Values and Implications. Springhouse, PA: Springhouse Corp, 1991.

Loeb S. Nurse's Handbook of Drug Therapy. Springhouse, PA: Springhouse Corp, 1993.

Lovejoy, NC, Rumley R. AIDS epidemiology and pathology. *Crit Care Nurs Clin North Am.* 1992;4:383–393.

Meredith T, Acierno L. Pulmonary complications of acquired immunodeficiency syndrome. *Heart Lung* 1988;17:173–178.

Murray JF, Garay SM, Hopewell PC, et al. Pulmonary complications of the AIDS: an update. *Am Rev Resp Dis* 1987;135:504–509.

Rieg LS. Metabolic alterations and nutritional management. *AACN Clin Issues Crit Care Nurs.* 1993;4:388–398.

Roberts SL. Disseminated intravascular coagulation. *Physiological Concepts and the Critically Ill Patient.* Englewood Cliffs, NJ: Prentice-Hall; 1985:386–413 [out of print].

Singer P, Askanazi J, Akiva L, et al. Reassessing intensive care for patients with the acquired immunodeficiency syndrome. *Heart Lung.* 1990;19:387–394.

Stillwell SB. *Mosby's Critical Care Nursing Reference.* St. Louis, MO: Mosby Year Book, 1992.

Swearingen PL, Keen JH. *Manual of Critical Care.* 2nd ed. St. Louis, MO: Mosby Year Book, 1992.

Tierney LM, McPhenn SJ, Papadakis MA, eds. *Current Medical Diagnosis and Treatment,* 33rd

ed. Norwalk, CT: Appleton & Lange, 1994; 1074–1097.

Tribett D. *Pneumocytis carinii* pneumonia in the patient with acquired immune deficiency syndrome. In: VonRueden KT, Walleck CA, eds. *Advanced Critical Care Nursing.* Rockville, MD: Aspen Publications; 1989:309–323.

Tribett D. Hematological data acquisition. In: Kinney MR, Packa DR, Dunbar SB, eds. *AACN's Clinical Reference for Critical Care Nursing.* 3rd ed. St. Louis, MO: Mosby Year Book; 1993: 975–983.

Tribett D. Hematological disorders. In Kinney MR, Packa DR, Dunbar SB, eds. *AACN's Clinical Reference for Critical Care Nursing.* 3rd ed. St. Louis, MO: Mosby Year Book; 1993: 985–1001.

Tribett D. The patient with human immunodeficiency virus (HIV). In: Kinney MR, Packa DR, Dunbar SB, eds. *AACN's Clinical Reference for Critical Care Nursing.* 3rd ed. St. Louis, MO: Mosby Year Book, 1993:1059–1076.

Timby BK. Pneumocystosis in patients with acquired immunodeficiency syndrome. *Crit Care Nurse.* 1992;12(7):64–71.

Walter, PH. Burn wound management. *AACN Clinical Issues Crit Care Nurs.* 1993;4:378–387.

Winkler JB, DiMola, MA, Woolen JA. Burns. In: Kinney MR, Packa DR, Dunbar SB, eds. *AACN's Clinical Reference for Critical Care Nursing.* 3rd ed. St. Louis, MO: Mosby Year Book, 1993;1195–1231.

Wilson RF, Wilson JA. Sepsis. In: Kinney MR, Packa DR, Dunbar SB, eds. *AACN's Clinical Reference for Critical Care Nursing.* 3rd ed. St. Louis, MO: Mosby Year Book; 1993: 1519–1555.

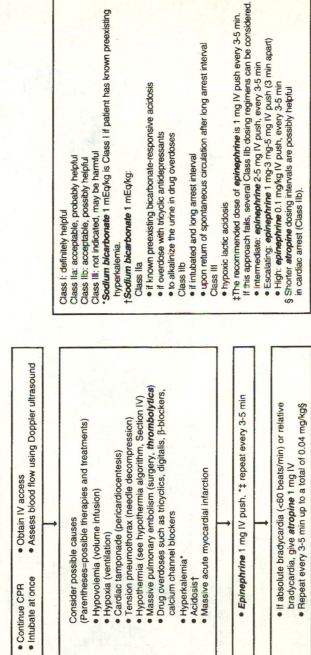

PEA includes
- Electromechanical dissociation (EMD)
- Pseudo-EMD
- Idioventricular rhythms
- Ventricular escape rhythms
- Bradyasystolic rhythms
- Postdefibrillation idioventricular rhythms

- Continue CPR
- Intubate at once
- Obtain IV access
- Assess blood flow using Doppler ultrasound

Consider possible causes
(Parentheses=possible therapies and treatments)
- Hypovolemia (volume infusion)
- Hypoxia (ventilation)
- Cardiac tamponade (pericardiocentesis)
- Tension pneumothorax (needle decompression)
- Hypothermia (see hypothermia algorithm, Section IV)
- Massive pulmonary embolism (surgery, *thrombolytics*)
- Drug overdoses such as tricyclics, digitalis, β-blockers, calcium channel blockers
- Hyperkalemia*
- Acidosis†
- Massive acute myocardial infarction

- *Epinephrine* 1 mg IV push, ‡ repeat every 3-5 min

- If absolute bradycardia (<60 beats/min) or relative bradycardia, give *atropine* 1 mg IV
- Repeat every 3-5 min up to a total of 0.04 mg/kg§

Class I: definitely helpful
Class IIa: acceptable, probably helpful
Class IIb: acceptable, possibly helpful
Class III: not indicated, may be harmful
Sodium bicarbonate 1 mEq/kg is Class I if patient has known preexisting hyperkalemia.
†*Sodium bicarbonate* 1 mEq/kg:
Class IIa
- if known preexisting bicarbonate-responsive acidosis
- if overdose with tricyclic antidepressants
- to alkalinize the urine in drug overdoses
Class IIb
- if intubated and long arrest interval
- upon return of spontaneous circulation after long arrest interval
Class III
- hypoxic lactic acidosis
‡The recommended dose of *epinephrine* is 1 mg IV push every 3-5 min.
If this approach fails, several Class IIb dosing regimens can be considered.
- intermediate: *epinephrine* 2-5 mg IV push, every 3-5 min
- Escalating: *epinephrine* 1 mg-3 mg-5 mg IV push (3 min apart)
- High: *epinephrine* 0.1 mg/kg IV push, every 3-5 min
§ Shorter *atropine* dosing intervals are possibly helpful in cardiac arrest (Class IIb).

Figure A–1. Algorithm for EMD. (From the American Heart Association Emergency Cardiac Care Committee Guidelines for cardiopulmonary resuscitation and emergency cardiac care. *Journal of the American Medical Association.* 1992;268:2217–2224.)

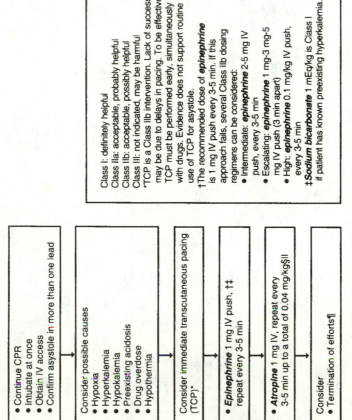

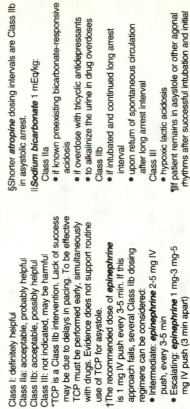

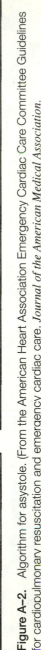

- Continue CPR
- Intubate at once
- Obtain IV access
- Confirm asystole in more than one lead

Consider possible causes
- Hypoxia
- Hyperkalemia
- Hypokalemia
- Preexisting acidosis
- Drug overdose
- Hypothermia

Consider immediate transcutaneous pacing (TCP),*

- *Epinephrine* 1 mg IV push, †‡ repeat every 3-5 min

- *Atropine* 1 mg IV, repeat every 3-5 min up to a total of 0.04 mg/kg§||

Consider
- Termination of efforts¶

Class I: definitely helpful
Class IIa: acceptable, probably helpful
Class IIb: acceptable, possibly helpful
Class III: not indicated, may be harmful
*TCP is a Class IIb intervention. Lack of success may be due to delays in pacing. To be effective TCP must be performed early, simultaneously with drugs. Evidence does not support routine use of TCP for asystole.
†The recommended dose of *epinephrine* is 1 mg IV push every 3-5 min. If this approach fails, several Class IIb dosing regimens can be considered:
- Intermediate: *epinephrine* 2-5 mg IV push, every 3-5 min
- Escalating: *epinephrine* 1 mg-3 mg-5 mg IV push (3 min apart)
- High: *epinephrine* 0.1 mg/kg IV push, every 3-5 min
‡*Sodium bicarbonate* 1 mEq/kg is Class I if patient has known preexisting hyperkalemia.

§Shorter *atropine* dosing intervals are Class IIb in asystolic arrest.
||*Sodium bicarbonate* 1 mEq/kg:
Class IIa
- if known preexisting bicarbonate-responsive acidosis
- if overdose with tricyclic antidepressants
- to alkalinize the urine in drug overdoses
Class IIb
- if intubated and continued long arrest interval
- upon return of spontaneous circulation after long arrest interval
Class III
- hypoxic lactic acidosis
¶If patient remains in asystole or other agonal rhythms after successful intubation and initial medications and no reversible causes are identified, consider termination of resuscitative efforts by a physician. Consider interval since arrest.

Figure A–2. Algorithm for asystole. (From the American Heart Association Emergency Cardiac Care Committee Guidelines for cardiopulmonary resuscitation and emergency cardiac care. *Journal of the American Medical Association.* 1992;268:2217–2224.)

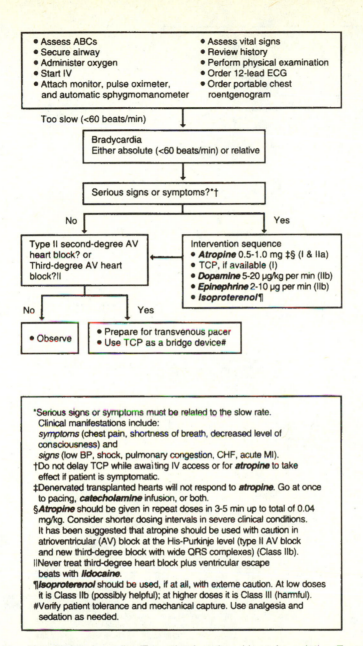

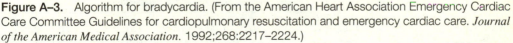

Figure A–3. Algorithm for bradycardia. (From the American Heart Association Emergency Cardiac Care Committee Guidelines for cardiopulmonary resuscitation and emergency cardiac care. *Journal of the American Medical Association.* 1992;268:2217–2224.)

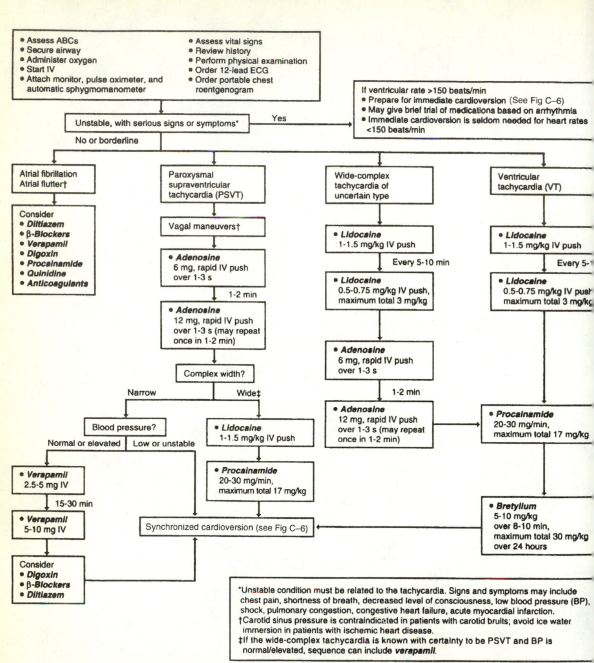

Figure A–4. Algorithm for paroxysmal supraventricular tachycardia. (From the American Heart Association Emergency Cardiac Care Committee Guidelines for cardiopulmonary resuscitation and emergency cardiac care. *Journal of the American Medical Association.* 1992;268:2217–2224.)

Ventricular Ectopy

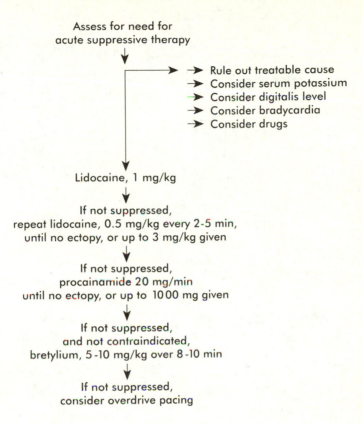

Assess for need for
acute suppressive therapy

→ → Rule out treatable cause
→ Consider serum potassium
→ Consider digitalis level
→ Consider bradycardia
→ Consider drugs

Lidocaine, 1 mg/kg

If not suppressed,
repeat lidocaine, 0.5 mg/kg every 2-5 min,
until no ectopy, or up to 3 mg/kg given

If not suppressed,
procainamide 20 mg/min
until no ectopy, or up to 1000 mg given

If not suppressed,
and not contraindicated,
bretylium, 5-10 mg/kg over 8-10 min

If not suppressed,
consider overdrive pacing

Once ectopy is resolved, maintain as follows:
After lidocaine, 1 mg/kg .... Lidocaine drip, 2 mg/min
After lidocaine, 1-2 mg/kg .... Lidocaine drip, 3 mg/min
After lidocaine, 2-3 mg/kg .... Lidocaine drip, 4 mg/min
After procainamide .... Procainamide drip, 1-4 mg/min
(Check blood level.)
After bretylium .... Bretylium drip, 2 mg/min

Ventricular ectopy: acute suppressive therapy. This sequence was developed to assist in teaching how to treat a broad range of patients with ventricular ectopy. Some patients may require care not specified herein. This algorithm should not be construed as prohibiting such flexibility. Such therapy has not been shown to improve mortality after MI.

Figure A–5. Algorithm for ventricular ectopy. (From the American Heart Association Emergency Cardiac Care Committee Guidelines for cardiopulmonary resuscitation and emergency cardiac care. *Journal of the American Medical Association.* 1992;268:2217–2224.)

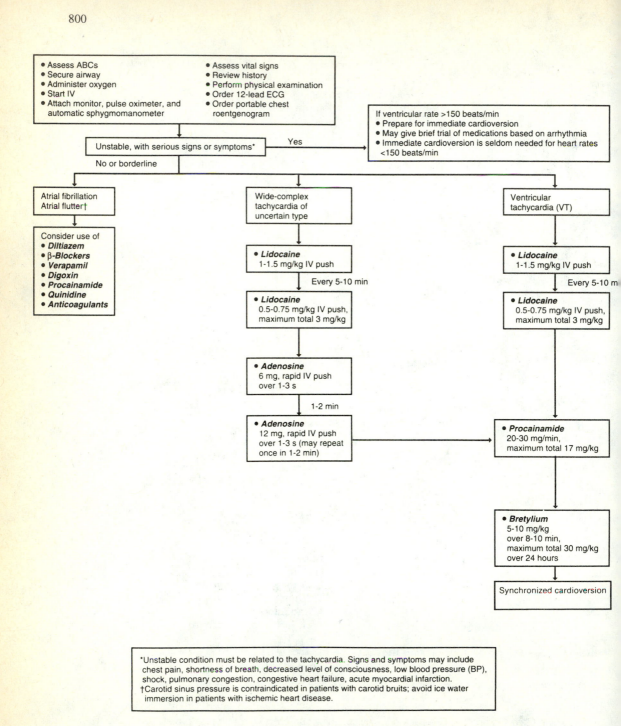

Figure A–6. Algorithm for sustained VT. (From the American Heart Association Emergency Cardiac Care Committee Guidelines for cardiopulmonary resuscitation and emergency cardiac care. *Journal of the American Medical Association.* 1992;268:2217–2224.)

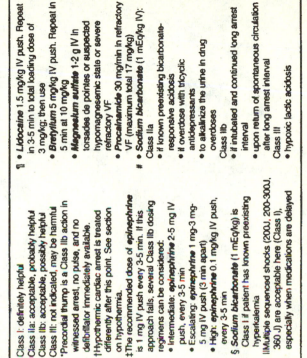

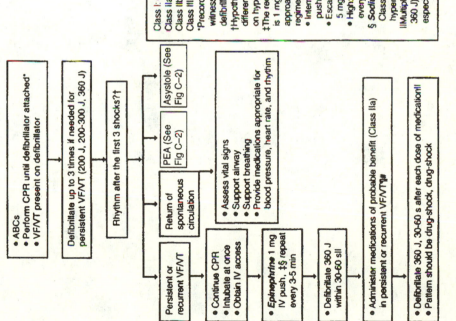

Figure A–7. Algorithm for VF and pulseless VT. (From the American Heart Association Emergency Cardiac Care Committee Guidelines for cardiopulmonary resuscitation and emergency cardiac care. *Journal of the American Medical Association.* 1992;268:2217–2224.)

Index

A page number followed by a *t* indicates tabular material.